Urine

pH	4.5-8 (av. 6)
Sodium	75-200 mg/24 hr
Potassium	25-100 mEq/L
Ammonia	20-70 mEq/L
Creatinine	1-2 g/24 hr
Urea	25-35 g/24 hr
Uric acid	0.6-1 g/24 hr
Glucose	0
Protein	0-150 mg/24 hr (trace)
Acetone	0
Bilirubin	0
Hemoglobin/cells	0
Casts	0
Bacteria	<10,000/ mL
Appearance	clear, pale yellow

Cerebrospinal Fluid (CSF)

Appearance	clear, colorless
Pressure	70-180 mm H_2O
Albumin	11-48 mg/100 mL
Glucose	50-75 mg/100 mL
Cells	occasional WBC
Bilirubin	0

HANDY TABLES

Blood Clotting Times

Bleeding time	4-8 minutes
Duke: earlobe	1-3 minutes
Clotting time	5-15 minutes (Lee White, room temperature)
INR	Values vary with lab technology and with anticoagulation therapy
Prothrombin time	11-16 seconds
Prothrombin/International normalized ratio (PT/INR)	1.5-2.5 seconds
Activated partial thromboplastin time (APTT)	25-38 seconds
Clot retraction time	begins in 30-60 minutes 50% complete in 2 hours

Blood Coagulation Factors

Factor	Name	Information
I	Fibrinogen	Plasma protein synthesized in liver: forms fibrin
II	Prothrombin	Plasma protein synthesized in liver (vitamin K required): forms thrombin
III	Tissue thromboplastin	Released from damaged tissue (extrinsic pathway) and platelets (intrinsic pathway); phospholipid involved in activation of clotting process
IV	Calcium ions	Required for many stages of coagulation process
V and VI	Proaccelerin; labile factor or accelerator globulin	Synthesized in liver: used in prothrombin activation
VII	Proconvertin; serum prothrombin conversion accelerator (SPCA)	Synthesized in liver (vitamin K required); used in extrinsic pathway
VIII	Antihemophilic factor (AHF)	Deficit causes hemophilia A
IX	Plasma thromboplastin component (PTC), Christmas factor, antihemophilic factor B	Synthesized in liver (vitamin K required)
X	Stuart factor	Synthesized in liver (vitamin K required); required for both extrinsic and intrinsic pathways
XI	Plasma thromboplastin antecedent (PTA), antihemophilic factor C	Synthesized in liver; used for activation of intrinsic pathway
XII	Hageman factor	Required in activation of intrinsic pathway
XIII	Fibrin stabilizing factor (FSF)	From platelets—cross-links fibrin to stabilize clot

pH Scale

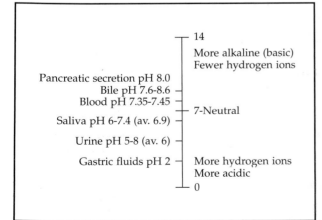

	— 14
	More alkaline (basic)
	Fewer hydrogen ions
Pancreatic secretion pH 8.0	
Bile pH 7.6-8.6 —	
Blood pH 7.35-7.45 —	
	— 7-Neutral
Saliva pH 6-7.4 (av. 6.9) —	
Urine pH 5-8 (av. 6) —	
Gastric fluids pH 2 —	More hydrogen ions
	More acidic
	— 0

Serum Enzymes and Isoenzymes and Markers

Alanine aminotransferase (ALT, formerly SGPT)	Elevated in damage to liver, heart, muscle, pancreas, kidneys
Prostatic acid phosphatase (PAP)	Elevated with metastatic prostatic cancer
Alkaline phosphatase (ALP)	Elevated in bone disease, liver damage
Aspartate aminotransferase (AST, formerly SGOT)	Elevated in damage to liver, heart, and muscle
C-reactive protein	Elevated with inflammation
Cardiac specific troponin	Elevated in myocardial infarction
Creatine kinase (CK, formerly CPK)	Elevated with heart and skeletal muscle damage
CK MB_2 (isoenzyme)	Elevated with MI
Gamma-glutamyl-transferase (GGT)	Elevated with liver damage due to alcohol
Lactate dehydrogenase (LDH)	Elevated with liver, heart, kidney, lung damage
LDH_1 and LDH_2 (isoenzymes)	Elevated with MI
Alpha-fetoprotein (AFP)	A marker for some ovarian tumors, some liver tumors
Carcinoembryonic antigen (CEA)	A marker for intestinal tumors
Prostate-specific antigen (PSA)	A marker for recurrent prostatic cancer

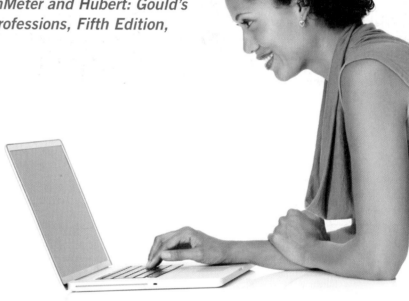

GOULD'S
Pathophysiology for the Health Professions

FIFTH EDITION

Karin C. VanMeter, PhD
Lecturer
Iowa State University
Department of Biomedical Sciences
College of Veterinary Medicine
Ames, Iowa

Robert J. Hubert, BS
Laboratory Coordinator
Iowa State University
Department of Animal Sciences
Ames, Iowa

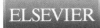

ELSEVIER
SAUNDERS

3251 Riverport Lane
St. Louis, Missouri 63043

Notices

Knowledge and best practice in this field are constantly changing. As new research and experience broaden our understanding, changes in research methods, professional practices, or medical treatment may become necessary.

Practitioners and researchers must always rely on their own experience and knowledge in evaluating and using any information, methods, compounds, or experiments described herein. In using such information or methods they should be mindful of their own safety and the safety of others, including parties for whom they have a professional responsibility.

With respect to any drug or pharmaceutical products identified, readers are advised to check the most current information provided (i) on procedures featured or (ii) by the manufacturer of each product to be administered, to verify the recommended dose or formula, the method and duration of administration, and contraindications. It is the responsibility of practitioners, relying on their own experience and knowledge of their patients, to make diagnoses, to determine dosages and the best treatment for each individual patient, and to take all appropriate safety precautions.

To the fullest extent of the law, neither the Publisher nor the authors, contributors, or editors, assume any liability for any injury and/or damage to persons or property as a matter of products liability, negligence or otherwise, or from any use or operation of any methods, products, instructions, or ideas contained in the material herein.

ISBN: 978-1-4557-5411-3

Content Manager: Billie Sharp
Content Development Specialist: Betsy McCormac
Publishing Services Manager: Julie Eddy
Senior Project Manager: Marquita Parker
Design Direction: Brian Salisbury

Printed in Canada

Last digit is the print number: 9 8 7 6 5 4 3

Working together
to grow libraries in
developing countries

www.elsevier.com • www.bookaid.org

We would like to dedicate this book to the memory of Barbara E. Gould, MEd. We hope that this book, the legacy of her work, will instill her passion for teaching and learning and will continue to inspire health profession students and educators worldwide.

Robert Hubert
Karin VanMeter

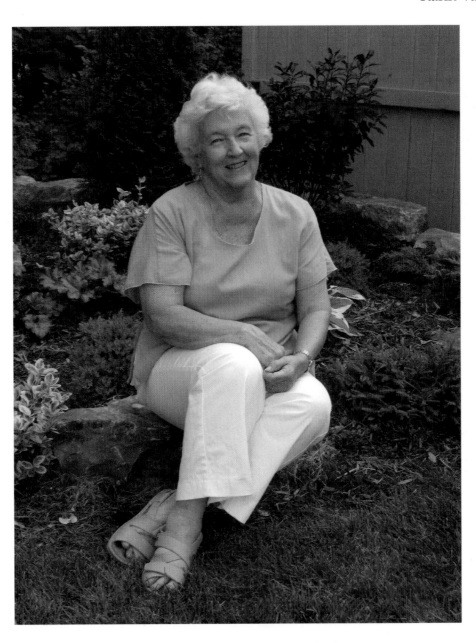

Reviewers

Teresa Cowan, DA, BS, MS
Program Director of Health Sciences
Baker College of Auburn Hills Michigan
Auburn Hills, Michigan

Kathleen A. Goei, PhD, MSN, RN
Assistant Professor
University of the Incarnate Word
San Antonio, Texas

Ecaterina Mariana Hdeib, MA, RDMS
Clinical Assistant Professor
Diagnostic Medical Ultrasound Program
University of Missouri
Columbia, Missouri

Stacy Lepsch, RN, MSN
Lecturer of Nursing
Mount Mercy University
Cedar Rapids, Iowa

Rachel J. Meyer, PhD
Assistant Professor of Biology
Midland University
Fremont, Nebraska

Laree Schoolmeesters, PhD, RN, CNL
Assistant Professor
Queens University of Charlotte
Charlotte, North Carolina

Trena Seago, RN, MSN
Assistant Professor
School of Nursing
Kentucky State University
Frankfort, Kentucky

Paula Denise Silver, BS, PharmD
Medical Instructor
ECPI University
Newport News, Virginia

William F. Simpson, PhD, CES, FACSM
Associate Professor, Director, Exercise Physiology Lab,
    Academic Program Director, Health and Wellness
    Management
University of Wisconsin-Superior
Superior, Wisconsin

Preface

This textbook provides an introduction to pathophysiology for students in a variety of academic programs for the health professions at colleges and universities. Major disorders are described as well as selected additional diseases with the intention of providing information on a broad spectrum of diseases with one or more distinguishing features for each. It is anticipated that additional information and resources pertinent to the individual's professional needs may be added to classroom presentations and assignments. We trust that students will enjoy studying these topics and proceed with enthusiasm to more detailed studies within their individual specialties.

Organization

The textbook is organized into five major sections followed by the appendices:

Section I—Basic Concepts of Disease Processes

- Introduction to pathophysiology includes medical terminology and basic cellular changes.
- Topics such as fluid, electrolyte, and acid-base imbalances, basic pharmacology and pain are covered.
- The core information for each topic is complemented by the inclusion of a specific disease/condition as an immediate clinical application at the end of each chapter.

Section II—Defense/Protective Mechanisms

- Topics such as inflammation and healing, infection, and immunity are covered.
- Specific areas included are a review of body defenses, healing involved in specific trauma such as burns, basic microbiology, review of the immune system components, and mechanisms.

Section III—Pathophysiology of Body Systems

- Selection of specific disorders is based on incidence and occurrence, as well as on the need to present a variety of pathophysiological processes and etiologies to the student.

- For major disorders, information is provided on pathophysiology, etiology, clinical manifestations, significant diagnostic tests, common treatment modalities, and potential complications.
- Other selected diseases are presented in less detail, but significant, unique features are highlighted.

Section IV: Biological Factors Contributing to Pathophysiology

- Normal physiological changes related to cancer, adolescence, pregnancy, and aging, with their relevance and affect on disease processes and the treatment of the affected individual, are described.
- Specific disorders associated with cancer and the developmental stages are discussed.

Section V: Environmental Factors and Pathophysiology

- Factors such as immobility, stress, substance abuse, and environmental hazards are the major components in this section.
- Affects of the various environmental factors on the various body systems and potential complications beyond physical pathologies are discussed.
- New research and data are included. as these are areas of increasing concern with regards to pathophysiology and patient health.

Appendices—additional information:

- Ready References include lists of anatomic terms, abbreviations and acronyms, a selection of diagnostic tests, an example of a medical history, a disease index, and drug index.
- A glossary and a list of additional resources complete this resource.

Format and Features

The basic format as well as the straightforward, concise approach remains unchanged from the previous editions. Some material has been reorganized to improve the flow of information and facilitate comprehension.

Many features related to the presentation of information in this textbook continue as before.

- Generic learning objectives are included in each chapter. Instructors may modify or add applicable objectives for a specific professional program.
- Cross-references are included, facilitating access to information.
- In the discussion of a particular disorder, the *pathophysiology* is presented *first* because this "sets the stage," describing the basic change(s) in the body. Once the student understands the essence of the problem, he or she can easily identify the role of predisposing factors or causes and relate the resulting signs and symptoms or complications. Diagnostic tests and treatment also follow directly from the pathophysiology.
- Changes at the *cellular* level are included when significant.
- Brief *reviews* of normal anatomy and physiology are presented at the beginning of each chapter, to remind students of the structures and functions that are frequently affected by pathological processes. A review of basic microbiology is incorporated into the chapter on infections. Additional review material, such as the pH scale or the location of body cavities, may be found in the Appendices.
- Numerous *illustrations,* including flow charts, schematic diagrams, and photographs, clarify and reinforce textual information, as well as offer an alternative visual learning mode, particularly when complex processes are involved. Illustrations are fully labeled, including anatomical structures and pathologic changes. Different colors may be used in a figure to distinguish between the various stages or factors in a process.
- *Tables* summarize information or offer comparisons, which are helpful to the student in selecting the more significant information and for review purposes.
- Brief reference to *diagnostic tests* and *treatment measures* promotes understanding of the changes occurring during a disease.
- *Questions* are found in boxes throughout the text to stimulate application and review of new concepts. "Apply Your Knowledge" questions are based on review of normal physiology and its application, "Think About" questions follow each small section of information, and "Study Questions" are located at the end of each chapter. Questions may relate to simple, factual information, potential applications, or the integration of several concepts. These questions are helpful in alerting a student to points initially overlooked and are useful for student self-evaluation before proceeding to the next section. These features may also serve as a tool for review and test preparation. Brief answers are provided on the Evolve website.
- Brief, adaptable *case studies* with questions are incorporated at the end of many chapters and are intended to provide a basis for discussion in a tutorial, an assignment, or an alternative learning mode. It is expected that specific clinical applications may be added by instructors for each professional group.
- Chapter summaries precede the review questions in each chapter.

What's New?

- Information on specific diseases has been updated throughout.
- The specific disorders for each body system have been expanded to reflect current trends and research.
- Neurological Disorders (acute and chronic) were combined into a single chapter; whereas, the Lymphatic System was broken out as its own chapter separate from the Blood Disorders.
- A broader emphasis on all allied health professions has been incorporated.
- Sections and chapters have been reorganized to present the student with a building block approach: basic science and how it relates to human biology, the body's various mechanisms that respond to the disorders/diseases, the general overview of body systems and their specific disorders, other biological factors outside of the physiology of each system that contribute to instances of disorders/disease and, finally, those environmental factors not directly attributed to a biological function or condition that may contribute to pathophysiology throughout a number of body systems.
- Figures have been updated with new photographs and illustrations to help in the recognition and identification of the various concepts and specific disorders.
- Tables have been updated with new information that has been made available since the previous edition.
- Additional resources at the end of each chapter have been expanded and updated.
- Study questions and Think About questions have been reviewed and updated to cover new material in the chapter. The Apply Your Knowledge questions have replaced the Challenge questions in the previous editions.
- The Study Guide associated with this text has been updated and many new visually-based questions have been added.

Guidelines for Users

Certain guidelines were developed to facilitate the use of this textbook by students with diverse backgrounds studying in various health science programs. As well as ongoing general changes, some professional groups have developed unique practice models and language. In some disciplines, rapid changes in terminology have occurred, creating difficulty for some students. For example, current terms such as *chemical dependency* or *cognitive impairment* have many synonyms, and some of these are included to enable students to relate to a more familiar phrase. To avoid confusion, the common, traditional terminology has been retained in this text.

- The recipient of care or service is referred to as a *patient*.
- When a disease entity refers to a group of related disorders, discussion focuses on either a typical representative of the group or on the general characteristics of the group.
- *Key terms* are listed at the beginning of the chapter. They are presented in **bold** print and defined when initially used in the chapter. Key terms are not indicated as such in subsequent chapters, but may be found in the glossary at the back of the book.
- *Italics* are used to emphasize significant words.
- It is assumed that students have studied anatomy and physiology prior to commencing a pathophysiology course.
- Concise, readable style includes sufficient scientific and medical terminology to help the student acquire a professional vocabulary and appropriate communication skills. An effort has been made to avoid overwhelming the student with a highly technical approach or impeding the learning process in a student who comes with little scientific background.
- The presence of numeric values within textual information often confuses students and detracts from the basic concepts being presented; therefore, specific numbers are included only when they promote understanding of a principle.
- Suggested diagnostic tests and treatments are not individualized or necessarily complete but are presented generally to assist the student's application of the pathophysiology. They are also intended to provide students with an awareness of the impact of certain diseases on a client and of possible modifications in the individualized care required. Diagnostic tests increase student cognizance of the extent of data collection and sifting that may be necessary before making a diagnosis, as well as the importance of monitoring the course of a disease or the response to treatment.
- A brief introduction to pharmacology is included in Section I and specific drugs are referred to during the discussion of certain disorders. Drugs are identified by *generic name*, followed by a trade name. Examples provided in the appropriate chapter are not recommendations, but are suggested only as frequently used representatives of a drug classification. A drug index with references to the applicable chapter is located in the appendices.
- Information regarding adverse effects of drugs or other treatment is included when there may be potential problems such as high risk for infection or special precautions required of members of the health care team.
- Every effort has been made to present current information and concepts simply but accurately. This content provides the practitioner in a health profession with the prerequisite knowledge to recognize and understand a client's problems and the limitations and implications of certain treatment measures; to reduce exacerbating factors; to participate in preventive programs; and to be an effective member of a health care team. The student will develop a knowledge base from which to seek additional information. Individual instructors may emphasize certain aspects or topics, as is most appropriate for students in a specialty area.

Resources

In the textbook:
- Selected additional resources are listed at the end of each chapter.
- *Reference tables* are located inside the front book cover. These comprise common normal values for blood, cerebrospinal fluid, and urine; a pH scale for body fluids; a list of blood clotting factors; and diagnostic tests.
- The chapter introducing pharmacology and therapeutics is limited in content, but combined with the brief references to treatments with individual disorders, is intended to complement the pathophysiology. This chapter also introduces a few traditional and non-traditional therapeutic modalities to facilitate the student's understanding of various therapies and of the impact of diverse treatments on the patient and on care by all members of the health care team. Also included are brief descriptions of a few selected forms of therapy, for example, physiotherapy, in hopes of clarifying the roles of different members of a health care team.
- The appendices at the back of the textbook are intended to promote effective use of study time. They include:
  - A brief review of anatomical terms describing *body cavities and planes* with accompanying illustrations as well as basic body movements
  - Selected numerical conversions for temperature, weights, and volumes
  - Lists of *anatomical terms* and combining forms, common *abbreviations*, and *acronyms*; because of the broad scope of pathophysiology, a medical dictionary is a useful adjunct for any student in the health-related professions
  - A brief description with illustrations of common diagnostic tests such as ultrasound and magnetic resonance imaging

- An example of a medical history, which can be modified to fit the needs of a particular professional group
- A disease index, with a brief description and references to the relevant chapter
- A drug index, identifying the principal action and references to the appropriate chapters
- A list of additional resources; websites consist primarily of health care groups or professional organizations that will provide accurate information and are likely to persist. Additional specific journals and websites are available for individual professions.
- A glossary, including significant terms used to describe diseases as well as key words
- Accompanying this textbook and developed for it, the ancillaries available include:

  A study guide for students provides learning activities such as complex test questions, matching exercises, crossword puzzles, diagrams to label, and other assignments

The interactive Evolve web site includes self-evaluation tools, and can be found at http://evolve.elsevier.com/VanMeter/Goulds/

We appreciate the time and effort of reviewers and users of this text, of sales representatives, and of the editors, who have forwarded comments regarding the first four editions. We have attempted to respond to these suggestions while recognizing that comments come from a variety of perspectives, and there is a need to respect the primary focus of this textbook, space constraints, and student concerns.

We hope that teachers and students will enjoy using this textbook, and that it will stimulate interest in the acquisition of additional knowledge in this dynamic field.

Robert Hubert
Karin VanMeter

Acknowledgments

The authors would like to acknowledge and dedicate this edition to the original author, Barbara E. Gould, who passed away. Dr. Gould always kept "student learning" in the forefront as the guideline for writing this book. We also would like to thank all the editorial and production staff at Elsevier for their support and encouragement. Furthermore, we would like to thank the reviewers for their valuable input.

I would first like to thank my co-author and friend Karin VanMeter. This is our third major project together and it is her continued dedication to education and professionalism that has contributed so much to the overall teamwork and fun working relationship that we enjoy. I would also like to thank Dr. Joan Cunnick and all of the faculty and staff in the microbiology program at Iowa State University for all of your encouragement and support. As with any and all challenges I have tackled in my life, I give my love and thanks to my family—my parents John and Ann and my sister Donna, for their unwavering love and support throughout my life. Finally, I lift up my thanks to Jesus Christ, my Lord and Savior who makes this all possible—to Him be the glory and honor forever.

Robert J. Hubert

My special thanks goes to my co-author Rob Hubert. He has been my friend and collaborator for many years and I am looking forward to many years of working together. Without him all the projects we have done together would have lacked his incredible insight into the topics we have addressed in this new addition. I also would like to thank my mother, Theresia, and my brother, Hermann, and his family for the love, support, and understanding. To my children, Christine and Andrew—thanks for your continuous love.

Karin C. VanMeter

Contents

CHAPTER **1**

Introduction to Pathophysiology

CHAPTER OUTLINE

What Is Pathophysiology and Why Study It?
Understanding Health and Disease
The Concept and Scope of Pathophysiology
Beginning the Process: A Medical History

New Developments and Trends
The Basic Terminology of Pathophysiology
The Disease Process
Causes of Disease
Characteristics of Disease
Disease Prognosis

Introduction to Cellular Changes
Terms Used for Common Cellular Adaptations
Cell Damage and Necrosis
Chapter Summary
Study Questions
Additional Resources

LEARNING OBJECTIVES

After studying this chapter, the student is expected to:

1. Explain the role of pathophysiology in the diagnosis and treatment of disease.
2. Use the terminology appropriate for pathophysiology.
3. Explain the importance of a patient's medical history.
4. Describe common cellular adaptations and possible reasons for the occurrence of each.

5. Identify precancerous cellular changes.
6. List the common causes of cell damage.
7. Describe the common types of cell necrosis and possible outcomes.

KEY TERMS

anaerobic
apoptosis
autopsy
biopsy
endogenous

exogenous
gangrene
homeostasis
hypoxia
iatrogenic

idiopathic
inflammation
ischemia
lysis
lysosomal

microorganisms
microscopic
morphologic
probability

What Is Pathophysiology and Why Study It?

Pathophysiology involves the study of *functional* or physiologic changes in the body that result from disease processes. This subject builds on knowledge of the normal structure and function of the human body. Disease development and the associated changes to normal anatomy and/or physiology may be obvious or may be hidden with its quiet beginning at the cellular level. As such, pathophysiology includes some aspects of *pathology*, the laboratory study of cell and tissue changes associated with disease.

Understanding Health and Disease

Disease may be defined as a deviation from the *normal* structure or function of any part, organ, system (or combination of these) or from a state of *wellness*. The World Health Organization includes physical, mental, and social well-being in its definition of health.

A state of health is difficult to define because the genetic differences among individuals as well as the many variations in life experiences and environmental influences create a variable base. The context in which health is measured is also a consideration. A person who is blind can be in good general health. Injury or surgery may create a temporary impairment in a specific area, but the person's overall health status is not altered.

Homeostasis is the maintenance of a relatively stable internal environment regardless of external changes. Disease develops when significant changes occur in the body, leading to a state in which homeostasis cannot be maintained without intervention. Under normal conditions homeostasis is maintained within the body with regard to such factors as blood pressure, body temperature, and fluid balance. As frequent minor changes occur in the body, the compensation mechanisms respond, and homeostasis is quickly restored. Usually the individual is not aware of these changes or the compensations taking place.

Steps to Heath (Box 1-1) are recommended to prevent disease.

When one is defining "normal" limits for health indicators such as blood pressure or pulse, the values used usually represent an *average* or a small *range*. These values represent what is expected in a typical individual but are not an absolute criterion. Among normal healthy individuals, the actual values may be adjusted for factors such as age, gender, genetics, environment, and activity level. Well-trained athletes often have a slower pulse or heart rate than the average person. Blood pressure usually increases slightly with age, even in healthy individuals. Also, small daily fluctuations in blood pressure occur as the body responds to minor changes in activity, body position, and even emotions. Therefore it is impossible to state a single normal value for blood pressure or pulse rate. It is also important to remember

BOX 1-1	Seven Steps to Health

1. Be a nonsmoker and avoid second-hand smoke.
2. Eat 5 to 10 servings of vegetables and fruit a day. Choose high-fiber, lower-fat foods. If you drink alcohol, limit your intake to one to two drinks a day.
3. Be physically active on a regular basis. This will also help you maintain a healthy body weight.
4. Protect yourself and your family from the sun.
5. Follow cancer screening guidelines.
6. Visit your doctor or dentist if you notice any change in your normal state of health.
7. Follow health and safety instructions at home and at work when using, storing, and disposing of hazardous materials.

that any one indicator or lab value must be considered within the total assessment for the individual client.

Likewise, a discussion of a specific disease in a text presents a general description of the typical characteristics of that disease, but some differences in the clinical picture can be expected to occur in a specific individual, based on similar variables.

Concept and Scope of Pathophysiology and Evidenced-Based Practice

Pathophysiology requires the use of knowledge of basic anatomy and physiology and is based on a loss of or a change in normal structure and function. This basis also saves relearning many facts! Many disorders affecting a particular system or organ, for example the liver, display a set of common signs and symptoms directly related to that organ's normal structure and function. For example, when the liver is damaged, many clotting factors cannot be produced; therefore, excessive bleeding results. Jaundice, a yellow color in the skin, is another sign of liver disease, resulting from the liver's inability to excrete bilirubin. Also, basic pathophysiologic concepts related to the causative factors of a disease, such as the processes of inflammation or infection are common to many diseases. Inflammation in the liver causes swelling of the tissue and stretching of the liver capsule, resulting in pain, as does inflammation of the kidneys. This cause and effect relationship, defined by signs and symptoms, facilitates the study of a specific disease.

In this text, in order to provide a comprehensive overview of disease processes, the focus is on major diseases. Other disorders are included when appropriate to provide exposure to a broad range of diseases. The principles illustrated by these diseases can then be applied to other conditions encountered in practice. In addition, a general approach is used to describe diseases in which there may be several subtypes. For example, only one type of glomerulonephritis, a kidney disease, is described in the text, acute poststreptococcal glomerulonephritis, which represents the many forms of glomerulonephritis.

Prevention of disease has become a primary focus in health care. The known causes of and factors predisposing to specific diseases are being used in the development of more effective preventive programs, and it is important to continue efforts to detect additional significant factors and gather data to further decrease the incidence of certain diseases. The Centers for Disease Control and Prevention in the United States have a significant role in collection of data about all types of disease and provide evidence based recommendations for prevention. Prevention includes such activities as maintaining routine vaccination programs and encouraging participation in screening programs such as blood pressure clinics and vision screening (Box 1-2). As more community health programs develop, and with the increase in information available on the internet, health care workers are becoming more involved in

responding to questions from many sources, and have an opportunity to promote appropriate preventive measures in their communities. A sound knowledge of pathophysiology is the basis for preventive teaching in your profession.

While studying pathophysiology, the student becomes aware of the complexity of many diseases, the difficulties encountered in diagnosis and treatment, and the possible implications arising from a list of signs and symptoms or a prognosis. Sophisticated and expensive diagnostic tests are now available. The availability of these tests, however, also depends on the geographic location of individuals, including their access to large, well-equipped medical facilities. More limited resources may restrict the number of diagnostic tests available to an individual, or a long waiting period may be necessary before testing and treatment are available. When a student understands the pathophysiology, comprehension of the manifestations and potential complications of a disease, and its treatment, usually follows. A solid knowledge base enables health care professionals to meet these increased demands with appropriate information.

Individuals working in health care have found that many new scientific developments have raised ethical, legal, and social issues. For example, the recent explosion in genetic information and related technologies has raised many ethical concerns (see Chapter 21). In relatively new areas of research such as genetics, discussion and resolution of the legal and ethical issues lag far behind the scientific advances. Health research is most often funded by commercial sources (up to 80% according to some studies) and new breakthrough therapies are often announced before the start of any clinical trials. This causes increased hope and immediate demand for such treatments often as much as a decade before they become available. Understanding the research process and the time required for clinical trials of new therapies is crucial in answering questions about new therapies.

The research process in the health sciences is a lengthy three-stage process that aims to demonstrate both the safety and effectiveness of a new therapy. The first stage in this process is often referred to as "basic science" in which researchers work to identify a technology that will work to limit or prevent the disease process. This stage is carried out in the laboratory and often requires the use of animals or cell cultures. The second stage involves a small number of human subjects to determine if the therapy is safe for humans. The third stage only takes place if the results of the previous research are positive; the majority of therapies do not make it to this point. In the third stage of research a large number of patients with the disease or at risk for the disease are enrolled in clinical trials. These are usually *double blind studies* in which the research subject and the person administering the treatment do not know if the subject is receiving a standard, proven therapy or the therapy

---

BOX 1-2 Primary, Secondary, and Tertiary Prevention

Primary Prevention
The goal is to protect healthy people from developing a disease or experiencing an injury in the first place. For example:
- Education about good nutrition, the importance of regular exercise, and the dangers of tobacco, alcohol, and other drugs
- Education and legislation about proper seatbelt and helmet use
- Regular exams and screening tests to monitor risk factors for illness
- Immunization against infectious disease
- Controlling potential hazards at home and in the workplace

Secondary Prevention
These interventions happen after an illness or serious risk factors have already been diagnosed. The goal is to halt or slow the progress of disease (if possible) in its earliest stages; in the case of injury, goals include limiting long-term disability and preventing re-injury. For example:
- Telling people to take daily, low-dose aspirin to prevent a first or second heart attack or stroke
- Recommending regular exams and screening tests in people with known risk factors for illness
- Providing suitably modified work for injured workers

Tertiary Prevention
This focuses on helping people manage complicated, long-term health problems such as diabetes, heart disease, cancer, and chronic musculoskeletal pain. The goals include preventing further physical deterioration and maximizing quality of life. For example:
- Cardiac or stroke rehabilitation programs
- Chronic pain management programs
- Patient support groups

From http://www.iwh.on.ca/wrmb/primary-secondary-and-tertiary-prevention.

being tested. The subject is identified by number only without the particular therapy administered. All results are recorded by the subject's identification number. The principal investigator is responsible for tracking data collected in trials with many patients often in several different health centers. The data are then analyzed to determine if the new therapy is more effective than the traditional therapy. In studies of vaccines or other preventive measures, data are collected about the occurrence of disease in both the control and the experimental group to determine if the new measure reduces the incidence of the specific disease. Research findings that demonstrate merit after this three-stage process are often referred to as "evidence-based research findings." The research data collected up to this point are then passed on to regulatory bodies such as the Food and Drug Administration for review. If the therapy is deemed safe and better than the standard therapy used in the past, the data will be approved for use for the specific disease identified in the research protocol.

Evidence-based research does not take into account cost, availability, or social and cultural factors that may influence use and acceptance of a therapy. These factors may be quite significant and affect the physician's or patient's acceptance of a therapy.

In some rare cases, stage three research trials will be stopped if there is a significant difference in the mortality rate for the experimental group versus the control group. Research on the first antiretroviral agent, AZT, was stopped 6 months early when the research showed a striking difference in survival rates. Those in the experimental group receiving AZT were outliving the control group in significant numbers. When the results were analyzed, trials stopped and all patients were given the option of receiving AZT.

Once a therapy is approved for use, it may show additional potential to treat a different disease. Such use is termed "off-label" use. For the manufacturer to advertise the drug or therapy for use in different diseases, it must go through stage three clinical trials in patients having the new disease. An example of this is research using the drug thalidomide to treat malignancies such as multiple myeloma.

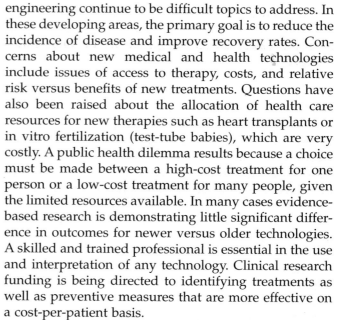

THINK ABOUT 1-1

a. What is the purpose of a double blind research trial?
b. What is a placebo and why is it used in some studies?

Other issues may affect professional practice. Current technology provides an opportunity to prolong life through the use of various machines, many advances in surgery, and the use of organ transplants. Legal and ethical issues about fetal tissue transplants, stem cell therapies, experimental drugs or treatments, and genetic

engineering continue to be difficult topics to address. In these developing areas, the primary goal is to reduce the incidence of disease and improve recovery rates. Concerns about new medical and health technologies include issues of access to therapy, costs, and relative risk versus benefits of new treatments. Questions have also been raised about the allocation of health care resources for new therapies such as heart transplants or in vitro fertilization (test-tube babies), which are very costly. A public health dilemma results because a choice must be made between a high-cost treatment for one person or a low-cost treatment for many people, given the limited resources available. In many cases evidence-based research is demonstrating little significant difference in outcomes for newer versus older technologies. A skilled and trained professional is essential in the use and interpretation of any technology. Clinical research funding is being directed to identifying treatments as well as preventive measures that are more effective on a cost-per-patient basis.

Many options other than traditional therapies are now available. Treatment by acupuncture or naturopathy may be preferred (see Chapter 3). These options may replace traditional therapies or may be used in conjunction with them. A patient may seek an alternative or complementary mode of treatment to supplement traditional care; thus knowledge of these complementary therapies is often needed. It is also recognized that such therapies and practices should be part of a health history for any client seeking care.

Beginning the Process: A Medical History

Many individuals in the health professions will be contributing to, completing, or updating a patient's medical or health history (see Ready Reference 6 for an example). This information is essential to identify any impact health care activities might have on a patient's condition, or how a patient's illness might complicate care. The assessment includes questions on current and prior illnesses, allergies, hospitalizations, and treatment. Current health status is particularly important, and should include specific difficulties and any type of therapy or drugs, prescription, nonprescription, and herbal items, including food supplements.

A basic form is usually provided for the patient to fill out, and then completed by the health professional asking appropriate follow-up questions to clarify the patient's current condition and identify any potential problems. Knowledge of pathophysiology is essential to developing useful questions, understanding the implications of this information, and deciding on the necessary precautions or modifications required to prevent complications. For example, a patient with severe respiratory problems or congestive heart failure would have difficulty breathing in a supine position. Reducing stress may be important for a patient with high blood pressure. Prophylactic medication may be necessary for some patients to prevent infection or excessive bleeding. In some cases, additional problems or undesirable effects of medications may be detected.

New Developments and Trends

Constant updating of information and knowledge is required by both students and practitioners. Developments in all areas of health care are occurring at a very rapid rate primarily due to changes in technologies. New causes of disease and more detail regarding the pathophysiology of a disorder are uncovered, diagnostic tests are improved, and more effective drugs are formulated. Technology has greatly altered many aspects of health care.

Extensive research projects continue in efforts to prevent, control, or cure many disorders. For example, research indicated that most cases of cervical cancer resulted from infection by human papillomavirus (HPV). The next step involved development of a vaccine effective against the most common strains of the virus. In clinical trials, use of the vaccine showed a reduction in the number of women developing cervical cancer. This vaccine is now available to young women to prevent cervical cancer in later years. It does not provide 100% prevention and other health prevention behaviors, such as routine screening, need to be maintained, but the number of actual cases of cervical cancer and the cost of treatment are expected to decline dramatically in the coming decades.

It is essential for the student and practitioner to continually check for new information, employing reliable, accurate resources such as professional web sites, journals, or seminars. It is anticipated that many changes in health care will occur in the near future as electronic devices are more frequently used. For example, sensors implanted under the skin may measure blood glucose levels in diabetic patients or release the amount of insulin appropriate to the patient's needs. The increased costs associated with technological advances then are balanced against the costs of hospitalization or chronic care.

Reports from health professionals are gathered by the World Health Organization (WHO), United States Public Health Service, the Centers for Disease Control and Prevention (CDC), and state and local authorities, as well as agencies in countries around the world. These data are organized and published, leading to new research efforts, tracking new or deadly diseases or in some cases, signaling a warning about predisposing conditions or current treatments. Awareness of deviations from the expected outcomes is a responsibility of those working in health care. Keeping up with new discoveries may sometimes feel like "information overload," but it is a critical part of professional practice.

> **APPLY YOUR KNOWLEDGE 1-1**
>
> Using the heart and the lungs, show how you can apply your prior knowledge of anatomy and physiology to your study of pathophysiology. (Hint: Change part of the normal structure and predict the resulting loss of function.)

Basic Terminology of Pathophysiology

Understanding basic terminology is the essential first step in learning a new subject. Second, a review of past learning in normal anatomy and physiology, along with the associated proper names and terms, is needed in the study of pathophysiology. Selected anatomical terms may be reviewed in Ready References 1 and 2 in the appendices at the back of the text. A firm foundation in anatomy and physiology is particularly important when a disease affects several organs or systems in the body. For example, kidney disease often affects cardiovascular function through the renin, angiotensin, and aldosterone mechanisms. The significance of these effects on another system can be more easily understood and remembered when prior knowledge of normal physiology can be quickly applied to the altered function.

A disease or abnormal condition usually involves changes at the organ or system (*gross*) level as well as at the cellular, or microscopic, level. Pathophysiology focuses on the effects of abnormalities at the organ level, but cellular changes are usually integral to a full understanding of these effects. Pathology laboratory studies, which are particularly useful in establishing the *cause* of a disease, examine tissue specimens from biopsy procedures (excision of very small amounts of living tissue), surgical specimens, or examination after death (autopsy). Analysis of body fluids is another essential diagnostic tool in a pathology laboratory. As indicated, the pathophysiologic changes at a particular site also include evidence of the basic cause of disease, whether it is an infection, a neoplasm, or a genetic defect.

The Disease Process

Following are a few terms frequently used in the discussion of disease processes. Not all of these terms are necessarily used when describing any one disorder.

- *Diagnosis* refers to the identification of a specific disease through evaluation of signs and symptoms, laboratory tests (see front inside cover and Ready Reference 5 in the Appendix) or other tools. More than one factor is usually required to verify a diagnosis. For example, a diagnosis of diabetes mellitus could be confirmed by a blood test following consideration of the patient's signs and a fractured leg bone is indicated by pain, swelling, perhaps the position of the leg, but it is confirmed by x-ray.
- *Etiology* concerns the causative factors in a particular disease. There may be one or several causative factors.

Etiologic agents include congenital defects, inherited or genetic disorders, microorganisms such as viruses or bacteria, immunologic dysfunction, metabolic derangements, degenerative changes, malignancy, burns and other trauma, environmental factors, and nutritional deficiencies.

Causes of Disease

When the cause of a disease is unknown, it is termed idiopathic. In some cases, a treatment, a procedure, or an error may cause a disease, which is then described as iatrogenic. Examples of iatrogenic disease are a bladder infection following catheterization, or bone marrow damage caused by a prescribed drug. In some cases, a difficult decision must be made about a treatment that does involve an additional serious risk, with careful assessment of the benefits versus the risks of a specific treatment. For example, certain forms of chemotherapy and radiation used in the treatment of cancer may cause other serious complications for the patient. In these situations, an informed choice must be made by the client and practitioner.

- *Predisposing factors* encompass the tendencies that promote development of a disease in an individual. A predisposing factor indicates a *high risk* for the disease but not certain development. Predisposing or high-risk factors may include age, gender, inherited factors, occupational exposure, or certain dietary practices. For example, insufficient calcium intake predisposes to osteoporosis. Exposure to asbestos is known to increase the risk of developing cancer. A high dietary intake of cholesterol and saturated fats, cigarette smoking, obesity, and a sedentary lifestyle are factors that increase the risk of heart attacks. By promoting avoidance of predisposing factors, the number of individuals developing the disorder could be greatly reduced.
- Prophylaxis measures designed to preserve health (as of an individual or society) and prevent the spread of disease. Prophylactic treatment for myocardial infarction for high-risk patients is a baby aspirin daily.
- *Prevention* of disease is closely linked to etiology and predisposing factors for a specific disease. Preventive measures include vaccinations, dietary or lifestyle modifications, removal of harmful materials in the environment, and cessation of potentially harmful activities such as smoking. The health professional can provide appropriate and reliable information about the activities that support the client's needs and allow him or her to make better decisions about his or her personal health.

Characteristics of Disease

In describing the characteristics of a particular disease, certain terms are standard:

- *Pathogenesis* refers to the development of the disease or the sequence of events involved in the tissue changes related to the specific disease process.
- The *onset* of a disease may be *sudden* and obvious or *acute*; for example, gastroenteritis with vomiting, cramps, and diarrhea; or the onset may be *insidious*, best described as a gradual progression with only vague or very mild signs. Hepatitis may manifest quietly in this way. There may be several stages in the development of a single disease.
- An *acute* disease indicates a short-term illness that develops very quickly with marked signs such as high fever or severe pain; for example, acute appendicitis.
- A *chronic* disease is often a milder condition developing gradually, such as rheumatoid arthritis, but it persists for a long time and usually causes more permanent tissue damage. Often a chronic disease is marked by intermittent acute episodes.
- A *subclinical* state exists in some conditions in which pathologic changes occur, but no obvious manifestations are exhibited by the patient, perhaps because of the great reserve capacity of some organs. For example, kidney damage may progress to an advanced stage of renal failure before symptoms are manifested.
- An initial *latent* or "silent" stage, in which no clinical signs are evident, characterizes some diseases. In infectious diseases this stage may be referred to as the *incubation* period, which is the time between exposure to the microorganism and the onset of signs or symptoms; it may last for a day or so or may be prolonged, perhaps for days or weeks. Often the disease agent may be communicable during this incubation period.
- The *prodromal* period comprises the time in the early development of a disease when one is aware of a change in the body, but the signs are nonspecific; for example, fatigue, loss of appetite, or headache. A sense of feeling threatened often develops in the early stage of infections. Laboratory tests are negative during the prodromal period; thus it is difficult to confirm a diagnosis.
- The *manifestations* of a disease are the clinical evidence or effects, the signs and symptoms, of disease. These manifestations, such as redness and swelling, may be *local*, or found at the site of the problem. Or signs and symptoms may be *systemic*, meaning they are general indicators of illness, such as fever.
- *Signs* are objective indicators of disease that are obvious to someone other than the affected individual. Examples of a sign are a fever or a skin rash.
- *Symptoms* are subjective feelings, such as pain or nausea. Both signs and symptoms are significant in diagnosing a particular problem.
- *Lesion* is the term used to describe a specific local change in the tissue. Such a change may be microscopic, as when liver cells are examined for

pathologic change, or highly visible, such as a blister or pimple observed on the skin.

- A *syndrome* is a collection of signs and symptoms, often affecting more than one organ, that usually occur together in response to a certain condition.
- *Diagnostic* tests are laboratory tests that assist in the diagnosis of a specific disease. The appropriate tests are ordered on the basis of the patient's manifestations and medical history, the clinical examination, and the patient's answers to specific questions. These tests may also be used for monitoring the response to treatment or the progress of the disease. Such tests may involve chemical analysis of body fluids such as blood, examination of tissues and cells from specimens (e.g., biopsies or body secretions), identification of microorganisms in body fluids or tissue specimens, or radiologic examination of the body. It is important that medical laboratories have a Quality Assurance (QA) program in place to ensure accurate test results. Also, it is often helpful for a patient to have any future or repeated tests done by the same laboratory to provide a more accurate comparison of results.
- *Remissions* and *exacerbations* may mark the *course* or progress of a disease. During a remission, the manifestations of the disease subside, whereas during an exacerbation the signs increase. Rheumatoid arthritis typically has periods of remission when pain and swelling are minimal, alternating with acute periods when swelling and pain are severe.
- A *precipitating* factor is a condition that triggers an acute episode, such as a seizure in an individual with a seizure disorder. Note that a precipitating factor differs from a predisposing factor. For example, a patient may be predisposed to coronary artery disease and angina because of a high-cholesterol diet. An angina attack can be precipitated by shoveling snow on a very cold day.
- *Complications* are new secondary or additional problems that arise after the original disease begins. For example, following a heart attack, a person may develop congestive heart failure, a complication.
- *Therapy* or therapeutic interventions are treatment measures used to promote recovery or slow the progress of a disease. These measures may include surgery, drugs, physiotherapy, alternative therapies or behavior modification (see Chapter 3).
- *Sequelae* describe the potential unwanted outcomes of the primary condition, such as paralysis following recovery from a stroke.
- *Convalescence* or *rehabilitation* is the period of recovery and return to the normal healthy state; it may last for several days or months.

Disease Prognosis

Prognosis defines the probability or likelihood for recovery or other outcomes. The probability figures used in prognosis are based on average outcomes, and there may be considerable variation among affected individuals. It is important to consider the basis of the statistics used to form such conclusions. How big was the clinical group? How long was the study? It is very difficult to state a prognosis for diseases that affect a very small group of clients or in which outcomes vary unpredictably.

- *Morbidity* indicates the disease rates within a group; this term is sometimes used to indicate the functional impairment that certain conditions such as stroke cause within a population.
- *Mortality* figures indicate the relative number of deaths resulting from a particular disease.
- *Epidemiology* is the science of tracking the pattern or occurrence of disease. Epidemiologic records include data on the transmission and distribution of diseases and are particularly important in the control of infectious diseases and environmentally related diseases. Data may be presented in graphs, tables, or on maps to provide a visible pattern. For example, epidemiologic information is used to determine the components of the influenza vaccine to be administered each year based on the currently active strains and geographic movement of the influenza virus. Major data collection centers are the World Health Organization (WHO) and the Centers for Disease Control and Prevention (CDC) in Atlanta, Georgia, and Ottawa, Canada. Notification and reporting of disease is required to provide data for epidemiologic studies and prevent occurrence of diseases.
- *Epidemics* occur when there are a higher than expected number of cases of an infectious disease within a given area, whereas *pandemics* involve higher numbers of cases in many regions of the globe (Fig. 1-1). Influenza may occur sporadically as well as in epidemic or pandemic outbreaks.
- The *occurrence* of a disease is tracked by recording two factors, the incidence and the prevalence. The *incidence* of a disease indicates the number of new cases in a given population noted within a stated time period (see Fig. 1-1). A significant increase or decrease in incidence of a specific disease may be analyzed to determine the responsible factors. *Prevalence* refers to the number of new and old or existing cases within a specific population and time period. Note that prevalence is always a larger figure than incidence.
- *Communicable* diseases are infections that can be spread from one person to another. Some of these must be reported to health authorities.
- *Notifiable* or *reportable* diseases must be reported by the physician to certain designated authorities. The authority varies with the local jurisdiction. The specific diseases required to be reported may change over time. The requirement of reporting is intended to prevent further spread of the disease and maintain public health. Such infections as measles, severe acute respiratory syndrome (SARS), and human immunodeficiency virus (HIV) or acquired

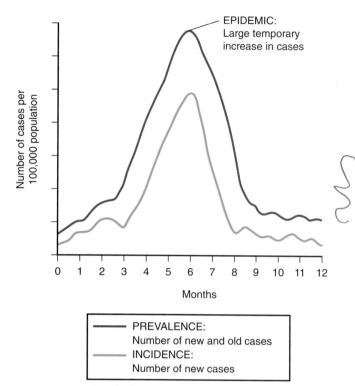

FIGURE 1-1 Graph illustrating the occurrence of disease.

immunodeficiency syndrome (AIDS) may be included in some jurisdictions.

- An *autopsy* or *postmortem examination* may be performed after death to determine the exact cause of death, or determine the course of the illness and effectiveness of treatment. An autopsy is an examination of all or part of the body by a pathologist. It includes gross and microscopic examination of tissues, organs, and fluids, and can include a variety of tests depending on individual circumstances.

THINK ABOUT   1-2

Rheumatoid arthritis is defined as a chronic systemic disorder with remissions and exacerbations, resulting in permanent joint damage. Describe this disease in terms of manifestations, etiology, predisposing factors, pathogenesis, and treatments.

Introduction to Cellular Changes

The cells have mechanisms by which they can adapt their growth and differentiation to altered conditions in the body. Some minor alterations, such as increases in breast and uterine tissue during pregnancy, are normal adaptations to change in the body. Tissues are frequently modified as a response to hormonal stimulation or environmental stimuli such as irritation. Frequently such changes are reversible after the stimulus is removed. However, disease may develop when cell

structure and function change and homeostasis cannot be maintained as a result. Irreversible changes in a cell signal a change in DNA structure or function. (See Fig. 21-2 for an illustration of DNA, the controlling nuclear material in a cell.) Abnormal changes are not necessarily a precursor to permanent tissue damage or the development of tumors or cancer, but it is important to determine the cause and monitor any abnormality to reduce the risk of serious consequences. Cells may be damaged or destroyed by changes in metabolic processes, reduced levels of adenosine triphosphate (ATP), altered pH in the cells, or damage to the cell membrane and receptors.

Terms Used for Common Cellular Adaptations

- *Atrophy* refers to a *decrease* in the *size* of cells, resulting in a reduced tissue mass (Fig. 1-2). Common causes include reduced use of the tissue, insufficient nutrition, decreased neurologic or hormonal stimulation, and aging. An example is the shrinkage of skeletal muscle that occurs when a limb is immobilized in a cast for several weeks.
- *Hypertrophy* refers to an *increase* in the *size* of individual cells, resulting in an enlarged tissue mass. This increase may be caused by additional work by the tissue, as demonstrated by an enlarged heart muscle resulting from increased demands (see Fig. 12-23). A common example of hypertrophy is the effect of consistent exercise on skeletal muscle, leading to an enlarged muscle mass. Excessive hormonal stimulation may also stimulate cell growth.
- *Hyperplasia* is defined as an increased *number* of cells resulting in an enlarged tissue mass. In some cases, hypertrophy and hyperplasia occur simultaneously, as in the uterine enlargement that occurs during pregnancy. Hyperplasia may be a compensatory mechanism to meet increased demands, or it may be pathologic when there is a hormonal imbalance. In certain instances there may be an increased risk of cancer when hyperplasia occurs.
- *Metaplasia* occurs when one mature cell type is replaced by a different mature cell type. This change may result from a deficit of vitamin A. Sometimes, metaplasia may be an adaptive mechanism that provides a more resistant tissue; for instance, when stratified squamous epithelium replaces ciliated columnar epithelium in the respiratory tracts of cigarette smokers. Although the new cells present a stronger barrier, they result in decreased defenses for the lungs because cilia are no longer present as a defense mechanism for the simpler squamous cells in the mucosa.
- *Dysplasia* is the term applied to tissue in which the cells vary in size and shape, large nuclei are frequently present, and the rate of mitosis is increased. This situation may result from chronic irritation

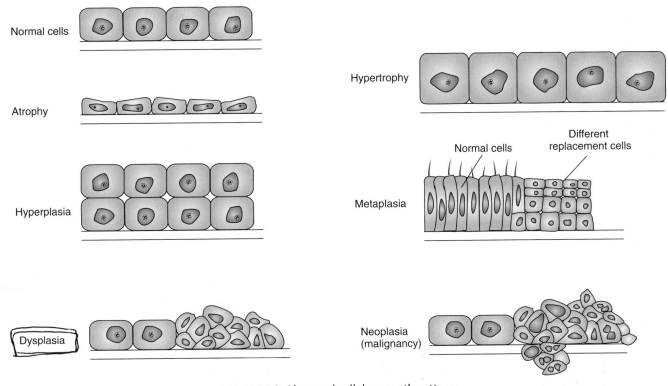

FIGURE 1-2 Abnormal cellular growth patterns.

infection, or it may be a precancerous change. Detection of dysplasia is the basis of routine screening tests for atypical cells such as the Pap smear (Papanicolaou test on cervical cells).

- *Anaplasia* refers to cells that are undifferentiated with variable nuclear and cell structures and numerous mitotic figures. Anaplasia is characteristic of cancer and is the basis for grading the aggressiveness of a tumor.
- Neoplasia means "new growth," and a neoplasm is commonly called a tumor. Tumors are of two types, benign and malignant (see Figs. 20-1 and 20-2). Malignant neoplasms are referred to as *cancer*. Benign tumors do not necessarily become malignant. Benign tumors are usually considered less serious because they do not spread and are not life threatening unless they are found in certain locations, such as the brain, where they can cause pressure problems. The characteristics of each tumor depend on the specific type of cell from which the tumor arises, resulting in a unique appearance and growth pattern. Neoplasms are discussed further in Chapter 20.

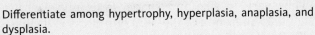

THINK ABOUT 1-3

Differentiate among hypertrophy, hyperplasia, anaplasia, and dysplasia.

Cell Damage and Necrosis

Apoptosis refers to programmed cell death, a normal occurrence in the body, which may increase when cell development is abnormal, cell numbers are excessive, or cells are injured or aged. Cells self-destruct, appearing to digest themselves enzymatically, and then disintegrate into fragments.

There are many ways of injuring cells in the body, including:

- Ischemia, a decreased supply of oxygenated blood to a tissue or organ, due to circulatory obstruction
- Physical agents, excessive heat or cold, or radiation exposure
- Mechanical damage such as pressure or tearing of tissue
- Chemical toxins
- Microorganisms such as bacteria, viruses, and parasites
- Abnormal metabolites accumulating in cells
- Nutritional deficits
- Imbalance of fluids or electrolytes

The most common cause of injury is ischemia or reduced blood supply to the tissue, which results in insufficient oxygen and reduced cellular metabolism. Decreased oxygen in the tissue may occur locally because of a blocked artery or systemically because of respiratory impairment. Cells with a high demand for oxygen, such as those of the brain, heart, and kidney, are quickly affected by hypoxia (reduced oxygen in the tissue). A severe oxygen deficit interferes with energy (ATP) production in the cell, leading to loss of the sodium pump at the cell membrane as well as loss of other cell functions. An increase in sodium ions inside the cell leads to swelling of the cell and eventually to rupture of the cell membrane. At the same time, in the absence of oxygen, anaerobic metabolism occurs in the cell, leading to a decrease in pH from build of lactic acid and further metabolic impairment. A deficit of other essential nutrients such as vitamins may also damage cells because normal metabolic processes cannot take place.

Another cause of cellular damage is physical injury related to thermal (heat) or mechanical pressures. These may impair blood supply to the cells or affect metabolic processes in the cells. Radiation exposure may damage cells by interfering with their blood supply or directly altering their chemical constituents, creating toxic materials inside the cells or changing DNA. Chemicals from both the environment (exogenous) and inside the body (endogenous) may damage cells, either by altering cell membrane permeability or producing other reactive chemicals, known as free radicals, which continue to damage cell components. Infectious diseases cause cell injury through the actions of microorganisms (living organisms too small to be seen with the naked eye) such as bacteria and viruses. Some genetic defects or inborn errors of metabolism can lead to abnormal metabolic processes. Altered metabolism leads to accumulation of toxic intermediary compounds inside the cells that ultimately destroy them.

Cell damage usually occurs in two stages. In general, the *initial* cell damage causes an alteration in a metabolic reaction, which leads to a *loss of function* of the cell. If the factor causing the damage is removed quickly, the cell may be able to recover and return to its normal state, and the damage is said to be reversible. As the amount of damage increases, detectable morphologic or structural changes occur in the nucleus and the cell as well. Cell death may take on a variety of forms. Generally these involve cellular swelling and rupture if the cell membrane is affected or accumulations of lipid inside the cell if metabolic derangements are present. If the noxious factor remains, the damage becomes irreversible and the cell dies.

Following cell death, the nucleus of the cell disintegrates. The cells undergo lysis or dissolution, releasing destructive lysosomal enzymes into the tissue, which cause inflammation (swelling, redness, and pain) as well as damage to nearby cells and reduced function (see Chapter 5). If a large number of cells have died, inflammation can be extensive, causing the destruction of additional cells. The enzymes released from the dead cells can diffuse into the blood, providing helpful clues in blood tests that indicate the type of cells damaged. Diagnostic tests for specific enzymes present in the blood may determine the site and source of the problem, for example, a heart attack, in which part of the heart muscle is destroyed.

Necrosis is the term used when a group of cells die. The process of cell death varies with the cause of the damage (Fig. 1-3).

- *Liquefaction necrosis* refers to the process by which dead cells liquefy under the influence of certain cell enzymes. This process occurs when brain tissue dies or in certain bacterial infections in which a cavity or ulcer may develop in the infected area.
- *Coagulative necrosis* occurs when the cell proteins are altered or denatured (similar to the coagulation that occurs when cooking eggs), and the cells retain some form for a time after death. This process typically occurs in a myocardial infarction (heart attack) when a lack of oxygen causes cell death.
- *Fat necrosis* occurs when fatty tissue is broken down into fatty acids in the presence of infection or certain enzymes (see Fig. 1-3C). These compounds may increase inflammation.
- *Caseous necrosis* is a form of coagulation necrosis in which a thick, yellowish, "cheesy" substance forms. Tuberculosis (TB) offers an interesting example of caseous necrosis (Fig. 1-4). When tuberculosis develops, the first stage is characterized by development of a granuloma, a small solid mass of macrophages and lymphocytes, often covered by connective tissue, which forms in some types of chronic inflammation (see Chapter 5). With TB, caseous necrosis can be seen inside this mass. The granuloma associated with tuberculosis is called a Ghon focus or complex, and it usually heals like a scar, containing the infection. If the infection continues to develop, this area may undergo liquefaction necrosis, forming a cavity. (See Chapter 13 for more details on tuberculosis.)
- *Infarction* is the term applied to an area of dead cells resulting from lack of oxygen (see Fig. 12-16B). When a large number of cells in an area die, the functional loss can be significant. For example, when part of the heart muscle is infarcted or dies, that area can no longer contract to pump blood (see Chapter 12). After tissue dies, it is eventually replaced either by tissue regenerated from nearby similar cells or connective tissue or scar tissue that fills the gap. Myocardial or heart muscle cells do not undergo mitosis; therefore scar tissue must replace the dead tissue.

Gangrene refers to an area of necrotic tissue that has been invaded by bacteria (see Fig. 1-3D). Necrotic tissue can provide a good medium for infection by microorganisms. Such an infection frequently occurs after an infarction in the intestines or in a limb in which blood supply is deficient and bacteria are normally present. Depending on its location, gangrene may be described as wet or dry. Gangrene may cause the buildup of gases within tissue and further reduce blood supply. Gangrenous tissue frequently must be removed surgically (e.g., by amputation) to prevent the spread of infection to other parts of the body.

NEUROSIS

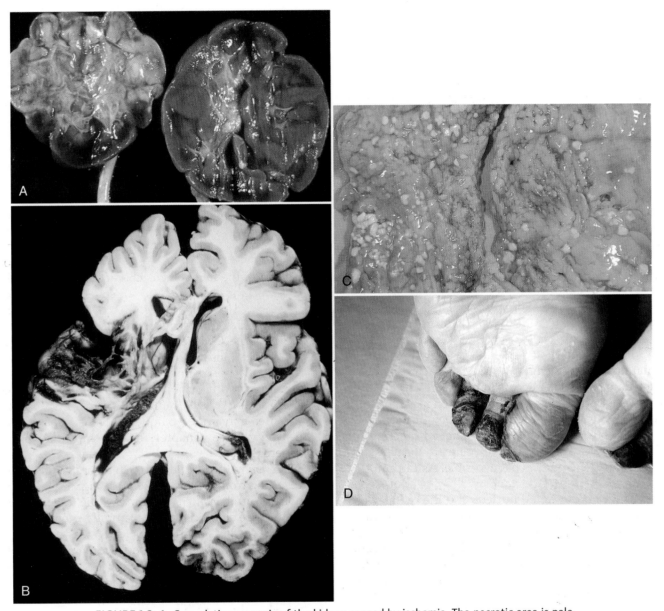

FIGURE 1-3 **A**, Coagulative necrosis of the kidney caused by ischemia. The necrotic area is pale yellow, in contrast to the normal reddish-brown tissue. **B**, Liquefaction necrosis following infarction in the brain, leading to destruction of tissue and cystic infarct. **C**, Fat necrosis in the mesentery. The areas of white chalky deposits represent calcium soap formation at sites of lipid breakdown. **D**, Dry gangrene of the toe. *(A, D From Damjanov I:* Pathology for the Health Professions, *ed 3, Philadelphia, 2006, WB Saunders. B, C From Kumar V, Abbas AK, Fausto M:* Robbins and Cotran Pathologic Basis of Disease, *ed 7, Philadelphia, 2005, WB Saunders.)*

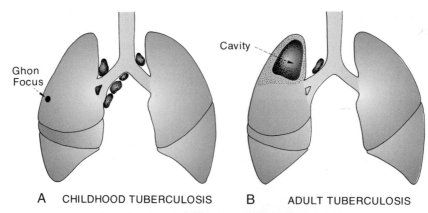

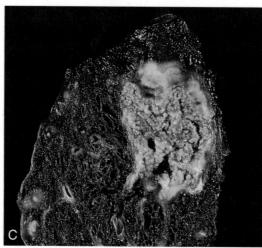

FIGURE 1-4 **A and B,** Pulmonary tuberculosis. *(Drawing by Margot Mackay, University of Toronto Faculty of Medicine, Department of Surgery, Division of Biomedical Communications, Toronto. Reprinted from Walter JB:* An Introduction to the Principles of Diseases, *ed 3, Philadelphia, 1992, WB Saunders.)* **C,** A tuberculous lung with a large area of caseous necrosis. *(From Kumar V, Abbas AK, Fausto M:* Robbins and Cotran Pathologic Basis of Disease, *ed 7, Philadelphia, 2005, WB Saunders.)*

THINK ABOUT 1-4

Describe the different types of necrosis and identify conditions in which amputation may be necessary.

Specific types of cells die at different rates. *Brain* cells die quickly (4-5 minutes) when deprived of oxygen, whereas *heart muscle* can survive for approximately 30 minutes. Formerly death of the body (*somatic death*) was assumed to occur when heart action and respiration ceased. Now because cardiac and respiratory function can be maintained artificially, the diagnosis of death is more complex. Currently *brain death* provides the criteria for somatic death. A diagnosis of brain death is made following a set protocol of tests and examinations including a lack of responses to stimuli, EEG changes, and decreased perfusion in the brain (see Chapter 14).

CHAPTER SUMMARY

- Disease is defined as a deviation from the individual's normal state of physical, mental, and social well-being, leading to a loss of homeostasis in the body. Pathophysiology is the study of the structural and functional changes related to disease processes.
- Effects of a specific disease depend on the organ or tissue affected and the cause of the disease; for example, infection or malignant tumor.
- Disease prevention campaigns or screening programs for early diagnosis are based on factors such as causes, predisposing factors, and incidence of specific disease.
- Health professionals need to be aware of the new information, diagnostic tests, and therapies that are constantly emerging. The allocation of resources for

health care and the ethical issues related to new technologies are concerns.

- The discussion of disease processes includes such topics as occurrence, diagnosis, or the identification of a disease; etiology or the cause of disease; pathologic changes in the tissues or organs, or signs and symptoms of disease; and prognosis, or the probable outcomes.
- Cell and tissue changes such as atrophy and hypertrophy are frequently linked to changes in demand or use of the tissue. Metaplasia often occurs as an adaptive change, replacing the normal cell with a more resistant cell. Dysplasia and anaplasia are connected to malignant changes.
- Cell damage for any reason may be reversible, causing temporary loss of function. Severe damage to a cell causes necrosis and loss of function.
- Causes of cell damage include ischemia or lack of oxygen, toxic substances, changes in pH, or microorganisms such as bacteria and viruses.

STUDY QUESTIONS

1. Choose a specific disease and prepare an appropriate list of six terms that you could use to describe this disease, and define each of the terms.
2. Define and give an example of:
   a. etiology
   b. incidence
   c. precipitating factor
   d. complication
   e. prognosis
   f. iatrogenic
   g. sequelae
3. Differentiate between the terms *metaplasia* and *malignant neoplasm*.
4. Describe the changes in a cell that lead to:
   a. loss of function
   b. necrosis
5. Define:
   a. apoptosis
   b. gangrene
6. What preventive practices can be used to reduce disease?
7. CJ is having surgery next week to remove a malignant breast tumor, following discovery of a lump in the breast and a biopsy. Her mother and aunt have had breast cancer. CJ is taking medication for high blood pressure.

   Match the significant information in the preceding question to the appropriate term: diagnosis, medical history, etiology, prognosis, benign neoplasm, iatrogenic, signs, complication, treatment, cancer, examination of living tissue. Some terms may not be used or may be used more than once.

ADDITIONAL RESOURCES

Dorland's Illustrated Medical Dictionary, ed 29, Philadelphia, 2009, WB Saunders.

Kumar V, Abbas AK, Fausto M: *Robbins and Cotran Pathologic Basis of Disease*, ed 7, Philadelphia, 2007, WB Saunders.

Mosby's Medical, Nursing & Allied Health Dictionary, ed 6, St Louis, 2009, Mosby.

CHAPTER 2

Fluid, Electrolyte, and Acid-Base Imbalances

CHAPTER OUTLINE

LEARNING OBJECTIVES

After studying this chapter, the student is expected to:

1. Explain the movement of water between body compartments that results in edema.
2. Describe the causes and effects of dehydration.
3. Explain the meaning of third-spacing.
4. Discuss the causes and signs of hyponatremia and hypernatremia.
5. Explain the causes and signs of hypokalemia and hyperkalemia.
6. Describe the causes and signs of hypocalcemia and hypercalcemia.
7. Describe the causes and effects of hypomagnesemia, hypophosphatemia, hypochloremia, and hyperchloremia.
8. Explain how metabolic acidosis, metabolic alkalosis, respiratory acidosis, and respiratory alkalosis develop and their effects on the body.
9. Explain how decompensation develops and its effects on the central nervous system.
10. Explain the normal function of atrial natriuretic peptide in maintaining fluid and electrolyte balance.

KEY TERMS

aldosterone	diffusion	hypervolemia	milliequivalent (mEq)
anion	diuretic	hypothalamus	nonvolatile metabolic acids
anorexia	dysrhythmia	hypotonic/hypo-osmolar	osmoreceptor
antidiuretic hormone (ADH)	electrocardiogram	hypovolemia	osmosis
ascites	extracellular	interstitial fluid	osmotic pressure
atrial natriuretic peptide	filtration	intracellular	paresthesias
capillary permeability	hydrogen ions	intravascular fluid	skin turgor
carpopedal spasm	hydrostatic pressure	isotonic/iso-osmolar	tetany
cation	hypertonic/hyper-osmolar	laryngospasm	transcellular

Fluid Imbalance

Review of Concepts and Processes

Water is a major component of the body and is found both within and outside the cells. It is essential to homeostasis, the maintenance of a relatively constant and favorable environment for the cells. Water is the medium within which metabolic reactions and other processes take place. It also comprises the transportation system for the body. For example, water carries nutrients into cells and removes wastes, transports enzymes in digestive secretions, and moves blood cells around the body. Without adequate fluid, cells cannot continue to function, and death results. Fluid also facilitates movement of body parts, for example, the joints and the lungs.

> **THINK ABOUT 2-1**
>
> Suggest several functions performed by water in the body and the significance of each.

Fluid Compartments

Although the body appears to be a solid object, approximately 60% of an adult's body weight consists of water, and an infant's body is about 70% water (Table 2-1). Female bodies, which contain a higher proportion of fatty tissue, have a lower percentage of water than male bodies. The elderly and the obese also have a lower proportion of water in their bodies. Individuals with less fluid reserve are more likely to be adversely affected by any fluid or electrolyte imbalance.

Fluid is distributed between the intracellular compartment (ICF), or fluid inside the cells, and the extracellular compartment (ECF). See Ready Reference 1 for a diagram showing fluid compartments of the body.

ECF includes the:
- Intravascular fluid (IVF) or blood
- Interstitial fluid (ISF) or intercellular fluid

TABLE 2-1	Fluid Compartments in the Body			
	Volume	Approximate Percentage of Body Weight		
	Adult Male (L)	Male (%)	Female (%)	Infant (%)
Intracellular fluid	28	40	33	40
Extracellular fluid	15	20	17	30
Plasma	(4.5)	(4)	(4)	(4)
Interstitial fluid	(10.5)	(15)	(9)	(25)
Other		(1)	(1)	(1)
Total water	43	60	50	70

Note: In elderly women, water content is reduced to approximately 45% of body weight.

- Cerebrospinal fluid (CSF)
- Transcellular fluids present in various secretions, such as those in the pericardial (heart) cavity or the synovial cavities of the joints

In an adult male, blood constitutes about 4% of body weight and interstitial fluid about 15%; the remaining transcellular fluids amount to about 1% of total body weight. Water constantly circulates within the body and moves between various compartments. For example, CSF forms continuously from the blood and is reabsorbed back into the general circulation. A large volume of water (up to 8 liters in 24 hours) is present in the digestive secretions entering the stomach and small intestine, and this fluid is reabsorbed in the colon, making up a very efficient *water-recycling* system.

> **THINK ABOUT 2-2**
>
> a. Which body compartment contains the most water?
> b. Suggest why diarrhea may cause a fluid deficit more rapidly than coughing and sneezing with a cold.

Movement of Water

To maintain a constant level of body fluid, the amount of water entering the body should equal the amount of water leaving the body. Fluid is added to the body through the ingestion of solid food and fluids and as a product of cell metabolism (Table 2-2). Fluid is lost in the urine and feces as well as through *insensible* (unapparent) losses through the skin (perspiration) and exhaled air.

Control of fluid balance is maintained by:
- The *thirst* mechanism in the hypothalamus, the osmoreceptor cells of which sense the internal environment, both fluid volume and concentration, and then promote the intake of fluid when needed
- The hormone, antidiuretic hormone (ADH), which controls the amount of fluid leaving the body in the urine (see Chapters 16 and 18); ADH promotes reabsorption of water into the blood from the kidney tubules
- The hormone aldosterone, which determines the reabsorption of both sodium ions and water from the kidney tubules; these hormones conserve more fluid when there is a fluid deficit in the body
- The hormone atrial natriuretic peptide (ANP) is a hormone synthesized and released by the myocardial cells in the atrium of the heart. Its role in homeostasis relates to reduction of workload on the heart by regulating fluid, sodium, and potassium levels. In the kidney ANP increases glomerular filtration rate (GFR) by altering pressure in the glomerular capillaries; it also reduces the reabsorption of sodium in the distal convoluted tubules through inhibition of antidiuretic hormone (ADH). Renin secretion is also reduced and thus the renin angiotensin system is inhibited. The result is fluid loss from the

TABLE 2-2	Sources and Losses of Water		
Sources (mL)		Losses (mL)	
Liquids	1200	Urine	1400
Solid foods	1000	Feces	200
Cell metabolism	300	Insensible losses	
		Lungs	400
		Skin	500
Total	2500		2500

extracellular compartment and lowered blood pressure. It also reduces aldosterone secretion, leading to retention of potassium. Research has shown that ANP is elevated in patients with congestive heart failure who have increased blood volume in the atria (see Chapter 12). Research is ongoing on this peptide and its possible use in the treatment of hypertension and congestive heart failure.

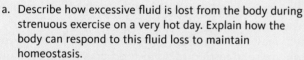

THINK ABOUT 2-3

a. Describe how excessive fluid is lost from the body during strenuous exercise on a very hot day. Explain how the body can respond to this fluid loss to maintain homeostasis.
b. What factors may limit such responses?

Fluid constantly circulates throughout the body and moves relatively freely, depending on the permeability of the membranes between compartments, by the processes of filtration or osmosis (Fig. 2-1). Water moves between the vascular compartment or blood and the interstitial compartment through the semipermeable capillary membranes, depending on the relative hydrostatic and osmotic pressures within the compartments (see Fig. 2-1). Proteins and electrolytes contribute to the osmotic pressure of a fluid and therefore are very important in maintaining fluid volumes in various compartments. Hydrostatic pressure may be viewed as the "push" force and osmotic pressure as the "pull" or attraction force in such fluid movements. Changes in either force will alter fluid movement and volume in the compartments.

At the arteriolar end of the capillary, the blood hydrostatic pressure (or blood pressure) exceeds the opposing interstitial hydrostatic pressure and the plasma colloid osmotic pressure of the blood, and therefore fluid moves out from (or is "pushed" out of) the capillary into the interstitial compartment. At the venous end of the capillary, the blood hydrostatic pressure is greatly decreased and osmotic pressure higher, and therefore fluid tends to shift (or is "pulled") back into the capillary. It is easier to remember the direction of movement if one thinks of the movement of nutrients and oxygen out of the arterial blood toward the cells and the flow of wastes and

carbon dioxide from the cell back into the venous blood. Excess fluid and any protein in the interstitial compartment is returned to the circulation through the lymphatic capillaries.

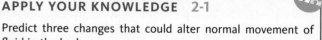

APPLY YOUR KNOWLEDGE 2-1

Predict three changes that could alter normal movement of fluid in the body.

Many cells have mechanisms to control intracellular volume. A major factor in the movement of water through cell membranes is the difference in osmotic pressure between the cell and the interstitial fluids. As the relative concentrations of electrolytes in the interstitial fluid and intracellular fluid change, the osmotic pressure also changes, causing water to move across the cell membrane by osmosis. For example, if an erythrocyte is placed in a dilute hypotonic solution (low osmotic pressure), water may enter the cell, causing it to swell and malfunction.

THINK ABOUT 2-4

a. Explain how a very high hydrostatic pressure in the venule end of a capillary affects fluid shift.
b. Explain how a loss of plasma protein affects fluid shift at the capillaries.
c. Explain how a high concentration of sodium ions in the interstitial fluid affects intracellular fluid levels.

Fluid Excess—Edema

Fluid excess occurs in the extracellular compartment and may be referred to as isotonic/iso-osmolar, hypotonic/hypo-osmolar, or hypertonic/hyperosmolar, depending on the cause. The osmolarity or the concentration of solute in the fluid, affects fluid shifts between compartments, including the cells.

Edema refers to an excessive amount of fluid in the interstitial compartment, which causes a swelling or enlargement of the tissues. Edema may be localized in one area or generalized throughout the body. Depending on the type of tissue and the area of the body, edema may be highly visible or relatively invisible, or not accurately reflect the amount of fluid hidden in the area; for example, facial edema is usually visible but edema of the liver or a limb may not be. Edema is usually more severe in *dependent* areas of the body, where the force of gravity is greatest, such as the buttocks, ankles, or feet of a person in a wheelchair. Prolonged edema interferes with venous return, arterial circulation, and cell function in the affected area.

Causes of Edema

Edema has four general causes (Fig. 2-2).
1. The first cause is *increased capillary hydrostatic pressure* (equivalent to higher BP or blood pressure), which

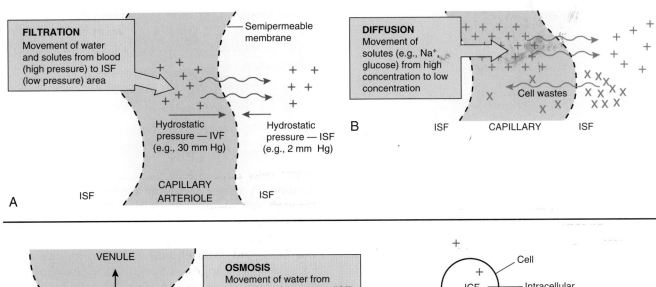

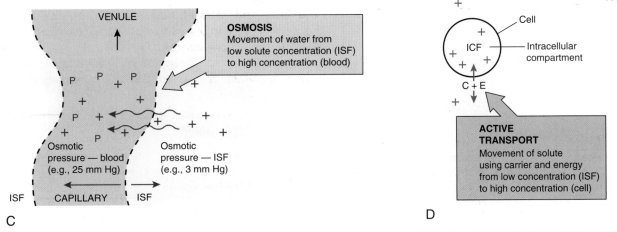

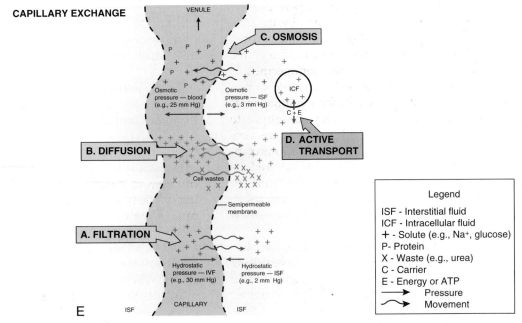

FIGURE 2-1 Movement of water and electrolytes between compartments.

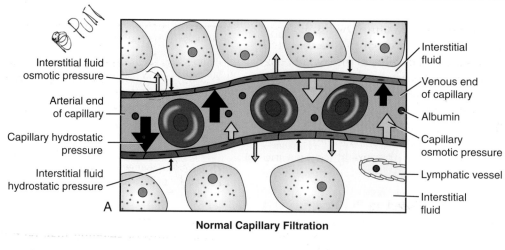
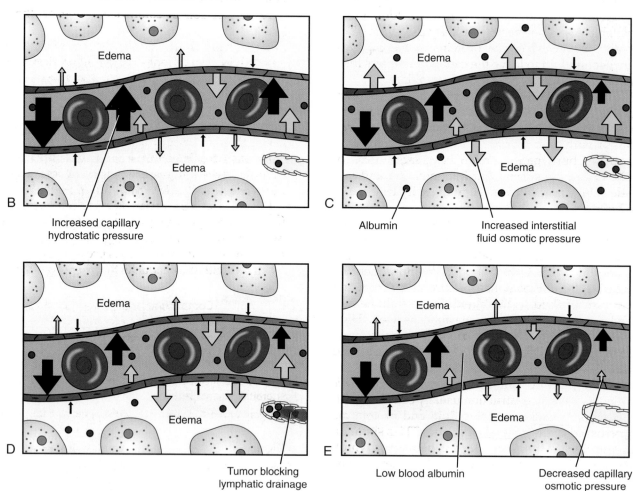

FIGURE 2-2 Causes of edema. **A,** Normal capillary filtration without edema. **B,** Edema due to increased capillary hydrostatic pressure. **C,** Edema due to increased interstitial fluid osmotic pressure from increased capillary permeability. **D,** Edema due to blocked lymphatic drainage. **E,** Edema due to decreased capillary osmotic pressure from hypoalbuminemia. *(From Copstead-Kirkorn LC:* Pathophysiology, *ed 4, St. Louis, 2009, Mosby.)*

prevents return of fluid from the interstitial compartment to the venous end of the capillary, or forces excessive amounts of fluid out of the capillaries into the tissues. The latter is a cause of pulmonary edema, in which excessive pressure, often due to increased

blood volume, can force fluid into the alveoli, interfering with respiratory function.

Specific causes of edema related to increased hydrostatic pressure include increased blood volume (hypervolemia) associated with kidney failure,

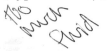

pregnancy, congestive heart failure, or administration of excessive fluids. In pregnancy, the enlarged uterus compresses the pelvic veins in the seated position and when a pregnant woman must stand still for long periods of time, the pressure in the leg veins can become quite elevated, causing edema in the feet and legs. In some people with congestive heart failure, the blood cannot return easily through the veins to the heart, raising the hydrostatic pressure in the legs and abdominal organs and causing ascites, or fluid in the abdominal cavity.

2. Second, edema may be related to the *loss of plasma proteins*, particularly albumin, which results in a decrease in plasma osmotic pressure. Plasma proteins usually remain inside the capillary and seldom move through the semipermeable capillary membrane. The presence of fewer plasma proteins in the capillary allows more fluid to leave the capillary and less fluid to return to the venous end of the capillary.

    Protein may be lost in the urine through kidney disease, or synthesis of protein may be impaired in patients with malnutrition and malabsorption diseases or with liver disease. Protein levels may drop acutely in burn patients who have large areas of burned skin; the subsequent inflammation and loss of the skin barrier allow protein to easily leak out of the body.

    Frequently *excessive sodium levels* in the extracellular fluid accompany the two causes just mentioned. When sodium ions are retained, they promote accumulation of fluid in the interstitial compartment by increasing the ISF osmotic pressure and decreasing the return of fluid to the blood. Blood volume and blood pressure are usually elevated as well. High sodium levels are common in patients with heart failure, high blood pressure, kidney disease, and increased aldosterone secretion.

3. Edema may result from *obstruction of the lymphatic circulation*. Such an obstruction usually causes a localized edema because excessive fluid and protein are not returned to the general circulation. This situation may develop if a tumor or infection damages a lymph node or if lymph nodes are removed, as they may be in cancer surgery.

4. The fourth cause of edema is *increased capillary permeability*. This usually causes localized edema and may result from an inflammatory response or infection (see Chapter 5). In this case, histamine and other chemical mediators released from cells following tissue injury cause increased capillary permeability and increased fluid movement into the interstitial area. Protein also leaks into the interstitial compartment, increasing the osmotic pressure in ISF and thus holding more fluid in the interstitial area. A general increase in capillary permeability can result from some bacterial toxins or large burn wounds, leading to both hypovolemia and shock.

loss of fluid

THINK ABOUT 2-5
a. In some cases of breast cancer, many of the axillary lymph nodes are removed. Why are injections not usually done on the affected arm?
b. Explain why severe kidney disease may cause generalized edema.
c. Explain why the feet may become swollen when one sits for long periods of time, but the swelling decreases when one lies recumbent in bed.
d. Explain how protein-calorie malnutrition results in ascites.

Effects of Edema

- A local area of swelling may be visible and may be very pale or red in color, depending on the cause (Table 2-3).
- *Pitting* edema occurs in the presence of excess interstitial fluid, which moves aside when firm pressure is applied by the fingers. A depression or "pit" remains after the finger is removed.
- In people with generalized edema there is a significant increase in *body weight*, which may indicate a problem before there are other visible signs (see Fig. 2-3).
- *Functional* impairment due to edema may occur, for example, when it restricts range of movement of joints. Edema of the intestinal wall may interfere with digestion and absorption. Edema or accumulated fluid around the heart or lungs impairs the movement and function of these organs.
- *Pain* may occur if edema exerts pressure on the nerves locally, as with the headache that develops in patients

| TABLE 2-3 | Comparison of Signs and Symptoms of Fluid Excess (Edema) and Fluid Deficit (Dehydration) |

Fluid Excess (Edema)	Fluid Deficit (Dehydration)
Localized swelling (feet, hands, periorbital area, ascites)	Sunken, soft eyes
Pale, gray, or red skin color	Decreased skin turgor, dry mucous membranes
Weight gain	Thirst, weight loss
Slow, bounding pulse; high blood pressure	Rapid, weak, thready pulse, low blood pressure, and orthostatic hypotension
Lethargy, possible seizures	Fatigue, weakness, dizziness, possible stupor
Pulmonary congestion, cough, rales	Increased body temperature
Laboratory values:	Laboratory values:
Decreased hematocrit	Increased hematocrit
Decreased serum sodium	Increased electrolytes (or variable)
Urine: low specific gravity, high volume	Urine: high specific gravity, low volume

Note: Signs may vary depending on the cause of the imbalance.

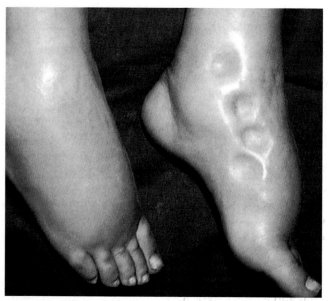

FIGURE 2-3 Pitting edema. Note the finger-shaped depressions that do not rapidly refill after an examiner has exerted pressure. *(From Bloom A, Ireland J: Color Atlas of Diabetes, ed 2, St. Louis, Mosby, 1992.)*

with cerebral edema. If cerebral edema becomes severe, the pressure can impair brain function because of ischemia and can cause death. When viscera such as the kidney or liver are edematous, the capsule is stretched, causing pain.

- With sustained edema the *arterial circulation* may be impaired. The increased interstitial pressure may restrict arterial blood flow into the area, preventing the fluid shift that carries nutrients into the cells. This can prevent normal cell function and reproduction and eventually results in tissue necrosis or the development of ulcers. This situation is evident in individuals with severe varicose veins in the legs—large, dilated veins that have a high hydrostatic pressure. Varicose veins can lead to fatigue, skin breakdown, and varicose ulcers (see Chapter 12). These ulcers do not heal easily because of the continued insufficient blood supply.
- In dental practice, it is difficult to take accurate impressions when the tissues are swollen; dentures do not fit well, and sores may develop that often are slow to heal and become infected because the blood flow is impaired to the gingival tissues.
- Edematous tissue in the skin is very susceptible to tissue breakdown from pressure, abrasion, and external chemicals. Proper skin care is essential to prevent ulceration, particularly in an immobilized patient (see Chapter 25).

THINK ABOUT 2-6

a. List three signs of local edema in the knee.
b. Explain why persistent edema in a leg could cause weakness and skin breakdown.

Fluid Deficit—Dehydration

Dehydration refers to insufficient body fluid resulting from inadequate intake or excessive loss of fluids or a combination of the two. Losses are more common and affect the extracellular compartment first. Water can shift within the extracellular compartments. For example, if fluid is lost from the digestive tract because of vomiting, water shifts from the vascular compartment into the digestive tract to replace the lost secretions. If the deficit continues, eventually fluid is lost from the cells, impairing cell function.

Fluid loss is often measured by a change in body weight; knowing the usual body weight of a person is very helpful in assessment of the extent of loss. As a general guide to extracellular fluid loss, a *mild* deficit is defined as a decrease of 2% in body weight, a *moderate* deficit as a 5% weight loss, and *severe* dehydration is a decrease of 8%. This figure should be adjusted for the individual's age, body size, and condition.

Dehydration is a more serious problem for infants and elderly people, who lack significant fluid reserves as well as the ability to conserve fluid quickly. Infants also experience not only greater insensible water losses through their proportionately larger body surface area but also an increased need for water owing to their higher metabolic rate. The vascular compartment is rapidly depleted in an infant (hypovolemia), affecting the heart, brain, and kidneys. This is indicated by decreased urine output (number of wet diapers), increased lethargy, and dry mucosal membranes.

Water loss is often accompanied by a loss of electrolytes and sometimes of proteins, depending on the specific cause of the loss. For example, sweating results in a loss of water and sodium chloride. Electrolyte losses can influence water balance significantly because electrolyte changes lead to osmotic pressure change between compartments. To restore balance, electrolytes as well as fluid must be replaced. Isotonic dehydration refers to a proportionate loss of fluid and electrolytes, hypotonic dehydration to a loss of more electrolytes than water, and hypertonic dehydration to a loss of more fluid than electrolytes. The latter two types of dehydration cause signs of electrolyte imbalance and influence the movement of water between the intracellular and extracellular compartments (see Electrolyte Imbalances).

THINK ABOUT 2-7

a. Explain why an infant is more vulnerable than a young adult to fluid loss.
b. If more sodium is lost from the extracellular fluid compartment than water, how will fluid move between the cell and the interstitial fluid compartment? Explain the result.

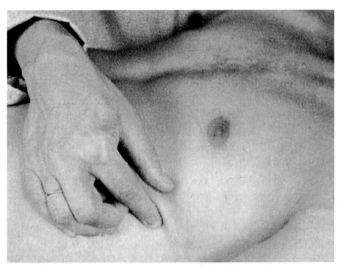

FIGURE 2-4 Testing for dehydration. Loss of skin elasticity or turgor is a sign of dehydration. Skin that does not return quickly to its normal shape after being pinched indicates interstitial water loss. *(From Patton KT, Thibodeau GA:* Anatomy & Physiology, *ed 8, St. Louis, 2013, Mosby.)*

Causes of Dehydration

Common causes of dehydration include:

1. Vomiting and diarrhea, both of which result in loss of numerous electrolytes and nutrients such as glucose, as well as water; drainage or suction of any portion of the digestive system can also result in deficits
2. Excessive sweating with loss of sodium and water
3. Diabetic ketoacidosis with loss of fluid, electrolytes, and glucose in the urine
4. Insufficient water intake in an elderly or unconscious person
5. Use of a concentrated formula in an attempt to provide more nutrition to an infant

Effects of Dehydration

Initially, dehydration involves a decrease in interstitial and intravascular fluids. These losses may produce *direct* effects such as:

- Dry mucous membranes in the mouth (see Table 2-3) Decreased skin turgor or elasticity (Fig. 2-4)
- Lower blood pressure, weak pulse, and a feeling of fatigue
- Increased hematocrit, indicating a higher proportion of red blood cells compared with water in the blood
- Decreasing mental function, confusion, and loss of consciousness, which develop as brain cells lose water and reduce function

The body attempts to *compensate* for the fluid loss by:

- Increasing thirst
- Increasing the heart rate
- Constricting the cutaneous blood vessels, leading to pale and cool skin

- Producing less urine and concentrating the urine, increasing the specific gravity, as a result of renal vasoconstriction and increased secretion of ADH and aldosterone

> **THINK ABOUT 2-8**
>
> Describe three signs or symptoms of dehydration that are direct effects, and three signs that indicate the compensation that is occurring in response to dehydration.

Third-Spacing: Fluid Deficit and Fluid Excess

Third-spacing refers to a situation in which fluid shifts out of the blood into a body cavity or tissue where it is no longer available as *circulating fluid*. Examples include peritonitis, the inflammation and infection of the peritoneal membranes, and burns. The result of this shift is a fluid deficit in the vascular compartment (hypovolemia) and a fluid excess in the interstitial space. Until the basic cause is removed, fluid remains in the "third space"—in the body, but is not a functional part of the circulating fluids. Simply weighing the patient will not reflect this shift in fluid distribution. Laboratory tests such as hematocrit and electrolyte concentrations will indicate third-spacing. In the case of burns, the third spacing is evident as edema in the area of the wounds.

> **THINK ABOUT 2-9**
>
> Based on the information given previously on fluid excess and fluid deficit, describe three signs and symptoms of third-spacing related to a large burn area.

Electrolyte Imbalances

Sodium Imbalance

Review of Sodium

Sodium (Na^+) is the primary cation (positively charged ion) in the extracellular fluid (Table 2-4). Diffusion of sodium occurs between the vascular and interstitial fluids. Sodium transport across the cell membrane is controlled by the sodium-potassium pump or active transport, resulting in sodium levels that are high in extracellular fluids and low inside the cell. Sodium is actively secreted into mucus and other body secretions. It exists in the body primarily in the form of the salts sodium chloride and sodium bicarbonate. It is ingested in food and beverages, usually in more than adequate amounts, and is lost from the body in perspiration, urine, and feces. Sodium levels in the body are primarily controlled by the kidneys through the action of aldosterone.

Sodium is important for the maintenance of extracellular fluid volume through its effect on osmotic pressure because it makes up approximately 90% of the solute in extracellular fluid. Sodium also is essential in the

TABLE 2-4	Distribution of Major Electrolytes	
Ions	Intracellular (mEq/L)	Blood (mEq/L)
Cations		
Sodium (Na)	10	142
Potassium (K)	160	4
Calcium (Ca)	Variable	5
Magnesium (Mg)	35	3
Anions		
Bicarbonate (HCO$_3^-$)	8	27
Chloride (Cl$^-$)	2	103
Phosphate (HPO$_4^-$)	140	2

Note: There are variations in "normal" values among individuals.
The concentration of electrolytes in plasma varies slightly from that in the interstitial fluid or other types of extracellular fluids.
The number of anions, including those present in small quantities, is equivalent to the concentration of cations in the intracellular compartment (or the plasma) so as to maintain electrical neutrality (equal negative and positive charges) in any compartment.

conduction of nerve impulses (Fig. 2-5) and in muscle contraction.

It is important to note the relative changes of electrolytes and fluids associated with the individual's specific problem to put the actual serum value in perspective. For example, excessive sweating may result in a low serum sodium level if proportionately more sodium is lost than water or if only water is used to replace the loss. If an individual loses more water than sodium in perspiration, the serum sodium level may be high.

Hyponatremia

Normal blood sodium levels are presented inside the front cover. Hyponatremia refers to a serum sodium concentration below 3.8 to 5 mmol per liter or 135 milliequivalent (mEq) per liter.

Causes of Hyponatremia

A sodium deficit can result from direct loss of sodium from the body or from an excess of water in the extracellular compartment, resulting in dilution of sodium. Common causes of low serum sodium levels include:

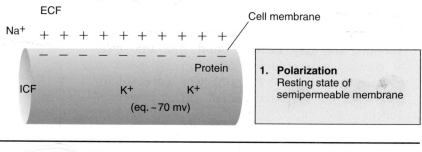

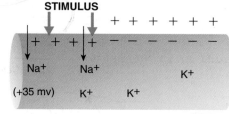

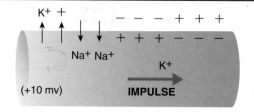

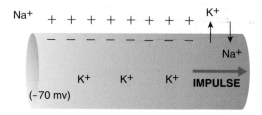

FIGURE 2-5 Role of sodium and potassium ions in the conduction of an impulse.

1. Losses from excessive sweating, vomiting, and diarrhea
2. Use of certain **diuretic** drugs combined with low-salt diets
3. Hormonal imbalances such as insufficient aldosterone, adrenal insufficiency, and excess ADH secretion
4. Early chronic renal failure
5. Excessive water intake

THINK ABOUT 2-10

a. A high fever is likely to cause deep, rapid respirations, excessive perspiration, and higher metabolic rate. How would this affect the fluid and electrolyte balance in the body?
b. List several reasons why drinking a fluid containing water, glucose, and electrolytes would be better than drinking tap water after vomiting.

Effects of Hyponatremia

- Low sodium levels impair nerve conduction and result in fluid imbalances in the compartments. Manifestations include fatigue, muscle cramps, and abdominal discomfort or cramps with nausea and vomiting (Table 2-5).
- Decreased osmotic pressure in the extracellular compartment may cause a fluid shift into cells, resulting in hypovolemia and decreased blood pressure (Fig. 2-6).
- The brain cells may swell, causing confusion, headache, weakness, or seizures.

Hypernatremia _(Too much)_

Hypernatremia is an excessive sodium level in the blood and extracellular fluids (more than 145 mEq per liter).

Causes of Hypernatremia

Excess sodium results from ingestion of large amounts of sodium without proportionate water intake or a loss of water from the body that is faster than the loss of sodium.

Specific causes include:

1. Insufficient ADH, which results in a large volume of dilute urine (diabetes insipidus)

TABLE 2-5	Signs of Sodium Imbalance
Hyponatremia	**Hypernatremia**
Anorexia, nausea, cramps	Thirst; tongue and mucosa are dry and sticky
Fatigue, lethargy, muscle weakness	Weakness, lethargy, agitation
Headache, confusion, seizures	Edema
Decreased blood pressure	Elevated blood pressure

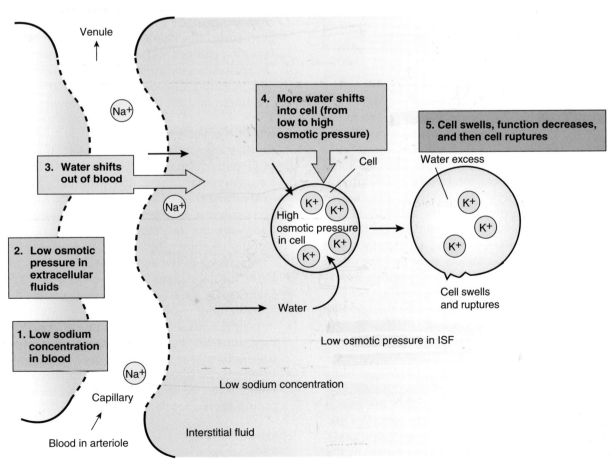

FIGURE 2-6 Hyponatremia and fluid shift into cells.

2. Loss of the thirst mechanism
3. Watery diarrhea
4. Prolonged periods of rapid respiration

> **THINK ABOUT   2-11**
>
> Hypernatremia accompanied by an elevated hematocrit value indicates what fact about body fluids?

Effects of Hypernatremia

The major effect of hypernatremia is a fluid shift out of the cells owing to the increased osmotic pressure of interstitial or extracellular fluid; this effect is manifested by:

- Weakness, agitation
- Firm subcutaneous tissues (see Table 2-5)
- Increased thirst, with dry, rough mucous membranes
- Decreased urine output because ADH is secreted

Note that the manifestations can change depending on the cause of the problem: If the cause of hypernatremia is fluid loss caused by lack of ADH, urine output is high.

> **THINK ABOUT   2-12**
>
> a. Compare the effects of aldosterone with those of ADH on serum sodium levels.
> b. List the signs and symptoms common to both hyponatremia and hypernatremia and also any signs that differentiate the two states.
> c. Explain how sodium imbalances affect cardiac function.

Potassium Imbalance

Review of Potassium   inside

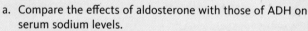

Potassium (K^+) is a major intracellular cation, and therefore serum levels are very low (3.5 to 5 mEq per liter or 3.5 to 5 mmol per liter) compared with the intracellular concentration that is about 160 mEq per liter (see Table 2-4). It is difficult to assess total body potassium by measuring the serum level. Potassium is ingested in foods and is excreted primarily in the urine under the influence of the hormone aldosterone. Foods high in potassium include bananas, citrus fruits, tomatoes, and lentils; potassium chloride tablets may be taken as a supplement. The hormone insulin also promotes movement of potassium into cells (see Chapter 16).

Potassium levels are also influenced by the *acid-base balance* in the body; acidosis tends to shift potassium ions out of the cells into the extracellular fluids, and alkalosis tends to move more potassium into the cells (Fig. 2-7). With acidosis, many hydrogen ions diffuse from the blood into the interstitial fluid because of the high hydrogen ion concentration in the blood. When these hydrogen ions move into the cell, they displace potassium out of the cell to maintain electrochemical neutrality. Then the excess potassium ions in the interstitial fluid diffuse into the blood, leading to

hyperkalemia. The reverse process occurs with alkalosis. Acidosis also promotes hydrogen ion excretion by the kidneys and retention of potassium in the body. Potassium assists in the regulation of intracellular fluid volume and has a role in many metabolic processes in the cell. It is also important in nerve conduction and contraction of all muscle types, determining the membrane potential (see Fig. 2-5). Most important, abnormal potassium levels, both high and low, have a significant and serious effect on the contractions of cardiac muscle causing changes in the electrocardiogram (ECG) and ultimately cardiac arrest or standstill.

Hypokalemia

In hypokalemia the serum level of potassium is less than 2 mmol per liter or 3.5 mEq per liter.

Causes of Hypokalemia

Low serum potassium levels may result from:

1. Excessive losses from the body due to diarrhea
2. Diuresis associated with certain diuretic drugs; patients with heart disease who are being treated with certain diuretic drugs such as furosemide may have to increase their intake of potassium in food or take a potassium supplement because hypokalemia may increase the toxicity of heart medications such as digitalis
3. The presence of excessive aldosterone or glucocorticoids in the body (in Cushing's syndrome, in which glucocorticoids have some mineralocorticoid activity, retaining sodium and excreting potassium)
4. Decreased dietary intake, which may occur with alcoholism, eating disorders, or starvation
5. Treatment of diabetic ketoacidosis with insulin

Effects of Hypokalemia

- Cardiac dysrhythmias are serious, showing typical ECG pattern changes (Fig. 2-8) that indicate prolonged repolarization, and eventually may lead to cardiac arrest (see Chapter 12).
- Hypokalemia interferes with neuromuscular function, and the muscles become less responsive to stimuli, as shown by fatigue and muscle weakness commencing in the legs (Table 2-6).
- Paresthesias such as "pins and needles" develop.
- Decreased digestive tract motility causes decreased appetite (anorexia) and nausea.
- In people with severe potassium deficits, the respiratory muscles become weak, leading to shallow respirations.
- In severe cases, renal function is impaired, leading to failure to concentrate the urine, and increased urine output (polyuria) results.

Hyperkalemia

In hyperkalemia the serum level of potassium is greater than 2.6 mmol per liter or 5 mEq per liter.

HYPOK = diuretic

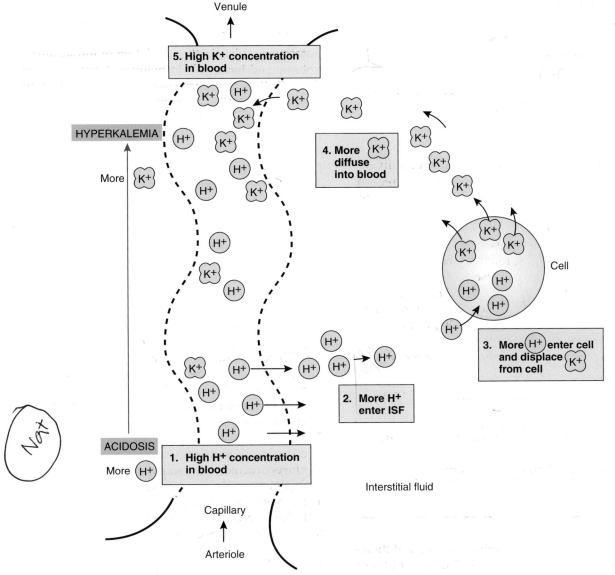

FIGURE 2-7 Relationship of hydrogen and potassium ions.

Causes of Hyperkalemia

Causes of high serum potassium levels include:

1. Renal failure
2. Deficit of aldosterone
3. Use of "potassium-sparing" diuretic drugs, which prevent potassium from being excreted in adequate amounts
4. Leakage of intracellular potassium into the extracellular fluids in patients with extensive tissue damage such as traumatic crush injuries or burns
5. Displacement of potassium from cells by prolonged or severe acidosis (see Fig. 2-7)

Effects of Hyperkalemia

- The ECG shows typical cardiac dysrhythmias (see Fig. 2-8), which may progress to cardiac arrest.

- Muscle weakness is common, progressing to paralysis as hyperkalemia advances and impairs neuromuscular activity (see Table 2-6).
- Fatigue, nausea, and paresthesias are also common.

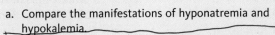

THINK ABOUT 2-13

a. Compare the manifestations of hyponatremia and hypokalemia.
b. Why is any small change in potassium level considered a serious problem?

Calcium Imbalance

Review of Calcium

Calcium (Ca^{++}) is a very important extracellular cation. Calcium is ingested in food, especially milk products,

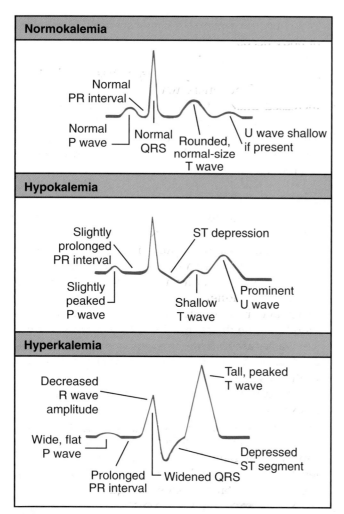

Normokalemia

Normal PR interval

Normal P wave

Normal QRS

Rounded, normal-size T wave

U wave shallow if present

Hypokalemia

Slightly prolonged PR interval

ST depression

Slightly peaked P wave

Shallow T wave

Prominent U wave

Hyperkalemia

Decreased R wave amplitude

Tall, peaked T wave

Wide, flat P wave

Prolonged PR interval

Widened QRS

Depressed ST segment

FIGURE 2-8 Electrocardiogram changes with potassium imbalance. From McCance KL, et al: Pathophysiology: The Biologic Basis for Disease in Adults and Children, ed 6, St. Louis, 2010, Elsevier.

TABLE 2-6   Signs of Potassium Imbalance

Hypokalemia	Hyperkalemia
Cardiac arrhythmias, cardiac arrest	Arrhythmias, cardiac arrest
Anorexia, nausea, constipation	Nausea, diarrhea
Fatigue, muscle twitch, weakness, leg cramps	Muscle weakness, paralysis beginning in legs
Shallow respirations, paresthesias	Paresthesias—fingers, toes, face, tongue
Postural hypotension, polyuria, and nocturia	Oliguria
Serum pH elevated—7.45 (alkalosis)	Serum pH decreased—7.35 (acidosis)

stored in bone, and excreted from the body in the urine and feces. Calcium balance is controlled by parathyroid hormone (PTH) and calcitonin (see Chapter 16), but is also influenced by vitamin D and phosphate ion levels. For example, low blood calcium levels stimulate the secretion of PTH, which increases calcium absorption

from the digestive tract and kidneys and promotes resorption from bone.

Vitamin D may be ingested or synthesized in the skin in the presence of ultraviolet rays, but then it must be activated in the kidneys. It promotes calcium movement from bone and intestines into blood. Most people living in northern climates have reduced vitamin D because of lack of exposure of the skin to the sun; dietary supplements are recommended to ensure adequate levels during cold weather. Sun blocking agents with an SPF greater than 15 appear to reduce vitamin D synthesis. There is also increasing evidence that vitamin D deficits may contribute to the development of multiple sclerosis and certain cancers.

Calcium and phosphate ions in the extracellular fluid have a reciprocal relationship. For example, if calcium levels are high, phosphate is low. The product of calcium and phosphate concentrations should be a constant value. If levels of both calcium and phosphate rise, crystals of calcium phosphate precipitate in soft tissue. The measured or biologically active form of calcium is the ionized form, which is not attached to plasma protein or bonded to other ions such as citrate. Alkalosis can decrease the number of free calcium ions, causing hypocalcemia.

Calcium has many important functions:
- It provides the structural strength essential for bones and teeth.
- Calcium ions maintain the stability of nerve membranes, controlling the permeability and excitability needed for nerve conduction.
- Calcium ions are required for muscle contractions.
- Calcium ions are necessary for many metabolic processes and enzyme reactions such as those involved in blood clotting.

THINK ABOUT 2-14

When nerve membranes become more permeable, is the nerve more or less easily stimulated?

Hypocalcemia

In hypocalcemia, the serum calcium level is less than 2.2 mmol per liter or below 4 mEq per liter.

Causes of Hypocalcemia

Causes of hypocalcemia include:
1. Hypoparathyroidism—decreased parathyroid hormone results in decreased intestinal calcium absorption
2. Malabsorption syndrome—resulting in decreased intestinal absorption of vitamin D or calcium
3. Deficient serum albumin
4. Increased serum pH—resulting in alkalosis

In renal failure, hypocalcemia results from retention of phosphate ion, which causes loss of calcium; also, vitamin D is not activated, thereby decreasing the intestinal absorption of calcium.

TABLE 2-7	Signs of Calcium Imbalance
Hypocalcemia	Hypercalcemia
Tetany—involuntary skeletal muscle spasm, carpopedal spasm, laryngospasm	Apathy, lethargy
	Anorexia, nausea, constipation
	Polyuria, thirst
Tingling fingers	Kidney stones
Mental confusion, irritability	Arrhythmias, prolonged strong cardiac contractions, increased blood pressure
Arrhythmias, weak heart contractions	

Note: Effects on bone depend on the cause of the calcium imbalance.

Effects of Hypocalcemia

- Low serum calcium levels increase the permeability and excitability of nerve membranes, leading to spontaneous stimulation of *skeletal muscle*. This leads to muscle twitching, carpopedal spasm (atypical contraction of the fingers), and hyperactive reflexes (Table 2-7). Chvostek's sign, spasm of the lip or face when the face is tapped in front of the ear, and Trousseau's sign, carpopedal spasm when a blood pressure cuff blocks circulation to the hand, both indicate low serum calcium and tetany, or skeletal muscle spasm. Severe calcium deficits may cause laryngospasm, which obstructs the airway. Paresthesias are common, as are abdominal cramps.
- *Heart* contractions become *weak* owing to insufficient calcium for muscle action, conduction is delayed, *arrhythmias* develop, and blood pressure drops.

Note that the effects of hypocalcemia on *skeletal muscle* and *cardiac muscle* differ. Skeletal muscle spasms result from the increased irritability of the nerves associated with the muscle fibers, whereas the weaker contraction of cardiac muscle (which lacks nerves) is directly related to the calcium deficit. Also, adequate calcium is stored in the skeletal muscle cells to provide for contractions, whereas contraction of cardiac muscle relies on available extracellular calcium ions passing through the calcium channels. This is the basis for action of one group of cardiac drugs.

THINK ABOUT 2-15

Explain the different effects of low serum calcium on skeletal muscle and cardiac muscle.

Hypercalcemia

In hypercalcemia the serum calcium is greater than 5 mEq per liter or greater than 2.5 mmol per liter.

Causes of Hypercalcemia

Excessive serum levels of calcium frequently result from:

1. Uncontrolled release of calcium ions from the bones due to neoplasms; malignant bone tumors may directly destroy the bone, and some tumors, such as bronchogenic carcinoma, may secrete PTH in excess of body needs
2. Hyperparathyroidism
3. Immobility, which may decrease stress on the bone, leading to demineralization
4. Increased intake of calcium due either to excessive vitamin D or to excess dietary calcium
5. Milk-alkali syndrome, associated with increased milk and antacid intake, which may also elevate serum calcium levels

Effects of Hypercalcemia

- High serum calcium levels depress neuromuscular activity, leading to muscle weakness, loss of muscle tone, lethargy, and stupor, often with personality changes, anorexia, and nausea (see Table 2-7).
- High calcium levels interfere with the function of ADH in the kidneys, resulting in less absorption of water and in polyuria. If hypercalcemia is severe, blood volume drops, renal function decreases, nitrogen wastes accumulate, and cardiac arrest may ensue.
- Cardiac contractions increase in strength, and dysrhythmias may develop.
- Effects on bone vary with the cause of hypercalcemia. If excess PTH is the cause, bone density will be decreased, and spontaneous (pathologic) fractures may occur, particularly in the weight-bearing areas, causing bone pain. If intake of calcium is high, PTH levels will be low, and more calcium will be stored in the bone, maintaining bone strength.

THINK ABOUT 2-16

Describe the effect of each of the following conditions on serum calcium levels and on bone density: (1) hyperparathyroidism, (2) renal failure, and (3) very large intake of vitamin D.

Other Electrolytes

Magnesium

Magnesium (Mg^{++}) is an intracellular ion that has a normal serum level of 0.7 to 1.1 mmol per liter. About 50% of total body magnesium is stored in bone. Serum levels are linked to both potassium and calcium levels. Magnesium is found in green vegetables and is important in many enzyme reactions as well as in protein and DNA synthesis. Magnesium imbalances are rare.

Hypomagnesemia results from malabsorption or malnutrition, often associated with chronic alcoholism. Low serum levels may also occur with the use of diuretics, diabetic ketoacidosis, hyperparathyroidism, and hyperaldosteronism.

Low serum magnesium leads to neuromuscular hyperirritability, with tremors or chorea (involuntary repetitive movements), insomnia, personality changes, and an increased heart rate with arrhythmias.

Hypermagnesemia usually occurs with renal failure. Excess magnesium depresses neuromuscular function, leading to decreased reflexes, lethargy, and cardiac arrhythmias.

Phosphate   *Bone & tooth*

Phosphate ions (HPO_4^{--} and $H_2PO_4^-$), are located primarily in the bone but circulate in both the intracellular and extracellular fluids. The serum level is normally 0.85 to 1.45 mmol per liter.

Phosphate is important:
- In bone and tooth mineralization
- In many metabolic processes, particularly those involving the cellular energy source, adenosine triphosphate (ATP)
- As the phosphate buffer system for acid-base balance, and it has a role in the removal of hydrogen ions from the body through the kidneys
- As an integral part of the cell membrane
- In its reciprocal relationship with serum calcium

Hypophosphatemia

Low serum phosphate levels may result from malabsorption syndromes, diarrhea, or excessive use of antacids. Alkalosis and hyperparathyroidism are other causes.

Neurologic function is impaired with low serum phosphate, causing tremors, weak reflexes (hyporeflexia), paresthesias, confusion and stupor, anorexia, and difficulty in swallowing (dysphagia).

The blood cells function less effectively—oxygen transport decreases, and clotting and phagocytosis decrease.

> **THINK ABOUT   2-17**
>
> Explain how serum calcium levels are affected by low phosphate levels.

Hyperphosphatemia

High serum phosphate often results from renal failure. Dialysis patients often take phosphate binders with meals to control their serum phosphate levels. Tissue damage or cancer chemotherapy may cause the release of intracellular phosphate. The manifestations of hyperphosphatemia are the same as those of hypocalcemia.

Chloride

Chloride ion (Cl^-) is the major extracellular **anion** with a normal serum level of 98 to 106 mmol per liter. Chloride ions tend to follow sodium because of the attraction between the electrical charge on the ions; therefore high sodium levels usually lead to high chloride levels.

Chloride and bicarbonate ions, both negatively charged, can exchange places as the blood circulates through the body to assist in maintaining acid-base balance (see Acid-Base Imbalance). As bicarbonate ions are used up in binding with metabolic acids, chloride ions diffuse out of the red blood cells into the serum to maintain the same number of negative ions in the blood (Fig. 2-9). The reverse situation can also occur when serum chloride levels decrease, and bicarbonate ions leave the erythrocytes to maintain electrical neutrality. Thus, low serum chloride leads to high serum bicarbonate, or alkalosis. This situation is referred to as a *chloride shift*.

Hypochloremia

Low serum chloride is usually associated with alkalosis in the early stages of vomiting when hydrochloric acid is lost from the stomach.

Excessive perspiration associated with fever or strenuous labor on a hot day can lead to loss of sodium chloride, resulting in hyponatremia and hypochloremia, and ultimately, dehydration.

Hyperchloremia

Excess chloride ion may develop with the excessive intake of sodium chloride, orally or intravenously, or hypernatremia due to other causes, leading to edema and weight gain.

> **THINK ABOUT   2-18**
>
> a. State one cause of hypomagnesemia.
> b. State one cause of hyperphosphatemia.
> c. List and describe two signs of hypophosphatemia.

Acid-Base Imbalance

Review of Concepts and Processes

Acid-base balance is essential to homeostasis because cell enzymes can function only within a very narrow pH range. *The normal serum pH range is 7.35 to 7.45.* Death usually results if serum pH is below 6.8 or above 7.8 (Fig. 2-10). For example, a pH of less than 7.35 depresses central nervous system function and decreases all cell enzyme activity.

When serum pH is less than 7.4, more hydrogen ions (H^+) are present, and acidosis results. A serum pH of greater than 7.4 is more basic, indicating alkalosis or the presence of fewer hydrogen ions. The body normally has a tendency toward acidosis, or a lower pH, because cell metabolism is constantly producing carbon dioxide (CO_2) or carbonic acid (H_2CO_3) and nonvolatile metabolic acids such as lactic acid, ketoacids, sulfates, or phosphates. Lactic acid results from the *anaerobic* (without oxygen) metabolism of glucose, ketoacids result from incomplete oxidation of fatty acids, and protein metabolism may produce sulfates or phosphates.

> **THINK ABOUT   2-19**
>
> a. When hydrogen ions are decreased, is the pH higher or lower?
> b. State the optimal range of serum pH and effects on normal cell function if serum pH is not in the optimal range.

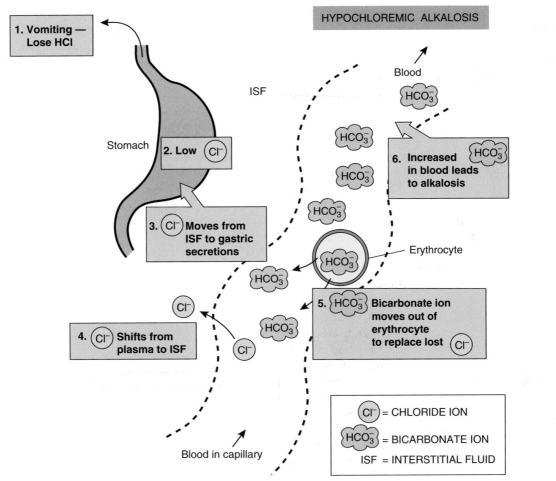

FIGURE 2-9 Schematic representation of chloride-bicarbonate shift with vomiting.

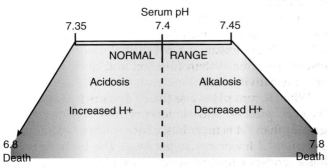

FIGURE 2-10 The hydrogen ion and pH scale.

Control of Serum pH

As the blood circulates through the body, nutrients diffuse from the blood into the cells, various metabolic processes take place in the cells using these nutrients, and metabolic wastes, including acids, diffuse from the cells into the blood (Fig. 2-11).

Three mechanisms control or compensate for pH:

1. The buffer pairs circulating in the blood respond to pH changes immediately.
2. The respiratory system can alter carbon dioxide levels (carbonic acid) in the body by changing the respiratory rate (see Chapter 13).

3. The kidneys can modify the excretion rate of acids and the production and absorption of bicarbonate ion (see Chapter 18).

Note that the lungs can change only the amount of carbon dioxide (equivalent to the amount of carbonic acid) in the body. The kidneys are slow to compensate for a change in pH but are the most effective mechanism because they can excrete all types of acids (volatile or gaseous and nonvolatile) and can also adjust serum bicarbonate levels.

> **THINK ABOUT 2-20**
>
> How does the respiratory rate change when more hydrogen ions enter the blood, and how does this change affect acid levels in the body?

Buffer Systems

To control serum pH, several buffer systems are present in the blood. A buffer is a combination of a weak acid and its alkaline salt. The components react with any acids or alkali added to the blood, neutralizing them and thereby maintaining a relatively constant pH.

The body has four major buffer pairs:

1. The sodium bicarbonate-carbonic acid system
2. The phosphate system

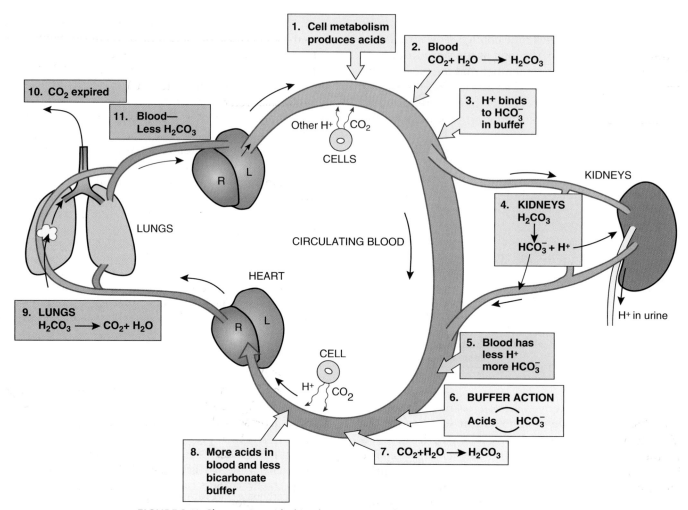

FIGURE 2-11 Changes in acids, bicarbonate ion, and serum pH in circulating blood.

3. The hemoglobin system

4. The protein system

The bicarbonate system is the major extracellular fluid buffer and is used clinically to assess a client's acid-base status. The principles of acid-base balance are discussed here using the bicarbonate pair. Specific numbers are not used because the emphasis is on understanding basic concepts and recognizing trends. Laboratory tests will report the specific values and state the implications of those values.

The Bicarbonate-Carbonic Acid Buffer System and Maintenance of Serum pH

The bicarbonate buffer system is composed of carbonic acid, which arises from the combination of carbon dioxide with water, and bicarbonate ion, which is present as sodium bicarbonate. The balance of bicarbonate ion (HCO_3^-), a *base*, and carbonic *acid* (H_2CO_3) levels is controlled by the respiratory system and the kidneys

(see Fig. 2-11). Cell metabolism produces carbon dioxide, which diffuses into the interstitial fluid and blood, where it reacts with water to form carbonic acid, which then dissociates immediately under the influence of the enzyme carbonic anhydrase to form three hydrogen ions and one bicarbonate ion per molecule of carbonic acid. This enzyme is present in many sites, including the lungs and the kidneys. In the *lungs*, this reaction can be reversed to form carbon dioxide, which is then expired along with water, thus reducing the total amount of carbonic acid or acid in the body. In the *kidneys*, the reaction needed to form more hydrogen ions is promoted by enzymes; the resultant hydrogen ions are excreted in the urine, and the bicarbonate ions are returned to the blood to restore the buffer levels.

To maintain serum pH within the normal range, 7.35 to 7.45, the *ratio* of bicarbonate ion to carbonic acid (or carbon dioxide) must be *20:1*. A 1:1 ratio will not maintain a pH of 7.4! The ratio is always stated with the H^+ component as one.

As one component of the ratio changes, the other component must change *proportionately* to maintain the 20:1 ratio and thus serum pH. For instance, if respiration is impaired, causing an increase in carbon dioxide in the blood, the kidneys must increase serum bicarbonate levels to compensate for the change. The actual concentrations are not critical as long as the proportions are sustained. It may help to remember that the bicarbonate part or alkali part of the buffer ratio is 20, the higher figure, because more bicarbonate base is required to neutralize the acids constantly being produced by the body cells.

> **THINK ABOUT 2-21**
>
> If bicarbonate ion is lost from the body, how will carbonic acid levels change?

Respiratory System

When serum carbon dioxide or hydrogen ion levels increase, chemoreceptors stimulate the respiratory control center to increase the respiratory rate, thus removing more carbon dioxide or acid from the body. When alkalosis develops, the respiratory rate decreases, thus retaining more carbon dioxide and increasing acid levels in the body.

Renal System

The kidneys can also reduce the acid content of the body by exchanging hydrogen for sodium ions under the influence of aldosterone and can remove H^+ by combining them with ammonia and other chemicals. The kidneys also provide the bicarbonate ion for the buffer pair as needed. Urine pH may range from 4.5 to 8.0 as the kidneys compensate for metabolic conditions and dietary intake.

$$lungs: CO_2 + H_2O \leftrightarrow H_2CO_3 \leftrightarrow H^+ + HCO_3^-: kidneys$$

$$lungs: \text{carbon dioxide} + \text{water} \leftrightarrow \text{carbonic acid} \leftrightarrow$$
$$\text{hydrogen ions} + \text{bicarbonate ions}: kidneys$$

> **THINK ABOUT 2-22**
>
> a. Reduced blood flow through the kidneys for a long time will have what effect on serum pH? Why?
> b. How would the lungs and kidneys respond to the ingestion of large quantities of antacids?
> c. How is the kidney more effective in maintaining serum pH than the lungs?

A number of laboratory tests can determine acid-base balance. These tests include arterial blood gases (ABGs), base excess or deficit, or anion gap, and details about them may be found in laboratory manuals. Some normal values are listed inside the front cover of this book.

Acid-Base Imbalance

There are four basic types of acid-base imbalance (Table 2-8). An increase in hydrogen ions or a decrease in serum pH results in acidosis, which can result either from an increase in carbon dioxide levels (acid) due to respiratory problems or from a decrease in bicarbonate ions (base) because of metabolic or renal problems. The first category is termed respiratory acidosis (increased carbon dioxide), and the second is called metabolic acidosis (decreased bicarbonate ions).

Alkalosis refers to an increase in serum pH or decreased hydrogen ions. It may be respiratory alkalosis if increased respirations cause a decrease in carbon dioxide (less acid), or metabolic alkalosis if serum bicarbonate increases.

Imbalances may be acute or chronic. In some situations, combinations of imbalances may occur; for example, metabolic acidosis and respiratory alkalosis can occur simultaneously.

> **THINK ABOUT 2-23**
>
> Name or state the category of the imbalance resulting from each of the following: (1) increased respiratory rate, (2) renal failure, and (3) excessive intake of bicarbonate, and state resulting change in the 20:1 ratio.

Compensation

The *cause* of the imbalance determines the first change in the ratio (Figs. 2-12 to 2-15). Respiratory disorders are always represented by an initial change in carbon dioxide. All other problems are metabolic and result from an initial change in bicarbonate ions.

The *compensation* is assessed by the subsequent change in the second part of the ratio (Table 2-9) and requires function by body systems *not* involved in the cause. For example, if a patient has a respiratory disorder causing acidosis, the lungs cannot compensate effectively, but the kidneys can. As long as the ratio of bicarbonate to carbonic acid is maintained at 20:1 and serum pH is normal, the imbalance is considered to be compensated. Compensation is limited and the patient must be monitored carefully if there is an ongoing threat to homeostasis.

Decompensation

If the kidneys and lungs cannot compensate adequately, the ratio changes, and serum pH moves out of the normal range, thus affecting cell metabolism and function. At this point, the imbalance is termed decompensation. Intervention is essential if homeostasis is to be regained. Examples of acid-base imbalance are given in Table 2-8.

> **THINK ABOUT 2-24**
>
> a. In an individual with very low blood pressure or circulatory shock, blood flow to the cells is very poor, resulting in increased lactic acid. Briefly describe the compensations that will take place.
> b. What changes in the bicarbonate ratio and serum pH indicate that decompensation has occurred?

TABLE 2-8 Acid-Base Imbalances

	Acidosis	Alkalosis
Respiratory		
Causes	Slow shallow respirations (e.g., drugs)	Hyperventilation (anxiety, aspirin overdose)
	Respiratory congestion	
Effect	Increased PCO_2	Decreased PCO_2
Compensation	Kidneys excrete more hydrogen ion and reabsorb more bicarbonate	Kidneys excrete less hydrogen ion and reabsorb less bicarbonate
Laboratory	Elevated PCO_2	Low PCO_2
	Elevated serum bicarbonate	Low serum bicarbonate
	Compensated—serum pH = 7.35 to 7.4	Compensated—serum pH = 7.4 to 7.45
	Decompensated—serum pH < 7.35	Decompensated—serum pH > 7.45
Metabolic		
Causes	Shock	Vomiting (early stage)
	Diabetic ketoacidosis	Excessive antacid intake
	Renal failure	
	Diarrhea	
Effect	Decreased serum bicarbonate ion	Increased serum bicarbonate ion
Compensation	Rapid, deep respirations	Slow, shallow respirations
	Kidneys excrete more acid and increase bicarbonate absorption	Kidneys excrete less acid and decrease bicarbonate absorption
Laboratory	Low serum bicarbonate	Elevated serum bicarbonate
	Low PCO_2	Elevated PCO_2
	Compensated—serum pH = 7.35 to 7.4	Compensated—serum pH = 7.4 to 7.45
	Decompensated—serum pH < 7.35	Decompensated—serum pH > 7.45

Acidosis

Causes of Acidosis

Respiratory acidosis, in which there is an increase in carbon dioxide levels, may occur under several conditions:

- Acute problems such as pneumonia, airway obstruction (aspiration or asthma), or chest injuries, and in those taking drugs such as opiates, which depress the respiratory control center
- Chronic respiratory acidosis, common in people with chronic obstructive pulmonary diseases (COPD) such as emphysema
- Decompensated respiratory acidosis, which may develop if the impairment becomes severe or if, for example, a patient with a chronic problem develops an additional infection

Metabolic acidosis is associated with a decrease in serum bicarbonate resulting from:

- Excessive loss of bicarbonate ions; for example, from diarrhea and loss of bicarbonate in the intestinal secretions
- Increased utilization of serum bicarbonate to buffer increased acids, when large amounts of acids are produced in the body because the buffer bicarbonate binds with such acids until they can be removed by the kidneys; for example, lactic acid may accumulate

if blood pressure decreases and insufficient oxygen is available to the cells, or diabetic patients may produce large amounts of ketoacids that use up bicarbonate ions (see Chapter 16)

- Renal disease or failure, in which both decreased excretion of acids and decreased production of bicarbonate ion occur (see Chapter 18). In people with renal failure, compensation by the lungs is inadequate because the lungs can only remove carbon dioxide, not other acids, nor can they produce bicarbonate; therefore a treatment such as dialysis is required to maintain serum pH.
- Decompensated metabolic acidosis, which may develop when an additional factor interferes with compensation. For example, a person with severe diarrhea may become so dehydrated that the kidneys receive little blood and cannot function adequately, causing decompensation. The same result is seen with cardiac arrest.

Effects of Acidosis

The direct effects of acidosis are manifested by the nervous system, in which function is impaired, leading to inadequate responses. Headache, lethargy, weakness, and confusion develop, leading eventually to coma and

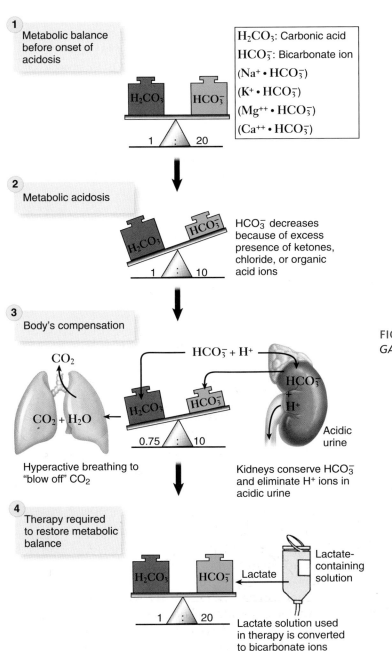

1 Metabolic balance before onset of acidosis

H_2CO_3: Carbonic acid
HCO_3^-: Bicarbonate ion
$(Na^+ \cdot HCO_3^-)$
$(K^+ \cdot HCO_3^-)$
$(Mg^{++} \cdot HCO_3^-)$
$(Ca^{++} \cdot HCO_3^-)$

H_2CO_3 HCO_3^-
1 : 20

2 Metabolic acidosis

HCO_3^- decreases because of excess presence of ketones, chloride, or organic acid ions

H_2CO_3 HCO_3^-
1 : 10

3 Body's compensation

CO_2
$HCO_3^- + H^+$
$CO_2 + H_2O$
H_2CO_3 HCO_3^-
$HCO_3^- + H^+$
Acidic urine
0.75 : 10

Hyperactive breathing to "blow off" CO_2

Kidneys conserve HCO_3^- and eliminate H^+ ions in acidic urine

4 Therapy required to restore metabolic balance

H_2CO_3 HCO_3^- Lactate
Lactate-containing solution
1 : 20

Lactate solution used in therapy is converted to bicarbonate ions in the liver

FIGURE 2-12 Metabolic acidosis. *(From Patton KT, Thibodeau GA: Anatomy & Physiology, ed 8, St. Louis, 2013, Mosby.)*

death. Compensations are manifested by deep, rapid breathing (Kussmaul's respirations) and secretion of urine with a low pH (e.g., 5).

Alkalosis

Alkalosis does not occur as frequently as acidosis. *Respiratory alkalosis* results from hyperventilation, usually caused by anxiety, high fever, or an overdose of aspirin (ASA). Head injuries or brainstem tumors may lead to hyperventilation. Stress-related alkalosis may develop rapidly. If the individual cannot quickly be calmed enough to hold his or her breath repeatedly, then it is best treated by rebreathing exhaled air containing

excreted carbon dioxide from a paper bag placed over the face. Even if renal compensation is not impaired it is slow to take place.

Metabolic alkalosis, in which there is an increase in serum bicarbonate ion, commonly follows loss of hydrochloric acid from the stomach either in the early stages of vomiting or with drainage from the stomach. Other potential causes are hypokalemia (see Electrolyte Imbalances) and excessive ingestion of antacids.

Effects of Alkalosis

Alkalosis increases the irritability of the nervous system, causing restlessness, muscle twitching, tingling and

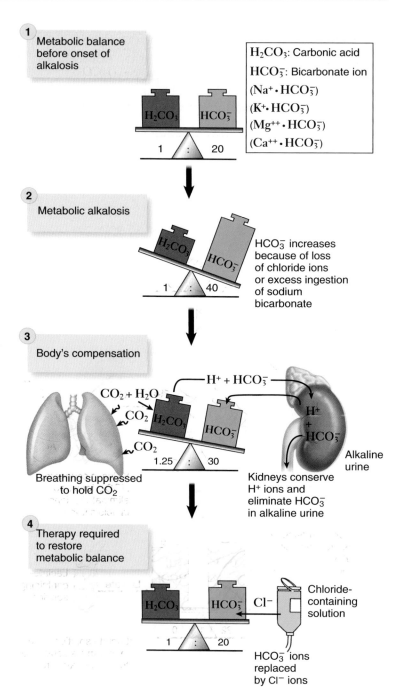

FIGURE 2-13 Metabolic alkalosis. *(From Patton KT, Thibodeau GA: Anatomy & Physiology, ed 8, St. Louis, 2013, Mosby.)*

numbness of the fingers, and eventually tetany, seizures, and coma.

Treatment of Imbalances

The underlying cause of the imbalance must be diagnosed and treated in addition to more immediate corrective measures such as fluid/electrolyte replacement or removal.

- Deficits can be reversed by adding fluid or the particular electrolyte to the body fluids. Excess amounts of either fluid or electrolytes must be removed. For example, a fluid deficit is returned to normal by the increased intake of fluid. Excess fluid is removed, perhaps by taking diuretic drugs to increase the excretion of fluid through the kidneys.
- Caution is required when adjusting fluid levels, to ensure that electrolyte balance is maintained. For example, when adding fluid to the body, it is

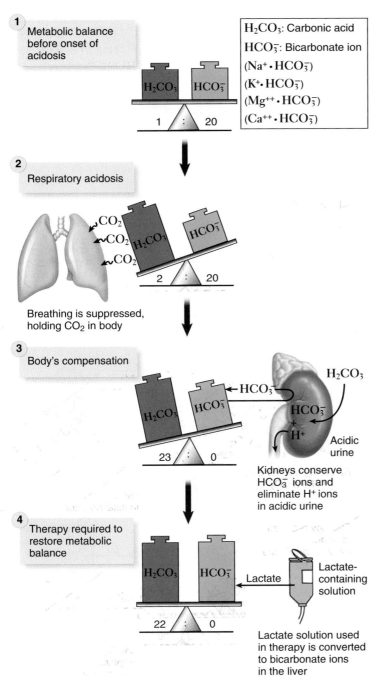

1 Metabolic balance before onset of acidosis

H_2CO_3: Carbonic acid
HCO_3^-: Bicarbonate ion
$(Na^+ \cdot HCO_3^-)$
$(K^+ \cdot HCO_3^-)$
$(Mg^{++} \cdot HCO_3^-)$
$(Ca^{++} \cdot HCO_3^-)$

H_2CO_3 HCO_3^-
1 : 20

2 Respiratory acidosis

CO_2
CO_2
CO_2
H_2CO_3 HCO_3^-
2 : 20

Breathing is suppressed, holding CO_2 in body

3 Body's compensation

H_2CO_3
HCO_3^-
HCO_3^-
H_2CO_3 HCO_3^-
HCO_3^- + H^+
23 : 0
Acidic urine

Kidneys conserve HCO_3^- ions and eliminate H^+ ions in acidic urine

4 Therapy required to restore metabolic balance

H_2CO_3 HCO_3^- Lactate
22 : 0
Lactate-containing solution

Lactate solution used in therapy is converted to bicarbonate ions in the liver

FIGURE 2-14 Respiratory acidosis. *(From Patton KT, Thibodeau GA: Anatomy & Physiology, ed 8, St. Louis, 2013, Mosby.)*

necessary to check electrolyte levels and perhaps add sodium or other electrolytes, to achieve normal levels of all components.

- Addition of bicarbonate to the blood will reverse acidosis; levels of bicarbonate need to be monitored because excess bicarbonate levels may occur.
- In some cases, diet may be modified to maintain better electrolyte balance.
- Other factors such as respiratory or kidney disorders and hormonal imbalances can have dramatic effects on the fluid/electrolyte balance.

THINK ABOUT 2-25

a. For each of the following situations, list the kind of acid-base imbalance likely to occur: (1) chest injury with fractured ribs, (2) infection with high fever, (3) diarrhea.

b. Describe the effect of metabolic acidosis on respiration and on the central nervous system.

c. In an elderly person with respiratory acidosis due to chronic respiratory congestion, why would decreased kidney function be so dangerous?

d. If serum pH decreases to 7.1 because of severe renal disease, explain the change that has occurred in the buffer pair and the effect of this change on the central nervous system.

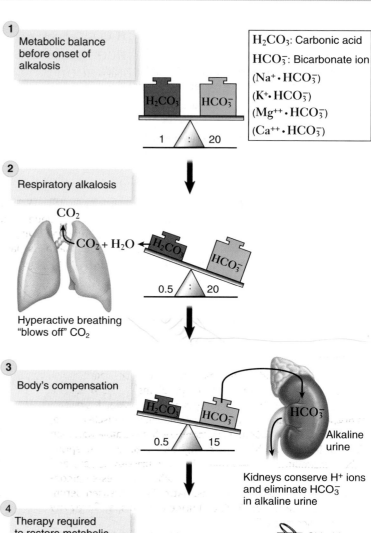

FIGURE 2-15 Respiratory alkalosis. *(From Patton KT, Thibodeau GA: Anatomy & Physiology, ed 8, St. Louis, 2013, Mosby.)*

TABLE 2-9   Examples of Acidosis

Respiratory Acidosis—Individual with Emphysema Retaining CO_2

Stage 1:	Kidneys compensate for slight increase in P_{CO_2} by increasing excretion of acids and production of bicarbonate	No change in serum levels
Stage 2:	Increased retention of CO_2. Respiratory acidosis	Elevated P_{CO_2}
Stage 3:	Compensation. Kidneys reabsorb more bicarbonate	Elevated serum ions. bicarbonate
Stage 4:	Compensated respiratory acidosis: Abnormal serum values indicate problem and compensation adequate to maintain ratio and normal serum pH.	Serum pH = 7.35
Stage 5:	Decompensated respiratory acidosis: Patient acquires pneumonia, and much more CO_2 is retained. Also, kidneys cannot maintain compensation. Ratio is no longer normal, CNS depression, coma, and serum pH drops below the normal range.	Serum pH = 7.31

TABLE 2-9	**Examples of Acidosis—cont'd**	
Metabolic Acidosis—Individual with Diabetic Ketoacidosis Owing to Insulin Deficit		
Stage 1:	Slight increase in production of ketoacids. Kidneys increase excretion of acids.	No change in serum values
Stage 2:	Metabolic acidosis: More ketoacids produced than kidneys can excrete quickly, and acids bind with or "use up" buffer bicarbonate.	Low serum bicarbonate
Stage 3:	Respirations become rapid and deep to remove CO_2. Kidneys compensate by excreting more acids and reabsorbing more bicarbonate but cannot keep up with the increasing ketoacids added to the blood.	Low P_{CO_2}
Stage 4:	Compensated metabolic acidosis: Abnormal serum values indicate the problem and compensation adequate to maintain ratio and normal serum pH.	Serum pH = 7.35
Stage 5:	Decompensated metabolic acidosis: Ketoacids continue to increase in the blood at a faster rate, and the kidneys have decreased function owing to dehydration. Therefore, the problem becomes more severe and compensation is inadequate. The ratio is not maintained, and serum pH drops below the normal range.	Serum pH = 7.31

CASE STUDY A

Vomiting

Mr. K.B. is age 81 and has had gastritis with severe vomiting for 3 days. He has a history of heart problems and is presently feeling dizzy and lethargic. His eyes appear sunken, his mouth is dry, he walks unsteadily, and he complains of muscle aching, particularly in the abdomen. He is thirsty but is unable to retain food or fluid. A neighbor has brought Mr. K.B. to the hospital, where examination shows that his blood pressure is low, and his pulse and respirations are rapid. Laboratory tests demonstrate elevated hematocrit, hypernatremia, decreased serum bicarbonate, serum pH 7.35, and urine of high specific gravity (highly concentrated).

This case study illustrates a combination of fluid, electrolyte, and acid-base imbalances. Specific laboratory values are not given so as to focus on the basic concepts. For clarity, this case study is discussed in three parts, the early stage, middle stage, and advanced stage of the imbalances. Further information about the specific problems involved is given in each part and is followed by a series of questions.

Part A: Day 1

Initially, Mr. K.B. lost water, sodium in the mucus content, and hydrogen and chloride ions in the hydrochloric acid portion of the gastric secretions.

Alkalosis develops for two reasons, the first being the direct loss of hydrogen ions and the second being the effects of chloride ion loss. When chloride ion is lost in the gastric secretions, it is replaced by chloride from the serum (see Fig. 2-9). To maintain equal numbers of cations and anions in the serum, chloride ion and bicarbonate ion can exchange places when needed. Therefore more bicarbonate ions shift into the serum from storage sites in the erythrocytes to replace the lost chloride ions. More bicarbonate ions in the serum raise serum pH, and the result is "hypochloremic alkalosis."

1. Which compartments are likely to be affected in this case by early fluid loss?
2. Explain how a loss of sodium ions contributes to dehydration.
3. Describe the early signs of dehydration in Mr. K.B.

4. What serum pH could be expected in Mr. K.B. after this early vomiting?
5. Describe the compensations for the losses of fluid and electrolytes that should be occurring in Mr. K.B.
6. Explain why Mr. K.B. may not be able to compensate for losses as well as a younger adult.

Part B: Days 2 to 3

As Mr. K.B. continues to vomit and is still unable to eat or drink any significant amounts, loss of the duodenal contents, which include intestinal, pancreatic, and biliary secretions, occurs. No digestion and absorption of any nutrients occurs.

Losses at this stage include water, sodium ions, potassium ions, and bicarbonate ions. Also, intake of glucose and other nutrients is minimal. Mr. K.B. shows elevated serum sodium levels.

7. Explain why serum sodium levels appear to be high in this case.
8. Explain how high serum sodium levels might affect the intracellular fluid.
9. Using your knowledge of normal physiology, explain how continued fluid loss is likely to affect:
   a. blood volume
   b. cell function
   c. kidney function
10. Given Mr. K.B.'s history, why might potassium imbalance have more serious effects on him?

Part C: Day 3: Admission to the Hospital

After a prolonged period of vomiting, metabolic acidosis develops. This change results from a number of factors:

- Loss of bicarbonate ions in duodenal secretions
- Lack of nutrients leading to catabolism of stored fats and protein with production of excessive amounts of ketoacids
- Dehydration and decreased blood volume leading to decreased excretion of acids by the kidney
- Decreased blood volume leading to decreased tissue perfusion, less oxygen to cells, and increased anaerobic metabolism with increased lactic acid
- Increased muscle activity and stress leading to increased metabolic acid production

These factors lead to an increased amount of acids in the blood, which bind with bicarbonate buffer and result in decreased serum bicarbonate and decreased serum pH or metabolic acidosis.

11. List several reasons why Mr. K.B. is lethargic and weak.
12. Predict the serum level of carbon dioxide or carbonic acid in this case.
13. If Mr. K.B. continues to lose body fluid, why might serum pH decrease below 7.35?
14. If serum pH drops below 7.35, what signs would be observed in Mr. K.B.?
15. Describe the effect of acidosis on serum potassium levels.
16. Mr. K.B. will be given replacement fluid therapy. Why is it important that sodium and potassium be given as well as water?

CASE STUDY B

Diarrhea

Baby C., 3 months old, has had severe watery diarrhea accompanied by fever for 24 hours. She is apathetic and responds weakly to stimulation. The condition has been diagnosed as viral gastroenteritis.

1. List the major losses resulting from diarrhea and fever.
2. List other signs or data that would provide helpful information.
3. Explain several reasons why infants become dehydrated very quickly.

CASE STUDY C

Nephrotic Syndrome

S.K., age 5, has idiopathic nephrotic syndrome (nephrosis). He has generalized edema with a puffy face, distended abdomen, and edematous legs. He has gained weight but has eaten very little during the past week and has been quite irritable and lethargic. His blood pressure is normal. Laboratory tests indicate high levels of albumin, lipids, and hyaline (protein) casts in the urine, which has a high specific gravity. Blood tests show hypoalbuminemia and elevated cholesterol levels.

1. State the cause of idiopathic nephrotic syndrome.
2. Describe the change in the nephron that leads to albuminuria.
3. Describe the characteristics of the blood and urine that distinguish nephrotic syndrome.
4. Explain how hypoalbuminemia causes generalized edema.
5. Explain why S.K. is retaining sodium and water.
6. Explain why skin breakdown is common in patients with prolonged edema.

CHAPTER SUMMARY

Water, electrolytes, and acids are constantly moving between compartments in the body, depending on intake, output, and variations in cell metabolism. Numerous mechanisms work to maintain a constant internal environment.

- Edema, local or general, results from excess fluid in the interstitial compartment due to increased capillary hydrostatic pressure, increased sodium ion concentration in ECF, decreased plasma osmotic pressure related to decreased plasma proteins, obstructed lymphatic circulation, or increased capillary permeability.
- Dehydration or fluid deficit in the body may be caused by decreased intake or excessive loss of water. Infants and elderly persons exhibit the greatest risk for dehydration.
- The signs of dehydration include thirst, dry oral mucous membrane and decreased skin turgor, fatigue, decreased urine output, and low blood pressure with rapid, weak pulse.
- Third-spacing refers to the movement of fluid out of the vascular compartment into a body cavity or tissue where it cannot circulate.
- Hyponatremia impairs conduction of nerve impulses, muscle contraction, and distribution of body fluids.
- Hypernatremia causes fluid to shift out of cells, affecting cell function.
- Both hyperkalemia and hypokalemia lead to cardiac arrhythmias and possible cardiac arrest.
- Calcium ion levels in the blood are affected by parathyroid hormone, calcitonin, vitamin D, phosphate ion levels, diet, digestive tract, and renal function.
- Hypocalcemia causes muscle twitching and tetany related to increased permeability and excitability of nerve fibers, but leads to weaker cardiac muscle contractions.
- Excessive parathyroid hormone leads to hypercalcemia and bone demineralization that may cause spontaneous fractures.
- Chloride and bicarbonate ions are important in acid-base balance.
- The buffer ratio of 20 parts bicarbonate ion (base) to 1 part CO_2 (carbonic acid) is essential to maintain serum pH in the normal range of 7.35 to 7.45.
- Respiratory acidosis or alkalosis is caused by respiratory impairment increasing P_{CO_2}, or hyperventilation decreasing P_{CO_2}, respectively. The kidneys compensate by altering bicarbonate ion levels to maintain the required ratio.
- Metabolic acidosis results from a deficit of bicarbonate ion, either due to excessive loss of acids (e.g., from diarrhea) or to excessive accumulated acids (e.g., diabetic ketoacidosis). Metabolic alkalosis is caused by increased bicarbonate ion levels, perhaps from increased antacid ingestion. The respiratory and renal systems compensate for these changes.
- Decompensation develops when serum pH moves outside the normal range, preventing the cell enzymes from functioning. This can happen when the kidneys

are damaged or when dehydration prevents adequate kidney function.

- Initially, vomiting causes loss of hydrochloric acid from the stomach and metabolic alkalosis. If vomiting is prolonged and severe, dehydration and metabolic acidosis develop.

- Diarrhea causes loss of fluid and bicarbonate ions, leading to metabolic acidosis.
- Generalized edema results from low levels of plasma proteins related to kidney or liver disease or malnutrition.

hyperkemia

hypo = impairs nerve
hyper = fluid shift

STUDY QUESTIONS

1. Describe the locations of intracellular and extracellular fluids.
2. Which makes up the higher proportion of body fluid, intracellular fluid or extracellular fluid?
3. How does the proportion of fluid in the body change with age?
4. Why does dehydration affect cell function?
5. What is the function of sodium ion in the body?
6. Describe the effect of hypernatremia on extracellular fluid volume and on intracellular fluid volume.
7. State the primary location (compartment) of potassium.
8. How are sodium and potassium levels controlled in the body?
9. Describe the signs and symptoms of hypocalcemia.
10. Describe how a deficit of vitamin D would affect:
    a. bones
    b. serum calcium level
11. Explain how hypochloremia affects acid-base balance.
12. State the normal range of pH for:
    a. blood
    b. urine
13. Describe how very slow, shallow respirations are likely to affect:
    a. P_{CO_2}
    b. serum pH
14. State three possible causes of metabolic acidosis.
15. A diabetic client is producing excess amounts of ketoacids.
    a. Describe the effects of this excess on serum bicarbonate levels and serum pH.
    b. Explain the possible compensations for this imbalance.
    c. Describe the signs of this compensation.

16. The respirations that accompany metabolic acidosis are frequently called Kussmaul's respirations or "air hunger." What is the purpose of such respirations?
17. A person is found unconscious. He is wearing a Medic-Alert bracelet for diabetes and his breath has the typical odor of acetone (ketoacids).
    a. Predict his serum pH and the rationale for this prediction.
    b. Predict his serum potassium level.
18. How does insulin administration affect serum potassium?
19. A person will probably become very dehydrated as ketoacidosis develops. What heart rate and pulse characteristics would you expect to be present in this dehydrated condition?
20. Prolonged strenuous exercise usually leads to an increase in lactic acid. Given your knowledge of normal circulation, explain why it is helpful to have a cool-down period with mild exercise rather than total rest immediately after strenuous exercise.
21. General anesthetics, presence of pain, and narcotic analgesics for pain often lead to slow, shallow respirations after surgery, circulation is frequently slow, and oxygen levels are somewhat reduced. Predict the effects on the partial pressure of carbon dioxide and, how this would affect serum pH.

parathyroid
hormone
↳ hypercalcemia

ADDITIONAL RESOURCES

Copstead LC, Banasik JL: *Pathophysiology*, ed 4, St. Louis, 2010, Saunders.

Damjanov I: *Pathology for the Health Professions*, ed 4, St Louis, 2011, Elsevier Saunders.

Guyton AC, Hall JE: *Textbook of Medical Physiology*, ed 11, Philadelphia, 2006, WB Saunders.

McCance KL, Huether SE: *Pathophysiology: The Biologic Basis for Disease in Adults and Children*, ed 5, St. Louis, 2005, Mosby.

Patton KT, Thibodeau GA: *Anatomy & Physiology*, ed 8, St Louis, 2013, Mosby.

CHAPTER 3

Introduction to Basic Pharmacology and Other Common Therapies

CHAPTER OUTLINE

LEARNING OBJECTIVES

After studying this chapter, the student is expected to:

1. Define common terms used in pharmacology.
2. Differentiate the types of adverse reactions.
3. Explain the factors that determine blood levels of a drug.
4. Compare the methods of drug administration.
5. Describe the role of receptor sites in drug action.
6. Differentiate a generic name from a trade name.
7. Explain the basis for the various legal restrictions on the sale of drugs listed in different schedules.
8. Describe the roles of specified members of the health care team, traditional and alternative.
9. Describe the basic concepts of Asian medicine.

KEY TERMS

acupoints
antagonism
compliance

holistic
idiosyncratic
meridians

parenteral
placebo
potentiation

synergism
synthesized

Pharmacology

Health professionals are required to record and maintain medical profiles for each patient including *all* medications, including over-the-counter drugs. An example of a general/simple medical history can be found in Ready Reference 6 at the back of the book. This chapter provides a brief overview of the basic principles of pharmacology and therapeutics.

Basic Principles

Pharmacology is an integrated medical science involving chemistry, biochemistry, anatomy, physiology, microbiology, and others. Pharmacology is the study of drugs, their actions, dosage, therapeutic uses (indications), and adverse effects. Drug therapy is directly linked to the pathophysiology of a particular disease. It is helpful for students to understand the common terminology and concepts used in drug therapy to enable them to look up and comprehend information on a specific drug. Medications frequently have an impact on patient care and have a part in emergency situations/care. It is important to recognize the difference between expected manifestations of a disease and the effects of a drug.

Drugs may come from natural sources such as plants, animals, and microorganisms such as fungi, or they may be synthesized. Many manufactured drugs originated as plant or animal substances. In time the active ingredient was isolated and refined in a laboratory and finally mass produced as a specific synthesized chemical or biologic compound.

A *drug* is a substance that alters biologic activity in a person. Drugs may be prescribed for many reasons, some of which are:
- To promote healing (e.g., an anti-inflammatory glucocorticoid)
- To cure disease (e.g., an antibacterial drug)
- To control or slow progress of a disease (e.g., cancer chemotherapy)
- To prevent disease (e.g., a vaccine)
- To decrease the risk of complications (e.g., an anticoagulant)
- To increase comfort levels (e.g., an analgesic for pain)
- As replacement therapy (e.g., insulin)
- To reduce excessive activity in the body (e.g., a sedative or antianxiety drug)

Pharmacology is organized into separate disciplines that deal with actions of drugs.
- Pharmacodynamics
  - Drug-induced responses of physiologic and biochemical systems in health and disease
- Pharmacokinetics
  - Drug amounts at different sites after administration
- Pharmacotherapeutics
  - Choice and drug application for disease prevention, treatment, or diagnosis
- Toxicology
  - Study of the body's response to drugs, their harmful effects, mechanisms of actions, symptoms, treatment, and identification
- Pharmacy
  - The preparation, compounding, dispensing, and record keeping of therapeutic drugs

Drug Effects

A drug may exert its *therapeutic* or desired action by stimulating or inhibiting cell function. Some drugs, such as antihistamines, block the effects of biochemical agents (like histamine) in the tissues. Other drugs have a physical or mechanical action; for example, some laxatives that provide bulk and increase movement through the gut. Drugs are classified or grouped by their primary pharmacologic action and effect, such as antimicrobial or anti-inflammatory. The *indications* listed for a specific drug in a drug manual provide the approved uses or diseases for which the drug has been proved effective. Off-label uses are those for which the drug has shown some effectiveness, but not the use for which the drug was approved by regulatory bodies. Listed *contraindications* are circumstances under which the drug usually should not be taken.

Generally drugs possess more than one effect on the body, some of which are undesirable, even at recommended doses. If these unwanted actions are mild, they are termed *side effects*. For example, antihistamines frequently lead to a dry mouth and drowsiness, but these effects are tolerated because the drug reduces the allergic response. On occasion, a side effect is used as the primary goal; for example, promethazine (Phenergan) has been used as an antiemetic or a sedative as well as an antihistamine. When the additional effects are dangerous, cause tissue damage, or are life threatening (e.g., excessive bleeding), they are called *adverse* or *toxic* effects. In such cases, the drug is discontinued or a lower dose ordered. In some cases, such as cancer chemotherapy, a choice about the benefits compared with the risks of the recommended treatment is necessary. Unfortunately, a long period of time may elapse before sufficient reports of toxic effects are compiled to warrant warnings about a specific drug, and in some cases its withdrawal from the marketplace. It is important to realize that undesirable and toxic effects can occur with over-the-counter (OTC) items as well as prescription drugs. For example, megadoses of some vitamins are very toxic, and excessive amounts of acetaminophen can cause kidney and liver damage. In late 2000, some cough and cold preparations as well as appetite suppressants containing phenylpropanolamine (PPA) were removed from the market because of a risk of hemorrhagic strokes in young women. Research continues into the development of "ideal" drugs with improved or more selective therapeutic effect, fewer (or no) side effects, and no toxic effects.

Several specific forms of adverse effects should be noted:
- *Hypersensitivity* or allergic reactions to drugs such as penicillin and local anesthetics are common. The reaction may be mild (e.g., a rash) or can result in anaphylaxis. The patient should stop taking the medication immediately and notify the physician. Generally a person is allergic to other structurally similar drugs and should avoid that group in the future.
- Idiosyncratic (also called paradoxic) reactions are unexpected or unusual responses to drugs; for example, excessive excitement after taking a sedative (sleep-inducing drug). These reactions occur in some elderly individuals. Some idiosyncratic reactions are used therapeutically; stimulants are used in ADHD to reduce distraction and increase concentration.

- *Iatrogenic* refers to a negative effect on the body caused by a medication error, drug overdose, or unusual response.
- *Teratogenic* or harmful effects on the fetus, leading to developmental defects, have been associated with some drugs. Fetal cells are particularly vulnerable in the first 3 months (see discussion of congenital defects in Chapter 21). This is an area in which research cannot be totally effective in screening drugs. It is recommended that pregnant women or those planning pregnancy avoid all medications.
- *Interactions* occur when a drug's effect is modified by combining it with another drug, food, herbal compounds, or other material. Interactions commonly occur with nonprescription drugs such as aspirin, antacids, or herbal compounds, as well as with alcohol. Even a healthy food such as grapefruit juice can cause changes in drug absorption. Interactions are a particular concern for elderly patients, who often take many drugs and consult several physicians.

The effect of the combination may be increased much more than expected (synergism) or greatly decreased (antagonism). Synergistic action can be life threatening; for example, causing hemorrhage or coma. It has been documented that the majority of drug overdose cases and fatalities in hospital emergency departments result from drug-drug or drug-alcohol combinations.

Alternatively, when synergism is established, it may be used beneficially to reduce the dose of each drug to achieve the same or more beneficial effects with reduced side effects. For example, this is an intentional advantageous action when combining drugs to treat pain.

The presence of an antagonist prevents the patient from receiving the beneficial action of a drug. In a patient with heart disease or a serious infection, this would be hazardous. On the other hand, antagonistic action is effectively used when an antidote is required for an accidental poisoning or overdose.

One other form of interaction involves potentiation, whereby one drug enhances the effect of a second drug. For example, the inclusion of epinephrine with local anesthetics is intended to prolong the effects of the local anesthetic, without increasing the dose. It causes vasoconstriction in the area, which decreases blood flow and thereby helps keep the anesthetic in the area longer because it will not be absorbed as quickly.

Administration and Distribution of Drugs

The first consideration with administration is the dosage of the medication. The *dose* of a drug is the amount of drug required to produce the specific desired effect in an adult, usually expressed by a weight or measure and a time factor such as twice a day. A child's dose is best calculated using the child's weight, not age. A proper measuring device should be used when giving medication because general household spoons and cups vary considerably in size.

In some circumstances, a larger dose may be administered initially, or the first dose may be given by injection, to achieve effective drug levels quickly. This "loading dose" principle is frequently applied to antimicrobial drugs, in which case it is desirable to have sufficient drug in the body to begin destruction of the infecting microbes as soon as possible. It is equally important not to increase the prescribed dose over a period of time (the "if one tablet is good, two or three are better" concept), nor to increase the frequency, because these changes could result in toxic blood levels of the drug.

The frequency of dosing is important in maintaining effective blood levels of the drug without toxicity, and directions regarding timing should be carefully followed (Fig. 3-1). Optimum dosing schedules are established for each drug based on factors such as absorption, transport in the blood, half-life of the particular drug, and biotransformation. Drugs usually should be taken at regular intervals over the 24-hour day, such as every 6 hours. Directions regarding timing related to meals or other daily events are intentional and should be observed. For example, insulin intake must match food intake. Sometimes the drug is intended to assist with food intake and digestion and hence should be taken before meals. In other cases, food may inactivate some of the drug or interfere with absorption, reducing the amount reaching the blood; therefore the drug must be taken well before a meal or certain foods must be avoided. Alternatively, it may be best to take the drug with or after the meal to prevent gastric irritation. A sleep-inducing drug is more effective if taken a half-hour before going to bed, rather than when getting into bed with the expectation that one will fall asleep immediately.

Actual blood levels of a drug are also dependent on such factors as the individual's:
- Circulation and cardiovascular function
- Age
- Body weight and proportion of fatty tissue
- Activity level/exercise
- Ability to absorb, metabolize, and excrete drugs (liver and kidney function)
- Food and fluid intake
- Genetic factors
- Health status, or presence of disease—chronic or acute

Therefore drug dosage and administration may have to be modified for some individuals, particularly young children and elderly people. It is sometimes difficult to determine exactly how much drug actually is effective at the site. A laboratory analysis can determine actual blood levels for many drugs. This may be requested if toxicity is suspected.

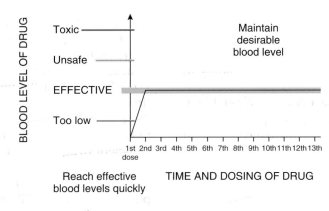

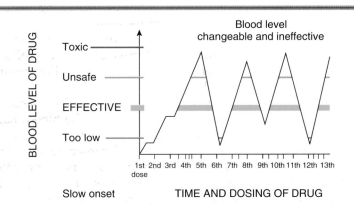

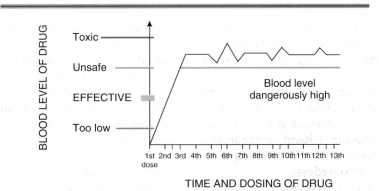

FIGURE 3-1 Factors affecting blood levels of drugs—amount of drug taken into the body, frequency of intake, and amount of drug excreted.

A drug enters the body by a chosen route, travels in the blood around the body, and eventually arrives at the site of action (e.g., the heart), exerts its effect, and then is metabolized and excreted from the body. For example, a drug taken orally is broken down and absorbed from the gastrointestinal tract into the blood (rather like ingesting food and drink!). Sometimes a drug is administered directly into an organ or tissue where it is expected to act. Another exception is the application of creams on skin lesions, where minimal absorption is expected.

Drugs can be administered for acting locally or having a systemic action:
- Local administration includes: skin, mucous membranes, orally; that is, antacids, inhalation for selected respiratory conditions, iontophoretically

• Systemic administration: transdermal therapeutic systems, orally, sublingual, rectal, inhalation, subcutaneous, intramuscular, intravenous intrathecal

The major routes for administration of drugs are oral and parenteral (injection). Table 3-1 provides a comparison of some common routes, with regard to convenience, approximate time required to reach the blood and the site of action, and the amount of drug lost. The common abbreviations for various routes may be found in Ready Reference 4. Drugs may also be administered by inhalation into the lungs (either for local effect, e.g., a bronchodilator, or for absorption into blood, e.g., an anesthetic), topical application through the skin or mucous membranes, and rectally, using a suppository for local effect or absorption into the blood. The transdermal (patch) method provides for long-term continuous absorption of drugs such as nicotine, hormones, or nitroglycerin through the skin into the blood. Variations on these methods are possible, particularly for oral medications. Time-release or long-acting forms are available (e.g., for cough and cold medications), which may contain three doses to be released over a 12-hour period.

Less frequent administration may be more efficient and increase patient compliance (adherence to directions) because of the convenience. Enteric-coated tablets (a special coating that prevents breakdown until the tablet is in the intestine) are prepared for drugs such as aspirin to prevent gastric ulcers or bleeding in persons who take large doses of this anti-inflammatory drug over prolonged periods of time.

Some drugs can only be taken by one route. However, insulin, which had to be injected in the past, can be given orally now (Generex Oral-lyn). A few drugs, such as glucocorticoids (e.g., cortisol or prednisone), can be administered in many ways, such as oral tablets, various types of injection, skin creams, and eye drops.

Oral medications are absorbed from the stomach or intestine, transported to the liver, and then released into the general circulation. This process takes time, and considerable drug may be lost in transit through the digestive tract and liver. Drugs injected intramuscularly are gradually absorbed into the blood, depending on the status of the circulation. For example, absorption could

TABLE 3-1	Various Routes for Drug Administration			
Route	Characteristics	Time to Onset and Drug Loss	Advantages	Disadvantages
Oral tablet, capsule, liquid ingested	Simple administration, easily portable	Long time to onset, e.g., 30-60 min More loss in digestive system	Tablets stable, cost varies, safe	Taste and swallowing problems; gastric irritation; uncertain absorption
Sublingual (e.g., nitroglycerin)	Very simple to use, portable	Immediate, directly into blood, little loss of drug	Convenient, rapid action	Tablets soft and unstable
Subcutaneous Injection (e.g., insulin)	Requires syringe, self-administer, portable	Slow absorption into blood Some loss of drug	Simplest injection Only small doses can be given	Requires asepsis and equipment Can be irritating
Intramuscular Injection (e.g., penicillin)	Requires syringe and technique (deltoid or gluteal muscle)	Good absorption into blood Some time lag and drug loss until absorption	Use when patient unconscious or nauseated Rapid, prolonged effect	Requires asepsis and equipment Short shelf-life Discomfort, especially for elderly
Intravenous Injection	Requires equipment and technique (directly into vein)	Immediate onset and no drug loss	Immediate effect, predictable drug level Use when patient unconscious	Costly, skill required No recovery of drug Irritation at site
Inhalation (into respiratory tract)	Portable inhaler (puffer) or machine and technique required	Rapid onset, little loss of drug.	Local effect or absorb into alveolar capillaries Rapid effect Good for anesthesia	Requires effective technique
Topical (skin or mucous membranes) gel, cream, ointment, patch, spray, liquid, or suppository	Local application, portable Also eye, ear, vaginal, rectal application	Onset rapid Some loss Absorption varies	Easy to apply Few systemic effects Useful local anesthetic	Can be messy Sometimes difficult application, e.g., eye
Intraperitoneal pump	Requires surgery	Excellent control of blood glucose levels	Immediate onset	Costly and may become infected

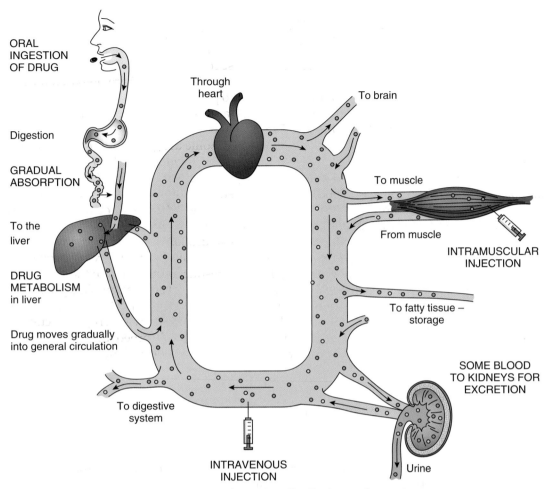

ORAL
INGESTION
OF DRUG

Through
heart

To brain

Digestion

GRADUAL
ABSORPTION

To muscle

To the
liver

From muscle

INTRAMUSCULAR
INJECTION

DRUG
METABOLISM
in liver

To fatty tissue –
storage

Drug moves gradually
into general circulation

SOME BLOOD
TO KIDNEYS FOR
EXCRETION

To digestive
system

INTRAVENOUS
INJECTION

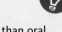 Urine

FIGURE 3-2 Drug absorption, distribution, and excretion.

be delayed for a person in shock, but occur more rapidly if the person is exercising.

The circulating blood picks up drugs and transports them, often bound to plasma proteins. Some of the drug may follow different pathways, branching off into different organs or tissues (Fig. 3-2). Depending on the specific characteristics of a drug, some may be lost temporarily in storage areas such as fatty tissue (e.g., anesthetics) or may be quickly metabolized. At some point during this movement through the body, the drug reaches the tissue or organ where it acts, passes into the interstitial fluid, and exerts its effect. Most drugs are gradually metabolized and inactivated in the liver and then excreted by the kidneys. A few drugs are excreted in bile or feces. Some anesthetics are expired through the lungs.

Some barriers to drug passage exist. Many drugs cannot pass the blood-brain barrier, a protection provided by tight junctions between cells surrounding the brain. However, at times, drugs are required in the brain, for example, anesthetics or antimicrobial drugs, and only a select few are able to pass through the blood-brain barrier. Likewise, the placental barrier protects the fetus.

THINK ABOUT 3-1

a. Explain why sublingual administration is faster than oral administration.
b. How would severe kidney or liver damage affect blood levels of a drug?
c. Describe three types of adverse reactions.

Drug Mechanisms and Receptors

Drugs possess different mechanisms for their actions. A common pharmacologic action is the drug-receptor interaction. Numerous receptors are present on or within cells in the body, responding to natural substances such as enzymes, natural hormones (e.g., estrogen), neurotransmitters (e.g., acetylcholine, norepinephrine, or GABA), or electrolytes (e.g., calcium ions). The drug classification may be named as such; for example, calcium-blocking drugs. Many medications act at these distinct receptor sites in cells or on cell membranes, either stimulating the receptor directly or blocking normal stimulating chemicals in the body (Fig. 3-3).

Depending on the uniqueness of the receptors, some drugs have very specific effects; others have a broad range of activity. The drug binds to one type of receptor and stimulates the same activity as the natural substance (an agonist). A different drug may bind to the same receptor, not stimulate it, but block entry of a natural substance and thus prevent the normal stimulus and inhibit the activity (an antagonist or blocking agent). For example, beta-adrenergic blocking agents bind to beta receptors (sympathetic nervous system) in the heart, preventing epinephrine from stimulating the heart to contract at a faster rate and increasing blood pressure. Similarly as different receptors have been identified, many drugs have been designed to stimulate or block certain activities in diverse areas of the body, including the brain and digestive tract. Research is focused on identifying particular receptors and synthesizing drugs that act only at those specific receptors in order to reduce the risk of side effects.

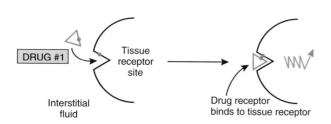

DRUG #1 STIMULATES INCREASED ACTIVITY

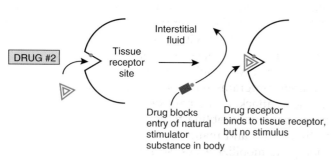

DRUG #2 DECREASES ACTIVITY

FIGURE 3-3 Receptors and drug action. Drugs may stimulate natural receptors, increasing activity, or may block receptors, decreasing activity.

Drug Classifications and Prescriptions

A prescription is a signed legal document that must include the patient's name and address and age if significant (e.g., the patient is a child); the prescriber's name, address, and identification; the date; the name and amount of the drug; the dosage, route, and directions for taking the drug; and permission for additional quantities. Abbreviations, taken from Latin words, are frequently used on prescriptions and physicians' orders in the hospital. Lists of common abbreviations and equivalent measures are found in Ready Reference 3 at the end of this book. The apothecary system of measurement (e.g., grains or drams) has largely been replaced by the metric system of mg and mL.

Chemical names for drugs tend to be very complex and difficult to remember and are therefore limited primarily to scientific or manufacturing groups. Each drug can be identified by two additional names. One is the *generic* name, a unique, official, simple name for a specific drug. This name is considered easy to remember accurately and is used in many circumstances. The other name is the trade, proprietary, or brand name, a trademark name assigned by a single manufacturer, and to be used only by that manufacturer. Many trade names may apply to one generic name, and they are considered equivalent. With the increase in new drugs some trade names sound very similar and this can lead to drug error. See Table 3-2 for examples of drug trade names.

Often members of a family of drugs with similar actions can be identified by the similarities in their generic names. For example, drugs classified as benzodiazepines, used as antianxiety agents, include diazepam, clonazepam, lorazepam, and oxazepam.

Trade names are always used for combinations of drugs in a single tablet or liquid. An exception to this pattern occurs with a few drugs that have been identified for many years by a common name, such as aspirin.

Many drug names are very similar in appearance and sound. This can lead to serious errors. It is important to match the drug name and its action with the patient's disease to prevent errors.

Legally, the Food and Drug Administration in the United States regulates the production, labeling, distribution, and other aspects of drug control. Similar agencies assume responsibility in other countries. Some

TABLE 3-2   Examples of Drug Nomenclature

Generic Name (Nonproprietary)	Trade Name (Proprietary)	Chemical Name
Diazepam	Valium, Vivol, Apo-Diazepam, Diastat	7-chloro-1,3-dihydro-1-methyl-5-phenyl-2H-1,4-benzodiazepin-2-one
Ibuprofen	Advil, Motrin, Ibren	2-(p-isobutyl phenyl)propionic acid
Hydrochlorothiazide	Hydro DIURIL, Esidrix, Hydro-Par, Oretic	6-chloro-3,4-dihydro-2H-1,2,4-benzothiadiazine-7-sulfonamide 1,1-dioxide

drugs are available without a prescription; termed *over-the-counter* or *OTC* items, such as aspirin, acetaminophen, antacids, and some cold medications, they are considered safe for open sale. When taking a drug history, it is wise to ask the patient specifically about OTC medications and any herbal products because individuals may feel they are not significant and not volunteer this information. However, for example, a drug such as aspirin may be important because it is likely to cause excessive bleeding. To prevent possible complications, it is recommended that a health professional *avoid* giving a patient any OTC drug for any reason, unless a physician or dentist so directs.

Other drugs, considered a greater risk, are classified in official schedules, according to their effects and potential for adverse effects, abuse, or dependency. Their sale is restricted, and prescription requirements are set accordingly. For example, certain narcotics such as morphine are under tighter control, requiring a written, signed prescription (not by telephone) without refill privileges. Another schedule contains drugs requiring prescription but that could be ordered by telephone. One schedule is very limited, listing drugs that can only be used for research. Drugs may be added or moved between schedules at any time. The Centers for Disease Control and Prevention (CDC) maintains a stock of drugs for rare infections. These drugs can only be obtained through consultation with the CDC.

Clinical research or trials of promising new drugs may be encountered in practice. The clinical research phase follows preliminary studies into efficacy and safety. Rules for this research have been established by government agencies, and committees oversee projects. Trials encompass a prolonged period of time. It usually takes a total of 10 to 15 years for the development of a new drug. Early trials involve a few selected patients; if successful, the trial group is greatly expanded. Researchers form a hypothesis and develop questions for their study based on the particular drug and trial requirements. A project design frequently involves dividing the patients randomly and anonymously into two groups, one to receive the standard drug therapy, the other group to receive the new therapy, in an effort to assess the effectiveness and safety of the new drug. On occasion, one group is given a placebo, a "sugar" pill lacking any active ingredient, to form a comparison for the new drug. A placebo may also be used for its psychological impact on certain patients.

THINK ABOUT 3-2

a. Explain why drugs are classified legally into different schedules.

b. What is the effect on patients when a breakthrough in scientific research is announced in the media?

Traditional Forms of Therapy

Many health professionals may be involved either directly or indirectly in the team approach to care of a patient who may be a hospital inpatient, an outpatient, or someone in the community. A few examples have been selected here to clarify roles and illustrate the multidisciplinary approach to providing therapeutic intervention. Therapies must address the pathophysiologic changes if a return to health is to result or function is to improve with minimal complications.

Physiotherapy

A physiotherapist assesses physical function and works to restore any deficit and prevent further physical dysfunction. Physiotherapy involves individualized treatment and rehabilitation as well as reduction in pain resulting from disease, surgery, or injury. Physiotherapy may include appropriate exercises, and use of ultrasound, transcutaneous electrical nerve stimulation (TENS), or other methods to alleviate pain and gain increased joint flexibility and mobility. Physiotherapists work with patients with acute neurologic, musculoskeletal, and cardiopulmonary disorders. Appropriate therapy is invaluable in preventing complications; for example, after a stroke. Infants with congenital defects or children with injuries affecting mobility require therapy as soon as possible to promote maximum development.

Other major areas for physiotherapy are rehabilitation and long-term care, in which the focus is on maximizing mobility and functional independence. Rehabilitation and long-term care involve working with amputees and those with acquired brain injury, spinal cord injuries, or strokes, as well as with group cardiac and respiratory rehabilitation programs. Cardiac rehabilitation programs have been quite successful following heart attack. Pulmonary rehabilitation has benefited many patients, enabling them to increase walking time without pain and maintain better oxygen levels. Chest therapy to mobilize excess secretions and aid lung function is useful for postoperative patients or those with chronic obstructive pulmonary disease (COPD) or bronchiectasis and cystic fibrosis. The benefits of appropriate physiotherapy to cancer patients undergoing chemotherapy and radiation are now being appreciated. Educating patients and families to assist with and maintain their individual programs is an important aspect of treatment. Physiotherapy aides or assistants may take on some responsibilities under supervision of a registered physiotherapist.

Occupational Therapy

Occupational therapists (OTs) provide a functional assessment of patient capabilities related to normal activities of daily living (ADLs). This assessment includes an evaluation of motor, cognitive, and visual-spatial ability. Guidance and practical assistance to maximize function and maintain independence are provided. Whereas the physiotherapist focuses on functional mobility and relief of pain, the occupational therapist integrates remediation of motor control, cognition, and visual-spatial perception, which is essential for client safety and productivity. Integration of functional activities is essential to continued independence and health.

In addition to remediation of functional capacities, the OT has expertise in teaching the client to use adaptations in meeting his or her needs. This includes assessment of technologies available in the marketplace, their effective use, and appropriateness for the particular client. In many cases, OTs work directly with technicians in the production of aids such as wheelchairs or walkers, as well as adaptive devices for food preparation, feeding, and personal hygiene. In the workplace setting, OTs work along with occupational health personnel to assess the workplace and essential tasks, identify appropriate accommodation, and instruct clients in the effective and safe use of supportive technologies.

OTs work in all health care settings within both institutions and the community. They may be observed working with children with developmental delays, seniors adapting to the challenges of aging and common disorders such as osteoarthritis, mentally ill clients, and recently disabled workers in the workplace.

Speech/Language Pathology

The speech/language pathologist is a specialist in the assessment and treatment of those with communication or swallowing problems. The patient could be an infant with swallowing and feeding problems, a child with a hearing deficit who is mute, an adult with aphasia after a stroke, or someone requiring a hearing assessment.

Nutrition/Diet

As an expert in foods and the nutritional needs of the body in health and illness, a nutritionist or dietitian offers advice to individuals or groups on the nutritional demands and food management best suited to a specific diagnosis; for example, diabetes. Dietitians supervise food services in hospitals and other health care institutions. They may be consulted regarding the dangers of extreme diets or eating disorders such as anorexia nervosa.

Registered Massage Therapy

Registered massage therapists (RMTs) use a variety of techniques to increase circulation, reduce pain, and increase flexibility for clients experiencing join pain or problems with body alignment. Registered massage therapists may also use soothing aromatics, acupuncture, or other modalities during therapy.

Osteopathy

Osteopaths are medical doctors who use all the traditional treatment methods such as surgery and drugs, but in addition, promote the body's natural healing processes by incorporating manipulations of the musculoskeletal system, both in diagnosis and treatment.

Chiropractic

Chiropractic medicine is based on the concept that one's health status is dependent on the state of the nervous system, which regulates all body functions to maintain homeostasis. Practice frequently involves manipulation of the vertebral column. Radiology may be used for diagnosis. Although no drugs or surgery are included in chiropractic therapy, acupuncture may be used.

Complementary or Alternative Therapies

Alternative therapies are those therapeutic practices considered to be outside the range of traditional Western medicine that also focus on alleviating disease and suffering. Included on the list of alternative therapies are acupuncture, aromatherapy, *shiatsu*, reflexology, and herbal medicine. Many of these therapies have roots in Asia, where more emphasis is placed on preserving a healthy lifestyle. The approach to disease and healing is generally holistic, a more comprehensive approach, recognizing the interrelationships of body, mind, and spirit, and the impact of pathophysiologic changes on all aspects of the individual, and treating the whole person.

Until recently, these therapies were viewed by some in the Western world to be "quackery" and by others simply to have a placebo effect, or at times even to be dangerous. Now they are accepted by more individuals and are termed *complementary*, to be used in conjunction with Western medical therapy. A few people have turned to one or more of the alternatives as a substitute for Western medical care. In some cases, alternative therapies have become a focus of last resort for individuals when traditional medicine could not achieve a cure. Current statistics show that almost half of the population uses some form of alternative therapy, and future trend predictions estimate this figure will continue to rise. Chinese medicine is now considered to be an independent system of thought and practice, including clinical observation, testing, and diagnosis.

Practitioners in these areas have varying degrees of training and professional regulation. As with traditional medicine, a patient should investigate the therapy and the individual practitioner to ensure safety and consistency with other treatment modalities. A few examples are described here.

Noncontact Therapeutic Touch

Many nurses, as well as other professionals, have trained in therapeutic touch since the 1970s. Energy is exchanged between people for relief of pain and anxiety and to promote healing. The first step in delivering touch therapy is to consciously form a positive *intent to heal*, a mindset both before and during the session. The practitioner is able to locate problem areas in the body by first scanning the body with the hands. Healing is promoted by lightly touching the skin or moving the hands just above the body surface. Imagery, light, or colors may be incorporated as a means of transferring healing energy to the patient, bringing comfort.

Naturopathy

Naturopathic treatment is based on promoting natural foods, massage, exercise, and fresh air as a way of life, thus enhancing health and preventing disease. Acupuncture, herbal medicines, nutrition, massage, and physical manipulations all have roles. Many alternative therapies are age-old home remedies that have stood the test of time to bring relief from human health complaints or promote good health. Naturopaths do not recommend any traditional drugs.

Homeopathy

Homeopathy has the goal of stimulating the immune system and natural healing power in the body through the use of plant, animal, and mineral products. A toxin or offending substance is identified for each disease state and following dilution by several thousand-fold, the toxin is administered to treat the problem.

Herbal Medicine

Medicinal herbs were first documented in ancient Egypt. Numerous groups throughout the world use herbs and plants for medicinal purposes. They are now freely available in many stores. There has been much publicity about the benefits of garlic in cardiovascular disease and other conditions. Echinacea is found in many cold remedies and used for prophylaxis. St. John's Wort contains compounds similar to standard antidepressant medications. Efforts are now being focused on providing standardized content, proving efficacy, and improving purity of herbal compounds. As with other medications, it is important to consult with a knowledgeable professional about safe dosage, interactions with other medications, and untoward effects with specific diseases.

Aromatherapy

Aromatherapy is enjoying increased popularity. Here essential oils that have therapeutic effects when rubbed on the skin and/or inhaled are extracted from plants. One oil can contain many substances. Oils may be absorbed through the skin into the general circulation, when bathing or with a massage, to exert a systemic effect. When inhaled, the essence influences physiologic functions through the olfactory system. For example, chamomile is used for its calming and sleep-inducing effect, lavender and peppermint oil soothe headache, and rosemary relieves muscle and joint disorders.

Asian Concepts of Disease and Healing

Asian therapies are based on the balance or imbalance of life energy called *qi* in Chinese medicine (also called ch'*i* or *chi*, pronounced *chee*) or *ki* in Japanese medicine. Disease is caused by a deficit or excess of *qi*, whereas healing restores the energy balance. *Qi* is derived from three sources: inherited or ancestral factors, the food ingested, and air breathed in. Imbalance or disharmony between *yin* (lack of *qi* or cold) and *yang* (excess of *qi* or heat) may be caused by changes in diet, stress, metabolism, activity, or environment, leading to disease.

In the body, the life force, *qi*, flows along specific channels called meridians, which join all organs and body parts together. Meridians are not to be confused with anatomic nerves or blood vessels. Each meridian has a name and function, and may be located some distance from the organ for which it is named. For example, the large intestine meridian begins on the surface of the index finger, travels past the wrist and shoulder, up the neck, and across the upper lip to the nose. Then the meridian goes internally to the lung, and finally to the large intestine. All meridians are bilateral except for one midline anterior (the conception vessel) and one midline posterior (the governor vessel). Along the meridians *qi* flows, and this flow may be accessed or altered at particular acupoints, or *tsubo* (Japanese). Each acupoint has very specific actions or properties, such as moving the *qi* or blood, pain reduction, heating, cooling, drying, or calming the emotions. A pattern of disharmony may involve a number of acupoints and meridians. The goal is to connect with the points that will normalize the flow of *qi* and restore the balance of *yin* and *yang*.

Acupuncture

Acupuncture is a Chinese therapeutic discipline over 3000 years old that involves inserting very fine needles into the various meridian acupoints that have potential to balance the body energy. There are classically 365 acupoints, or *tsubo* (Japanese), but today the commonly used points number only 150. Each point has a specific and a more generalized therapeutic action, and the points are often used in combinations. Acupuncture may be performed on extra points not related to meridians, and also on *ashi* or "ouch points" anywhere. Acupuncture deals with pain relief and also with balancing energy to restore health by using superficial meridian acupoints. Current theory suggests that acupuncture works to decrease pain because it causes the release of endorphins in the brain.

An acupuncture treatment on average uses 5 to 15 needles, which should be sterile, stainless steel, and disposable. The needles may be rotated or connected to low-level electric current or laser for a period of 30 to 45 minutes. The needle may only be laid on the acupoint on the surface of the skin without actually being inserted, but most often the needles are inserted into the skin to depths ranging from 1 to 2 mm on the face and ears to up to 3 inches in the heavily muscled buttocks. Instead of needles, ultrasonic waves or laser may be used over acupoints.

Moxibustion is a form of acupuncture that specifically treats cold or deficiency patterns by burning moxa to produce pure *yang* energy that penetrates deeply into the body tissues to bring about relief. The heating medium is *Artemisia vulgaris*, or common mugwort, whose dried and purified leaves produce moxa wool. The benefit of moxa is that when it is burned in a cone shape, the heat produced penetrates the body much the same way as a laser concentrates light to a concentrated beam of light energy.

Recently medical schools have begun to offer continuing education in acupuncture for health care professionals. The curricula include both traditional Chinese medicine theories and practice, as well as acupuncture based on allopathic knowledge of pain pathways. Such practice is often termed *medical acupuncture* and is offered by a variety of regulated practitioners.

Shiatsu

Shiatsu (Japanese: finger pressure) is the Japanese refined version of Chinese *anma* massage, or acupuncture without needles. There are two main forms of *shiatsu*, one using only thumbs, and the Zen *shiatsu*, the more traditional form that uses fingers, thumbs, palms, elbows, and knees to deliver slow, deep, but gentle pressure by a relaxed therapist to access the *tsubo*, or acupoints. The patient remains clothed, usually supine on a mat on the floor. This therapy provides a whole-body treatment in which all meridians are treated, from their beginning to their end, followed by the area of complaint, taking approximately 1 hour. Initially assessment is performed by palpating the meridians and the *hara*, the area below the ribs and above the pubic bone. *Shiatsu* therapists give clients exercises or other techniques that are self-administered at home between treatment sessions.

Shiatsu is recommended for stress-related illness and back pain because it provides relaxation. Zen *shiatsu* puts an emphasis upon the psychologic/emotional causes of disharmony. The therapist also adopts the "intent to heal" attitude before and during the treatment, using the power of touch.

Yoga

Yoga is an ancient Indian discipline of various forms that combines physical activity in the form of body stretching postures (*asanas*) with meditation. Practice with stretching, meditation, and special breathing techniques serves to improve the flow of *prana*, the Indian equivalent to Chinese *qi*. *Prana* circulates through the body via channels or *nadis* to connect to seven *chakras* or energy centers running up the midline. Regular practice opens these *chakras*, improves flexibility, muscle tone, endurance, and overall health, and reduces stress. Often a diet of simple (unrefined), pure food, possibly vegetarian in nature, is recommended. The practice relieves pain and anxiety in some individuals with chronic disease.

Reflexology

Reflexology, a therapy from ancient China and Egypt, relates points on the feet (mainly) and the hands to 10 longitudinal zones in the body. When the foot is stimulated with massage, this can elicit changes in distant organs or structures in the body through meridians similar to those of acupuncture. For example, areas of the great toe represent head and brain activities, and the medial arch (bilaterally) influences the vertebral column.

The practitioner applies varying degrees of pressure to the standard rotating thumb massage technique and may include slight vibration directed to various foot reflex areas. The session may conclude with essential oils being massaged into the feet. This relieves stress and muscle tension.

Craniosacral Therapy

Craniosacral therapy was first published as a scientific research paper by Dr. W. Sutherland, an osteopathic physician, in the 1930s. This system is used by a wide variety of health care practitioners: physiotherapists, occupational therapists, acupuncturists, chiropractors, medical doctors, osteopathic physicians, and dentists. The therapy deals with the characteristic ebb and flow pulsing rhythm of the meninges and cerebrospinal fluid around the brain and spinal cord. Gentle palpation and manipulation of the skull bones and vertebrae are thought to rebalance the system.

Ayurveda

This system of medicine originated in India and is still practiced today. Its goal is to balance body *dosas* or factors so that a healthy mind and body result. Special dietary plans, yoga, and herbal remedies are commonly used in Ayurvedic medicine.

THINK ABOUT 3-3

Describe three ways in which Asian medicine differs from the Western medical practices.

Emergency Assessment and Aid

Emergency care can be provided by any member of the health care team within the standards and scope of practice in their profession. Regardless of the circumstances and the responder's background, a simple assessment is the first step in any emergency situation. The format used by different groups may vary somewhat, but the same principles apply. The effectiveness of emergency response depends on the initial assessment. Using an organized checklist and keeping accurate notes of observations and care are critical elements in emergency care.

CASE STUDY A

Therapies for Pain

Where possible, the following case study should be considered from the professional standards of your studies.

While taking her health history, Ms. Z. reports severe pain in her lower back.

1. What questions would you include in your history taking for Ms. Z.? Provide a rationale for each question.

   Ms. Z. reports using herbal remedies to help her sleep, and herbal compresses during the day to reduce pain. Her doctor has prescribed acetaminophen with codeine to relieve pain. She thinks that she usually takes two "extra-strong" acetaminophen tablets every 4 hours and a Tylenol 3 tablet whenever the pain is severe.
2. What sources would you use to find information on herbal compounds and drugs?
3. What should Ms. Z. understand about the dosage of acetaminophen she is taking?
4. How can Tylenol 3 tablets assist Ms. Z to fall asleep?
5. How may the Tylenol 3 tablets interfere with sleep in some individuals?
6. What other measures can Ms. Z. use to control her pain and reduce her need for acetaminophen?
7. What therapeutic help can you provide Ms. Z. in controlling her pain? Does this therapy affect drug action?

CHAPTER SUMMARY

Drug therapy as well as other therapeutic modalities may have an impact on the course of a disease, patient well-being, or patient care by any member of the health care team.

- Drugs may have mild side effects, such as nausea, or serious toxic effects, such as bone marrow depression, in the body in addition to the beneficial or therapeutic effect. Other potential unwanted outcomes of drug treatment include hypersensitivity reaction, idiosyncratic response, or teratogenic effects.
- The route of administration, dosing schedule, distribution in the individual's body, and timing of elimination of the drug determine the effective blood level of the drug.
- Drugs may be used to stimulate or block specific natural receptor sites in the body so as to alter certain activities, such as heart rate.
- Drug interactions with other drugs, foods, or alcohol may result in synergistic or antagonistic effects.
- Physiotherapists assess physical functions and select therapy to improve mobility and/or relieve pain. Occupational therapists assist patients with ADLs, maximizing independent function.
- Alternative or complementary therapies may be provided by alternative practitioners such as osteopaths, naturopaths, and homeopaths. Treatments may be offered as replacement or in conjunction with traditional medicine.
- Asian healing is based on restoring the balance of life energy in the body (*qi* in Chinese medicine or *ki* in Japanese therapy) using specific points or meridians in the body. Therapeutic measures include acupuncture, shiatsu, and reflexology.
- The first steps in a general emergency assessment include evaluation of level of consciousness, airway function, breathing pattern, and circulatory status.

STUDY QUESTIONS

1. Compare a generic name with a trade name.
2. Explain why one drug is taken every 3 hours, but another drug is taken once daily.
3. Compare the advantages and disadvantages of:
   a. oral administration
   b. intravenous administration
4. Explain how synergism can be:
   a. dangerous
   b. beneficial
5. Explain why some drug is lost following administration and not used in the body.
6. Which group of therapists could best:
   a. assist with fitting a wheelchair?
   b. assist a young child with a swallowing problem?
7. Compare the therapies used by osteopathic physicians and chiropractors.
8. Compare the similarities and differences between acupuncture and *shiatsu*.

ADDITIONAL RESOURCES

Burnham TH Sr, editor: *Drug Facts and Comparisons*, St. Louis, 2009, Facts and Comparisons, a drug index updated monthly.

Mosby's Dental Drug Reference, ed 8, St. Louis, 2008, Mosby.

Hogan RW: *The PDR Guide to Prescription Drugs: Physicians' Desk Reference*, ed 62, Montvale, NJ, 2009, Thomson Healthcare.

Mosby's Drug Consult 2006, St. Louis, 2006, Mosby.

PDR for Nonprescription Drugs and Dietary Supplements, Montvale, NJ, 2009, Thomson Healthcare.

Skidmore-Roth L: *Mosby's Handbook of Herbs and Natural Supplements*, ed 3, St. Louis, 2006, Mosby.

Spratto G: *PDR Nurse's Drug Handbook*, Montvale, NJ, 2009, Thomson Healthcare.

Web Sites

http://www.nlm.nih.gov/medlineplus/druginformation.html *Drugs, Supplements, and Herbal Information*

http://nccam.nih.gov *NIH National Center for Complementary and Alternative Medicine*

http://www.cancer.gov/clinicaltrials *National Cancer Institute; information on clinical trials*

http://www.ccnm.edu *Canadian College of Naturopathic Medicine/Robert Schad Naturopathic Clinic*

http://www.health.harvard.edu *Harvard Health Publications*

Pain

CHAPTER OUTLINE

LEARNING OBJECTIVES

After studying this chapter, the student is expected to:

1. State the causes of pain.
2. Describe the pain pathway.
3. Relate the methods of pain control to the gate-control theory.
4. Discuss the signs and symptoms of pain in adults and young children.
5. Compare referred and phantom pain.
6. Explain the factors that may alter pain perception.
7. Compare acute and chronic pain.
8. Discuss the types of headache.
9. Describe methods of pain management.

KEY TERMS

afferent fibers
analgesic
bradykinin
cordotomy
dermatome
efferent

endogenous
histamine
intractable
ischemia
neurotransmitter
nociceptors

opioids
parenterally
prostaglandin
reticular activating system
  (RAS)
reticular formation

rhizotomy
sedatives
substance P
tachycardia

Pain is an unpleasant sensation, a feeling of discomfort resulting from stimulation of pain receptors in the body when tissue damage occurs or is about to occur. Pain is a body *defense* mechanism and is a warning of a problem, particularly when it is acute. It is difficult to define because it can have many variable characteristics, and it is a subjective feeling, impossible to accurately measure. However, subjective scales have been developed to facilitate comparison of pain levels over time. In cases of trauma, the danger may be obvious, but in other situations the cause may be hidden deep inside the body. Pain involves very complex mechanisms, many of which are not totally understood by scientists or health care workers.

Etiology and Sources of Pain

Pain stimuli may occur for many reasons. Pain may be felt because of inflammation, infection, ischemia and tissue necrosis, stretching of tissue, chemicals, or burns. In skeletal muscle, pain may result from ischemia or hemorrhage. Many organs such as the liver, kidney, or brain are characterized by pain receptors in the covering capsule, and pain is felt when the capsule is stretched by inflammation. Stretching of tendons, ligaments, and joint capsules also elicits pain; these effects may occur secondary to inflammation or muscle spasm to guard a joint or painful body part. In the stomach and intestines, pain may result from inflammation of the mucosa, ischemia, distention, or muscle spasm.

Somatic pain may arise from the skin (cutaneous) or from deeper structures such as bone or muscle, to be conducted by sensory nerves. Visceral pain originates in the organs and travels by sympathetic fibers. Depending on the cause, pain may be sudden and short-term,

marked primarily by a reflex withdrawal. For example, if one touches a hot object, the hand is involuntarily jerked away from the source of injury. Or pain may be relatively continuous, as when infection or swelling is present.

Structures and Pain Pathways

Pain receptors or nociceptors are free sensory nerve endings that are present in most tissues of the body (Fig. 4-1). These sensory nerves may be stimulated by thermal, chemical, or physical means. Thermal means refer to extremes of temperature, mechanical means could refer to pressure, and chemical sources could include acids or compounds produced in the body, such as bradykinin, histamine, or prostaglandin.

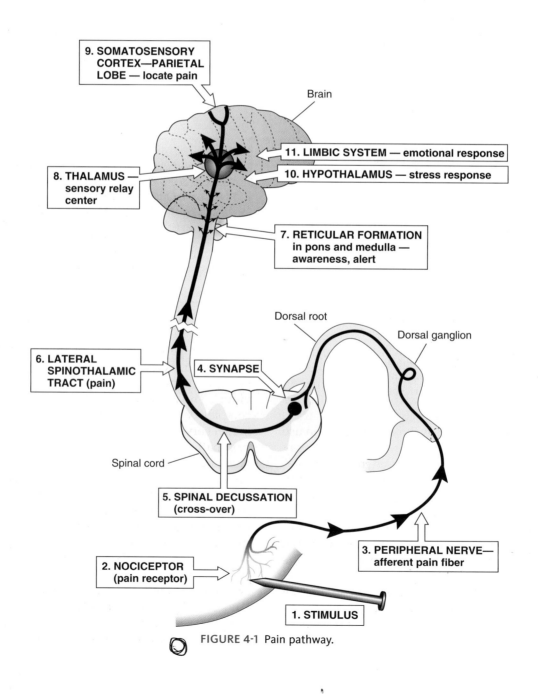

FIGURE 4-1 Pain pathway.

The *pain threshold* refers to the level of stimulation required to activate the nerve ending sufficiently for the individual to perceive pain. The associated nerve fibers then transmit the pain signal to the spinal cord and brain. The pain threshold is relatively constant over time and between individuals. The ability to withstand pain or the perception of its intensity is referred to as pain tolerance; this varies considerably with past pain experience and overall state of health.

Two types of afferent fibers conduct pain impulses: The myelinated A delta fibers that transmit impulses very rapidly and the unmyelinated C fibers that transmit impulses slowly. Acute pain—the sudden, sharp, localized pain related to thermal and physical stimuli primarily from skin and mucous membranes—is transmitted by the A delta fibers, whereas chronic pain—often experienced as a diffuse, dull, burning or aching sensation—is transmitted by C fibers. C fibers receive thermal, physical, and chemical stimuli from muscle, tendons, the myocardium, and the digestive tract as well as from the skin. The peripheral nerves transmit the afferent pain impulse to the dorsal root ganglia and then into the spinal cord through the dorsal horn or substantia gelatinosa (see Chapter 14).

Each spinal nerve conducts impulses from a specific area of the skin called a dermatome (see Fig. 14-22, which illustrates the areas of the skin innervated by each spinal nerve), and the somatosensory cortex is "mapped" to correspond to areas of the body so that the source of the pain can be interpreted in the brain (see Fig. 14-3 for a map of the brain). The dermatomes can be used to test for areas of sensory loss or pain sensation and thus determine the site of damage after spinal cord injuries.

At the spinal cord synapse, a *reflex response* to sudden pain results in a motor, or efferent, impulse back to the muscles that initiates an involuntary muscle contraction to move the body away from the source of pain. After the sensory impulse reaches the synapse, connecting neurons also transmit it across the spinal cord to the ascending tracts to the brain. There are two types of tracts in the spinothalamic bundle: The fast impulses for acute sharp pain travel in the neospinothalamic tract, whereas the slower impulses for chronic or dull pain use the paleospinothalamic tract. This double pathway explains the two stages of pain one often experiences with an injury to the skin, the initial sharp severe pain, followed by a duller but persistent throbbing or aching pain. These tracts connect with the reticular formation in the brain stem, hypothalamus, thalamus, and other structures as they ascend to the somatic sensory area in the cerebral cortex of the parietal lobe of the brain. It is here that the location and characteristics of the pain are perceived. The many branching connections from the ascending tracts provide information to other parts of the brain, forming the basis for an integrated response to pain.

THINK ABOUT   4-1

Trace the pathway of a pain impulse originating from stubbed toe by drawing a simple diagram and labeling the parts.

The arousal state of the reticular activating system (RAS) in the reticular formation in the pons and medulla influences the brain's awareness of the incoming pain stimuli. In clinical practice, many drugs depress the RAS, thereby decreasing the pain experienced. The hypothalamus plays a role in the response to pain through its connections with the pituitary gland and sympathetic nervous system. Response to pain usually involves a stress response (see Chapter 26) as well as an emotional response such as crying, moaning, or anger. There may be a physical response, perhaps rigidity, splinting, or guarding of an area of the body. The thalamus processes many types of sensory stimuli as they enter the brain and is important in the emotional response to pain through the limbic system.

THINK ABOUT   4-2

a. Describe your response to a sudden severe pain in your own experience; for example, an injury. Describe your physical response and your emotional reactions.
b. Using your knowledge of normal physiology, list the effects of increased sympathetic nervous system stimulation on body function and muscle tone.
c. Suggest how monitoring for sympathetic nervous system changes assists you in evaluating a person's level of pain.

Physiology of Pain and Pain Control

Pain is a highly complex phenomenon that is not fully understood. There are many variables in its source and perception and in the response to it in a specific individual. The *gate-control theory* has been modified as the complexity of pain is better realized, but the simple model serves as a useful tool and visual explanation of pain pathways that can be related to many concepts of pain and pain control. According to this theory, control systems, or "gates," are built into the normal pain pathways in the body that can modify the entry of pain stimuli into the spinal cord and brain. These gates at the nerve synapses in the spinal cord and brain can be *open*, thus permitting the pain impulses to pass from the peripheral nerves to the spinothalamic tract and ascend to the brain (Fig. 4-2). Or they may be *closed*, reducing or modifying the passage of pain impulses. Gate closure can occur in response to other sensory stimuli along competing nerve pathways that may diminish the pain sensations or by modulating or inhibitory impulses

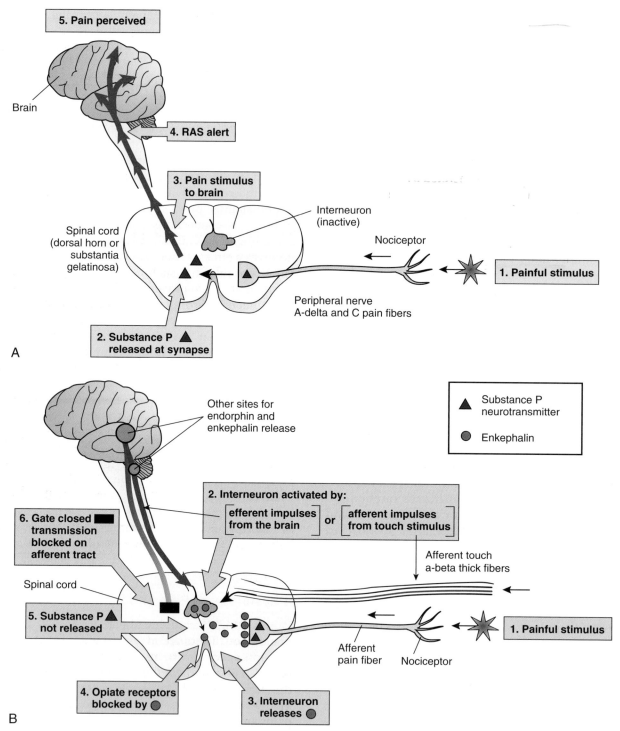

FIGURE 4-2 Pain control. **A,** Gate open—pain stimulus transmitted. **B,** Gate closed—pain stimulus blocked.

from higher centers in the brain. For example, application of ice to a painful site may reduce pain because one is more aware of the cold than the pain. Transcutaneous electrical nerve stimulation (TENS) is a therapeutic intervention that increases sensory stimulation at a site, thus blocking pain transmission. Alternatively, the brain can inhibit or modify incoming pain stimuli by producing efferent or outgoing transmissions through the reticular formation. Many factors can activate this built-in control system, including prior conditioning, the emotional state of the affected person, or distraction by other events. This last phenomenon has been observed in many individuals who feel no pain when injured suddenly but do experience delayed onset of pain once they are no longer distracted by the immediate emergency situation.

The key to this analgesia system, or the blocking of pain impulses to the brain, is the release of a number of opiate-like chemicals (opioids) secreted by interneurons within the central nervous system. These substances block the conduction of pain impulses into the central nervous system. They resemble the drug morphine, which is derived from opium and is used as an analgesic, and are therefore called *endorphins* or *endogenous morphine*. Endorphins include enkephalins, dynorphins, and beta-lipotropins. Figure 4-2 illustrates how enkephalin is released in the spinal cord and is attached to opiate receptors on the afferent neuron, thus blocking release of the neurotransmitter substance P at the synapse. This process prevents transmission of the pain stimulus into the spinal cord. *Serotonin* is another chemical released in the spinal cord that acts on other neurons in the spinal cord to increase the release of enkephalins. Clients with clinical depression often report chronic pain due to reduction in serotonin levels in the brain. In addition, natural *opiate receptors* are found in many areas of the brain, as are secretions of endorphins, which can block pain impulses at that level. The body has its own endogenous analgesic or pain control system that explains some of the variables in pain perception and can be used to assist in pain control.

THINK ABOUT   4-3

Briefly describe three methods of "closing the gate" and reducing pain.

Characteristics of Pain

Signs and Symptoms

Pain is a real sensation but a subjective symptom perceived by each individual. There are many variations in the clinical picture of pain as well as the verbal reports of pain.

Possible details that may be helpful in diagnosing the severity and cause of pain include:
- The location of the pain
- The use of many descriptive terms, such as aching, burning, sharp, throbbing, widespread, cramping, constant, periodic, unbearable, or moderate
- The timing of the pain or its association with an activity such as food intake or movement, or with pressure applied at the site

- Physical evidence of pain, when the patient may demonstrate a stress response with physical signs such as pallor and sweating, high blood pressure, or tachycardia
- Nausea and vomiting or fainting and dizziness, which may occur with acute pain
- Anxiety and fear, which are frequently evident in people with chest pain but may be present in other situations as well
- Clenched fists or rigid faces; restless or constant motion, or lack of movement; often protecting, or "guarding" the affected area

Young Children and Pain

For many years it was thought that newborn infants, because of their immature nervous systems, did not perceive or experience pain. It has now been established that a young infant does perceive pain and responds to it physiologically, with tachycardia and increased blood pressure as well as characteristic facial expressions. Infants with their eyes tightly closed, their eyebrows low and drawn together, and their mouths open and square are probably in pain.

There is great variation in the developmental stages and coping mechanisms of children. A range of behavior that may not accurately reflect the severity of pain should be expected. Older children may flail their legs and arms and resist comfort measures, or they may become physically rigid. Children may find it difficult to describe their pain verbally. However, drawings of happy or sad faces, mechanical scales, or multicolored symbols can be used by children to better describe their feelings. Withdrawal and lack of communication are often the result of pain in older children and teens.

Referred Pain

Sometimes the source of a pain stimulus can be localized to a specific area. In other cases the pain is generalized, and the source is difficult to determine. Sometimes the pain is perceived at a site distant from the source. This is called *referred* pain. Generalized and referred pains are characteristic of visceral damage in the abdominal organs. In some conditions, such as acute appendicitis, the characteristics of the pain may change as pathologic changes occur.

Referred pain occurs when the sensations of pain are identified in an area some distance from the actual source (Fig. 4-3). Usually the pain originates in a deep organ or muscle and is perceived on the surface of the body in a different area. For example, pain in the left neck and arm is characteristic of a heart attack or ischemia in the heart. Pain in the shoulder may be due to stretching of the diaphragm. Multiple sensory fibers from different sources connecting at a single level of the

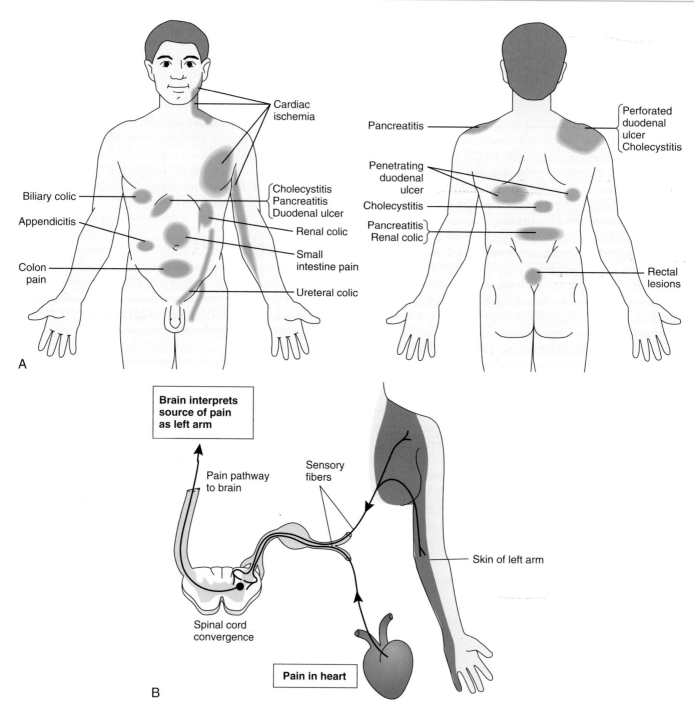

FIGURE 4-3 **A,** Locations of referred pain. **B,** Proposed mechanism for referred pain. (**A,** *From Copstead-Kirkorn LC: Pathophysiology, ed 4, St. Louis, 2009, Mosby.*)

spinal cord make it difficult for the brain to discern the actual origin of the pain.

Phantom Pain

Pain or another sensation such as itching or tingling occurs in some individuals, usually adults, after an amputation. Pain is perceived by the person as occurring in the lost limb and usually does not respond to usual pain therapies. The pain may resolve within weeks to months. Although the phenomenon is not fully understood, it appears that the brain "understands" the limb is still present when processing incoming stimuli. Research suggests that a history of prolonged or severe chronic pain before surgery increases the probability of phantom pain developing.

Pain Perception and Response

Pain tolerance is the degree of pain, either its intensity or its duration, which is endured before an individual takes some action. Tolerance may be increased by endorphin release or reduced by other factors such as fatigue or stress. Tolerance does not necessarily depend on the severity of the pain. Rather, it varies among people and different situations.

Pain perception and response are subjective and depend on the conditioning of the individual. Factors such as age, culture, family traditions, and prior experience with pain shape one's perception and response to pain. For example, in certain groups it is customary to approach pain with stoic acceptance, whereas in other groups the proper response would include loud crying and wailing. Prior unpleasant experiences and anticipatory fear or anxiety can lower pain tolerance, magnifying the extent of the pain and the victim's response.

An individual's temperament and personality can influence his or her response to pain, and the circumstances existing at the time of the incident may affect perception of it. Anxiety, fear, and stress can increase the severity of pain because in these circumstances the central nervous system is at a higher level of awareness. Fatigue, hunger, and the presence of other pathologies or problems may magnify a person's response. Likewise, the specific cause of the pain and its implications with respect to body image, family relationships, or employment responsibilities might alter the person's perception of pain and his or her response to it.

> **THINK ABOUT   4-4**
>
> a. From your own experience, describe a sharp pain, an aching pain, and a cramping pain.
> b. List factors that often make pain seem more severe.
> c. Differentiate pain threshold from pain tolerance.

Basic Classifications of Pain

Acute Pain

- Acute pain is usually sudden and severe, but short term.
- It indicates tissue damage and decreases once the cause has been treated.
- It may be localized or generalized.
- Acute pain usually initiates a physiologic stress response with increased blood pressure and heart rate; cool, pale, moist skin; increased respiratory rate; and increased skeletal muscle tension (see Chapter 26).
- Vomiting may occur.
- In addition, there may be a strong emotional response, as indicated by facial or verbal expression and a high anxiety level.

Chronic Pain

Long-term pain leads to different and often negative effects such as loss of employment or interference with personal relationships.

- Chronic pain is usually more difficult to treat effectively than acute pain, and the prognosis may be less certain.
- Chronic pain is often perceived by the patient as being more generalized, and it is difficult to discern an exact location.
- Because a specific cause may be less apparent to the person experiencing the pain, the pain is more difficult to deal with and can be quite debilitating.
- It is impossible to sustain a stress response over a long period of time, and the individual with chronic pain frequently is fatigued, irritable, and depressed.
- Sleep disturbances are common, and appetite may be affected, leading to weight gain or loss.
- Constant pain frequently affects daily activities and may become a primary focus in the life of the individual, thus complicating any measures to affect pain control by medication or other methods. Effective support from the health care team and a caring approach that does not minimize the person's pain may significantly reduce the client's focus on controlling pain.
- Periods of acute pain may accompany exacerbations of chronic disease, making it more difficult for the patient to participate effectively in a pain management program.
- Long-term pain usually reduces tolerance to any additional injury or illness.
- Table 4-1 provides a brief comparison of acute and chronic pain.

> **THINK ABOUT   4-5**
>
> Compare the characteristics of acute and chronic pain.

Headache

Headache is a very common type of pain. There are many categories of headache associated with different causes, and some have specific locations and characteristics.

1. Headaches associated with congested sinuses, nasal congestion, and eyestrain are located in the eye and forehead areas. Sinus headaches can be quite severe. These headaches are usually steady and relieved when the cause is removed.
2. Headaches associated with muscle spasm and tension result from emotional stress and cause the neck muscles to contract to a greater degree, pulling on the scalp. Sometimes when people work for long periods of time in one position, contraction and spasm of the

TABLE 4-1 General Comparison of Acute and Chronic Pain

Acute Pain	Chronic Pain
Type	
A warning: fast, localized	Slow, diffuse, prolonged
Stimuli	
Injury: mechanical, thermal	Existing, chemical
Pathway	
Fast A-delta myelinated fibers	Slow unmyelinated C fibers
Neospinothalamic tract	Paleospinothalamic tract
Response	
Sudden, short-term	Long-term, disabling
Stress response; increased pulse and blood pressure: cool, moist skin; nausea/vomiting	Fatigue, depression, irritability
Emotion	
Anxiety	Loss of hope, depression, anger
Treatment	
If cause is identified, treatment is effective	Difficult to treat effectively

neck muscles also result, causing a dull, constant ache usually in the occipital area. Tension headaches tend to persist for days or weeks.

3. Headache in the temporal area is often associated with temporomandibular joint (TMJ) syndrome, in which the underlying cause is a malocclusion involving the jaw or inflammation of the joint due to arthritis or poor body alignment which causes muscle tension in the neck that is transferred to the jaw.

4. *Migraine* headaches are related to abnormal changes in blood flow and metabolism in the brain, but the exact mechanism is not yet fully understood. Research has suggested that migraines may be caused by the following reactions:

   a. Increased neural activity spreads over areas of the brain initiating pain stimuli in the trigeminal system, which are then conducted to the thalamus and pain centers in the sensory cortex.

   b. An accompanying reduction in serotonin is observed during migraine headaches and may cause the release of *neuropeptides*, which travel to the meninges covering the brain.

   c. These neuropeptides act on the smooth muscle of the blood vessels in the meninges, causing stretching and inflammation. The result is severe vascular pain.

   There are many precipitating factors, including atmospheric changes, stress, menstruation, dietary choices, and hunger.

The pain associated with a migraine is usually throbbing and severe and is often incapacitating. Characteristically, migraine headaches begin unilaterally in the temple area but often spread to involve the entire head. The pain is often accompanied or preceded by visual disturbances and dizziness, nausea and abdominal discomfort, and fatigue. These headaches may last up to 24 hours, and there is often a prolonged recovery period. Mild migraine may be treated with nonsteroidal anti-inflammatory drugs (NSAIDs) such as ibuprofen (Advil, Motrin, and others) and acetaminophen (Tylenol and others). Moderate migraine pain often responds to a combination of acetaminophen, codeine, and caffeine, or acetaminophen, aspirin, and caffeine (Excedrin migraine).

Treatment of severe migraine pain is difficult, although ergotamine can be effective if it is administered *immediately* after the onset of the headache. Newer forms of ergotamine are available in a soluble tablet to be placed under the tongue, thus providing a more readily available and rapid-acting form of the drug and a combination of ergotamine and caffeine can also be used. The drugs of choice for severe migraine are the triptans that act on some 5-HT (5-hydroxytryptamine) receptors to block the vasodilation and release of vasoactive peptides in the brain. These drugs relieve the nausea and light sensitivity as well as pain and nausea. Commercial examples of this family of drugs are almotriptan (Axert), rizatriptan (Maxalt), sumatriptan (Imitrex), naratriptan (Amerge), zolmitriptan (Zomig), frovatriptan (Frova), and eletriptan (Relpax). In severe cases, opiates such as codeine may be used but due to the habit-forming nature of these narcotics, they are considered a last resort measure.

Preventive medication may be used by some patients on a daily basis or just before a known migraine trigger. These drugs include several cardiovascular drug groups usually used for hypertension, the beta-blockers and calcium channel blockers (see Chapter 12). The older tricyclic antidepressants such as amitriptyline (Elavil) may be helpful because they raise serotonin and norepinephrine levels. Migraine clinics are researching the hereditary factors as well as individual exacerbating factors.

5. *Intracranial* headaches result from increased pressure inside the skull. Any space-occupying mass stretches the cerebral vascular walls or the meninges covering the brain. Causes of increased pressure include trauma with edema or hemorrhage, tumors, infections such as meningitis, or inflammation resulting from toxins such as alcohol. Headaches may be occipital or frontal in location depending on the site of the problem. Usually other indicators of increased intracranial pressure accompany the headache (see Chapter 14).

THINK ABOUT 4-6

Compare the signs of a migraine headache with those of a tension headache.

Central Pain

Central pain is pain that is caused by dysfunction or damage to the brain or spinal cord. A lesion such as abscess, infarction, hemorrhage, tumor, or damage resulting from direct injury may cause central pain. This type of pain can be very localized or can involve a large area of the body. It is persistent, irritating, and can cause considerable suffered over an extended period of time.

Neuropathic Pain

Neuropathic pain is caused by trauma or disease involving the peripheral nerves. This type of pain can vary from a tingling to a burning or severe shooting pain. Movement can stimulate this pain as well as injured nerves that can become hyperexcitable and some neurons with low thresholds for thermal, mechanical or chemical stimuli may spontaneously fire. Neuralgias are examples of extremely painful conditions that are a result of damage to peripheral nerves caused by infection or disease. Causalgia is a type of neuralgia that involves severe burning pain that can be triggered by normally "nontraumatic" stimuli such as a light touch, sound or cold.

Ischemic Pain

Ischemic pain results from a profound, sudden loss of blood flow to an organ or tissues in a specific area of the body. The decreased blood supply results in hypoxia, which leads to tissue damage and the release of inflammatory and pain-producing substances. The description of the pain may vary from aching, burning, or prickling to a strong shooting pain (particularly in an extremity). The exact symptoms depend on the location of the hypoxic tissue and can be characterized as either acute or chronic pain. Atherosclerotic disorders that cause blocking of arterial flow can cause ischemic pain, particularly in the lower extremities. Improving blood flow and preventing/reducing tissue hypoxia can do much to manage ischemic pain.

Cancer-Related Pain

Cancer is very often associated with pain, usually chronic pain. This pain has been broken down into several categories: pain caused by the advance of the disease and resultant damage to the body, pain associated with the treatment of the disease, and pain that is the result of a coexisting disease unrelated to the cancer.

The most common category encountered in cancer-related pain is that which is caused by the advance of the disease. As the tumors grow, they can cause infections and inflammation, which in turn cause increased pressure on nerve endings, stretching of tissues, or obstruction of vessels, ducts, or the intestines. This type of pain may be characterized as acute with sudden onset, intermittent, or chronic persisting over a long period of time.

Aspirin - blood thinner & ↓ inflammation

Pain Control

Methods of Managing Pain

Pain can be managed in a number of ways in addition to removing the cause as soon as possible. The most common method is the use of analgesic medications to relieve pain. These drugs may be administered in a variety of ways, including orally or parenterally (by injection) or transdermal patch. New drugs are constantly being developed to improve the efficacy of treatment and reduce side effects. Analgesics are frequently classified by their ability to relieve mild, moderate, or severe pain (Table 4-2).

Mild pain is usually managed with acetaminophen (Tylenol) or acetylsalicylic acid (ASA, aspirin), which act primarily at the peripheral site. The latter is particularly useful when inflammation is present, whereas the former is popular because it has fewer side effects. Acetylsalicylic acid also acts as a platelet inhibitor, reducing blood clotting. NSAIDs, such as naproxen and ibuprofen, are widely used to treat both acute and chronic pain, particularly when inflammation is present (see Chapter 5 for more information on inflammation and drugs). In addition, these drugs possess antipyretic action, lowering body temperature in case of fever. Even in high doses, this group of drugs is not effective for severe pain.

For *moderate* pain, codeine is commonly used, either alone, or more frequently, in combination with acetaminophen or aspirin. Codeine is a narcotic, a morphine derivative, acting at the opiate receptors in the central nervous system. Codeine exhibits some adverse effects, causing nausea, constipation, and in high doses, respiratory depression. Taking the drug with food or milk reduces gastric irritation. Another choice is oxycodone, a synthetic narcotic combined with acetaminophen or aspirin (Percocet or Percodan). This drug affects the perception of pain and emotional response, promoting relaxation and a sense of well-being, predisposing to dependency. Oxycodone abuse has become a significant problem (see Chapter 27).

For *severe* pain, morphine, hydromorphone, or other narcotics are favored. These drugs block the pain pathways in the spinal cord and brain and also alter the perception of pain in a positive manner. In long-term use, tolerance often develops, requiring a higher dose to

TABLE 4-2	Analgesic Drugs		
Use	Name	Action	Adverse Effects
For Mild Pain			
	ASA* Acetaminophen NSAIDs*	Decreases pain at peripheral site All are antipyretic ASA and NSAIDs are anti-inflammatory	ASA and NSAIDs have many adverse effects (nausea, gastric ulcers, bleeding, allergies)
For Moderate Pain			
	Codeine Oxycodone Percocet Vicodin	Acts on central nervous system and affects perception	Narcotic (opium)—often combined with ASA/acetaminophen High dose may depress respiration
For Severe Pain			
	Morphine Demerol Methadone Meperidine Oxycodone	Acts on central nervous system; euphoria and sedation	Narcotic—Tolerance and addiction High dose depresses respiration; nausea, constipation common.

*ASA, acetylsalicylic acid (aspirin); NSAIDs, nonsteroidal anti-inflammatory drugs.

be effective or an alternative drug. Narcotics have a number of adverse effects, and concern is often expressed about addiction with long-term use. However, addiction does not always develop, and in most cases it is more important to ensure that pain is managed effectively. Meperidine is helpful for short-term pain, but its brief duration of action as well as continuous usage, which results in a buildup of a toxic metabolite, prevents its use for severe chronic pain.

Sedatives and antianxiety drugs (minor tranquilizers such as lorazepam) are popular adjuncts to analgesic therapy because they promote rest and relaxation and reduce the dosage requirement for the analgesic. The muscle relaxation that is a side effect of the medication is also helpful in relieving or preventing muscle spasm associated with pain.

In patients with chronic and increasing pain, such as occurs in some cases of cancer, pain management requires a judicious choice of drugs used in a stepwise fashion to maximize the reduction of pain. Usually tolerance to narcotic drugs develops in time, requiring an increase in dosage to be effective. Eventually a new drug may be required.

Many patients with severe pain administer their own medications as needed, using *patient-controlled analgesia (PCA)*. Small pumps are attached to vascular access sites, and the patient either receives a dose of analgesic such as morphine when needed or maintains a continuous infusion. This has been a highly successful approach and has been found to lessen the overall consumption of narcotics.

Other pain control methods may accompany the use of medications. Pain management clinics offer a variety of therapeutic modalities for the individual. Such measures include stress reduction and relaxation therapy, distraction, applications of heat and cold, massage,

Intractable = No Meds

physiotherapy modalities, exercise, therapeutic touch, hypnosis imaging, and acupuncture (see Chapter 3). These measures may act in the spinal cord at the "gate" or may modify pain perception and response in the brain. Many of these strategies are believed to increase the levels of circulating endorphins that elevate the pain tolerance. Also, maintenance of basic nutrition and activity levels as well as adequate rest assist people in coping with pain. Specialized clinics deal with certain types of pain such as chronic back pain or temporal mandibular joint pain.

For intractable pain that cannot be controlled with medications, surgical intervention is a choice. Procedures such as rhizotomy or cordotomy to sever the sensory nerve pathway in the spinal nerve or cord may be done. Injections can be given with similar effects. These procedures carry a risk of interference with other nerve fibers and functions, particularly when the spinal cord is involved.

Anesthesia

Local anesthesia may be injected or applied topically to the skin or mucous membranes (Table 4-3). Local anesthetics may be used to block transmission of pain stimuli from a specific small area. For example, an injection of lidocaine may be given before performing a tooth extraction, removal of a skin lesion, or a diagnostic procedure that is likely to be painful. A long-acting, localized block may be used to reduce pain after some surgeries.

Spinal or *regional anesthesia* may be administered to block pain impulses from the legs or abdomen. Spinal anesthesia involves administering a local anesthetic into the epidural space or the cerebrospinal fluid in the subarachnoid space at an appropriate level, blocking all nerve conduction at and below that level.

TABLE 4-3	Anesthetics		
Type	Example	Effects	Purpose
1. Local anesthetic	Lidocaine; injected or topical; may add epinephrine	Blocks nerve conduction (sensory) in a peripheral nerve	Removal of a skin lesion; tooth extraction
2. General anesthetic	Intravenous—thiopental sodium Inhalation (gas)—nitrous oxide	Affects brain—partial or total loss of consciousness	General surgery, no pain/awareness when combined with analgesic
Relative or neurolept-anesthesia	Diazepam or droperidol	Can respond	
3. Spinal anesthesia	Local anesthetic injected into subarachnoid or epidural space around lower spinal cord	Blocks nerve conduction (sensation) at and below level of injection	Surgery on lower part of body: labor and delivery

General anesthesia involves administering a gas to be inhaled such as nitrous oxide or injecting a barbiturate such as sodium pentothal intravenously. Loss of consciousness accompanies general anesthesia. Analgesics are required with these drugs. *Neuroleptanesthesia* is a type of general anesthesia in which the patient can respond to commands but is relatively unaware of the procedure or of any discomfort. For example, diazepam can be administered intravenously in combination with a narcotic analgesic such as meperidine or morphine. Droperidol (a neuroleptic) and fentanyl (a narcotic analgesic) are a popular combination (e.g., Innovar) that is administered by intravenous or intramuscular injection.

CASE STUDY A

Acute Pain

L.Y. is a healthy 13-year-old who had all her wisdom teeth removed 6 hours ago and is experiencing significant pain. She has been prescribed acetaminophen and codeine for pain relief and is at home recovering. Her mother wants her to rest and stop text messaging her friends about her dental surgery.

1. How do acetaminophen and codeine act to reduce pain? What is a side effect of high levels of each drug? Why has the dentist prescribed only a limited supply of the medication?
2. How does L.Y.'s text messaging behavior affect her perception of pain?
3. Does L.Y. need to rest in bed quietly to reduce pain?
4. L.Y. becomes increasingly irritated with her mother and tells her to "get off my case." How does L.Y.'s stress affect pain perception?

CASE STUDY B

Chronic Pain

Ms. J. is a 30-year-old healthy single mother with two children. She has worked as a paramedic in her community for 6 years. She and her partner responded to a call involving a man who had been drinking heavily at a family party and who was partially conscious. When she and her partner attempted to transfer the 100-kg man to a stretcher, the man grabbed her neck, causing her severe pain. Ms. J.'s doctor diagnosed a spinal injury and completed papers for Ms. J. to be absent from work. He recommended rest and application of heat and cold to the neck. One week later, Ms. J. saw him again, reporting continuing pain. She was referred to a specialist who told her she had a herniated disk in the cervical area of her neck and would require ongoing care and rehabilitation. Ms. J. has been on disability leave for 6 months, during which she has continued to have severe neck, jaw, and back pain. She takes acetaminophen with codeine as required, and sees a physiotherapist and a registered massage therapist routinely in an attempt to control chronic pain. She is worried that her disability benefits will cease before she can return to work and has incurred debts during her leave. She also finds it difficult to care for her two children and keep the house clean.

1. What factors are significant in Ms. J.'s perception of pain? How might each be reduced?
2. Why has Ms. J.'s doctor not prescribed stronger narcotic medication?
3. Why does Ms. J. experience pain in her jaw and lower back when the injury was to her neck?
4. Where in the pain pathway do massage therapy and physiotherapy act to alleviate pain?
5. Ms. J. is concerned about maintaining her physical fitness and decides to attend exercise classes in her community pool. She finds this gives her more energy and reduces her pain. How does appropriate exercise affect pain perception? What precautions does Ms. J. need to observe when exercising?
6. Ms. J. hears about acupuncture as a help for back pain and does some research on the Internet before making an appointment for treatment. How could acupuncture act to block impulses for pain?
7. After 8 months, Ms. J. is cleared to return to work on a part-time basis, which she manages well. Why does she not return to full-time work immediately?
8. What can Ms. J. expect in the future as a result of this injury?

CHAPTER SUMMARY

Pain serves as one of the body's defense mechanisms, resulting from stimulation of nociceptors by ischemia, chemical mediators, or distention of tissue.

- The pain pathway may be interrupted at many points, including the receptor site, a peripheral nerve, the spinal cord, or the brain.
- The gate control theory recognizes the role of synapses serving as open or closed gates at points in the pain pathway in the central nervous system. These gates may close under the influence of natural endorphins or other stimuli, thus inhibiting the passage of pain impulses to the brain.
- Descriptions of pain are subjective evaluations by an individual.

- Referred pain occurs when an individual locates the pain at a site other than the actual origin.
- An individual's perception of and response to pain depend on prior conditioning and experiences.
- Acute pain is usually sudden and severe but short term. Chronic pain is milder but long lasting. The person with chronic pain is often fatigued and depressed.
- There are many types of headaches, among them tension, sinus, and migraine, each with different characteristics.
- Analgesics are rated for the severity of pain controlled by the drug; for example, aspirin for mild pain and morphine for severe pain.
- Anesthesia may be classified as local, spinal or regional, or general.

STUDY QUESTIONS

1. Describe the characteristics and role of each of the following in the pain pathway:
   a. nociceptor
   b. C fibers
   c. spinothalamic tract
   d. parietal lobe
   e. reticular formation
   f. endorphins and enkephalins

2. Define and give an example of referred pain.
3. Differentiate the characteristics of acute and intractable pain.
4. List several factors that can alter the perception of pain and the response to pain.
5. Briefly describe six possible methods of pain control.

ADDITIONAL RESOURCES

Mosby's Drug Consult 2006, St. Louis, 2006, Mosby.

Web Sites

http://www.ampainsoc.org *American Pain Society*
http://www.mayoclinic.com *Mayo Clinic*

http://www.webmd.com/pain-management/default.htm
http://www.webmd.com/pain-management/
    guide/11-tips-for-living-with-chronic-pain
http://www.cancer.org/ssLINK/pain-control-toc

CHAPTER 5

Inflammation and Healing

CHAPTER OUTLINE

LEARNING OBJECTIVES

After studying this chapter, the student is expected to:

1. Explain the role of normal defenses in preventing disease.
2. Describe how changes in capillary exchange affect the tissues and the blood components.
3. Compare normal capillary exchange with exchange during the inflammatory response.
4. Describe the local and systemic effects of inflammation.
5. Explain the effects of chronic inflammation.
6. Discuss the modes of treatment of inflammation.
7. Describe the types of healing and the disadvantages of each.
8. List the factors, including a specific example for each, that hasten healing.
9. Identify the classifications of burns and describe the effects of burns.
10. Describe the possible complications occurring in the first few days after a burn.
11. Explain three reasons why the healing of a burn may be difficult.

KEY TERMS

abscess	fibrinogen	isoenzymes	pyrogens
adhesions	fibrinous	leukocyte	regeneration
angiogenesis	fibroblast	leukocytosis	replacement
anorexia	glucocorticoids	macrophage	resolution
chemical mediators	granulation tissue	malaise	scar
chemotaxis	granuloma	neutrophil	serous
collagen	hematocrit	osmotic pressure	stenosis
contracture	hematopoiesis	perforation	ulcer
diapedesis	hydrostatic pressure	permeability	vasodilation
erythrocyte sedimentation	hyperemia	phagocytosis	
rate (ESR)	interferons	purulent	
exudate	intra-articular	pyrexia	

Review of Body Defenses

Mechanical Barriers

Defense mechanisms used by the body to protect itself from any injurious agent may be specific or nonspecific. One nonspecific or general defense mechanism is the mechanical barrier such as skin or mucous membrane (often called the first line of defense) that blocks entry of bacteria or harmful substances into the tissues (Fig. 5-1). Associated with these mechanical barriers are body secretions such as saliva or tears that contain enzymes or chemicals that inactivate or destroy potentially damaging material.

Nonspecific Mechanisms

The second line of defense includes the nonspecific processes of phagocytosis and inflammation. Phagocytosis is the process by which neutrophils (a leukocyte) and macrophages," randomly engulf and destroy bacteria, cell debris, or foreign matter (see Fig. 5-2). Inflammation involves a sequence of events intended to limit the effects of injury or a dangerous agent in the body. Interferons are nonspecific agents that protect uninfected cells against viruses (see Chapter 6).

Specific Mechanisms

The third line of defense is the *specific* defense mechanism in the body (see Chapter 7). It provides protection by stimulating the production of unique antibodies or sensitized lymphocytes following exposure to specific substances. In recent years much effort has been expended on research on the immune system in an effort to increase understanding of the process of the immune response and to create ways to strengthen this defense mechanism.

> **APPLY YOUR KNOWLEDGE   5-1**
>
> Predict three ways that the normal defense systems in the body can fail.

> **APPLY YOUR KNOWLEDGE   5-2**
>
> Predict three factors that can change and interfere with normal capillary exchange.

Review of Normal Capillary Exchange

Usually all capillaries are not open in a particular capillary bed unless the cells' metabolic needs are not being met by the blood supply to the area, or an accumulation of wastes (byproduct of metabolism) occurs. Precapillary sphincters composed of smooth muscle restrict blood flow through some channels. Movement of fluid, electrolytes, oxygen, and nutrients out of the capillary at the arteriolar end is based on the *net* hydrostatic pressure. See Chapter 2 and Figure 2-1 for a detailed explanation of fluid shifts between body compartments. The net hydrostatic pressure is based on the difference between the hydrostatic pressure within the capillary (essentially arterial pressure) as compared with the hydrostatic pressure of the interstitial fluid in the tissues as well as the relative osmotic pressures in the blood and interstitial fluid (Fig. 5-2). Differences in concentrations of dissolved substances in the blood and interstitial fluid promote diffusion of electrolytes, glucose, oxygen, and other nutrients across the capillary membrane. Blood cells and plasma proteins (albumin, globulin, and fibrinogen) normally remain inside the capillary.

At the venous end of the capillary hydrostatic pressure is decreased due to the previous movement of fluid into the interstitial fluid space, and osmotic pressure in the vessels is relatively high because plasma proteins remain within the capillaries. This arrangement facilitates the movement of fluid, carbon dioxide, and other wastes into the blood. Excess fluid and any proteins are recovered from the interstitial area by way of the lymphatic system and eventually returned to the general circulation.

Physiology of Inflammation

The inflammatory response is a protective mechanism and an important basic concept in pathophysiology.

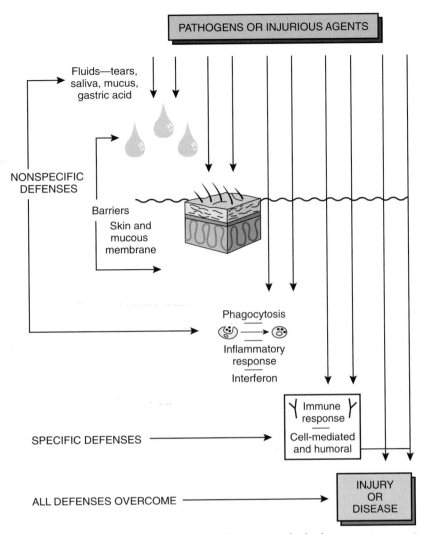

FIGURE 5-1 Defense mechanisms in the body.

Inflammation is a normal defense mechanism in the body and is intended to localize and remove an injurious agent, whatever it may be. You have probably observed the inflammatory process resulting from a cut, an allergic reaction, an insect bite, an infection, or a small burn on your body. The general signs and symptoms of inflammation serve as a *warning* of a problem, which may be hidden within the body.

Inflammation is not the same as infection, although infection is one cause of inflammation. With infection, microorganisms such as a bacteria, viruses, or fungi are always present at the site, causing the inflammation. This microbe can be identified and appropriate treatment instituted to reduce the infection, and the inflammation will subside. When inflammation is caused by an allergy or a burn, no microbes are present.

Definition

Inflammation is the body's nonspecific response to tissue injury, resulting in redness, swelling, warmth,

and pain, and perhaps loss of function. Disorders are named using the ending *-itis* for inflammation. The root word is usually a body part or tissue; for example, pancreatitis, appendicitis, laryngitis, or ileitis.

THINK ABOUT   5-1

a. What term would indicate inflammation of the stomach? the liver? the large intestine? a tendon? the heart muscle?

b. Explain the relationship between inflammation and infection.

Causes

Inflammation is associated with many different types of tissue injury. Causes include direct physical damage such as cuts or sprains, caustic chemicals such as acids or drain cleaners, ischemia or infarction, allergic reactions, extremes of heat or cold, foreign bodies such as splinters or glass, and infection.

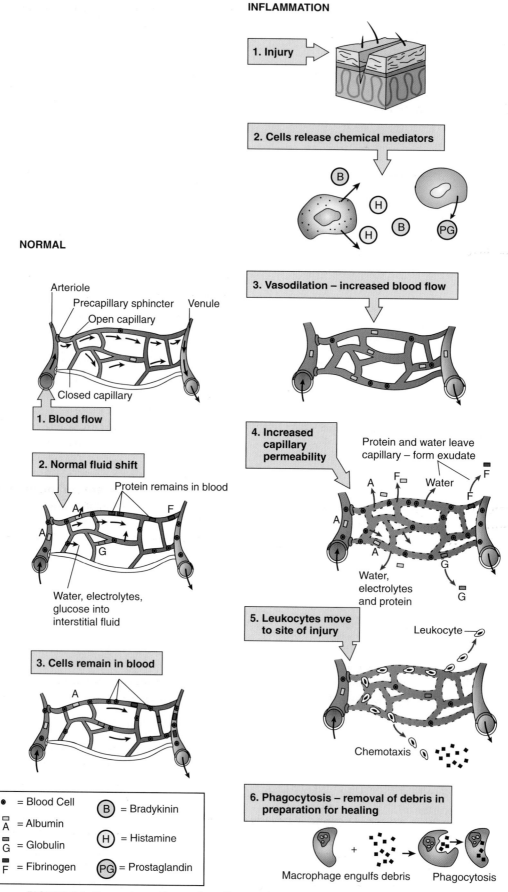

INFLAMMATION

1. Injury

2. Cells release chemical mediators

NORMAL

Arteriole
Precapillary sphincter   Venule
Open capillary
Closed capillary

1. Blood flow

3. Vasodilation – increased blood flow

2. Normal fluid shift

Protein remains in blood

Water, electrolytes, glucose into interstitial fluid

4. Increased capillary permeability

Protein and water leave capillary – form exudate

Water

Water, electrolytes and protein

3. Cells remain in blood

5. Leukocytes move to site of injury

Leukocyte

Chemotaxis

6. Phagocytosis – removal of debris in preparation for healing

Macrophage engulfs debris   Phagocytosis

● = Blood Cell   Ⓑ = Bradykinin
A = Albumin
G = Globulin   Ⓗ = Histamine
F = Fibrinogen   ⒫ = Prostaglandin

FIGURE 5-2 Comparison of normal capillary exchange and the inflammatory response.

Steps of Inflammation

An injury to capillaries and tissue cells will result in the following reactions:

- Bradykinin is released from the insured cells.
- Bradykinin activates pain receptors.
- Sensation of pain stimulates mast cells and basophils to release histamine.
- Bradykinin and histamine cause capillary dilation.
  - This results in an increase of blood flow and increased capillary permeability.
- Break in skin allows bacteria to enter the tissue.
  - This results in the migration of neutrophils and monocytes to the site of injury.
- Neutrophils phagocytize bacteria.
- Macrophages leave the bloodstream and phagocytose microbes.

Acute Inflammation

Pathophysiology and General Characteristics

The inflammatory process is basically the same regardless of the cause. The timing varies with the specific cause. Inflammation may develop immediately and last only a short time; it may have a delayed onset (e.g., a sunburn), or it may be more severe and prolonged. The severity of the inflammation varies with the specific cause and duration of exposure.

When tissue injury occurs, the damaged mast cells and platelets release chemical mediators including histamine, serotonin, prostaglandins, and leukotrienes into the interstitial fluid and blood (Table 5-1). These chemicals affect blood vessels and nerves in the damaged area. Cytokines serve as communicators in the tissue fluids, sending messages to lymphocytes and macrophages, the immune system, or the hypothalamus to induce fever.

Chemical mediators such as histamine are released immediately from granules in mast cells and exert their effects at once. Other chemical mediators such as leukotrienes and prostaglandins must be synthesized from arachidonic acid in mast cells before release and, therefore, are responsible for the later effects, prolonging the inflammation. Many of these chemicals also intensify the effects of other chemicals in the response. Note that many anti-inflammatory drugs and antihistamines reduce the effects of some of these chemical mediators.

Although nerve reflexes at the site of injury cause immediate transient vasoconstriction, the rapid release of chemical mediators results in local vasodilation (relaxation of smooth muscle causing an increase in the diameter of arterioles), which causes hyperemia, increased blood flow in the area. Capillary membrane permeability also increases, allowing plasma proteins to move into the interstitial space along with more fluid (see Fig. 5-2). The increased fluid dilutes any toxic material at the site, while the globulins serve as antibodies, and fibrinogen forms a fibrin mesh around the area in an attempt to localize the injurious agent. Any blood clotting will also provide a fibrin mesh to wall off the area. Vasodilation and increased capillary permeability make up the vascular response to injury.

During the cellular response, leukocytes are attracted by chemotaxis to the area of inflammation as damaged cells release their contents. Several chemical mediators at the site of injury act as potent stimuli to attract leukocytes. Leukocytes and their functions are summarized in Table 5-2. First neutrophils (polymorphonuclear

TABLE 5-1   Chemical Mediators in the Inflammatory Response

Chemical	Source	Major Action
Histamine	Mast cell granules	Immediate vasodilation and increased capillary permeability to form exudate
Chemotactic factors	Mast cell granules	For example, attract neutrophils to site
Platelet-activating factor (PAF)	Cell membranes of platelets	Activate neutrophils Platelet aggregation
Cytokines (interleukins, lymphokines)	T lymphocytes, Macrophages	Increase plasma proteins, ESR Induce fever, chemotaxis, leukocytosis
Leukotrienes	Synthesis from arachidonic acid in mast cells	Later response: vasodilation and increased capillary permeability, chemotaxis
Prostaglandins (PGs)	Synthesis from arachidonic acid in mast cells	Vasodilation, increased capillary permeability, pain, fever, potentiate histamine effect
Kinins (e.g., bradykinin)	Activation of plasma protein (kinogen)	Vasodilation and increased capillary permeability, pain, chemotaxis
Complement system	Activation of plasma protein cascade	Vasodilation and increased capillary permeability, chemotaxis, increased histamine release

TABLE 5-2	Function of Cellular Elements in the Inflammatory Response	
Leukocytes	**Activity**	
Neutrophils	Phagocytosis of microorganisms	
Basophils	Release of histamine leading to inflammation	
Eosinophils	Numbers are increased in allergic responses	
Lymphocytes	**Activity**	
T lymphocytes	Active in cell-mediated immune response	
B lymphocytes	Produce antibodies	
Monocytes	Phagocytosis	
Macrophages	Active in phagocytosis. These are mature monocytes that have migrated into tissues from the blood.	

leukocytes [PMNs]) and later monocytes and macrophages collect along the capillary wall and then migrate out through wider separations in the wall into the interstitial area. This movement of cells is termed *diapedesis*. There the cells destroy and remove foreign material, microorganisms, and cell debris by phagocytosis, thus preparing the site for healing. When phagocytic cells die at the site, lysosomal enzymes are released and damage the nearby cells prolonging inflammation. If an immune response (see Chapter 7) or blood clotting occurs, these processes also enhance the inflammatory response.

As excessive fluid and protein collects in the interstitial compartment, blood flow in the area decreases as swelling leads to increased pressure on the capillary bed, and fluid shifts out of the capillary are reduced. Severely reduced blood flow can decrease the nutrients available to the undamaged cells in the area and prevent the removal of wastes. This may cause additional damage to the tissue.

There are naturally occurring defense or control mechanisms in the form of enzymes that inactivate chemical mediators and prevent the unnecessary spread or prolongation of inflammation.

THINK ABOUT 5-2

a. List the local signs and symptoms of inflammation.
b. Consider the last time you experienced tissue injury. Describe the cause of the injury and how inflammation developed.

Local Effects

The *cardinal* signs of inflammation are redness (rubor or erythema), heat, swelling, and pain:

• Redness and warmth are caused by increased blood flow into the damaged area (Fig. 5-3).

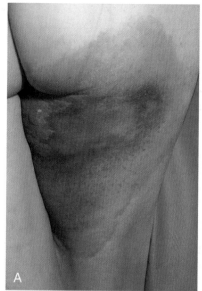
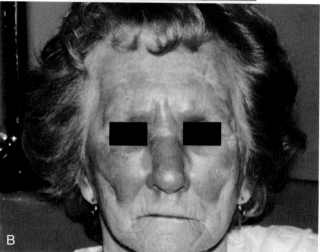

FIGURE 5-3 **A,** Erysipelas (cellulitis). *(From Lookingbill D, Marks J: Principles of Dermatology, ed 3, Philadelphia, 2000, WB Saunders.)* **B,** Erysipelas of the face caused by group A Streptococcus. *(From Mahon CR, Lehman DC, Manuselis G: Textbook of diagnostic microbiology, ed 3, St. Louis, 2007, Saunders.)*

• Swelling or edema is caused by the shift of protein and fluid into the interstitial space.
• Pain results from the increased pressure of fluid on the nerves, especially in enclosed areas, and by the local irritation of nerves by chemical mediators such as bradykinins.
• Loss of function may develop if the cells lack nutrients or swelling interferes mechanically with function, as happens in restricted joint movement.

Exudate refers to a collection of interstitial fluid formed in the inflamed area. The characteristics of the exudate vary with the cause of the trauma:

• *Serous* or watery exudates consist primarily of fluid with small amounts of protein and white blood cells. Common examples of serous exudates occur with allergic reactions or burns.

- **Fibrinous** exudates are thick and sticky and have a high cell and fibrin content. This type of exudate increases the risk of scar tissue in the area.
- **Purulent** exudates are thick, yellow-green in color, and contain more leukocytes and cell debris as well as microorganisms. Typically, this type of exudate indicates bacterial infection, and the exudate is often referred to as "pus."
- An **abscess** is a localized pocket of purulent exudate or pus in a solid tissue (e.g., around a tooth or in the brain).
- A hemorrhagic exudate may be present if blood vessels have been damaged.

Systemic Effects

Other general manifestations of inflammation include mild fever, malaise (feeling unwell), fatigue, headache, and anorexia (loss of appetite).

Fever or pyrexia (low grade or mild) is common if inflammation is extensive. If infection has caused the inflammation, fever can be severe, depending on the particular microorganism. However, high fever can be beneficial if it impairs the growth and reproduction of a pathogenic organism. Fever results from the release of pyrogens, or fever-producing substances (e.g., interleukin-1), from white blood cells (WBCs) or macrophages (Fig. 5-4). Pyrogens circulate in the blood and cause the body temperature control system (the thermostat) in the hypothalamus to be reset at a higher level. Heat production mechanisms such as shivering are activated to increase cell metabolism. Involuntary cutaneous vasoconstriction characterized by pallor and cool skin reduces heat loss from the body. Voluntary actions such as curling up or covering the body conserve heat. These mechanisms continue until the body temperature reaches the new, higher setting. Following removal of the cause, body temperature returns to normal by reversing the mechanisms.

> **THINK ABOUT 5-3**
>
> a. What are the physiologic changes that occur when the cause of a fever is removed?
> b. Explain the differences among serous, fibrinous, and purulent exudates.

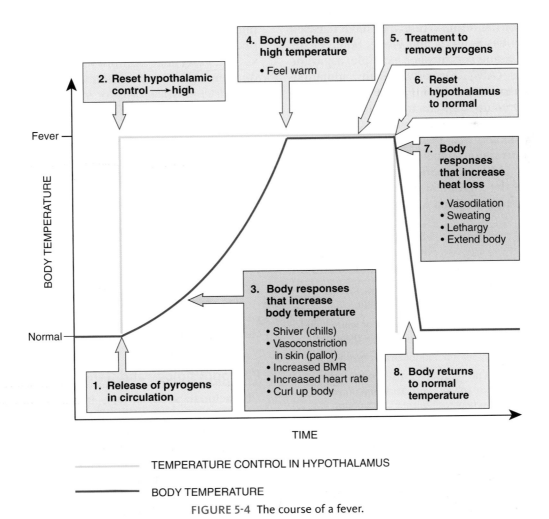

FIGURE 5-4 The course of a fever.

Diagnostic Tests

Refer to the *normal values* shown on the inside front cover of this book.

Leukocytosis (increased white blood cells in the blood), elevated serum C-reactive protein (CRP), an elevated erythrocyte sedimentation rate or ESR, and increased plasma proteins and cell enzymes in the serum are nonspecific changes (Table 5-3); they do not indicate the particular cause or site of inflammation. They provide helpful screening and monitoring information when a problem is suspected or during treatment. In patients with leukocytosis, there is often an increase in *immature* neutrophils, commonly referred to as "a shift to the left." A *differential* count (the proportion of each type of WBC) may be helpful in distinguishing viral from bacterial infection. Allergic reactions commonly produce eosinophilia. Examination of a peripheral blood smear may disclose significant numbers of abnormal cells, another clue as to the cause of a problem. Increased circulating plasma proteins (fibrinogen, prothrombin, and alpha-antitrypsin) result from an increase in protein synthesis by hepatocytes.

Cell enzymes and more specific isoenzymes may be elevated in the blood in the presence of severe inflammation and necrosis. These may be helpful in locating the site of the necrotic cells that have released the enzymes into tissue fluids and blood. Some of the enzymes are not tissue specific. For example, aspartate aminotransferase (AST, formerly serum glutamic-oxaloacetic transaminase [SGOT]) is elevated in liver disease and in the acute stage of a myocardial infarction (heart attack). However, the isoenzyme CK-MB (isoenzyme of creatine kinase with myocardial component) is specific for myocardial infarction. The enzyme alanine aminotransferase (ALT) is specific for the liver.

If the cause of the inflammatory response is a brief exposure to a damaging agent, for instance, touching a hot object, the response often subsides in approximately 48 hours. Vascular integrity is regained, and excess fluid and protein are recovered by the lymphatic capillaries and returned to the general circulation. The manifestations of inflammation gradually decrease. Otherwise inflammation persists until the causative agent is removed (Fig. 5-5).

The amount of necrosis that occurs depends on the specific cause of the trauma and the factors contributing to the inflammatory response. Extensive necrosis may lead to ulcers or erosion of tissue. For example, gingivitis or stomatitis in the oral cavity often leads to painful ulcerations in the mouth, and inflammation in the stomach may result in peptic ulcers.

Potential Complications

Local complications depend on the site of inflammation. For example, inflammation in the lungs may impair the expansion of the lungs, decreasing the diffusion of oxygen. Inflammation of a joint may affect its range of movement.

Infection may develop in an inflamed tissue because microorganisms can more easily penetrate when the skin or mucosa is damaged and the blood supply is impaired (see Fig. 5-14). Foreign bodies often introduce microbes directly into the tissue. Some microbes resist phagocytosis, and the inflammatory exudate itself provides an excellent medium for microorganism to reproduce and colonize the inflamed area.

Skeletal muscle spasms or strong muscle contractions may be initiated by inflammation resulting from musculoskeletal injuries such as sprains, tendinitis, or fractures. A spasm is likely to force the bones of a joint out of normal alignment, thus causing additional pressure on the nerves and increasing the pain.

Chronic Inflammation

Chronic inflammation may develop following an *acute* episode of inflammation when the cause is not completely eradicated. Or inflammation may develop insidiously owing to *chronic* irritation such as smoking, certain bacteria, or long-term abnormal immune responses.

Pathophysiology and General Characteristics

Characteristics of chronic inflammation include less swelling and exudate but the presence of more lymphocytes, macrophages, and fibroblasts (connective tissue cells) than in acute inflammation. Frequently more tissue destruction occurs with chronic inflammation. More collagen is produced in the area, resulting in more fibrous scar tissue forming. A granuloma, a small mass of cells with a necrotic center and covered by connective

TABLE 5-3	Changes in the Blood with Inflammation
Leukocytosis	Increased numbers of white blood cells, especially neutrophils
Differential count	Proportion of each type of white blood cell altered, depending on the cause
Plasma proteins	Increased fibrinogen and prothrombin
C-reactive protein	A protein not normally in the blood, but appears with acute inflammation and necrosis within 24-48 hours
Increased ESR	Elevated plasma proteins increase the rate at which red blood cells settle in a sample
Cell enzymes	Released from necrotic cells and enter tissue fluids and blood: may indicate the site of inflammation

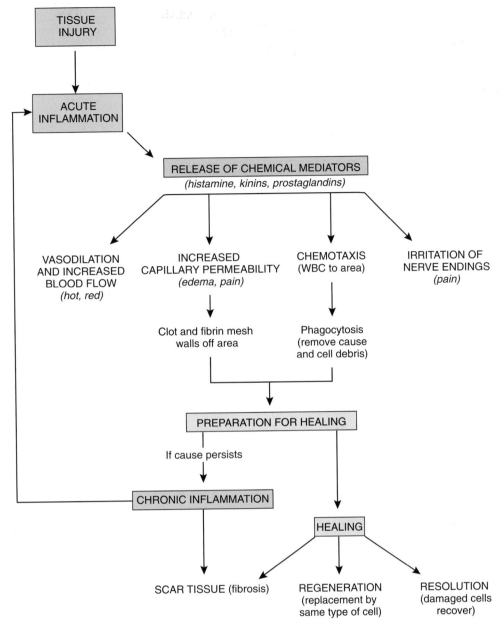

FIGURE 5-5 The course of inflammation and healing.

tissue, may develop around a foreign object such as a splinter, or as part of the immune response in some infections such as tuberculosis.

Potential Complications

Disorders such as rheumatoid arthritis are characterized by chronic inflammation with periodic exacerbations of acute inflammation. Deep *ulcers* may result from severe or prolonged inflammation because cell necrosis and lack of cell regeneration cause erosion of tissue. This in turn can lead to complications such as perforation (erosion through the wall) of viscera or development of extensive scar tissue.

THINK ABOUT 5-4

a. Describe three differences between acute and chronic inflammation.

b. Describe three changes in the blood with acute inflammation.

Treatment of Inflammation

Drugs

Acetylsalicylic acid (aspirin, ASA) has long been used as an anti-inflammatory agent, sometimes in very large doses (Table 5-4). This drug decreases prostaglandin

[handwritten annotations: "Blood thinner", "Tylenol", "Non inflammatory yes", "proven", "not inflammatory", "Aspirin", "fever"]

Actions	ASA	Acetaminophen	NSAID	Glucocorticoid	COX-2
Antiinflammatory	Yes	No	Yes	Yes	Yes
Analgesia	Yes	Yes	Yes	No	Yes
Antipyretic	Yes	Yes	Yes	No	No
Adverse Effects					
Allergy*	Yes	No	Yes	No	Yes
Delays blood clotting	Yes	No	Yes	No	No
Risk of infection	No	No	No	Yes	No
GI distress	Yes	No	Yes	Yes	May occur
Stomach ulceration	Yes	No	Yes	Yes	May occur
Edema or Increased BP	No	No	No	Yes	May occur
MI or CVA	No	No	No	No	May occur
Liver damage	No	No	No	No	May occur

TABLE 5-4   Comparison of Drugs Used to Treat Inflammation

*Note allergic reactions may occur with administration of any drug.

synthesis at the site of inflammation, reducing the inflammatory response. Acetylsalicylic acid reduces pain (analgesic effect) and fever (antipyretic effect), which are often helpful. However, ASA is never recommended for children with viral infections because the combination of ASA and a viral infection is believed to contribute to the development of Reye's syndrome, a serious complication involving the brain and liver, which may be fatal. Many individuals are allergic to ASA and similar anti-inflammatory drugs. For others, the drug may cause irritation and ulcers in the stomach. An enteric-coated tablet (the tablet coating does not dissolve until it reaches the small intestine) is available, as are drugs to reduce acid secretion in the stomach to reduce this risk. Anti-inflammatory drugs also interfere with blood clotting by reducing platelet adhesion, and therefore cannot be used in all conditions. Also it is usually necessary to discontinue taking ASA for 7 to 14 days before any surgical procedure to prevent excessive bleeding.

Acetaminophen (Tylenol or Paracetamol) decreases fever and pain, but does not diminish the inflammatory response.

THINK ABOUT 5-5

a. Based on your knowledge of the normal physiology of the stomach, explain why intake of food or milk with a drug reduces the risk of nausea and irritation of the stomach?

b. Why might an individual taking large quantities of ASA need to be monitored for the presence of blood in the feces?

Nonsteroidal anti-inflammatory drugs (NSAIDs) such as ibuprofen (Advil or Motrin), piroxicam (Feldene), or diclofenac sodium (Arthrotec) are now used extensively to treat many types of inflammatory conditions. These drugs have anti-inflammatory, analgesic, and antipyretic activities. They act by reducing production of prostaglandins. They are used to treat inflammation in the musculoskeletal system, both acute injuries and long-term problems, such as rheumatoid arthritis. Also, they have become the treatment of choice for many dental procedures when an analgesic and anti-inflammatory are required. Ibuprofen has been recommended for many disorders, including menstrual pain and headache. The side effects are similar to those of aspirin, but are less severe. These drugs are available as oral medications, and some, such as ibuprofen, are available in small doses without a prescription.

A newer type of NSAID is celecoxib (Celebrex), which appears to be effective without unwanted effects on the stomach. This group of drugs (COX-2 inhibitors) is currently under further investigation following the withdrawal from the market of one drug in this class (rofecoxib, Vioxx). This followed reports of serious side effects such as increased incidence of heart attacks. This is an example of the necessity for long-term data collection from a large population to determine all the facts about new drugs or medical procedures.

Corticosteroids or steroidal anti-inflammatory drugs, are synthetic chemicals that are related to the naturally occurring glucocorticoids (hydrocortisone), hormones produced by the adrenal cortex gland in the body (see Chapter 16). These drugs are extremely valuable in the short-term treatment of many disorders, but also have significant undesirable effects that may affect health care.

The beneficial anti-inflammatory effects of glucocorticoids include:

• Decreasing capillary permeability and enhancing the effectiveness of the hormones epinephrine and norepinephrine in the system; thus, the vascular system is stabilized

- Reducing the number of leukocytes and mast cells at the site, decreasing the release of histamine and prostaglandins
- Blocking the immune response, a common cause of inflammation

The chemical structure of the drug has been altered slightly to enhance its anti-inflammatory action and reduce the other, less desirable effects of the hormone. These drugs can be administered as oral tablets, creams and ointments for topical application, or injections, both local and systemic. Examples include prednisone (oral), triamcinolone (topical), methylprednisolone (intra-articular—into joint), dexamethasone (intramuscular [IM] or intravenous [IV] injections), and beclomethasone dipropionate (Beclovent [inhaler]).

However, with long-term use and high dosages of glucocorticoids, marked *side effects* occur, similar to Cushing's disease (see Chapter 16). These side effects (or adverse effects) should be considered when taking a medical history from a patient because they may complicate the care of the person.

The adverse effects of glucocorticoids include:

- Atrophy of lymphoid tissue and reduced numbers of WBCs, leading to an increased risk of infection and a decreased immune response
- Catabolic effects (increased tissue breakdown with decreased protein synthesis and tissue regeneration), including osteoporosis (bone demineralization), muscle wasting, and a tendency to thinning and breakdown of the skin and mucosa (e.g., peptic ulcer)
- Delayed healing
- Delayed growth in children
- Retention of sodium and water, often leading to high blood pressure and edema
  - Increases gluconeogenesis causing a rise is blood sugar

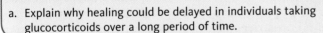

THINK ABOUT 5-6

a. Explain why healing could be delayed in individuals taking glucocorticoids over a long period of time.

One additional consideration with the long-term use of steroids involves the effect of increased intake of glucocorticoids on the normal feedback mechanism in the body, leading to a reduction of the normal secretion of the natural hormones and atrophy of the adrenal gland. Therefore, sudden cessation of the administration of glucocorticoid drugs or the presence of increased stress may cause adrenal crisis (similar to shock) because insufficient glucocorticoids are available in the body.

To lessen the risk of serious side effects, it is best to limit use of glucocorticoids to minimal dosages in the treatment of acute episodes. Intermittent drug-free time periods (drug holidays) are recommended during long-term therapy. Whenever the drug is discontinued, the dosage should be gradually decreased over a period of days to allow the body's natural hormone secretions to increase to normal levels. Adrenocorticotropic hormone (ACTH) therapy is used for long-term therapy in some patients because it stimulates the patient's glands to produce more cortisol. The risk of adrenal shock is less because glandular atrophy does not occur.

A brief comparison of drugs used to treat inflammation is shown in Table 5-4.

Other drugs, such as analgesics for pain, antihistamines, and antibiotics to prevent secondary infection may be required, depending on the cause of the inflammation.

First Aid Measures

First aid directives for injury-related inflammation frequently recommend the RICE approach: Rest, Ice, Compression, and Elevation. Cold applications are useful in the early stage of acute inflammation. Application of cold causes local vasoconstriction, thereby decreasing edema and pain. The use of hot or cold applications during long-term therapy and recovery periods depends on the particular situation. In some instances, for example, acute rheumatoid arthritis, heat, and moderate activity may improve the circulation in the affected area, thereby removing excess fluid, pain-causing chemical mediators, and waste metabolites, as well as promoting healing.

Other Therapies

It is often helpful to keep an inflamed limb elevated to improve fluid flow away from the damaged area. Compression using elastic stockings or other supports may reduce the accumulation of fluid.

Mild-to-moderate exercise is useful in cases of many chronic inflammatory conditions in which improved blood and fluid flow is beneficial and mobility could be improved.

Other treatment measures, including physiotherapy and/or occupational therapy, may be necessary to maintain joint mobility and reduce pain, although splints may be required during acute episodes to prevent contractures, and fixed abnormal joint positions. Rest and adequate nutrition and hydration are also important.

Healing

Types of Healing

Healing of a wound area can be accomplished in several ways.

- Resolution is the process that occurs when there is minimal tissue damage. The damaged cells recover, and the tissue returns to normal within a short period of time; for example, after a mild sunburn.

- Regeneration is the healing process that occurs in damaged tissue in which the cells are capable of mitosis. Some types of cells (e.g., epithelial cells) are constantly replicating, whereas other cells such as hepatocytes in the liver are able to undergo mitosis when necessary. The damaged tissue is thus replaced by identical tissue from the proliferation of nearby cells. This type of healing may be limited if the organization of a complex tissue is altered. For instance, sometimes fibrous tissue develops in the liver, distorting the orderly arrangement of cells, ducts, and blood vessels. Although nodules of new cells form, they do not contribute to the overall function of the liver.

THINK ABOUT 5-7

a. Which types of cells can regenerate? Name three types that cannot regenerate.
b. Explain why it is often advisable to elevate an inflamed limb.

- Replacement by connective tissue (scar or *fibrous tissue* formation) takes place when there is extensive tissue damage or the cells are incapable of mitosis; for example, the brain or myocardium. The wound area must be filled in and covered by some form of tissue. Chronic inflammation or complications such as infection result in more fibrous material.

Healing by first intention refers to the process involved when the wound is clean, free of foreign material and necrotic tissue, and the edges of it are held close together, creating a minimal gap between the edges. This type of healing is seen in some surgical incisions. Healing by second intention refers to a situation in which there is a large break in the tissue and consequently more inflammation, a longer healing period, and formation of more scar tissue. A compound fracture would heal in this manner.

The Healing Process

The process of tissue repair begins following injury when a *blood clot* forms and seals the area. Inflammation develops in the surrounding area (Fig. 5-6). After 3 to 4 days, foreign material and cell debris have been removed by phagocytes, monocytes, and macrophages, and then granulation tissue grows into the gap from nearby connective tissue.

Granulation tissue is highly vascular and appears moist and pink or red in color. It contains many new capillary buds from the surrounding tissue. This tissue is very fragile and is easily broken down by microorganisms or stress on the tissue (Fig. 5-7).

THINK ABOUT 5-8

What often happens if you pull a scab off a wound too early? Describe the appearance of the tissue.

At the same time as the wound cavity is being filled in, nearby *epithelial* cells undergo mitosis, extending across the wound from the outside edges inward. Shortly, fibroblasts, connective tissue cells, enter the area and produce collagen, a protein that is the basic component of scar tissue and provides strength for the new repair. As well, fibroblasts and macrophages produce growth factors (cytokines) in the area for the purpose of attracting more fibroblasts, which act as mitogens to stimulate epithelial cell proliferation and migration, and promote development of new blood vessels (angiogenesis) in the healing tissue.

Gradually cross-linking and shortening of the collagen fibers promote formation of a tight, strong scar. The capillaries in the area decrease, and the color of the scar gradually fades. It is important to remember that scar tissue is not normal, functional tissue, nor does it contain any specialized structures such as hair follicles or glands. It merely fills the defect or gap in the tissue. As scar tissue matures over time, it gains strength, but may also contract, causing increased tension on normal tissues.

THINK ABOUT 5-9

a. Which would heal more rapidly, a surgical incision in which the edges have been stapled closely together, or a large, jagged tear in the skin and subcutaneous tissue? Why?
b. Even after a long period of healing, explain how the scar tissue from a wound will be different from the surrounding undamaged tissue.

One area of current research is "tissue engineering," the search for new methods of replacing damaged tissue where regeneration is not possible; for example, extensive burns, deep ulcers, or cardiac muscle death. Biosynthetic skin is now available and research on other tissues uses a scaffold of synthetic material on which new cells can grow in an organized fashion. Growth factors and mitogens are released from the scaffolding as cells begin to metabolize nutrients in the scaffolding. Cells to populate the engineered tissue may be from a person's own stem cells, cord blood that has been stored, or a stem cell line maintained by the laboratory. Research is progressing, but to date (2012) no solid organs have been produced and used in clinical practice to replace a damaged organ. Ethical concerns regarding cost and access to commercially produced organs are important and need to be addressed before commencing therapies with this technology.

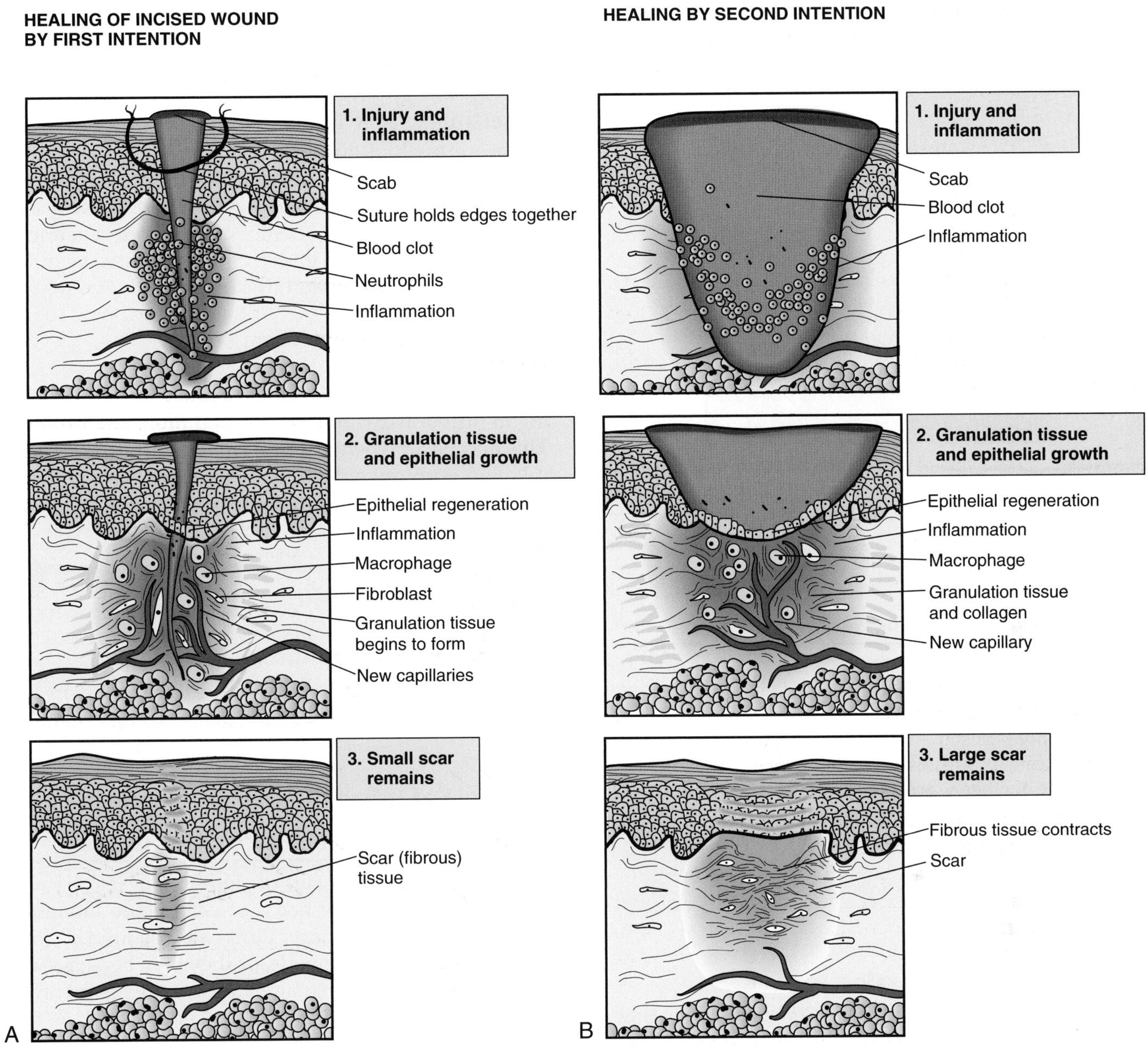

**HEALING OF INCISED WOUND
BY FIRST INTENTION**

HEALING BY SECOND INTENTION

1. Injury and inflammation
- Scab
- Suture holds edges together
- Blood clot
- Neutrophils
- Inflammation

2. Granulation tissue and epithelial growth
- Epithelial regeneration
- Inflammation
- Macrophage
- Fibroblast
- Granulation tissue begins to form
- New capillaries

3. Small scar remains
- Scar (fibrous) tissue

1. Injury and inflammation
- Scab
- Blood clot
- Inflammation

2. Granulation tissue and epithelial growth
- Epithelial regeneration
- Inflammation
- Macrophage
- Granulation tissue and collagen
- New capillary

3. Large scar remains
- Fibrous tissue contracts
- Scar

A   B

FIGURE 5-6 The healing process.

Factors Affecting Healing

A small gap in the tissue results in complete healing within a short period of time and with minimal scar tissue formation. A large or deep area of tissue damage requires a prolonged healing time and results in a large scar.

Many factors can promote healing or delay the process (Boxes 5-1 and 5-2).

Complications due to Scar Formation

Loss of Function

Loss of function results from the loss of normal cells and the lack of specialized structures or normal organization in scar tissue. For example, if scar tissue replaces normal

BOX 5-1   Factors Promoting Healing

- Youth
- Good nutrition: protein, vitamins A and C
- Adequate hemoglobin
- Effective circulation
- Clean, undisturbed wound
- No infection or further trauma to the site

skin, that area will lack hair follicles, glands, and sensory nerve endings. In a highly organized organ such as the kidney, it is unlikely that the new tissue will fit the pattern of blood vessels, tubules, and ducts of the normal kidney; therefore the replacement tissue will not provide normal function.

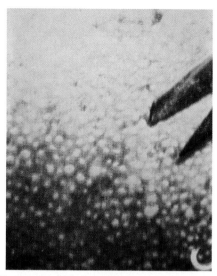

FIGURE 5-7 An example of granulation tissue in a burn wound. *(Courtesy of Judy Knighton, Clinical Nurse Specialist, Ross Tilley Burn Center, Sunnybrook and Women's College Health Center, Toronto, Ontario, Canada.)*

BOX 5-2	Factors Delaying Healing

- Advanced age, reduced mitosis
- Poor nutrition, dehydration
- Anemia (low hemoglobin)
- Circulatory problems
- Certain chronic diseases, such as diabetes
- Presence of other disorders such as diabetes or cancer
- Irritation, bleeding, or excessive mobility
- Infection, foreign material, or exposure to radiation
- Chemotherapy treatment
- Prolonged use of glucocorticoids

Contractures and Obstructions

Scar tissue is nonelastic and tends to shrink over time. This process may restrict the range of movement of a joint and eventually may result in fixation and deformity of the joint, a condition known as contracture. Fibrous tissue may also limit movement of the mouth or eyelids. Physiotherapy or surgery may be necessary to break down the fibrous tissue and improve mobility. Shrinkage of the scar tissue may also cause shortening or narrowing (stenosis) of structures, particularly tubes or ducts. For example, if the esophagus is shortened, malposition of the stomach (hiatal hernia) or a narrowed esophagus causing obstruction during swallowing (Fig. 5-8) can result.

Adhesions

Adhesions are bands of scar tissue joining two surfaces that are normally separated. Common examples are adhesions between loops of intestine (see Fig. 5-8B) or between the pleural membranes. Such adhesions usually result from inflammation or infection in the body cavities. Adhesions prevent normal movement of the structures and may eventually cause distortion or twisting of the tissue.

Hypertrophic Scar Tissue

An overgrowth of fibrous tissue consisting of excessive collagen deposits may develop, leading to hard ridges of scar tissue or keloid formation (Fig. 5-9). These masses are disfiguring and frequently cause more severe contractures. Skin and the underlying tissue may be pulled out of the normal position by the shortening of the scar tissue.

Ulceration

Blood supply may be impaired around the scar, resulting in further tissue breakdown and possible ulceration. This may occur when scar tissue develops in the stomach following surgery or healing of an ulcer. This scar tissue interferes with blood flow in nearby arteries.

THINK ABOUT 5-10

a. Describe three ways scar tissue on the thumb can interfere with normal function.
b. Explain how the characteristics of scar tissue can actually lead to new potential infections in the affected area.

Example of Inflammation and Healing

Burns

A burn is a thermal (heat) or nonthermal (electrical or chemical) injury to the body, causing acute inflammation and tissue destruction. Burns may be mild or cover only a small area of the body, or they may be severe and life threatening, as when an extensive area is involved. Burns may be caused by direct contact with a heat source such as flames or hot water (a scald), by chemicals, radiation, electricity, light, or friction. Most burns occur in the home. Any burn injury causes an acute inflammatory response and release of chemical mediators, resulting in a major fluid shift, edema, and decreased blood volume. Major burns constitute a medical emergency requiring specialized care as quickly as possible.

The severity of the burn depends on the cause of the burn, and the temperature, duration of the contact, as well as the extent of the burn surface and the site of the injury. Young children with their thin skin frequently receive severe burns from immersion in excessively hot water in a bathtub. The elderly also have thinner skin; therefore they can suffer much deeper burn injuries than younger adults. Skin thickness varies over the body, with facial skin being much thinner than the skin on the palms and soles. Thus, facial burns are more often more damaging than burns to the soles of the feet.

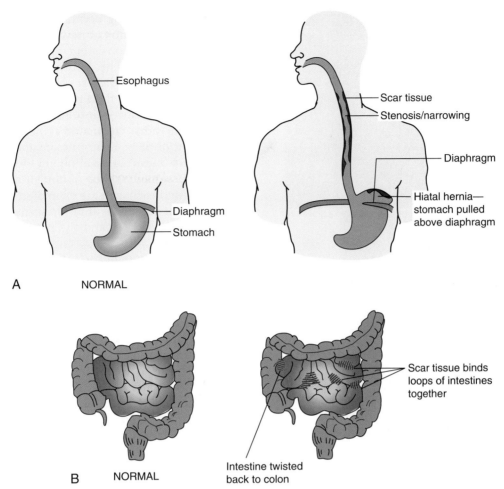

A   NORMAL

B   NORMAL   Intestine twisted
back to colon

FIGURE 5-8 Effects of scar tissue. **A,** Esophageal scarring and obstruction. **B,** Adhesions and twisting of the intestines.

> ### THINK ABOUT 5-11
>
> From your own experience and the information just given, describe the appearance and sensation over time of a thermal burn (e.g., a burn resulting from touching a hot object).

Classifications of Burns

Burns are classified by the depth of skin damage and the percentage of body surface area involved. *Partial-thickness* burns involve the epidermis and part of the dermis (Fig. 5-10). Superficial partial-thickness burns (formerly known as first-degree burns) damage the epidermis and may involve the upper dermis. They usually appear red and painful but heal readily without scar tissue. Examples include sunburn or a mild scald.

Deep partial-thickness burns (formerly second-degree burns) involve the destruction of the epidermis and part of the dermis (Fig. 5-11). The area is red, edematous, blistered, and often hypersensitive and painful during the inflammatory stage. In severe cases, the skin appears waxy with a reddened margin. The dead skin gradually sloughs off, and healing occurs by regeneration from the edges of the blistered areas and from epithelium lining the hair follicles and glands. If the area is extensive, healing may be difficult, and complications occur. Grafts may be necessary to cover larger areas. These burns easily become infected, causing additional tissue destruction and scar tissue formation.

Full-thickness burns (formerly third- and fourth-degree burns) result in destruction of all skin layers and often underlying tissues as well (see Fig. 5-11C). The burn wound area is coagulated or charred and therefore is hard and dry on the surface. This damaged tissue (eschar) shrinks, causing pressure on the edematous tissue beneath it. If the entire circumference of a limb is involved, treatment (escharotomy—surgical cuts through this crust) may be necessary to release the pressure and allow better circulation to the area. This procedure may also be required when a large area of the chest is covered by eschar, impairing lung expansion. Initially the burn area may be painless because of destruction of the nerves, but it becomes very painful as adjacent tissue becomes inflamed due to chemical mediators released by the damaged tissues. Full-thickness burns require

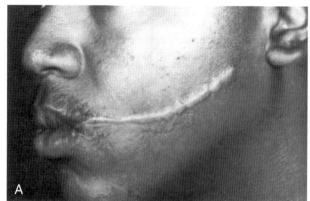

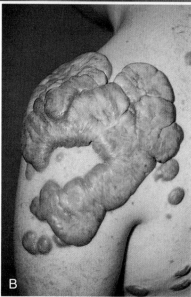

FIGURE 5-9 Complications of scar tissue. **A,** Example of scar tissue that may shrink and distort facial features in time. **B,** Example of a keloid. *(From Callen J, Greer K, Hood A, et al: Color Atlas of Dermatology, Philadelphia, 1993, WB Saunders.)*

skin grafts for healing because there are no cells available for the production of new skin. Many burn injuries are mixed burns, consisting of areas of partial burns mixed with full-thickness burns.

The percentage of *body surface area (BSA)* burned provides a guideline for fluid replacement needs as well as other therapeutic interventions. Complicated charts are provided in burn treatment centers for the accurate assessment of BSA. The "rule of nines" (Fig. 5-12) is a method for rapid calculation. In this estimate, body parts are assigned a value of nine or a multiple of nine. The head and each arm are estimated at 9%. Each leg is calculated at 18%. The anterior surface of the trunk is given a value of 18%, and the posterior surface is also 18%. The groin area at 1% brings the total BSA to 100%. The parts can be subdivided also; for example, the distal part of the arm (elbow to hand) accounts for 4.5% of the BSA. These figures are approximations and can be revised; for example, because a young child has a larger head and shorter limbs than an adult, an adjustment is required. The Lund and Browder chart provides a more detailed calculation for children.

Minor burns to a small area can be treated in a physician's office. Major burns, as classified by the American Burn Association, are best treated in a center specializing in burn wound care. Major burns include burns involving a large surface area, young children, or the elderly; burns to hands, feet, face, ears, or genitalia; inhalation injury; chemical burns; or cases in which other injuries or complications are present. Electrical injuries are always considered serious because there is immediate interference with the normal conduction of electrical impulses in the body, often causing cardiac arrest, and extensive unseen damage to blood vessels and organs. (An electric current travels on the path of

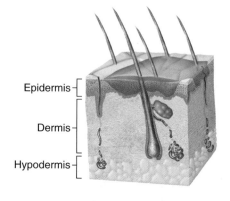

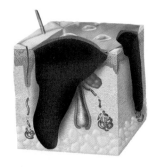

| Partial-thickness burns | First-degree burn: Damaged epidermis and edema | Second-degree burn: Damaged epidermis and dermis | Full-thickness burns | Third-degree burn: Deep tissue damage |

Epidermis
Dermis
Hypodermis

FIGURE 5-10 Classification of burns. Partial-thickness burns include first- and second-degree burns. Full-thickness burns include third-degree burns. Fourth-degree burns involve tissues under the skin, such as muscle or bone. *(From Patton KT, Thibodeau GA: Anatomy & Physiology, ed 8, St. Louis, 2013, Mosby.)*

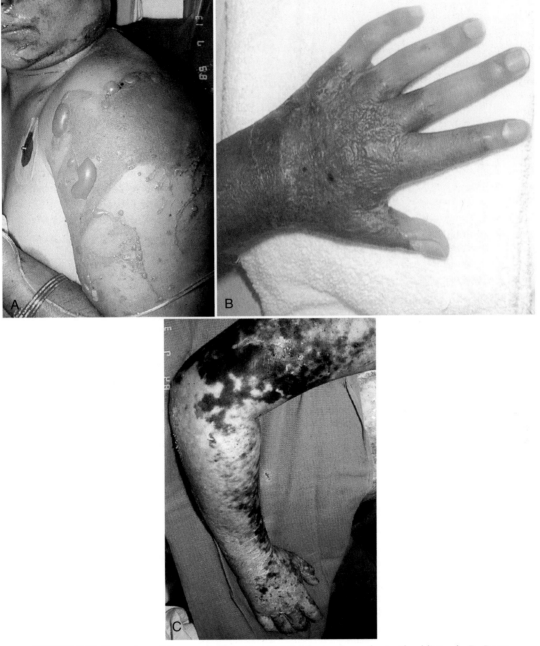

FIGURE 5-11 Examples of burns. **A**, Deep partial-thickness burn (note the blisters). **B**, Deep partial-thickness burn (note the edema). **C**, Full-thickness burn (note the dark color). *(All photos courtesy of Judy Knighton, Clinical Nurse Specialist, Ross Tilley Burn Center, Sunnybrook and Women's College Health Center, Toronto, Ontario, Canada.)*

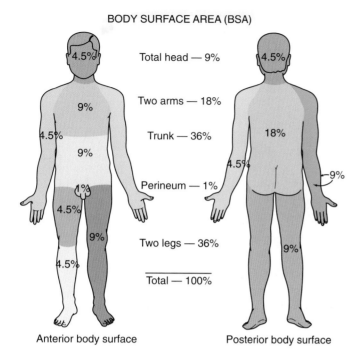

BODY SURFACE AREA (BSA)

Total head — 9%

Two arms — 18%

Trunk — 36%

Perineum — 1%

Two legs — 36%

Total — 100%

Anterior body surface   Posterior body surface

FIGURE 5-12 Assessment of burn area using the rule of nines.

least resistance, such as along the blood vessels, coagulating and obstructing blood supply.)

EMERGENCY CARE FOR BURNS

Stop, Drop, and Roll!

- When clothes are on fire, stop what you are doing, drop to the floor, cover up if possible, and roll to extinguish flames.
- Call emergency services (911) if the burn appears to be extensive or a major burn.
- Ensure that electrical power is off before caring for an electrical burn injury!
- Cool the burned area by soaking it with cool or tepid water. Remove nonsticking clothing if possible, and continue with cool water. Do not apply lotions, fats, or lubricants!
- Cover loosely with a clean cloth (e.g., the inside of a folded sheet) or sterile gauze.
- For a chemical burn, remove any affected clothing and flush the burn area well with cool water, then cover with a clean cloth.

THINK ABOUT   5-12

a. Using the rule of nines, calculate the approximate area of partial-thickness burn in an adult with burns to the right arm and chest area.
b. State two reasons why full-thickness burns are considered more serious than partial-thickness burns.
c. Why does sunburn usually heal readily?

Effects of Burn Injury

Serious burns have many effects, both local and systemic, in addition to the obvious damage to the skin. The burn wound is debrided during treatment, removing all foreign material and damaged tissue, in preparation for healing. A temporary covering is then applied.

Following is a brief description of additional effects, to be expanded upon in subsequent chapters.

Shock

No bleeding occurs with a burn injury (tissue and blood are coagulated or solidified by the heat). Under the burn surface an inflammatory response occurs. Where the burn area is large, the inflammatory response results in a massive shift of water, protein, and electrolytes into the tissues, causing fluid excess or edema (see Chapter 2) (Fig. 5-13). Loss of water and protein from the blood leads to decreased circulating blood volume, low blood pressure, and hypovolemic shock (see Chapter 12), as well as an increased hematocrit (the percentage of red blood cells in a volume of blood) due to hemoconcentration. The fluid imbalance is aggravated by the protein shift out of the capillaries and the resulting lower osmotic pressure in the blood, making it difficult to maintain blood volume until the inflammation subsides. Prolonged or recurrent shock may cause kidney failure or damage to other organs. Fluid and electrolytes as well as plasma expanders (a substitute for lost protein) are replaced intravenously using formulas designed to treat burn patients. In some cases of severe shock, particularly with extensive full-thickness burns, acute renal failure may develop (see Chapter 18).

THINK ABOUT   5-13

a. Explain how an increased hematocrit indicates a fluid shift.
b. How do reduced protein levels in the blood affect tissue metabolism and healing?
c. How does the reduction in blood flow through the burn promote infection and make an infection harder to treat should one develop?

Respiratory Problems

An immediate concern in the case of a burn patient is the inhalation of toxic or irritating fumes. Inspiration of carbon monoxide is dangerous because this gas preferentially binds to hemoglobin, taking the place of needed oxygen. The increasing presence of synthetic materials in the environment has increased the risk of exposure to toxic gases such as cyanide during a fire. These gases are particularly dangerous when an individual has been trapped in an enclosed space, such as a room or an automobile. High levels of oxygen are administered and the patient is observed for signs of respiratory impairment following such a burn.

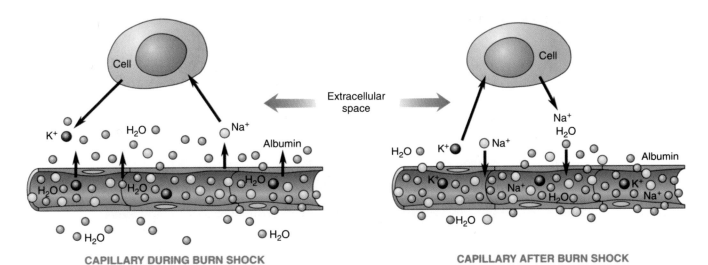

FIGURE 5-13 Direction of fluid and electrolyte shifts associated with burn shock. During burn shock, K^+ is moving out of the cell, and Na^+ and H_2O are moving in. After burn shock, K^+ moves in, and Na^+ and H_2O move out. *(From Copstead-Kirkorn LC:* Pathophysiology, *ed 4, St. Louis, 2009, Mosby.)*

If flame, hot air, steam, or irritating chemicals have been inhaled, damage to the mucosal lining of the trachea and bronchi may occur, and patients are observed for indications of inflammation and obstruction developing in the airway. Facial burns may be present, wheezing, and coughing up sputum containing black particles. Ventilation may be limited by eschar or pain. Pneumonia, a lung infection, is a threat, because of inflammation in the respiratory tract and immobility (see Chapter 13).

Pain

Burns are very painful injuries throughout the treatment process until healing is complete. The original injury, body movements, and application of grafts and other treatments contribute to pain. Analgesics (pain killers) are required.

Infection

Infection is a major concern in patients with burns. Infection of burn injuries increases tissue loss in the area, often converting a partial-thickness burn to a full-thickness burn. Because microbes are normally present deep in glands and hair follicles (see Chapter 8), there is a ready-made source of infection in the injured area. Also, opportunistic bacteria and fungi (see Chapter 6) are waiting to invade open areas, when defensive barriers and blood flow are reduced. Common microbes involved in burn injury infections include *Pseudomonas aeruginosa*, *Staphylococcus aureus* (including drug-resistant strains), *Klebsiella*, and *Candida* (Fig. 5-14). Antimicrobial drugs are usually administered only after specific microorganisms from the wound have been cultured and identified. Excessive or incorrect use of antimicrobial drugs increases the risk of emergence of drug-resistant microorganisms (see Chapter 6). When serious infection develops, there is risk of microorganisms or toxins spreading throughout the body, causing septic shock and other complications. Treatment involves rapid excision or removal of the damaged and infected tissue, application of antimicrobial drugs, and replacement with skin grafts or a substitute covering.

> **THINK ABOUT 5-14**
>
> a. Suggest three potential sources of infection in a burn patient.
> b. Other than skin damage, explain what other dangerous effects can result from burns.

Metabolic Needs

Hypermetabolism occurs during the healing period, and increased dietary intake of protein and carbohydrates is required. There is considerable heat loss from the body until the skin is restored; the patient with burns tends to feel chilled and is sensitive to air movement. Therefore the ongoing need to produce more body heat and replace tissue demands increased nutrients. Also, protein continues to be lost in exudate from the burn site until healing is complete. The stress response contributes to an increased metabolic rate and demand for nutrients. Anemia or a low hemoglobin concentration in the blood develops because many erythrocytes are destroyed or damaged by the burn injury, and often bone marrow functioning is depressed by compounds released from damaged tissues, reducing hematopoiesis (the production of blood cells in bone marrow).

Healing of Burns

An immediate covering of a clean wound is needed to protect the burned area and prevent infection. Nonstick

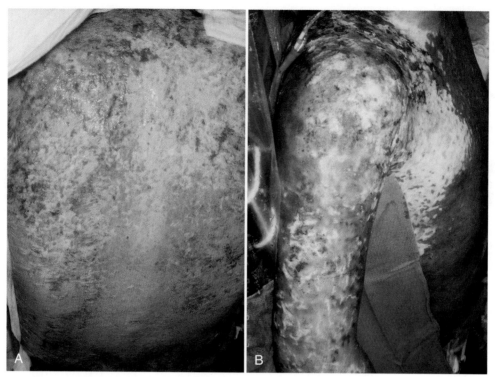

FIGURE 5-14 Infections in a burn wound. **A,** Purulent exudate (to be cultured to identify microbes). **B,** Blue-green color indicates infection by *Pseudomonas aeruginosa.* (*Courtesy of Judy Knighton, Clinical Nurse Specialist, Ross Tilley Burn Center, Sunnybrook and Women's College Health Center, Toronto, Ontario, Canada.*)

dressings are satisfactory for small areas or superficial burns. When a piece of skin is to be grafted over the burn wound, it may be "stretched" as a *mesh* to cover a greater area (Fig. 5-15A). In some cases, a small section of skin from the patient is cultured, producing a large piece of skin in several weeks. Alternative protection for the burn area may involve temporary substitute coverings, such as pig skin or cadaver skin, which will be rejected in time. In most serious burn cases, few epithelial cells are available in the burn area for healing.

Large burn centers are now using biosynthetic skin substitutes (e.g., Integra or TransCyte), particularly where severely burned patients lack sufficient healthy skin to graft (Fig. 5-15B). These coverings consist of two layers: A synthetic "epidermis" that can be removed easily as healing occurs, and underneath, a framework of proteins, collagen, and growth factors to stimulate healing. Some types contain living human cells. They are strong but elastic to conform to body structure. Research is proceeding to provide improvements to these materials. A very thin skin graft can then be applied with less scar tissue developing. Healing is more rapid, the number of surgical procedures and grafts are reduced, there is less risk of infection, and scarring is decreased when stable coverage of the burn wound can be quickly accomplished.

In a major burn, healing is a prolonged process, taking perhaps months. *Scar tissue* occurs even with skin grafting and impairs function as well as appearance.

Hypertrophic scar tissue is common. Long-term use of elasticized garments and splints may be necessary to control scarring. In Figure 5-16, a burn survivor is being measured for an elastic pressure sleeve, a process that may be repeated many times.

Physiotherapy and occupational therapy are often necessary to reduce the effects of scar tissue and increase functional use of the area. In some cases, surgery may be necessary to release restrictive scar tissue or contractures. Severe burns require long-term team treatment because complications are frequent. The length of treatment has a major impact on a burn survivor, considering the psychological and practical effects on physical appearance and function, family, and job.

Children

The *growth of children* is often affected during the acute phase of burn recovery, when metabolic needs are compromised and stress is great. Often at a later time, additional surgery or grafts may be required to accommodate growth and ease the effects of scarring.

THINK ABOUT 5-15

a. Explain why healing is a particularly slow process in burn patients.
b. Explain what particular problems a child would encounter in any case where they have suffered an injury that has resulted in a considerable amount of scar tissue.

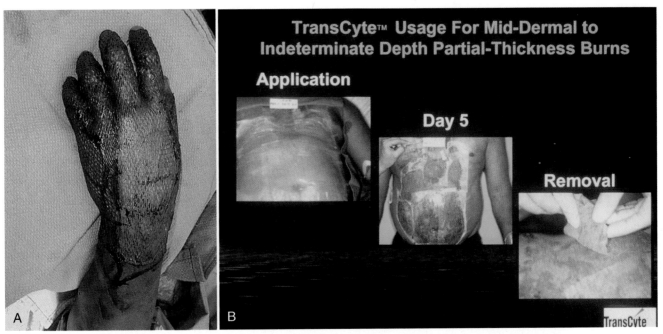

FIGURE 5-15 **A**, Example of a mesh skin graft. *(Courtesy of Judy Knighton, Clinical Nurse Specialist, Ross Tilley Burn Center, Sunnybrook and Women's College Health Center, Toronto, Ontario, Canada.)* **B**, Biosynthetic Covering (TransCyte). *Top:* A temporary dermal substitute "skin" is placed on a clean, partial-thickness burn wound. *Bottom:* The covering is removed after new epithelial tissue has formed. *(From Advanced Healing, Inc.)*

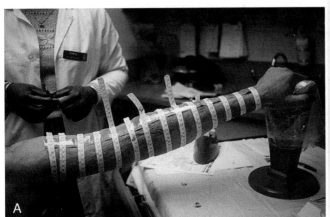

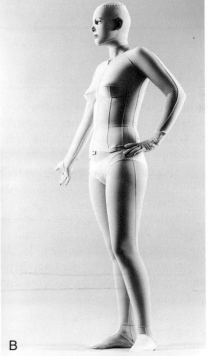

FIGURE 5-16 **A.** Measurement for an elastic garment to control scar tissue from a burn. *(Courtesy of Judy Knighton, Clinical Nurse Specialist, Ross Tilley Burn Center, Sunnybrook and Women's College Health Center, Toronto, Ontario, Canada.)* **B.** The custom-fitted antiscar support garment modeled here effectively provides pressure therapy over wounds, which helps to minimize the development of hypertrophic scarring. *(From Black JM, Matassarin-Jacobs E, editors:* Medical-Surgical Nursing: Clinical Management for Positive Outcomes, *ed 7, Philadelphia, 2005, Saunders, p 1356. Courtesy Medical Z, San Antonio, Texas.)*

CASE STUDY A

Trauma

M.H., age 6, fell while running down stairs and hurt his wrist and elbow. His arm was scraped and bleeding slightly, and the elbow became red, swollen, and painful. Normal movement was possible, although painful.

1. Explain why the elbow is red and swollen.
2. Suggest several reasons why movement is painful.
3. State two reasons why healing may be slow in the scraped area on the arm, and two factors that encourage healing in this boy.

CASE STUDY B

Burns

While trying to light a barbecue, the propane tank exploded, burning the face, arms, and chest of P.J., age 28. He had mixed burns to most areas except for his hands and face, which were full-thickness burns.

1. Why would this be considered a major burn?
2. Describe the process taking place in the burned area during the first hours after the injury.
3. P.J. was wheezing, coughing up mucus, and short of breath. Explain why this has likely developed.
4. P.J. developed a bacterial infection on his right hand. Explain three predisposing factors to this.
5. How will this burn injury affect P.J.'s ability to work? What are some of the social needs in this case?

CHAPTER SUMMARY

The inflammatory response is one of the nonspecific defense mechanisms in the body. Other defenses include: first, the barriers, skin, mucous membrane, and secretions such as tears and saliva; second, phagocytosis; and third, the specific defense, the immune response.

- The inflammatory response is the response to any cell or tissue injury by any agent.
- The acute inflammatory response consists of a sequence of events: the release of chemical mediators from damaged mast cells and platelets, local vasodilation and increased capillary permeability, formation of exudate, movement of leukocytes to the site, and phagocytosis for removal of the offending agent and debris.
- The signs of acute inflammation are redness, warmth, swelling, pain, and, frequently, loss of function.
- With extensive inflammation, systemic signs may present, including mild fever, headache, fatigue, and leukocytosis.
- Chronic inflammation results in formation of fibrotic or scar tissue.
- Anti-inflammatory drugs include aspirin (ASA) and the nonsteroidal anti-inflammatory drugs (NSAIDs), which block prostaglandin production at the site. These drugs also have antipyretic and analgesic activity. The glucocorticoids such as hydrocortisone are effective anti-inflammatory and antiallergenic agents, but significant adverse effects develop with long-term use.
- Healing may take place by regeneration, if cells are capable of mitosis and the damaged area is small.
- Fibrotic or scar tissue, consisting primarily of collagen fibers, replaces normal tissue when damage is extensive or cells are incapable of mitosis. Scar tissue lacks normal function and is nonelastic, tending to shrink over time, possibly causing contractures, deformity, or strictures at a later time.
- Factors promoting healing include youth, good circulation and nutrition, and lack of infection or other disease.
- Burns, an example of inflammation and healing, are classified by the percentage of body surface area damaged and the depth of the skin damage in the burn area. Partial-thickness burns involve the epidermis and part of the dermis. Full-thickness burns destroy all skin layers; thus, a skin graft is required for healing. In some cases, eschar restricts circulation or ventilation.
- Following severe burns, shock frequently occurs because of fluid and protein loss from the burn wound. Infection is a threat because the protective skin barrier has been lost. Inhalation of toxic or irritating fumes may cause respiratory impairment. Hypermetabolism and the increased demand for nutrients for healing require dietary supplements.
- Healing of burns is a prolonged process, and multiple skin grafts may be required. Biosynthetic wound coverings have promoted healing in many cases.

STUDY QUESTIONS

In answering these questions, the student is expected to use knowledge of normal anatomy and physiology.

Inflammation

1. a. Explain why a cast placed around a fractured leg in which extensive tissue damage has occurred might be too tight after 24 hours.
   b. Explain why such a cast might become loose in 3 weeks.
2. List specific reasons why the inflammatory response is considered a body defense mechanism.
3. a. Explain the rationale for each of the following with acute inflammation: (i) warmth, (ii) fever.
   b. State three systemic signs of inflammation.

4. Explain why leukocytosis, a differential count, and elevated ESR are useful data but are of limited value.
5. a. Explain how acute inflammation predisposes to development of infection.
   b. Classify each as inflammation or infection: (i) sunburn, (ii) skin rash under adhesive tape, (iii) common cold, (iv) red, swollen eye with purulent exudate.
6. How does the presence of thick, cloudy, yellowish fluid in the peritoneal cavity differ from the normal state?
7. If a large volume of fluid has shifted from the blood into the peritoneal cavity, how would this affect blood volume and hematocrit?
8. Explain how acute inflammation impairs movement of a joint.
9. Explain two mechanisms used to increase body temperature as a fever develops.
10. Why might a client be advised to avoid taking ASA a few days before extensive oral surgery (e.g., multiple tooth extractions)?
11. Explain why a young child taking prednisone (glucocorticoid) for chronic kidney inflammation is at high risk for infection and might need prophylactic antibiotics.

Healing

12. a. When part of the heart muscle dies, how does it heal?
    b. How would the new tissue affect the strength of the heart contraction?

13. Suggest several reasons why healing is slow in the elderly.
14. Explain how scar tissue could affect the function of the:
    a. small intestine
    b. brain
    c. cornea of the eye
    d. mouth
    e. lungs (try to find more than one point!)

Burns

15. a. Explain the rationale for pain and redness accompanying a burn.
    b. Explain three reasons why protein levels in the body are low after a major burn.
16. a. Explain why immediate neutralization or removal of a chemical spilled on the hand minimizes burn injury.
    b. Describe some of the factors that would promote rapid healing of this burn.
17. Describe three potential complications of a full-thickness burn covering 30% of the body, including the legs and back.
18. If the face receives a full-thickness burn, describe three ways function could be impaired after healing.

ADDITIONAL RESOURCES

Applegate EJ: *The Anatomy and Physiology Learning System,* ed 2, Philadelphia, 2006, WB Saunders.
Kumar V, Abbas AK, Fausto M: *Robbins and Cotran Pathologic Basis of Disease,* ed 7, Philadelphia, 2009, WB Saunders.
Mosby's Drug Consult 2006. St. Louis, 2006, Mosby.

Web Sites

http://www.nlm.nih.gov/medlineplus/burns.html *Medline Plus: Burns.*
http://www.aaem.org/jem/ *Journal of Emergency Medicine* (American Academy of Emergency Medicine).

Infection

CHAPTER OUTLINE

LEARNING OBJECTIVES

After studying this chapter, the student is expected to:

1. Describe the basic characteristics of bacteria, viruses, chlamydiae, rickettsiae, mycoplasmas, fungi, prions, and helminths.
2. Discuss the locations, advantages, and disadvantages of resident (normal) flora.
3. Describe the modes of transmission of microbes.
4. Describe the factors determining host resistance.
5. Explain the factors contributing to pathogenicity and virulence of microbes.
6. Discuss methods of preventing and controlling infection.
7. Describe the stages in the development and course of an infection.
8. Describe typical, local, and systemic signs of infection.
9. State the common diagnostic tests for infection and the purpose of each.
10. Describe the mechanisms of action of common antimicrobial drugs.
11. Explain the basic guidelines for use of antimicrobial drugs.
12. Describe the respiratory infection influenza, including the cause, transmission, immunization, incidence, manifestations, and possible complications.

KEY TERMS

antiseptics	infection	nosocomial	seizures
autoclaving	leukocytosis	obligate	septicemia
culture	leukopenia	parasite	sterilization
disinfectants	lymphadenopathy	pathogens	toxins
endemic	monocytosis	pili	unicellular
epidemics	mutation	prions	
fimbriae	neutropenia	prosthetic	

Review of Microbiology

Microorganisms

Microbiology refers to the study of microorganisms or microbes, very small living forms that are visible only with a microscope. Microorganisms include bacteria, fungi, protozoa, and viruses (Fig. 6-1). Detailed classifications of organisms with their proper names are available in microbiology references (e.g., *Bergey's Manual*). Selected examples of microorganisms are examined briefly here.

Bacteria are classified as prokaryotic cells because they are very simple in structure—lacking even a nuclear membrane—but they function metabolically and reproduce. They also have a complex cell wall structure. By comparison, eukaryotic cells are nucleated cells found in higher plants and animals, including humans. They lack cell walls (except in plants) but their DNA is enclosed in a nuclear membrane and the cell membrane has a complex structure.

Many microorganisms are classified as nonpathogenic because they do not usually cause disease; in fact, they are often beneficial. Pathogens are the disease-causing microbes often referred to as "germs." Infectious diseases result from invasion of the body by microbes and multiplication of these microbes, followed by damage to the body. These agents and their ability to cause disease vary widely. In the 18th and 19th centuries, scientists experimented on fermentation and spoilage of foods. This resulted in the concept of the "germ theory of disease" as well as explanations of how wine and other foods became unfit for consumption. The transmission of pathogens and infection through hands, surfaces, water, and the air was documented, and the practices of asepsis were begun.

Microorganisms vary widely in their growth needs, and their specific requirements often form the basis for identification tests. Many microbes can be grown in a laboratory using an appropriate environment and a suitable culture medium in a Petri dish (Fig. 6-2A) or a test tube. The culture medium provides the required nutrients for specific microbial groups. The culture base may be synthetic or a broth base with additives. The need for oxygen, carbohydrates, a specific pH or temperature, or a living host depends on the needs of the particular microbe. Those microbes that require living cells in which to survive are particularly difficult to identify without specialized laboratory techniques such as cell culture, immunoassays, or electron microscopy. The specific growth factors play a role in determining the site of infection in the human body. For example, the organism causing tetanus is an anaerobic bacterium that thrives in the absence of oxygen and therefore can easily cause infection deep in the tissue.

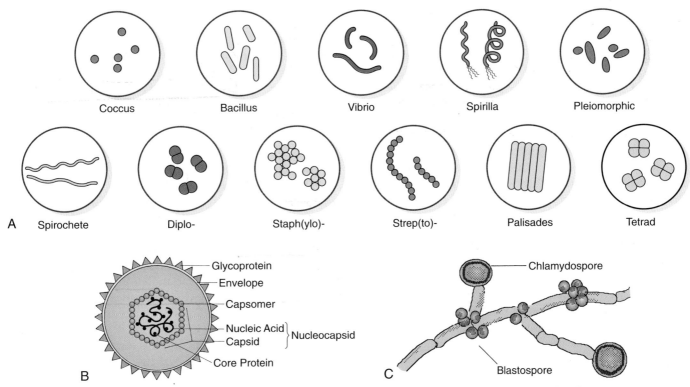

FIGURE 6-1 **A**, Bacterial cell morphology. *(From VanMeter K, Hubert R: Microbiology for the Healthcare Professional, ed 1, St. Louis, 2010, Mosby.)* **B**, Virus. **C**, Fungus.

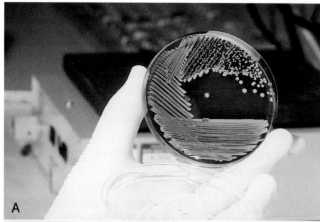

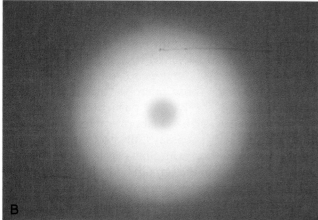

FIGURE 6-2 A, Culture plate growing *Staphylococcus aureus*. *(From Stepp CA, Woods M: Laboratory Procedures for Medical Office Personnel, Philadelphia, 1998, WB Saunders.)* **B,** Culture plate with hemolytic streptococcus destroying erythrocytes (colorless area). *(From De la Maza LM, Pezzlo MT, Baron EJ: Color Atlas of Diagnostic Microbiology, St. Louis, 1997, Mosby.)*

Types of Microorganisms

Bacteria

Bacteria are unicellular (single cell) organisms that do not require living tissue to survive. They vary in size, shape, and arrangement and are classified and named accordingly (see Fig. 6-1). These obvious characteristics may assist in rapid identification of microbes.

The major groups of bacteria based on cellular shape are:

- *Bacilli*, or rod-shaped organisms, which include vibrio (curved rods) and pleomorphic (variable or indistinct shape).
- *Spirals*, which include spirochetes and spirilla, displaying a coiled shape or "wavy line" appearance. These two classifications of bacterial shape differ in that the spirochete contains a structure called an axial filament, whereas the spirilla have flagella. Both of these structures facilitate cell movement.
- *Cocci*, or spherical forms.

Bacterial cells can further be categorized by their characteristic groupings or arrangement.

- Diplo- prefix, indicating pairs
- Strep(to)- prefix, indicating chains
- Staph(ylo)- prefix, indicating irregular, grapelike clusters
- Tetrads- refers to cells grouped in a packet or square of four cells
- Palisade- refers to cells lying together with the long sides parallel

The basic structure of bacteria includes:

1. An outer rigid *cell wall* protects the microbe and provides a specific shape (Fig. 6-3). A bacterium has one of two types of cell walls, *gram-positive* or *gram-negative*, which differ in their chemical composition. This difference can be quickly determined in the laboratory using a *Gram stain* and provides a means of identification and classification for bacteria. This classification is useful in selecting appropriate antimicrobial therapy; for instance, penicillin acts on the cell wall of gram-positive bacteria. Targeting cell wall structure and function is important because human cells do *not* have cell walls. A drug such as penicillin thus does not damage human cells but is effective against gram-positive bacteria.

2. A *cell membrane* is located inside the bacterial cell wall. This semipermeable membrane selectively controls movement of nutrients and other materials in and out of the cell. Metabolic processes also take place in the cell membrane.

3. An external *capsule* or *slime layer* is found on *some*, but not all, bacteria. This layer is found outside the cell wall and offers additional protection to the organism. It also interferes with the phagocytosis by macrophages and WBCs in the human body.

4. One or more rotating *flagellae* attached to the cell wall provide motility for some species.

5. Pili or fimbriae are tiny hairlike structures found on some bacteria, usually in the gram-negative class. Pili assist in attachment of the bacterium to tissue and also in transfer of genetic material (DNA) to another bacterium, thus leading to greater genetic variation.

6. Bacteria contain *cytoplasm*, which contains the chromosome (composed of one long strand of DNA), ribosomes and RNA, and plasmids, which are DNA fragments that are important in the exchange of genetic information with other bacteria. Plasmids commonly contain genetic information conveying drug resistance; thus such resistance can be shared with many other types of bacteria. The cellular components provide for the metabolism, growth, reproduction, and unique characteristics of the bacterium. Drugs often target a particular pathway in bacterial metabolism.

7. Some bacteria secrete *toxic substances*, toxins, and enzymes. Toxins consist of two types, exotoxins and endotoxins.

   - *Exotoxins* are usually produced by gram-positive bacteria and diffuse through body fluids. They

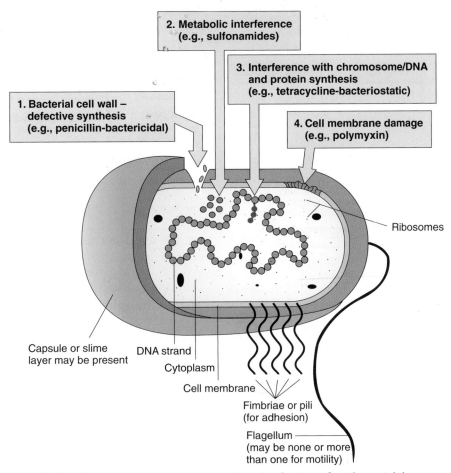

2. Metabolic interference
(e.g., sulfonamides)

3. Interference with chromosome/DNA
and protein synthesis
(e.g., tetracycline-bacteriostatic)

1. Bacterial cell wall –
defective synthesis
(e.g., penicillin-bactericidal)

4. Cell membrane damage
(e.g., polymyxin)

Ribosomes

Capsule or slime
layer may be present

DNA strand

Cytoplasm

Cell membrane

Fimbriae or pili
(for adhesion)

Flagellum
(may be none or more
than one for motility)

FIGURE 6-3 Structure of a bacterium and mode of action of antibacterial drugs.

have a variety of effects, often interfering with nerve conduction, such as the *neurotoxin* from the tetanus bacillus. Other toxins termed *enterotoxins* may stimulate the vomiting center and cause gastrointestinal distress. Exotoxins stimulate antibody or antitoxin production, which after being processed to reduce the toxic effect, can be used as toxoids to induce an immune response (see Chapter 7).

- *Endotoxins* are present in the cell wall of gramnegative organisms and are released after the bacterium dies. Endotoxins may cause fever and general weakness, or they may have serious effects on the circulatory system, causing increased capillary permeability, loss of vascular fluid, and endotoxic shock.

- *Enzymes* are produced by some bacteria and are a source of damage to the host tissues or cells. For example, hemolysin is produced by bacteria called "hemolytic streptococcus." This enzyme destroys red blood cells, as seen on a culture medium containing red blood cells (see Fig. 6-2*B*). Other enzymes assist the bacteria to invade tissue by breaking down components. For example, collage-

nase breaks down collagen, and streptokinase dissolves blood clots.

8. Several species can form *spores,* a latent form of the bacterium with a coating that is highly resistant to heat and other adverse conditions (Fig. 6-4). These bacteria can survive long periods in the spore state, but they cannot reproduce when in spore form. Later, when conditions improve, the bacteria resume a vegetative state and reproduce. Tetanus and botulism are two examples of dangerous infections caused by spores in the soil entering the body, where they return to the vegetative state and reproduce.

Bacteria duplicate by a simple process called binary fission (see Fig. 6-4), a division of the cell to produce two daughter cells identical to the parent bacterium. The generation time or rate of replication varies from a few minutes to many hours, depending on the particular microbe. If binary fission occurs rapidly, a large colony of bacteria can develop very quickly, and this leads to the rapid onset of infection. The limiting factors to bacterial growth include insufficient nutrients and oxygen, the effects of increased metabolic wastes in the area, and changes in pH or temperature, all of which cause microbes to die faster than they can divide. Thus the

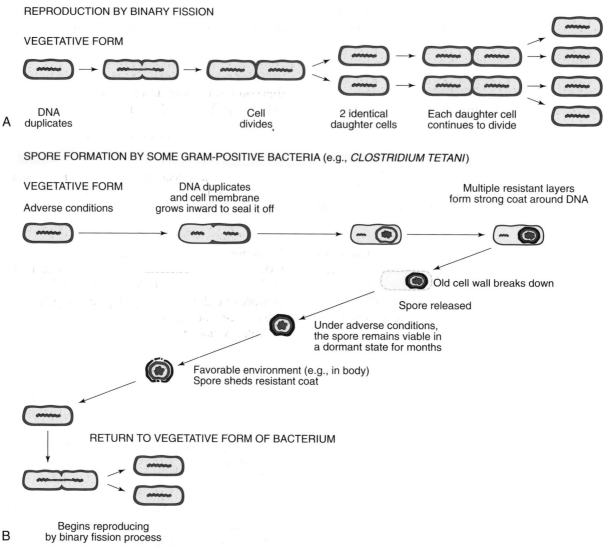

FIGURE 6-4 Bacteria—binary fission and spore formation.

colony eventually self-destructs, but pathogenic bacteria may cause life-threatening damage to tissues before self-destruction.

APPLY YOUR KNOWLEDGE   6-1

1. Describe three similarities and three differences between bacteria and human cells.
2. Explain how some bacterial cells may be just as dangerous when they are dead as when they are alive.

Viruses

There are several types of viruses, many of which include numerous subtypes. Table 6-1 lists some types of viruses and common pathogens causing disease in humans. A virus is a very small obligate intracellular parasite that requires a *living* host cell for replication. The need of viruses for living tissue complicates any laboratory procedure to grow or test viruses. When it is extracellular, a virus particle is called a *virion*. It consists of a *protein* coat, or capsid, and a core of *either* DNA or RNA (see Fig. 6-1B). The protein coat comes in many shapes and sizes and undergoes change relatively quickly in the evolution of the virions. The nucleic acid content and its form provide methods of classification of viruses. A retrovirus such as HIV, the human immunodeficiency virus, contains RNA only, plus an enzyme to convert RNA into DNA, a process activated when the virus enters the host cell. Most viruses contain DNA. Some viruses have an additional outer protective *envelope*.

When a virus infects a person, it attaches to a host cell, and the viral genetic material enters the cell. Viral DNA or RNA takes over control of the host cell, using the host's capacity for cell metabolism to synthesize protein, producing many new viral components (Fig. 6-5). The new viruses are assembled, then released by lysis of the host cell or by budding from the host cell membrane (see Fig. 7-14 and Fig. 6-5D)—usually with destruction of the host cell—and the new viruses in turn infect nearby cells.

Some viruses remain in a *latent stage*; they enter host cells and replicate very slowly or not at all until sometime later. Viruses can also insert their capsid proteins into the cell membrane of the host cells; these cells are then recognized as viral invaders and are attacked by the body's immune system.

Frequently one type of virus exists in many similar forms or strains, and viruses tend to *mutate*, or change slightly, during replication (e.g., the cold or influenza viruses). Some viruses such as the influenza virus are composed of nucleic acids from differing viral strains in animals and humans. Influenza H1N1 has components from both swine influenza and human influenza; these mixtures can change rapidly, leading to new combinations. These factors make it difficult for a host to develop adequate immunity to a virus, either by effective antibodies or vaccines. Because of their unique characteristics, viruses are difficult to control. They can hide inside human cells, and they lack their own metabolic processes or structures that might be attacked by drugs.

TABLE 6-1 Common Viral Diseases

Type of Virus	RNA or DNA	Example of Disease
Orthomyxoviruses	RNA	Influenza A, B, and C
Paramyxoviruses	RNA	Mumps, measles
Togavirus	RNA	Rubella virus (German measles), Hepatitis C virus
Herpesvirus	DNA	Herpes simplex, Infectious mononucleosis, Varicella (chickenpox)
Flaviviruses	RNA	West Nile virus, Encephalitis
Picornaviruses	RNA	Poliovirus, Hepatitis A virus
Hepadnaviruses	DNA	Hepatitis B virus
Papovaviruses	DNA	Warts, cancer (human papillomavirus/HPV)
Retrovirus	RNA	Human immunodeficiency viruses

Certain intracellular viruses may also alter host cell chromosomes, thus leading to the development of malignant cells or cancer. Several strains of the human papillomavirus (HPV) have been shown to be a major cause of cervical cancer. A vaccine is now available for this common cancer and is approved for use in females entering puberty to prevent later cancer.

THINK ABOUT 6-1

a. Compare three characteristics of a bacterium and a virus.
b. Why are viruses so hard to control?

Chlamydiae, Rickettsiae, and Mycoplasmas

These three groups of microorganisms have some similarities to both bacteria and viruses (Table 6-2). They replicate by binary fission, but they lack some basic component; therefore they require the presence of living cells for reproduction.

- Chlamydiae are considered very primitive forms related to bacteria that lack many enzymes for metabolic processes. They exist in two forms. One, the elementary body (EB) is infectious, possessing a cell wall and the ability to bind to epithelial cells. The other form, the reticulate body (RB) is noninfectious, but uses the host cell to make ATP and reproduce as an obligate intracellular organism (Fig. 6-6A). After large numbers of new microbes are produced inside the host cells, the new RBs change into EBs, rupturing the host cells' membranes and dispersing to infect more cells. Chlamydial infection is a common sexually transmitted disease that causes pelvic inflammatory disease and sterility in women. Infants born to infected mothers may develop eye infections or pneumonia.
- Rickettsiae are tiny gram-negative bacteria that live inside a host cell (obligate intracellular parasites). They are transmitted by insect vectors, such as lice or ticks, and cause diseases such as typhus fever and Rocky Mountain spotted fever. They attack blood vessel walls, causing a typical rash and small hemorrhages.

TABLE 6-2 Comparison of Common Microorganisms

	Bacteria	Virus	Fungi	Protozoa	Mycoplasma
Cell wall	Yes	No	Yes	No	No
Obligate intracellular parasite	No	Yes	No	Some	No
DNA and RNA	Yes	No	Yes	Yes	Yes
Reproduction	Binary fission	Use host cell to replicate components and for assembly	Budding, and spores and extend hyphae	Varies	Binary fission
Drug used to treat	Antibacterial	Antiviral	Antifungal	Selective	Selective

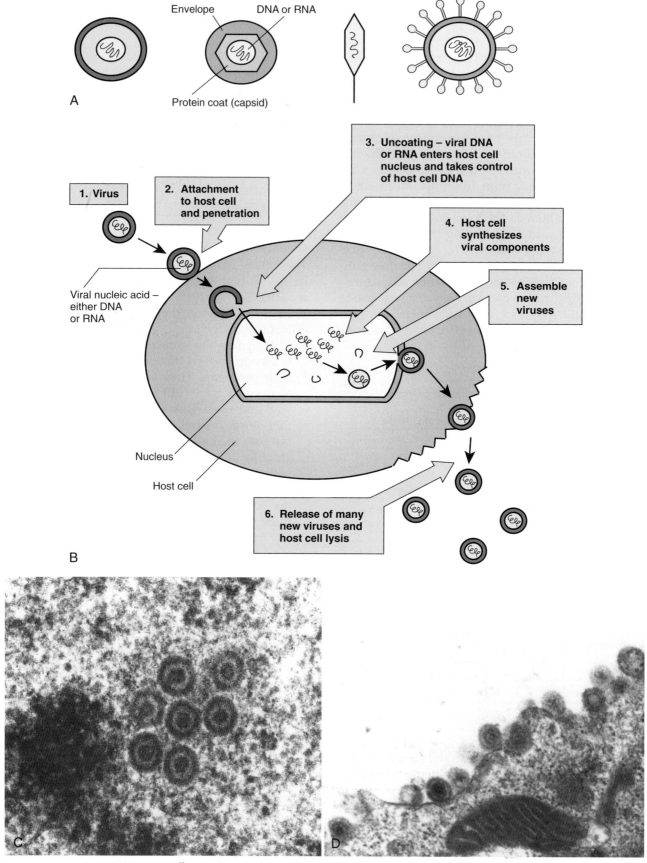

FIGURE 6-5 **A,** Different shapes of viruses. **B,** Viral replication. **C** and **D,** Herpesvirus particles and budding. Herpes simplex virus using electron microscopy; HSV consists of a core containing DNA in an icosahedral capsid surrounded by a granular zone, within an external envelope. The particles form in the host cell nucleus (Fig. 6-5C), but the envelope is acquired during budding through the host cell membrane (Fig. 6-5D). *(**C** and **D** from De la Maza LM, Pezzlo MT, Baron EJ: Color Atlas of Diagnostic Microbiology, St. Louis, 1997, Mosby.)*

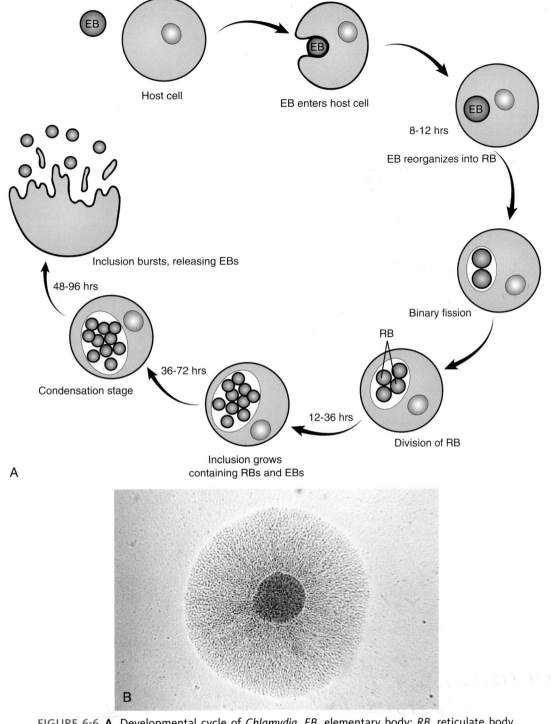

Host cell

EB enters host cell

8-12 hrs

EB reorganizes into RB

Binary fission

RB

Division of RB

12-36 hrs

Inclusion grows
containing RBs and EBs

Condensation stage

36-72 hrs

48-96 hrs

Inclusion bursts, releasing EBs

A

B

FIGURE 6-6 A, Developmental cycle of *Chlamydia. EB,* elementary body; *RB,* reticulate body. *(From Stepp CA, Woods M:* Laboratory Procedures for Medical Office Personnel, *Philadelphia, 1998, WB Saunders.)* **B,** *Mycoplasma. Mycoplasma hominis* colonies viewed through a light microscope. Mycoplasmas are the smallest free-living organisms. Unlike bacteria they lack a cell wall and behave as parasites on the surface of the host cells but are not intracellular. Complex media and tissue culture techniques are used for their isolation. *(From De la Maza LM, Pezzlo MT, Baron EJ:* Color Atlas of Diagnostic Microbiology, *St. Louis, 1997, Mosby.)*

- Mycoplasmal infection is a common cause of pneumonia (Fig. 6-6*B*) (see Chapter 13). These microbes lack cell walls—therefore are not affected by many antimicrobial drugs—and they can appear in many shapes. They are the smallest cellular microbe.

Fungi

Fungi are found everywhere, on animals, plants, humans, and foods. Growth of various types of fungi can be observed easily on cheese, fruit, or bread. They are often found on dead organic material such as plants.

Fungal or mycotic infection results from single-celled yeasts or multicellular molds. These organisms are classified as eukaryotic and consist of single cells or chains of cells, which can form a variety of structures (see Fig. 6-1). Fungal growth is promoted by warmth and moisture. Fungi are frequently considered beneficial because they are important in the production of yogurt, beer, and other foods, as well as serving as a source of antibiotic drugs.

The long filaments or strands of a fungus are hyphae, which intertwine to form a mass called the mycelium, the visible mass. Fungi reproduce by budding, extension of the hyphae, or producing various types of spores. Spores can spread easily through the air and are resistant to temperature change and chemicals. Inhaled spores can stimulate an allergic reaction in humans.

Only a few fungi are pathogenic, causing infection on the skin or mucous membranes. Infections such as *tinea pedis* (athlete's foot) result from the fungus invading the superficial layers of the skin. *Tinea pedis* infection is often transmitted in public pools, showers, or gymnasiums.

Candida is a harmless fungus normally present on the skin (Fig. 6-7). However, it may cause infection in the oral cavity (see Fig. 17-5*B*), sometimes called thrush in infants, and is a common cause of vaginal infection. In immunodeficient individuals, *Candida* frequently becomes opportunistic, causing extensive chronic infection (see Fig. 7-17*C*) and perhaps spreading to cause serious systemic infection. *Histoplasma* is a fungus causing a lung infection that may become disseminated through the body in immunosuppressed patients. Histoplasmosis is transmitted by inhaling contaminated dust or soil particles.

It is not always easy to clearly classify microorganisms because microbes may demonstrate characteristics of more than one group. For example, *Pneumocystis carinii*, an opportunist causing pneumonia, has some characteristics of fungi and some of protozoa. It was once considered a fungus, then a protozoon, but now may be classified as a fungus again (see Fig. 7-17*A*).

Protozoa

Protozoa are eukaryotic or more complex organisms. They are unicellular, motile, and lack a cell wall, but occur in a number of shapes, sometimes within the life cycle of a single type. Many live independently, some

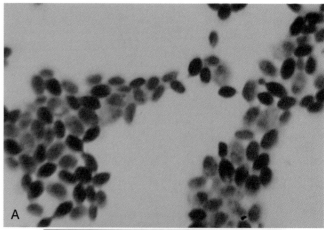

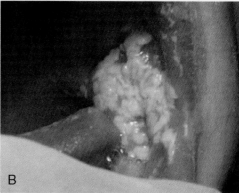

FIGURE 6-7 Thrush. **A,** Micrograph of the fungus *Candida albicans* in the yeast form (this fungus can also form filamentous mycelia) that is responsible for an oral infection called *thrush. Candida albicans* can also cause vaginal infections in women. **B,** Oral candidiasis illustrating the white plaques. (**A,** *from VanMeter K, Hubert R:* Microbiology for the Healthcare Professional, *St. Louis, 2010, Mosby.* **B,** *From Zitelli BJ, Davis HW:* Atlas of pediatric physical Diagnosis, *ed 4. St. Louis, 2002, Mosby.)*

live on dead organic matter, and others are parasites living in or on another living host. As in other microbial classifications, protozoa are divided into a number of subcategories.

The pathogens are usually parasites. Some diseases caused by protozoan infection include trichomoniasis, malaria, and amebic dysentery.

Trichomonas vaginalis is distinguished by its flagella (Fig. 6-8*A*). It causes a sexually transmitted infection of the reproductive tracts of men and women, attaching to the mucous membranes and causing inflammation (see Chapter 19).

The causative agents for malaria, the *Plasmodium* species, belong to a group of nonmotile protozoa called sporozoa. *Plasmodium vivax* is found in temperate climates such as the southern United States (Fig. 6-8*B*). Clinically these microbes are found in the red blood cells, where they undergo several stages in their life cycle. The red blood cells become large and eventually rupture and release new microbes and toxins into the blood, causing acute illness. The microbe is transmitted

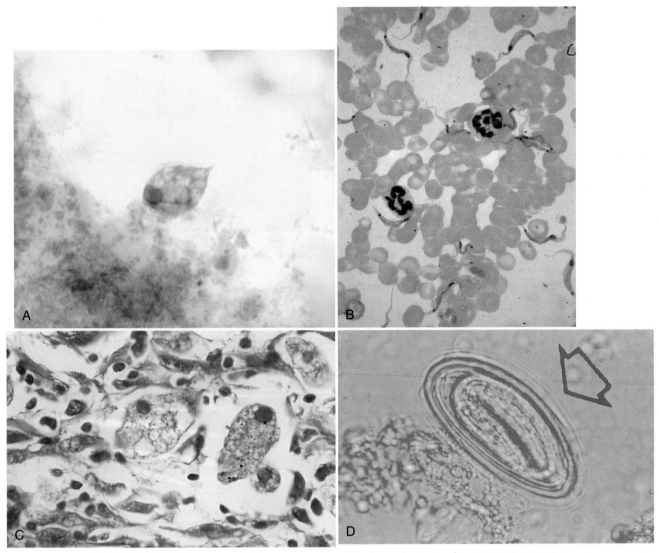

FIGURE 6-8 **A**, Trichomonas. **B**, Trypanosoma in a blood sample. **C**, Ameba. **D**, Pinworm ova in a fecal smear. *(A from De la Maza LM, Pezzlo MT, Baron EJ: Color Atlas of Diagnostic Microbiology. St Louis, Mosby, 1997; B From VanMeter K, Hubert R: Microbiology for the Healthcare Professional, ed 1, St. Louis, 2010, Mosby. C from Cotran RS, Kumar V, Collins T: Robbins Pathologic Basis of Disease, 6th ed. Philadelphia, WB Saunders, 1999; D from Stepp CA, Woods M: Laboratory Procedures for Medical Office Personnel. Philadelphia, 1998, WB Saunders.)*

by a blood-sucking insect, the female *Anopheles* mosquito. One form of malarial parasite, *Plasmodium falciparum*, is extremely virulent and has become resistant to almost all antimalarial drugs. It is expected that global warming will put more of the world's population at risk of malaria in the future as the *Anopheles* mosquito extends its range and infects nonimmune individuals.

The *amebas* are a motile group of protozoa, moving by extending part of their cytoplasm and flowing forward (ameboid movement). They engulf food in the same manner. The important pathogen in this group is *Entamoeba histolytica*, a parasite in the large intestine that causes amebic dysentery, a severe form of diarrhea, and liver abscesses if it penetrates into the portal circulation (Fig. 6-8C). These organisms exist in two forms. One

form is actively pathogenic and is termed the *trophozoite*. Trophozoites secrete proteolytic enzymes, which break down the intestinal mucosa, causing flask-shaped ulcers. Trophozoites may invade blood vessels and spread to other organs, such as the liver. The organism also forms *cysts*, which are resistant to environmental conditions and are excreted in feces. *Entamoeba histolytica* infection is spread by the fecal-oral route. Although the infection is more common in less developed areas of the world, people may become infected and transmit the infection to family members and associates if proper handwashing is not employed. Simple treatment of water with chlorine or other halogens does not destroy the cysts; filtration and/or boiling of water are necessary to prevent infection when water has been fecally contaminated.

Other Agents of Disease

Helminths

Helminths or worms are not microorganisms, but are often included with microbes because they are parasites and cause infections in humans throughout the world. They are multicellular, eukaryotic organisms that are divided into many subgroups, depending on their physical characteristics. They may be very small, barely visible, or up to 1 meter in length. Their life cycle consists of at least three stages, ovum (egg), larva, and adult. The ova or larvae may be ingested in contaminated food or water, or may enter through the skin or be transmitted by infected insects. They are often found in the intestine but can inhabit the lung or blood vessels during parts of their life cycle.

Helminths are usually diagnosed by observation of ova or eggs in stool specimens (Fig. 6-8D). Helminth infections are more commonly found in young children and in North America include pinworms (Fig. 6-9), hookworms, tapeworms (Fig. 6-10), and *Ascaris* or giant roundworms. When large numbers of worms are present in the body, systemic effects may develop, such as severe anemia.

Prions

Prions are protein-like agents that are transmitted by consumption of contaminated tissues such as muscle or the use of donor tissues contaminated with the protein. There is a great deal that is not known about prion disorders and some researchers question whether prions are actually the agent of diseases. The following information is from current publications of the Centers for Disease Control and Prevention (CDC).

A prion is an abnormal molecule that is transmissible in tissues or blood of animals or humans. It induces proteins within the brain of the recipient to undergo abnormal folding and change of shape. This renders the protein molecule non-functional and causes degenerative disease of the nervous system. Prion diseases in humans include Creutzfeldt-Jakob disease and variant Creutzfeldt-Jakob disease (see Chapter 14). These are rapidly progressive and fatal. It is thought that variant Creutzfeldt-Jakob disease is caused by consumption of meat that has been contaminated with nervous tissue from an infected animal such as beef cattle. In areas where bovine spongiform encephalopathy (BSE), the animal prion infection, is prevalent, consumption of ground meats, sausages, or offal should be avoided.

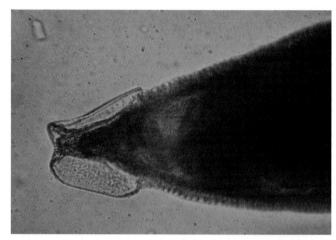

FIGURE 6-9 Pinworm. This micrograph shows the mouth structure of the pinworm *Enterobius vermicularis*, which causes the disease enterobiasis. (*From VanMeter K, Hubert R:* Microbiology for the Healthcare Professional, *St. Louis, 2010, Mosby.*)

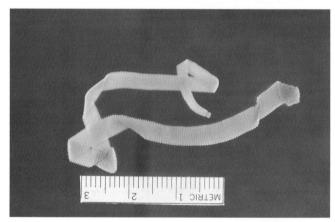

FIGURE 6-10 Tapeworm. Two main features of the tapeworm are the scolex, which has muscular suckers surrounded by hooks for attachment, and the individual body segments called *proglottids*. (*From VanMeter K, Hubert R:* Microbiology for the Healthcare Professional, *St. Louis, 2010, Mosby.*)

Algae

Algae are eukaryotic microorganisms widespread in fresh and marine waters; they are a main component of plankton and are usually not a concern for human disease. Medical concerns involving algae include: human consumption of marine animals that have fed on algae and accumulated toxins produced by the algae and recent disorders attributed to the algae *Pfiesteria piscicida*.

Resident Flora (Indigenous Normal Flora, Resident Microbiota)

Many areas of the body, such as the skin, nasal cavity, and mouth, have a resident population of mixed microorganisms, primarily bacteria. Different sites host different species. For example, streptococci, *Haemophilus*, and

TABLE 6-3	Location of Resident Flora
Resident Flora Present	Sterile Area
Skin	Blood, cerebrospinal fluid
Nose, pharynx	Lungs
Mouth, colon, rectum	
Vagina	Uterus, fallopian tubes, ovary
Distal urethra and perineum	Bladder and kidney

staphylococci are a few of the microbes found in the upper respiratory tract; staphylococcus and *Candida*, among others, occur on the skin. Some areas of the body such as the lungs, bladder, and kidneys lack resident flora or are sterile under normal circumstances, and properly obtained specimens from these areas should not contain microorganisms (Table 6-3).

Certain microbes in the intestinal tract are of great benefit to the host in the synthesis of vitamin K and in some digestive processes. These microbes are not pathogenic under normal circumstances but may cause disease if they are transferred to another location in the body, or if the balance among the species is not maintained (e.g., one variety becomes dominant), or if the body's defenses are impaired (e.g., in immunodeficiency states). Such infections are termed *opportunistic*.

Resident flora are usually helpful in preventing other organisms from establishing a colony. For example, some antibacterial drugs intended to treat infection elsewhere in the body, will destroy part of the normal flora in the intestine, thus allowing for an imbalance in growth there or invasion by other microbes, causing opportunistic infection and diarrhea.

Principles of Infection

An infection occurs when a microbe or parasite is able to reproduce in or on the body's tissues. Infectious diseases may occur sporadically in single individuals, localized groups, and epidemics or worldwide pandemics. Certain infections are endemic to an area, consistently occurring in that population. Others may occur outside their normal geographic range or in higher than expected numbers; these infections are referred to as epidemics. Knowledge of the modes of transmission of microorganisms and methods of control is essential for the prevention and control of infection within the community.

Transmission of Infectious Agents

A chain of events occurs during the transmission of infecting organisms from one person to another (Fig. 6-11). The *reservoir*, or source of infection, may be a person with an obvious active infection in an acute stage, or a person who is asymptomatic and shows no clinical signs or symptoms. The latter may be in the early incubation stage of infection, or the person may be a *carrier* of the organism and never develop infection. Hepatitis B is an example of an infection that is often transmitted by unknown carriers or persons who have a *subclinical* form of infection that is very mild, with few or no manifestations. The reservoir also may be an animal or contaminated water, soil, food, or equipment.

The mode of transmission from the reservoir to the new host may be:

- *Direct* contact with no intermediary, such as touching an infectious lesion or sexual intercourse. Microbes may be in the blood, body secretions, or a lesion. Not all microorganisms can cross the blood-brain barrier or placental barriers. However, some microbes that can cross the placenta have serious effects on fetal development and health. *Treponema pallidum*, the cause of syphilis, can lead to multiple defects or death in the fetus, and *Toxoplasma gondii*, the cause of toxoplasmosis, results in many neurologic deficits.
- *Indirect* contact involving an intermediary such as a contaminated hand or food, or a *fomite*, an inanimate object such as instruments or bed linen that carries organisms. In some cases, there are several stages in transmission. For example, shellfish can be contaminated by human feces in the water. The microorganisms in the shellfish are then ingested and cause infection in another human.
- *Droplet* transmission (oral or respiratory) occurring when respiratory or salivary secretions containing pathogens such as tuberculosis bacteria are expelled from the body. The organisms from these secretions may be inhaled directly by another person close by or fall on nearby objects to be transmitted indirectly.
- *Aerosol* transmission involving small particles from the respiratory tract that remain suspended in the air and travel on air currents, infecting any new host who inhales the particles.
- *Vector*-borne, when an insect or animal serves as an intermediary host in a disease such as malaria.

Hands are considered a major culprit in spreading infection from many sources, in health care facilities, the home, office, or school. Frequent, proper handwashing is essential in infection control and has been shown to be the most commonly ignored procedure in maintaining personal and public health.

Nosocomial infections are infections that occur in health care facilities, including hospitals, nursing homes, doctors' offices, and dental offices. The CDC estimates that 10% to 15% of patients acquire an infection in the hospital. Reasons for these infections include the presence of many microorganisms in these settings, patients with contagious diseases, overcrowding, use of contaminated instruments, immunocompromised and weakened patients, the chain of transmission through staff, diagnostic procedures, and equipment, therapeutic aids, and food trays. Also, many microbes in health

SOURCE

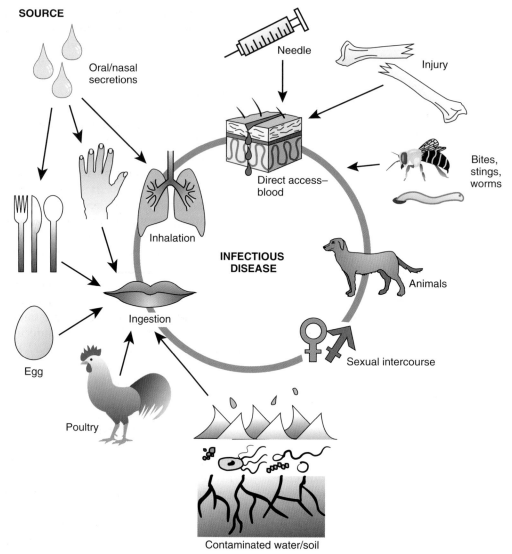

FIGURE 6-11 Transmission of infectious agents.

care settings are resistant to several drugs. Common nosocomial infections include urinary tract infections (the highest number), pneumonia, diarrhea, and surgical wound infection. Most infections in health care facilities are spread by direct contact between persons or contaminated objects. Recently there have been several outbreaks of infection in hospitals by a more dangerous strain of the bacterium, *Clostridium difficile* (c-diff), particularly in intensive care units where most individuals are taking antimicrobial drugs. The resulting disruption of normal flora allows *C. difficile* to multiply and cause severe diarrhea and many deaths. Methicillin-resistant *Staphylococcus aureus* (MRSA) infections are also increasingly seen as a source of nosocomial infection that is very challenging to treat (this is in the community, not just the hospital). The importance of obtaining a complete and accurate health history with respect to hospitalization and prior infections cannot be overstated.

Host Resistance

The healthy individual is quite resistant to infection. With some infections, such as tuberculosis, host resistance is a primary factor in determining the risk of active infection following exposure (Box 6-1).

Interferons are proteins produced by human host cells in response to viral invasion of the cell. These interferons then influence the activity of nearby host cells, increasing their resistance to viral invasion and interfering with viral replication. Interferons also stimulate the immune system and are used in cancer treatment for this reason. Unfortunately, they have not proved to be as beneficial in the widespread treatment of cancer or other immune-based diseases as expected.

Factors that *decrease* host resistance include:
- Age (infants and the elderly)
- Genetic susceptibility
- Immunodeficiency of any type
- Malnutrition

BOX 6-1	**Host Resistance and Microbial Virulence**
Host Resistance	**Increased Microbial Virulence**
Intact skin and mucous membrane	Production of exotoxins and endotoxins
Body secretions—stomach acid, tears	Production of destructive enzymes
Nonspecific phagocytosis	Spore formation
Effective inflammatory response	Entry of large number of organisms into body
Absence of disease	Presence of bacterial capsule and pili
Effective immune system	
Interferon production (virus)	

- Chronic disease, including cardiovascular disease, cancer, and diabetes
- Severe physical or emotional stress
- Inflammation or trauma affecting the integrity of the skin or mucosa, including burns, lack of protective secretions, bladder catheters, or other invasive procedures. Sometimes infection occurs easily because of a very small break in the skin or mucous membrane, or in an area of inflammation. As discussed in Chapter 5, the loss of skin and other defenses in a burn patient often results in secondary infection at the site.
- Impaired inflammatory response, for example, due to long-term glucocorticoid medication
- Severe or multiple infections are very common in homeless individuals, in whom multiple factors decrease host resistance. For example, poor nutrition, open lesions, inadequate hygiene, fatigue, lack of access to health care, and possible drug or alcohol abuse combine to create a high risk of infections such as tuberculosis.

Prophylactic antimicrobial medication may be required by any individuals with low resistance before exposure to possible infecting microbes, for example, before an invasive procedure.

Virulence and Pathogenicity of Microorganisms

Pathogenicity refers to the capacity of microbes to cause disease. Nonpathogens can become pathogens. When a member of the resident flora is introduced into another area of the body, it may become an opportunistic pathogen. For example, if *Escherichia coli* from the colon enter the urinary tract, they will cause infection. (This microbe is the most common cause of cystitis.)

Virulence is the degree of pathogenicity of a specific microbe, based on:
- Invasive qualities, allowing it to directly damage host cells and tissues and spread
- Toxic qualities, including production of enzymes, exotoxins, and endotoxins that damage host cells or interfere with a host function such as nerve conduction

- Adherence to tissue by pili, fimbriae, capsules, or specific membrane receptor sites. Certain organisms tend to establish infection in particular areas of the body, considered hospitable to that microbe; for example, streptococci are common in respiratory and ear infections.
- Ability to avoid host defenses (e.g., the presence of a capsule or mutation with altered antigenicity). Microorganisms undergo frequent mutation. Slight changes in the organism may occur spontaneously or in response to environmental conditions, including the presence of drugs. When bacteria or viruses mutate, antibodies that matched the earlier form are no longer effective, so the individual is no longer protected. Vaccines or drugs are unlikely to be effective against the new form. This is why a new influenza vaccine must be developed and administered each year.

Virulence is often expressed in the *case fatality rate*, the percentage of deaths occurring in the number of persons who develop the disease. In parasitic infections host resistance and the ability of a microbe to cause disease often coexist in a delicate balance.

New Issues Affecting Infections and Transmission

There has been increasing concern and fear about new emerging diseases and "superbugs," microbes that have caused very serious illness in otherwise healthy individuals or do not respond to any drugs. Emerging infectious diseases are identified by a new or unique set of signs or symptoms, or by increased spread. Careful monitoring and collection of data are essential to identify new threats so that preventive measures may be put in place. The severe acute respiratory syndrome (SARS) epidemic in the Toronto area was well established before information about cases occurring in travelers from Southeast Asia was received. In some cases the incubation period is so short that it is difficult to prevent an epidemic even if health statistics are collected, for example, in cholera infections. In such situations the focus must be on preventing the spread of infection to the wider community. Increased global travel, changing environments and global weather patterns, and changes in food and water supplies are some of the factors leading to altered disease patterns. Epidemiologists at the CDC, World Health Organization (WHO), as well as a greater number of local agencies collect and analyze reports on new diseases and other trends. They also update the list of notifiable diseases, approximately 60 diseases that must be reported to public health agencies. The CDC reports are published in *Morbidity and Mortality Weekly Report.* The United Nations (UN) has also assumed a role in a number of global issues related to infectious diseases such as AIDS, tuberculosis, and malaria.

Following the SARS threat (see Chapter 13) in 2003, these agencies cooperated to quickly identify a previously unknown microbe, a coronavirus, and work on controlling the spread of the infection. As more deaths occurred and a second wave of infection developed, they were able to identify factors in the transmission of the virus.

The CDC and WHO have published guidelines for health care facilities to manage the screening procedures, rapid containment, and treatment of serious infectious diseases that may lead to a pandemic. These measures have proved effective in several recent outbreaks, such as the influenza A H1N1 outbreak in Mexico in 2009. Precautions were instituted in several countries, and at the time of writing these precautions appear to have been successful in preventing a full-blown pandemic. Health care workers in all settings were required to screen clients and put respiratory precautions in place for those who were symptomatic.

In some cases, organisms such as the Ebola virus are spreading and have become highly virulent and have the power to cause serious infection, even in a healthy host. At this time, there are no drugs available to control this and related viral infections. Certain strains of a common microorganism, such as E. coli, a normal part of resident intestinal flora, have suddenly developed new strains that have caused life-threatening infections. The so-called flesh-eating bacteria are specific strains of a beta-hemolytic streptococcus that are highly invasive, secreting proteases, enzymes that break down tissue, resulting in the life-threatening disease necrotizing fasciitis. These bacteria also produce a toxin-causing shock.

The effectiveness of immunizations over long time periods is difficult to assess. It appears that some vaccines are losing their protective qualities over time. The increasing incidence of pertussis (whooping cough), mumps, and measles appears related to decreasing immunity from vaccines given in childhood. This indicates a need for booster immunization and the importance of continued monitoring of all infectious diseases, including those in which routine immunizations are in place. Many jurisdictions now offer re-immunization with MMR vaccine in the teen years. The recommended immunization schedules for children 0 to 6 and 7 to 18 as well as a catch-up schedule are updated regularly and approved by the American Academy of Pediatrics, the Advisory Committee on Immunization Practices of the CDC, and the American Academy of Family Physicians.

The other issue to be addressed is the increasing number of microbes that are resistant to several drug groups, thus making infection control much more difficult. The multi-drug resistant microbes include strains of *Mycobacterium tuberculosis*, *Plasmodium falciparum*, *Streptococcus pneumoniae*, *Haemophilus influenzae*, *Staphylococcus aureus*, and *Neisseria gonorrhoeae*. Currently there is much more emphasis on reduced use of antibacterial drugs to treat minor infections or as prophylactics to lessen the problem. It is important for health care workers to remain up to date on current recommendations about infection control measures in their scope of practice.

Control of Transmission and Infection

Isolation of infected persons is rarely carried out on a large scale, and there are fewer diseases that must be reported to government bodies. It is not feasible to test every client or patient for the presence of infection before initiating care. Therefore infection control, understanding the transmission, and breaking the chain of infection (Fig. 6-12) become much more important, particularly to health professionals, who must protect themselves, their families, and the community as well as their patients.

Universal precautions provide the basic guidelines by which all blood, body fluids, and wastes are considered "infected" in *any* client regardless of the client's apparent condition. There are two levels, one general for all individuals, and one specific to known infections at specific sites in the body, for example, the intestines. Gloves and appropriate protective apparel are then used to reduce the transmission of organisms in either direction, that is, from patient to caregiver and from caregiver to patient. Guidelines have been established for the disposal of such potentially dangerous items as needles, tissue, and waste materials. The CDC can be consulted for appropriate and up-to-date information.

To break the cycle and minimize the risk of infection:
- The reservoir or sources of infection must be located and removed. *Sources and contacts* must be identified in some situations, especially when asymptomatic carriers may be involved, or when travelers may be infected:
  - *Contaminated food or water or carrier food handlers* should be identified to prevent continued transmission or epidemics of infectious disease. As a precaution, some institutions test stool specimens from food handlers so as to identify carriers. Some intestinal pathogens can survive in feces outside the body for long periods of time and increase the risk of contaminating food or water.
  - In some cases, infection can be transmitted before clinical signs are evident in the infected person, and this permits widespread contamination if the incubation period is prolonged. For example, there is a prolonged "window" of time before hepatitis or human immunodeficiency virus (HIV) infection can be identified in persons. In institutions, infection such as Hepatitis A can spread very rapidly, particularly when the patient's health status is already compromised.
  - Infected travelers should refrain from travel to prevent spreading infectious diseases into new areas, and travelers who become ill should seek prompt health care and share their specific travel history with health care workers.

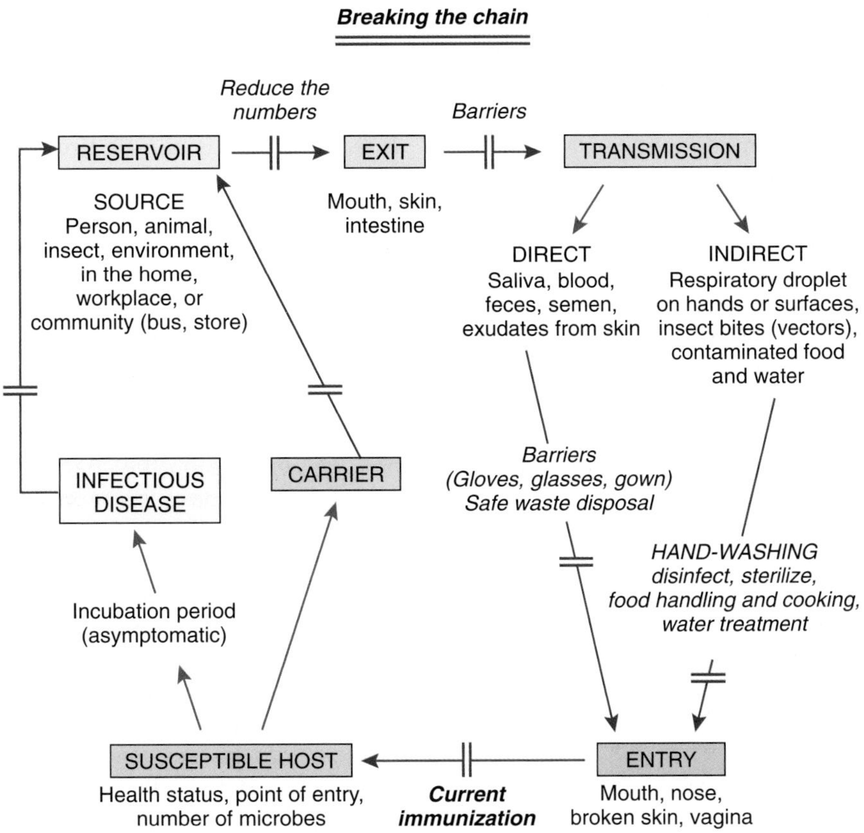

Breaking the chain

FIGURE 6-12 Infection cycle and breaking the chain.

- The portal of exit (secretions, e.g., blood, saliva, urine) of microbes from the reservoir should be blocked. This includes minimizing the effects of coughing and sneezing when the infected person is in close contact with other people. However, it is now evident that contaminated oral and nasal secretions are more dangerous when they are on the hands or on tissues than when they are airborne, so proper disposal of contaminated items is essential. It is advisable for anyone with or without an infection to use general universal precautions to prevent transmission by body fluids.
- Knowledge of the mode (droplet, fecal-oral) or modes of transmission of specific infections is essential to block transmission. Precautions must be undertaken in a prescribed manner; for example, the use of appropriate condoms following recommended guidelines is essential to prevent the spread of sexually transmitted disease during intimate sexual activity. Using disposable equipment, proper sterilization and cleaning, good ventilation, and frequent handwashing are some ways to reduce transmission:
  - Portals of entry and exit should be blocked by covering the nose and mouth with a mask and placing barriers over breaks in the skin or mucous membranes.

- Reduce host susceptibility (increase host resistance) by maintaining immunizations and boosters according to guidelines. Proper nutrition to maintain skin and mucous membranes is also essential in reducing host susceptibility.

Additional techniques to reduce transmission include:
1. Adequate cleaning of surroundings and clothing.
2. Sterilization of fomites by exposure to heat using several methods, such as autoclaving. Time, packaging, and temperature are critical to success. Moist heat is preferable, because it penetrates more efficiently and can destroy microbes at lower temperatures. Incineration (burning) and autoclaving are also effective methods of destroying microbes in waste.
3. Disinfectants are chemical solutions that are known to destroy microorganisms or their toxins on inanimate objects. The literature on these solutions must be carefully checked to determine the limitations of the specific chemicals as well as the instructions for use. For example, few chemicals destroy spores. Adequate exposure time and concentration of the chemical are required to kill some viruses, such as hepatitis B. Other potential problems include inactivation of some chemicals by soap or protein (mucus, blood) or damage to metals or latex materials on instruments by the disinfectant. One of the more effective

disinfectants at present is *glutaraldehyde.* Flushing certain equipment and tubing (e.g., in a dental office), with disinfectant and water is a recommended daily activity.

4. Antiseptics are chemicals applied to the body that do not usually cause tissue damage, such as isopropyl alcohol-70%, which is the active ingredient in hand sanitizers. The chemical affects only surface organisms and does not penetrate crevices. Antiseptics reduce the number of organisms in an area but do not destroy all of them. Also, they may be diluted or removed quickly by body secretions. Some antiseptics, such as iodine compounds, may cause allergic reactions in some individuals.

THINK ABOUT 6-3

a. Explain why, when using an antiseptic, killing all the bacteria may not be the desired result.
b. Given that every client cannot be fully screened for infections, what precautions are essential to limit the transmission of microbes that are agents of disease? Relate your answer to your specific scope of practice.

Physiology of Infection

Onset and Development

Infectious agents can be present in the body for some time before any clinical signs are apparent. The microorganisms must gain entry to the body, choose a hospitable site, establish a colony, and begin reproducing (Fig. 6-13). Only if the host defenses are insufficient to destroy all the pathogens during this process will infection be established.

The *incubation period* refers to the time between entry of the organism into the body and appearance of clinical signs of the disease. Incubation periods vary considerably, depending on the characteristics of the organism, and may last days or months. During this time the organisms reproduce until there are sufficient numbers to cause adverse effects in the body.

The *prodromal period,* which is more evident in some infections than others, follows. This is the time when the infected person may feel fatigued, lose appetite, or have a headache, and usually senses that "I am coming down with something."

Next comes the *acute period,* when the infectious disease develops fully, and the clinical manifestations

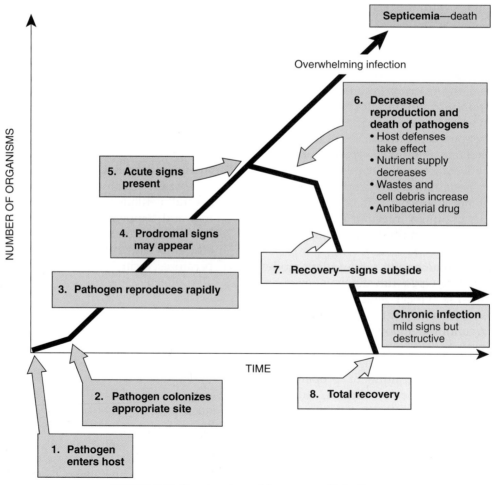

FIGURE 6-13 Onset and possible courses of infection.

reach a peak. The *onset* of a specific infection may be insidious with a prolonged prodromal period, or sudden or acute with the clinical signs appearing quickly with severe manifestations.

The length of the acute period depends on the virulence of the particular pathogen and host resistance. In many cases the acute period ends when host resistance, perhaps the immune system, becomes effective at destroying the pathogen. It may end when sufficient nutrients for the numbers of microbes decline, or when they are affected by wastes from dead organisms and necrotic tissue, thus decreasing their reproductive rate. The acute phase is followed by the recovery or convalescent period, when signs subside and body processes return to normal.

Patterns of Infection

Infections have varied patterns as defined by their characteristics and/or location.

- Local infections—organism enters the body and remains confined to a specific location
- Focal infections—pathogen spreads from a local infection to other tissues
- Systemic infections—infection spreads to several sites and tissue fluids, typically through the circulatory system
  - Septicemia—caused by multiplication of pathogens in the blood. This condition is the cause of sepsis, a toxic inflammatory condition arising from the spread of microbes
  - Bacteremia—presence of bacteria in the blood
  - Toxemia—presence of toxins in the blood
  - Viremia—presence of viruses in the blood
- Mixed Infections—several infectious agents concurrently establish themselves at the same site
- Acute infections—appear rapidly with severe symptoms but are short lived
- Chronic infections—less severe symptoms than acute but persist for a long period
- Primary infections—initial infection followed by complications caused by another microbe
- Secondary infections—follows a primary infection and is caused by a microbe other than that causing the primary infection. Opportunistic pathogens are often the cause of a secondary infection.
- Subclinical infections—does not cause and apparent signs or symptoms, although it may persist over long periods of time.

THINK ABOUT 6-4

a. Compare the prodromal period with the acute period of infection, using your own experience as an example (perhaps the last time you had a cold).
b. Compare subclinical infection and chronic infection.
c. Explain three reasons why infection may not occur after microbes enter the body.

Signs and Symptoms of Infection

Local Signs

The local signs of infection are usually those of inflammation: pain or tenderness, swelling, redness, and warmth (Fig. 6-14). If the infection is caused by bacteria, a purulent exudate, or pus, is usually present, whereas a viral infection results in serous, clear exudates. The color and other characteristics of the exudates and tissue may help to identify the microorganism. Figure 5-13 illustrates infection of a burn wound by two different microorganisms. Tissue necrosis at the site is likely as well. Lymphadenopathy occurs and is manifest by swollen and tender lymph nodes (Table 6-4).

Other local signs depend on the site of infection. For instance, in the respiratory tract, local signs probably include coughing or sneezing and difficulty in breathing. In the digestive tract, local signs might include vomiting or diarrhea.

Systemic Signs

Systemic signs include signs and symptoms common to significant infections in any area of the body. Fever, fatigue and weakness, headache, and nausea are all commonly associated with infection. The characteristics of *fever (pyrexia)* may vary with the causative organism. The body temperature may be very high or spiking and

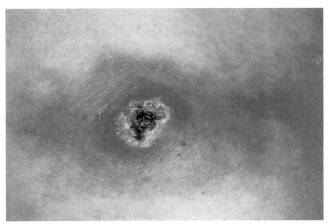

FIGURE 6-14 Staphylococcus abscess. *(From Braverman IM: Skin Signs of Systemic Disease, ed 3, Philadelphia, 1998, Saunders.)*

TABLE 6-4 Local and Systemic Signs of Bacterial Infection

Local Signs	Systemic Signs
Swelling	Fever
Erythema (redness)	Leukocytosis
Pain and tenderness	Elevated ESR
Lymphadenopathy	Fatigue, weakness, anorexia
Exudate, purulent	Headache, arthralgia

ESR, erythrocyte sedimentation rate.

may be accompanied by chills (see Chapter 5), or it may be elevated only slightly. In some viral infections the temperature is subnormal. With severe infection the nervous system may be affected, resulting in confusion or disorientation, seizures (convulsions), or loss of consciousness.

THINK ABOUT 6-5

List three local signs of infection and three systemic signs and explain what is causing these signs.

Methods of Diagnosis

Organisms can be identified by *culture and staining* techniques, using specific specimens such as sputum in patients in whom tuberculosis is suspected. It is important that specimens be procured carefully and examined quickly to achieve an accurate result. Many organisms can be grown easily on specific culture media in the laboratory, whereas other organisms such as viruses require a living host. Blood cultures may be examined to check the distribution or possible spread of the infecting agent. Frequently drug sensitivity tests, such as the Kirby Bauer method (Disc Diffusion Method) and the Minimum Inhibitory Concentration (MIC) method (Fig. 6-15), are also instituted. Drug therapy is often ordered immediately based on preliminary data and knowledge of the common infections occurring at the particular site, but it is helpful to establish the most effective therapy as soon as possible, particularly if there may be serious consequences to continued infection. Any test that calls for a culture requires several days.

- *Blood tests,* particularly variations in the numbers of leukocytes, are another general indicator of infection. With bacterial infections, leukocytosis, or an increase in white blood cells, is common, whereas viral infections often cause leukopenia, a reduction in the number of leukocytes in the blood. Changes in the distribution of types of leukocytes occur as well (differential count), depending on the organism, for example, monocytosis or neutropenia. Neutrophils tend to increase with acute infections, but lymphocytes and monocytes increase with chronic infection. C-reactive protein and erythrocyte sedimentation rate are usually elevated and are a general indicator of inflammation (see Chapter 5).

Blood tests also are useful in detecting antibodies and confirming a diagnosis, particularly in the case of viral infection. None of these factors by themselves provides a diagnosis, but they contribute to a final diagnosis. In hepatitis B infections, such tests can also be used to monitor the course of the infection because different antibodies form at various points in the course of this infection.

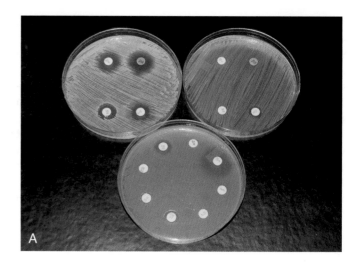

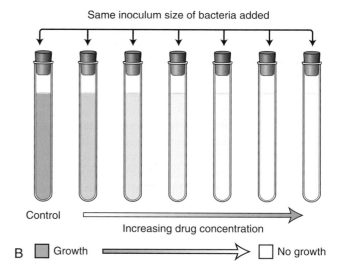

FIGURE 6-15 **A,** Disk diffusion (Kirby-Bauer method). The clear areas surrounding the antibiotic disks are called the *zones of inhibition.* The size of these zones can be used to determine the effectiveness of the antibiotic against the selected bacterium. **B,** Minimal inhibitory concentration. The minimal inhibitory concentration (MIC) for a specific agent is indicated by the absence of growth in the tube containing the lowest drug concentration. *(From VanMeter K, Hubert R:* Microbiology for the Healthcare Professional, *St. Louis, 2010, Mosby.)*

- In addition, *radiologic* examination may be used to identify the site of the infection and may assist in the identification of the agent. For example, lung congestion localized in one lobe (consolidation) usually indicates pneumococcal pneumonia.

Treatment and Antimicrobial Drugs

Guidelines for Use

It is not always necessary to use drugs to treat an infection because the body's normal defenses are often adequate to limit the infection. Also the usual growth pattern of the microbes is self-limiting as the colony uses up nutrients and produces more wastes. Current guidelines attempt to limit the use of antimicrobial drug so that the development of drug resistance can be reduced.

Increased use of antimicrobials has resulted in resistance of many organisms to certain drugs. Through mutations, *drug resistance* has developed in several ways as some bacteria have had changes in their metabolism allowing them to block drug action.

Improper use of an antibiotic can allow resistant organisms to dominate an infection that may have had very few resistant organisms at the onset. Improper use may result in an inadequate concentration of the drug being in contact for too short a time to be effective on all the organisms. In this case the weaker organisms will be killed, whereas stronger organisms with resistance mutations will survive, thrive and eventually dominate the infection.

Antimicrobial drugs may be administered prophylactically, before any invasive procedure, in high-risk clients (e.g., immunosuppressed patients). In treating an acute infection, frequently a *loading* or larger dose is administered initially to achieve effective blood levels quickly; this is often paired with a shorter duration of treatment.

Guidelines for effective drug therapy include:
1. The drug should be taken at regular, evenly spaced intervals over 24 hours to maintain blood levels that are adequate to control and destroy the organisms.
2. Antimicrobial drugs should be taken until the prescribed medication is completely used (usually 5 to 10 days), even if the symptoms have subsided, to ensure that the infection is completely eradicated and prevent the development of resistant organisms.
3. It is important to follow directions for administration with respect to food or fluid intake because drugs may be inactivated or drug absorption impaired if consumed with certain foods.
4. It is best to identify the specific organism and choose the most effective antibiotic that has the least effect on resident flora and human tissue.
5. Because many individuals have drug allergies, obtaining a complete drug history is essential, keeping in mind that an allergy usually includes all members of the chemically related drug group.
6. In viral infections, antiviral agents do not destroy the virus but merely inhibit its reproduction, providing an opportunity for host defenses to remove the virus. Antibacterial agents (antibiotics) are *not* effective against viruses. Antibacterials block synthesis of a bacterial cell wall or interfere with bacterial metabolism, but because viruses lack these components, antibacterials have no effect on them. Antibacterial drugs may be given in viral infection to reduce the risk of secondary bacterial infection in particularly vulnerable clients, but this is not a common practice. Use of an antimicrobial drug for a viral illness such as the common cold usually makes the person feel worse without any benefit.

Classification

Antimicrobials may be grouped in many ways in addition to their chemical classification. This section provides an overview of their classification, but a pharmacology reference should be consulted for details.
- *Antibiotic* is an older term and can be misleading. *Antibiotics* are drugs derived from organisms, such as penicillin from mold. Now many drugs are synthetic.
- *Antimicrobials* may be classified by the type of microbe against which the drug is active, such as antibacterials, antivirals, and antifungals. These drugs are unique to the type of organism and are not interchangeable.
- *Bactericidal* refers to drugs that destroy organisms, whereas *bacteriostatic* applies to drugs that decrease the microbe's rate of reproduction and rely on the host's defenses to destroy the organisms.
- *Broad spectrum* refers to antibacterials that are effective against both gram-negative and gram-positive organisms; *narrow spectrum* agents act against either gram-negative or gram-positive organisms, but not both. Narrow spectrum drugs are often preferred because they are less likely to upset the balance of resident flora in the body, which may result in an overgrowth of one organism and secondary or *superinfection.* For example, after a prolonged course of tetracycline, clients may develop a fungal (*Candida*) infection in the mouth, and women may develop vaginal candidiasis.
- The terms *first-generation and second-generation* drug now appear in texts, first generation referring to the original drug class, second generation referring to a later, improved version of the same drug group.

Mode of Action

Most antibacterial drugs may act in one of four ways:
1. Interference with bacterial cell wall synthesis is a bactericidal mechanism and is seen in drugs such as penicillin (see Fig. 6-3). Large doses of such drugs are usually safe in humans because human cells lack cell walls and are not directly affected by the drug.
2. A second mechanism is to increase the permeability of the bacterial cell membrane, allowing leakage of bacterial cell contents; this mechanism is exemplified by polymyxin.
3. Some drugs, such as tetracycline, interfere with protein synthesis and cell reproduction. These have significant effects on the developing fetus and young child.
4. Another group, including the sulfonamides, interferes with the synthesis of essential metabolites.

The common problems with antibacterial drugs are *allergic* reactions, both mild and severe, and digestive tract discomfort. Penicillin and its related compounds may cause anaphylaxis. Digestive tract discomfort may result from irritation of the stomach or the change in the

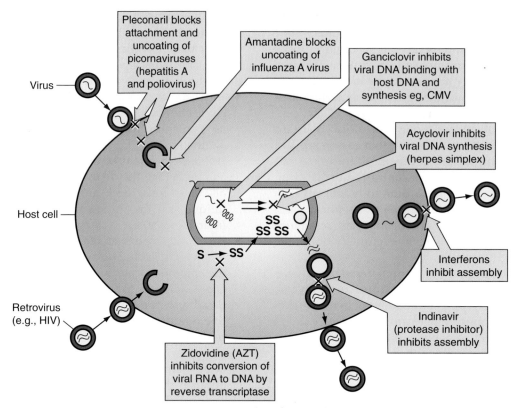

FIGURE 6-16 Examples of antiviral agents.

intestinal resident flora caused by the antibacterial action, often leading to diarrhea. Secondary infections, particularly fungal, may develop as the balance of resident flora is disturbed.

THINK ABOUT 6-6

a. Describe two mechanisms by which antibacterial drugs act on microorganisms.
b. Why do most antibacterial drugs not destroy human cells?
c. Explain the benefit of narrow spectrum over broad spectrum drugs.
d. Explain why a drug may have to be changed if an infection persists.

One drug, cefotaxime, is a third-generation cephalosporin and is related to the penicillin family. It has been developed to be more active against gram negative microbes and multi-drug resistant organisms. This drug can pass through the blood-brain barrier, thus it is more effective in treating some forms of meningitis as well.

Antiviral agents decrease the reproduction of viruses inside the host cell but cannot destroy the virus. They control but do not cure infection. In some cases the drugs are effective only against actively replicating viruses, not against those in the latent stage. These drugs may interfere with attachment of the virus to the host cell, with the shedding of the protein coat, with the action of enzymes such as reverse transcriptase required for synthesis of DNA and RNA or with protein synthesis (Fig. 6-16). The drugs may be virus specific; for example, acyclovir is effective against herpes simplex viruses. Antiviral drugs tend to have significant adverse effects on the host because they alter viral interaction within the host cell.

Genomics is the basis for several new types of antiviral drugs as the search continues for drugs targeting Hepatitis B and/or C, enteroviruses, HIV, and other viral pathogens. One type of drug is based on blocking segments of viral DNA or RNA with *antisense molecules*, rendering the nucleic acid incapable of expression or replication. Ribozymes are enzymes that split DNA or RNA into segments and inhibit replication of viral genes in the cell. These new agents appear to be active against several types of viruses; a few drugs are in clinical trials.

Antifungal agents may interfere with mitosis in fungi (e.g., griseofulvin), or they may increase fungal membrane permeability; amphotericin B may be administered intravenously for systemic infections. Because fungi are eukaryotic cells with many similarities to animal/human cells, systemic antifungal agents are often toxic to the animal/human cells and treatment with these agents usually requires strict medical supervision. Most antifungal agents are administered topically to skin or mucous membranes.

Antiprotozoal agents have a similar characteristic to the antifungal agents in that the targets are eukaryotic cells and can be toxic to human cells. Many pathogenic protozoa also have several stages in their life cycles that require treatment with different agents at different stages. With exception of quinine, most antiprotozoal agents are synthetic, such as metronidazole and pyrimethamine.

Antihelminthic agents have a variety of modes of action. These agents share the same drawback as the antifungal and antiprotozoal agents as they are attacking eukaryotic organisms. Some are designed to suppress a metabolic process that is more important to the helminth than the host while others inhibit the movement of the worm and/or prevent it from remaining in the specific organ. Some examples of these agents are piperazine (paralyzes muscles in the worm's body wall), niclosamide (prevents ATP formation) and ivermectin (blocks nerve transmission).

Example of Infection: Influenza (Flu)

Influenza is a viral infection that may affect both the upper and the lower respiratory tracts. Annually on average 10% to 20% of the population is affected in North America. Although the influenza infection itself may be mild, it is frequently complicated by secondary bacterial infections such as pneumonia. The mortality rate from complications can be high, particularly in those older than 65 years and those with chronic cardiovascular or respiratory disease. Influenza may occur sporadically, in epidemics or pandemics, usually during colder weather. Serious pandemics occurred in 1918 to 1919 (Spanish flu) with a very high mortality rate, again in 1957 (Asian flu), and in 1968 (Hong Kong flu). In 1997 there was an outbreak in Hong Kong of an avian flu transmitted from chickens to humans, and this potential crossover to a new species host is being closely monitored. Epidemiologists predict that serious pandemics will occur in the future.

The influenza viruses are classified as RNA viruses of the myxovirus group. There are three subgroups of the influenza virus—type A, the most prevalent pathogen, type B, and type C. Types A and B cause epidemics and pandemics that tend to occur in cycles. The influenza virus, particularly type A, is difficult to control because it undergoes frequent mutations leading to antigenic shifts or variations. This limits the ability of individuals to develop long-term immunity to the virus and requires the preparation of new vaccines annually to match the predicted new strains of the virus for the coming year. Unfortunately, new strains may emerge during the winter months, creating a slightly different infection. Some years the epidemic has occurred at an earlier time and individuals have not yet received their immunization. Technology to produce a new type of vaccine using viruses grown in a cell culture rather than in eggs is being developed. This process would permit more rapid production to meet an increased demand for vaccines.

In the spring of 2009 a new variant of type A influenza was identified in Mexico. This form of influenza was subsequently named 2009 type A H1N1 influenza. It was highly contagious and caused significant morbidity and mortality in children less than 18 and pregnant women. It is thought that those older than 65 may have some immunity to the virus from earlier outbreaks of similar viruses. The H1N1 influenza virus is genetically and antigenically similar to the virus that caused the Spanish flu pandemic in 1918. It contains genetic material from avian, pig, and human influenza types and is expected to mutate rapidly. The designation H1N1 refers to the specific type of antigens on the viral capsule (Fig. 6-17).

Some children developed severe acute respiratory syndrome and died quickly from the infection in 2009. At the time of writing it is unclear how the H1N1 virus causes this response in young children and teens particularly because most had no other health problems at the time of infection. Possible explanations being researched include formation of pulmonary emboli or altered capillary exchange in the alveoli of the lung. H1N1 flu reemerged in North America and Europe in late September of 2009. Immunization programs specific for H1N1 were begun but vaccine shortages and public resistance to vaccines may lead to high rates of morbidity and mortality in at risk populations.

The constituents of each multivalent vaccine, currently three in number, are specifically designated each year. WHO monitors the incidence and movement of the infection worldwide. Most new strains evolve in Southeast Asia. World Health Organization scientists collect and analyze specimens worldwide, then check the incidence of each strain so as to determine the most effective vaccine components. For example, one antigen might be called A/New Caledonia/20/99, which indicates the type (A), the geographic origin (New Caledonia), the strain number (20), and the year of isolation (1999) for a particular viral strain.

The vaccine may be administered as an intranasal spray (live vaccine) or intramuscular injection (inactivated or killed). It is now recommended that all individuals be immunized annually between November and February. For many health care providers immunization is a condition of employment. The vaccine that remains effective from 2 to 4 months reduces the severity of the infection in cases in which it does not provide total prevention.

The influenza virus was first isolated and identified in 1933. It is transmitted directly by respiratory droplet or indirectly by contact with a contaminated object. The virus can survive at room temperature as long as 2 weeks. It is destroyed by heat and some disinfectants such as ethanol and detergents.

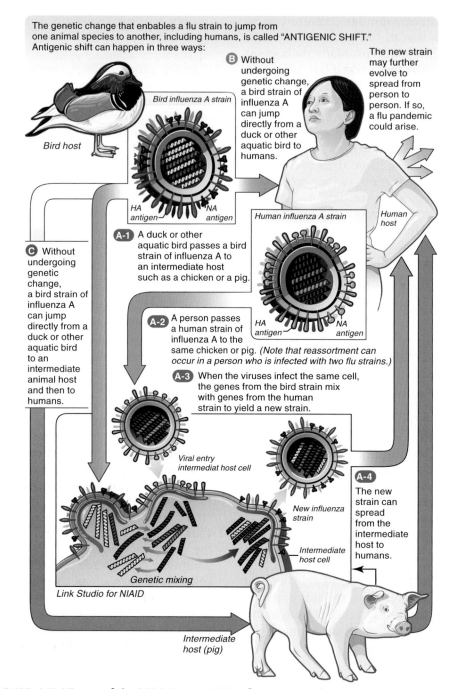

FIGURE 6-17 History of the 2009 Type A H1N1 influenza virus showing antigenic shift. *(From National Institute of Allergy and Infectious Disease [NIAID].)*

The virus enters the cells in the respiratory mucosa, replicates, and causes inflammation and necrosis of the tissue as well as shedding of the virus into the secretions and adjacent cells. The inflammation may also involve the sinuses, pharynx, and auditory tube, causing congestion and obstruction. The widespread necrosis of the respiratory mucosa typical of influenza leaves the area vulnerable to secondary infection by bacteria, which are often resident flora of the upper respiratory tract. The virus may extend into the lungs and cause viral pneumonia.

Influenza usually has a sudden, acute onset with fever and chills, marked malaise, headache, general muscle aching, sore throat, unproductive or dry cough, and nasal congestion. The infection is often self-limiting, although fatigue may persist for several weeks afterward. Continued fever or other signs usually indicate complications, such as the development of bacterial pneumonia.

Treatment is symptomatic and supportive unless bacterial infection or respiratory complications occur. Certain antiviral drugs such as oseltamivir (Tamiflu) if given promptly, may reduce the symptoms in some cases. The CDC recommended the use of oseltamivir (Tamiflu) or zanamivir (Relenza) for the 2008 to 2009 flu season. Other antiviral treatment has been tried, but adverse effects have occurred.

THINK ABOUT 6-7

a. Explain why influenza continues to be a common infection in North America.
b. State three ways the incidence might be reduced.
c. Explain why secondary bacterial infection is common in persons with influenza.

CASE STUDY A

Viral Gastroenteritis

G.B., 15 months old, had severe vomiting and diarrhea for 12 hours and no intake of fluid or food. She began vomiting blood and was quite dehydrated and lethargic. She was taken to the hospital, admitted, and treated with intravenous fluid, electrolytes, and glucose. A fecal specimen was submitted to the laboratory for diagnosis.

The report indicated an infection with rotavirus, an RNA virus and member of the reovirus class. This virus causes gastroenteritis. The incubation period is 1 to 2 days, and the virus is transmitted by the fecal-oral route, probably at G.B.'s nursery school, where several children have been ill. The virus replicates in the epithelial cells at the tip of villi in the small intestine. This cell damage results in lack of absorption of fluid and nutrients.

1. Explain, using the pathophysiology, how the virus could cause bleeding.
2. Using your knowledge of normal physiology, explain how the vomiting and diarrhea as well as the lack of intake could affect the child physiologically.
3. Describe several factors probably contributing to transmission in this case. How long before the vomiting began was the child probably exposed to the virus?
4. What does the classification "RNA virus" mean?
5. Why is it necessary to determine the specific cause of the vomiting and diarrhea? Is any other treatment for rotavirus infection indicated?

CASE STUDY B

Upper Respiratory Infection

K.W., age 9, suddenly developed a fever with very sore throat, headache, and malaise. When examined, her pharynx was red and her tonsils enlarged with pus on the surface and in the crypts. Her cervical lymph nodes were also enlarged. The physician suspected a bacterial infection, and therefore took a throat swab for examination and prescribed a course of penicillin so as to prevent complications.

Laboratory examination confirmed streptococcal infection, and continued treatment with penicillin. This microbe is gram-positive and it adheres to epithelial cells in the pharynx. It produces several exotoxins and resists phagocytosis. It is spread by oral droplet.

1. Suggest several precautions to prevent further transmission in this case.
2. What factor indicated this was a bacterial infection rather than viral?
3. Describe the typical appearance of *Streptococcus* under a microscope.
4. Explain the meaning of gram-positive and how this classification is helpful.
5. K.W. wanted to stop her medication several days later when the headache and fever disappeared. State two reasons why this is not advisable.

CHAPTER SUMMARY

- Infections are caused by pathogenic microorganisms. They may be classified and identified by their characteristics, such as size, shape, component parts, and requirements for growth and reproduction.
- Bacteria are single-cell organisms enclosed within a cell wall and sometimes an outer capsule. They reproduce by binary fission. They may secrete exotoxins, endotoxins, or enzymes that damage the human host cells.
- A virus is an intracellular parasite requiring a living host cell for reproduction. Each viral particle contains either DNA or RNA. They cause disease by destroying human cells during replication or by altering human cell DNA.
- Only a few fungi are pathogenic; *Candida* is an example of an opportunistic member of resident flora in the human body.
- Helminths are parasitic worms that can infect the gut, liver, bloodstream, or lungs.
- Prions are protein-like molecules that cause deformation of proteins within the central nervous system. Their mode of action is not well understood. Prions are transmitted by ingestion of undercooked meat contaminated with prions or by organ donation from an infected donor.
- Resident or normal flora refers to the large variety of nonpathogenic microbes normally present in diverse sites in the body, such as skin, mouth, nose and pharynx, intestines, and vagina.
- The degree of virulence of a specific pathogen determines the severity of the resulting infection.
- Transmission of pathogens may occur by direct or indirect contact, including oral or respiratory droplet, sexual contact, fomite, or vector.
- The infection cycle may be broken by reducing the reservoir of microbes, blocking transmission, or increasing host resistance.

- Universal precautions, as outlined by the CDC, assume that blood and body fluids from any person may be a source of infection; therefore appropriate preventive measures must be taken with all individuals.
- Signs of infection are not apparent until sufficient numbers of microorganisms are established and reproducing in the body. Local signs of infection include inflammation and necrosis of tissue. Systemic signs include fever, headache, fatigue, anorexia, and malaise.
- Infection may be eradicated without drug treatment when the microbial colony becomes limited in growth, perhaps because of insufficient nutrients, or when host defenses destroy the invader.
- Antibacterial drugs are classified by their activity (bactericidal or bacteriostatic, narrow or broad spectrum) and mechanism (e.g., interference with protein or cell wall synthesis).
- Adverse effects of antibacterial agents are allergic reactions, secondary infections, and increasing numbers of drug-resistant microbes.
- Antiviral drugs limit viral replication, thus reducing the active stage, but do not kill the virus or cure the infection.
- Influenza is a respiratory infection caused by a virus that frequently mutates, preventing long-term immunity by vaccination or experiencing the infection. Epidemics are common. Secondary bacterial infections such as pneumonia are common, particularly in the elderly.

STUDY QUESTIONS

1. Explain how each of the following contributes to the virulence of bacteria:
   a. production of endotoxin
   b. spore formation
   c. presence of a capsule
2. Predict how each of the following could reduce host resistance to infection:
   a. bone marrow damage
   b. circulatory impairment
   c. puncture wound
3. Explain two benefits of resident flora.
4. Differentiate infection from inflammation.
5. Describe three ways of reducing transmission of a respiratory infection.
6. Explain each of the following:
   a. why the clinical signs of infection are not present immediately after the microorganism enters the body
   b. why infection can often be cured without drug treatment
   c. why antibacterial agents might be prescribed for an infection
7. Explain why it is important to take the complete course of antimicrobial medication prescribed.
8. Explain why viral infections are difficult to treat.
9. State two local and two systemic signs of influenza.
10. Explain why a new influenza vaccine is prepared each year and consists of several components.

ADDITIONAL RESOURCES

Bergquist LM, Pogosian B: *Microbiology: Principles and Health Science Applications*, Philadelphia, 2000, WB Saunders.

Chin J: *Control of Communicable Diseases Manual*, ed 17, Washington, DC, 2000, American Public Health Association.

Greenwood D, Slack RCB, Peutherer JF: *Medical Microbiology*, ed 18, St. Louis, 2007, Churchill Livingstone.

Heymann D, editor: *Control of Communicable Diseases Manual*, ed 18, Washington, DC, 2004, American Public Health Association.

Holt J, Krieg N, Sneath P, Staley J, Williams S: *Bergey's Manual of Determinative Bacteriology*, ed 9, Philadelphia, 2000, Lippincott Williams & Wilkins.

Mosby's Drug Consult 2006, St. Louis, 2006, Mosby.

VanMeter K, VanMeter W, Hubert R: *Microbiology for the Healthcare Professional*, St. Louis, 2010, Mosby.

Web Sites

http://www.cdc.gov Centers for Disease Control and Prevention.

http://www.cdc.gov/mmwr Morbidity and Mortality Weekly Report.

http://www.asm.org American Society for Microbiology.

http://www.nlm.nih.gov National Library of Medicine.

http://www.nlm.nih.gov/medlineplus/infections.html Health Information.

http://www.niaid.nih.gov National Institute of Allergy and Infectious Diseases.

http://www.merck.com/mmhe/index.html.

http://www.who.int.

CHAPTER 7

Immunity

CHAPTER OUTLINE

LEARNING OBJECTIVES

After studying this chapter, the student is expected to:

1. Describe the normal immune response.
2. List the components of the immune system and the purpose of each.
3. Explain the four methods of acquiring immunity.
4. Discuss tissue transplant rejection and how it is treated.
5. Describe the mechanism and clinical effects of each of the four types of hypersensitivity reactions.
6. Explain the effects of anaphylaxis.
7. Discuss the mechanism of autoimmune disorders.
8. Describe the disorder systemic lupus erythematosus, its pathophysiology, clinical manifestations, diagnostic tests, and treatment.
9. Explain the causes and effects of immunodeficiency.
10. Describe the cause, modes of transmission, and implications for health professionals of acquired immunodeficiency syndrome.
11. Describe the course, effects, and complications of HIV-AIDS.

KEY TERMS

antibiotic
antimicrobial
antiviral
autoantibodies
bronchoconstriction
colostrum
complement
cytotoxic

encephalopathy
erythema
fetus
glycoprotein
hypogammaglobulinemia
hypoproteinemia
mast cells
monocytes

mononuclear phagocytic
  system
mutate
opportunistic
placenta
polymerase chain reaction
prophylactic
pruritic

replication
retrovirus
splenectomy
stem cells
thymus
titer
vesicles

Review of the Immune System

The immune system is responsible for the body's defenses. The system has a nonspecific response as shown in Chapter 5 and a specific response mechanism discussed in this chapter. In specific defense the immune system is responding to particular substances, cells, toxins, or proteins, which are perceived as foreign to the body and therefore unwanted or potentially dangerous. The specific immune response is intended to recognize and remove undesirable material from cells, tissues, and organs.

Components of the Immune System

The immune system consists of lymphoid structures, immune cells, tissues concerned with immune cell development, and chemical mediators. The lymphoid structures, including the lymph nodes, the spleen and tonsils, the intestinal lymphoid tissue, and the lymphatic circulation, form the basic structure within which the immune response can function (Fig. 7-1). The immune cells, or lymphocytes, as well as macrophages provide the specific mechanism for the identification and removal of foreign material. All immune cells originate in the bone marrow, and the bone marrow and thymus have roles in the maturation of the cells. The

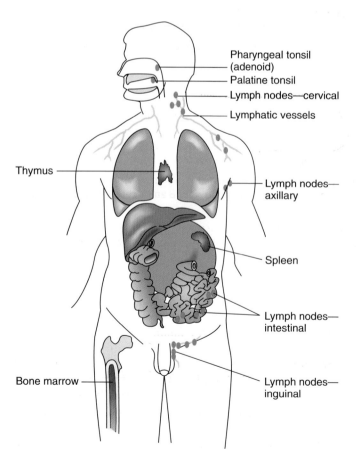

FIGURE 7-1 Structures in the immune system.

thymus is significant during fetal development in that it programs the immune system to ignore self-antigens. When this process is faulty, the body may attack its own tissues as non–self. The blood and circulatory system provide a major transportation and communication network for the immune system. The major components of the immune system and their functions are summarized in Table 7-1.

Elements of the Immune System

Antigens

Antigens (or immunogens) are either foreign substances or human cell surface antigens that are unique (except in identical twins) in each individual. They are usually composed of complex proteins or polysaccharides, or a combination of molecules such as glycoproteins. Antigens activate the immune system to produce *specific* produce *specific antibodies.*

The antigens representing *self* are present on an individual's plasma membranes. These antigen molecules are coded by a group of genes inherited from the parents, called major histocompatibility complex (MHC) located on chromosome 6. Owing to the large number of possible combinations of genes that may be inherited from the parents, it is unlikely that two individuals would ever have the same antigens, with the exception of identical twins. Major histocompatibility complex has an essential role in the activation and regulation of the immune response as well as intercellular communications. Major histocompatibility complex molecules are useful in detecting changes in cell membranes altered by viruses or cancerous changes and alerting the immune system to their presence. Human MHC is also known as human leukocyte antigen (HLA), because it was first detected on the cell membranes of leukocytes. These antigens are also used to provide the close match for a tissue transplant; the immune system will be activated by the presence of cells with different MHC molecules. The immune system generally *tolerates* self-antigens on its cells, thus no immune response is initiated against the own cells. Autoimmune diseases are an exception in which the immune system no longer recognizes self from non–self and begins to attack its own cells/structures or organs.

Cells

The *macrophage* is critical in the initiation of the immune response. Macrophages develop from monocytes (see Chapter 10), part of the mononuclear phagocytic system that was formerly known as the reticuloendothelial system. Macrophages occur throughout the body in such tissues as the liver, lungs, and lymph nodes. They are large phagocytic cells that intercept and engulf foreign material and then process and display the antigens from the foreign material on their cell membranes; the lymphocytes respond to this display, thus

TABLE 7-1	Major Components of the Immune System and Their Functions
Antigen	Foreign substance, microbes or component of cell that stimulates immune response
Antibody	Specific protein produced in humoral response to bind with antigen
Autoantibody	Antibodies against self-antigen; attacks body's own tissues
Thymus	Gland located in the mediastinum, large in children, decreasing size in adults. Site of maturation and proliferation of T lymphocytes
Lymphatic tissue and organs	Contain many lymphocytes. Filter body fluids, remove foreign matter, immune response
Bone marrow	Source of stem cells, leukocytes, and maturation of B lymphocytes
Cells	
Neutrophils	White blood cells for phagocytosis; nonspecific defense; active in inflammatory process
Basophils	White blood cells: bind IgE, release histamine in anaphylaxis
Eosinophils	White blood cells: participate in allergic responses and defense against parasites
Monocytes	White blood cells: migrate from the blood into tissues to become macrophages
Macrophages	Phagocytosis; process and present antigens to lymphocytes for the immune response
Mast cells	Release chemical mediators such as histamine in connective tissue
B lymphocytes	Humoral immunity-activated cell becomes an antibody-producing plasma cell or a B memory cell
Plasma cells	Develop from B lymphocytes to produce and secrete specific antibodies
T lymphocytes	White blood cells: cell-mediated immunity
Cytotoxic or killer T cells	Destroy antigens, cancer cells, virus-infected cells
Memory T cells	Remember antigen and quickly stimulate immune response on reexposure
Helper T cells	Activate B and T cells; control or limit specific immune response
NK lymphocytes	Natural killer cells destroy foreign cells, virus-infected cells, and cancer cells
Chemical Mediators	
Complement	Group of inactive proteins in the circulation that, when activated, stimulate the release of other chemical mediators, promoting inflammation, chemotaxis, and phagocytosis
Histamine	Released from mast cells and basophils, particularly in allergic reactions. Causes vasodilation and increased vascular permeability or edema, also contraction of bronchiolar smooth muscle, and pruritus
Kinins (e.g., bradykinin)	Cause vasodilation, increased permeability (edema), and pain
Prostaglandins	Group of lipids with varying effects. Some cause inflammation, vasodilation and increased permeability, and pain
Leukotrienes	Group of lipids, derived from mast cells and basophils, which cause contraction of bronchiolar smooth muscle and have a role in development of inflammation
Cytokines (messengers)	Includes lymphokines, monokines, interferons, and interleukins; produced by macrophages and activated T-lymphocytes; stimulate activation and proliferation of B and T cells, communication between cells; involved in inflammation, fever, and leukocytosis
Tumor necrosis factor (TNF)	A cytokine active in the inflammatory and immune responses; stimulates fever, chemotaxis, mediator of tissue wasting, stimulates T cells, mediator in septic shock (decreasing blood pressure), stimulates necrosis in some tumors
Chemotactic factors	Attract phagocytes to area of inflammation

initiating the immune response (Fig. 7-2). Macrophages also secrete chemicals such as monokines and interleukins (see Table 7-1) that play a role in the activation of additional lymphocytes and in the inflammatory response, which accompanies a *secondary* immune response.

The primary cell in the immune response is the *lymphocyte,* one of the *leukocytes* or white blood cells produced by the bone marrow (see Chapter 11). Mature lymphocytes are termed *immunocompetent* cells—cells that have the special function of recognizing and reacting with antigens in the body. The two groups of lymphocytes, B lymphocytes and T lymphocytes, determine which type of immunity will be initiated, either cell-mediated immunity or humoral immunity, respectively.

T lymphocytes (T cells) arise from stem cells, which are incompletely differentiated cells held in reserve in the

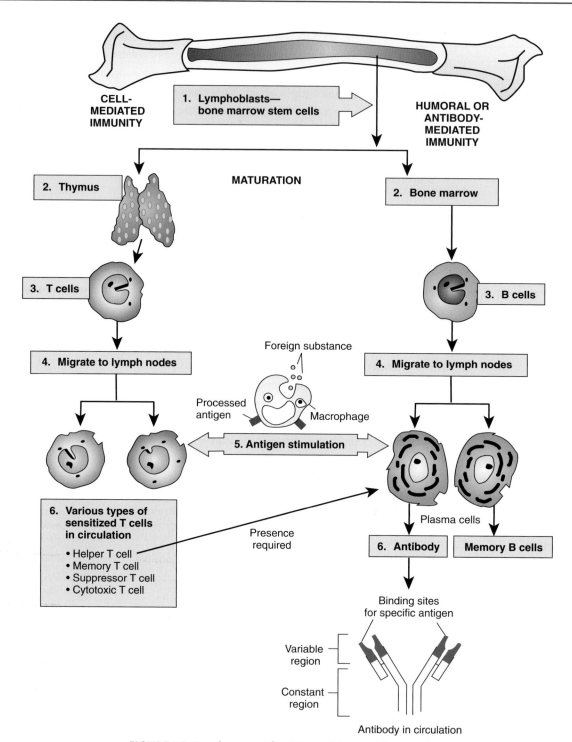

FIGURE 7-2 Development of cellular and humoral immunities.

bone marrow and then travel to the thymus for further differentiation and development of cell membrane receptors. *Cell-mediated immunity* develops when T lymphocytes with protein receptors on the cell surface recognize antigens on the surface of target cells and directly destroy the invading antigens (Fig. 7-2). These specially programmed T cells then reproduce, creating an "army" to battle the invader, and they also activate other T and B lymphocytes. T cells are primarily effective against virus-infected cells, fungal and protozoal

infections, cancer cells, and foreign cells such as transplants. There are a number of subgroups of T cells, marked by different surface receptor molecules, each of which has a specialized function in the immune response (see Table 7-1). The cytotoxic *CD8 positive* T-killer cells destroy the target cell by binding to the antigen and releasing damaging enzymes or chemicals, such as monokines and lymphokines, which may destroy foreign cell membranes or cause an inflammatory response, attract macrophages to the site, stimulate the proliferation of more lymphocytes, and stimulate hematopoiesis. Phagocytic cells then clean up the debris. The *helper CD4 positive* T cell facilitates the immune response. A subgroup, the *memory* T cells, remains in the lymph nodes for years, ready to activate the response again if the same invader returns.

Two subgroups of T cells have gained prominence as markers in patients with acquired immunodeficiency syndrome (AIDS). T-helper cells have "CD4" molecules as receptors on the cell membrane, and the killer T cells have "CD8" molecules. These receptors are important in T-cell activation. Although the CD8+ killer cells are primarily cytotoxic, CD4+ T cells regulate *all* the cells in the immune system, the B and T lymphocytes, macrophages, and natural killer (NK) cells, by secreting the "messenger" cytokines. The human immunodeficiency virus (HIV) destroys the CD4 cells, thus crippling the entire immune system. The ratio of CD4 to CD8 T cells (normal ratio, 2:1) is closely monitored in people infected with HIV as a reflection of the progress of the infection.

The *B lymphocytes* or *B cells* are responsible for *humoral immunity* through the production of *antibodies* or *immunoglobulins*. B cells are thought to mature in the bone marrow and then proceed to the spleen and lymphoid tissue. After exposure to antigens, and with the assistance of T lymphocytes, they become antibody-producing plasma cells (see Fig. 7-2). B lymphocytes act primarily against bacteria and viruses that are outside body cells. B-memory cells that provide for repeated production of antibodies also form in humoral immune responses.

Natural killer cells are lymphocytes distinct from the T and B lymphocytes. They destroy, without any prior exposure and sensitization, tumor cells and cells infected with viruses.

APPLY YOUR KNOWLEDGE 7-1

Predict three reasons why the immune system might not respond correctly to foreign material in the body.

Antibodies or Immunoglobulins

Antibodies are a specific class of proteins termed immunoglobulins. Each has a unique sequence of amino acids (*variable* portion, which binds to antigen) attached to a common base (*constant* region that attaches to macrophages). Antibodies bind to the specific matching antigen, destroying it. This specificity of antigen for antibody, similar to a key opening a lock, is a significant factor in the development of immunity to various diseases. Antibodies are found in the general circulation, forming the globulin portion of the plasma proteins, as well as in lymphoid structures. Immunoglobulins are divided into five classes, each of which has a special structure and function (Table 7-2). Specific

TABLE 7-2	Immunoglobulins and Their Functions	
Characteristic	Structure	Function
IgG	Monomer	Most common antibody in the blood; produced in both primary and secondary immune responses; activates complement; includes antibacterial, antiviral, and antitoxin antibodies. Crosses placenta, creates passive immunity in newborn
IgM	Pentamer	Bound to B lymphocytes in circulation and is usually the first to increase in the immune response; activates complement; forms natural antibodies; is involved in blood ABO type incompatibility reaction
IgA	Monomer, dimer	Found in secretions such as tears and saliva, in mucous membranes, and in colostrum to provide protection for newborn child
IgE	Monomer	Binds to mast cells in skin and mucous membranes; when linked to allergen, causes release of histamine and other chemicals, resulting in inflammation
IgD	Monomer	Attached to B cells; activates B cells

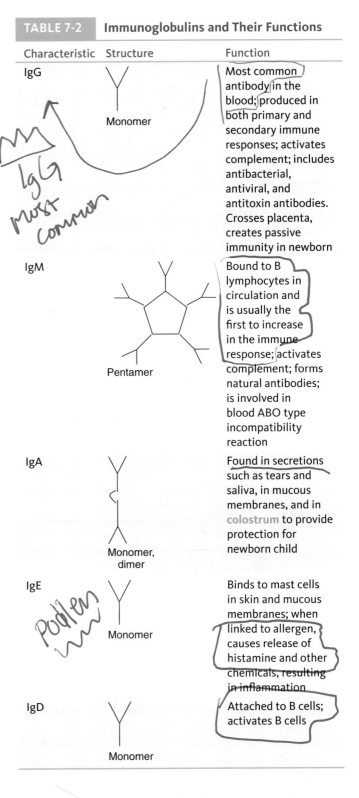

immunoglobulins may be administered to treat diseases such as Guillain-Barré syndrome an autoimmune disease that attacks the peripheral nervous system that can cause progressive paralysis.

Complement System

The complement system is frequently activated during an immune reaction with IgG or IgM class immunoglobulins. Complement involves a group of inactive proteins, numbered C1 to C9, circulating in the blood. When an antigen–antibody complex binds to the first complement component, C1, a sequence of activating steps occurs (similar to a blood clotting cascade). Eventually this activation of the complement system results in the destruction of the antigen by lysis when the cell membrane is damaged, or some complement fragment may attach to a microorganism, marking it for phagocytosis. Complement activation also initiates an inflammatory response.

Chemical Mediators

A number of chemical mediators such as histamine or interleukins may be involved in an immune reaction, depending on the particular circumstances. These chemicals have a variety of functions, such as signaling a cellular response or causing cellular damage (see Chapter 5). A brief summary is provided in Table 7-1.

THINK ABOUT 7-1

a. Describe two differences between B and T lymphocytes.
b. Where is IgG found in the body?
c. Which lymphocyte has a role in both cell-mediated and humoral immunity?
d. Describe the development of antibodies to a specific antigen.

The Immune Response

Because of unique antigens, often a protein, on the surface of an individual's cells, that person's immune system can distinguish *self* from *non–self* (foreign) and can thus detect and destroy unknown material. Normally the immune system ignores "self" cells, demonstrating *tolerance*. When the immune system *recognizes* a *specific* non–self-antigen as foreign, it develops a specific *response* to that particular antigen and stores that particular response in its *memory* cells for future reference if the antigen reappears in the body. It is similar to a surveillance system warning of attack and the subsequent mobilization of an army for defense. For example, lymphoid tissue in the pharynx, such as tonsils and adenoids, can capture antigens in material that is inhaled or ingested and process the immune response. Note that a person must have been exposed to the specific foreign antigen and must have developed specific immunity to it (such as antibodies) before this defense is effective. This response is usually repeated each time the person is exposed to a particular substance (antigen) because the immune system has memory cells. Immune responses that occur after the first introduction of the antigen are usually more rapid and intense than the initial response. In destroying foreign material, the immune system is assisted by nonspecific defense

mechanisms such as phagocytosis and the inflammatory response. By removing the foreign material, the immune system also plays a role in preparing injured tissue for healing.

When the plasma membrane of malignant neoplastic cells is abnormal, the immune system may be able to identify these cells as "foreign" and remove them, thus playing an important role in the prevention of cancer (see Chapter 20). It has been noted that individuals frequently develop cancer when the immune system is depressed as with an infection or increased stress. However, not all cancer cells are identifiable as foreign; therefore the immune system may not remove them. The immune system directs the response to an antigen, but also has built-in controls to prevent excessive response. Two limiting factors are the removal of the causative antigen during the response, and the short lifespan of the chemical messengers. Tolerance to self-antigens prevents improper responses.

THINK ABOUT 7-2

a. Explain why the immune system is considered a *specific* defense.
b. Explain why the immune system must distinguish between *self* and *non–self.*

Diagnostic Tests

Many new and improved techniques are emerging, and more details on these techniques may be found in reference works on serology or diagnostic methods.

Tests may assess the levels and functional quality (qualitative and quantitative) of serum immunoglobulins or the titer (measure) of specific antibodies. Identification of antibodies may be required for such purposes as detecting Rh blood incompatibility (indirect Coombs' test) or screening for HIV infection (by enzyme-linked immunosorbent assay [ELISA]). Pregnant women are checked for levels of antibodies, particularly for German measles to establish their potential for complications if they are exposed to this disease while pregnancy which could result in fetal death. During hepatitis B infection, changes in the levels of antigens and antibodies take place, and these changes can be used to monitor the course of the infection and level of immunity (see Chapter 17). The number and characteristics of the lymphocytes in the circulation can be examined as well. Extensive HLA (MHC) typing is required to complete tissue matching before transplant procedures.

The Process of Acquiring Immunity

Natural immunity is species specific. For example, humans are not usually susceptible to infections common to many other animals. *Innate* immunity is gene specific and is related to ethnicity, as evident from the increased susceptibility of North American aboriginal people to tuberculosis.

The immune response consists of two steps:

- A *primary* response occurs when a person is first exposed to an antigen. During exposure the antigen is recognized and processed, and subsequent development of antibodies or sensitized T lymphocytes is initiated (Fig. 7-3). This process usually takes 1 to 2 weeks and can be monitored by testing serum antibody titer. Following the initial rise in seroconversion the level of antibody falls.
- A *secondary* response results when a repeat exposure to the same antigen occurs. This response is much more rapid and results in higher antibody levels than the primary response. Even years later the memory cells very quickly stimulate production of large numbers of the matching antibodies or T cells.

When a single strain of bacteria or virus causes a disease, the affected person usually has only one episode of the disease because the specific antibody is retained in the memory. Young children are subject to many infections until they establish a pool of antibodies. As one ages, the number of infections declines. However, when there are many strains of bacteria or viruses causing a disease, for example, the common cold (which has more than 200 causative organisms, each with slightly different antigens), an individual never develops antibodies to all the organisms, and therefore he or she has recurrent colds. The influenza virus, which affects the respiratory tract, has several antigenic forms, for example, type A and type B. These viruses have various strains that mutate or change slightly over time. For this reason, a new influenza vaccine is manufactured each year, its composition based on the current antigenic forms of the virus most likely to cause an epidemic of the infection.

THINK ABOUT 7-3

a. Predict why a person usually has chickenpox only once in a lifetime but may have influenza many times.
b. Explain how the secondary response to an antigen is faster and greater than the primary response.

Immunity is acquired four ways (Table 7-3). Active immunity develops when the person's own body develops antibodies or T cells in response to a specific antigen introduced into the body. This process takes a few weeks, but the result usually lasts for years because memory B and T cells are retained in the body.

- *Active natural immunity* may be acquired by direct exposure to an antigen, for example, when a person has an infection and then develops antibodies.
- *Active artificial immunity* develops when a specific antigen is purposefully introduced into the body, stimulating the production of antibodies. For example, a *vaccine* is a solution containing dead or weakened (attenuated) organisms that stimulate the immune system to produce antibodies but does not result in the disease itself. Work continues on the development of vaccines using antigenic fragments of microbes or genetically altered forms.

A long list of vaccines is available, including those for protection against polio, diphtheria, measles, and chickenpox. Infants begin a regular schedule of

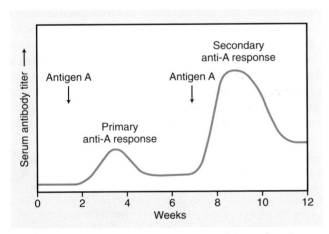

FIGURE 7-3 Graph illustrating primary and secondary immune responses. *(Adapted from Abbas AK, Lichtman AH: Cellular and Molecular Immunology, ed 5, Philadelphia, 2003, Saunders.)*

TABLE 7-3	Types of Acquired Immunity			
Type	Mechanism		Memory	Example
Natural active	Pathogens enter body and cause illness; antibodies form in host		Yes	Person has chickenpox once
Artificial active	Vaccine (live or attenuated organisms) is injected into person. No illness results, but antibodies form		Yes	Person has measles vaccine and gains immunity
Natural passive	Antibodies passed directly from mother to child to provide temporary protection		No	Placental passage during pregnancy or ingestion of breast milk
Artificial passive	Antibodies injected into person (antiserum) to provide temporary protection or minimize severity of infection		No	Gammaglobulin if recent exposure to microbe

immunizations/vaccines shortly after birth to reduce the risk of serious infections and in hopes of eradicating some infectious diseases. Immunization recommendations for all age groups are published by the CDC. A *toxoid* is an altered or weakened bacterial *toxin* that acts as an antigen in a similar manner. A *booster* is an additional immunization given perhaps 5 or 10 years after initial immunization that "reminds" the immune system of the antigen and promotes a more rapid and effective secondary response. Booster immunizations are currently used for tetanus.

Outcome of Infectious Disease

The occurrence of many infectious diseases, such as polio and measles, has declined where vaccination rates have been high, creating "herd immunity"—a phenomenon in which a high percentage of a population is vaccinated, thus decreasing chances of acquiring and spreading an infectious disease. Believing smallpox (variola) had been eradicated in many countries by the mid-1950s, the United States discontinued the smallpox vaccine in 1972. The WHO worked toward worldwide eradication and the last case of naturally occurring smallpox was recorded in 1977.

Polio vaccination was implemented in 1954, and cases are a rare occurrence today in developed areas of the world. Recent outbreaks of measles and mumps in North America are the result of inadequate revaccination of teens.

The search continues for additional vaccines against AIDS and malaria, tuberculosis, and other widespread infections. Research is also continuing on genetic vaccines, in which only a strand of bacterial DNA forms the vaccine, thus reducing any risks from injection of the microorganism itself. Immunotherapy is an expanding area of cancer research in the search for new and more specific therapies.

Emerging and Re-emerging Infectious Diseases and Immunity

Emerging infectious diseases are those newly identified in a population. Re-emerging infectious diseases were previously under control but unfortunately not all individuals participate in immunization programs; therefore infectious disease outbreaks persist. These infectious diseases are on the rise due to globalization, drug resistance, and many other factors.

Bioterrorism

Biological warfare and bioterrorism use biological agents to attack civilians or military personnel. Concern continues about the possibility of bioterrorism using altered antigenic forms of common viruses or bacteria. Such bioweapons would have widespread impact on

populations because current immunizations do not protect against such agents. It is important to recognize that large outbreaks of diseases formerly controlled by vaccines may represent acts of bioterrorism. Such outbreaks should be reported to the local authorities as soon as they are recognized.

> **APPLY YOUR KNOWLEDGE 7-2**
>
> a. Predict reasons why antibodies might not form in response to an antigen.
> b. Suggest reasons why individuals might not want vaccinations.

Passive immunity occurs when antibodies are transferred from one person to another. These are effective immediately, but offer only temporary protection because memory has not been established in the recipient, and the antibodies are gradually removed from the circulation. There are also two forms of passive immunity:

- *Passive natural immunity* occurs when IgG is transferred from mother to fetus across the placenta. Breast milk also supplies maternal antibodies. These antibodies protect the infant for the first few months of life.
- *Passive artificial immunity* results from the injection of antibodies from a person or animal into a second person. An example is the administration of rabies antiserum or snake antivenom. Sometimes immunoglobulins are administered to an individual who has been exposed to an organism but has not been immunized to reduce the effects of the infection (for example, hepatitis B).

> **THINK ABOUT 7-4**
>
> a. Explain why a newborn infant is protected from infection by the measles virus immediately after birth but later will be given the measles vaccine.
> b. Explain the differences between active artificial immunity and passive natural immunity.

Tissue and Organ Transplant Rejection

Replacement of damaged organs or tissues by healthy tissues from donors is occurring more frequently as the success of such transplants improves. Skin, corneas, bone, kidneys, lungs, hearts, and bone marrow are among the more common transplants. Transplants differ according to donor characteristics, as indicated in Table 7-4. In most cases transplants, or grafts, involve the introduction of foreign tissue from one human, the donor, into the body of the human recipient (*allograft*). Because the genetic makeup of cells is the same only in identical twins, the obstacle to complete success of

TABLE 7-4	Types of Tissue or Organ Transplants
Allograft (homograft)	Tissue transferred between members of the same species but may differ genetically; e.g., one human to another human
Isograft	Tissue transferred between two genetically identical bodies; e.g., identical twins
Autograft	Tissue transferred from one part of the body to another part on the same individual; e.g., skin or bone
Xenograft (heterograft)	Tissue transferred from a member of one species to a different species; e.g., pig to human

transplantation has been that the immune system of the recipient responds to the HLAs (MHCs) in foreign tissue, *rejecting* and destroying the graft tissue.

Rejection Process

Rejection is a complex process, primarily involving a type IV cell-mediated hypersensitivity reaction (see the next section on hypersensitivity reactions), but also involving a humoral response, both of which cause inflammation and tissue necrosis. The rejection process eventually destroys the organ, so that transplanted organs often must be replaced after a few years. Survival time of a transplant is increased when the HLA match is excellent, the donor is living (less risk of damage to donor tissue), and immunosuppressive drugs are taken on a regular basis. Corneas and cartilage lack a blood supply; therefore rejection is not a problem with these transplanted tissues. With improved surgical techniques and better drug therapy, transplants are now lasting a longer time and significantly prolonging the recipient's life.

It now appears that neonates and young infants can receive heart transplants from donors *without* a good tissue match. Rejection does not occur because the infant's immune system is not yet mature and does not respond to the foreign tissue. The long-term effects are not known, but the results to date are encouraging. Because heart transplants in infants are limited by organ size as well as organ availability, the removal of the HLA restrictions would make more heart transplants available when needed and more donor hearts could be used rather than wasted.

One type of rejection occurs when the host, or recipient's, immune system rejects the graft (host-versus-graft disease [HVGD]), a possibility with kidney transplants. The other type of rejection that occurs is when the graft tissue contains T cells that attack the host cells (graft-versus-host disease [GVHD]), as may occur in bone marrow transplants.

Rejection may occur at any time:

- *Hyperacute* rejection occurs immediately after transplantation as circulation to the site is re-established.

This is a greater risk in patients who have pre-existing antibodies, perhaps from prior blood transfusions. The blood vessels are affected, resulting in lack of blood flow to the transplanted tissue.
- *Acute* rejection develops after several weeks when unmatched antigens cause a reaction.
- *Chronic* or late rejection occurs after months or years, with gradual degeneration of the blood vessels.

Treatment and Prevention

Immunosuppression techniques are used to reduce the immune response and prevent rejection. The common treatment involves drugs such as cyclosporine, azathioprine (Imuran), and prednisone, a glucocorticoid (see Chapter 5). The drugs must be taken on a continuous basis and the patient monitored for signs of rejection. The use of cyclosporine has been very successful in reducing the risk of rejection, but the dosage must be carefully checked to prevent kidney damage. Many new drugs are also under investigation in clinical trials. The major concern with any immunosuppressive drug is the high risk of *infection*, because the normal body defenses are now limited. Infections are often caused by opportunistic microorganisms, microbes that usually are harmless in healthy individuals (see Chapter 6). Persons with diabetes frequently require transplants of kidneys and other tissues, and this group of patients is already at risk for infection because of vascular problems (see Chapter 16). Loss of the surveillance and defense functions of the immune system has also led to increased risk of lymphomas, skin cancers, cervical cancer, and colon cancer in those taking antirejection drugs. Dental professionals should be aware of the high incidence of gingival hyperplasia in patients taking cyclosporine. (See Fig. 14-27 for a photograph of gingival hyperplasia.)

THINK ABOUT 7-5

Explain why immunosuppressive drugs should be taken on a regular and permanent basis following a transplant.

Hypersensitivity Reactions

Hypersensitivity or allergic reactions are unusual and perhaps damaging immune responses to normally harmless substances. These reactions stimulate an inflammatory response. There are four basic types of hypersensitivities (Table 7-5), which differ in the mechanism causing tissue injury. The World Allergy Organization has developed a standard nomenclature to identify allergic problems and differentiate them from similar conditions; for example, allergic rhinitis, allergic asthma, and allergic contact dermatitis.

TABLE 7-5	**Types of Hypersensitivities**		
Type	Example	Mechanism	Effects
I	Hay fever; anaphylaxis	IgE bound to mast cells; release of histamine and chemical mediators	Immediate inflammation and pruritus
II	ABO blood incompatibility	IgG or IgM reacts with antigen on cell–complement activated	Cell lysis and phagocytosis
III	Autoimmune disorders: SLE, glomerulonephritis	Antigen–antibody complex deposits in tissue–complement activated	Inflammation, vasculitis
IV	Contact dermatitis: transplant rejection	Antigen binds to T-lymphocyte; sensitized lymphocyte releases lymphokines	Delayed inflammation

SLE, systemic lupus erythematosus.

Type I: Allergic Reactions

Allergies are very common and appear to be increasing in incidence and severity, particularly in young children. Allergic reactions take many forms, including skin rashes, hay fever, vomiting, and anaphylaxis. A tendency toward allergic conditions is inherited, and the manifestation of such an allergy in a family is referred to as an *atopic* hypersensitivity reaction. The antigen is often called an *allergen.* The specific allergen may be a food, a chemical, pollen from a plant, or a drug. One person may be allergic to a number of substances, and these may change over time. Common allergenic foods include shellfish, nuts, and strawberries. Hypersensitivities occur frequently with drugs such as ASA (aspirin), penicillin, sulfa, and local anesthetics. Cross-allergies are common; therefore an allergy to one form of penicillin means that an individual is likely allergic to all drugs in the penicillin family.

There has been a significant increase in the number of children who experience severe type I hypersensitivity reactions. Most of these reactions occur when the child is exposed to a particular food, such as peanuts or other members of the legume family. The reactions may be severe enough to result in anaphylaxis. Once diagnosed, the child carries an emergency injector or EpiPen, which can be administered to prevent severe anaphylaxis resulting in bronchospasm and hypovolemia.

Causative Mechanism

Type I hypersensitivity begins when an individual is exposed to a specific allergen and for some reason develops IgE antibodies from B lymphocytes. These antibodies attach to mast cells in specific locations (Fig. 7-4), creating *sensitized* mast cells. Mast cells are connective tissue cells that are present in large numbers in the mucosa of the respiratory and digestive tracts. On re-exposure to the same allergen, the allergen attaches to the IgE antibody on the mast cell, stimulating the release of chemical mediators such as histamine from granules within the mast cells (see Table 7-1). These chemical mediators cause an inflammatory reaction involving vasodilation and increased capillary permeability at the site (e.g., the nasal mucosa), resulting in swelling and redness of the tissues. This initial release of histamine also irritates the nerve endings, causing itching or mild pain.

Other chemical mediators, including prostaglandins and leukotrienes, are released at the site in a second phase of the reaction, and these cause similar effects. If the sensitized mast cells are located in the nasal mucosa, the antigen–antibody reaction causes the typical signs of hay fever. If sensitization occurs in the respiratory mucosa in the lungs, the chemical mediators also cause bronchoconstriction (contraction of the bronchiolar smooth muscle and narrowing of the airway) and release of mucus in the airways, resulting in obstruction of the airways, or asthma.

Clinical Signs and Symptoms

The signs and symptoms of an allergic reaction occur on the second or any subsequent exposure to the specific allergen because the first exposure to the allergen causes only the formation of antibodies and sensitized mast cells. The target area becomes red and swollen, there may be vesicles or blisters present, and usually the area is highly pruritic or itchy.

Hay Fever or Allergic Rhinitis

An allergic reaction in the nasal mucosa causes frequent sneezing, copious watery secretions from the nose, and itching. Because the nasal mucosa is continuous with the mucosa of the sinuses and the conjunctiva of the eyelid, the eyes are frequently red, watery, and pruritic as well. Hay fever, or allergic rhinitis, is usually seasonal because it is related to plant pollens in the air, but some people are susceptible to multiple allergens such as molds or dusts and can exhibit signs at any time of year.

Food Allergies

Food allergies may be manifested in several ways. When an inflammatory reaction occurs in the mucosa of the digestive it results in nausea, vomiting, and/or diarrhea. In some cases, food allergies may cause a rash on the skin

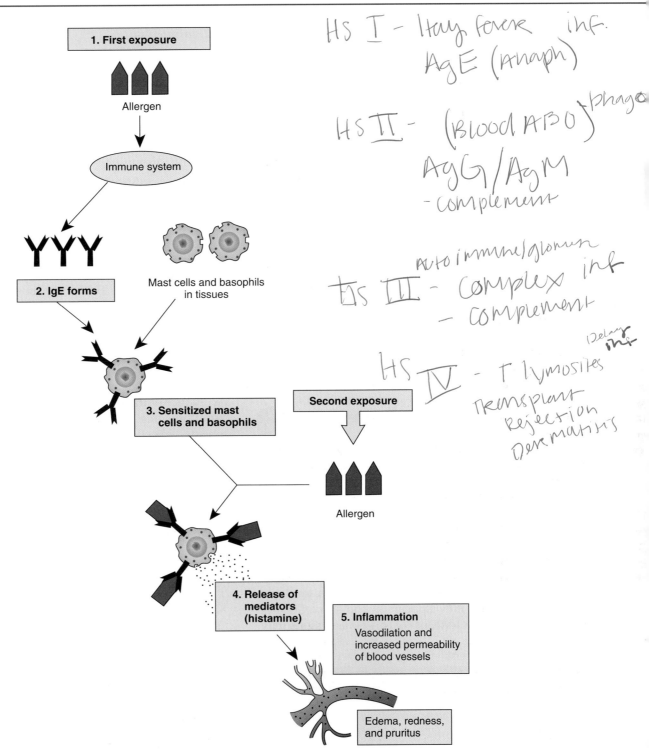

FIGURE 7-4 Type I hypersensitivity, allergic reaction.

called hives, which are large, hard, raised red masses that are highly pruritic. In severe cases, these hives also occur on the pharyngeal mucosa and may obstruct airflow; therefore it is important to watch for respiratory difficulty associated with any allergenic skin rash.

Atopic Dermatitis or Eczema

Eczema or atopic dermatitis is a chronic skin condition, often with a genetic component, common in infants and young children. The skin rash may occur on the face, trunk, or extremities (see Chapter 8). It is associated with ingested foods, irritating fabrics, and a dry atmosphere. There may be remissions as the child develops, but the condition may recur in adulthood.

Asthma

A lung disorder, asthma may result from an allergic response in the bronchial mucosa that interferes with airflow. Asthma is covered in more detail in Chapter 13. Frequently a triad of atopic conditions including hay fever, eczema, and asthma occurs in family histories.

Anaphylaxis or Anaphylactic Shock

Anaphylaxis is a severe, life-threatening, systemic hypersensitivity reaction resulting in decreased blood pressure, airway obstruction, and severe hypoxia. Commonly caused by exposure to latex materials such as gloves, insect stings, ingestion of nuts or shellfish, administration of penicillin, or local anesthetic injections, the reaction usually occurs within minutes of the exposure.

■ *Pathophysiology*

Large amounts of chemical mediators are released from mast cells into the general circulation very quickly, resulting in two serious problems. General or systemic vasodilation occurs with a sudden, severe decrease in blood pressure. In the lungs, edema of the mucosa and constriction of the bronchi and bronchioles occur, obstructing airflow (Fig. 7-5). The marked lack of oxygen that results from both respiratory and circulatory impairment causes loss of consciousness within minutes.

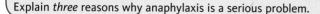

THINK ABOUT 3-6

Explain *three* reasons why anaphylaxis is a serious problem.

■ *Signs and Symptoms*

The initial manifestations of anaphylaxis include a generalized itching or tingling sensation over the body, coughing, and difficulty in breathing. This is quickly followed by feelings of weakness, dizziness or fainting, and a sense of fear and panic (Table 7-6). Edema may be observed around the eyes, lips, tongue, hands, and feet. Hives, or urticaria, may appear on the skin. General collapse soon follows with loss of consciousness, usually within minutes.

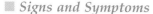

EMERGENCY TREATMENT FOR ANAPHYLAXIS

- Inject epinephrine immediately if it is available. Persons who have experienced acute allergic or anaphylactic reactions often carry an injectable epinephrine (EpiPen) with them because there are only seconds or minutes between the exposure to the allergen and the body's collapse. Epinephrine acts to increase blood pressure by stimulating the sympathetic nervous system; it causes vasoconstriction and increases the rate and strength of the heartbeat. This drug also relaxes the bronchial smooth muscle, opening the airway.
- If available, oxygen should be administered immediately along with an injectable antihistamine.
- Seek emergency help as soon as possible by dialing 911.
- Treat for shock, keeping the person warm.
- Cardiopulmonary resuscitation (CPR) should be initiated if necessary.

■ *Treatment*

It is essential that an epinephrine injection be administered immediately. This acts in the same way as the natural hormone epinephrine.

Antihistamine drugs (diphenhydramine [Benadryl] or chlorpheniramine [Chlor-Trimeton]) are useful in the early stages of an allergic reaction because they block the response of the tissues to the released histamine (blocking histamine-1 receptors on cells). Glucocorticoids or cortisone derivatives may be used for severe or prolonged reactions because they reduce the immune response and stabilize the vascular system. Glucocorticoids can be administered by injection or by mouth, or they can be applied topically to the skin (see Chapter 5).

Skin tests can be performed to determine the specific cause of an allergy. This procedure involves scratching the skin and dropping a small amount of purified antigen on the scratch. The site is observed for erythema or redness, which indicates a positive skin reaction. In many cases, the person with an allergy can determine the contributing factors by observation and keep a log of daily exposure to foods, pollens, and other allergens. Avoidance of the suspected antigen will keep the person symptom free. Desensitization treatments involving repeated injections of very small amounts of antigen to create a blocking antibody may reduce the allergic response.

THINK ABOUT 7-7

a. Explain the importance of determining the specific causes of allergic reactions.
b. Explain the purpose of including allergies in a health history.

Type II: Cytotoxic Hypersensitivity

In type II hypersensitivity, often called cytotoxic hypersensitivity, the antigen is present on the cell membrane (Fig. 7-6). The antigen may be a normal body component or foreign. Circulating IgG antibodies react with the antigen, causing destruction of the cell by phagocytosis or by releasing cytolytic enzymes related to complement activation. An example of this reaction is the response to an incompatible blood transfusion (see Chapter 10). A person with type A blood has A antigens on his red blood cells and anti-B antibodies in his blood. A person with type B blood has anti-A antibodies. If type B blood from a donor is added to the recipient's type A blood, the antigen–antibody reaction will destroy the red blood cells (hemolysis) in the type A blood (see Fig. 7-6). Another type of blood incompatibility involves the Rh factor, which is discussed in Chapter 22.

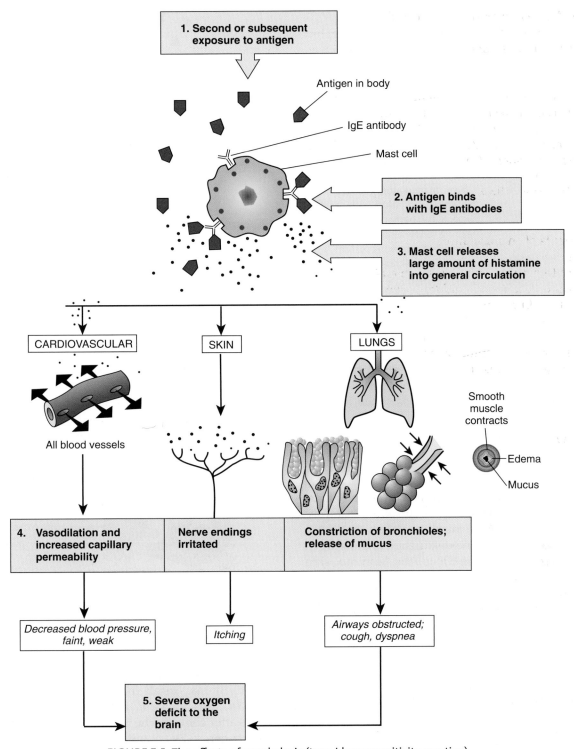

FIGURE 7-5 The effects of anaphylaxis (type I hypersensitivity reaction).

Type III: Immune Complex Hypersensitivity

In this type of reaction, the antigen combines with the antibody, forming a complex, which is then deposited in tissue, often in blood vessel walls, and also activates complement (Fig. 7-7). This process causes inflammation and tissue destruction. A number of diseases are now thought to be caused by immune complexes, including glomerulonephritis (see Chapter 18) and rheumatoid arthritis (see Chapter 9). *Serum sickness* refers to the systemic reaction that occurs when immune complex deposits occur in many tissues. With reduced use of animal serum for passive immunization, serum sickness is much less common today. An *Arthus* reaction is a localized inflammatory and tissue necrosis that

TABLE 7-6	Signs and Symptoms of Anaphylaxis
Manifestation	Rationale
Skin: pruritus, tingling, warmth, hives	Histamine and chemical mediators irritate sensory nerves
Respiration: difficulty in breathing, cough, wheezing, tight feeling	Chemical mediators cause contraction of smooth muscle in bronchioles, edema, and increased secretions, leading to narrow airways and lack of oxygen
Cardiovascular: decreased blood pressure	Chemical mediators cause general vasodilation, with rapid, weak pulse, perhaps irregular leading to low blood pressure; sympathetic nervous system responds by increasing rate
Central nervous system: anxiety and fear (early); weakness, dizziness, and loss of consciousness	Early, sympathetic response; later, lack of oxygen to the brain because of low blood pressure and respiratory obstruction

results when an immune complex lodges in the blood vessel wall, causing vasculitis. One example is "farmer's lung," a reaction to molds inhaled when an individual handles moldy hay.

Type IV: Cell-Mediated or Delayed Hypersensitivity

This type of hypersensitivity is a delayed response by sensitized T lymphocytes to antigens, resulting in release of lymphokines or other chemical mediators that cause an inflammatory response and destruction of the antigen (Fig. 7-8). The tuberculin test (e.g., the Mantoux skin test) uses this mechanism to check for prior exposure to the organism causing tuberculosis. Once in the body, this mycobacterium has the unusual characteristic of causing a hypersensitivity reaction in the lungs, even when an active infection does not develop (see Chapter 13). When a small amount of antigen is injected into the skin of a previously sensitized person, an area of inflammation develops at the injection site, indicating a positive test. This positive reaction does not necessarily indicate active infection, but it does indicate exposure of the body to the tuberculosis organism at some prior time. An x-ray and sputum culture will determine the absence or presence of active tuberculosis. As mentioned previously in this chapter, organ transplant rejection belongs in this category.

Contact dermatitis, or an allergic skin rash, is caused by a type IV reaction to direct contact with a chemical. Such chemicals include cosmetics, dyes, soaps, and metals. Other examples include skin reactions to plant toxins such as poison ivy. These skin reactions usually do not occur immediately after contact; these reactions usually take more than 24 hours.

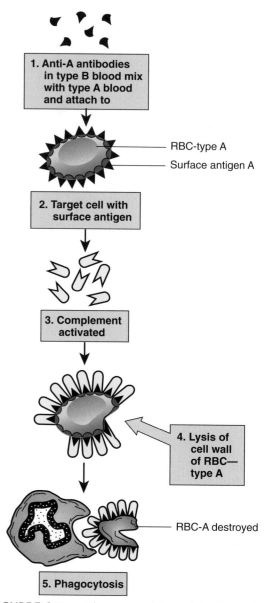

1. Anti-A antibodies in type B blood mix with type A blood and attach to

RBC-type A
Surface antigen A

2. Target cell with surface antigen

3. Complement activated

4. Lysis of cell wall of RBC—type A

RBC-A destroyed

5. Phagocytosis

FIGURE 7-6 Type II hypersensitivity, cytotoxic reaction.

Of importance to health workers is the high frequency of sensitivity to rubber and latex products, particularly with the increased use of latex gloves. Latex sensitivity may result from type I or type IV reactions. In most cases, a type IV reaction causes a rash, 48 to 96 hours after contact. The type I response is more rare but also more serious, manifested as asthma, hives, or anaphylaxis. Contact with latex proteins may occur through skin or mucous membranes, by inhalation, or by internal routes. More severe reactions often occur when mucous membranes are involved, such as the mouth or vagina of latex-sensitive individuals. Also metals such as nickel, which are frequently found in instruments or equipment used by health care professionals, can trigger an immune response. Such sensitivities are usually indicated by the location of the rash. The skin is red and pruritic, and vesicles and a serous exudate may be present at the site.

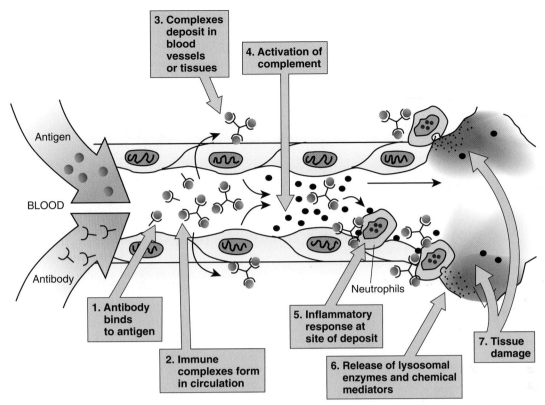

FIGURE 7-7 Type III hypersensitivity, immune complex reaction.

Autoimmune Disorders

Autoimmune disorders occur when the immune system cannot distinguish between self and non–self-antigens. The exact causes of autoimmune diseases/disorders are still unknown.

Mechanism

Autoimmune disorders occur when individuals develop antibodies to their own cells or cellular material and these antibodies then attack the individual's tissues (Fig. 7-9). The term autoantibodies refers to antibodies formed against self-antigens. There is greater recognition as well as better diagnosis and treatment of autoimmune disorders now due to advances in diagnostic procedures. Some of these disorders affect single organs or tissues, for example, Hashimoto's thyroiditis, and some are generalized, such as systemic lupus erythematosus. Other examples are rheumatic fever, myasthenia gravis, scleroderma, pernicious anemia, and hyperthyroidism (Graves' disease).

Self-antigens are usually tolerated by the immune system, and there is no reaction to one's own antigens. When self-tolerance is lost, the immune system is unable to differentiate self from foreign material. The autoantibodies then trigger an immune reaction leading to inflammation and necrosis of tissue. Some individuals may lose their immune tolerance following tissue destruction and subsequent formation of antibodies to the damaged cell components. Aging may lead to loss of tolerance to self-antigens. There also appears to be a genetic factor involved in autoimmune diseases, as evidenced by increased familial incidence.

Example: Systemic Lupus Erythematosus

Systemic lupus erythematosus (SLE) is a chronic inflammatory disease that affects a number of systems; therefore it can be difficult to diagnose and treat. The name of this systemic disorder is derived from the characteristic facial rash, which is erythematous and occurs across the nose and cheeks, resembling the markings of a wolf (lupus) (Fig. 7-10). The rash is now often referred to as a "butterfly rash," reflecting its distribution. The condition is becoming better known and more cases are identified in the early stages, improving the prognosis. Certain drugs may cause a lupus-like syndrome, which usually disappears when the drug is discontinued. *Discoid lupus erythematosus* is a less serious version of the disease affecting only the skin.

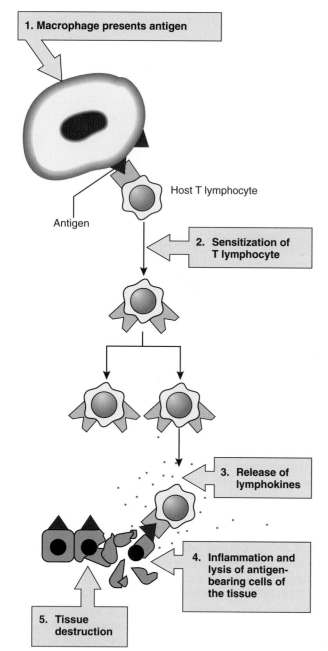

1. **Macrophage presents antigen**

Host T lymphocyte

Antigen

2. **Sensitization of T lymphocyte**

3. **Release of lymphokines**

4. **Inflammation and lysis of antigen-bearing cells of the tissue**

5. **Tissue destruction**

FIGURE 7-8 Type IV hypersensitivity, cell-mediated delayed hypersensitivity.

Occurrence is uncertain because many cases are probably not diagnosed in the early stages. Systemic lupus erythematosus affects primarily women and becomes manifest between the ages of 20 and 40 years. The incidence is higher in African Americans, Asians, Hispanics, and Native Americans.

The specific cause has not been established, but it appears to be multifactorial and includes genetic, hormonal (estrogen levels), and environmental (ultraviolet light exposure) factors. A single lupus gene has not been identified, but genes increasing susceptibility to autoimmune disorders have been identified. A number of research projects are in process, including studies of the complement system and immune systems in affected individuals and their families. Another focus concerns identification of a possible genetic defect interfering with normal apoptosis and removal of damaged cells, leaving cell contents such as nucleic acids in the tissues.

■ Pathophysiology

Systemic lupus erythematosus is characterized by the presence of large numbers of circulating autoantibodies against DNA, platelets, erythrocytes, various nucleic acids, and other nuclear materials (antinuclear antibodies [ANAs]). Immune complexes, especially those with anti-DNA antibody, are deposited in connective tissues anywhere in the body, activating complement and causing inflammation and necrosis. Vasculitis, or inflammation of the blood vessels, develops in many organs, impairing blood supply to the tissue. The resulting ischemia (inadequate oxygen for the cells) leads to further inflammation and destruction of the tissue. This process usually takes place in several organs or tissues. Common sites include the kidneys, lungs, heart, brain, skin, joints, and digestive tract. Diagnosis is based on the presence of multiple system involvement (a minimum of four areas) and laboratory data showing the presence of autoantibodies.

■ Clinical Signs and Symptoms

The clinical presentation of SLE varies greatly because different combinations of effects develop in each individual, often making it difficult to diagnose the disorder. Many persons present initially with skin rash or joint inflammation, then progress to lung or kidney involvement. Common signs and symptoms are listed in Table 7-7. The course is progressive and is marked by remissions and exacerbations.

■ Diagnostic Tests

The presence of numerous ANAs, especially anti-DNA, as well as other antibodies in the serum is indicative of SLE. Lupus erythematosus (LE) cells, mature neutrophils containing nuclear material (Fig. 7-11) in the blood are a positive sign. Complement levels are typically low, and the erythrocyte sedimentation rate (ESR) is high, indicating the inflammatory response. Frequently counts of erythrocytes, leukocytes, lymphocytes, and platelets are low. Additional immunologic tests for various antibodies may be required to confirm the diagnosis. Also, all organs and systems need to be examined for inflammation and damage.

■ Treatment

Systemic lupus erythematosus is usually treated by a rheumatologist. Frequently prednisone, a glucocorticoid, is the drug used to reduce the immune response and subsequent inflammation (see Chapter 5). High doses may be taken during an exacerbation or periods of stress, but the dose should be reduced when the

NORMAL IMMUNE RESPONSE

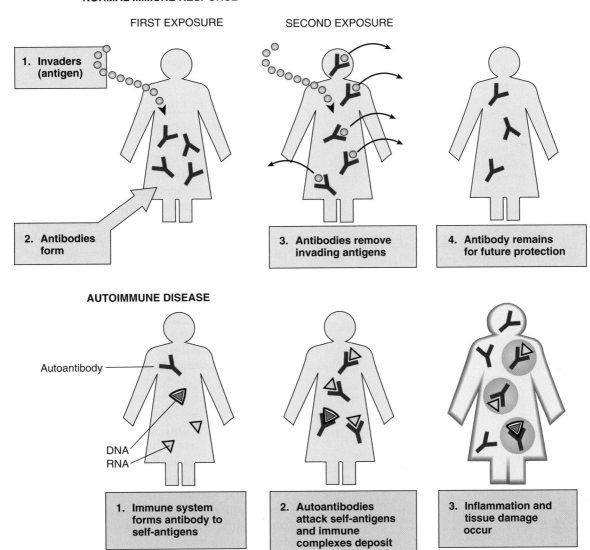

FIRST EXPOSURE   SECOND EXPOSURE

1. Invaders (antigen)

2. Antibodies form

3. Antibodies remove invading antigens

4. Antibody remains for future protection

AUTOIMMUNE DISEASE

Autoantibody

DNA
RNA

1. Immune system forms antibody to self-antigens

2. Autoantibodies attack self-antigens and immune complexes deposit

3. Inflammation and tissue damage occur

FIGURE 7-9 The autoimmune process.

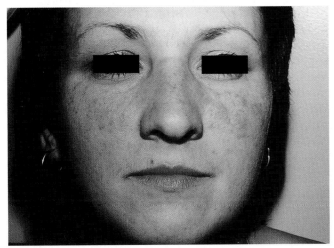

FIGURE 7-10 "Butterfly rash" with distribution on the cheeks and over the nose associated with systemic lupus erythematosus. *(Courtesy of Dr. M. McKenzie, Toronto, Ontario, Canada.)*

patient is in remission to minimize the side effects of the drug. Nonsteroidal anti-inflammatory drugs are also useful. The antimalarial drug, hydroxychloroquine, appears to reduce exacerbations. Additional therapy may be required for specific system involvement. Limiting damage to vital organs improves quality of life. One research effort continues to seek drugs that block only the B-lymphocyte response to antigens, reducing antibody formation.

Minimizing exacerbations by avoiding aggravating factors and by promptly treating acute episodes is a major goal. Avoidance of sun exposure and excessive fatigue assists in preventing flare-ups. Warning signs of exacerbations include increasing fatigue, rash, pain, fever, and headache.

The prognosis for SLE is much improved now with early diagnosis and careful treatment, providing most individuals with an active life and normal lifespan.

TABLE 7-7	Common Manifestations of Systemic Lupus Erythematosus
Joints	Polyarthritis, with swollen, painful joints, without damage; arthralgia
Skin	Butterfly rash with erythema on cheeks and over nose or rash on body; photosensitivity—exacerbation with sun exposure; ulcerations in oral mucosa; hair loss
Kidneys	Glomerulonephritis with antigen–antibody deposit in glomerulus, causing inflammation with marked proteinuria and progressive renal damage
Lungs	Pleurisy—inflammation of the pleural membranes, causing chest pain
Heart	Carditis—inflammation of any layer of the heart, commonly pericarditis
Blood vessels	Raynaud's phenomenon—periodic vasospasm in fingers and toes, accompanied by pain
Central nervous system	Psychoses, depression, mood changes, seizures
Bone marrow	Anemia, leukopenia, thrombocytopenia

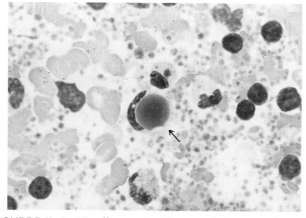

FIGURE 7-11 An LE cell present with systemic lupus erythematosus. Note the large LE mass that has been phagocytized by the neutrophil (*arrow*) and is taking up most of the cytoplasm of the cell. The cell nucleus has been pushed to the side. (*From Stevens ML:* Fundamentals of Clinical Hematology, *Philadelphia, 1997, Saunders.*)

THINK ABOUT 7-9

a. Define the term and describe the autoantibodies present in SLE.
b. Explain why it is important to reduce the number of exacerbations.
c. Explain why SLE may be difficult to diagnose and treat.

Immunodeficiency

Immunity is the body's capacity to fight foreign substances. Immunodeficiency will result in a compromised or lack of an immune response.

Causes of Immunodeficiency

Immunodeficiency results from a loss of function, partial or total, of one or more components of the immune system leading to increased risk of infection and cancer. Examples are presented in Table 7-8. The problem may be acute and short-term or chronic. Deficits may be classified by etiology or component. *Primary* deficiencies involve a basic developmental failure somewhere in the system (for example, in the bone marrow's production of stem cells), the thymus, or the synthesis of antibodies. Many defects result from a genetic or congenital abnormality and are first noticed in infants and children. There may be associated problems that affect other organs and systems in the body. Examples include an inherited X-linked hypogammaglobulinemia (low antibody levels because of a B-cell defect) or a developmental defect known as DiGeorge syndrome (hypoplasia of the thymus).

Secondary or acquired immunodeficiency refers to loss of the immune response resulting from specific causes and may occur at any time during the lifespan. Loss of the immune response can occur with infection, particularly viral infection, splenectomy (removal of the spleen), malnutrition or liver disease (hypoproteinemia—low serum protein level), use of *immunosuppressive* drugs in clients with organ transplants, and radiation and chemotherapy for cancer treatment. Immunodeficiency associated with cancer is a result of malnutrition and blood loss as well as the effects of treatment, all of which depress bone marrow production of leukocytes (see Chapter 20). Glucocorticoid drugs such as prednisone, a common long-term treatment for chronic inflammatory diseases as well as for cancer, cause decreased leukocyte production, atrophy of lymph nodes, and suppression of the immune response (see Chapter 5). Also it is thought that severe stress, physical or emotional, may cause a temporary immunodeficiency state owing to high levels of glucocorticoid secretion in the body. Another well-known cause of secondary immunodeficiency is AIDS or HIV infection, affecting T-helper cells, discussed later in this chapter.

Effects of Immunodeficiency

Immunodeficiency states predispose patients to the development of *opportunistic* infections by normally harmless microorganisms. This may involve multiple organisms and be quite severe. These infections are difficult to treat successfully. They often arise from resident

TABLE 7-8	Examples of Immunodeficiency Disorders	
Deficit	Primary	Secondary
B cell (humoral)	Hypogammaglobulinemia (congenital)	Kidney disease with loss of globulins
T cell (cell-mediated)	Thymic aplasia	Hodgkin's disease (cancer of the lymph nodes)
DiGeorge syndrome	AIDS (HIV infection); temporary with some viruses	
B and T cell	Inherited combined immunodeficiency syndromes (CIDS)	Radiation, immunosuppressive drugs, cytotoxic drugs (cancer chemotherapy)
Phagocytes	Inherited chronic granulomatous diseases (CGDs)	Immunosuppression (glucocorticoid drugs, neutropenia); diabetes (decreased chemotaxis)
Complement	Inherited deficit of one or more systems	Malnutrition (decreased synthesis), components liver disease—cirrhosis

flora of the body; for example, fungal or candidal infection in the mouth of someone whose normal defenses are impaired. Sometimes severe, life-threatening infections result from unusual organisms that are normally not pathogenic or disease causing in healthy individuals, such as *Pneumocystis carinii.*

It is essential that prophylactic antimicrobial drugs (preventive antibiotics) be administered to anyone in an immunodeficient state before undertaking an invasive procedure that carries an increased risk of organisms entering the body. The immune-compromised host is vulnerable to microorganisms not usually considered harmful (opportunistic infection). This includes any procedure in which there is direct access to blood or tissues, for example, a tooth extraction, and especially procedures in areas in which normal flora are present (see Chapter 6). There also appears to be an increased incidence of cancer in persons who have impaired immune systems, probably related to the decrease in the body's immune surveillance and the failure of the immune system to destroy malignant cells quickly.

▓ *Treatment*

Replacement therapy for antibodies using gamma globulin may be helpful. Depending on the cause, bone marrow or thymus transplants are possible, but success with these has been limited.

THINK ABOUT 7-10

Explain why a person whose blood test shows an abnormally low leukocyte count should be given an antimicrobial drug before a tooth extraction.

Acquired Immunodeficiency Syndrome

Acquired immunodeficiency syndrome (AIDS) is a chronic infectious disease caused by HIV, which destroys helper T-lymphocytes, causing loss of the immune response and increased susceptibility to secondary infections and cancer. It is characterized by a prolonged latent period followed by a period of active infection (Fig. 7-12). An individual is considered *HIV-positive* when the virus is known to be present in the body, but few if any clinical signs have developed. *Acquired immunodeficiency syndrome* is the stage of *active* infection, with marked clinical manifestations and multiple complications. An individual may be HIV positive for many years before he or she develops AIDS.

Current therapy has extended the time before development of symptomatic AIDS; however, eventually the active stage develops. The infection may not be diagnosed in the early stages because of this latent asymptomatic period; this contributes to greater spread of the disease. If a patient presents with an unusual infection such as *Pneumocystis carinii* pneumonia or a cancer such as Kaposi's sarcoma (termed an AIDS indicator disease) and no other pathology, this often marks the presence of active HIV infection and signals the need for HIV testing.

History

The first case of AIDS was recognized in 1981, although there is evidence that there were earlier, sporadic cases. Acquired immunodeficiency syndrome is now considered a worldwide pandemic, and cases still are multiplying, particularly in sub-Saharan Africa and Asia. Many cases are not diagnosed or recorded; therefore the estimates may not reflect the true extent of the infection. It is no longer a disease of homosexual men; more women and children are now infected. In 1995, AIDS was the leading cause of death in the 25- to 40-year-old group; now, with treatment, the lifespan has been greatly extended from the original 6 months to many years, and AIDS is considered to be a chronic disease.

The CDC reports for 2006 indicated there were 1 million cases in North America, including 35,000 newly infected, of which 27% of the adults were women. Race/ethnicity of persons newly diagnosed in the United States in 2006 shows:
- 49% African American (Black)
- 30% Caucasian (White)

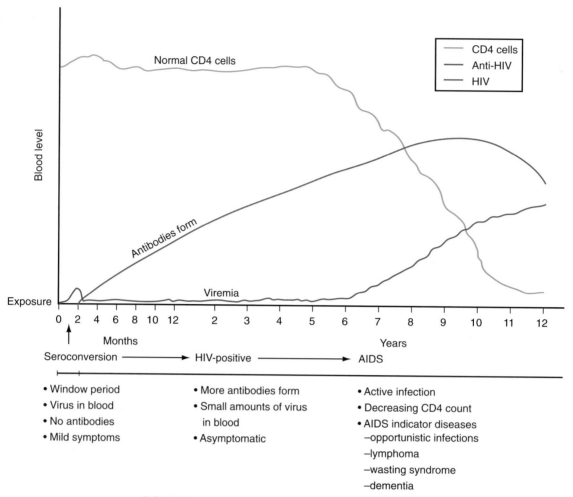

FIGURE 7-12 Typical stages in the development of AIDS.

- 18% Hispanic (Latino)
- 1% Asian or Pacific Islander
- <1% American Indian or Alaskan indigenous

The same report shows the highest incidence of new cases in adult males for 2006 occurred as a result of male-to-male sexual transmission, with injection drug use and high-risk heterosexual transmission being about equal in rate of infection. Newly diagnosed cases in adult females related to high-risk heterosexual sex were fourfold higher than those in women who injected drugs. Seventy-three percent of cases were in teens (age 13+) and adults under the age of 45. Children accounted for 1% of new cases in 1996.

Globally the UN reports for 2007 include about 33 million persons infected. Sub-Saharan Africa reports 22 million infected persons (more than 50% are women). Numbers of newly infected cases in Asia continue to rise, particularly in India and China. In 2007, the UN reported that 90% of HIV-infected persons were not receiving appropriate antiretroviral drug treatment. The global mortality from AIDS was 2 million in 2007; this estimate includes both children and adults. Only 30% of pregnant women had access to antiretroviral agents, although it is known that these drugs reduce the risk of

infection of the fetus. Among HIV-infected people diagnosed with TB, only 30% received drugs for both conditions on a consistent basis.

These numbers must be viewed with the knowledge that in many areas reporting of new cases is sporadic or absent, thus the numbers are likely much higher than actual incidence of infection. In 2003 the UN launched the 3 by 5 initiative to provide a combination of three less expensive drugs along with educational materials to 3 million infected persons living in Africa and other countries lacking access to these materials. The goal was to be achieved by 2005; in fact, the 2008 report on the global AIDS epidemic by the UNAIDS program characterizes progress on reducing the HIV epidemic as a "stable rate of transmission at unacceptably high levels."

According to the CDC 1.2 million people in the United States are infected with HIV. In addition 20% of those infected are unaware of their infections. Despite these facts the annual number of new HIV infections as remained relatively stable.

Since the beginning of the epidemic in the United States an estimated 1,129,127 people have been diagnosed with AIDS. An estimated 17,774 patients with

AIDS died in 2009 and an estimated 619,400 people died with AIDS in the United States since the epidemic began (information from the CDC).

In addition the number of persons aged 50 years and older infected with HIV or having AIDS has been increasing in the recent years. This increase is partially due to the increased life expectance because of active antiviral therapy and also due to new diagnosed cases for persons over the age of 50. Compared with Whites, the rates of HIV/AIDS among persons over 50 is suggested to be 12 times as high among Blacks and five times as high among Hispanics.

The Agent

Human immunodeficiency virus refers to human immunodeficiency virus (type 1 or 2), a retrovirus, which contains RNA. (See Chapter 6 for general information on viruses and infections.) The virus is a member of a subfamily, lentivirus, so called because infection develops slowly. HIV-1 is the major cause of AIDS in the United States and Europe and appears to have originated in central Africa, although it now occurs worldwide. Human immunodeficiency virus-2 (HIV-2) is found primarily in central Africa. It is thought that the virus crossed from chimpanzees to humans as chimpanzees were hunted and prepared for food. New research has indicated that this likely happened between 1894 and 1924 in Central Africa. Initially the infection was sporadic, but with the development of industry and movement to crowded urban centers with workers migrating seasonally between village and city, the rate of infection increased dramatically.

As indicated earlier in the chapter, the virus primarily infects the CD4 T-helper lymphocytes, leading to a decrease in function and number of these cells, which play an essential role in both humoral and cell-mediated immune responses. Also, HIV attacks macrophages and central nervous system cells. At an early stage, the virus invades and multiplies in lymphoid tissue, the lymph nodes, tonsils, and spleen, using these tissues as a reservoir for continued infection.

The core of HIV contains two strands of RNA and the enzyme reverse transcriptase, and the coat is covered with a lipid envelope studded with "spikes" of glycoproteins that the virus uses to attach to human cells (Fig. 7-13). Once inside the human host cell, the viral RNA must be converted by the viral enzyme into viral DNA, which is then integrated with the human DNA. The virus then controls the human cell and uses its resources to produce more virus particles, and subsequently the host cell dies. The new viruses can be seen "budding" out of the host cell in Figure 7-14. A number of subtypes and recombinants have been identified.

There is a delay or "window" before the antibodies to the virus appear in the blood; the delay may be from 2 weeks to 6 months but averages 3 to 7 weeks. Antibodies form more rapidly following direct transmission into

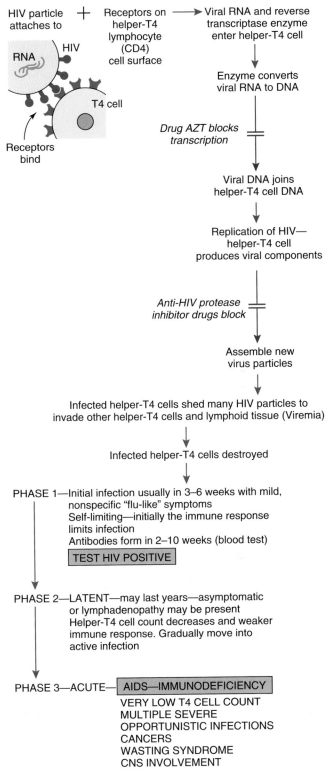

FIGURE 7-13 The course of HIV-AIDS.

blood and more slowly from sexual transmission. This likely reflects a differing dose rate received through the differing routes.

Antibodies form the basis for routine testing for the presence of HIV, and this delay creates difficulty in detecting the infection following exposure. In areas

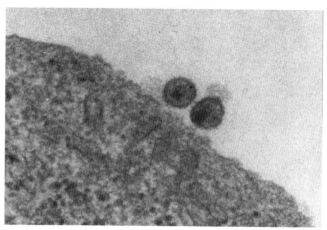

FIGURE 7-14 HIV budding from a host cell surface. *(From De la Maza LM, Pezzlo MT, Baron EJ: Color Atlas of Diagnostic Microbiology, St. Louis, 1997, Mosby.)*

where infection is less than 10%, three-stage testing is required. In highly endemic areas with an infection rate greater than 10%, a two-stage testing protocol is used. The viral RNA or DNA can be identified in the blood and lymphocytes in about 5 days using polymerase chain reaction (PCR) technology to rapidly replicate the genetic material in the laboratory. With this technology a small amount of the nucleic acids to be tested or analyzed is introduced into a solution of enzymes and nucleotides in the presence of heat; the result is thousands of copies of the nucleic acid that can then be compared with a reference sample.

In developed areas of the world with medical laboratories, diagnosis of AIDS is based on the absolute number of CD4 T-helper cells. Infection is shown when the CD4 T-helper lymphocyte count is less than 200 cells per cubic milliliter of blood. Where a suitable equipped laboratory is not available, a modified case definition is recommended by the WHO based on the presence of opportunistic infections, tumors such as Kaposi's sarcoma, weight loss, or *Pneumocystis carinii* pneumonia (PCP).

Early in the infection, large numbers of viruses are produced, followed by a reduction as the antibody level rises. The failure of the antibodies to destroy all the viruses is not totally understood, but the factors include:
- The virus is hidden safely inside host cells in the lymphoid tissue during the latent phase.
- There appear to be frequent slight mutations in the viral envelope, making the antibodies less effective.
- Progressive destruction of the T-helper cells and macrophages gradually cripples the entire immune system.

Transmission

When transmitted, the virus must find entry into the circulating blood of the recipient. The virus is transmitted in body fluids, such as blood, semen, and vaginal secretions. Blood contains the highest concentration of virus, with semen next. Human immunodeficiency virus may be present in small numbers in other secretions, such as saliva, but transmission in such cases has not been established. There is a slight risk that blood donated by newly infected persons will not test positive for antibodies during the "window" period; therefore blood products are now tested for the virus and treated when possible. This has reduced the risk for hemophiliacs and others who must have repeated treatment with blood products. Infected organ donors can also transmit the infection. Individuals who have a history of high-risk activities such as IV drug use, unprotected sex, or untreated sexually transmitted diseases are not accepted as organ or blood donors to reduce the possibility of transmitting the virus.

Health care workers should assume there is a risk of some infection (there is a higher risk of transmitting other infections such as hepatitis B or C) from contact with body fluids from any individual and follow universal precautions (see Chapter 6). Patients infected with HIV are not isolated or labeled because such information may not include those infected and in the "window period." All clients must be treated as though they may be infected if transmission by blood and body fluids is to be prevented. Where transmission is suspected, the health care worker should immediately seek counseling and postexposure prophylaxis. Testing for HIV antibodies will be carried out using the three-stage testing procedure.

In cases in which it is known that a client has HIV infection, appointments for invasive procedures may be scheduled at the end of the clinic day before daily disinfection of the clinic. Judgment must be used to balance the needs of the immunocompromised client and others in the clinic. Special precautions may be required in preparing the body of a patient who has died of AIDS to prevent transmission before cremation or burial.

People who are high-risk sources of HIV include intravenous drug users (shared needles) and those with multiple sexual partners. Unprotected sexual intercourse with infected persons (heterosexual as well as homosexual) provides another mode of transmission, particularly in the presence of associated tissue trauma and other sexually transmitted infections that promote direct access to the blood.

Currently the greatest increase in cases of HIV infection is occurring in women, either by heterosexual contact or intravenous drug use. Infected women may also transmit the virus to a fetus in the uterus, particularly if AIDS is advanced. Administration of azidothymidine (AZT, zidovudine) to pregnant women has greatly decreased the risk of infant infection. Many infants carry the mother's antibodies for the first few months, appearing infected, but eventually they convert to test negative. The child may become infected during delivery through contact with secretions in the birth canal and should receive drug treatment after a vaginal birth. Delivery by cesarean section can reduce this risk. Also, breast milk can transmit the virus. In developing countries, this creates a dilemma, because breast milk protects infants from so many other potentially fatal infections, and infant formula is not readily available.

Human immunodeficiency virus is *not transmitted* by casual contact (touching or kissing an infected person), sneezing and coughing, fomites such as toilet seats or eating utensils, or insect bites.

Studies have shown the virus may survive up to 15 days at room temperature, but is inactivated at temperatures greater than 60° C. It is inactivated by 2% glutaraldehyde disinfectants, autoclaving, and many disinfectants, such as alcohol and hypochlorite (household bleach).

■ Diagnostic Tests

The presence of HIV infection is determined by using a blood test for HIV antibodies, using HIV antigen from recombinant HIV or ELISA for the primary test. A positive result is followed by the more sensitive Western blot test, which is used for confirmation. Tests for the virus itself, both RNA and DNA, include PCR typing of viral RNA and DNA from the blood. Polymerase chain reaction typing is used to check the status of a newborn child who may carry the mother's antibodies but not be infected. It is essential for testing blood donations and to monitor the viral load in the blood as the disease progresses. A new rapid, noninvasive test (20 minutes) using saliva is now available, but the more complex testing is necessary to confirm a positive result. The ease of this new test may facilitate diagnosis in more individuals.

A diagnosis of AIDS depends on a major decrease in CD4+ T-helper lymphocytes in the blood (see Fig. 7-13) and a change in the CD4+ to CD8+ ratio in the presence of opportunistic infection or certain cancers. B lymphocytes remain normal, and IgG is increased. Additional tests depend on the particular effects of AIDS in the individual. The CDC has established case definition criteria using the indicator diseases, opportunistic infections, and unusual cancers, and has provided a classification for the phases of the infection.

THINK ABOUT 7-11

a. Explain the problem when a virus attacks T-helper cells.
b. Why are the infections and cancers that accompany AIDS significant?
c. Differentiate among HIV exposure, HIV infection, and AIDS.

■ Clinical Signs and Symptoms

The clinical effects of HIV infection vary among individuals, and differences are also apparent among men, women, and children. During the first phase, a few weeks after exposure, viral replication is rapid and there may be mild, generalized flulike symptoms such as low fever, fatigue, arthralgia, and sore throat. These symptoms disappear without treatment. Many persons are asymptomatic. In the prolonged second, or latent, phase, many patients demonstrate no clinical signs, whereas some have a generalized lymphadenopathy or enlarged lymph nodes. It appears that viral replication is reduced during this time.

The final acute stage, when immune deficiency is evident, is marked by numerous serious complications. The categories include general manifestations of HIV infection, gastrointestinal effects, neurologic effects, secondary infections, and malignancies. Secondary infections and cancer are caused by the immunodeficiency. Each patient may demonstrate more effects in one or two categories as well as minor changes in the other systems (Fig. 7-15).

- Generalized effects include lymphadenopathy, fatigue and weakness, headache, and arthralgia. Gastrointestinal effects seem to be related primarily to opportunistic infections, including parasitic infections. The signs include chronic severe diarrhea, vomiting, and ulcers on the mucous membranes. Necrotizing periodontal disease is common, with inflammation, necrosis, and infection around the teeth in the oral cavity. Severe weight loss, malnutrition, and muscle wasting frequently develop.

- Human immunodeficiency virus encephalopathy (general brain dysfunction), sometimes called AIDS dementia, refers to the direct infection of brain cells by HIV. This is often aggravated by malignant tumors, particularly lymphomas, and by opportunistic infections such as herpesvirus, various fungi, and toxoplasmosis in the brain. Nutritional deficits, particularly of vitamins, are a contributing factor. Encephalopathy is reflected by confusion, progressive cognitive impairment, including memory loss, loss of coordination and balance, and depression. Eventually the person cannot talk or move and seizures or coma may develop.

- Secondary infections are common with AIDS and are the primary cause of death. They are frequently multiple, and more extensive and severe than usual. Drug treatment of secondary infection is often ineffective. In the lungs, *Pneumocystis carinii*, now considered a fungus, is a common cause of severe pneumonia (see Chapter 13) and is frequently the cause of death (Fig. 7-16A). Herpes simplex, a virus causing cold sores, is common (see Fig. 28-8), and *Candida*, a fungus, involves the mouth and often extends into the esophagus (see Fig. 37-17C). The incidence of tuberculosis in AIDS patients is quite high and climbing rapidly.

- There is an increased incidence of all cancers in persons with AIDS, but unusual cancers are a marker

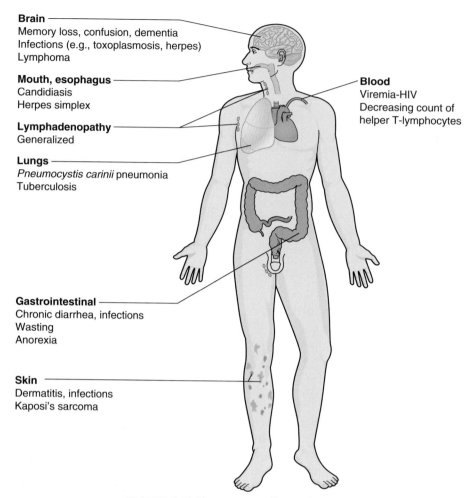

Brain
Memory loss, confusion, dementia
Infections (e.g., toxoplasmosis, herpes)
Lymphoma

Mouth, esophagus
Candidiasis
Herpes simplex

Lymphadenopathy
Generalized

Lungs
Pneumocystis carinii pneumonia
Tuberculosis

Gastrointestinal
Chronic diarrhea, infections
Wasting
Anorexia

Skin
Dermatitis, infections
Kaposi's sarcoma

Blood
Viremia-HIV
Decreasing count of
helper T-lymphocytes

FIGURE 7-15 The common effects of AIDS.

for AIDS. Kaposi's sarcoma affects the skin, mucous membranes, and internal organs (see Fig. 7-16*B*). Skin lesions of Kaposi's sarcoma appear purple or brown, are nonpruritic (not itchy), painless patches that eventually become nodular. Non-Hodgkin's lymphomas are another frequent form of malignancy in AIDS patients (see Chapter 11).

Women with AIDS

Although AIDS in women is clinically similar to the disease in men in many ways, Kaposi's sarcoma is much rarer in women than in men. It appears that women with AIDS have a higher incidence of severe and resistant vaginal infections and pelvic inflammatory disease (PID) than women without AIDS (see Chapter 19), as well as more oral *Candida* and herpes infections. Sexually transmitted diseases are more severe in women with AIDS than in unaffected women, and infected women show a high incidence of cervical cancer.

Children with AIDS

Two positive PCR tests are required to confirm HIV infection in young children. Some children are seriously

ill and die within the first or second year. In others, the effects develop gradually over some years. Infants born with AIDS are usually smaller in size and exhibit failure to thrive, developmental delays, and neurologic impairment such as spastic paralysis early in life. Seizures and poor motor skills are common. Malignancies are rare in children. The life and health care of an infected child are frequently complicated by the illness and perhaps death of the parents. *Pneumocystis carinii* pneumonia is often the cause of death in children and prophylactic antimicrobial drugs are often prescribed.

People over 50 with HIV/AIDS

Persons over the age of 50 have the many of the same risk factors for HIV infections than the younger population. The challenges for prevention in this age group include but are not limited to:

- Older persons are sexually active but may not practice safe sex
- Drug injections or smoking of crack cocaine may occur
- Late testing because of stigma
- Misdiagnosis because of normal symptoms of aging

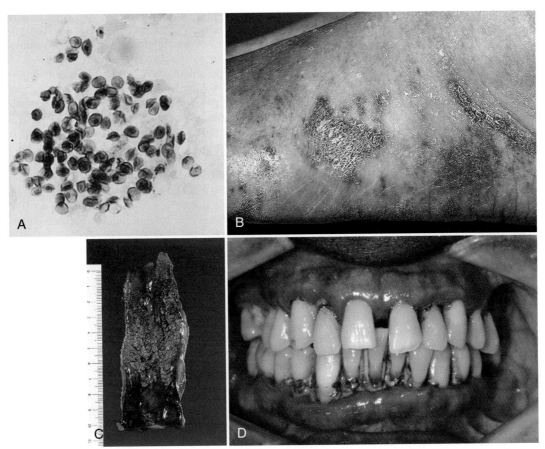

FIGURE 7-16 Complications of AIDS. **A**, *Pneumocystis carinii* organisms within a sputum sample from an AIDS patient. **B**, Kaposi's sarcoma. (***A*** and ***B*** *from Kumar V, Abbas AK, Fausto M: Robbins and Cotran Pathologic Basis of Disease, ed 7, Philadelphia, 2005, Saunders.*) **C**, Candida esophagitis. The thick greenish membrane is composed of *Candida hyphae* and purulent exudate. (*From Cooke RA, Stewart B: Colour Atlas of Anatomical Pathology, ed 3, Sydney, 2004, Churchill Livingstone.*) **D**, Necrotizing periodontal disease with inflammation, necrosis, and infection around the teeth. (*Courtesy of Evie Jesin, RRDH, BSc, George Brown College, Toronto, Ontario, Canada.*)

▓ Treatment

Antiviral drugs can reduce the replication of viruses, but they do not kill the virus, and thus are not a cure. There also are significant side effects, especially with higher drug dosages. The virus mutates as well, becoming resistant to the drug, particularly when single drugs are administered. Azidothymidine (or zidovudine) is the best-known drug. Several newer protease inhibitors drugs that block protein synthesis, including saquinavir and ritonavir, are now being used routinely in developed countries. Recently approved drugs are viral integrase inhibitors (raltegravir) that block the incorporation of viral DNA into the host chromosomes, entry inhibitors such as maraviroc, which is the first drug to block entry proteins on uninfected WBCs, and fusion inhibitors (Enfuvirtide), which block the fusion of the viral membrane with the membrane of the healthy host cell. The latter drug has shown effectiveness against drug-resistant forms of HIV.

Combinations of three to five drugs in a "cocktail" are being used successfully to prolong the latent phase as well as reduce the viral load during the final phase. For example, two viral reverse transcriptase inhibitors, such as zidovudine and lamivudine, plus a protease inhibitor such as indinavir form one such combination. This approach reduces drug-resistant mutations of the virus and the drugs are chosen to attack the virus from several points (see Fig. 6-16). The drugs must be taken continually on a rigid schedule. A "one pill daily" combination of three drugs (Atripla) is available to improve patient adherence to their drug protocol. Currently highly active antiretrovirus (HAART) therapy has been very effective at controlling the virus, reducing the viral load in the blood, and returning CD4 cell counts to near-normal levels.

A primary focus of treatment is on minimizing the effects of complications, such as infections or malignancy, by prophylactic medications and immediate treatment. Tuberculosis is reactivated in 50% of HIV+ patients and is often a systemic form requiring intensive drug treatment. In many cases tuberculosis (TB) is resistant to drugs that have been used in the past.

Antidiarrheal medication may also be required on a long-term basis. Even though safer and more effective drugs are available in many parts of the world, there continues to be an uneven distribution of such drugs. Concerns continue with respect to the toxicity of drugs, particularly for pregnant women, and the development of drug resistance in various strains of HIV.

The prognosis at the present time is much improved because persons with HIV infection are living longer with improved drug treatment. Without treatment, death occurs within several years as opposed to decades.

Treatment should start when the following have occurred:

- Severe symptoms
- CD4 count is under 500
- Pregnancy
- HIV-related kidney disease
- When treated for hepatitis B

CASE STUDY A

Hypersensitivity

M.C., a 23-year-old woman, has developed a skin rash as well as nausea and vomiting, after taking an antimicrobial drug for a short time. The skin rash is red and quite itchy and is spreading over her entire body. The physician stops the medication because of this allergic reaction. The patient has a history of skin rashes, both eczema and contact dermatitis, since infancy. She has had hay fever during the summer and fall for the past few years.

1. Why would the physician consider this an allergic reaction to a drug?
2. What kind of hypersensitivity is hay fever, and what are the signs of it?

anaphylaxis was suspected. He was given an epinephrine injection and oxygen then was transported to hospital. There he was given intravenous glucocorticoids. He recovered consciousness and was able to talk. The diagnosis was anaphylaxis resulting from multiple insect stings.

1. Describe the type of hypersensitivity reaction involved here.
2. Is it likely that J.A. had experienced a sting at some previous time?
3. Explain the rationale for: (a) pruritus (itchy skin), (b) difficulty talking and breathing, and (c) feeling faint.
4. Why was this condition difficult for emergency personnel to diagnose?
5. Explain how epinephrine and glucocorticoids would help reduce the manifestations of anaphylaxis.

J.A. was expecting to be discharged from the hospital that evening. However, the doctor noted a rash developing on his back. This continued to spread over his entire body and his neck was swollen, therefore he remained in the hospital. Intravenous glucocorticoids were continued as well as the antihistamine diphenhydramine (Benadryl). The rash began to subside in 48 hours. By the third day, the area where the stings occurred on the leg had turned a dark purple color.

6. What likely caused this rash to develop?

J.A. was finally discharged from the hospital and directed to continue the medications oral prednisone and diphenhydramine for a week. He returned for testing, which indicated allergy to hornets and honeybees.

He continues to take desensitizing injections. Each of these causes swelling, itchiness, and pain on the arm. He also carries an EpiPen and Benadryl with him at all times, as well as avoiding situations in which a sting could occur.

7. Why is it important for this patient to carry an EpiPen with him and wear a Medic-Alert bracelet? Suggest several situations to avoid, thus reducing the risk of future stings.

CASE STUDY B

Anaphylaxis

Mr. J.A., age 32, with no prior history of allergies, was mowing grass around the noon hour when he felt a sharp pain in his lower right leg. It was later determined that the lawn mower hit a hornets' nest in the ground. He continued cutting the grass for a moment, and then felt itchy all over his body. It was a very hot day and the air was heavy with dust and grass fragments. He jumped in the swimming pool to cool off, but immediately felt exhausted and climbed out. He lay down, feeling faint, and tried to call for help. However he could not talk clearly and was having difficulty breathing. Shortly, a family member appeared and called 911. At this time he couldn't swallow and was feeling nauseated. When emergency services arrived, J.A. could not talk or provide information to assist with a diagnosis. Finally one paramedic could detect a mark on his leg, but no swelling at the site. He was losing consciousness and had cold, moist skin. His blood pressure was falling, so

CASE STUDY C

Systemic Lupus Erythematosus

Ms. A.S., age 31, has been diagnosed with systemic lupus erythematosus. She had her first signs and symptoms 2 years ago. At this time she is having an exacerbation, which includes a facial rash, joint pains, and chest pain. She also has protein in her urine, indicating a kidney abnormality.

1. Explain the basic pathophysiology of this disease.
2. Describe three factors that would assist in making the diagnosis.
3. Describe the typical rash Ms. A.S. would have at this time.
4. Her chest pain is due to inflammation of the pleural membranes. Explain why this pain would be more severe during inspiration.
5. Her dose of prednisone, a glucocorticoid, has been increased. Briefly explain why she will return to a lower dose after the exacerbation ends.
6. Explain why moderate exercise would be helpful.

CASE STUDY D

HIV and AIDS

Ms. C.W. is a college student with an active social life. She is in a relationship with a fellow classmate who says that he has not had many relationships before theirs. After a party, they engage in unprotected sex, although they usually use a condom. She believes she will be safe because he shows no signs of AIDS and comes from a nice home. Several weeks later her friend tells her he has just tested HIV+. She immediately seeks advice and testing from the campus health center and is told that three tests over several months will be done. She is offered zidovudine (AZT) as a preventive medication that may reduce infectivity.

1. Why does the health care center recommend more than one test for HIV antibody status?
2. What is the action of zidovudine (AZT) in preventing infection with HIV?

   Ms. C.W.'s second test shows presence of HIV antibodies and she is diagnosed as HIV+. Although this is a great shock to her, her physician and counselor help her to accept the fact that she is HIV+ and can most likely live several years if she takes a combination of antiretroviral drugs. Ms. C.W.'s CD4 helper cell count rises and remains in a healthy range. She pursues a career and meets a man whom she marries.

3. What is the risk of transmission of HIV to men versus women? What are considered very high-risk sexual practices?
4. What factors might the couple consider in deciding whether to have a child?

   Ms. C.W. becomes pregnant and seeks information from her specialist about the risks of transmission of HIV to her unborn child.

5. What is the risk of transmission of HIV during pregnancy and labor and delivery?
6. How can the risk of infection be reduced before birth, during delivery, and after birth?
7. Why is blood testing of her newborn daughter for HIV not done until 3 to 6 months after birth?
8. Ms. C.W. wants to breastfeed her daughter, but is told by her doctor that she should not do so. Why should she not breastfeed?

   Ms. C.W.'s daughter is not infected and grows into a healthy toddler. Six years later, Ms. C.W. develops a chronic cough, overwhelming fatigue, recurrent diarrhea, and a sore mouth. Her physician diagnoses AIDS with PCP pneumonia, oral thrush, and infectious diarrhea. Blood tests show a significant reduction in CD4 helper T cells. Ms. C.W. is admitted to hospital for treatment.

9. There is no notice on Ms. C.W.'s room that she is HIV+. Why is this not done to reduce infection of the staff by HIV?
10. What is the significance of a reduction in CD4 helper T cells?
11. Ms. C.W. remains antibody positive for HIV; why don't the antibodies reduce viral load?
12. What is the cause of her pneumonia and oral infection?
13. What is the prognosis for Ms. C.W. if these infections cannot be controlled and if her CD4 helper T cell count does not return to more normal levels?

CHAPTER SUMMARY

The immune response is a specific defense mechanism in the body. When a foreign antigen enters the body, specific matching antibodies (humoral immunity) or sensitized T-lymphocytes (cell-mediated immunity) form, which then can destroy the matching foreign antigen. Specialized memory cells ensure immediate recognition and destruction of that antigen during future exposures.

- Active immunity is acquired by exposure to the antigen, for example, infectious bacteria or intentional immunization before exposure.
- Passive immunity provides only temporary protection.
- Hypersensitivity reactions are abnormal immune responses to harmless substances.
- Type I hypersensitivity (allergies) refers to responses to allergens, ingested, inhaled, or by direct contact, with subsequent development of IgE antibodies.
- Anaphylaxis is a severe, systemic, life-threatening allergic reaction characterized by rapidly decreasing blood pressure and respiratory obstruction.
- Type II, cytotoxic, hypersensitivity involves a reaction with IgG and cell antigens, such as occurs with incompatible blood transfusion.
- Type III, immune complex, hypersensitivity occurs when antigen–antibody complexes are deposited in tissues, causing inflammation, the basis of some diseases such as glomerulonephritis.
- Type IV, cell-mediated, hypersensitivity involves a delayed response by sensitized T lymphocytes, as may be seen with a tuberculin skin test.
- Autoimmune diseases develop when antibodies form in response to self-antigens, elements of the person's cells or tissues. Systemic lupus erythematosus is an example, in which antibodies to nuclear material such as DNA form, causing inflammatory responses in various organs and tissues.
- Immunodeficiency occurs in many forms, resulting from a deficit of any component of the immune response.
- Acquired immunodeficiency syndrome, is an example in which the human immunodeficiency virus (HIV) destroys T-helper lymphocytes, preventing both humoral and cell-mediated immunity. A diagnosis of HIV+ means the virus and its antibodies are present in the blood. A diagnosis of AIDS means active disease is present, with frequent opportunistic infections, malignant tumors, or AIDS encephalopathy. More women and children are now affected by HIV. Life expectancy has been prolonged by the administration of HAART, using combinations drugs and by prophylactic antimicrobial drugs. Women and children present a different clinical picture than men.
- Human immunodeficiency virus is transmitted by blood, tissues, or sexual contact, not by casual contact. It also may be transmitted by infected mothers to infants before, during, or after birth.

STUDY QUESTIONS

1. Describe the role of the macrophage in the immune response.
2. State the origin and purpose of lymphocytes.
3. Compare active natural immunity and passive artificial immunity, describing the causative mechanism and giving an example.
4. What is the purpose of a booster vaccination?
5. Describe the purpose of gamma globulins.
6. Where is IgA found in the body?
7. Describe how type III hypersensitivity develops.
8. Explain the process by which an attack of hay fever follows exposure to pollen.
9. Explain why anaphylaxis is considered life threatening.
10. Describe the pathophysiology of a type III hypersensitivity reaction.
11. Define an autoimmune disease, and explain how the causative mechanism differs from a normal defense.
12. Describe two factors that promote a successful organ transplant.
13. Differentiate between a diagnosis of being HIV+ and a diagnosis of having AIDS.
14. Why are opportunistic infections common with AIDS?
15. State three methods of transmitting HIV and three methods by which the virus is not transmitted.
16. Describe two common complications associated with AIDS.

ADDITIONAL RESOURCES

Applegate EJ: *The Anatomy and Physiology Learning System Textbook*, ed 3, Philadelphia, 2006, Saunders.

Greenwood D, Slack RCB, Peutherer JF: *Medical Microbiology*, ed 17, London, 2007, Churchill Livingstone.

Guyton AC, Hall JE: *Textbook of Medical Physiology*, ed 11, Philadelphia, 2005, Saunders.

Journal of Allergy and Clinical Immunology. American Academy of Allergy, Asthma, and Immunology, Washington, DC, and http://www.aaaai.org/members/jaci.stm

Kumar V, Abbas AK, Fausto M: *Robbins and Cotran Pathologic Basis of Disease*, ed 8, Philadelphia, 2007, Saunders.

Miller-Keane, O'Toole M: *Miller-Keane Encyclopedia & Dictionary of Medicine, Nursing & Allied Health*, ed 7, Philadelphia, 2005, Saunders.

Purtilo R: *Ethical Dimensions in the Health Professions*, ed 4, Philadelphia, 2005, Saunders.

Web Sites

http://www.aarda.org American Autoimmune Related Diseases Association

http://www.cdc.gov/mmwr Morbidity and Mortality Weekly Report

http://www.clinicaltrials.gov National Library of Medicine

http://familydoctor.org/online/famdocen/home/healthy/safety/work/004. Occupational Exposure to HIV: Advice for Health Care Workers

http://library.med.utah.edu/WebPath/TUTORIAL/AIDS/AIDS.html AIDS Tutorial

http://www.niams.nih.gov National Institute of Arthritis and Musculoskeletal and Skin Diseases

http://www.rheumatology.org American College of Rheumatology

http://www.transweb.org A Resource on Transplantation and Donation

Information on Vaccinations or on HIV/AIDS

http://www.cdc.gov/travel Information on disease outbreaks and medications for foreign travel

http://www.nih.gov National Institutes of Health

http://www.who.int/en World Health Organization

http://www.who.int/hiv HIV/AIDS information

CHAPTER 8

Skin Disorders

CHAPTER OUTLINE

LEARNING OBJECTIVES

After studying this chapter, the student is expected to:

1. Describe common skin lesions.
2. Describe the causes, typical lesions, and location of contact dermatitis, urticaria, and atopic dermatitis.
3. Describe the cause and lesions associated with the inflammatory conditions psoriasis erythematosus, pemphigus, and scleroderma.
4. Distinguish between the bacterial infections impetigo and furuncles.
5. Describe the effects of *Streptococcus pyogenes* on connective tissue in acute necrotizing fasciitis.
6. Describe the affects and treatment of leprosy.
7. Describe the viral infections herpes simplex and warts.
8. Describe the forms of tinea, a fungal infection.
9. Describe the agent, the infection, and manifestations of scabies and pediculosis.
10. Compare the skin cancers, describing the lesion, predisposing factors, and spread of squamous cell carcinoma, malignant melanoma, and Kaposi's sarcoma.

KEY TERMS

albinism
atopic
autoinoculation

denuded
excoriations

keratin
larvae

lichenification
sebum

Review of the Skin

As the largest organ in the body, the skin plays significant roles in both the function of the body physically and in how we are perceived in society. The skin, or integument, consists of two layers, the epidermis and the underlying dermis, along with their associated appendages, such as hair follicles and glands (Fig. 8-1). The *epidermis* consists of five layers, which vary in thickness at different areas of the body. For example, facial skin is relatively thin, but the soles are protected by a thick layer of skin (primarily stratum corneum). There are *no blood vessels or nerves* in the epidermis. Nutrients and fluid diffuse into it from blood vessels located in the dermis.

The innermost layer of the epidermis is the stratum basale, located on the basement membrane. New squamous epithelial cells form by mitosis in the stratum basale (the only layer of the epidermis where mitosis occurs), and one of each pair of cells then moves upward, forming, in turn, the stratum spinosum, the stratum granulosum, and the stratum lucidum (which is present primarily in thick skin), eventually being shed from the outer layer, the stratum corneum. Although these cells are in the stratum granulosum, keratin, a protein found in skin, hair, and nails, is deposited in them. Keratin prevents both loss of body fluid through the skin and entry of excessive water into the body, as when swimming. The epithelial cells become flatter as they progress upward away from the dermis, and they eventually die from lack of nutrients. Thus, the stratum corneum, the top or outer layer of the epidermis, consists of many layers of dead, flat, keratinized cells that are constantly sloughed from the surface a few weeks after being formed in the basal layer.

The epidermis also contains melanocytes, specialized pigment-producing cells. The amount of *melanin*, or dark pigment, produced by these cells determines skin color. Melanin production depends on multiple genes as well as environmental factors such as sun exposure (ultraviolet light). African Americans rarely develop skin cancer as a result of ultraviolet light exposure because of increased melanin in the skin, which acts as a protection from the sun's rays.

Albinism results from a recessive trait leading to a lack of melanin production. A person with this trait has white skin and hair and lacks pigment in the iris of the eye. This individual must avoid exposure to the sun. *Vitiligo* refers to small areas of hypopigmentation which may gradually spread to involve larger areas. *Melasma*, or *chloasma*, refers to patches of darker skin, often on the face, that may develop during pregnancy. An additional pigment, carotene, gives a yellow color to the skin. Pink tones in the skin are increased with additional vascularity or blood flow in the dermis.

The *dermis* is a thick layer of connective tissue that includes elastic and collagen fibers and varies in thickness over the body. These constituents provide both flexibility and strength in the skin and support for the nerves and blood vessels passing through the dermis. Many sensory receptors for pressure or texture, pain, heat, or cold are found in the dermis. The junction of the dermis with the epidermis is marked by papillae, irregular projections of dermis into the epidermal region. More capillaries are located in the papillae to facilitate diffusion of nutrients into the epidermis. Blood flow is controlled by the sympathetic nervous system.

Embedded in the skin are the *appendages,* or accessory structures—the hair follicles, sweat and sebaceous glands, and nails.

- The *hair follicles* are lined by epidermis that is continuous with the surface, the stratum basale producing the hair. Each hair follicle has smooth muscle attached to it, the arrector pili, controlled by sympathetic nerves. These may be stimulated by emotion or exposure to cold, causing the hairs to stand upright ("on end") or creating small elevations on the skin ("goose bumps").
- *Sebaceous glands* may be associated with hair follicles or may open directly onto the skin. These glands produce an oily secretion, sebum, which keeps the hair and skin soft and retards fluid loss from the skin. Secretions of sebum increase at puberty under the influence of the sex hormones.
- *Sweat glands* are of two types:
  - *Eccrine*, or merocrine, glands are located all over the body and secrete sweat through pores onto the skin in response to increased heat or emotional stress (SNS control).
  - *Apocrine* sweat glands are located in the axillae, scalp, face, and external genitalia, and the ducts of these glands open into the hair follicles.

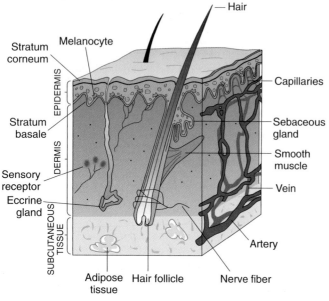

Stratum corneum
Melanocyte
Hair
EPIDERMIS
Capillaries
Stratum basale
DERMIS
Sebaceous gland
Smooth muscle
Sensory receptor
Vein
Eccrine gland
SUBCUTANEOUS TISSUE
Artery
Adipose tissue   Hair follicle   Nerve fiber

FIGURE 8-1 Diagram of the skin.

The secretion, sweat or perspiration, is odorless when formed, but bacterial action by normal flora on the constituents of sweat often causes odor to develop.

Beneath the dermis is the *subcutaneous tissue* or *hypodermis*, which consists of connective tissue, fat cells, macrophages, fibroblasts, blood vessels, nerves, and the base of many of the appendages.

A complex mix of *resident (normal) flora* is present on the skin, and the components differ in various body areas (see Chapter 6). Microbes residing under the fingernails may infect inflammatory lesions or breaks in the skin, particularly when one scratches the skin. Microbes, primarily bacteria and fungi, are also present deep in the hair follicles and glands of the skin and may be a source of opportunistic infections when there is injury such as burns (see section on burns in Chapter 5) or other inflammatory lesion. Infection may spread systemically from skin lesions.

APPLY YOUR KNOWLEDGE   8-1

Explain how excessive handwashing may in some cases increase the potential for a bacterial skin infection.

Skin has many functions:

- When unbroken, it provides the *first line of defense* against invasion by microorganisms and other foreign material. The sebaceous glands produce sebum which is acidic and inhibits bacterial growth. The resident flora of the skin is a deterrent to invading organisms.
- Skin prevents excessive fluid loss.
- It is important in controlling body temperature, using two mechanisms: cutaneous vasodilation, which increases peripheral blood flow, and increased secretion and evaporation of sweat—both have a cooling effect on the body
- Sensory perception provided by the skin is important as a defense against environmental hazards, as a learning tool, and as a means of communicating emotions.
- Another important function of the skin is the synthesis and activation of vitamin D on exposure to small amounts of ultraviolet light.

The skin is prone to damage as it is in constant contact with the external environment which includes such threats as toxic chemicals, direct trauma, or animal bites/stings. Systemic disorders additionally may affect the skin. Also, the skin changes with aging, showing loss of elasticity, thinning, and loss of subcutaneous tissue (see Chapter 24). Minor abrasions or cuts of the skin heal quickly with mitosis of the epithelial cells (see Chapter 5 for the healing process). When large areas of the skin are damaged, appendages may be lost, function impaired, and fibrous scar tissue forms, often restricting mobility

of joints. See the discussion on burns in Chapter 5 for information on biosynthetic wound coverings or "artificial skin," useful when large areas of skin are damaged.

THINK ABOUT   8-1

a. Describe three ways in which the dermis differs from the epidermis.
b. Explain how the basal layer of the epidermis is nourished.
c. Describe the role of sebaceous glands and eccrine glands.
d. Explain three ways the skin acts as a defense mechanism.

Skin Lesions

The characteristics of skin lesions are frequently helpful in making a diagnosis. Skin lesions may be caused by systemic disorders such as liver disease, systemic infections such as chickenpox (typical rash), or allergies to ingested food or drugs, as well as by localized factors such as exposure to toxins. Common types of lesions are illustrated in Figure 8-2 and defined in Table 8-1. The location, length of time the lesion has been present, and any changes occurring over time are significant. Physical appearance, including color, elevation, texture, type of exudate, and the presence of pain or pruritus (itching) are also important considerations. Some lesions, such as tumors, usually are neither painful nor pruritic and therefore may not be noticed. A few skin disorders, such as herpes, cause painful lesions.

TABLE 8-1	Description of Some Skin Lesions
Macule	Small, flat, circumscribed lesion of a different color than the normal skin
Papule	Small, firm, elevated lesion
Nodule	Palpable elevated lesion; varies in size
Pustule	Elevated, erythematous lesion, usually containing purulent exudate
Vesicle	Elevated, thin-walled lesion containing clear fluid (blister)
Plaque	Large, slightly elevated lesion with flat surface, often topped by scale
Crust	Dry, rough surface or dried exudate or blood
Lichenification	Thick, dry, rough surface (leather-like)
Keloid	Raised, irregular, and increasing mass of collagen resulting from excessive scar tissue formation
Fissure	Small, deep, linear crack or tear in skin
Ulcer	Cavity with loss of tissue from the epidermis and dermis, often weeping or bleeding
Erosion	Shallow, moist cavity in epidermis
Comedone	Mass of sebum, keratin, and debris blocking the opening of a hair follicle

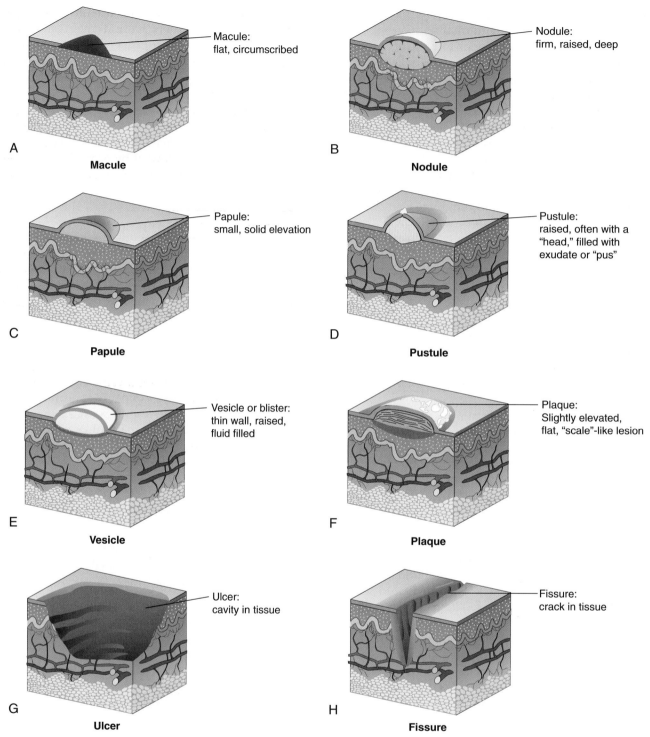

FIGURE 8-2 Common skin lesions.

Pruritus is associated with allergic responses, chemical irritation due to insect bites, or infestations by parasites such as scabies mites. The mechanisms producing pruritus are not totally understood. It is known that release of histamine in a hypersensitivity response causes marked pruritus (see Chapter 7). Pruritus also may result from mild stimulation of pain receptors by irritants. The most common manifestations include redness, and itchiness. Scratching a pruritic area usually increases the inflammation and may lead to secondary infection. Infection results from breaking the skin barrier, thus allowing microbes on the fingers (under the nails) or on the surrounding skin to invade the area. Infection may then produce scar tissue in the area.

■ *Diagnostic Tests*

Bacterial infections may require culture and staining of specimens for identification. Skin scrapings for microscopic examination, sample culturing, direct observation of the infected area and other specific procedures (e.g., ultraviolet light, Wood's lamp) are necessary to detect fungal or parasitic infections.

Biopsy is an important procedure in the detection of malignant changes in tissue and provides a safeguard prior to or following removal of any skin lesion.

Blood tests may be helpful in the diagnosis of conditions due to allergy or abnormal immune reactions. Patch or scratch tests are used to screen for allergens and may be followed up by diet restrictions to identify specific food allergens. Drug reactions are assessed utilizing specific antigen–antibody testing.

■ *General Treatment Measures*

Pruritus may be treated by antihistamines or glucocorticoids, administered topically or orally. Identification and avoidance of allergens reduce the risk of recurrence. With many skin disorders, extremes of heat or cold and contact with certain rough materials such as wool aggravate the skin lesions. Soaks or compresses using solutions such as Burow's solution (aluminum acetate) or colloidal oatmeal (Aveeno) may cool the skin and reduce itching. Some topical skin preparations contain a local anesthetic to reduce itching and burning sensations. Infections may require appropriate topical antimicrobial treatment. If the infection is severe, systemic medication may be preferred.

Precancerous lesions may be removed, by surgery, laser therapy, electrodesiccation (heat), or cryosurgery (e.g., freezing by liquid nitrogen).

> ### THINK ABOUT 8-2
>
> a. Describe each of the following: (1) macule; (2) vesicle; and (3) pustule.
> b. Explain two causes of pruritus.
> c. List four potential causes of skin lesions.
> d. Explain why cellular components of all resected skin lesions should be evaluated by a pathologist.

There are a large number of skin disorders. Only a small number of representative dermatologic conditions are included here.

Inflammatory Disorders

Burns cause an acute inflammatory response. This topic is covered in Chapter 5 along with the processes of healing.

Contact Dermatitis

Contact dermatitis may be caused by exposure to an allergen or by direct chemical or mechanical irritation of the skin. *Allergic* dermatitis may result from exposure to any of a multitude of substances, including metals, cosmetics, soaps, chemicals, and plants. Sensitization occurs on the first exposure (type IV cell-mediated hypersensitivity—see Chapter 7), and on subsequent exposures, manifestations such as a pruritic rash develop at the site a few hours after exposure to that allergen. The location of the lesions is usually a clue to the identity of the allergen (Fig. 8-3). For example, poison ivy may cause lesions, often linear, on the ankles or hands, or a necklace may cause a rash around the neck. Typical allergic dermatitis is indicated by a pruritic, erythematous, and edematous area, which is often covered with small vesicles.

Direct *chemical* irritation does not involve an immune response but is an inflammatory response caused by direct exposure to substances such as soaps and cleaning materials, acids, or insecticides. The skin is usually red and edematous and may be pruritic or painful. Removal of the irritant as soon as possible and reduction of the inflammation with topical glucocorticoids are usually effective treatment.

Urticaria

Urticaria (hives) results from a type I hypersensitivity reaction, commonly caused by ingested substances such as shellfish or certain fruits or drugs. The subsequent release of histamine causes the eruption of hard, raised erythematous lesions on the skin, often scattered all

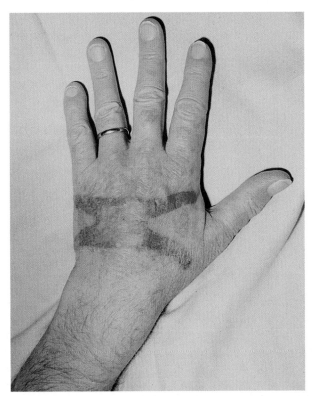

FIGURE 8-3 Contact dermatitis resulting from adhesive tape. Note how the location and shape of the rash indicate the causative agent. *(Courtesy of Dr. M. McKenzie, Toronto, Canada.)*

over the body (Fig. 8-4). The lesions are highly pruritic. Occasionally hives also develop in the pharyngeal mucosa and may obstruct the airway, causing difficulty with breathing. In this case, medical assistance should be sought as quickly as possible.

Atopic Dermatitis

Atopic dermatitis (eczema) is a common problem in infancy and may persist into adulthood in some persons. Atopic refers to an inherited tendency toward allergic

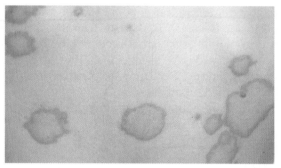

FIGURE 8-4 Urticaria (hives). *(From Dorland's Illustrated Medical Dictionary, ed 32, St. Louis, 2012, Saunders.)*

conditions. Frequently the family history includes individuals with eczema, allergic rhinitis or hay fever, and asthma, indicating a genetic component. Chronic inflammation results from the response to allergens (Fig. 8-5). Eosinophilia and increased serum IgE levels indicate the allergenic basis for atopic dermatitis (type I hypersensitivity).

In infants, the pruritic lesions are moist, red, vesicular, and covered with crusts. Involved areas are usually located symmetrically on the face, neck, extensor surfaces of the arms and legs, and buttocks.

In adults, the affected skin appears dry and scaling with lichenification (thick and leathery patches), although it may be moist and red in the skin folds. Pruritus is common. Areas affected include the flexor surfaces of the arms and legs (e.g., antecubital areas) and the hands and feet. Potential complications include secondary infections due to scratching and disseminated viral infections such as herpes. Affected areas also become more sensitive to many irritants such as soaps and certain fabrics. Marked changes in temperature and humidity tend to aggravate the dermatitis, leading to more exacerbations in patients living in areas with dry winter months or hot, humid summers.

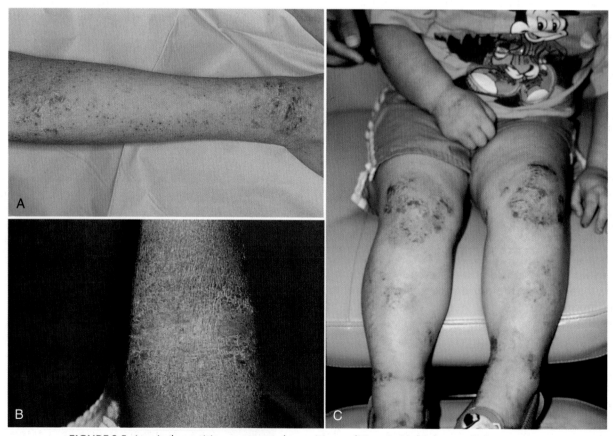

FIGURE 8-5 Atopic dermatitis—an extremely pruritic condition. **A,** Multiple excoriations, vesiculation, and marked lichenification are seen in this patient. **B,** Minute excoriations with marked lichenification in the antecubital fossa. *(From Callen JP, et al: Color Atlas of Dermatology, Philadelphia, 1993, Saunders, p 192.)* **C,** Atopic dermatitis. Characteristic lesions with crusting from irritation and scratching over knees and around ankles. *(From McCance KL, et al: Pathophysiology, ed 6, St. Louis, 2010, Mosby. Courtesy Department of Dermatology, School of Medicine, University of Utah.)*

Identification and elimination of the aggravating agents and the use of topical glucocorticoids are helpful. Antihistamines may reduce pruritus, and avoidance of skin irritants such as strong detergents or wool, a change to a hypoallergenic diet, and adequate moisturizing of the skin may reduce the inflammation. In severe cases, topical glucocorticoids may be used when severe pruritus interferes with sleeping and eating, particularly in infants, when the condition further exacerbates irritability and stress.

Psoriasis

Psoriasis is a chronic inflammatory skin disorder that affects 1% to 3% of the population and is considered to be genetic in origin following recent research studies in mice. Onset usually occurs in the teen years, and the course is marked by remissions and exacerbations. Cases vary in severity and psoriatic arthritis is associated with psoriasis in some cases.

Psoriasis results from the abnormal activation of T cells and an associated increase in cytokines in affected tissues. These immunologic changes then lead to excessive proliferation of keratinocytes and the symptoms of the disease. Animal studies have shown that a reduction in T-cell activity leads to regression of skin changes in a short period of time.

The rate of cellular proliferation is greatly increased, leading to thickening of the dermis and epidermis. Epidermal shedding may occur in 1 day rather than the normal 2-week turnover period. The lesion begins as a small red papule that enlarges. A silvery plaque forms while the base remains erythematous because of inflammation and vasodilation. (Figure 8-6 illustrates the acute inflammatory stage and the chronic lesion.) If the plaque is removed, small bleeding points are apparent. Lesions are commonly found on the face, scalp, elbows, and knees and may be accompanied by itching or burning sensation. The fingernails may be thickened, pitted or ridged.

Treatments that reduce cell proliferation include glucocorticoids, tar preparations, and, in severe cases, the antimetabolite methotrexate. Exposure to ultraviolet light is frequently part of the treatment regimen. Research on new treatments related to immunologic changes in psoriasis is underway.

Pemphigus

Pemphigus is an *autoimmune* (see Chapter 7) disorder that comes in several forms: pemphigus vulgaris, pemphigus foliaccus, and pemphigus erythematosus. The severity of the disease varies among individuals.

The autoantibodies disrupt the cohesion between the epidermal cells, causing blisters to form. In the most common form, pemphigus vulgaris, the epidermis separates above the basal layer. Blisters form initially in the

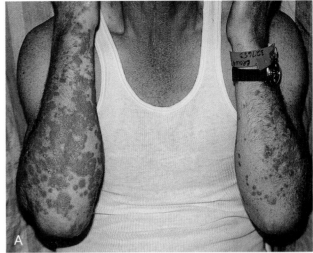

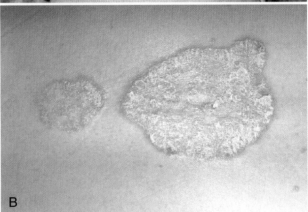

FIGURE 8-6 **A**, Psoriasis—acute inflammatory stage. *(Courtesy of Dr. M. McKenzie, Toronto, Canada.)* **B**, Psoriasis. *(From Lookingbill DP, Marks JG:* Principles of Dermatology, *ed 3, Philadelphia, 2000, Saunders.)*

oral mucosa or scalp and then spread over the face and trunk during the ensuing months. The vesicles become large and tend to rupture, leaving large denuded areas of skin covered with crusts.

Systemic glucocorticoids such as prednisone and other immunosuppressants are used to treat pemphigus.

Scleroderma

Scleroderma may occur as a skin disorder, or it may be systemic, affecting the viscera. The primary cause is not known but increased collagen deposition is observed in all cases. Collagen deposition in the arterioles and capillaries reduces blood flow to the skin and/or internal organs.

Collagen deposits, inflammation, and fibrosis with decreased capillary networks develop in the skin, leading to hard, shiny, tight, immovable areas of skin. The fingertips are narrowed and shortened, and Raynaud's phenomenon may be present, further predisposing the individual to ulceration and atrophy in the

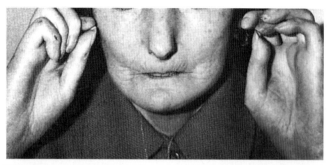

FIGURE 8-7 Scleroderma. *(From Odom RB, James WD, Berger TG: Andrews' Diseases of the Skin, ed 9, Philadelphia, 2000, Saunders.)*

fingers. The facial expression is lost as the skin tightens, and movement of the mouth and eyes may be impaired (Fig. 8-7). The cutaneous form may also affect the microcirculation of various organs, eventually causing renal failure, intestinal obstruction, or respiratory failure due to pulmonary hypertension.

THINK ABOUT 8-3

a. Describe the typical lesions of atopic dermatitis in the infant and adult in terms of their location and characteristics.

b. Explain the pathologic changes in the skin that occur with psoriasis.

c. Describe the development of the skin lesions of pemphigus vulgaris.

d. Explain how the deposition of collagen in scleroderma may lead to tissue/organ damage.

e. Name two findings in the evaluation of a blood sample that would indicate the allergenic basis for atopic dermatitis.

Skin Infections

Infections occur frequently in the skin. They may be caused by bacteria, viruses, fungi, or other types of microorganisms as well as parasites. Pathogens or opportunistic microbes may penetrate the skin through minor abrasions or cuts as well as through inflamed areas. When serious infections develop, it is essential to culture the exudate to identify the causative organism and determine appropriate treatment.

Bacterial Infections

Bacterial infections of the skin are common. They may be primary, often caused by resident flora, or they may be secondary, developing in wounds or pruritic lesions. Some infections are superficial; others can involve deeper tissues (abscesses).

Acne, a staphylococcal infection common in young adults, is covered in Chapter 23 (see Fig. 23-5).

Cellulitis

Cellulitis (erysipelas) is an infection of the dermis and subcutaneous tissue, usually arising secondary to an injury, a furuncle (boil), or an ulcer (see Fig. 5-3). The causative organism is usually *Staphylococcus aureus*, or occasionally Streptococcus.

It frequently occurs in the lower trunk and legs, particularly in individuals with restricted circulation in the extremities or those who are immunocompromised and the area becomes red, swollen, and painful. Red streaks running along the lymph vessels proximal to the infected area may develop. Systemic antibiotics are usually necessary to treat the infection along with analgesics for pain.

Furuncles

A furuncle (boil) is an infection, usually by *S. aureus*, which begins in a hair follicle (folliculitis) and spreads into the surrounding dermis (Fig. 8-8A). Common locations are the face, neck, and back. Initially, the lesion is a firm, red, painful nodule, which develops into a large, painful mass called an abscess that frequently drains large amounts of purulent exudate (pus). Pus is composed of leukocytes, cellular debris from dead blood cells and bacteria and a thin protein rich fluid component.

Squeezing boils can result in the spread of infection by autoinoculation (transfer, perhaps by fingers, of microbes from one site of infection on the body to another site) to other areas of the skin, cause cellulitis, or can force the bacteria in the abscess deeper into the dermis or subcutaneous tissue. Also, compression of furuncles in the nasal area may lead to thrombi or infection that spreads to the brain if the infected material reaches the cavernous sinus (a collecting point for venous blood from the face and brain) in the facial bones.

Carbuncles are a collection of furuncles that coalesce to form a large infected mass, which may drain through several sinuses or develop into a single large abscess.

Impetigo

Impetigo is a common infection in infants and children but can also occur in adults. *Staphylococcus aureus* may cause highly contagious infections in neonates, which is a threat in neonatal nurseries. In older children, infection results primarily from *S. aureus* but, alternatively, may be caused by group A beta-hemolytic streptococci. The infection is easily spread by direct contact with the hands, eating utensils, or towels. Activities involving close physical contact or contact with infected fomites can cause a rapid spread of this infection. Impetigo has often been seen spreading through individual members of wrestling teams and other full contact sports in which the mats or equipment may serve to spread the infection from one person to the next.

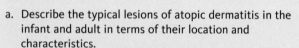

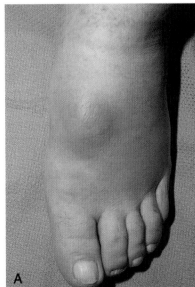

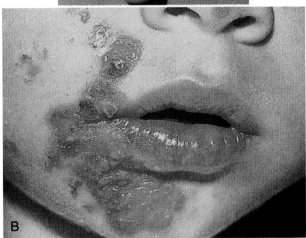

FIGURE 8-8 **A**, Furuncle. *(From Lookingbill D, Marks J:* Principles of Dermatology, *ed 2, Philadelphia, 1993, Saunders.)* **B**, Impetigo. Note the yellowish pustules with brownish crust, the inflammation, and the spreading lesions on the face. *(Courtesy of Dr. M. McKenzie, Toronto, Canada.)*

Lesions commonly occur on the face and begin as small vesicles, which rapidly enlarge and rupture to form yellowish-brown crusty masses (see Fig. 8-8B). Underneath this characteristic crust, the lesion is red and moist and exudes a honey-colored liquid. Additional vesicles develop around the primary site by auto-inoculation with hands, towels, or clothes. Pruritus is common, leading to scratching and further spread of infection.

Topical antibiotics may be used in the early stages, but systemic administration of these drugs is necessary if the lesions are extensive. Unfortunately, the number of antibiotic-resistant strains of *S. aureus* is increasing, resulting in local outbreaks of infection. Another concern with impetigo due to certain strains of streptococci or staphylococci is glomerulonephritis, which can develop if treatment is not instituted promptly (see Chapter 18).

Acute Necrotizing Fasciitis

It has been termed *flesh-eating disease* because of the extremely rapid tissue invasion resulting from reduced blood supply to the tissues and the secretion of protease enzymes that destroy tissue Although a mixture of aerobic and anaerobic microbes is frequently present at the site, the fulminant course with severe inflammation and tissue necrosis appears primarily to result from the actions of a highly virulent strain of gram-positive, group A, beta-hemolytic *Streptococcus* (*S. pyogenes*, also responsible for "strep throat"). This strain also produces a toxin causing toxic shock (see Chapter 12). Although relatively rare, there has been an increase in cases during the past few years and the cases seem to increase in frequency in the cold months.

There is often a history of minor trauma or infection in the skin and subcutaneous tissue of an extremity. The superficial fascia in the subcutaneous tissue and fascia surrounding the skeletal muscle, as well as other soft tissues, become edematous and necrotic, with occlusion of small blood vessels leading to gangrene. The infected area appears markedly inflamed and very painful, rapidly increases in size, and dermal gangrene is apparent.

Systemic toxicity develops with fever, tachycardia, hypotension, mental confusion, and disorientation, and possibly organ failure.

Diagnosis during the early stages of this infection is sometimes difficult as the signs/symptoms can be very similar to cellulitis. This delay in diagnosis and subsequent treatment is extremely dangerous as this infection progresses so rapidly.

Treatment includes aggressive antimicrobial therapy, fluid replacement, excision of all infected tissue, treatment with high oxygen flow in hyperbaric chambers and possibly amputation to prevent further spread of infection. Delays in treatment result in greater tissue loss, potential amputation, and higher probability of mortality. Case fatality rates are estimated by the CDC to be 20% to 30%.

Leprosy

Leprosy (Hansen's disease) is caused by the bacterium *Mycobacterium leprae* and in the past has affected millions of people worldwide. According to data from the World Health Organization, the global number of new cases has decreased dramatically although it is still a problem in parts of Africa, Asia, the South Pacific, and some areas of South America. The organism is not highly contagious, and extended contact with a source is required for infection.

This chronic disease is classified into three major types. The clinical signs and symptoms vary but generally affect the skin, mucous membranes, and peripheral nerves. In addition to the formation of characteristic skin lesions or macules, the loss of feeling due to nerve damage results in a situation where the person may damage or destroy tissue through injury but not know it immediately. This damage can lead to the loss of limbs or other extremities due to irreparable damage and/or infection and eventual tissue necrosis.

The actual mechanism of pathogenicity of *Mycobacterium leprae* is largely unknown because this organism cannot easily be grown of culture media, which makes laboratory studies very difficult.

The method of diagnosis involves microscopic examination of a skin biopsy to identify the presence of the bacterium.

Treatment of leprosy primarily involves the use of antibiotics to control the causative organism as well as treat any secondary infections, rehabilitation, and education.

Viral Infections

Herpes Simplex

Herpes simplex (cold sores) virus type 1 (HSV-1) is the most common cause of cold sores or fever blisters, which occur on or near the lips. Herpes simplex type 2 (genital herpes) is considered in Chapter 19, Herpes zoster or shingles is presented in Chapter 14, and herpetic stomatitis is covered in Chapter 17. Both types of Herpes simplex virus cause similar effects and type 2 may cause oral as well as genital lesions.

The primary infection may be asymptomatic, but the virus remains in a latent stage in the sensory nerve ganglion of the trigeminal nerve, from which it may be reactivated, causing the skin lesion (Fig. 8-9). Recurrence may be triggered by infection such as a common cold, sun exposure, or stress. Reactivation usually is indicated by a preliminary burning or tingling sensation along the nerve and at the site on the lips, followed by development of painful vesicles, which then rupture and form a crust. Spontaneous healing occurs in 2 to 3 weeks. The acute stage and viral shedding and spreading may be reduced by the topical application of antiviral drugs such as acyclovir (Zovirax).

The virus is spread by direct contact with fluid from the lesion. Viral particles may be present in the saliva for some weeks following healing of the lesion and therefore can spread the infection to others or to the fingers; for example, if there is a break in the skin. A potential complication is spread of the virus to the eyes, causing keratitis (infection and ulceration of the cornea). Another complication is herpetic whitlow, a very painful infection of the fingers, which can pose a risk for dental personnel (see Fig. 17-6).

Verrucae

Warts (verrucae) are caused by human papillomaviruses (HPVs). There are many types of these viruses, associated with a variety of diseases. Common plantar warts, discussed here, are caused by HPV types 1 through 4. They frequently develop in children and young adults and are annoying but relatively harmless. Genital warts (HPV types 6 and 11) are described in Chapter 19, as is cervical cancer, associated with HPV types 16 and 18.

Plantar warts are common, occurring on the soles, with a similar variety affecting the hands or fingers (dorsal surface) and face. Warts appear first as a firm, raised papule, and then they develop a rough surface (Fig. 8-10). They are white or tan in color and often are multiple. The infection spreads by viral shedding of the surface skin. They may be painful if pressure is applied, especially on the feet.

Warts tend to persist even with treatment. Sometimes they resolve spontaneously within several years. A variety of local treatments are available, including laser, freezing with liquid nitrogen, and topical medications with ASA compounds.

Fungal Infections

Fungal infections (mycoses) are diagnosed from scrapings of the skin processed with potassium hydroxide to accentuate the spores and hyphae (filaments) of the fungal growth, which then becomes fluorescent in ultraviolet light. Microscopic examination and culturing of samples can also be used to aid in identification. Most fungal infections are superficial, because the fungi live off the dead, keratinized cells of the epidermis (dermatophytes). Specific antifungal agents are required to treat these infections. Candidal infections are discussed in Chapter 17 (see Fig. 17-5, oral candida or thrush) and in Chapter 19 (vaginal infection). *Candida* also occurs frequently in clients with diabetes (see Fig. 16-8*B*).

Tinea

Tinea may cause several types of superficial skin infections (dermatophytoses or *ringworm*), depending on the area of the body affected.

Tinea capitis is an infection of the scalp that is common in school-aged children (Fig. 8-11*A*). The infection may result from *Microsporum canis*, transmitted by cats and dogs, or by *Trichophyton tonsurans*, transmitted by humans. It manifests as a circular bald patch as hair is broken off above the scalp. Erythema or scaling may be apparent. Oral antifungal agents such as griseofulvin are recommended.

Tinea corporis is a fungal infection of the body, particularly the nonhairy parts (Fig. 8-11*B*). The lesion is a round, erythematous ring of vesicles or papules with a clear center (ringworm) scattered over the body. Pruritus or a burning sensation may be present. Topical antifungal medications such as tolnaftate or ketoconazole are effective.

Tinea pedis, or athlete's foot, involves the feet, particularly the toes. *Trichophyton mentagrophytes* or *Trichophyton rubrum* are the usual causative organisms. This condition may be associated with swimming pools and

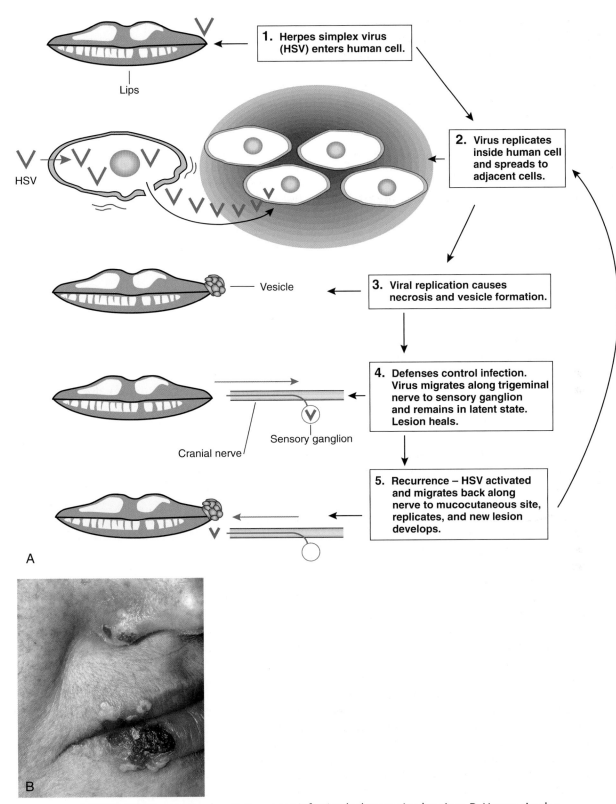

1. Herpes simplex virus (HSV) enters human cell.

Lips

HSV

2. Virus replicates inside human cell and spreads to adjacent cells.

Vesicle

3. Viral replication causes necrosis and vesicle formation.

4. Defenses control infection. Virus migrates along trigeminal nerve to sensory ganglion and remains in latent state. Lesion heals.

Sensory ganglion

Cranial nerve

5. Recurrence – HSV activated and migrates back along nerve to mucocutaneous site, replicates, and new lesion develops.

A

B

FIGURE 8-9 Herpes simplex. **A,** Recurrent infection by herpes simplex virus. **B,** Herpes simplex on the face. *(Courtesy of Dr. M. McKenzie, Toronto, Canada.)*

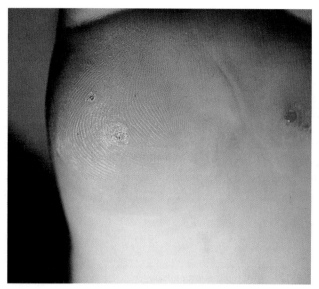

FIGURE 8-10 Plantar warts on sole of foot. *(Courtesy of Dr. M. McKenzie, Toronto, Canada.)*

gymnasia if appropriate precautions are not in place (e.g., wearing sandals, changing to clean, dry socks). The organisms may be normal flora that become opportunists or that spread easily from lesions under conditions of excessive warmth and moisture. The skin between the toes becomes inflamed and macerated, with painful and pruritic fissures (Fig. 8-11C). The feet may have a foul odor. Secondary bacterial infection is common, adding to the inflammation and necrosis. Topical tolnaftate is usually effective.

Tinea unguium, or onychomycosis, is an infection of the nails, particularly the toenails. Infection begins at the tip of one or two nails, the nail turning first white and then brown. The nail then thickens and cracks, and the infection tends to spread to other nails.

Other Infections

Scabies

Scabies is the result of an invasion by a mite, *Sarcoptes scabiei*. The female mite burrows into the epidermis, laying eggs over a period of several weeks as she moves along in the stratum corneum (Fig. 8-12). The male dies after fertilizing the female, and the female dies after

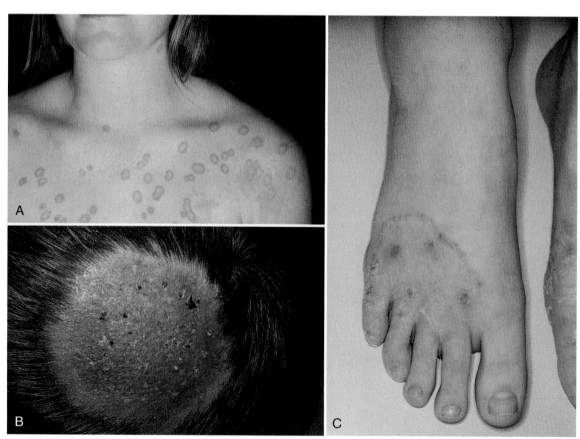

FIGURE 8-11 **A,** Tinea corporis. Annular scaly plaques in superficial basal cell epithelioma. **B.** Tinea capitis, localized patch. **C.** Tinea pedis. *(From Callen JP, et al: Color Atlas of Dermatology, Philadelphia, 1993, Saunders.)*

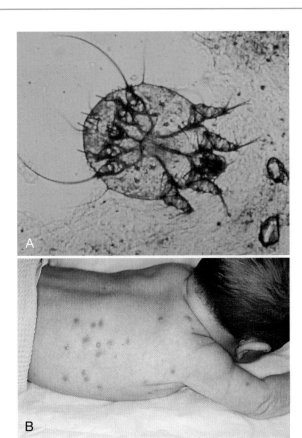

FIGURE 8-12 Scabies. **A,** Scabies mite, as seen clinically when removed from its burrow. **B,** Characteristic scabies bites. *(From McCance KL, et al: Pathophysiology, ed 6, St. Louis, 2010, Mosby. Courtesy Department of Dermatology, School of Medicine, University of Utah.)*

laying the eggs. The larvae emerging from the eggs migrate to the skin surface and then burrow into the skin in search of nutrients. As the larvae mature into adults, the cycle is repeated. The burrows appear on the skin as tiny, light brown lines, often with small vesicles and erythema. The inflammation and pruritus that result are caused by the damage done to the skin by the burrowing and the presence of mite fecal material in the burrow.

Common sites include the areas between the fingers, the wrists, the inner surfaces of the elbow, and the waistline. Topical treatment with lindane is effective. Mites can survive for only a short time away from the human host and are usually spread only by close contact.

Pediculosis

Pediculosis (lice) can take three forms in humans. *Pediculus humanus corporis* is the body louse, *Pediculus pubis* is the pubic louse, and *Pediculus humanus capitis* is the head louse (cooties). Lice are small, brownish parasites that feed off human blood (humans are hosts only to human lice, not to animal lice) and cannot survive for long without the human host.

Female lice lay eggs on hair shafts, cementing the egg firmly to the hair close to the scalp (Fig. 8-13). The egg, or *nit*, appears as a small, whitish shell attached to a hair. After hatching, the louse bites the human host, sucking blood for its survival. The site of each bite is demonstrated by a macule or papule, which is highly pruritic owing to the mite saliva. The excoriations that result from scratching and the visible nits provide evidence of infestation; the adult lice usually are not visible.

Topical permethrin, malathion, or pyrethrin is used to treat lice, although resistance to these drugs is widespread. A fine-toothed comb can be used to remove empty nits from the hair. Clothing, linen, and the surrounding area need to be carefully cleaned to prevent reinfection.

THINK ABOUT 8-4

a. Distinguish between tinea pedis and tinea capitis by location and lesion.
b. State one significant identifying feature of the lesions of: (1) impetigo, and (2) herpes simplex.
c. State the causative organism of: (1) scabies, (2) ringworm, and (3) pediculosis.
d. Explain why herpes simplex tends to recur.

Skin Tumors

Keratoses

Keratoses are benign lesions that are usually associated with aging or skin damage. *Seborrheic keratoses* result from proliferation of basal cells, leading to an oval elevation that may be smooth or rough and is often dark in color. This type of keratosis is often found on the face or upper trunk. *Actinic keratoses* occur on skin exposed to ultraviolet radiation and commonly arise in fair-skinned persons. The lesion appears as a pigmented, scaly patch. Actinic keratoses may develop into squamous cell carcinoma.

There is increasing concern regarding the continued rise in skin lesions related to sun exposure. Recent estimates indicate that one in seven persons will develop skin cancer. Skin cancers currently represent 50% of all cancers diagnosed in the United States. In recent years, increased exposure to harmful ultraviolet rays is a result of more participation in outdoor sports, clothes that expose more skin along with the desire to have a fashionable tan, and increased use of tanning salons, as well as depletion of the protective ozone layer around the earth. The danger is evidenced by the increased incidence of tumors in those who have experienced severe sunburns, those who work or spend considerable time outdoors in the sun, or those who have blond hair and light-colored skin containing less melanin.

Guidelines to reduce the risk of skin cancers have been developed. They include:
• Reducing sun exposure at midday and early afternoon

Head louse
(Pediculus humanus capitis)

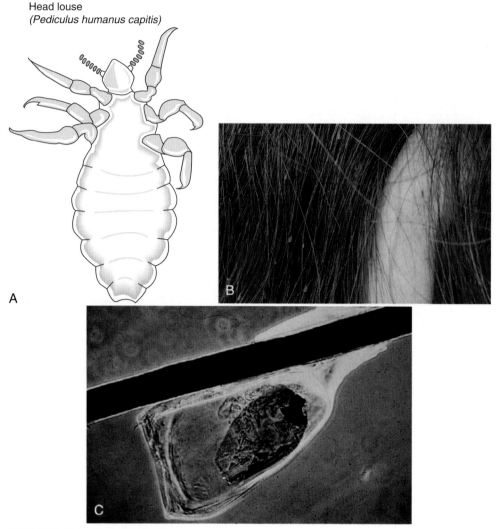

FIGURE 8-13 Pediculosis. **A,** Schematic representation of a louse. **B,** Lice in hair. *(From Callen JP, et al: Color Atlas of Dermatology, Philadelphia, 1993, Saunders.)* **C,** Nit (egg case) of head louse attached to hair shaft. *(From Kumar V, Abbas AK, Fausto M: Robbins and Cotran Pathologic Basis of Disease, ed 7, Philadelphia, 2005, Saunders.)*

- Covering up with clothing, remaining in shade, and wearing broad-brimmed hats to protect face and neck
- Applying sunscreen or sunblock, minimum SPF-15 (sun protection factor), broad spectrum, to protect from UVA and UVB rays

- Protecting infants and children from exposure and sun damage to skin that may lead to skin cancer (see Chapter 20).

Squamous Cell Carcinoma

Skin cancer is easy to detect and accessible for treatment and when identified in the early stages should have a good prognosis. Squamous cell carcinoma is similar to the common basal cell carcinoma in many respects (see Chapter 20 and Fig. 20-11). Both of these malignant tumors have an excellent prognosis when the lesion is removed within a reasonable time.

Squamous cell carcinoma is a painless, malignant tumor of the epidermis; sun exposure is a major contributing factor. The lesions are found most frequently on exposed areas of the skin, such as the face and neck (Fig. 8-14). Smokers also have a higher incidence of

---

⚠ WARNING SIGNS OF SKIN CANCER

1. A sore that does not heal
2. A change in shape, size, color, or texture of a lesion, especially an expanding, irregular circumference or surface
3. New moles or odd-shaped lesions that develop
4. A skin lesion that bleeds repeatedly, oozes fluid, or itches

It is recommended that individuals routinely check skin, particularly exposed areas, moles, lesions resulting from sun damage, dark spots, or keratoses. Photodynamic therapy for keratoses and skin cancer involves a light-sensitive drug in a cream that is absorbed by the tumor cells. A laser then destroys the cells containing the chemical.

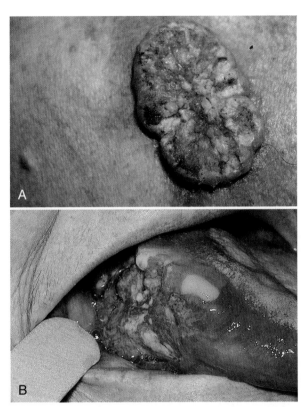

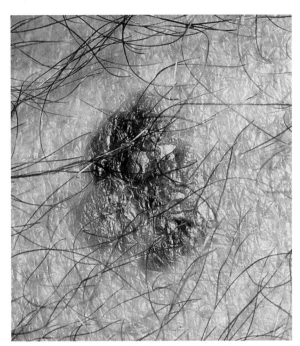

FIGURE 8-15 Malignant melanoma. *(Courtesy of Dr. M. McKenzie, Toronto, Canada.)*

FIGURE 8-14 Squamous cell carcinoma. **A**, Skin. *(From Callen JP, et al: Color Atlas of Dermatology, Philadelphia, 1993, Saunders.)* **B**, Squamous cell carcinoma at the base of the tongue. *(From Cooke RA, Stewart B: Colour Atlas of Anatomical Pathology, ed 3, Sydney, 2004, Churchill Livingstone.)*

BOX 8-1	"ABCD" Signs That a Mole or Nevus May be Melanoma

Area of the mole is increased
Border is irregular
Color is changed in mole
Diameter of the mole is increased

squamous cell carcinoma in the lower lip region and mucous membranes of the mouth. Scar tissue is also a source of carcinoma, particularly in the African-American population. Actinic keratoses predispose to in situ or intraepidermal squamous cell carcinoma, which usually remains limited to the epidermis for a long time.

The invasive type of squamous cell carcinoma arises from premalignant conditions such as leukoplakia. This carcinoma develops as a scaly, slightly elevated, reddish lesion with an irregular border and central ulceration. The tumor grows relatively slowly in all directions, invading surrounding tissues, and then spreads to the regional lymph nodes. It rarely metastasizes to distant sites.

Malignant Melanoma

This much more serious form of skin cancer develops from the melanocytes and is increasing in incidence. The development of malignant melanoma depends on genetic factors, exposure to ultraviolet radiation, and hormonal influences.

Melanomas arise from melanocytes in the basal layer of the epidermis or from a nevus (mole), a collection of melanocytes. There are many types of nevi, most of which do not become malignant. Nevi that grow; change shape, color, size, or texture; or bleed are to be suspected (Box 8-1). Malignant melanoma often appears as a multicolored lesion with an irregular border (Fig. 8-15). Melanomas grow quickly, extending down into the tissues, then metastasize quickly to the regional lymph nodes and then to other organs, leading to a poor prognosis in many cases. When they are surgically removed, an extensive amount of tissue around and below the lesion is excised as well to ensure that all the malignant cells are removed. Additional radiation and chemotherapy now provides a 5-year survival rate of approximately 99% in cases of localized tumors and 7% to 70% in cases in which the tumor has invaded or metastasized, depending on what tissues have been invaded and the extent of the metastasis. In the United States 80% of melanomas are identified in the localized stage.

Kaposi's Sarcoma

This formerly rare type of skin cancer has come into prominence in recent years because of its association with human immunodeficiency virus (HIV) infection or acquired immunodeficiency syndrome (AIDS) (see Chapter 7). Kaposi's sarcoma was a relatively rare cancer that occurred in older men originating from Eastern Europe or the Mediterranean area before the HIV pandemic. The disease is also endemic in Africa and affects younger individuals. Cases are still seen in individuals who are not HIV positive.

In immunosuppressed patients, the cancer is quite common and may affect the viscera as well as the skin. Herpesvirus #8 (kSHV) forms part of the etiology of these tumors. The malignant cells arise from the endothelium in small blood vessels. The multiple skin lesions commence as purplish macules, often on the face, scalp, oral mucosa, or lower extremities. Initially, the lesions are nonpruritic and nonpainful. These lesions progress to form large, irregularly shaped plaques or nodules, which may be darker in color, purplish or brownish (see Fig. 7-17B). In immunocompromised patients, the lesions develop rapidly over the upper body and may become painful. A combination of radiation, chemotherapy, surgery, and biologic therapy constitute the common treatment.

THINK ABOUT 8-5

a. Explain why squamous cell carcinoma has a better prognosis than malignant melanoma.
b. List skin disorders to which exposure to sunlight is a predisposing factor.
c. List the signs of possible malignant changes in a skin lesion.
d. Compare the characteristics of the typical lesion of squamous cell carcinoma, melanoma, and Kaposi's sarcoma.
e. List the four warning signs of skin cancer.

CASE STUDY A

Atopic Dermatitis

J.W., at age 5 months, had a moist, erythematous rash on the cheeks, chest, and extensor surfaces of the arms, caused by atopic dermatitis. She had a secondary bacterial infection on one cheek.

1. State the factors in the family history that may support a genetic predisposition to atopic dermatitis in this infant.
2. Explain why a secondary bacterial infection has probably developed.
3. List four factors that tend to aggravate atopic dermatitis.
4. Explain two ways in which administration of an antihistamine could help J.W. sleep.

   Two years later, eczema has persisted, although controlled partially by use of moisturizers and hydrocortisone cream. The skin in some areas is thick and rough in texture.
5. Explain how hydrocortisone cream may reduce the inflammation and skin damage.

CASE STUDY B

Malignant Melanoma

Mr. P.X. age 45, had been swimming and was sitting on the beach when a friend commented on a dark reddish-black "pimple" with a rough surface on it on his upper back. Mr. P.X. said he had numerous moles on his body and it was not of concern. However, later he thought about the comment and saw his physician, who thought the lesion was suspicious and should be checked. The border and surface of the mass were irregular, and it appeared to be quite thick. A similar small lesion was located nearby. The lesion was diagnosed as a superficial spreading malignant melanoma, and surgery was scheduled. Surgery revealed that the melanoma had penetrated through the dermis and had spread to the regional lymph nodes.

1. Explain the factors that make this lesion suspicious for cancer.
2. List the possible predisposing factors in this patient.
3. Predict the prognosis and the reasons for it in this case.

CHAPTER SUMMARY

The skin or integument has many important functions, particularly in protecting the body from the environment. Secondary effects of many skin lesions include infection or scar tissue. Skin lesions may be distinguished by their physical characteristics, location, exudate if any, and the presence of pruritus or pain.

- *Contact dermatitis* may be caused by an irritant or an allergen, often identifiable by the location of the lesion.
- *Urticaria* (hives) results from a type I hypersensitivity to ingested food or drugs.
- *Atopic dermatitis* (eczema) is a familial hypersensitivity beginning in infancy and often associated with hay fever and asthma.
- *Psoriasis* is a chronic inflammatory disorder characterized by accelerated cell proliferation. The typical lesion is a silvery plaque covering an erythematous base.
- *Staphylococcus aureus* is a common cause of skin infections, including *cellulitis* (in the legs and lower trunk), *furunculosis* (in hair follicles), and *impetigo* (on the faces of young children).
- *Acute necrotizing fasciitis* is characterized by bacterial invasion with rapid tissue destruction and septic shock.
- *Herpes simplex virus type 1* (cold sores) causes recurrent painful vesicles around the mouth. It may be transmitted in the exudate or the saliva. Between exacerbations the virus remains in a latent form in a nearby sensory ganglion.
- *Mycoses* are fungal infections such as *tinea*, which may affect the feet (athlete's foot), the scalp, or the body.

- *Pediculosis* (lice) may infect the scalp or body, thriving on human blood.
- There is increasing evidence of sun damage to skin predisposing patients to malignant tumors.

- *Squamous cell carcinoma* is a slow-growing tumor common to exposed areas.
- *Malignant melanoma*, arising from a nevus, grows quickly and metastasizes early.

STUDY QUESTIONS

1. Describe the structure of a hair follicle, including any gland associated with it.
2. Describe the location of resident or normal flora related to the skin and its appendages.
3. State the location of nerves and blood vessels in the skin.
4. List the functions of the skin.
5. Define the terms *papule*, *ulcer*, and *fissure*.
6. Explain how glucocorticoids may reduce pruritus, and give examples of conditions for which these drugs may be helpful.
7. Compare the mechanisms and possible causes of allergic and irritant contact dermatitis.
8. Describe the manifestations of each of the following and state the causative agents for each:
   a. shingles
   b. boils
   c. scabies
   d. scleroderma
9. Prepare a list of contagious skin disorders.
10. Suggest a preventive measure that could reduce the risk of skin cancer.
11. Explain why allergic responses tend to recur.
12. Compare the characteristics of the exudate found in a furuncle and in herpes simplex.
13. Explain why Kaposi's sarcoma is more common in immunocompromised patients.
14. Explain the specific cause of pruritus with:
    a. scabies
    b. pediculosis
    c. contact dermatitis

ADDITIONAL RESOURCES

Gawkrodger D: *Dermatology: An Illustrated Colour Text*, ed 4, New York, 2008, Churchill Livingstone.

Graham-Brown R, Bourke J, Cunliffe T: *Dermatology: Fundamentals of Practice*. St. Louis, 2008, Mosby.

Habib T: *Clinical Dermatology*, ed 4, Philadelphia, 2004, Saunders.

Thibodeau G, Patton K: *Anatomy and Physiology*, ed 7, St. Louis, 2010, Mosby.

Web Sites

http://www.aad.org American Academy of Dermatology
http://www.niams.nih.gov National Institute of Arthritis and Musculoskeletal and Skin Diseases

http://www.cancer.org/docroot/cri/content/cri_2_4_1x_what_is_kaposis_sarcoma_21.asp American Cancer Society—Information on Kaposi's sarcoma
http://www.cancer.org/docroot/CRI/CRI_2x.asp?sitearea=&dt=39 American Cancer Society—Information on skin cancer—melanoma

CHAPTER 9

Musculoskeletal System Disorders

CHAPTER OUTLINE

Review of the Musculoskeletal System
Bone
Skeletal Muscle
Joints
Diagnostic Tests
Trauma
Fractures
Factors Affecting the Healing of Bone
Dislocations
Sprains and Strains
Other Injuries
Muscle Tears
Repetitive Strain Injury

Bone Disorders
Osteoporosis
Rickets and Osteomalacia
Paget's Disease (Osteitis Deformans)
Osteomyelitis
Abnormal Curvatures of the Spine
Bone Tumors
Disorders of Muscle, Tendons, and Ligaments
Muscular Dystrophy
Primary Fibromyalgia Syndrome

Joint Disorders
Osteoarthritis
Rheumatoid Arthritis
Juvenile Rheumatoid Arthritis
Infectious (Septic) Arthritis
Gout (Gouty Arthritis)
Ankylosing Spondylitis
Other Inflammatory Joint Disorders
Case Studies
Chapter Summary
Study Questions
Additional Resources

LEARNING OBJECTIVES

After studying this chapter, the student is expected to:

1. Describe the general structure and function of bone and joints.
2. Describe the general structure and function of skeletal muscle.
3. Describe the types of fractures, the healing process in bone, and potential complications.
4. Compare dislocations, sprains, and strains.
5. Describe the pathophysiology of osteoporosis, the predisposing factors, and possible complications.
6. Compare the causes and effects of rickets, osteomalacia, and Paget's disease.

7. Describe the common bone tumors.
8. Describe the characteristics of Duchenne's muscular dystrophy.
9. Describe the effects of fibromyalgia.
10. Compare osteoarthritis, rheumatoid arthritis, and ankylosing spondylitis with regard to pathophysiology, etiology, manifestations, and possible complications.
11. Describe the distinguishing features of infectious (septic) arthritis.
12. State the etiology and common signs of gout.

KEY TERMS

anabolic steroids
ankylosis
arthroscopy
articulation
crepitus
diaphysis

electromyograms
endosteum
epiphysis
fascia
hyperuricemia
kyphosis

lordosis
medullary cavity
metaphysis
motor unit
neuromuscular junction
osteoblasts

osteoclast
osteocytes
periosteum
pseudohypertrophic
scoliosis
uveitis

Review of the Musculoskeletal System

Bone

The skeletal system provides rigid support for the body, particularly when it is in an upright position or is in motion. The skeletal framework determines the basic size and proportions of the body. Protection is provided for the viscera, such as the heart and lungs, and for fragile structures such as the spinal cord and brain. Bone also has important metabolic functions related to calcium metabolism and storage and the bone marrow, which serves as the area where new blood cells are produced by a process called hematopoiesis.

Bones may be classified by *shape*:

- Long bones, such as the humerus and femur, consist of a long, hollow shaft with two bulbous ends.
- Short bones are generally square-like in shape and are found in the wrist and ankle.
- Flat bones occur in the skull and are relatively thin and often curved.
- Irregular bones, which have many projections and vary in shape, are represented by the vertebrae and the mandible.

Individual bones have unique markings, which may be lines, ridges, processes, or holes. Such landmarks provide for attachment of tendons or passage of nerves and blood vessels.

Bone is special connective tissue consisting of an intercellular matrix and bone cells. The matrix is organized in microscopic structural units called *Haversian systems* or osteons, in which rings of matrix (lamellae) surround a Haversian canal containing blood vessels (Fig. 9-1). The matrix is composed of collagen fibers and calcium phosphate salts (e.g., hydroxyapatite crystals), which provide a very strong and rigid structure. Mature bone cells, or osteocytes, lie between the rings of matrix in spaces called *lacunae*. Small passages termed canaliculi provide communication between the Haversian canals and the lacunae.

- A dynamic equilibrium is maintained between new bone, which is constantly being produced by osteoblasts, and the resorption of bone by osteoclast activity, in accordance with the various hormonal levels and the degree of stress imposed on the bone substance. Osteoblast and osteoclast activity provide the homeostasis of bone. Osteoprogenitor cells differentiate into osteoblasts.
  - Osteoprogenitor cells are derived from embryonic mesenchymal cells.
- Osteoblasts are responsible for secreting the matrix of bone.
- Osteoclasts are derivatives of macrophage progenitor cells.
- Osteoblast and osteoclast activity depend on two hormones: calcitonin and parathyroid hormone.

- Calcitonin stimulates osteoblasts.
- Parathyroid hormone stimulates osteoclasts.

Bone tissue consists of two types, which differ in density. *Compact* bone is formed when many Haversian systems are tightly packed together, producing a very strong, rigid structure that forms the outer covering of bones. *Cancellous* or *spongy* bone is less dense and forms the interior structure of bones. Spongy bone lacks Haversian systems but is made up of plates of bone bordering cavities that contain marrow.

A typical long bone consists of the diaphysis, a thin shaft, between two larger ends or epiphyses (see Fig. 9-1B). The diaphysis is formed of compact bone surrounding a medullary cavity containing marrow. The metaphysis is the area where the shaft broadens into the epiphysis. The epiphysis is made up of spongy bone covered by compact bone. The end of each epiphysis is covered by hyaline cartilage (articular cartilage), which facilitates movement at points of articulation between bones.

The epiphyseal cartilage or plate ("growth" plate) is the site of longitudinal bone growth in children and adolescents, such growth being promoted by growth hormone and sex hormones. Longitudinal bone growth ceases when the epiphyseal plate ossifies during adolescence or early adulthood depending on the specific bone. The epiphyseal plate is referred to as the epiphyseal line following ossification or closure. No bone growth in length occurs after the epiphyseal plate becomes the epiphyseal line.

However, bone may change in density or thickness at any time under the influence of hormones such as growth hormone, parathyroid hormone, or cortisol. The stress (weight-bearing or muscle tension) placed on the bone also affects the balance between osteoblastic and osteoclastic activity. With aging, bone loss is accentuated, resulting in decreased bone mass and density. *Osteoporosis, loss of bone density due to loss of calcium salts*, is common in older people, particularly women (see Chapter 24). Except for the surface of the bone covered by articular cartilage, the bone is covered by periosteum, a fibrous connective tissue. The periosteum contains osteoblasts, blood vessels, nerves, and lymphatics, some of which penetrate into the canals in the bone. When the periosteum is stretched or torn, severe pain results.

The medullary cavity is lined with endosteum, also containing osteoblasts. These osteoblasts are required for bone repair and remodeling as needed. At birth the medullary cavity in most bones contains red bone marrow in which *hematopoiesis* takes place. Gradually, yellow (fatty) bone marrow replaces red bone marrow in the long bones. In adults, red bone marrow is found in the cranium, bodies of the vertebrae, ribs, sternum, and ilia, the last two being the usual sites of bone marrow aspiration used in the diagnosis and monitoring of leukemias and blood dyscrasias.

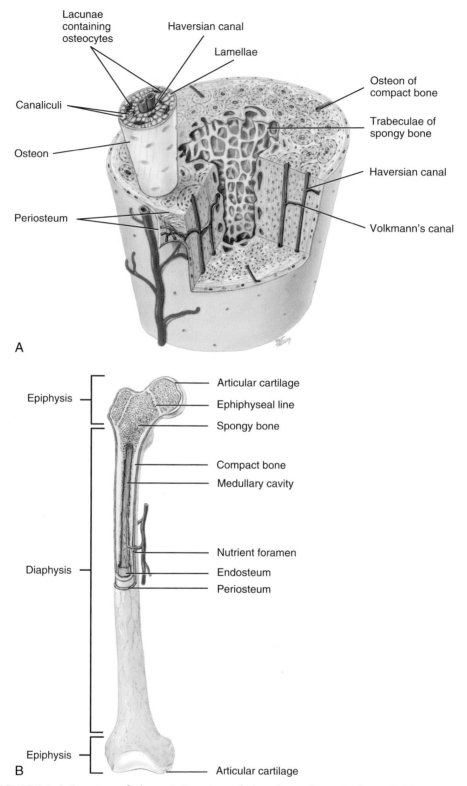

FIGURE 9-1 A, Structure of a bone. **B**, Structure of a long bone. *(From Applegate EJ: The Anatomy and Physiology Learning System, Philadelphia, 2000, Saunders.)*

THINK ABOUT 9-1

a. Describe the functions of bone.
b. Differentiate compact bone from cancellous bone in terms of structure and function.
c. Describe the characteristics of the: (1) periosteum; (2) epiphyseal plate; and (3) metaphysis.

Skeletal Muscle

Skeletal muscle has four basic functions:
1. To facilitate body movement by muscle contraction
2. To maintain body position by continuing *muscle tone*
3. To stabilize the joints and prevent excessive movement
4. To maintain body temperature by producing heat through muscle contraction

Skeletal muscle is considered to be under voluntary control, although some muscle activities occur without deliberate intent, such as respiratory movements, postural reflexes, blinking, shivering, or certain facial expressions.

Skeletal is *striated* muscle that consists of bundles of muscle fibers (cells) covered by connective tissue. The striated or striped appearance results from the arrangement of the actin and myosin filaments within the muscle fibers.

Connective tissue coverings of skeletal muscles are:
- Epimysium—surrounding the entire muscle
- Perimysium—surrounding the fascicles
- Endomysium—surrounding the individual muscles fibers (cells)

Muscle tissue is well supplied with nerves and blood vessels, necessary to fulfill its function. Each muscle fiber is an elongated muscle multinucleated cell containing many mitochondria that supply energy for the contraction process. A muscle is stimulated to contract when an efferent impulse is conducted along a motor neuron to a muscle. The axon of the motor nerve branches as it penetrates a muscle so that each muscle fiber in the muscle receives a stimulus to contract at the same time. The motor neuron of the spinal cord and all the muscle fibers it stimulates are referred to as the motor unit. At the neuromuscular junction, where the synapse between the end of the motor nerve and the receptor site in the muscle fiber is located, the chemical transmitter *acetylcholine* is released (Fig. 9-2). Following its release and the subsequent muscle contraction, acetylcholine is inactivated by the enzyme acetylcholinesterase (AChE). Skeletal muscle relaxing drugs may act by blocking acetylcholine at the muscle receptor sites,

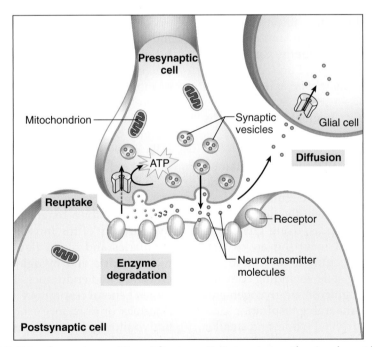

FIGURE 9-2 Fate of neurotransmitters. After synaptic transmission, the signal must be stopped by removing neurotransmitters from the synaptic cleft. Many neurotransmitters are immediately transported back into the presynaptic neuron in a process called reuptake. Some neurotransmitters are broken down by enzymes in the synaptic cleft, and the resulting molecules are transported back into the presynaptic neuron for recycling. Some neurotransmitter molecules may diffuse out of the synapse and be transported into a nearby glial cell (which may return an altered form of the molecule to the presynaptic neuron). *(From Patton KT, Thibodeau GA: Anatomy & Physiology, ed 8, St. Louis, 2013, Mosby.)*

whereas muscle activity may be promoted by drugs that interfere with cholinesterase activity.

Each muscle cell contains myofibrils, which in turn are made up of smaller myofilaments consisting of the proteins actin and myosin. Actin and myosin filaments are the contractile elements of the muscle fiber.

The mechanism of muscle contraction starts at the neuromuscular junction and ends with the actual contraction of the skeletal muscle fibers.

- An action potential from the motor neuron arrives at the presynaptic terminal.
- The arrival of the action potential results in the depolarization of the presynaptic terminal.
- The depolarization is followed by a calcium influx into the presynaptic terminal.
- The calcium influx results in the exocytosis of the neurotransmitter (Ach) into the synaptic cleft.
- Diffusion of the neurotransmitter to the postsynaptic receptor results in a muscle action potential.
- The muscle action potential travels down the t-tubules to cause a second messenger activation.
- Calcium is released from the sarcoplasmic reticulum and causes the power stroke—contraction of the muscle fiber.
- During muscle relaxation calcium is transported back into the sarcoplasmic reticulum.
- Both muscle contraction and relaxation require cellular energy (adenosine triphosphate, ATP).

During exercise, the blood vessels in the muscles are dilated to promote greater blood flow into the muscle, thus increasing the supply of oxygen and nutrients (glucose and fatty acids) to provide energy for the contraction and remove metabolic wastes. Limited amounts of oxygen can be bound to *myoglobin* and stored in muscle fibers. Myoglobin is a red oxygen-binding protein, similar in structure to hemoglobin, which is present in muscle cells. *Glycogen*, a source of glucose, is also stored in muscle.

Aerobic respiration to produce ATP can be maintained in muscle fibers as long as adequate oxygen is made available from the myoglobin and the circulating blood. If the supply of oxygen does not meet the demand, the process of *anaerobic respiration* begins, using glucose as the primary energy source and incurring an oxygen debt (the amount of oxygen required to restore the muscle cell to its normal resting state, including converting lactic acid to pyruvic acid, glucose, or glycogen and replenishing stores of ATP). Anaerobic respiration produces lactic acid rather than carbon dioxide, and smaller amounts of ATP. This state of acidosis leads to the increased respirations commonly observed during exercise. These respirations operate as a compensatory mechanism to reduce acidosis by decreasing carbon dioxide levels in the blood (see Chapter 2).

The accumulated lactic acid may cause local muscle pain and cramping during and immediately after exercise. A muscle *cramp* is pain resulting from a strong muscle contraction or spasm, usually caused by local irritation from metabolic wastes. Muscle spasm reduces blood flow, thus leading to ischemic pain. Muscle soreness and pain that appear a day or so after strenuous exercise are often due to minor damage to muscle cells and subsequent inflammation. Also, during periods of strenuous physical activity and anaerobic metabolism, excessive lactic acid diffuses into the blood, lowering serum pH and causing metabolic acidosis.

A muscle may be attached directly to the periosteum of a bone, but more often the connective tissue covering the muscle (perimysium) extends to form a cordlike structure or *tendon*, which attaches each end of the muscle to the two bones that articulate at a joint. At a joint, one bone remains fixed, forming the *origin* of the muscle. The other bone attached to the same muscle is moved by the muscle contraction and is called the *insertion*. *Ligaments* form a direct attachment between two bones. Tendons and ligaments are composed of collagen fibers arranged in bundles, a structure that can withstand considerable stress. At the insertion point of tendons or ligaments there is a gradual transition from the connective tissue to the bone or cartilage. Tendons and ligaments have little blood supply; therefore healing of these structures is difficult and slow.

Muscles may work singly or in groups to perform a specific movement. Also, muscles at a site may be designated as *antagonists* because one muscle opposes the action of another, allowing movement in either direction. For example, at the elbow, the triceps brachii muscle functions as an extensor muscle, whereas the biceps brachii is a flexor muscle. Antagonistic muscles prevent excessive movement and provide better control of movements.

Skeletal muscle cells do not undergo mitosis; therefore that process cannot be used to enhance muscle activity or replace damaged muscle. However, muscle cells may undergo *hypertrophy* (increased size of the muscle cell) when the demands are increased, such as with regular exercise. *Aerobic* or *endurance* exercise, such as swimming or running, increases the muscle's capacity to work for a longer time without causing marked hypertrophy of the muscle. Such exercise increases the capillaries and blood flow in a muscle as well as the mitochondria and myoglobin content, thus improving efficiency and endurance. This type of exercise also promotes general respiratory and cardiovascular function. *Anaerobic* or resistance exercise, such as weight lifting or bodybuilding, focuses on increasing muscle strength by increasing muscle mass (hypertrophy). It is helpful for those persons interested in developing strong muscles to incorporate some aerobic exercise into the training program to improve cardiopulmonary fitness as well as strength.

Anabolic steroids are synthetic hormones similar to testosterone, the male sex hormone. They are used by some athletes, bodybuilders, and others interested in changing the body image to *build up* muscle strength and mass. Speed and endurance do not appear to be affected. These synthetic hormones (e.g., methenolone [Primobolan]) have been developed to increase the anabolic effects, or protein synthesis, and decrease the androgenic or male characteristics produced by these chemicals. Serious and sometimes life-threatening side effects are associated with the use of these substances, such as liver damage, cardiovascular disease, personality changes, emotional lability, and sterility. Unfortunately, this type of steroid is abused by many adolescents and young adults, including those involved in sports, those with eating disorders, and those with psychological problems related to body image and poor self-esteem. The use of anabolic steroids by participants in athletic competition has been banned by many organizations.

Skeletal muscle also may *atrophy*, in which muscle cell size is decreased, when the muscle is not used (see Chapter 1). Atrophied muscle becomes weak and flaccid. Atrophy may occur within a short period of time when a fractured limb is placed in a cast or the pain of arthritis limits movement. Such *disuse atrophy* is also associated with immobilization and chronic illness (see Chapter 25). Atrophy may be secondary to nerve injury, with resultant flaccid paralysis. Also, nutritional deficiencies, particularly protein, secondary to disorders such as anorexia or Crohn's disease, lead to atrophy. Skeletal muscle may also become weak owing to degenerative changes involving accumulations of fatty or fibrous tissue. With aging, muscle mass decreases owing to both a decrease in number of muscle cells and a decrease in size (diameter) of the fibers. Muscle strength generally diminishes as well, although this may vary with the individual's degree of activity and general health status.

Muscle twitch or *tetany* usually results from increased irritability of the motor nerves supplying the muscle. For example, hypocalcemia causes increased permeability of the nerve membrane and therefore increased or spontaneous stimulation of the skeletal muscle fibers, causing a contraction or spasm of the muscle. Note that sufficient calcium is stored and returned to storage in the skeletal muscle cell following contraction, and therefore hypocalcemia does not directly affect skeletal muscle function, but rather its innervation.

THINK ABOUT 9-2

a. Explain why skeletal muscle cells contain many mitochondria.
b. Explain the purpose of shivering when one is cold.
c. What electrolyte is required for skeletal muscle contraction and what is its source?
d. Differentiate muscle hypertrophy from atrophy and give a cause of each.
e. Explain how an anticholinesterase drug affects skeletal muscle function.
f. When does anaerobic metabolism occur in skeletal muscle and what are the effects of this?

Joints

Joints or articulations between bones vary in the degree of movement allowed:

- *Synarthroses*, represented by the sutures in the skull, are immovable joints.
- *Amphiarthroses*, slightly movable joints, are joints in which the bones are connected by fibrocartilage or hyaline cartilage. Examples of this type of joint include the junction of the ribs and sternum and the symphysis pubis.
- *Diarthroses* or *synovial* joints are freely movable joints and are the most common type of joint in the body.

Different types of diarthroses allow a variety of movements. For example, a hinge joint, providing flexion and extension, is found at the elbow, whereas a ball-and-socket joint at the shoulder provides a wide range of motion, including rotation. Both hinge and gliding movements are found in the temporomandibular joint (TMJ), controlling the opening of the mouth. Common body movements are illustrated in Ready Reference 1 (see Fig. RR 1-6).

In a synovial joint, the ends of the bone are covered with *articular* (hyaline) *cartilage*, providing a smooth surface and a slight cushion during movement (see Fig. 9-13*A*). With aging, the cartilage in joints tends to degenerate and become thin, leading to difficulty with movement and potential changes in the alignment of bones.

The joint cavity or space between the articulating ends of the bones is filled with a small amount of *synovial fluid*, which facilitates movement. The synovial fluid prevents the articular cartilage on the two surfaces from damaging each other and also provides nutrients to the articular cartilage. The synovial fluid is produced by the *synovial membrane* (synovium), which lines the joint capsule to the edge of the articular cartilages. The synovial membrane is well supplied with blood vessels.

The *articular capsule* is composed of the synovial membrane and its outer covering, the *fibrous capsule*, a tough protective material that extends into the periosteum of each articulating bone (Sharpey's fibers). The capsule is reinforced by *ligaments*, straps across the joint that link the two bones, which support the joint and prevent excessive movement of the bones.

In a few joints there are some variations in structure. The knee has additional moon-shaped fibrocartilage pads, termed lateral and medial *menisci*, which act to stabilize the joint. *Bursae* are fluid-filled sacs composed of synovial membrane and located between structures such as tendons and ligaments; they act as additional cushions in the joint. The TMJ, the only movable joint in the skull and face, has two synovial cavities and a central articular cartilage of dense collagen tissue.

The *nerves* supplying a joint are those supplying the muscles controlling the joint. These motor fibers are accompanied by sensory fibers from *proprioceptors* in the tendons and ligaments that respond to the changing tensions related to movement and posture. The joint capsule and ligaments are supplied with pain receptors.

THINK ABOUT 9-3

a. Name and describe the type of joint found in the skull.
b. Describe two structures in a joint that facilitate movement.
c. Describe the location and purpose of the synovial membrane.

Diagnostic Tests

In persons in whom trauma, tumors, or metabolic disease are suspected, bone abnormalities may be evaluated using x-rays (radiographs) and bone scans.

Electromyograms (EMGs) measure the electrical charge associated with muscle contraction and are helpful in differentiating muscle disorders from neurologic disease. Also, the strength of individual muscle groups can be determined. Muscle biopsy is required to confirm the presence of some muscular disorders, such as muscular dystrophy. Joints may be visualized by arthroscopy (insertion of a lens directly into the joint) or by magnetic resonance imaging (MRI), a noninvasive imaging procedure. Synovial fluid may be aspirated and analyzed to ascertain whether inflammation, bleeding, or infection is present.

Serum calcium, phosphate, and parathyroid hormone levels may indicate metabolic changes, perhaps secondary to renal disease or parathyroid hormone imbalance. Muscle disorders may be checked by determining levels of components such as serum creatine kinase (CK), which is elevated in persons with many muscle diseases. Creatine kinase, an enzyme with an essential role in energy storage, leaks out of damaged muscle cells into body fluids.

Trauma

Fractures

A fracture is a break in the rigid structure and continuity of a bone (Fig. 9-3). Fractures can be classified in several ways:

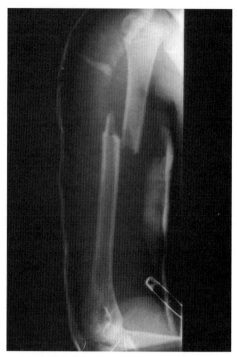

FIGURE 9-3 Fracture of the midshaft of the humerus. *(Courtesy of Dr. Mercer Rang, The Hospital for Sick Children, Toronto, Ontario, Canada.)*

- Complete-incomplete. A *complete fracture* occurs when the bone is broken to form two or more separate pieces, whereas in an *incomplete fracture* the bone is only partially broken. An example of the latter is a *greenstick* fracture, common in the softer bones of children, in which the shaft of the bone is bent, tearing the cortical bone (outer layer of compact bone) on one side but not extending all the way through the bone.
- Open-closed. An *open* or compound fracture results when the skin is broken (Fig. 9-4). The bone fragments may be angled and protrude through the skin. In open fractures there is more damage to soft tissue, including the blood vessels and nerves, and there is also a much higher risk of infection. In a *closed* fracture the skin is not broken at the fracture site.
- Number of fracture lines:
  - *Simple* fracture, a single break in the bone in which the bone ends maintain their alignment and position
  - *Comminuted* fracture, in which there are multiple fracture lines and bone fragments
  - *Compression* fracture, common in the vertebrae, occurring when a bone is crushed or collapses into small pieces
- Other types:
  - *Impacted* fracture occurs when one end of the bone is forced or telescoped into the adjacent bone; for example, the neck of the femur is crushed against the pelvis.

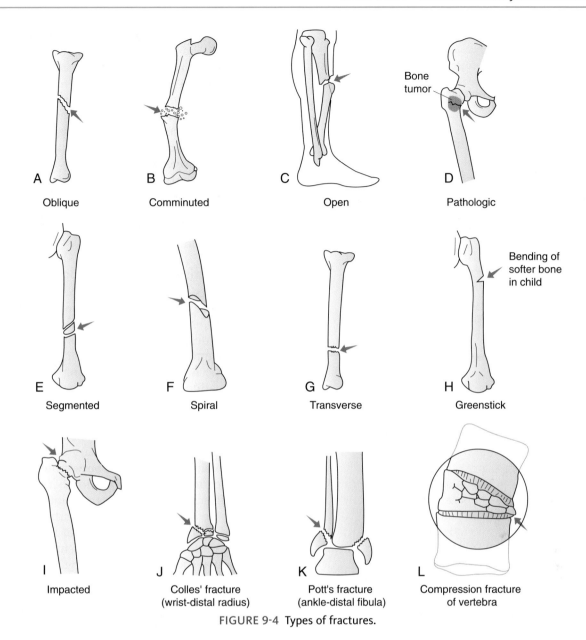

A Oblique   B Comminuted   C Open   D Pathologic

Bone tumor

E Segmented   F Spiral   G Transverse   H Greenstick

Bending of softer bone in child

I Impacted   J Colles' fracture (wrist-distal radius)   K Pott's fracture (ankle-distal fibula)   L Compression fracture of vertebra

FIGURE 9-4 Types of fractures.

- *Pathologic* fracture results from a weakness in the bone structure due to conditions such as a tumor or osteoporosis. The break occurs spontaneously or with very little stress on the bone.
- *Stress* fractures (fatigue fractures) result from repeated excessive stress, commonly in the tibia, femur, or second and third metatarsals.
- *Depressed* fracture occurs in the skull when the broken section is forced inward on the brain.
- Direction of the fracture line; for example:
  - A fracture across the bone is a *transverse* fracture.
  - A break along the axis of the bone is a *linear* fracture.
  - A break at an angle to the diaphysis of the bone is an *oblique* fracture.
  - A break that angles around the bone, usually due to a twisting injury, is a *spiral* fracture.

- Unique names for certain types of fractures; for example:
  - Colles' fracture is a break in the distal radius at the wrist, commonly occurring when a person attempts to break a fall by extending the arm and open hand. Sometimes the ulna is also damaged.
  - Pott's fracture refers to a fracture of the lower fibula due to excessive stress on the ankle; for example, when stepping down with force. The tibia may be damaged as well.

■ *Pathophysiology*

When a bone breaks, bleeding occurs from the blood vessels in the bone and periosteum. Bleeding and inflammation also develop around the bone because of soft tissue damage. This *hematoma* or clot forms in the medullary canal, under the periosteum, and between

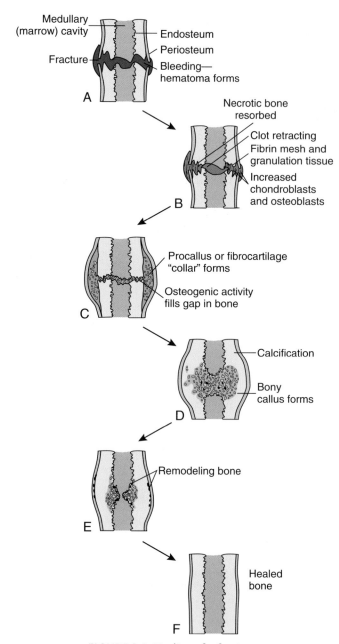

FIGURE 9-5 Healing of a fracture.

the ends of the bone fragments (Fig. 9-5). Necrosis occurs at the ends of the broken bone because the torn blood vessels are unable to continue delivery of nutrients. An inflammatory response develops as a reaction to the trauma and the presence of debris at the site.

At fracture sites, the hematoma serves as the basis for a fibrin network into which granulation tissue grows. Many new capillaries extend into this tissue, and phagocytic cells (for removing debris) and fibroblasts (for laying down new collagen fibers) migrate to it. Also, chondroblasts begin to form cartilage. Thus, the two bone ends become splinted together by a *procallus* or *fibrocartilaginous callus* (collar). This structure is *not* strong enough to bear weight, but constitutes the preliminary bridge repair in the bone.

Osteoblasts from the periosteum and endosteum begin to generate new bone to fill in the gap. Gradually the fibrocartilaginous callus is replaced by bone through extensive osteogenic activity, which forms a *bony callus*. Note that damaged bone is repaired by new bone formation, not by scar tissue. During subsequent months the repaired bone is *remodeled* by osteoblastic and osteoclastic activity in response to mechanical stresses on the bone. The excessive bone in the callus is removed, more compact bone is laid down, and eventually the bone assumes a normal appearance.

To summarize, the five stages of bone healing are hematoma, granulation tissue, procallus (fibrocartilage), bony callus, and remodeling.

Factors Affecting the Healing of Bone

Many factors affect the *healing process* in bone. In children fractures usually heal in approximately 1 month; in adults the process requires 2 or more months. A fracture in an elderly person may require many months.

- The amount of local damage done to the bone and soft tissue is a major determining factor. Prolonged inflammation or extensive damage to the periosteum or blood vessels impairs healing.
- The more closely approximated the ends of the bone are, the smaller the gap to be filled and the faster the healing process. When necessary to promote healing and prevent deformity, the bones must be realigned (reduced) in the proper position before healing can begin. It is most important to maintain immobilization of the bones to prevent disturbance or damage to the developing fragile bridge of tissue.
- Any secondary problem such as foreign material or infection at the site delays healing.
- Numerous systemic factors also affect the healing process in bone. For example, fracture repair is delayed in older persons and individuals with circulatory problems, anemias, diabetes mellitus, or nutritional deficits as well as in those taking drugs such as glucocorticoids (see Chapter 5).

Complications may affect healing in patients who sustain severe injuries:

1. Muscle spasm may occur as local pain and irritation cause strong muscle contractions at the fracture site. This muscle spasm pulls the bone fragments further out of position, causing angulation (deformity), rotation of a bone, or overriding of the bone pieces. Such abnormal movement of the bone causes more soft tissue damage, bleeding, and inflammation.
2. *Infections* such as tetanus or osteomyelitis (see Chapters 6 and 23) are a threat in persons with compound fractures or when surgical intervention is required. In such cases, precautions include wound débridement, application of a windowed cast, tetanus booster shots, and prophylactic antimicrobial therapy.
3. *Ischemia* is a complication that develops in a limb following treatment as edema increases during the first

48 hours after the trauma and casting. If the peripheral area (e.g., the toes or fingers) becomes pale or cold and numb or if the peripheral pulse has decreased or is absent, it is likely that the cast has become too tight and is compromising the circulation in the limb. The cast must be released quickly to prevent secondary tissue damage. During the later stages of healing it is also important that the cast not become too loose as edema decreases and muscle atrophies because the newly formed procallus may break down if there is any bone movement.

4. *Compartment syndrome* may develop shortly after the fracture occurs when there is more extensive inflammation, such as with crush injuries. Increased pressure of fluid within the fascia, the nonelastic covering of the muscle, compresses the nerves and blood vessels, causing severe pain and ischemia or necrosis of the muscle. The pressure effects may be aggravated by a cast.

5. *Fat emboli* are a risk when fatty marrow escapes from the bone marrow into a vein within the first week after injury. Fat emboli are more common in patients with fractures of the pelvis or long bones such as the femur, particularly when the fracture site has not been well immobilized during transportation immediately after the injury.

　　Fat emboli travel to the lungs (see Chapter 13), where they cause obstruction, extensive inflammation, and respiratory distress syndrome, and they may disseminate into the systemic circulation as well. Frequently the first indications of a fat embolus are behavioral changes, confusion, and disorientation associated with cerebral emboli, in combination with respiratory distress and severe hypoxia.

6. Nerve damage may occur with severe trauma or tearing of the periosteum.

7. Failure to heal (nonunion) or healing with deformity (malunion) may result if the bone is not stabilized with ends closely approximated and aligned.

8. Fractures in or near the joint may have long-term residual effects, such as osteoarthritis or stunted growth if the epiphyseal plate is damaged in a child.

Signs and Symptoms

In some cases a fracture is clearly present, as in patients with compound fractures or an obvious deformity. Swelling, tenderness at the site, or altered sensation is present but may occur with any type of injury. Inability to move the broken limb is apparent. Crepitus, a grating sound, may be heard if the ends of the bone fragments move over each other. (The limb should *not* be moved to test for this!)

Pain usually occurs immediately after the injury. In some cases, particularly with compound or multiple fractures, pain is delayed when nerve function at the site is lost temporarily. Pain results from direct damage to the nerves by the trauma and from pressure and irritation due to the accumulated blood and inflammatory response. Severe pain may cause shock with pallor, diaphoresis, hypotension, and tachycardia. Nausea and vomiting sometimes occur.

Diagnostic Tests

X-ray films are used to confirm the presence of a fracture.

Treatment

Immediate splinting and immobilization of the fracture site is essential to minimize the risk of complications.

If necessary, *reduction* of the fracture is performed to restore the bones to their normal position. *Closed* reduction is accomplished by exerting pressure and traction; *open* reduction requires surgery. During surgery, devices such as pins, plates, rods, or screws may be placed to fix the fragments in position; any necrotic or foreign material is removed, and the bone ends are aligned and closely approximated. Immobilization is attained by applying a cast or splints or by using traction.

Traction involves the application of a force or weight pulling on a limb that is opposed by body weight. This force maintains the alignment of the bones, prevents muscle spasm, and immobilizes the limb. During the healing period, exercises are helpful to limit muscle atrophy in the immobilized area, maintain good circulation, and minimize joint stiffness or contractures.

EMERGENCY TREATMENT FOR FRACTURES

1. Cover open wounds with sterile or clean dressing material.
2. Splint for support and immobilize for transport, including joints above and below the fracture.
3. Elevate the limb slightly and apply cold if possible. Check pulse and sensory function distal to the fracture.
4. Keep patient warm. Check for signs of shock.

Dislocations

A dislocation is the separation of two bones at a joint with loss of contact between the articulating bone surfaces (Fig. 9-6). Usually one bone is out of position, while the other remains in its normal location. For example, the humerus is displaced from the shoulder joint. If the bone is only partially displaced, with partial loss of contact between the surfaces, the injury is termed *subluxation.*

Trauma, such as a fall, is usually the cause of dislocations. In some cases, a fracture is associated with a dislocation, whereas in others, an underlying disorder such as a muscular disease or rheumatoid arthritis, or other damage such as torn ligaments, may predispose the individual to dislocation.

Dislocations cause considerable soft tissue damage, including damage to the ligaments, nerves, and blood

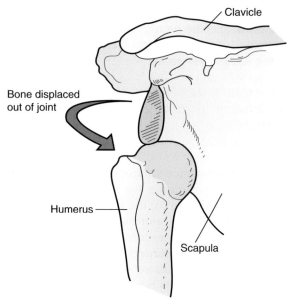

FIGURE 9-6 Dislocation.

vessels as the bone is pulled away from the joint. Bleeding and inflammation result. Severe pain, swelling, and tenderness develop. Deformity and limited movement are usually evident. The diagnosis is confirmed by x-rays. Treatment consists of reduction to return the dislocated bone to its normal position, immobilization during healing, and therapy to maintain joint mobility. Healing is slow if the ligaments and soft tissue are extensively damaged.

Sprains and Strains

A tear in a *ligament* is called a *sprain*, and a tear in a *tendon* is referred to as a *strain*. Ligaments and tendons support the bones in a joint and can easily be torn when excessive force is exerted on a joint. In some cases, the ligaments or tendons can be completely separated from their bony attachments, a problem known as *avulsion*. Sprains and strains are quite painful and are accompanied by tenderness, marked swelling, and often discoloration due to hematoma formation. Bleeding into the joint capsule delays healing. Strength and range of movement in the joint are limited. Diagnosis requires x-rays and other tests to rule out the presence of a fracture and determine the extent of the damage.

After a tear occurs, inflammation and then granulation tissue develop at the site. Collagen fibers are formed that create links with the remaining tendon or ligament, and eventually the healing mass is bound together with fibrous tissue. A tendon or ligament requires approximately 6 weeks before it is strong again. Stress on a tendon in the early stage will reopen the tear and lead to the development of excessive fibrous tissue in the tendon and thus less strength, shortening, and decreased

flexibility at the joint. With severe damage to the tendons and ligaments, surgical repair may be necessary.

Other Injuries

The number of traumatic and overuse injuries has been increasing with the rising numbers of adults and children participating in fitness and recreational activities. Some of the predisposing factors include inappropriate or inadequate equipment, training, or warm-up techniques; more aggressive approaches to sports (e.g., skiing); and failure to allow minor injuries to heal completely before resuming activity. Minor injuries resulting from excessive use or abuse, particularly of joints, are also increasing; for example, tennis elbow, in which inflammation develops at the junction of the forearm muscles with the humerus. Muscle tears are more common, leading to hematoma and scar tissue formation.

Muscle Tears

Muscle tears are tears along the muscle itself or at points of attachment. They can occur as a result of a direct trauma or overexertion/overstressing of the muscle. There are three degrees of muscle tears:
- First degree—usually involves only a small percentage of the muscle. Pain is usually mild and does not result in any appreciable loss in strength or range of motion.
- Second degree—a larger tear than involves much of the muscle but stops short of being a complete tear. Pain is usually severe and the muscle can be partially contracted with a substantial loss of strength and range of motion.
- Third degree—a complete tear across the width of the muscle. The muscle will be unable to contract, there will be a great deal of internal bleeding and may require surgery for proper healing.

As soon as a tear occurs, activity involving the use of the muscle should stop, cold should be applied to help reduce internal bleeding, a compression bandage should be applied, and the limb or affected area should be elevated. In third-degree tears surgery may be necessary to repair the tear. An example of a third degree requiring surgery may be tearing of the gastrocnemius (the "hamstring"). In all cases, any scar tissue that forms will reduce the flexibility and strength of the muscle

Repeated injuries eventually result in fibrous scar tissue replacing normal structures, hindering mobility, as well as permanent joint damage and development of osteoarthritis. For example, repeated tears in the knee ligaments appear to cause early development of osteoarthritis. Shoulder pain and damage to the rotator cuff can result from excessive swinging motions, particularly with force (as in golf, tennis, hockey, and painting walls and ceilings), leading to tendinitis.

Repetitive Strain Injury

Repetitive strain injury (RSI) is a term referring to disorders affecting muscles, tendons, and nerves that develops over a period of time. The cause seems to be repeated forceful or precision movements, many of which are associated with work-related activities, although sports such as golf and certain exercises are also common causes. It appears that rapid repetition of certain movements interferes with circulation to the area and damages soft tissues, with cumulative effects. Most injuries affect the upper body. Higher stress levels increase the risk. Those affected are primarily in the 30 to 50 year range, and the incidence is increasing. Work such as repetitive lifting of merchandise, pivoting on an assembly line, or retrieving and shelving library materials are examples that are associated with a higher risk of RSI. The result is pain, weakness, and numbness, causing disability and interference with sleep. Examples include tendinitis, inflammation or injury of the tendon and sheath, or compression of a peripheral nerve, seen in carpal tunnel syndrome. In the latter, the median nerve is compressed at the wrist between tendons and the transverse carpal ligament.

Diagnosis requires a history, x-rays, and perhaps arthroscopic examination. Common treatment includes rest, applications of cold or heat, use of nonsteroidal anti-inflammatory drugs, and physiotherapy. Occupational therapy is helpful in identifying ergonomic changes in work that will lessen damage or reduce strain and pain. Surgery may be required to repair tears, remove damaged tissue, or replace joints. Sports medicine clinics can provide evaluation, education and preventive measures, assistive devices, and rehabilitation programs.

THINK ABOUT 9-4

a. Define each type of fracture: (1) compound; (2) comminuted; and (3) transverse.
b. List the three degrees of muscle tears and the steps in the treatment of a third-degree tear.
c. Differentiate a dislocation from a sprain.

Bone Disorders

Osteoporosis

Osteoporosis is a common metabolic bone disorder characterized by a decrease in bone mass and density, combined with loss of bone matrix and mineralization (see Fig. 24-1). Estimates for prevalence run as high as 10 million in the United States, with many more having low bone mass, and therefore increased risk. Although women have a higher risk of osteoporosis, a significant number of men also have been diagnosed. Osteoporosis is a factor in an estimated 1.5 million fractures annually, of which 300,000 involve the hip. Regular bone mass density tests are recommended for all individuals more than 50 years of age. This procedure requires resting on the scanner table for 10 to 15 minutes and is noninvasive.

Osteoporosis occurs in two forms: primary, including postmenopausal, senile, or idiopathic osteoporosis, and secondary, affecting men and women, following a specific primary disorder such as Cushing's syndrome.

■ *Pathophysiology*

During the continuous bone remodeling process, bone resorption exceeds bone formation, leading to thin, fragile bones that are subject to spontaneous fracture, particularly in the vertebrae (see Fig. 24-2). Although bone density and mass are reduced, the remaining bones are normal. Osteoporosis affects the bones consisting of higher proportions of cancellous bone, such as the vertebrae and femoral neck. The early stages of the condition are asymptomatic, but can be diagnosed using various bone density scans and x-rays to demonstrate the bone changes.

■ *Etiology*

Bone mass normally peaks in young adults, and then gradually declines, depending on genetic factors (such as vitamin D receptors), nutrition, weight-bearing activity, and hormonal levels. It appears that calcium intake in the child and young adult is critical to maintenance of bone mass later in life. A number of factors predispose people to osteoporosis. These include:

- Aging:
  - Osteoporosis is common in older individuals, particularly postmenopausal women with estrogen deficiency (see Chapter 24).
  - Osteoblastic activity is less effective with advancing age.
- Decreased mobility or a sedentary lifestyle:
  - Mechanical stress on bone by muscle activity is essential for osteoblastic activity. Decreased mobility is a factor with aging, but also if a patient is on bed rest for a prolonged time with a chronic illness, or has limited activity due to rheumatoid arthritis.
  - One limb or area of the body may be affected by osteoporosis when it is immobilized because of conditions such as a fracture (disuse osteoporosis).
- Hormonal factors such as hyperparathyroidism, Cushing's syndrome, or continued intake of catabolic glucocorticoids such as prednisone
- Deficits of calcium, vitamin D, or protein related to diet or history of deficits in childhood or malabsorption disorders
- Cigarette smoking

- Small, light bone structure, as in Asian and Caucasian persons
- Excessive caffeine intake

Signs and Symptoms

Compression fractures of the vertebrae have several obvious effects. Back pain is a common sign of osteoporosis, associated with the altered vertebrae causing pressure on the nerves. Kyphosis and scoliosis, abnormal curvatures of the spine with accompanying loss of height, are characteristic of the spinal changes seen with osteoporosis (see Figs. 23-2 and 23-3). Spontaneous fractures involving the head of the femur or pelvis are frequent occurrences. Healing of the fractures is slow.

Treatment

Usually bone cannot be restored to normal structural levels, but therapy can retard further bone loss. In addition to treating any underlying problem, therapeutic measures may include:

- Dietary supplements of calcium and vitamin D or protein. It is currently recommended that premenopausal women need at least 1000 mg of calcium, whereas postmenopausal women require more than 1500 mg. Intake of vitamin D should be 400 to 800 IU daily.
- Fluoride supplements to promote bone deposition
- Bisphosphonates such as alendronate (Fosamax) can be used as a short-term option to inhibit osteoclast activity and bone resorption.
- Calcitonin (Miacalcin nasal spray)
- Injected human parathyroid hormone to decrease bone resorption (helpful for some individuals)
- Regular weight-bearing exercise program such as walking or weight lifting
- Raloxifene (Evista) or tamoxifen, classed as selective estrogen receptor modulator drugs; recommended in specific cases because there is less effect on uterine and breast tissue. (The use of estrogen replacement therapy for osteoporosis has been questioned because of the possible risk of cancer.)
- Other newer medications under investigation, including strontium ranelate that appears to decrease bone resorption and increase bone formation as well as antibody preparations that bind to osteoclasts, preventing bone resorption
- Surgery to reduce kyphosis and realign the vertebral column

Research continues into new methods to stabilize bones and prevent fractures.

Rickets and Osteomalacia

These conditions result from a deficit of vitamin D and phosphates required for bone mineralization. They occur with dietary deficits, malabsorption, prolonged intake of phenobarbital (for seizures), or lack of sun exposure. The result is soft bone and rickets in children. Vitamin D is required for the absorption of calcium, and the lack of calcification of the cartilage forming at the epiphyseal plate leads to weak bones, often deformities, and the typical "bow legs" (rickets). The child's height is usually below normal. Osteomalacia occurs in adults in whom poor absorption of vitamin D or sometimes calcium causes soft bones and resulting compression fractures. "Renal rickets" refers to osteomalacia associated with severe renal disease (see Chapter 18).

Paget's Disease (Osteitis Deformans)

Paget's disease is a progressive bone disease that occurs in adults older than 40 years. The cause has not yet been established; however, childhood infection with a virus has been implicated and there is evidence of a genetic factor. Excessive bone destruction occurs, with replacement of bone by fibrous tissue and abnormal bone. Structural abnormalities, evident on x-rays, and enlargement (or thickening) are apparent in the long bones, vertebrae, pelvis, and skull. In some cases, the disease is asymptomatic. Pathologic fractures are common. When the vertebrae are affected, compression fractures and kyphosis result. Skull involvement leads to signs of increased pressure such as headache and compression of cranial nerves. Paget's disease also causes cardiovascular disease and heart failure. Treatment goals are to reduce the risk of fractures and deformity.

Osteomyelitis

Pathophysiology and Etiology

Osteomyelitis is a bone infection usually caused by bacteria and sometimes fungi. The microorganisms can enter the blood from an infection anywhere in the body and spread to the bones. An infection can also occur as result of surgery, particularly when a pin or structural insert is involved.

Signs and Symptoms

As with most infections there can be both local and systemic manifestations. These may include:
- Local inflammation and bone pain
- Fever and excessive sweating
- Chills
- General malaise

Treatment

As with other infections, use of antibiotics are the primary treatment used to eliminate the infection. If the infection is prolonged and significant damage has occurred in the bone tissue, surgery may be required to remove and repair the damaged tissue. If an insert or mechanical implant is involved, surgery may also be necessary to remove the device.

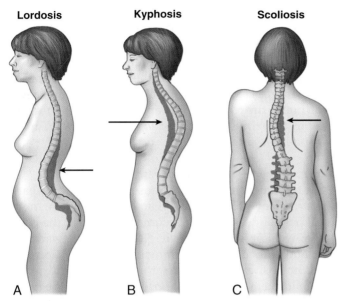

Lordosis   **Kyphosis**   **Scoliosis**

A   B   C

FIGURE 9-7 Abnormal spine curvatures. **A**, Lordosis. **B**, Kyphosis. **C**, Scoliosis. Black arrows highlight areas of abnormal curvature. *(From Patton KT, Thibodeau GA:* Anatomy & Physiology, *ed 8, St. Louis, 2013, Mosby.)*

Abnormal Curvatures of the Spine

The curves formed by the vertebrae help the spine absorb the stress of body movement and the action of gravity. When abnormalities occur, the curves may become misaligned or exaggerated, resulting in three main types of curvature disorders: lordosis, kyphosis, and scoliosis (Fig. 9-7).

■ *Pathophysiology and Etiology*

The three types share some common causes such as osteoporosis or arthritis, but other causes are specific to the disorder. These abnormalities can also develop during adolescence and are covered in Chapter 23.

Lordosis, also referred to as *swayback*, is characterized by the spine curving significantly inward at the lower back. Some of the specific causes of lordosis include:

- Achondroplasia
- Obesity
- Discitis
- Slipping forward of the vertebrae

Kyphosis, also referred to as *hunchback* or *humpback*, is characterized by an abnormally rounded upper back. Some specific causes of kyphosis include:

- Poor posture
- Spina bifida
- Congenital defects
- Spinal tumors or infections
- Scheuermann's disease

Scoliosis is characterized by either an S- or C-shaped sideways curve to the spine. The specific causes of the most common form of this abnormality are generally not known; however, scoliosis tends to run in families, and some more general causes such as disease,

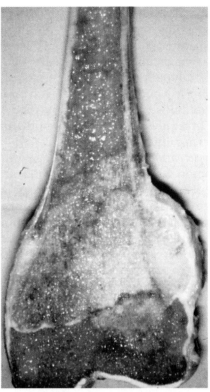

FIGURE 9-8 Osteosarcoma. The tumor *(white area)* has grown through the cortex of the bone and elevated the periosteum. *(From Kumar V, Cotran RS, Robbins SL:* Basic Pathology, *ed 8, Philadelphia, 1997, WB Saunders.)*

trauma, or congenital defects are also believed to be implicated.

Bone Tumors

The majority of primary bone tumors are malignant. Bone is also a common site of secondary tumors, particularly in the spine and pelvis. Metastatic bone tumors usually are secondary to malignant tumors in the breast, lung, or prostate.

Osteosarcoma (osteogenic sarcoma) is a primary malignant neoplasm that usually develops in the metaphysis of the femur, tibia, or fibula in children or young adults, particularly males (Fig. 9-8). *Ewing's* sarcoma is another malignant neoplasm common in adolescents that occurs in the diaphysis of long bones.

Both types of tumor grow quickly and metastasize to the lungs in the early stages of tumor development. Sometimes the tumor is revealed by pathologic fracture. Bone pain is the common symptom, a constant steady pain at rest as well as with activity that gradually increases in severity. An individual often feels the increased pain at night. Treatment involves surgical amputation or excision of the tumor, followed by chemotherapy. Some clinics have used adjuvant chemotherapy before localized surgery without the need for amputation. Adjuvant chemotherapy appears to increase the survival rates in most patients. Survival rates vary greatly depending on the stage of the cancer and the histologic features of the tumor. Tumors localized to the bone at the time of diagnosis have a survival rate of 70%. Many bone tumors have already metastasized at diagnosis, leading to a poorer prognosis, with approximately 30% survival rates. Newer surgical methods have been successful in removing secondary tumors from the lung and preserving lung tissue.

Chondrosarcomas arise from cartilage cells and are more common in adults older than 30 years. These tumors develop more gradually in the pelvic bone or shoulder girdle at the points of muscle attachment and eventually metastasize to the lung. Pain does not develop until late, and the tumors may remain silent until they are well advanced. Surgery is the primary treatment for chondrosarcomas.

THINK ABOUT 9-5

a. Describe four contributing factors to osteoporosis in older women.
b. Explain how osteoporosis leads to loss of height.

Disorders of Muscle, Tendons, and Ligaments

Muscular Dystrophy

Muscular dystrophy (MD) is a group of inherited disorders characterized by degeneration of skeletal muscle. The disorders differ in type of inheritance, area affected, age at onset, and rate of progression. Common types are summarized in Table 9-1.

Duchenne's or pseudohypertrophic muscular dystrophy is the most common type, affecting young boys, with a prevalence of about 3/100,000 males. X-linked inheritance has been demonstrated in most cases of Duchenne's muscular dystrophy. Some cases appear to be spontaneous gene mutations. Serum CK is elevated in many but not all carriers of the abnormal gene and appears before the first signs.

■ *Pathophysiology*

The basic pathophysiology is the same in all types of muscular dystrophy. A metabolic defect, a deficit of dystrophin (a muscle cell membrane protein) leads to degeneration and necrosis of the cell. Skeletal muscle fibers are replaced by fat and fibrous connective tissue (leading to the hypertrophic appearance of the muscle; see Fig. 9-9). Muscle function is gradually lost. Cardiomyopathy is common.

■ *Signs and Symptoms*

With the Duchenne type of muscular dystrophy, early signs appear at around 3 years of age, when motor weakness and regression become apparent in the child. Initial weakness in the pelvic girdle causes a waddling gait and difficulty with climbing stairs or attaining an upright position. The "Gower's maneuver," in which the child pushes to an erect position by using the hands to climb up the legs, is a typical manifestation (see Fig. 9-9). The weakness spreads to other muscle groups and eventually to the shoulder girdle. Tendon reflexes are reduced. Vertebral deformities such as kyphoscoliosis and various contractures develop. Respiratory insufficiency and infections are common. The majority of patients with muscular dystrophy develop cardiac abnormalities and mental retardation.

■ *Diagnostic Tests*

Diagnosis is based on identification of common genetic abnormalities, elevated creatine kinase levels (which are raised before clinical signs appear), electromyography, and muscle biopsy. Female carriers in a family can be identified by the presence of defective dystrophin in the blood. Chorionic villus testing can be performed on the fetus at 12 weeks' gestation.

Because no specific treatment is available, the goal is to maintain motor function as much as possible with moderate exercise and the use of supportive appliances. Occupational therapists play a significant role in support, assessment, and provision of appropriate assistive devices as the client's status and needs change. Death usually results by age 20 from respiratory or cardiac failure. If the patient chooses to use a ventilator

---

TABLE 9-1	Types of Muscular Dystrophy			
Type	Inheritance	Age of Onset	Distribution	Progress
Duchenne's (variant-Becker type)	X-linked recessive (affects males)	2-3 years	Hips, legs, shoulder girdle (ascending)	Rapid
Fascioscapulohumeral (Landouzy)	Autosomal dominant	Before age 20	Shoulder, neck, face	Slow to moderate
Myotonic	Autosomal dominant (chromosome 19)	Birth to 50 years	Face, hands	Slow
Limb girdle	Autosomal recessive	All ages	Shoulders, pelvis	Varies

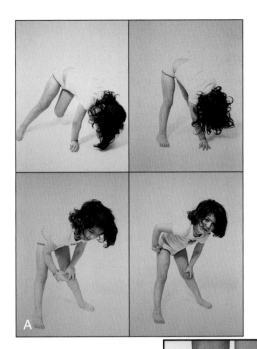

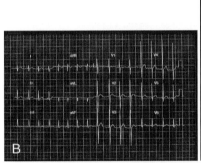

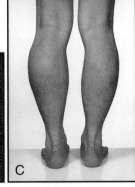

FIGURE 9-9 **A**, Gower's maneuver. **B**, Electrocardiogram in Duchenne's muscular dystrophy. **C**, Calf hypertrophy in Becker's muscular dystrophy. *(From Perkin GD: Mosby's Color Atlas and Text of Neurology, ed 2, London, 2002, Mosby.)*

in the event of respiratory failure, the lifespan can be prolonged substantially. Research on muscular dystrophy in mice has identified genetic therapies that alter the expression of MD genes and prevent dystrophic changes in young mice. This research is promising, but human applications will not be available for at least a decade.

THINK ABOUT 9-6

a. Describe the pathophysiologic changes in muscular dystrophy.
b. Explain how vertebral deformities develop in muscular dystrophy.

Primary Fibromyalgia Syndrome

Primary fibromyalgia syndrome is a group of disorders characterized by pain and stiffness affecting muscles,

tendons, and surrounding soft tissues (not joints). Eighteen specific tender or trigger points, where pain and tenderness may be stimulated, have been identified in tendons and ligaments in the neck and shoulder area, trunk, and limbs, and these trigger points may be used in diagnosis. There are no obvious signs of inflammation or degeneration in the tissues. The cause is not known, but it appears to be related to altered central neurotransmission, resulting in increased soft tissue sensitivity to substance P, a neurotransmitter involved in pain sensation.

The incidence is higher in women 20 to 50 years of age. There is often a history of prior trauma or osteoarthritis. Aggravating factors include sleep deprivation, stress, and fatigue. Generalized aching pain is accompanied by marked fatigue, sleep disturbances, and depression. In some individuals, irritable bowel syndrome or urinary symptoms due to interstitial cystitis may accompany the chronic pain. Men tend to have localized fibromyalgia, including jaw pain or headache. Treatment includes stress reduction, regular early morning exercise, rest as needed, local applications of heat or massage as needed, and low doses of antidepressants, such as the tricyclic antidepressants or selective serotonin-norepinephrine reuptake inhibitors (SSNRIs). A new drug, Lyrica (pregabalin), has been approved for fibromyalgia and mediates the pain pathway. Nonsteroidal anti-inflammatory drugs (NSAIDs) have been helpful to some individuals. Massage therapy is helpful as is occupational therapy to identify strategies to deal with pain and fatigue.

Joint Disorders

Arthritis occurs in many forms that impair joint function, leading to various types of disability in all age groups.

Osteoarthritis

Osteoarthritis (OA) may be called a degenerative, or "wear and tear," joint disease. The incidence of osteoarthritis is increasing. It is estimated that one in three adults in the United States has some degree of osteoarthritis. Men are affected more often than women. It is a major cause of disability and absence from the workplace.

■ *Pathophysiology*
In this condition:
1. The articular cartilage, of weight-bearing joints in particular (e.g., hips, knees), is damaged and lost through structural fissures and erosion resulting from excessive mechanical stress (Fig. 9-10), or breaks down for unknown reasons.
2. The surface of the cartilage becomes rough and worn, interfering with easy joint movement.

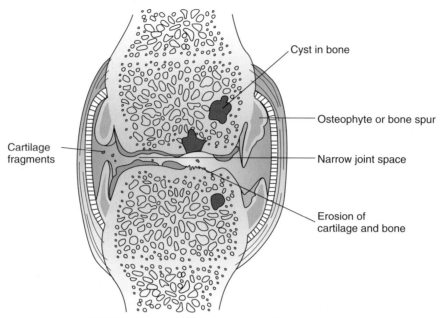

Cyst in bone

Osteophyte or bone spur

Narrow joint space

Erosion of
cartilage and bone

Cartilage
fragments

FIGURE 9-10   Pathologic changes with osteoarthritis.

3. Tissue damage appears to cause release of enzymes from the cells, which accelerates the disintegration of the cartilage.
4. Eventually the subchondral bone may be exposed and damaged, and cysts and *osteophytes* or new bone spurs develop around the margin of the bone.
5. Pieces of the osteophytes and cartilage break off into the synovial cavity, causing further irritation.
6. The joint space becomes narrower (easily seen on x-rays).
7. There may be secondary inflammation of the surrounding tissues in response to altered movement and stress on the joint. No systemic effects are present with osteoarthritis.

■ *Etiology*

The primary form of osteoarthritis is associated with obesity and aging, whereas the secondary type follows injury or abuse. Genetic changes in joint cartilage have been identified in research studies now underway. These genetic changes result in accelerated breakdown of articular cartilage.

Osteoarthritis often develops in specific joints because of injury or excessive wear and tear on a joint. This is a common consequence of participation in sports and certain occupations. Congenital anomalies of the musculoskeletal system may also predispose a patient to osteoarthritis. Once the cartilage is damaged, joint alignment or the frictionless surface of the articular cartilage is lost. A vicious cycle ensues, because uneven mechanical stress is then applied to other parts of the joint and to other joints. The large weight-bearing joints (e.g., the knees and hips) that are subject to injury or occupational stress are frequently affected.

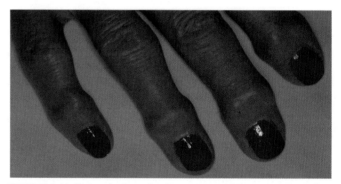

FIGURE 9-11   Heberden's node. (*From Lemmi FO, Lemmi CAE:* Physical Assessment Findings CD-ROM, *Philadelphia, 2000, Saunders*).

■ *Signs and Symptoms*

The pain of osteoarthritis, which is often mild and insidious initially, is an aching that occurs with weight bearing and movement. Pain becomes more severe as the degenerative process advances. It may be unilateral in some cases.

Joint movement is limited. Frequently the joint appears enlarged and hard as osteophytes develop. Walking becomes difficult if the joint is unstable, and the muscles atrophy, causing a predisposition to falls, particularly in older individuals. When the temporomandibular joint (TMJ) is involved, mastication becomes difficult, there is difficulty opening the mouth to speak or yawn, and preauricular pain may be quite severe. In some cases, the hands are involved with bony enlargement of the distal interphalangeal joints (Heberden's nodes; Fig. 9-11). Usually little soft tissue swelling is seen.

Crepitus may be heard as the cartilages become irregular, grating against each other. In some cases, other joints are affected as the individual exerts more stress on normal joints to protect the damaged joints.

Osteoarthritis is not a systemic disorder; therefore there are no systemic signs or changes in serum levels. Diagnosis is based on exclusion of other disorders and radiographic evidence of joint changes consistent with the clinical signs. Radiographic evidence often shows lesser progression of joint changes than the clinical effects of disease.

■ *Treatment*

Any undue stress on the joint should be minimized and adequate rest and additional support provided to facilitate movement. Ambulatory aids such as canes or walkers are helpful. Orthotic inserts in the shoes reduce the risk of deformity and help to maintain function. Physiotherapy and massage therapy help to reduce spasm in adjacent muscles due to pain. This results in maintenance of joint function and muscle strength. Occupational therapy is important in providing assistive devices such as joint splints and teaching alternate practices to reduce pain and deal with stiffness. Individuals with early OA may find pain relief and improved flexibility with the use of glucosamine-chondroitin compounds. Research studies on the use of static magnets to reduce pain have not shown significant results in rigorous double-blinded studies. Intra-articular injection of synthetic synovial fluid may reduce pain and facilitate movement. Glucocorticoids may be helpful. Analgesics or NSAIDs may be required for pain. Surgery is available to repair or replace joints such as the knee or hip with prostheses (Fig. 9-12). Success of such arthroplasty also depends on full participation in a rehabilitation program following surgery.

Rheumatoid Arthritis

Rheumatoid arthritis (RA) is considered an autoimmune disorder causing chronic systemic inflammatory disease. It affects more than 1% of the population, and is a major cause of disability. Rheumatoid arthritis has a higher incidence in women than men and increases in older individuals.

■ *Pathophysiology*

Remissions and exacerbations lead to progressive damage to the joints. The disease often commences rather insidiously with symmetric involvement of the small joints such as the fingers, followed by inflammation and destruction of additional joints (e.g., wrists, elbows, knees). Many individuals also have involvement of the upper cervical vertebrae and TMJ. The severity of the condition varies from mild to severe, reflecting the number of joints affected, the degree of inflammation, and the rapidity of progression.

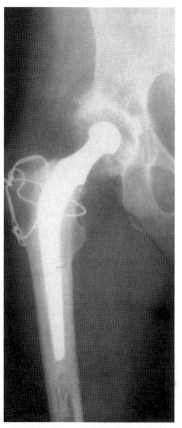

FIGURE 9-12 Hip arthroplasty. Radiograph shows hip after Charnley total hip arthroplasty (replacement of the femoral head and acetabulum with prosthesis cemented into bone). *(From Petty W: Total Joint Replacement, Philadelphia, 1991, Saunders.)*

In the affected joints, the first step in the development of rheumatoid arthritis is an abnormal immune response, causing inflammation of the synovial membrane with vasodilation, increased permeability, and formation of exudate, causing the typical red, swollen, and painful joint. This *synovitis* appears to result from the immune abnormality. *Rheumatoid factor (RF)*, an antibody against immunoglobulin G, as well as other immunologic factors, is present in the blood in the majority of persons with rheumatoid arthritis. Rheumatoid factor is also present in synovial fluid. After the first period of acute inflammation, the joint may appear to recover completely.

During subsequent exacerbations, the process continues:

1. Synovitis—Inflammation recurs, synovial cells proliferate.
2. Pannus formation—Granulation tissue from the synovium spreads over the articular cartilage. This granulation tissue, called *pannus*, releases enzymes and inflammatory mediators, destroying the cartilage (Fig. 9-13).
3. Cartilage erosion—Cartilage is *eroded* by enzymes from the pannus, and in addition, nutrients that are normally supplied by the synovial fluid to the

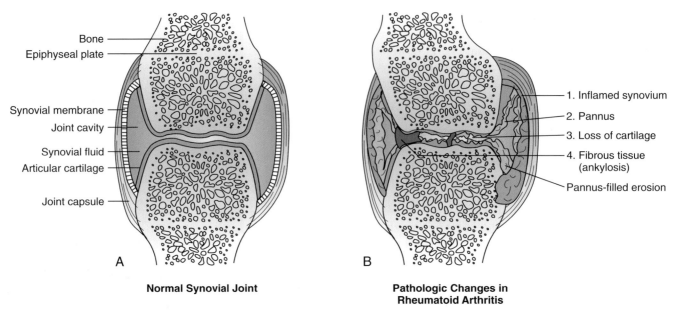

FIGURE 9-13 Pathologic changes with rheumatoid arthritis.

cartilage are cut off by the pannus. Erosion of the cartilage creates an unstable joint.

4. Fibrosis—In time, the pannus between the bone ends becomes fibrotic, limiting movement. This calcifies and the joint space is obliterated.

5. Ankylosis—Joint fixation and deformity develop.

During each exacerbation or acute period, inflammation and further damage occur in joints previously affected, and additional joints become affected by synovitis.

During this process, other changes frequently occur around the joint:

- Atrophy of muscles—The acute inflammation leads to disuse atrophy of the muscles and stretching of the tendons and ligaments, thus decreasing the supportive structures in the unstable joint.
- The alignment of the bones in the joint shifts, depending on how much cartilage has been eroded and the balance achieved between muscles.
- Inflammation and pain may cause muscle spasm, further drawing the bones out of normal alignment.
- Contractures and deformity with subluxation develop. Various contractures and deformities, such as ulnar deviation, swan neck deformity, or boutonniere deformity, may occur in the hands (Fig. 9-14), depending on the degree of flexion and hyperextension in the joints.

Mobility is greatly impaired as the various joints become damaged and deformed. Walking becomes very difficult when the knees or ankles are affected.

The inflammatory process has other effects on the body. Rheumatoid or subcutaneous nodules may form on the extensor surfaces of the ulna. Nodules also may form on the pleura, heart valves, or eyes. These are small granulomas on blood vessels.

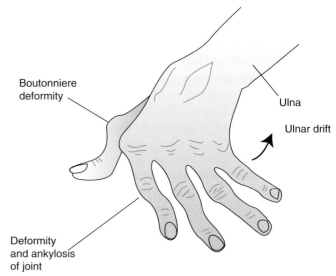

FIGURE 9-14 Typical deformity in a hand with rheumatoid arthritis.

Systemic effects are thought to arise from the circulating immune factors, causing marked fatigue, depression and malaise, anorexia, and low-grade fever. Iron deficiency anemia with low serum iron levels is common; when it results from rheumatoid arthritis, this anemia is resistant to iron therapy.

Etiology

Although rheumatoid arthritis is considered an autoimmune disorder, the exact nature of the abnormality has not been fully determined. A genetic factor is present, with familial predisposition. The abnormality seems to be linked to several viral infections. Rheumatoid factor is not present in all patients with rheumatoid arthritis, yet it may be present in certain other disorders as well. Rheumatoid arthritis is more common in women than men, and the incidence increases with aging.

■ Signs and Symptoms

Rheumatoid arthritis is insidious at onset, often becoming manifest as mild general aching and stiffness.

Inflammation may be apparent first in the fingers or wrists. It affects joints in a symmetric (bilateral) fashion, and usually more than one pair of joints is involved.

The joints appear red and swollen and often are very sensitive to touch as well as painful. Joint stiffness occurs following rest, which then eases with mild activity as circulation through the joint improves.

Joint movement is impaired by the swelling and pain. Frequently, daily activities become difficult, including dressing, food preparation, and oral hygiene. Malocclusion of the teeth may develop from TMJ involvement as the condyle is damaged.

With each exacerbation of disease, the function of the affected joints is further impaired as joint damage progresses. Eventually the joint is no longer inflamed but is fixed and deformed ("burned out").

The College of Rheumatology has established criteria for diagnosis based on four out of seven of the manifestations on their list, for example, swelling of three joints for a minimum of 6 weeks.

Systemic signs are marked during exacerbations and include fatigue, anorexia, mild fever, generalized lymphadenopathy, and generalized aching.

■ Diagnostic Tests

Synovial fluid analysis demonstrates the inflammatory process. Rheumatoid factor may be present in serum but is not specific for diagnosis.

■ Treatment

- A balance between rest and moderate activity is suggested to maintain mobility and muscle strength while preventing additional damage to the joints. Physical therapy and occupational therapy are important parts of any treatment regimen. Both assist in reducing pain and maintaining function. Occupational therapy also teaches adaptive practices to reduce effort and fatigue.
- For pain control, relatively high doses of the anti-inflammatory analgesic aspirin (ASA) or NSAIDs may be required (see Chapter 4). In more severe cases, glucocorticoids may be prescribed, and administered either orally or as intra-articular injections. Patients like the effects of glucocorticoids because the drug does promote a feeling of well-being and improves the appetite. However, there are a number of potential complications with long-term use of these drugs, so they should be used only during acute episodes or taken on alternate days at the lowest effective dose (see Chapter 4). Other drugs, such as gold compounds and immunosuppressants (methotrexate), are used in more resistant cases.

A newer group of NSAIDs, the COX-2 (cyclooxygenase-2) inhibitors, such as celecoxib (Celebrex) act to inhibit prostaglandins during inflammation. They appear to be quite effective in rheumatoid arthritis; at this time they are under further investigation because of the increased incidence of heart attacks and strokes associated with their use.

Disease-modifying antirheumatic drugs (DMARDs), including gold salts, methotrexate, and hydroxychloroquine have proved useful in some cases.

Newer biologic response modifying agents (such as infliximab [Remicade]) block tumor necrosis factor an inflammatory cytokine present in RA. Beta cell–depleting agents (rituximab [Rituxan]) and Interleukin-1 antagonists (anakinra [Kineret]) seem to be effective in cases of severe pain and improving joint function.

- The use of heat and cold modalities can be very effective when they are used correctly.
- During acute episodes, joints may require splinting to prevent excessive movement and maintain alignment. Appropriate body positioning and body mechanics when walking or moving also help to maintain function.
- Assistive devices such as wrist supports or padded handles with straps are available to help the patient cope with daily activities and reduce contractures.
- Surgical intervention to remove pannus, replace damaged tendons, reduce contractures, or replace joints may be necessary to improve function. This is particularly important in the treatment of RA in the hands.

Most individuals are subject to periodic exacerbations. If the number and severity of recurrences can be minimized, mobility can be maintained. About 10% of individuals incur severe disability.

Juvenile Rheumatoid Arthritis

Juvenile rheumatoid arthritis (JRA) occurs in several different types. In some respects, JRA differs from the adult form of rheumatoid arthritis (see Chapter 23). For example, the onset is usually more acute than the adult form. Systemic effects are more marked, but rheumatoid nodules are absent. The large joints are frequently affected. Rheumatoid factor is not usually present, but other abnormal antibodies such as antinuclear antibodies (ANAs) may be present. The systemic form, sometimes referred to as Still's disease, develops with fever, rash, lymphadenopathy, and hepatomegaly as well as joint involvement. A second form of JRA causes polyarticular inflammation similar to that seen in the adult form. A third form of JRA involves four or fewer joints but causes uveitis, inflammation of the iris, ciliary body, and choroid (uveal tract) in the eye.

Infectious (Septic) Arthritis

Infectious or septic arthritis usually develops in a *single* joint. The joint is red, swollen, and painful, with decreased range of movement. The synovium is swollen, and a purulent exudate forms. Aspiration of synovial fluid followed by culture and sensitivity tests confirms the diagnosis. Blood-borne bacteria such as gonococcus or staphylococcus are the source of infection in many cases, although anaerobic bacteria are becoming increasingly common. In some cases there is a history of trauma, surgery, or spread from a nearby infection such as osteomyelitis (see Chapter 23).

Lyme disease, caused by a spirochete and transmitted by ticks, is characterized by a migratory arthritis and rash developing several weeks to months after the tick bite. The knee and other large joints are most often involved. A vaccine for Lyme disease is now available.

In cases of infectious arthritis, immediate, aggressive antimicrobial treatment is necessary to prevent excessive cartilage destruction and fibrosis of the joint.

Gout (Gouty Arthritis)

This form of joint disease is common in men older than 40 years. Gout results from deposits of uric acid and urate crystals in the joint that then cause an acute inflammatory response (Fig. 9-15). Uric acid is a waste product of purine metabolism, normally excreted through the kidneys. Hyperuricemia may develop if renal excretion is not adequate or a metabolic abnormality, often a genetic factor such as a deficit of the enzyme uricase, leading to elevated levels of uric acid (primary gout) is present.

A sudden increase in serum uric acid levels usually precipitates an attack of gout. Gout often affects a single joint, such as in the big toe. When acute inflammation develops from uric acid deposits, the articular cartilage is damaged. The inflammation causes redness and swelling of the joint and severe pain. Attacks occur

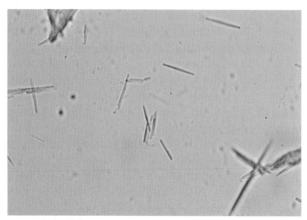

FIGURE 9-15 Gout. Urate crystals in synovial fluid cause inflammation in the joint. *(From Stevens ML: Fundamentals of Clinical Hematology, Philadelphia, 1997, Saunders.)*

intermittently. Diagnosis is confirmed by examination of synovial fluid and blood tests.

A *tophus* is a large, hard nodule consisting of urate crystals that have been precipitated in soft tissue or bone, causing a local inflammatory reaction. Tophi usually occur a few years after the first attack of gout and may develop at joint bursae, on the extensor surfaces of the forearm, or on the pinnae of the ear.

Treatment consists of reducing serum uric acid levels by drugs and dietary changes, depending on the underlying cause. Increasing fluid intake and increasing the pH of the urine promotes excretion of excess uric acid. Colchicine may be used during an acute episode, and allopurinol is used as a preventive maintenance treatment. Normalization of serum uric acid levels is important because uric acid kidney stones are a threat in anyone with chronic hyperuricemia. Also, relief of the inflammation and pain associated with acute attacks by NSAIDs should be achieved as soon as possible.

Ankylosing Spondylitis

Ankylosing spondylitis is a chronic progressive inflammatory condition that affects the sacroiliac joints, intervertebral spaces, and costovertebral joints of the axial skeleton. Women tend to have peripheral joint involvement to a greater extent than men, although the disorder is more common in men. It usually develops in persons 20 to 30 years of age and varies in severity. Remissions and exacerbations mark the course.

The cause has not been fully determined, but it is deemed an autoimmune disorder with a genetic basis, given the presence of HLA-B27 antigen in the serum of most patients.

◼ *Pathophysiology*

In patients with ankylosing spondylitis:
1. The vertebral joints first become inflamed.
2. Fibrosis and calcification or fusion of the joints follows. The result is ankylosis or fixation of the joints and loss of mobility (Fig. 9-16).
3. Inflammation begins in the lower back at the sacroiliac joints and progresses up the spine, eventually causing a typical "poker back."
4. Kyphosis develops as a result of postural changes necessitated by the rigidity and loss of the normal spinal curvature.
5. Osteoporosis is common and may contribute to kyphosis because of pathologic compression fractures of the vertebrae.
6. Lung expansion may be limited at this stage, as calcification of the costovertebral joints reduces rib movement.

◼ *Signs and Symptoms*

Initially low back pain and morning stiffness are evident. Pain is often more marked when lying down, and may

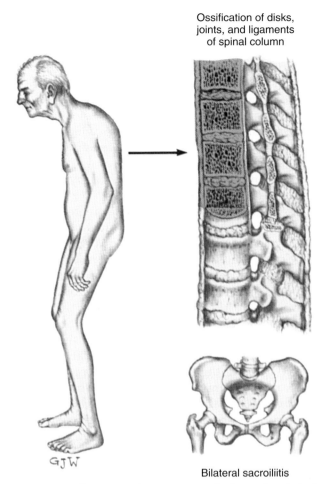

Ossification of disks, joints, and ligaments of spinal column

Bilateral sacroiliitis

FIGURE 9-16 Characteristic posture and sites of ankylosing spondylitis. *(From Mourad L:* Orthopedic Disorders, *St. Louis, 1991, Mosby).*

radiate to the legs similar to sciatic pain. The discomfort is relieved by walking or mild exercise.

As calcification develops, the spine becomes more rigid, and flexion, extension, and rotation of the spine are impaired.

Some individuals (about one third of patients) develop systemic signs such as fatigue, fever, and weight loss. Uveitis, particularly iritis (inflammation in the eye), is a common additional problem.

Treatment is directed at relief of pain and maintenance of mobility. Sleeping in a supine position reduces the tendency to flexion, and an appropriate daily exercise program promotes muscle support and proper posture. Anti-inflammatory drugs, as described, are useful during exacerbations of disease.

Other Inflammatory Joint Disorders

Bursitis is an inflammation of the bursae associated with bones, muscles, tendons, and ligaments of various joints. The bursae are small fluid-filled sacs that act as cushions at or near the structures of the joint. The most common causes of this inflammation are repetitive motions or positions that physically irritate the bursae at a specific joint. These include actions such as throwing a baseball repeatedly or washing floors frequently on hands and knees. Bursitis is primarily diagnosed by physical examination in which the joint appears swollen, red, achy, or stiff and pain with joint motion. Other methods for diagnosis may include imaging such as ultrasound or MRI and analysis of the fluid in the bursae to detect underlying problems such as an infection. The first step in treatment involves rest, application of cold compresses, and pain relievers. If the condition persists or worsens treatments include anti-inflammatory drugs, physical therapy, antibiotics in cases in which an infection is a cause, and in severe cases the bursae can be surgically drained.

Synovitis is an inflammation of the synovial membrane lining the joint. Movement of the joint is restricted and painful due to swelling as the synovial sac fills with fluid. The joint becomes swollen, red, and warm and can also be diagnosed by analyzing the synovial fluid for signs of infection or crystals indicating gout. Treatment includes use of anti-inflammatory drugs and treatment for underlying causes such as in cases of infection.

Tendinitis is the irritation or inflammation of the tendon. It is usually characterized by a dull ache at the site of tendon attachment, tenderness, and mild swelling. Although tendinitis can be caused by a single, sudden trauma, it is more likely the result of repetitive motions/actions. Diagnosis is done by physical examination. The first line of treatment involves rest, application of ice, and pain relievers. If the condition persists or worsens, treatments include anti-inflammatory drugs and physical therapy. In cases in which there has been significant injury to the tendon, surgery may be required.

THINK ABOUT 9-7

a. Compare osteoarthritis and rheumatoid arthritis with respect to pathophysiology, common joints affected, and characteristics of pain.

b. Describe two unique characteristics of septic arthritis.

c. Explain how the pathophysiologic changes in ankylosing spondylitis differ from those of rheumatoid arthritis.

CASE STUDY A

Fracture

J.R., age 17, has a compound fracture of the femur and is undergoing surgical repair.

1. Describe a compound fracture.
2. Give several reasons why it is important in this case to have immobilized the femur well before transporting J.R. to the hospital.
3. Explain why there is an increased risk of osteomyelitis in this case.
4. Explain why there is severe pain with this type of fracture.

The day after surgery J.R.'s toes are numb and cold.
5. Explain the possible causes of the cold, numb toes.
6. Explain why appropriate exercise is important during healing of the fracture.
7. List four factors that would promote healing of this fracture.
8. Explain why the leg should be elevated during recovery.
9. Explain why, following the removal of the cast, J.R. can expect to feel some weakness and stiffness in the leg.

CASE STUDY B

Rheumatoid Arthritis

Ms. W.P. is 42 years old and has had rheumatoid arthritis for 6 years. Her fingers are stiff and show slight ulnar deviation. She is now experiencing an exacerbation, and her wrists are red and swollen. She finds clothing or a touch on the skin over her wrists very painful. Her elbows and knees are also stiff and painful, especially after she has been resting. She is feeling extremely tired and depressed and has not been eating well.
1. Explain the reasons for the appearance and the pain occurring at her wrists.
2. Describe the factors contributing to the stiff, deformed fingers.
3. Explain why some activity relieves the pain and stiffness of rheumatoid arthritis.
4. Describe several factors contributing to the systemic symptoms noted in Ms. W.P.
5. Explain how each of the following drugs acts in the treatment of rheumatoid arthritis (see Chapter 5): (1) NSAIDs; (2) glucocorticoids; (3) disease-modifying agents; and (4) biologic agents.
6. Predict the possible course of this disease in Ms. W.P.

CHAPTER SUMMARY

Muscles, bones, and joints form the framework of the body, providing support and protection as well as a mechanism for movement. Any damage to the parts of this system is likely to impair mobility.

- The type of *fracture*, such as open, closed, or comminuted, is defined by the characteristics of the bone fragments.
- Fractures heal in four stages, the hematoma, fibrocartilaginous callus, bony callus, and remodeling.
- Dislocations, sprains, and strains cause soft tissue damage at joints.
- *Osteoporosis* is a common disorder, in which decreased bone mass and density predispose patients to fractures.
- *Rickets* and *osteomalacia* are caused by deficits of vitamin D and phosphate.
- *Osteosarcoma* and *Ewing's* sarcoma are malignant tumors, commonly occurring in the long bones of young adults. Constant bone pain is typical.
- *Duchenne's* muscular dystrophy is one of a group of progressive degenerative muscle disorders, often inherited as an X-linked recessive trait, affecting boys.
- *Primary fibromyalgia syndrome* causes generalized aching pain, severe fatigue, and depression.
- *Osteoarthritis* is a progressive degenerative disorder often affecting the large weight-bearing joints. Pain increases with movement and weight bearing.
- *Rheumatoid arthritis* is a progressive systemic inflammatory disease that usually affects the small joints initially and progresses symmetrically. The pathologic process in an affected joint includes synovitis, pannus formation, cartilage erosion, fibrosis, and ankylosis, leading to contractures and loss of function.
- *Infectious* or *septic arthritis* usually involves a single joint. Early treatment is required to prevent permanent damage.
- *Gout* is a form of inflammatory arthritis caused by deposits of uric acid and urates in a joint.
- *Ankylosing spondylitis* is a progressive inflammatory disorder of the vertebral joints that leads to a rigid spine.

STUDY QUESTIONS

1. Describe each of the following structures in a bone:
   a. endosteum
   b. medullary cavity
   c. diaphysis of a long bone
2. Define an irregular bone and give an example.
3. Where is red bone marrow found in adults? What is the purpose of red marrow?
4. a. Describe the sources of energy for skeletal muscle contraction.
   b. Explain the effect of a cholinergic blocking agent on skeletal muscle contraction (see Chapter 14).

   c. Explain how anabolic steroid drugs affect skeletal muscle.
   d. Describe the purpose and structure of a tendon.
   e. Describe the outcome after part of a muscle has died.
5. a. Describe the structures that stabilize and support a joint.
   b. What type of joint is needed for the articulation between the ribs and sternum? What kind of mobility does it have?
   c. Explain the meaning of the term *origin* as related to muscles at a joint.

6. a. Describe each type of fracture: (1) compression fracture, (2) pathologic fracture, and (3) spiral fracture.
   b. Differentiate the procallus from the bony callus in the healing of a fracture.
7. Compare the changes and effects of a strain and a subluxation.
8. Compare the pathophysiology of osteoporosis, osteomalacia, and Paget's disease.
9. a. Explain why the muscles of the legs of a child with Duchenne's muscular dystrophy appear large.
   b. Explain why only boys are affected by Duchenne's muscular dystrophy.
   c. Explain why a child with muscular dystrophy pulls himself up a flight of stairs.
10. Describe the characteristics of synovial fluid in:
    a. rheumatoid arthritis
    b. gout
    c. septic arthritis
    d. osteoarthritis
11. Explain why eating and coughing may be difficult in a person with severe ankylosing spondylitis.

ADDITIONAL RESOURCES

Applegate EJ: *The Anatomy and Physiology Learning System Textbook*, ed 3, Philadelphia, 2006, Saunders.
Beers MH, Berkow R, editors: *The Merck Manual of Diagnosis and Therapy*, ed 18, Rahway, NJ, 2006, Merck Research Laboratories.
Kumar V, Abbas AK, Fausto M: *Robbins and Cotran Pathologic Basis of Disease*, ed 8, Philadelphia, 2007, Saunders.

Web Sites

http://www.arthritis.org *Arthritis Foundation*
http://www.niams.nih.gov *National Institute of Arthritis and Musculoskeletal and Skin Diseases*

http://www.ninds.nih.gov/disorders/md/md.htm *National Institute of Neurological Disorders and Stroke*
http://www.nof.org *National Osteoporosis Foundation*
http://www.osteo.org *The NIH Osteoporosis and Related Bone Diseases—National Resource Center*
http://www.rheumatology.org *American College of Rheumatology*

CHAPTER 10

Blood and Circulatory System Disorders

CHAPTER OUTLINE

LEARNING OBJECTIVES

After studying this chapter, the student is expected to:

1. Define the terms describing abnormalities in the blood.
2. Describe and compare the pathophysiology, etiology, manifestations, diagnostic tests, and treatment for each of the selected anemias: iron-deficiency, pernicious, aplastic, sickle cell, and thalassemia.
3. Differentiate between primary and secondary polycythemia, and describe the effects on the blood and circulation.
4. Describe hemophilia A: its pathophysiology, signs, and treatment.

5. Discuss the disorder disseminated intravascular coagulation: its pathophysiology, etiology, manifestations, and treatment.
6. Discuss the myelodysplastic syndrome and its relationship to other blood disorders.
7. Compare acute and chronic leukemia: the incidence, onset and course, pathophysiology, signs, diagnostic tests, and treatment.

KEY TERMS

achlorhydria	ferritin	leukocytosis	pallor
agglutination	gastrectomy	leukopenia	pancytopenia
autoregulation	glossitis	leukopoiesis	petechiae
bilirubin	hemarthrosis	macrocytes	phlebotomy
cyanotic	hematocrit	macrophages	plasma
demyelination	hematopoiesis	malabsorption	plethoric
deoxyhemoglobin	hemolysis	megaloblasts	reticulocyte
diapedesis	hemoptysis	microcytic	serum
dyscrasia	hemosiderin	morphology	splenomegaly
dyspnea	hemostasis	myelotoxins	stomatitis
ecchymoses	hepatomegaly	myelodysplastic	syncope
erythrocytosis	hypochromic	neutropenia	tachycardia
erythropoietin	interleukin	oxyhemoglobin	thrombocytopenia

Review of the Circulatory System and Blood

Anatomy, Structures, and Components

As any student of anatomy and physiology quickly discovers, although distinct in their specific structures and functions, all the systems of the human body are intricately interrelated and must interact constantly in order to maintain the proper functioning of the body. One component upon which all systems depend is blood that: transports essential oxygen to all tissues along with nutrients required for cellular metabolism, provides for the necessary removal of many cell wastes, plays a critical role in the body's defenses/immune system and serves in maintaining body homeostasis. Blood and lymph, another essential body fluid, are transported throughout the body via a complex system of vessels and the pumping action of the heart. Due to the complexity and distinct features involved in the production and circulation of blood and lymph, this chapter examines blood itself along with a basic review of the vessels involved in the distribution of blood throughout the body and the associated blood disorders. Chapter 11 presents an examination of the lymphatic system and associated disorders. Chapter 12 presents a detailed examination of the cardiovascular system with specific emphasis on the heart and associated disorders along with disorders of the blood vessels themselves.

Blood Vessels

The arteries, capillaries, and veins constitute a closed system for the distribution of blood throughout the body. Major blood vessels, most of which are paired left and right, are shown in Figures 10-1 and 10-2.

To review the components of the circulatory system:

- There are two separate circulations—the pulmonary circulation allows the exchange of oxygen and carbon dioxide in the lungs, and the systemic circulation provides for the exchange of nutrients and wastes between the blood and the cells throughout the body.
- Arteries transport blood away from the heart into the lungs or to body tissues.
- Arterioles are the smaller branches of arteries that control the amount of blood flowing into the capillaries in specific areas through the degree of contraction of smooth muscle in the vessel walls (vasoconstriction or dilation).
- Capillaries are very small vessels organized in numerous networks that form the microcirculation. Blood flows very slowly through capillaries, and precapillary sphincters determine the amount of blood flowing from the arterioles into the individual capillaries, depending on the metabolic needs of the tissues.
- Small venules conduct blood from the capillary beds toward the heart.
- Larger veins collect blood draining from the venules. Normally a high percentage of the blood (approximately 70%) is located in the veins at any one time; hence, the veins are called capacitance vessels. Blood flow in the veins depends on skeletal muscle action, respiratory movements, and gravity. *Valves* in the larger veins in the arms and legs have an important role in keeping the blood flowing toward the heart. Respiratory movements assist the movement of blood through the trunk.

The walls of arteries and veins are made up of three layers.

1. The tunica intima, an endothelial layer, is the inner layer.
2. The tunica media, a layer of *smooth muscle* that controls the diameter and lumen size (diameter) of the blood vessel, is the middle layer.
3. The tunica adventitia, or externa, is the outer connective tissue layer and contains *elastic* and collagen fibers.

The vasa vasorum consists of tiny blood vessels that supply blood to the tissues of the wall itself. Normally the large arteries are highly elastic in order to adjust to the changes in blood volume that occur during the cardiac cycle. For example, the aorta must expand during systole to prevent systolic pressure from rising too high, and during diastole the walls must recoil to maintain adequate diastolic pressure. Veins have thinner walls than arteries and less smooth muscle (Fig. 10-3).

Localized vasodilation or vasoconstriction in arterioles is controlled by autoregulation, a reflex adjustment in a small area of a tissue or an organ, which varies depending on the needs of the cells in the area. For example, a decrease in pH, an increase in carbon dioxide, or a decrease in oxygen leads to local vasodilation. Release of chemical mediators such as histamine or an increase in temperature at a specific area can also cause vasodilation. These local changes do not affect the systemic blood pressure.

Norepinephrine and epinephrine increase systemic vasoconstriction by stimulating alpha$_1$-adrenergic receptors in the arteriolar walls. Angiotensin is another powerful systemic vasoconstrictor. At all times, even at rest, vascular or vasomotor tone is maintained by constant input from the SNS that results in partial vasoconstriction throughout the body to ensure continued circulation of blood.

Capillary walls consist of a single endothelial layer to facilitate the exchange of fluid, oxygen, carbon dioxide, electrolytes, glucose and other nutrients, and wastes between the blood and the interstitial fluid. Capillary exchange and abnormal electrolyte shifts are discussed in Chapter 2.

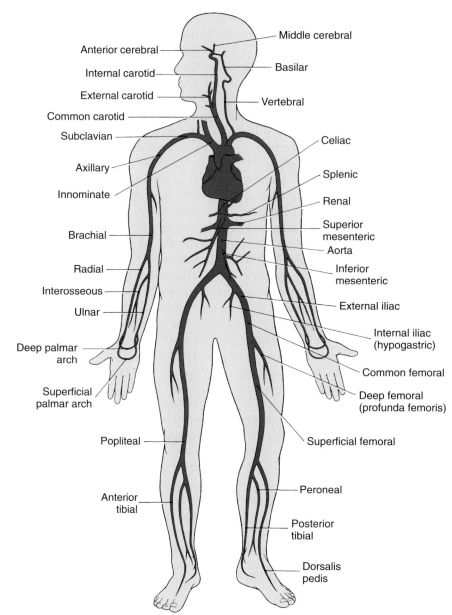

FIGURE 10-1 Anatomy of major arteries. *(From Fahey VA: Vascular Nursing, ed 4, Philadelphia, 2004, Saunders.)*

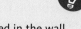

THINK ABOUT   10-1

a. Explain why a high elastic content is required in the wall of the aorta.
b. Explain the function of smooth muscle in the arterioles.
c. Predict those organs that would be expected to have a large capillary network. What criteria did you use in making this prediction?
d. Explain how venous return increases with exercise and the purpose of such action.

Blood

Blood provides the major transport system of the body for essentials such as oxygen, glucose and other nutrients, hormones, electrolytes, and cell wastes. It serves as a critical part of the body's defenses, carrying antibodies and white blood cells for the rapid removal of any foreign material. As a vehicle promoting homeostasis, blood provides a mechanism for controlling body temperature by distributing core heat throughout the peripheral tissues. Blood is the medium through which body fluid levels and blood pressure are measured and adjusted by various controls, such as hormones. Clotting factors in the circulating blood are readily available for hemostasis. Buffer systems in the blood maintain a stable pH of 7.35 to 7.45 (see discussion of acid-base balance in Chapter 2).

Composition of Blood

The adult body contains approximately 5 liters of blood. Blood consists of water and its dissolved solutes, which

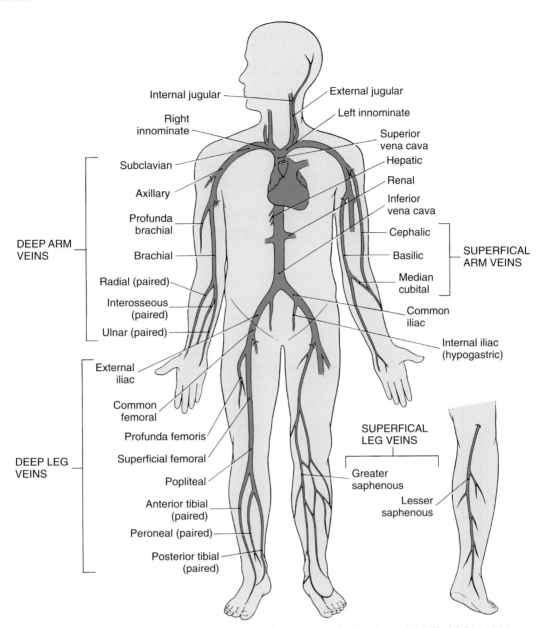

FIGURE 10-2 Anatomy of major veins. *(From Fahey VA:* Vascular Nursing, *ed 4, Philadelphia, 2004, Saunders.)*

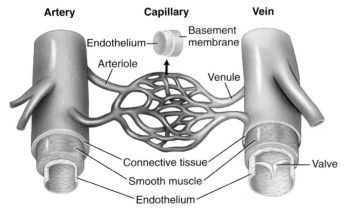

FIGURE 10-3 Cardiovascular system overview. The cardiovascular system consists of the heart and the blood and blood vessels. *(From VanMeter K, Hubert R:* Microbiology for the Healthcare Professional, *St. Louis, 2010, Elsevier.)*

make up about 55% of the whole blood volume; the remaining 45% is composed of the cells or formed elements, the erythrocytes, along with leukocytes, and thrombocytes or platelets. Hematocrit refers to the proportion of cells (essentially the erythrocytes) in blood and indicates the viscosity of the blood. Males have a higher hematocrit, average 42% to 52%, than females, 37% to 47%. An elevated hematocrit could indicate dehydration (loss of fluid) or excess red blood cells. A low hematocrit might result from blood loss or anemia. Plasma is the clear yellowish fluid remaining after the cells have been removed, and serum refers to the fluid and solutes remaining after the cells and fibrinogen have been removed. The plasma proteins include albumin, which maintains osmotic pressure in the blood;

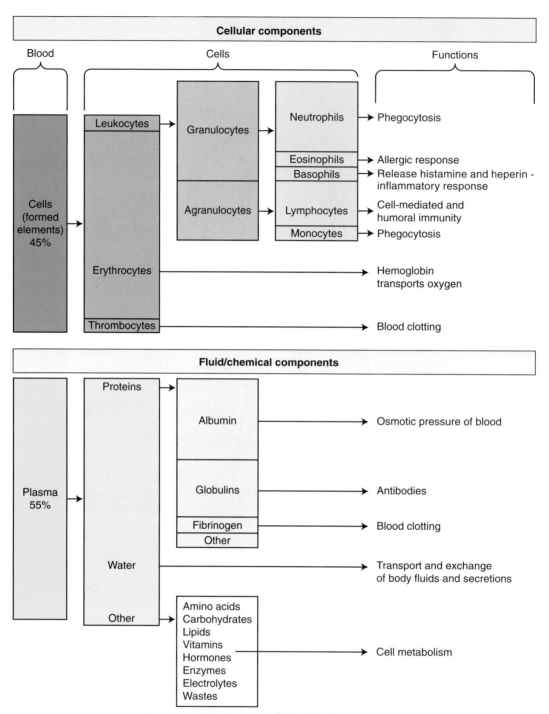

FIGURE 10-4 Components of blood and their functions.

globulins or antibodies; and fibrinogen, which is essential for the formation of blood clots.

The components of blood and their functions are summarized in Figure 10-4. Normal values for blood components are found inside the front cover of this book.

Blood Cells and Hematopoiesis

All blood cells originate from the red bone marrow. In the adult, red bone marrow is found in the flat and irregular bones, ribs, vertebrae, sternum, and pelvis. The iliac crest in the pelvic bone is a common site for a bone marrow aspiration for biopsy. The various blood cells develop from a single stem cell (pluripotential hematopoietic stem cell) during the process of hemopoiesis or hematopoiesis (Fig. 10-5). From this basic cell, the differentiation process forms committed stem cells for each type of blood cell. These cells then proliferate and mature, providing the specialized functional cells needed by the body. A pathological condition of the

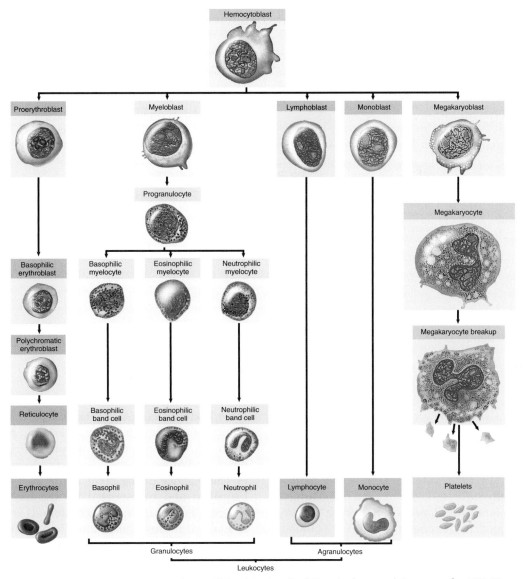

FIGURE 10-5 Hematopoiesis. *(From Shiland BJ:* Medical Terminology and Anatomy for ICD-10 Coding. *St. Louis, 2012, Mosby.)*

blood that usually refers to disorders involving the cellular components of blood is called dyscrasia. A number of specific blood dyscrasias are addressed later in the chapter.

Erythrocytes or *red blood cells* (RBCs) are biconcave, flexible discs (like doughnuts but with thin centers rather than holes) that are *non-nucleated* when mature and contain hemoglobin (Fig. 10-6). The size and structure are essential for easy passage through small capillaries. The hormone erythropoietin, originating from the kidney, stimulates erythrocyte production in the red bone marrow in response to tissue *hypoxia*, or insufficient oxygen available to cells. Normally RBCs (4.2 to 6.2 million/mm^3) constitute most of the cell volume in blood. Adequate RBC production and maturation depend on the availability of many raw materials, including amino acids, iron, vitamin B$_{12}$, vitamin B$_6$, and folic acid.

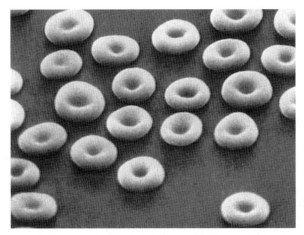

FIGURE 10-6 Normal biconcave non-nucleated red blood cells. *(From Rodak BR:* Hematology: Clinical Principles and Applications, *ed 2, Philadelphia, 2002, Saunders.)*

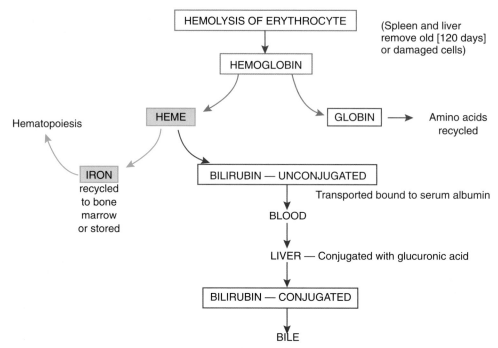

FIGURE 10-7 Breakdown of hemoglobin.

Hemoglobin consists of the globin portion, two pairs of amino acid chains, and four heme groups, each containing a ferrous iron atom, to which the oxygen molecule (O_2) can attach (see Fig. 10-16A). Heme provides the red color associated with hemoglobin. Normally hemoglobin becomes fully saturated with oxygen in the lungs. Oxyhemoglobin is a bright red color, which distinguishes arterial blood from venous blood. As the blood circulates through the body, oxygen dissociates from hemoglobin, depending on local metabolism (see Fig. 13-6). Deoxygenated hemoglobin (deoxyhemoglobin or reduced hemoglobin) is dark or bluish-red in color and is found in venous blood.

Only a small proportion of the carbon dioxide (CO_2) in blood is carried by hemoglobin (carbaminohemoglobin) attached to nitrogen in an amino acid group at a *different* site from that for oxygen. Most carbon dioxide is transported in blood as *bicarbonate ion* (in the buffer pair). Oxygen can easily be displaced from hemoglobin by carbon monoxide, which binds tightly to the iron, thus causing a fatal hypoxia (deficit of oxygen). Carbon monoxide poisoning can be recognized by the bright cherry-red color in the lips and face.

The lifespan of a normal RBC is approximately 120 days. As it ages, the cell becomes rigid and fragile and finally succumbs to phagocytosis in the spleen or liver and is broken down into globin and heme (Fig. 10-7). Globin is broken down into amino acids, which can be recycled in the amino acid pool, and the iron can be returned to the bone marrow and liver to be reused in the synthesis of more hemoglobin. Excess iron can be stored as ferritin or hemosiderin in the liver, blood, and other body tissues. A genetic disorder, *hemochromatosis*, otherwise known as iron overload, results in large amounts of hemosiderin accumulating in the liver, heart, and other organs, causing serious organ damage.

The balance of the heme component is converted to bilirubin and transported by the blood to the liver, where it is conjugated (or combined) with glucuronide to make it more soluble, and then excreted in the bile. Excessive hemolysis or destruction of RBCs may cause elevated serum bilirubin levels, which result in *jaundice*, the yellow color in the sclera of the eye and of the skin.

Hematopoiesis

Leukocytes, which number 5 to 10,000/mm^3, make up only about 1% of blood volume. They are subdivided into three types of granulocytes and two types of agranulocytes. All types develop and differentiate from the original stem cell in bone marrow (see Fig. 10-5). Leukopoiesis, or production of white blood cells (WBCs), is stimulated by colony-stimulating factors (CSFs) produced by cells such as macrophages and T lymphocytes. For example, granulocyte CSF or multi-CSF (interleukin-3 [IL-3]) may be produced to increase certain types of WBCs during an inflammatory response (see Chapter 5). White blood cells may leave the capillaries and enter the tissues by diapedesis or *ameboid* action (movement through an intact capillary wall) when they are needed for defensive purposes.

The five types of *leukocytes* vary in physical characteristics and functions (see Fig. 10-4). Some examples of WBCs are visible as large, nucleated cells (purple stain) in the blood smear in Figure 10-8.

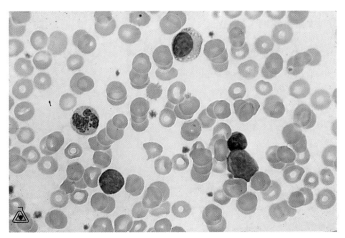

FIGURE 10-8 Normal blood cells. Note the many erythrocytes, discs with concave (faded) centers; the leukocytes, larger size with nuclei; stained purple, various types; thrombocytes, the small dark pieces. *(From Stepp C, Woods M:* Laboratory Procedures for Medical Office Personnel, *Philadelphia, 1998, Saunders.)*

- Lymphocytes make up 30% to 40% of the WBCs. The roles of B and T lymphocytes in the immune response are reviewed in Chapter 7. Some T cells are designated natural killer cells and are significant in immunity.
- Neutrophils (also called polys, segs, or PMNs) are the most common leukocyte, comprising 50% to 60% of WBCs, but they survive only 4 days. They are the first to respond to any tissue damage and commence phagocytosis. An immature neutrophil is called a band or stab, and these are increased in numbers by bacterial infection. The laboratory reports note this as a "shift to the left" in the pattern of leucocytes seen.
- Basophils appear to migrate from the blood and enter tissue to become mast cells that can release histamine and heparin. They may be fixed in tissues or wandering.
- Eosinophils tend to combat the effects of histamine. They are increased by allergic reactions and parasitic infections.
- Monocytes can enter the tissue to become *macrophages*, which act as phagocytes when tissue damage occurs.

A *differential count* indicates the proportions of specific types of WBCs in the blood and frequently assists in making a diagnosis. For example, a bacterial infection or inflammatory condition stimulates an increase in neutrophils, whereas allergic reactions or parasitic infections increase the eosinophil count.

Thrombocytes, also called platelets, are an essential part of the blood-clotting process or hemostasis (Fig. 10-9). Thrombocytes are not cells; rather, they are very small, irregularly shaped, non-nucleated fragments from large megakaryocytes (see Fig. 10-8). Platelets stick to damaged tissue as well as to each other to form a

platelet plug that seals small breaks in blood vessels, or they can adhere to rough surfaces and foreign material. The common drug ASA (aspirin) reduces this adhesion and can lead to an increased bleeding tendency. Thrombocytes can also initiate the coagulation process.

APPLY YOUR KNOWLEDGE 10-1

Predict three possible problems that could arise in the production of blood and blood cells and explain the cause of each.

Blood Clotting

Hemostasis consists of three steps.

- First, the immediate response of a blood vessel to injury is vasoconstriction or vascular spasm. In small blood vessels, this decreases blood flow and may allow a platelet plug to form.
- Second, thrombocytes tend to adhere to the underlying tissue at the site of injury and, if the blood vessel is *small*, can form a platelet plug in the vessel.
- The blood-clotting or coagulation mechanism is required in *larger* vessels, by which the clotting factors that are present in inactive forms in the circulating blood are activated through a sequence of reactions (see Fig. 10-9). Recent evidence indicates additional overlap in factor activity between the intrinsic and extrinsic pathways, but the cascade of reactions is the basis for coagulation.

Clot formation (coagulation) requires a sequence or cascade of events as summarized:

1. Damaged tissue and platelets release factors that stimulate a series of reactions involving numerous clotting factors, finally producing *prothrombin activator (PTA)*.
2. *Prothrombin* or factor II (inactive in the plasma) is converted into *thrombin*.
3. *Fibrinogen* (factor I) is converted into *fibrin* threads.
4. A *fibrin mesh* forms to trap *cells*, making up a solid clot, or *thrombus*, and stopping the flow of blood (Fig. 10-10).
5. The clot gradually shrinks or *retracts*, pulling the edges of damaged tissue closer together and sealing the site.

The circulating clotting factors are produced primarily in the liver. Their numbers relate to the order of their discovery, not to the step in the clotting process. *Vitamin K*, a fat-soluble vitamin, is required for the synthesis of most clotting factors. *Calcium* ions are essential for many steps in the clotting process.

Other measures can be used by a person to facilitate this clotting process. For example, applying pressure and cold (a vasoconstrictor) to the site reduces blood flow in the area, or thrombin solution can be applied directly to speed up clotting.

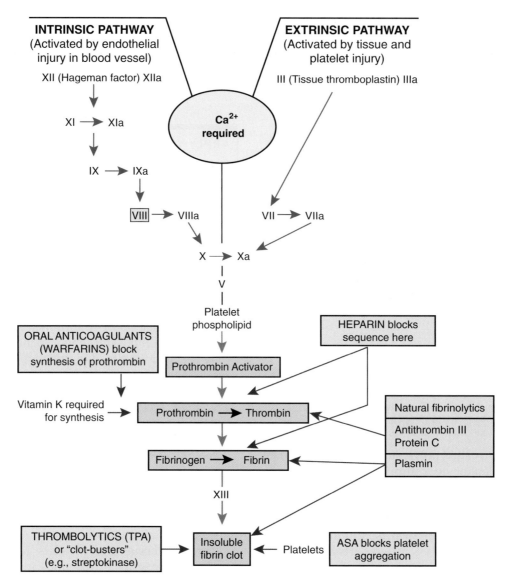

FIGURE 10-9 Hemostasis and anticoagulant drugs.

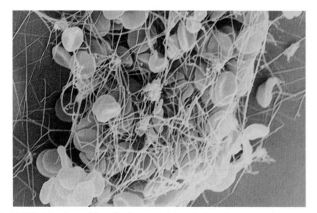

FIGURE 10-10 A blood clot or thrombus, showing blood cells trapped by fibrin strands (scanning electron microscope photograph). *(From Stevens ML: Fundamentals of Clinical Hematology, Philadelphia, 1997, Saunders.)*

Fibrinolysis

A delicate balance is always necessary between the tendency to clot to prevent blood loss and the tendency to form clots unnecessarily and cause infarctions. Some individuals tend to form clots very readily; others are predisposed to excessive bleeding. To prevent inappropriate thrombus formation, coagulation inhibitors such as antithrombin III circulate in the blood. Through thrombin, a prostaglandin is released to prevent platelets sticking to nearby undamaged tissue. Heparin, an anticoagulant, is released from basophils or mast cells in the tissues and exerts its major action by blocking thrombin. Heparin, as a drug, may be administered intravenously to patients at risk for thrombus formation. It does not dissolve clots, but will prevent further growth of the thrombus.

Also, there is a natural fibrinolytic process that can break down newly formed clots. Inactive plasminogen circulates in the blood. Following injury, it can be converted by tissue plasminogen activator (tPA) and streptokinase through a sequence of reactions, into plasmin. The product, plasmin, then breaks down fibrin and fibrinogen. This fibrinolysis is a localized event only, because plasmin is quickly inactivated by plasmin inhibitor. These numerous checks and balances are essential in the regulation of defense mechanisms. Application of this mechanism with "clot-buster" drugs such as streptokinase (Streptase) is proving very successful in minimizing the tissue damage resulting from blood clots causing strokes (cardiovascular accidents, CVAs) and heart attacks (myocardial infarctions, MIs). However, constant monitoring of blood-clotting times and careful administration technique are essential to prevent excessive bleeding or hematoma formation. New protocols for anticoagulant medications are under development in the United States to ensure greater safety for patients.

APPLY YOUR KNOWLEDGE 10-2

Predict three ways that normal blood clotting could be impaired. Predict three ways that inappropriate blood clotting could be promoted.

Antigenic Blood Types

An individual's blood type (e.g., ABO and Rh groups) is determined by the presence of specific antigens on the cell membranes of that person's erythrocytes. *ABO* groups are an inherited characteristic that depends on the presence of type A or B *antigens* or agglutinogens (Table 10-1). Shortly after birth, antibodies that can react with different antigens on another person's RBCs form in the blood of the newborn infant. Such an antigen–antibody reaction would occur with, for example, an incompatible blood transfusion, resulting in agglutination (clumping) and hemolysis of the recipient's RBCs (Fig. 10-11).

Blood types of both donor and recipient are carefully checked before transfusion. Persons with type O blood

TABLE 10-1 ABO Blood Groups and Transfusion Compatibilities

Blood Group	RBC Antigens	Antibodies in Plasma	For Transfusion, Can Receive Donor Blood Group
O	None	Anti-A and anti-B	O
A	A	Anti-B	O or A
B	B	Anti-A	O or B
AB	A and B	None	O, A, B, or AB

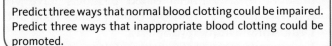

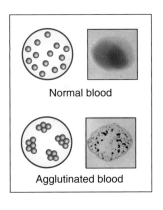

Recipient's blood		Reactions with donor's blood			
RBC antigens	Plasma antibodies	Donor type O	Donor type A	Donor type B	Donor type AB
None (type O)	Anti-A Anti-B				
A (type A)	Anti-B				
B (type B)	Anti-A				
AB (type AB)	(None)				

FIGURE 10-11 Results of (cross-matching) different combinations (types) of donor and recipient blood. The left columns show the antigen and antibody characteristics that define the recipient's blood type, and the top row shows the donor's blood type. Cross-matching identifies either a compatible combination of donor-recipient blood (no agglutination) or an incompatible combination (agglutinated blood). Photo inset shows drops of blood showing appearance of agglutinated and nonagglutinated red blood cells. *(From Belcher AE: Blood Disorders, St. Louis, 1993, Mosby.)*

lack A and B antigens and therefore are considered *universal donors*. Persons with type AB blood are universal recipients. Signs of a transfusion reaction include a feeling of warmth in the involved vein, flushed face, headache, fever and chills, pain in the chest and abdomen, decreased blood pressure, and rapid pulse.

Another inherited factor in blood is the Rh factor, which may cause blood incompatibility if the mother is Rh-negative and the fetus is Rh positive (see Fig. 22-2). Rh blood incompatibility between maternal and fetal blood is reviewed in Chapter 22.

Plasma or colloidal volume-expanding solutions can be administered without risk of a reaction because they are free of antigens and antibodies.

Diagnostic Tests

The basic diagnostic test for blood is the complete blood count (CBC), which includes total RBCs, WBCs, platelet counts, and morphology (size and shape), a differential count for WBCs, hemoglobin, and hematocrit values (see normal values inside the front cover of this book). These tests are useful screening tools. For example, leukocytosis, an increase in WBCs in the circulation, is often associated with inflammation or infection. Leukopenia, a decrease in leukocytes, occurs with some viral infections as well as with radiation and chemotherapy. An increase in eosinophils is common with allergic responses. The characteristics of the individual cells observed in a blood smear, including size and shape, uniformity, maturity, and amount of hemoglobin, are very important. Different types of anemia are distinguished by the characteristic size and shape of the cell, and presence of a nucleus in the RBC. More specialized tests are available. A summary of the most common diagnostic tests is provided in Ready Reference 5.

The hematocrit shows the percentage of blood volume composed of RBCs and indicates fluid and cell content. It may be an indicator of anemia, a low RBC count. Hemoglobin is measured, and the amount of hemoglobin per cell is shown by the mean corpuscular volume (MCV). MCV indicates the oxygen-carrying capacity of the blood.

Bone marrow function can be assessed by the reticulocyte (immature non-nucleated RBC) count, plus a bone marrow aspiration and biopsy.

Chemical analysis of the blood can determine the serum levels of such components as iron, vitamin B_{12} and folic acid, cholesterol, urea, glucose, and bilirubin. The results can indicate metabolic disorders and disorders within various other body systems.

Blood-clotting disorders can be differentiated by tests such as bleeding time (measures platelet function—the time to plug a small puncture wound); prothrombin time or INR International Normalized Ratio (measures the extrinsic pathway); and partial thromboplastin time (PTT—intrinsic pathway), which measure the function of various factors in the coagulation process. They are also used to monitor anticoagulant therapy. The reference values for these tests are best established for individual patients based on their health history.

Blood Therapies

- Whole blood, packed red blood cells, or packed platelets may be administered when severe anemia or thrombocytopenia develops.
- Plasma or colloidal volume-expanding solutions can be administered without risk of a reaction because they are free of antigens and antibodies.
- Artificial blood products are available, but none can perform all the complex functions of normal whole blood. They are compatible with all blood types. Hemolink is made from human hemoglobin, whereas Hemopure is made from cow hemoglobin. Oxygent is a synthetic, genetically engineered blood substitute. Other agents, such as MP4, which is undergoing clinical trials, is combined with blood to improve the oxygen transfer from RBCs to tissues. Polyethylene glycol (PEG) is also being tested by various companies to bind and stabilize hemoglobin molecules, thus decreasing the problem of the disassociation of hemoglobin that occurs in storage. Although promising, none of these artificial blood products have yet received approval from the United States Food and Drug Administration (USFDA).
- Epoetin alfa (Procrit, Eprex) is a form of erythropoietin produced through the use of recombinant DNA technology. It may be administered by injection to stimulate production of red blood cells before certain surgical procedures (e.g., hip replacement) and for patients with anemia related to cancer or chronic renal failure. This reduces the risks of infection or immune reaction associated with multiple blood transfusions.
- Bone marrow or stem cell transplants are used to treat some cancers, severe immune deficiency, or severe blood cell diseases. For success, a close match in tissue or human leukocyte antigen (HLA) type is required. The marrow stem cells are extracted from the donor's pelvic bone, filtered, and infused into the recipient's vein. Normal cells should appear in several weeks. In cases of malignant disease, pretreatment with chemotherapy or radiation is required to destroy tumor cells before the transplant.
- For patients suffering from a lack of blood clotting capability, there are drugs available to aid in the clotting process. Nplate is a drug that has been recently approved by the FDA that directly stimulates platelet production by the bone marrow. NovoSeven is a drug developed primarily to treat hemophiliacs, but it has been adapted for use in treating combat trauma. Although these drugs are in use today, problems with unintentional clots that may form during their use continues to be a dangerous problem that must be considered.

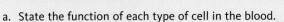

Blood Dyscrasias

The Anemias

Anemias cause a reduction in oxygen transport in the blood due to a decrease in hemoglobin content. The low hemoglobin level may result from declining production of the protein, a decrease in the number of erythrocytes, or a combination of these factors. Anemias may be classified by typical cell characteristics such as size and shape (morphology) or by etiology, for example, the hemolytic anemias.

The oxygen deficit leads to a sequence of events:
- Less energy is produced in all cells; cell metabolism and reproduction are diminished.
- Compensation mechanisms to improve the oxygen supply include tachycardia and peripheral vasoconstriction.
- These changes lead to the general signs of anemia, which include fatigue (excessive tiredness), pallor (pale face), dyspnea (increased effort to *breathe*), and tachycardia (rapid heart rate).
- Decreased regeneration of epithelial cells causes the digestive tract to become inflamed and ulcerated, leading to stomatitis (ulcers in the oral mucosa), inflamed and cracked lips, and dysphagia (difficulty swallowing); the hair and skin may show degenerative changes.
- Severe anemia may lead to angina (chest pain) during stressful situations if the oxygen supply to the heart is sufficiently reduced. Chronic severe anemia may cause congestive heart failure.

Anemias may occur when there is a deficiency of a required nutrient, bone marrow function is impaired, or blood loss or excessive destruction of erythrocytes occurs. This section of the chapter covers a few examples of different types of anemias.

Iron Deficiency Anemia
Pathophysiology

Insufficient iron impedes the synthesis of hemoglobin, thereby reducing the amount of oxygen transported in the blood (see Fig. 10-16*A* for a diagram showing four heme groups). This results in microcytic (small cell), hypochromic (less color) erythrocytes owing to a low concentration of hemoglobin in each cell (see Fig. 10-12). Iron deficiency anemia is very common; it ranges from mild to severe and occurs in all age groups. An

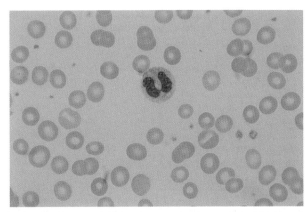

FIGURE 10-12 Iron deficiency anemia shown in a blood smear. *(From Stevens ML:* Fundamentals of Clinical Hematology, *Philadelphia, 1997, Saunders.)*

estimated one in five women is affected, and the proportion increases for pregnant women. Because iron deficiency anemia is frequently a sign of an underlying problem, it is important to determine the specific cause of the deficit. There is also a reduction in stored iron, as indicated by decreased serum ferritin, decreased hemosiderin, and decreased iron-containing histiocytes in the bone marrow.

Etiology
An iron deficit can occur for many reasons:
- Dietary intake of iron-containing vegetables or meat may be below the minimum requirement, particularly during the adolescent growth spurt or during pregnancy and breastfeeding, when needs increase. Normally, only 5% to 10% of ingested iron is absorbed, but this can increase to 20% when there is a deficit.
- Chronic blood loss from a bleeding ulcer, hemorrhoids, cancer, or excessive menstrual flow is a common cause of iron deficiency. Continuous blood loss, even small amounts of blood, means that less iron is recycled to maintain an adequate production of hemoglobin (Fig. 10-13).
- Duodenal absorption of iron may be impaired by many disorders, including malabsorption syndromes such as regional ileitis and achlorhydria (lack of hydrochloric acid in the stomach).
- Severe liver disease may affect both iron absorption and iron storage. An associated protein deficit would further impede hemoglobin synthesis.
- In the form of iron deficiency anemia associated with some infections and cancers, iron is present but is not well used, leading to low hemoglobin levels but high iron storage levels.

Signs and Symptoms
Mild anemias are frequently asymptomatic. As the hemoglobin value drops, the general signs of anemia become apparent:

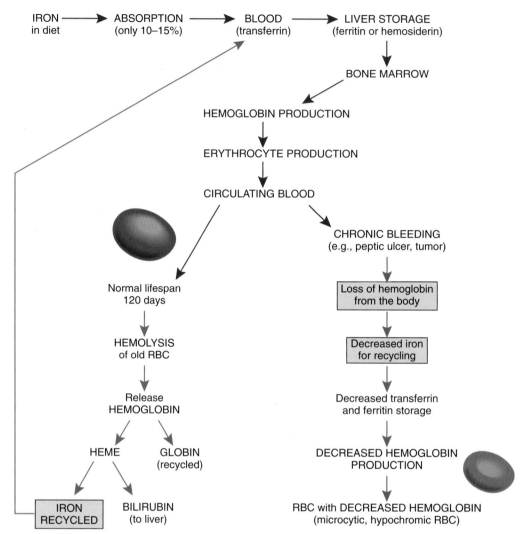

FIGURE 10-13 Iron deficiency anemia related to blood loss.

- Pallor of the skin and mucous membranes related to cutaneous vasoconstriction
- Fatigue, lethargy, and cold intolerance as cell metabolism decreases
- Irritability, a central nervous system response to hypoxia
- Degenerative changes, such as brittle hair, spoon-shaped (concave) and ridged nails
- Stomatitis and glossitis, inflammation in the oral mucosa and tongue, respectively
- Menstrual irregularities
- Delayed healing
- Tachycardia, heart palpitations, dyspnea, and perhaps syncope (fainting) as the anemia becomes more severe

Diagnostic Tests

Laboratory tests demonstrate low values for hemoglobin, hematocrit, mean corpuscular volume and mean corpuscular hemoglobin, serum ferritin and serum iron, and transferrin saturation. On microscopic examination the erythrocytes appear hypochromic and microcytic.

Treatment

The underlying cause must be identified and resolved if possible. The treatment and prognosis depend on the cause. Iron-rich foods or iron supplements in the least irritating and most easily absorbable forms for the individual may be given. It is advisable to take iron with food to reduce gastric irritation and nausea. Iron supplements usually lead to constipation. Liquid iron mixtures stain teeth and dentures, and therefore a straw should be used for drinking the medication.

THINK ABOUT 10-3

a. Explain how chronic bleeding leads to iron deficiency anemia.
b. Explain the signs of anemia that indicate compensation for hypoxia is occurring.
c. Explain how the destruction of acid-producing cells in the stomach can lead to iron deficiency anemia.

Pernicious Anemia-Vitamin B₁₂ Deficiency (Megaloblastic Anemia)

Megaloblastic anemias, as the name implies, are characterized by very large, immature, nucleated erythrocytes. This type of anemia usually results from a deficit of folic acid (vitamin B_9) or vitamin B_{12} (cyanocobalamin). Vitamin deficiencies usually develop gradually. There is now an increased interest in the folic acid deficiency that may occur during the first 2 months of pregnancy, resulting in an increased risk of spina bifida and other spinal abnormalities in the child. It is recommended that women in the childbearing years take folic acid supplements. Folic acid deficits are usually diet related.

The prototype of megaloblastic anemia in this chapter is pernicious anemia, a vitamin B_{12} deficiency.

■ Pathophysiology

Pernicious anemia is the common form of megaloblastic anemia that is caused by the malabsorption of vitamin B_{12} owing to a lack of intrinsic factor (IF) produced in the glands of the gastric mucosa (Fig. 10-14). Intrinsic factor must bind with vitamin B_{12} to enable absorption of the vitamin in the lower ileum. An additional problem occurs with the atrophy of the mucosa because the parietal cells can no longer produce hydrochloric acid. Achlorhydria interferes with the early digestion of protein in the stomach and with the absorption of iron; thus, an iron deficiency anemia may be present as well.

A deficit of vitamin B_{12} leads to impaired maturation of erythrocytes owing to interference with DNA synthesis. The RBCs are very large (megaloblasts or macrocytes) and contain nuclei (Fig. 10-15). These large erythrocytes are destroyed prematurely, resulting in a low erythrocyte count, or anemia. The hemoglobin in the RBCs is normal and is capable of transporting oxygen. Often the maturation of granulocytes is also affected, resulting in development of abnormally large hypersegmented neutrophils. Thrombocyte levels may be low. In addition, lack of vitamin B_{12} is a direct cause of demyelination of the peripheral nerves and eventually of the spinal cord. Loss of myelin interferes with conduction of nerve impulses and may be irreversible. Sensory fibers are affected first, followed by motor fibers.

■ Etiology

- Dietary insufficiency is rarely a cause of this anemia because very small amounts of vitamin B_{12} are required. Because the source of the vitamin is animal foods, vegetarians and vegans must ensure they include a source in their daily intake.
- The most common cause of vitamin B_{12} deficiency is malabsorption, which may result from an autoimmune reaction, particularly in older individuals; from chronic gastritis, which is common in alcoholics and causes atrophy of the gastric mucosa; or from inflammatory conditions such as regional ileitis.

- The condition may also be an outcome of such surgical procedures as gastrectomy (removal or resection of part of the stomach), in which the parietal cells are removed, or resection of the ileum, which is the site of absorption.

■ Signs and Symptoms

The basic manifestations of anemia are listed earlier. In addition, pernicious anemia has the following distinctive signs:

1. The tongue is typically enlarged, red, sore, and shiny.
2. The decrease in gastric acid leads to digestive discomfort, often with nausea and diarrhea.
3. The neurologic effects include tingling or burning sensations (paresthesia) in the extremities or loss of coordination and ataxia.

■ Diagnostic Tests

- The erythrocytes appear macrocytic or megaloblastic and nucleated on microscopic examination and are reduced in number in the peripheral blood.
- The bone marrow is hyperactive, with increased numbers of megaloblasts. Granulocytes are hypersegmented and are decreased in number.
- The vitamin B_{12} level in the serum is below normal. In Schilling's test, an oral dose of radioactive vitamin B_{12} is used to measure absorption.
- The presence of hypochlorhydria or achlorhydria confirms the presence of gastric atrophy.

■ Treatment

Oral supplements are recommended as prophylaxis for pregnant women and vegetarians. Vitamin B_{12} is administered by injection as replacement therapy for people with pernicious anemia. Prompt diagnosis and treatment of pernicious anemia prevents cardiac stress and neurologic damage.

THINK ABOUT 10-4

a. Explain why individuals with pernicious anemia have a low hemoglobin level.
b. Explain how pernicious anemia can cause a neurologic effect such as a tingling sensation in extremities or loss of coordination.
c. Why is oral administration of vitamin B_{12} not effective as a treatment for pernicious anemia?

Aplastic Anemia

■ Pathophysiology

Aplastic anemia results from impairment or failure of bone marrow, leading to loss of stem cells and pancytopenia, the decreased numbers of erythrocytes, leukocytes, and platelets in the blood. These deficits lead to many serious complications. In addition the bone

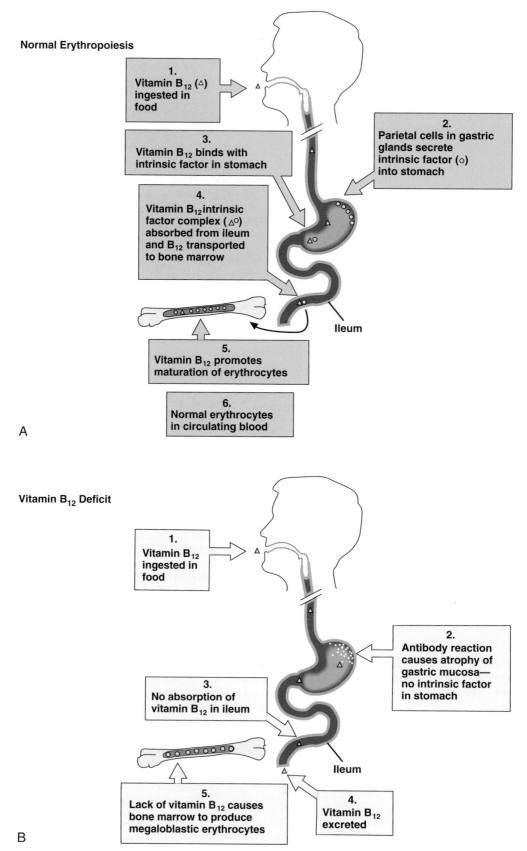

Normal Erythropoiesis

1. Vitamin B$_{12}$ ($\triangle$) ingested in food

2. Parietal cells in gastric glands secrete intrinsic factor ($\circ$) into stomach

3. Vitamin B$_{12}$ binds with intrinsic factor in stomach

4. Vitamin B$_{12}$ intrinsic factor complex ($\triangle\circ$) absorbed from ileum and B$_{12}$ transported to bone marrow

5. Vitamin B$_{12}$ promotes maturation of erythrocytes

6. Normal erythrocytes in circulating blood

Ileum

A

Vitamin B$_{12}$ Deficit

1. Vitamin B$_{12}$ ingested in food

2. Antibody reaction causes atrophy of gastric mucosa— no intrinsic factor in stomach

3. No absorption of vitamin B$_{12}$ in ileum

4. Vitamin B$_{12}$ excreted

5. Lack of vitamin B$_{12}$ causes bone marrow to produce megaloblastic erythrocytes

Ileum

B

FIGURE 10-14 Development of pernicious anemia.

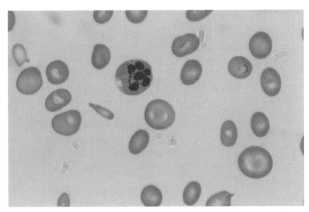

FIGURE 10-15 Vitamin B$_{12}$ deficiency with macrocytes and a neutrophil with hypersegmented nucleus in a peripheral blood smear. *(From Stevens ML: Fundamentals of Clinical Hematology, Philadelphia, 1997, Saunders.)*

marrow exhibits reduced cell components and increased fatty tissue.

■ *Etiology*

Aplastic anemia may be a temporary or permanent condition depending on the cause.

- In approximately half the cases, the patients are middle-aged, and the cause is unknown or idiopathic (primary type).
- Myelotoxins, such as radiation, industrial chemicals (e.g., benzene), and drugs (e.g., chloramphenicol, gold salts, phenylbutazone, phenytoin, and antineoplastic drugs) may damage the bone marrow. In these cases it is important to detect and remove the causative factor quickly to allow the marrow to recover. When severe aplastic anemia due to cancer treatment is a risk, the patient's stem cells may be harvested before treatment and then transfused later when needed.
- Viruses, particularly hepatitis C, may cause aplastic anemia.
- Autoimmune disease such as systemic lupus erythematosus (SLE) may affect the bone marrow.
- Genetic abnormalities such as myelodysplastic syndrome or Fanconi's anemia may also affect bone marrow function.

■ *Signs and Symptoms*

In the majority of cases, the onset is insidious. Because the entire bone marrow is affected, manifestations include those of:

1. Anemia (pallor, weakness, and dyspnea)
2. Leukopenia, such as recurrent or multiple infections
3. Thrombocytopenia (petechiae—flat, red, pinpoint hemorrhages on the skin [Fig. 10-19]—and a tendency to bleed excessively, particularly in the mouth)

As blood counts diminish, particularly WBCs and platelets, uncontrollable infection and hemorrhage are likely.

■ *Diagnostic Tests*

Blood counts indicate pancytopenia. A bone marrow biopsy may be required to confirm the cause of the pancytopenia. The erythrocytes are often normal in appearance.

■ *Treatment*

Prompt treatment of the underlying cause and removal of any bone marrow suppressants are essential to recovery of the bone marrow. Blood transfusion may be necessary if stem cell levels are very low.

Bone marrow transplantation may be helpful in younger patients; its success depends on the accuracy of the tissue match using human leukocyte antigen (HLA). Chemotherapy and radiation are used to prepare the recipient's bone marrow for transplantation of stem cells (taken from the marrow of the pelvic bone of a suitable donor). Newer techniques allow harvesting of stem cells from the peripheral blood, not the marrow. The donor stem cells are infused intravenously into the blood of the recipient; they migrate to the bone marrow and provide a new source of blood cells after several weeks. Antirejection drugs are required for a year, but unlike the situation with other transplants, these drugs can then be discontinued. Common complications include damage to the digestive tract from the preparatory treatment, infection resulting from immune suppression, and rejection reactions.

THINK ABOUT 10-5

a. Explain why bone marrow damage can result in multiple, recurring infections.
b. Explain why excessive bleeding occurs with aplastic anemia.
c. Explain why it is necessary to treat the bone marrow recipient with chemotherapy and radiation before transplant.

Hemolytic Anemias

Hemolytic anemias result from excessive destruction of RBCs, or hemolysis, leading to a low erythrocyte count and low total hemoglobin. They have many causes, including genetic defects affecting structure, immune reactions, changes in blood chemistry, the presence of toxins in the blood, infections such as malaria, transfusion reactions, and blood incompatibility in the neonate (erythroblastosis fetalis). Two examples follow.

Sickle Cell Anemia

■ *Pathophysiology*

Sickle cell anemia is representative of a large number of similar hemoglobinopathies. In this anemia, an inherited characteristic leads to the formation of abnormal hemoglobin, hemoglobin S (HbS). In HbS, one amino

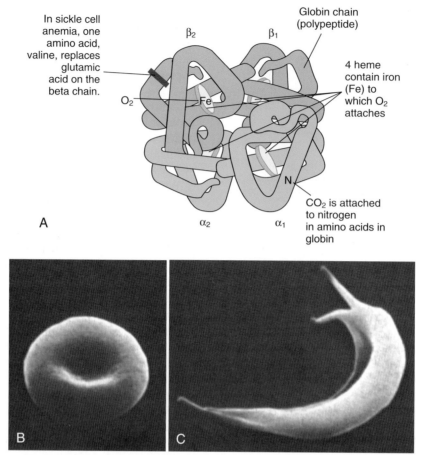

FIGURE 10-16 **A,** Structure of hemoglobin. **B,** An oxygenated sickle cell erythrocyte. **C,** A deoxygenated sickle cell erythrocyte. (*B and C courtesy of Dr. James White.*)

acid in the pair of beta-globin chains has been changed from the normal glutamic acid to valine (Fig. 10-16). When this altered hemoglobin is deoxygenated, it crystallizes and changes the shape of the RBC from a disc to a crescent or "sickle" shape. The cell membrane is damaged, leading to hemolysis, and the cells have a much shorter lifespan than normal, perhaps only 20 days, instead of the normal 120 days. Initially the sickling may be reversible when increased oxygen is available, but after several episodes, the damage to the RBC is irreversible and hemolysis occurs. Hemoglobin S can transport oxygen in the normal fashion, but the erythrocyte count is very low, resulting in a low hemoglobin level in the blood.

A major problem resulting from the sickling process is the obstruction of the small blood vessels by the elongated and rigid RBCs, resulting in thrombus formation and repeated multiple infarctions, or areas of tissue necrosis, throughout the body (Fig. 10-17). The deoxygenation of hemoglobin may occur in the peripheral circulation as the oxygen content of the blood is gradually reduced, leading to repeated minor infarctions. A serious crisis may occur in individuals with lung infection or dehydration when basic oxygen levels are reduced. During a sickling crisis, many larger blood

vessels may be involved, and multiple infarctions occur throughout the body, affecting the brain, bones, or organs. In time, significant damage and loss of function occur in many organ systems.

In addition to the basic anemia, the high rate of hemolysis leads to hyperbilirubinemia, jaundice, and gallstones (see Fig. 10-7 and Chapter 17).

■ *Etiology*

The gene for HbS is recessive and is very common in individuals from Africa and the Middle East. In homozygotes, most of the normal hemoglobin (hemoglobin A [HbA]) is replaced by HbS, resulting in clinical signs of sickle cell *anemia* (Fig. 10-18). Individuals vary greatly in the severity of the anemia and the number of sickling crises. In heterozygotes, less than half the hemoglobin is the abnormal HbS; therefore clinical signs occur only with severe hypoxia under unusual circumstances, for example, pneumonia or at high altitudes; this condition is termed the sickle cell *trait.* It is estimated that 1 in 12 African Americans have the trait and about 1 in 500 have sickle cell anemia. It is interesting that the carrier population in Africa is very high, evidently owing to a decreased incidence of malaria in those with HbS.

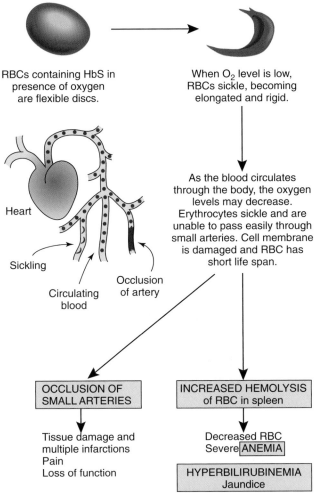

RBCs containing HbS in presence of oxygen are flexible discs.

When O₂ level is low, RBCs sickle, becoming elongated and rigid.

Heart

Sickling

Circulating blood

Occlusion of artery

As the blood circulates through the body, the oxygen levels may decrease. Erythrocytes sickle and are unable to pass easily through small arteries. Cell membrane is damaged and RBC has short life span.

OCCLUSION OF SMALL ARTERIES

INCREASED HEMOLYSIS of RBC in spleen

Tissue damage and multiple infarctions
Pain
Loss of function

Decreased RBC
Severe ANEMIA

HYPERBILIRUBINEMIA
Jaundice

FIGURE 10-17 Sickle cell anemia—the effects of sickling.

■ *Signs and Symptoms*

Clinical signs of sickle cell anemia do not appear until the child is about 12 months of age, when fetal hemoglobin (HbF) has been replaced by HbS. The proportion of HbS in the erythrocytes determines the severity of the condition.

- Severe anemia causes pallor, weakness, tachycardia, and dyspnea.
- Hyperbilirubinemia is indicated by jaundice, the yellowish color being most obvious in the sclerae of the eyes. The high bilirubin concentration in the bile may cause the development of gallstones (see Chapter 17).
- Splenomegaly, enlargement of the spleen, is common in young people because sickled cells cause congestion, but in adults the spleen is usually small and fibrotic owing to recurrent infarction.
- Vascular occlusions and infarctions lead to periodic painful crises and permanent damage to organs and tissues. Such damage may be manifested as ulcers on the legs and feet, areas of necrosis in the bones or kidneys, or seizures or hemiplegia resulting from cerebral infarctions (strokes). Pain can be quite intense.
- In the lungs, occlusions and infection cause acute chest syndrome with pain and fever. It can be diagnosed by x-ray. It is a frequent cause of death.
- Occlusions in the smaller blood vessels of the hands or feet cause hand-foot syndrome. Pain and swelling are often early signs in children.
- Growth and development are delayed. Late puberty is common. Tooth eruption is late, and hypoplasia is common. Intellectual development is usually impaired.

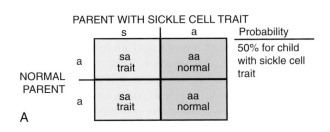

PARENT WITH SICKLE CELL TRAIT

	s	a	Probability
a	sa trait	aa normal	50% for child with sickle cell trait
a	sa trait	aa normal	

NORMAL PARENT

A

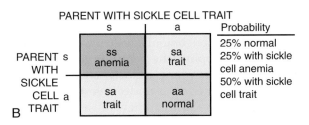

PARENT WITH SICKLE CELL TRAIT

	s	a	Probability
PARENT WITH SICKLE CELL TRAIT — s	ss anemia	sa trait	25% normal
a	sa trait	aa normal	25% with sickle cell anemia
			50% with sickle cell trait

B

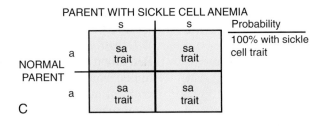

PARENT WITH SICKLE CELL ANEMIA

	s	s	Probability
a	sa trait	sa trait	100% with sickle cell trait
a	sa trait	sa trait	

NORMAL PARENT

C

KEY
aa = normal: HbA
ss = sickle cell anemia: HbS
sa = sickle cell trait: mixed HbA and HbS

FIGURE 10-18 Inheritance of sickle cell anemia.

- Congestive heart failure may develop owing to constant efforts to improve the supply of oxygen and the increased peripheral resistance caused by the obstructions.
- Frequent infections occur because of the decreased defenses when the damaged spleen can no longer adequately filter the blood, the presence of necrotic tissues, and poor healing capabilities. Pneumonia is a common cause of death in children. Infections tend to cause more sickling, and a vicious cycle develops.

■ Diagnostic Tests

Carriers of the defective gene can be detected by a simple blood test (hemoglobin electrophoresis). This identification is useful in alerting those with sickle cell trait to avoid severe hypoxia and sickling episodes (e.g., with severe anemia, surgery, or at high altitudes), as well as in assisting prospective parents in decision making about the risk of having an affected child (see Chapter 21).

Prenatal diagnosis can be checked by DNA analysis of the fetal blood. In children more than 1 year of age, the diagnosis can be confirmed by the presence of sickled cells in peripheral blood and the presence of HbS. The bone marrow is hyperplastic, and more reticulocytes (immature RBCs) are released into the circulation.

■ Treatment

The search continues for more effective drugs to reduce sickling. The use of hydroxyurea (Hydrea) has reduced the frequency of crises and prolonged the lifespan for many, but is not effective for all patients. Dietary supplementation with folic acid (folate) is recommended even during asymptomatic periods. Avoidance of strenuous activity or high altitudes is helpful. Other supportive measures are utilized to prevent dehydration, acidosis, infection, or exposure to cold, all of which increase the sickling tendency and painful crises. Children should be immunized against pneumonia, influenza, and meningitis. Continued prophylactic penicillin may be necessary for two groups, young children and adults with severe cases. Gene therapy is under investigation. Bone marrow transplant is effective, but because of the limited number of African-American potential donors on bone marrow registries, it may be very difficult to find a match. In the past, patients rarely lived past their twenties, but recent improvements in care have extended the lifespan into middle age for many patients.

THINK ABOUT 10-6

a. Explain why vascular occlusions are common in patients with sickle cell disease.
b. Compare sickle cell trait and sickle cell anemia in terms of the genetic factor involved, the amount of HbS present, and the presence of clinical signs.

Thalassemia
■ Pathophysiology

This anemia results from a genetic defect in which one or more genes for hemoglobin are missing or variant. When two genes are involved, thalassemia is moderate to severe. This abnormality interferes with the production of the globin chains, and therefore, the *amount* of hemoglobin synthesized and the number of RBCs is reduced. Hemoglobin is normally composed of four globin chains, two alpha and two beta (see structure in Fig. 10-16A). Thalassemia *alpha* refers to a reduction in or lack of alpha chains. Thalassemia *beta* refers to a decrease or lack of beta chains. In either case, less normal hemoglobin can be made. In addition to missing chains, there is an accumulation of the other available chains, damaging the RBCs. For example, when a beta chain is missing, the extra alpha chains collect in RBCs and damage the cell membrane, leading to hemolysis and anemia. Homozygotes have thalassemia major (Cooley's anemia) a severe form of the anemia; heterozygotes have thalassemia minor and exhibit mild signs of anemia. In severe cases, increased hemolysis of RBCs aggravates the anemia and causes splenomegaly, hepatomegaly, and hyperbilirubinemia. The bone marrow is hyperactive, trying to compensate.

■ Etiology

Thalassemia is the most common genetic disorder in the world and it occurs in two common forms. Thalassemia beta (autosomal dominant inheritance) occurs frequently in people from Mediterranean countries such as Greece or Italy, and thalassemia beta is the more common form. The alpha form is found in those of Indian, Chinese, or Southeast Asian descent. Because more than one gene is involved, there are many possible gene mutations with varied effects on hemoglobin synthesis and the severity of the resultant anemia.

■ Signs and Symptoms

The usual signs of anemia and increased hemolysis are present as described earlier. The child's growth and development are impaired directly by the hypoxia and indirectly by the fatigue and inactivity. Hyperactivity in the bone marrow leads to invasion of bone and impairs normal skeletal development. Heart failure develops as a result of the compensation mechanism increasing cardiac work load.

■ Diagnostic Tests

Red blood cells are microcytic, often varying in size, and hypochromic (low hemoglobin). There is an increase in erythropoietin levels. Often an iron overload exists. Prenatal diagnosis can be done by chorionic villus assay at 12 weeks or by amniocentesis at 16 weeks.

■ Treatment

Blood transfusions are the only treatment available at this time. Iron chelation therapy may be necessary to

TABLE 10-2	Comparison of Selected Anemias		
Anemia	Characteristic RBC	Etiology	Additional Effects
Iron deficiency anemia	Microcytic, hypochromic Decreased hemoglobin production	Decreased dietary intake, malabsorption, blood loss	Only effects of anemia
Pernicious anemia	Megaloblasts (immature nucleated cells) Short lifespan	Deficit of intrinsic factor owing to immune reaction	Neurologic damage Achlorhydria
Aplastic anemia	Often normal cells Pancytopenia	Bone marrow damage or failure	Excessive bleeding and multiple infections
Sickle cell anemia	RBC elongates and hardens in "sickle" shape when O_2 levels are low—short lifespan	Recessive inheritance	Painful crises with multiple infarctions Hyperbilirubinemia

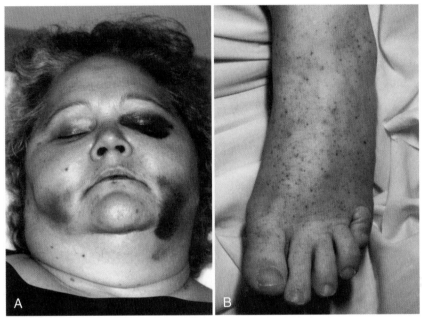

FIGURE 10-19 **A**, Facial ecchymoses. **B**, Petechiae. *(From Young NS: Bone Marrow Failure Syndromes, Philadelphia, 2000, Saunders.)*

remove the excess iron from numerous transfusions. Administration of folate is also recommended. Bone marrow transplants have been curative in some children and are in clinical research trials. Patients with mild forms of the disease have a normal lifespan, and those with moderate to severe disease live into their thirties with transfusions and chelation therapy. Those with very severe anemia may die in childhood.

Characteristics of the selected anemias are compared in Table 10-2.

Blood-Clotting Disorders

Spontaneous bleeding or excessive bleeding following minor tissue trauma often indicates a blood-clotting disorder. Note: The following warning signs may also be caused by *other factors*, such as infections and damaged or fragile blood vessels (e.g., vitamin C deficit).

WARNING SIGNS OF EXCESSIVE BLEEDING AND POSSIBLE BLOOD-CLOTTING DISORDERS

- Persistent bleeding from the gums (around the teeth) or repeated nosebleeds
- Petechiae—pinpoint flat red spots on skin or mucous membranes (like a rash); result from bleeding from a capillary or small arteriole (see Fig. 10-19B)
- Frequent purpura and ecchymoses—large, purplish red or greenish areas on the skin (bruises) (see Fig. 10-19A)

More persistent bleeding than warranted by a trauma

- Bleeding into a joint—hemarthroses—swollen, red, and painful
- Coughing up blood—hemoptysis—bright red flecks in sputum
- Vomiting blood—hematemesis—often coarse brown particles (coffee grounds); may be red
- Blood in feces—often black (tarry) or occult (hidden)
- Anemia
- Feeling faint and anxious, low blood pressure, rapid pulse

Excessive bleeding has many causes:

- Thrombocytopenia may be caused by acute viral infections in children (usually resolves in 6 months) or autoimmune reactions in adults (chronic idiopathic thrombocytopenic purpura). The chronic form occurs primarily in adults, especially in young women when thrombocytes are destroyed by antibodies. Human immunodeficiency virus infection, hepatomegaly and splenomegaly, and certain drugs also lead to thrombocytopenia.
- Chemotherapy, radiation treatments, and cancers such as leukemia also reduce platelet counts, causing bleeding.
- Defective platelet function is associated with uremia (end-stage kidney failure) and ingestion of aspirin (ASA). Anyone with a bleeding disorder should avoid ASA or ASA-containing drugs, as well as nonsteroidal anti-inflammatory drugs because all these interfere with platelet adhesion.
- Vitamin K deficiency may cause a decrease in prothrombin and fibrinogen levels. Vitamin K is a fat-soluble vitamin produced by the intestinal bacteria and is present in some foods as well. A deficiency of vitamin K may occur in patients with liver disease, accompanied by a decrease in bile production, and in those with malabsorption problems. However, vitamin K is a useful antidote when an excess of warfarin (Coumadin), an oral anticoagulant, causes bleeding.
- Liver disease reduces the available proteins and vitamin K, and thus interferes with the production of clotting factors in the liver and reduces the available proteins and vitamin K.
- Inherited defects cause bleeding disorders resulting from a deficiency of one of the clotting factors. Serum factor analysis and more specific tests are useful here. These include PT to measure the extrinsic pathway, activated partial thromboplastin time (APTT) to measure the intrinsic pathway, and thrombin time for the final stage, fibrinogen to fibrin.
- Hemorrhagic fever viruses such as Ebola virus cause excessive bleeding and acute illness, affecting many organs.

- Anticoagulant drugs such as warfarin (Coumadin) are often prescribed on a long-term basis and the patient's hemostatic ability requires close monitoring (see Fig. 10-6 for site of action of anticoagulant drugs). The difference between a helpful therapeutic drug level and a blood level that causes bleeding is very small. Also, many foods, drugs, and herbal compounds can alter the effects of anticoagulant drugs, creating a dangerous situation.

When a patient with any bleeding disorder is at risk for hemorrhage because of an invasive procedure, it is best to be prepared by using laboratory tests to check the current blood-clotting status and to administer prophylactic medications if needed. Personnel should be ready and supplies should be available for any emergency, including the application of pressure, cold dressings, and absorbable hemostatic packing agents such as Gelfoam or Oxycel and styptics.

Hemophilia A

■ *Pathophysiology*

Hemophilia A, or classic hemophilia, is a deficit or abnormality of clotting factor VIII (see Fig. 10-9) and is the most common inherited clotting disorder. Ninety percent of hemophiliac patients have type A. The defect causing hemophilia A is transmitted as an X-linked recessive trait (Fig. 10-20); therefore, it is manifest in men but is carried by women, who are asymptomatic (see Chapter 21). With improved treatment and a longer lifespan for men, this pattern could change. An affected man and a carrier woman could produce a female child who inherits the gene from both parents.

Hemophilia B (Christmas disease) is similar and involves a deficit of factor IX; hemophilia C (Rosenthal's hemophilia) is a milder form resulting from a decrease in factor XI. Some cases of hemophilia result from a spontaneous gene mutation in a person with no previous family history of the disease.

There are approximately 18,000 to 20,000 cases of hemophilia in the United States and an estimated 400 infants are born each year with hemophilia. There are varying degrees of severity of hemophilia, depending on the amount of the factor present in the blood. In mild

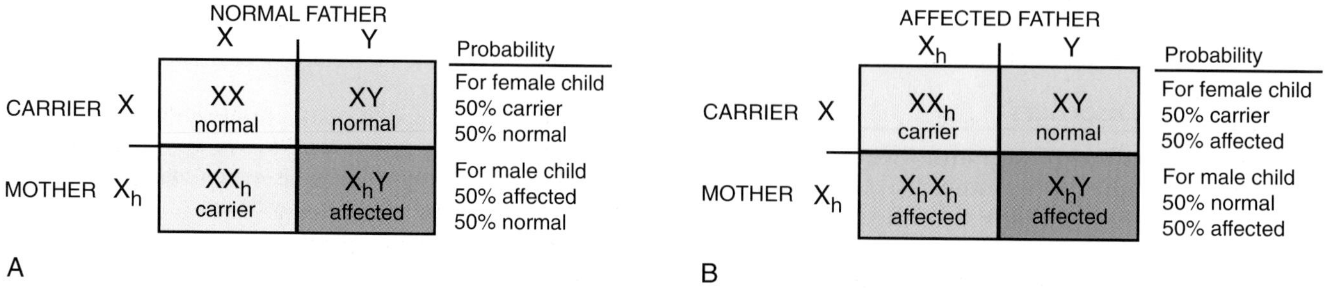

FIGURE 10-20 Inheritance of hemophilia A.

forms (more than 5% factor VIII activity), excessive bleeding occurs only after trauma, whereas frequent spontaneous bleeding is common in people with severe deficiencies (less than 1% factor VIII activity). About 70% of affected individuals have the severe form.

▓ *Signs and Symptoms*

Prolonged or severe hemorrhage occurs following minor tissue trauma. Persistent oozing of blood after minor injuries and hematomas is common. Spontaneous hemorrhage into joints (hemarthrosis) may occur, eventually causing painful and crippling deformities resulting from recurrent inflammation. Blood may appear in the urine (hematuria) or feces because of bleeding in the kidneys or digestive tract.

▓ *Diagnostic Tests*

Bleeding time and PT are normal, but the PTT, APTT, and coagulation time are prolonged. Serum levels of factor VIII are low. Thromboplastin generation time differentiates between deficits of factor VIII and factor IX.

▓ *Treatment*

All precautions mentioned earlier should be followed. Treatment with desmopressin (DDAVP) may raise clotting factor levels in some clients. This drug stimulates the endothelium lining blood vessels to release stored factor VIII. Replacement therapy for factor VIII is available for intravenous administration at regular intervals and especially before any surgical or dental procedure. Unfortunately, hepatitis and HIV have been transmitted through blood products. Although blood is now treated to destroy known viruses, a risk remains that some unknown infection may be acquired by such treatment. Some individuals have developed immune reactions to repeated replacement therapy. A newer recombinant DNA product (Advate), produced through genetic engineering, does not contain any material such as protein from human or animal blood, therefore reducing the risk of immune responses. A new drug Nplate has recently been approved by the USFDA that stimulates platelet production in bone marrow. Research continues into gene therapy.

von Willebrand Disease

▓ *Pathophysiology*

This is the most common hereditary blood clotting/bleeding disorder. This disease is caused by a deficiency of the von Willebrand factor, a clotting factor that helps platelets clump and stick to the walls of blood vessels where damage has occurred. There are three major types of this disease which have signs/symptoms similar to, but much milder than hemophilia.

▓ *Signs and Symptoms*

Depending on the type of the disease, signs and symptoms typically include: skin rashes, frequent nosebleeds, easy bruising, bleeding of the gums, and abnormal menstrual bleeding.

▓ *Diagnostic Tests*

Although sometimes hard to diagnose due to nonspecific signs and symptoms, the tests that may be done to diagnose this disease include: bleeding time, blood typing, factor VIII levels, platelet count and aggregation test, ristocetin cofactor test, and von Willebrand factor specific tests.

▓ *Treatment*

Treatment is based on the type of von Willebrand disease and its severity. Because most cases of this disease are relatively mild, treatment may only be required in cases such as surgery, tooth extraction, or accident trauma. The manmade hormone desmopressin can be used to treat milder cases. The injection or nasal spray of this hormone causes increased release of von Willebrand factor and factor VIII into the bloodstream. These factors can also be directly injected into a vein as a replacement therapy and are used in the more severe types of the disease. Antifibrinolytic drugs that help prevent the breakdown of blood clots are often used after minor surgery or injury. In addition to these drugs, women with an abnormal menstrual flow caused by this disease can be treated with birth control pills as these also cause an increase in release of the clotting factors.

Disseminated Intravascular Coagulation

▓ *Pathophysiology*

Disseminated intravascular coagulation (DIC) is a condition, often life threatening, that involves both excessive bleeding and excessive clotting. It occurs as a complication of numerous primary problems, which activate the clotting process in the microcirculation throughout the body (Fig. 10-21). Clotting may be induced by the release of tissue thromboplastin or by injury to the endothelial cells, causing platelet adhesion. The process causes multiple thromboses and infarctions but also consumes the available clotting factors and platelets and stimulates the fibrinolytic process. The resulting consumption of clotting factors and fibrinolysis then leads to hemorrhage and eventually to hypotension or shock.

Chronic DIC is a milder form and may be difficult to diagnose: Blood counts may be normal or abnormal. It is usually caused by chronic infection, and thromboembolism is the dominant feature.

▓ *Etiology*

A variety of disorders can initiate DIC. It may result from an obstetric complication such as toxemia, amniotic fluid embolus, or abruptio placentae, in which tissue thromboplastin is released from the placenta (see Chapter 22). Infection, particularly gram-negative infection, leads to endotoxins that cause endothelial damage or stimulate the release of thromboplastin from

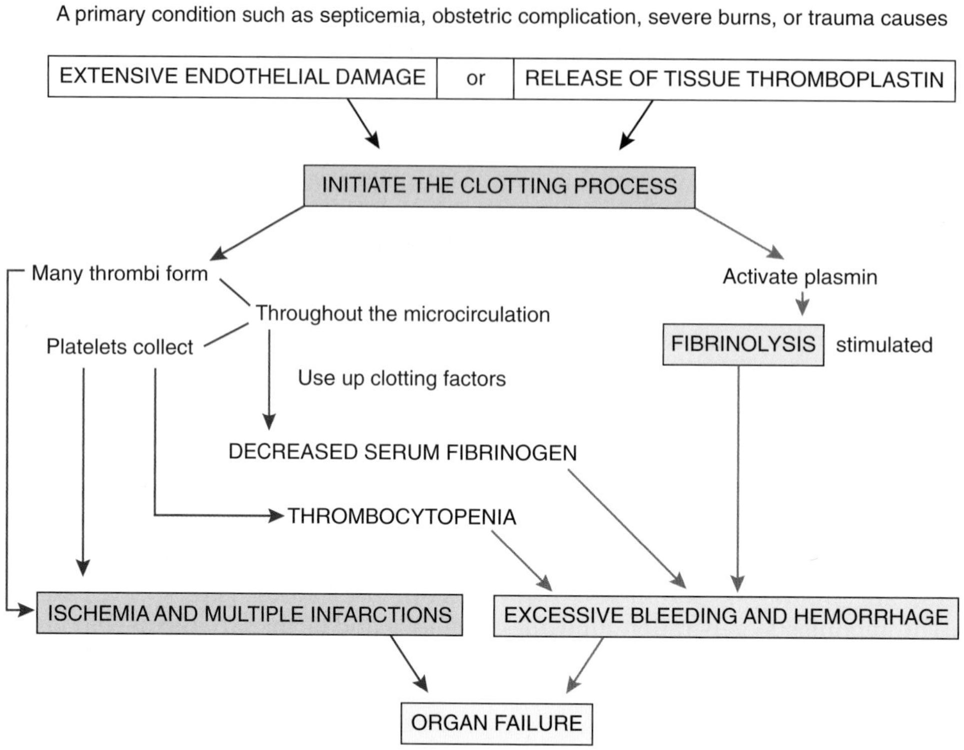

A primary condition such as septicemia, obstetric complication, severe burns, or trauma causes

| EXTENSIVE ENDOTHELIAL DAMAGE | or | RELEASE OF TISSUE THROMBOPLASTIN |

INITIATE THE CLOTTING PROCESS

Many thrombi form

Throughout the microcirculation

Platelets collect

Use up clotting factors

Activate plasmin

FIBRINOLYSIS stimulated

DECREASED SERUM FIBRINOGEN

THROMBOCYTOPENIA

ISCHEMIA AND MULTIPLE INFARCTIONS

EXCESSIVE BLEEDING AND HEMORRHAGE

ORGAN FAILURE

FIGURE 10-21 Disseminated intravascular coagulation.

monocytes. Many carcinomas release substances that trigger coagulation. Major trauma, such as burns or crush injuries, and widespread deposits of antigen–antibody complexes result in endothelial damage, releasing thromboplastin and initiating the process.

■ *Signs and Symptoms*

Whether hemorrhage or thrombosis dominates, the clinical effects depend somewhat on the underlying cause. Obstetric patients usually manifest increased bleeding, whereas cancer patients tend to have more thromboses. More often, hemorrhage is the critical problem. This is indicated by low plasma fibrinogen level, thrombocytopenia, and prolonged bleeding time, PT, APTT, and thrombin time. Accompanying hemorrhage are the effects of low blood pressure or shock. Multiple bleeding sites are common, petechiae or ecchymoses may be present on the skin or mucosa, mucosal bleeding is common, and hematuria may develop (see Fig. 10-19). Vascular occlusions are frequently present in small blood vessels but occasionally affect the large vessels as well, causing infarcts in the brain or other organs.

Respiratory impairment is evident as difficulty in breathing and cyanosis. Neurologic effects include seizures and decreased responsiveness. Acute renal failure with oliguria often accompanies shock.

■ *Treatment*

A fine balance is required to treat the coagulation imbalance, particularly in life-threatening cases. Treatment is

difficult, dependent on whether hemorrhages or thromboses are dominant. The underlying cause, such as infection, must be treated successfully, as well as the major current problem, whether it is excessive clotting or hemorrhage. The prognosis depends on the severity of the primary problem.

Thrombophilia

■ *Pathophysiology*

Thrombophilia is group of inherited or acquired disorders that increase the risk of the development of abnormal clots in the veins or arteries. Abnormal clotting events can result in conditions such as a deep venous thrombosis, pulmonary embolism, or peripheral vascular disease.

Inherited thrombophilias are a result of mutations among the genes responsible for producing the coagulation proteins in the blood. Acquired thrombophilias commonly occur during events such as surgery, injury, or other medical conditions that allow for an increase of the amount of clotting factors in the blood or an accumulation of antibodies.

■ *Signs and Symptoms*

The signs and symptoms of an abnormal clotting event are not specific and can affect any organ or system in which the clot may lodge and cut off the blood supply. In cases in which the clot lodges in the heart or vessels of the lung, the result can be a myocardial infarction or an acute stroke.

■ *Diagnosis*

Tests to diagnose thrombophilia involve blood testing for clotting factor levels and abnormal antibody levels.

■ *Treatment*

In cases in which the disorder has been provoked by another underlying medical condition, the causative condition should be treated to decrease the potential of acquired thrombophilia. In those cases in which the disorder is not provoked by another condition, anticoagulants such as warfarin (Coumadin) may be prescribed to reduce the risk of abnormal clot formation. The use of these types of medication must be weighed with the risks for excessive bleeding due to the interruption of the normal coagulation capability of the blood.

THINK ABOUT 10-7

a. State the probability that a child with a carrier mother will have hemophilia A.
b. Describe briefly three causes of excessive bleeding other than hemophilia.
c. Explain how a deep vein thrombosis in a large vein in the leg can result in a life-threatening condition such as a stroke or myocardial infarction.

Myelodysplastic Syndrome

Myelodysplastic syndrome (MDS) is the term used for diseases that involve inadequate production of cells by the bone marrow. It excludes disorders such as aplastic anemias and deficiency dyscrasias. Myelodysplastic diseases may be idiopathic or can often occur following chemotherapy or radiation treatment for other cancers. Several different types are described, including anemias and pancytopenias in which all cell types or reduced. Diagnosis is based on the patient's history, standard blood tests, and bone marrow biopsy. Treatment measures depend on the type of deficiency and include transfusion replacements, chelation therapy to reduce iron levels, and supportive therapies to prevent complications. Low level chemotherapy may be used with growth factors to stimulate more normal bone marrow function. Bone marrow transplants are curative, but often the patient's health will not allow this treatment. The prognosis for patients with MDS is dependent on age of onset, past treatment with chemotherapy or radiation, and response to treatment. Myelodysplastic syndrome may progress to chronic or acute leukemia in some cases if treatment is not effective in normalizing the blood picture.

Neoplastic Blood Disorders

Polycythemia

■ *Pathophysiology*

Primary polycythemia, or polycythemia vera, is a condition in which there is an increased production of erythrocytes and other cells in the bone marrow. It is considered a neoplastic disorder. Serum erythropoietin levels are low. Secondary polycythemia, or erythrocytosis, is an increase in RBCs that occurs in response to prolonged hypoxia and increased erythropoietin secretion. Usually the increase in RBCs is not as marked in secondary polycythemia, and more reticulocytes appear in the peripheral blood.

In polycythemia vera, there is a marked increase in erythrocytes and often in granulocytes and thrombocytes as well, resulting in increased blood volume and viscosity. Blood vessels are distended and blood flow is sluggish, leading to frequent thromboses and infarctions throughout the body, especially when platelet counts are high. Blood pressure is elevated and the heart hypertrophied. Hemorrhage is frequent in places where the blood vessels are distended. The spleen and liver are congested and enlarged, and the bone marrow is hypercellular.

In some patients, the bone marrow eventually becomes fibrotic, hematopoiesis develops in the spleen, and anemia follows. In a few patients, acute myeloblastic leukemia develops in the later stages, especially if treatment has involved chemotherapy.

■ *Etiology*

Primary polycythemia is a neoplastic disorder of unknown origin that commonly develops between the ages of 40 and 60 years, although younger individuals can be affected. Secondary polycythemia may be a compensation mechanism intended to provide increased oxygen transport in the presence of chronic lung disease or heart disease or from living at high altitudes. Some cases result from erythropoietin-secreting tumors such as renal carcinoma.

■ *Signs and Symptoms*

The patient appears plethoric and cyanotic, with the deep bluish-red tone of the skin and mucosa resulting from the engorged blood vessels and sluggish blood flow. Hepatomegaly, an enlarged liver, and splenomegaly are present. Pruritus is common. Blood pressure increases, the pulse is full and bounding, and dyspnea, headaches, or visual disturbances are common. Thromboses and infarctions may affect the extremities, liver, or kidneys as well as the brain or the heart. Congestive heart failure frequently develops because of the increased work load resulting from the increased volume and viscosity of blood. High levels of uric acid resulting from cell destruction result in severe joint pain.

■ *Diagnostic Tests*

Cell counts are increased, as are hemoglobin values, and hematocrit is elevated. In polycythemia vera, the malignant or abnormal cell is the erythrocyte. Bone marrow is hypercellular, with the red marrow replacing some fatty marrow. Hyperuricemia is present because of the high cell destruction rate.

Treatment

Drugs or radiation may be used to suppress the activity of the bone marrow. There is significant risk that fibrosis or leukemia may develop with these methods. Periodic phlebotomy, or removal of blood, may be used to minimize the possibility of thromboses or hemorrhages.

THINK ABOUT   10-8

Compare the general effects of anemia and polycythemia in terms of hemoglobin level, hematocrit, general appearance, and possible complications.

The Leukemias

The leukemias are a group of neoplastic disorders involving the white blood cells. The estimated number of new cases of leukemia each year is 31,000 including 2500 children. Of these cases, 11,000 are lymphoid, 15,000 are myelogenous, and 5000 fall into other categories. Although some types of leukemia respond well to chemotherapy, overall survival is about 45% with much higher survival rates seen in lymphoid types in children.

Pathophysiology

One or more of the leukocyte types are present as undifferentiated, immature, nonfunctional cells that multiply uncontrollably in the bone marrow and large quantities are released as such into the general circulation (Fig. 10-22). As the numbers of leukemic cells increase, they infiltrate the lymph nodes, spleen, liver, brain, and other organs. Acute leukemias are characterized by a high proportion of very immature, nonfunctional cells (blast cells) in the bone marrow and peripheral circulation; the onset usually is abrupt, with marked signs and complications. Chronic leukemias have a higher proportion of

mature cells (although they may have reduced function), with an insidious onset, mild signs, and thus a better prognosis.

Depending on the particular stem cell affected, both acute and chronic leukemias can be further differentiated according to the cell type involved; for example, lymphocytic leukemia. The four major types are acute lymphocytic leukemia (ALL), chronic lymphocytic leukemia (CLL), acute myelogenous leukemia (AML), and chronic myelogenous leukemia (CML). Most cases of ALL involve the precursors to B-lymphocytes. Myelogenous leukemia affects one or more of the granulocytes. The neoplastic stem cell may, in some cases of myelogenous leukemia, involve all blood cells. The major groups are then further differentiated; for example, acute monoblastic leukemia, which is a type of myelogenous leukemia. In some severe forms of acute leukemias, only undifferentiated stem cells can be identified. When the cells are primitive, the term *blast* may be used in the name. Several detailed classifications for the leukemias are available. A brief summary can be found in Table 10-3.

The proliferation of leukemic cells in the bone marrow suppresses the production of other normal cells, leading to anemia, thrombocytopenia, and a lack of normal functional leukocytes (Fig. 10-23). The rapid turnover of cells leads to hyperuricemia and a risk of kidney stones and kidney failure, especially in patients who are receiving chemotherapy. The crowding of the bone marrow causes severe bone pain resulting from pressure on the nerves in the rigid bone and the stretching of the periosteum. As the malignancy progresses, the increased numbers of leukemic cells cause congestion and enlargement of lymphoid tissue, lymphadenopathy, splenomegaly, and hepatomegaly. Death usually results from a complication such as overwhelming infection or hemorrhage.

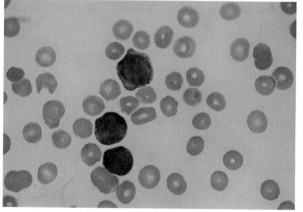

FIGURE 10-22 Acute lymphocytic leukemia, common in young children. Blood smear shows small lymphocytes and normocytic anemia. *(From Stevens ML: Fundamentals of Clinical Hematology, Philadelphia, 1997, Saunders.)*

TABLE 10-3	Types of Leukemias	
Type	Malignant Cell	Primary Age Group
Acute lymphocytic leukemia (ALL)	B-lymphocytes	Young children
Acute myelogenous (or myelocytic) leukemia (AML)	Granulocytic stem cells	Adults
Chronic lymphocytic leukemia	B-lymphocytes	Adults greater than 50 years
Chronic myelogenous leukemia (CML)	Granulocytic stem cells	Adults 30-50
Acute monocytic leukemia	Monocytes	Adults
Hairy cell leukemia	B-lymphocytes	Males greater than 50 years

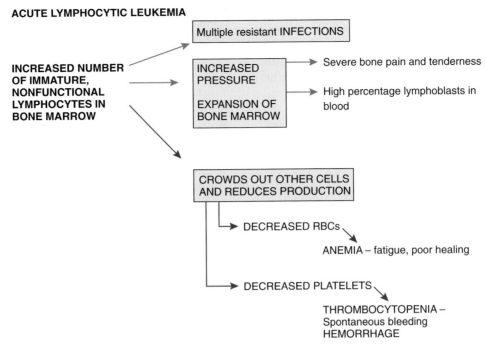

FIGURE 10-23 Effects of acute lymphocytic leukemia.

Etiology

Chronic leukemias are more common in older people, whereas acute leukemias occur primarily in children and younger adults. Acute lymphocytic leukemia (ALL), the most common childhood cancer, usually begins between the ages of 2 and 5 years and constitutes 80% of childhood leukemia cases. The cause in children has not been established. Acute myelogenous leukemia (AML) is common in adults. A number of factors have been shown to be associated with leukemia in adults, including exposure to radiation, chemicals such as benzene, and certain viruses. It may develop years after a course of chemotherapy, particularly those protocols incorporating alkylating agents.

There also appears to be an association of leukemia, particularly ALL, with chromosomal abnormalities, particularly translocations; this factor is evident in the increased incidence of leukemia in children with Down syndrome. Of interest is the fact that many adults with chronic myeloblastic leukemia have the Philadelphia chromosome (#22), a specific abnormal chromosomal translocation that serves as a marker in the diagnosis of chronic myeloblastic leukemia.

Signs and Symptoms

The onset of acute leukemia is usually marked by infection that is unresponsive to treatment or by excessive bleeding, and these problems persist through the active stages of the disease and may be life threatening.

- Multiple infections often develop because of the nonfunctional WBCs.
- Severe hemorrhage (in the brain or digestive tract) occurs because of thrombocytopenia.

- The signs of anemia develop as the erythrocyte count drops.
- Bone pain is severe and steady, continuing during rest.
- Weight loss and fatigue result from the hypermetabolism associated with neoplastic growth, from anorexia caused by infection, from pain, and from the effects of chemotherapy.
- Fever may result from hypermetabolism or infection.
- The lymph nodes, spleen, and liver are often enlarged and may cause discomfort.
- If leukemic cells infiltrate the central nervous system, headache, visual disturbances, drowsiness, or vomiting follows.

Chronic leukemia tends to have a more insidious onset, with milder signs, and may be diagnosed during a routine blood check. Early signs include fatigue, weakness, and frequent infections.

Diagnostic Tests

Peripheral blood smears show the immature leukocytes and the altered numbers of WBCs, which are usually greatly increased. A high percentage of the WBCs are immature and appear abnormal. Numbers of RBCs and platelets are decreased. Bone marrow biopsy confirms the diagnosis.

Treatment

Chemotherapy is administered (see Chapter 20). Some types of leukemia, such as ALL in young children, respond well to drugs, and the prognosis is excellent, with many children enjoying a cure. The best prognosis is found in children between 1 and 9 years of age, infants and adolescents respond less positively to chemotherapy. The more rapid the response to drugs, the more positive is the outlook. Chemotherapy is less successful in adults with AML, although remissions may be achieved. Biologic therapy, such as interferon, to stimulate the immune system, has been used in cases of CML. Even with treatment, the course of CML may accelerate in some cases to an acute stage. Individuals with chronic leukemia may live up to 10 years with treatment. The prognosis is often related to the WBC count and the proportion of blast cells present at the time of diagnosis.

It is important to try to maintain the proper level of nutrition and hydration, particularly if high uric acid levels develop. Alkalinizing the urine by ingesting antacids may help prevent the formation of uric acid kidney stones. Chemotherapy may have to be temporarily discontinued if the blood cell counts drop too low, for example, in marked thrombocytopenia or neutropenia (a reduction in circulating neutrophils). Transfusions of platelets and/or blood cells may be required.

Bone marrow transplantation may be tried when chemotherapy is ineffective. Any tumor cells must be eradicated in the recipient's bone marrow, and a suitable donor must be located before transplantation is attempted (see earlier section on Aplastic Anemia).

THINK ABOUT 10-9

a. Compare and contrast the characteristics of acute and chronic leukemias, including the age groups involved, onset, and typical blood cell characteristics.

b. Why are multiple opportunistic infections common in patients with leukemia?

c. Explain why it is best to defer (if possible) any invasive procedures in leukemic patients, including dental treatment, until the blood counts become normal.

d. The mouth and mucosa of the digestive tract are usually inflamed and ulcerated because of anemia, the effects of chemotherapy, and the presence of infections, such as candidiasis. Explain how this situation would affect food and fluid intake and list some possible subsequent effects on the patient with leukemia.

CASE STUDY A

Acute Lymphocytic Leukemia

P.M., aged 4 years, has returned to the family physician because of a recurrent sore throat and cough. Her mother mentions unusual listlessness and anorexia. The physician notices several bruises on her legs and arms and one on her back. The physician orders blood tests and a course of antibacterial drugs. Test results indicate a low hemoglobin level, thrombocytopenia, and a high lymphocyte count, with abnormally high numbers

of blast cells. Following a bone marrow aspiration, a diagnosis of ALL is confirmed.

1. Describe the pathophysiology of ALL.
2. State the rationale for each of P.M.'s signs.
3. Explain the significance of blast cells in the peripheral blood.
4. Describe the effects of hypermetabolism in leukemia.
5. Explain how chemotherapy aggravates the effects of leukemia (refer to Chapter 20).
6. Describe the possible effects if leukemic cells infiltrate the brain.
7. Describe the pain associated with leukemia and explain the reason for it.

CHAPTER SUMMARY

Blood serves many purposes in the body. Abnormalities involving blood cells, plasma proteins, or blood clotting factors frequently have widespread and possibly life-threatening effects on the body. When lymphatic disorders interfere with the immune response, serious consequences may result.

- Anemias may be caused by many factors, including dietary deficits, malabsorption syndromes, genetic defects, damage to the bone marrow, or blood loss.
- Chronic blood loss causes iron-deficiency anemia with production of hypochromic, microcytic RBCs.
- Pernicious anemia is a megaloblastic anemia resulting from a deficit of intrinsic factor required for the absorption of vitamin B_{12}. Peripheral nerve degeneration and hypochlorhydria accompany the anemia.
- Pancytopenia characterizes aplastic anemia, with impaired production of all blood cells.
- Sickle cell anemia and thalassemia are caused by inherited defects in hemoglobin synthesis. These result in excessive hemolysis and a low erythrocyte count.
- Polycythemia may occur as a primary or secondary problem. Increased RBCs cause vascular congestion.
- Hemophilia A is a genetic blood-clotting disorder related to a deficit of factor VIII. Replacement therapy is now available. Infections such as hepatitis B and HIV have been transmitted through transfusions to many of these patients.
- When DIC develops as a complication of trauma, infection, or other primary problems, generalized blood clotting occurs, using up available blood clotting factors, and subsequently causing hemorrhage. The balance between coagulation and hemorrhage varies with the individual patient, the underlying problem, and the difficulty in treating the combination of problems.
- Myelodysplastic syndrome is comprised of a number of conditions in which the bone marrow does not

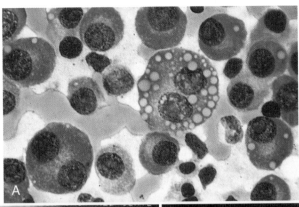

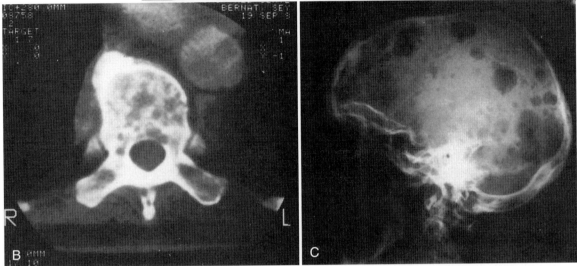

FIGURE 10-24 **A,** Bone marrow aspirate from a patient with multiple myeloma showing a large number of abnormal plasma cells with multiple nuclei and cytoplasmic droplets. *(From Kumar V, et al, editors:* Robbins Basic Pathology, *ed 8, Philadelphia, 2007, Saunders, p 455.)* Vertebral body **(B)** and skull **(C)** radiographs showing the characteristic "honeycomb" appearance of demineralized bone associated with multiple myeloma. *(Courtesy Marvin J. Stone, MD, Sammons Cancer Center, Baylor University Medical Center, Dallas. From Copstead LE, Banasik J:* Pathophysiology, *ed 5, St. Louis, 2013, Mosby.)*

produce adequate cellular elements for the blood. It may be related to prior history of chemotherapy or radiation.

- Leukemias may be acute or chronic. They are named by the specific neoplastic cell that is proliferating excessively in the bone marrow. The malignant cells are immature and nonfunctional, increasing the risk of infection. Thrombocytopenia and anemia are also present.

STUDY QUESTIONS

1. Name six substances that are transported in the blood and the function of each.
2. Explain the importance/function for each of the following:
   a. High elastic fiber content in the aorta
   b. Smooth muscle in the arterioles
   c. Extensive capillaries in the liver and lungs
   d. Valves in the leg veins
3. Explain the cause of incompatible blood transfusion.
4. List three types of clotting problems.
5. Explain how pernicious anemia may develop from chronic gastritis.
6. For which conditions could secondary polycythemia develop as compensation? VSD, CHF, chronic lung disease, aplastic anemia, multiple myeloma
7. Explain how DIC develops and state two signs of its development.
8. Explain why severe bone pain occurs with leukemia.

ADDITIONAL RESOURCES

Guyton AC, Hall JE: *Textbook of Medical Physiology*, ed 12, Philadelphia, 2007, Saunders.

Kliegman RM, Marcdante K, Jenson HB, Behrman RE: *Nelson Essentials of Pediatrics*, 5th ed. Philadelphia, Saunders, 2006.

Kumar V, Abbas AK, Fausto M: *Robbins and Cotran Pathologic Basis of Disease*, ed 8, Philadelphia, 2007, Saunders.

Patton KT, Thibodeau GA: *Anatomy and Physiology*, ed 7, St. Louis, 2010, Mosby.

Web Sites

http://www.cancer.gov *National Cancer Institute, U.S. National Institutes of Health*

http://www.lls.org *The Leukemia & Lymphoma Society*

http://www.mayoclinic.com *Mayo Clinic*

http://www.nlm.nih.gov/medlineplus *U.S. National Library of Medicine and National Institutes of Health*

http://www.mskcc.org *Memorial Sloan-Kettering Cancer Center*

http://www.nhlbi.nih.gov/health/public/blood *National Heart, Lung and Blood Institute, National Institutes of Health*

http://www.vasculardisease.org

Lymphatic System Disorders

CHAPTER OUTLINE

LEARNING OBJECTIVES

After studying this chapter, the student is expected to:

1. Identify the structures that comprise the lymphatic system and their general functions.
2. Differentiate between the vessels of the lymphatic system and blood vessels based on structure, function, and general circulation.
3. Compare and contrast Hodgkin's and non-Hodgkin's lymphomas based on pathophysiology, signs and symptoms, diagnosis, and treatment.

4. Describe the pathophysiology, signs and symptoms, and treatment of multiple myeloma.
5. Identify and describe those disorders resulting from obstruction of the flow of lymph in the lymphatic circulation.
6. Describe the pathophysiology, signs and symptoms, and treatment of Castleman disease

KEY TERMS

Ann Arbor staging system
Castleman disease
fascia
filaria

hydrocele
lymph
lymphedema

lymphoma
myeloma
Reed-Sternberg cell

spleen
thymus gland
tonsils

Review of the Lymphatic System

Structures and Function

The lymphatic system consists of lymphatic vessels, lymphoid tissue, which includes the palatine and pharyngeal tonsils, lymph nodes the spleen, and the thymus gland (Fig. 11-1). The system functions to return excess interstitial fluid and protein to the blood, to filter and destroy unwanted material from the body fluids, and to initiate an immune response.

Lymphatic vessels originate as microscopic capillaries that are in direct contact with tissue cells and the interstitial fluid surrounding the cells (Fig. 11-2). These capillaries in turn form branches, then trunks, and finally ducts. These ducts empty into the left and right subclavian veins. Although similar in structure to veins, lymphatic vessels have thinner walls, more valves, and contain nodes at certain intervals. The thinner walls allow an increased degree of permeability allowing large molecules and some particulate matter to be removed from the interstitial spaces. Proteins that eventually accumulate in the interstitial fluids can only be returned to the blood system through the lymphatic vessels. Any condition that might affect normal return from lymphatic vessels to the blood vessels could have a dramatic effect on blood protein concentration and osmotic pressure with serious or fatal results. Lymph capillaries in the villi of the small intestines are called lacteals and have the important function in the absorption of fats and other nutrients that are produced as a result of digestion.

The lymph nodes and lymphoid tissue act as a defense system, removing foreign or unwanted material

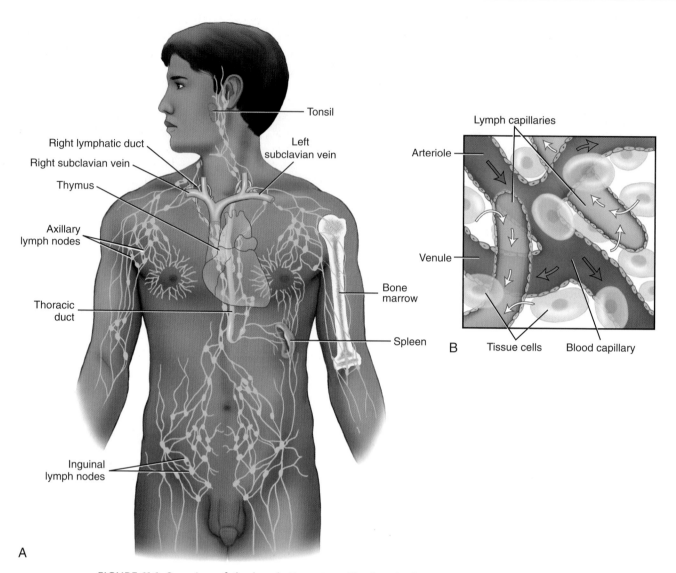

FIGURE 11-1 Overview of the lymphatic system. The lymphatic system consists of lymphatic vessels, lymphoid tissue and cells, and lymphatic organs. *(From VanMeter K, Hubert R:* Microbiology for the Healthcare Professional, *St. Louis, 2010, Elsevier.)*

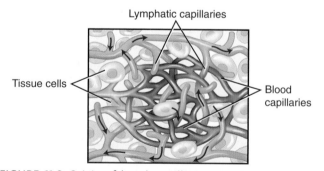

FIGURE 11-2 Origin of lymph capillaries. Lymph capillaries are microscopic blind-ended vessels originating in the capillary beds of tissues. *(From VanMeter K, Hubert R:* Microbiology for the Healthcare Professional, *St. Louis, 2010, Elsevier.)*

from the lymph fluid before it enters the general circulation. When infection is present, the regional lymph nodes are often swollen and tender; for example, upper respiratory infection causes enlarged nodes in the neck area. Lymph nodes containing many lymphocytes and macrophages are situated along all lymphatic and blood vessels, ensuring constant filtration and surveillance of body fluids. As well, the lymph nodes are essential to the immune response and the sensitization of B and T lymphocytes (see Chapter 7).

The palatine and pharyngeal tonsils are composed of lymphoid tissue and are located in a ring under the mucous membrane of the mouth and at the back of the throat. These tonsils function as protection against bacterial infection in the area of the openings between the nasal and oral cavities. The tonsils are truly the first line of defense from invasion by external organisms and are therefore often subject to infections such as tonsillitis.

Removal of the tonsils when infected has been a controversial topic due to the important immunological role that is played by lymphoid tissue.

The spleen is located on the left side of the abdominopelvic cavity directly below the diaphragm. As with other lymphoid organs, the spleen is surrounded by a fibrous capsule and internally it is divided into compartments (see Fig. 11-2).

The spleen has many functions: defense, hematopoiesis, and red blood cell and platelet destruction, as well as serving as a reservoir for blood.

As part of the body's defense, the blood passes through the spleen, where macrophages remove microorganisms from the blood and destroy them through phagocytosis.

In the role of hematopoiesis, monocytes and lymphocytes mature and become activated in the spleen and before birth erythrocytes are also formed in the spleen. After birth the spleen is responsible for red blood cell formation only in extreme cases of hemolytic anemia.

The function of red blood cell and platelet destruction is carried out by macrophages that destroy old blood cells and platelets through phagocytosis. These cells also break down the hemoglobin molecules from the destroyed RBCs and salvage the iron and globin portion of the hemoglobin, where they are then returned to the blood circulation for storage in the liver and bone marrow.

Finally, as a blood reservoir the spleen contains a large amount of blood in the pulp and venous sinuses. This blood can be quickly returned to the circulatory system if needed. This large reservoir of blood also damages the spleen, in the form of severe trauma, a serious problem that can result in rapid death; for instance, if a rib punctures the spleen with its significant volume of stored blood.

The thymus gland consists of two lobes and is located in the mediastinum, lying in front of the top half of the heart and extending up the neck to the bottom of the thyroid gland. The thymus is covered by a fibrous capsule that extends inward to subdivide the lobes into small lobules (Fig. 11-3).

The thymus plays a critical role as part of the immunity mechanism against infections. In this role it has at

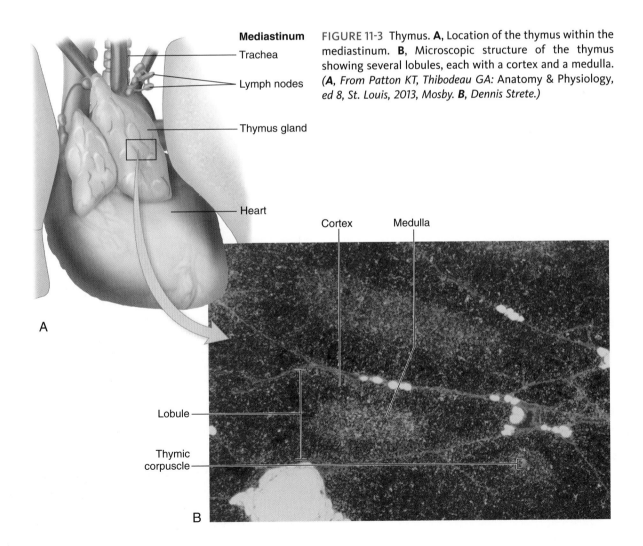

Mediastinum
— Trachea
— Lymph nodes
— Thymus gland
— Heart

A

FIGURE 11-3 Thymus. **A,** Location of the thymus within the mediastinum. **B,** Microscopic structure of the thymus showing several lobules, each with a cortex and a medulla. (**A,** *From Patton KT, Thibodeau GA:* Anatomy & Physiology, *ed 8, St. Louis, 2013, Mosby.* **B,** *Dennis Strete.*)

Cortex   Medulla

Lobule —
Thymic corpuscle —

B

least two primary functions: the final site of lymphocyte development before birth and the secretion of hormones after birth, which enable lymphocytes to develop into mature T cells (Fig. 11-4). Because of the T cell's functions in attacking foreign or abnormal cells and as regulators of immune function, the role of the thymus is extremely important as part of the immune mechanism of the body.

Composition and Production of Lymph

Lymph is the clear, watery, isotonic fluid that is circulated in the lymphatic vessels. Lymph and interstitial fluid (see Chapter 2) are almost chemically identical when taken from the same part of the body. Both also closely resemble blood plasma; however, they usually contain a lower protein percentage than plasma except in the thoracic duct. Here in the thoracic duct, the lymph is protein rich as a result of the outflow into the duct from the liver and small intestine. Interstitial fluid that is not absorbed by the cells or the capillaries tends to accumulate in the interstitial spaces and as this fluid builds it will drain into the lymphatic vessels and become lymph.

Lymphatic Circulation

The lymphatic circulation functions as follows:

1. It begins with blind-ending capillaries containing one-way minivalves at the terminus, into which excess interstitial fluid flows as pressure builds up in the tissues (Fig. 11-5).
2. The lymphatic capillaries join to form larger vessels with valves to ensure a one-way flow of fluid, similar to the network of veins. Flow depends on pressure arising from movement of surrounding skeletal muscle and organs (Fig. 11-6).
3. Lymphatic vessels are interrupted periodically by lymph nodes, at which point the lymph is filtered and more lymphocytes may enter the lymph en route to the general circulation.
4. The vessels of the upper right quadrant of the body empty into the right lymphatic duct, which returns the lymph into the general circulation via the right subclavian vein.
5. The remainder of the lymphatic vessels drain into the thoracic duct in the upper abdomen and thoracic cavity. This duct drains into the left subclavian vein.
6. Lymphatic capillaries in the intestinal villi absorb and transport most lipids as chylomicrons.

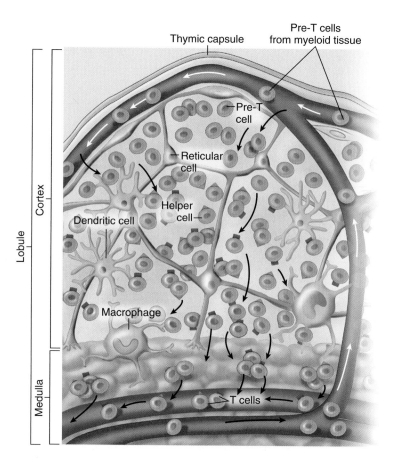

FIGURE 11-4 T-cell development in the thymus. This diagram shows part of a lobule, with the cortex at the top and the medulla at the bottom. Pre-T cells derived from hematopoietic stem cells in red bone marrow (myeloid tissue) travel through the bloodstream to the cortex of the thymus. Under the influence of thymosin and other regulators, the pre-T cells divide and mature as they migrate toward the medulla. Along the way, the developing T cells (T lymphocytes) are tested for immune capability against various lymphoid immune cells, such as dendritic cells and macrophages. Only about 5% of the cells pass these tests and are released into the bloodstream to defend the body. *(From Patton KT, Thibodeau GA: Anatomy & Physiology, ed 8, St. Louis, 2013, Mosby.)*

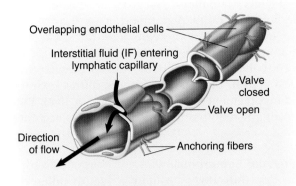

Overlapping endothelial cells

Interstitial fluid (IF) entering lymphatic capillary

Valve closed

Valve open

Direction of flow

Anchoring fibers

FIGURE 11-5 Structure of a typical lymphatic capillary. Notice that interstitial fluid enters through clefts between overlapping endothelial cells that form the wall of the vessel. Valves ensure one-way flow of lymph out of the tissue. Small fibers anchor the wall of the lymphatic capillary to the surrounding extracellular matrix and cells, thus holding it open to allow entry of fluids and small particles. *(From Patton KT, Thibodeau GA:* Anatomy & Physiology, *ed 8, St. Louis, 2013, Mosby.)*

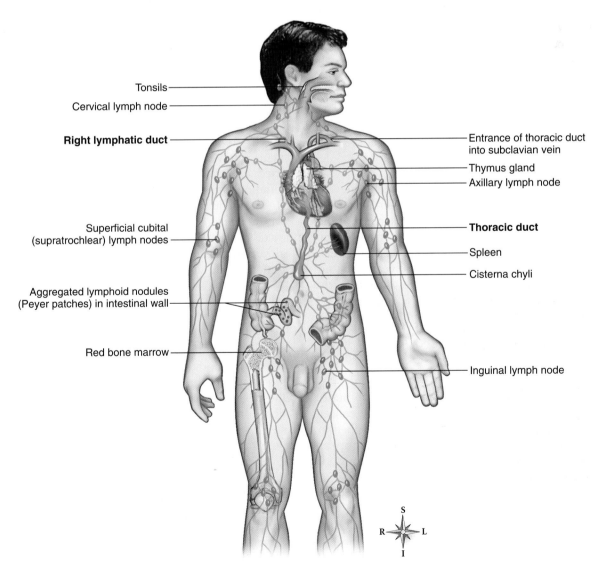

Tonsils

Cervical lymph node

Right lymphatic duct

Superficial cubital (supratrochlear) lymph nodes

Aggregated lymphoid nodules (Peyer patches) in intestinal wall

Red bone marrow

Entrance of thoracic duct into subclavian vein

Thymus gland

Axillary lymph node

Thoracic duct

Spleen

Cisterna chyli

Inguinal lymph node

FIGURE 11-6 Principal organs of the lymphatic system. *(From Patton KT, Thibodeau GA:* Anatomy & Physiology, *ed 8, St. Louis, 2013, Mosby.)*

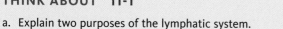

THINK ABOUT 11-1

a. Explain two purposes of the lymphatic system.
b. Predict the result of destruction of the lymph nodes in a specific region.
c. Under what circumstances might lymph nodes be surgically removed?

Lymphatic Disorders

A common infection involving the lymphatic system, infectious mononucleosis, is covered in Chapter 23.

Lymphomas

Lymphomas are malignant neoplasms involving lymphocyte proliferation in the lymph nodes. The two main disorders, Hodgkin's lymphoma and non-Hodgkin's lymphoma, actually a group of lymphomas, are differentiated by lymph node biopsy. Many research projects have focused on characterizing new types of lymphoma and determining a classification system. One component of the latter relates to how rapidly growing or aggressive the tumor is. Specific causes of lymphomas have not been identified, but there is a higher incidence in adults who received radiation treatments during childhood.

Hodgkin's Disease/Hodgkin's Lymphoma

The incidence of Hodgkin's lymphoma has declined in recent years; it was estimated that approximately 9290 new cases would be diagnosed in 2013. The onset of the disease occurs primarily in adults 20 to 40 years of age, with equal numbers in men and women. A second peak occurrence is found in those more than 50 years old, but primarily in men. The prognosis for patients in the early stages of disease, when the malignancy is *localized*, is excellent; many are considered cured with survival rates well beyond 5 years.

■ *Pathophysiology*

The malignancy initially involves a single lymph node, frequently in the neck area (Fig. 11-7). Later the cancer spreads to *adjacent nodes in an orderly fashion* and then to organs via the lymphatics. The T lymphocytes appear to be defective, and the lymphocyte count is decreased. The atypical cell used as a marker for diagnosis of Hodgkin's lymphoma is the Reed-Sternberg cell, a giant cell present in the lymph node (Fig. 11-8). Hodgkin's disease can be subdivided into four subtypes based on the cells found at biopsy.

Various staging systems are available. Staging for Hodgkin's lymphoma uses the diaphragm as the differential landmark (Fig. 11-9). The Ann Arbor staging system generally defines a stage I cancer as affecting a single lymph node or region and stage II as affecting two or more lymph node regions on the same side of the diaphragm or in a relatively localized area. Stage III cancer involves nodes on both sides of the diaphragm and the spleen. Stage IV represents diffuse extralymphatic involvement such as bone, lung, or liver. Extensive testing is required to stage lymphomas accurately.

■ *Signs and Symptoms*

- The first indicator is usually a lymph node, often cervical, that is large, *painless*, and *nontender*.
- Later splenomegaly and enlarged lymph nodes at other locations may cause pressure effects; for example, enlarged mediastinal nodes may compress the esophagus.
- General signs of cancer, such as weight loss, anemia, low-grade fever and night sweats, and fatigue may develop.
- Generalized pruritus is common.
- Recurrent infection is common because the abnormal lymphocytes interfere with the immune response.

■ *Treatment*

Radiation, chemotherapy, and surgery are used with much greater success now than formerly. Although many newer drugs and combinations have been tried, one of the most effective remains the ABVD combination illustrated in Figure 20-10. For a patient in stage II, three courses of chemotherapy at 4-week intervals would be suggested, and then the patient's status evaluated. In the advanced stages, remissions are common, although secondary cancers have occurred in some patients following extensive treatment.

Non-Hodgkin's Lymphomas

Non-Hodgkin's lymphomas are increasing in incidence, partly due to the numbers associated with HIV infection. Non-Hodgkin's lymphomas are similar to Hodgkin's lymphoma only in some ways. About 80% of the cases involve B lymphocytes. The initial manifestation is an enlarged, painless lymph node. The clinical signs, staging, and treatment are similar to Hodgkin's lymphoma.

Non-Hodgkin's lymphoma is distinguished by multiple node involvement scattered throughout the body and a nonorganized pattern of widespread metastases, often present at diagnosis. Intestinal nodes and organs are frequently involved in the early stage. It is more difficult to treat when the tumors are not localized, but the survival rates have risen to 65% from the previous 30%.

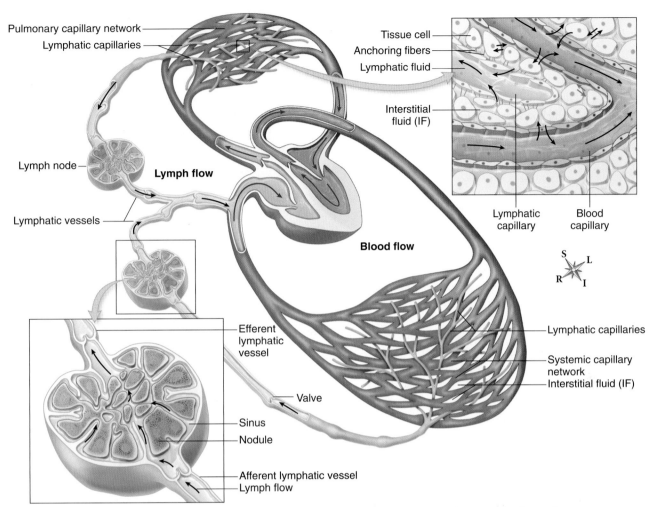

Pulmonary capillary network
Lymphatic capillaries

Lymph node
Lymph flow

Lymphatic vessels

Blood flow

Tissue cell
Anchoring fibers
Lymphatic fluid

Interstitial
fluid (IF)

Lymphatic
capillary

Blood
capillary

S
L
R
I

Efferent
lymphatic
vessel

Lymphatic capillaries

Systemic capillary
network
Interstitial fluid (IF)

Valve

Sinus
Nodule

Afferent lymphatic vessel
Lymph flow

FIGURE 11-7 Circulation plan of lymphatic fluid. This diagram outlines the general scheme for lymphatic circulation. Fluids from the systemic and pulmonary capillaries leave the bloodstream and enter the interstitial space, thus becoming part of the interstitial fluid (IF). The IF also exchanges materials with the surrounding tissues. Often because less fluid is returned to the blood capillary than had left it, IF pressure increases, causing IF to flow into the lymphatic capillary. The fluid is then called lymph (lymphatic fluid) and is carried through one or more lymph nodes and finally to large lymphatic ducts. The lymph enters a subclavian vein, where it is returned to the systemic blood plasma. Thus fluid circulates through blood vessels, tissues, and lymphatic vessels in a sort of "open circulation." *(From Patton KT, Thibodeau GA: Anatomy & Physiology, ed 8, St. Louis, 2013, Mosby.)*

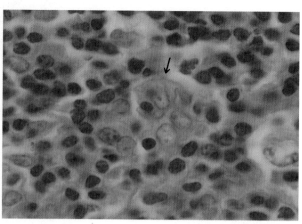

FIGURE 11-8 A Reed-Sternberg cell (*arrow*) diagnostic for Hodgkin's lymphoma. This lymphocyte is large with an irregular nucleus. *(From Stevens ML: Fundamentals of Clinical Hematology, Philadelphia, 1997, Saunders.)*

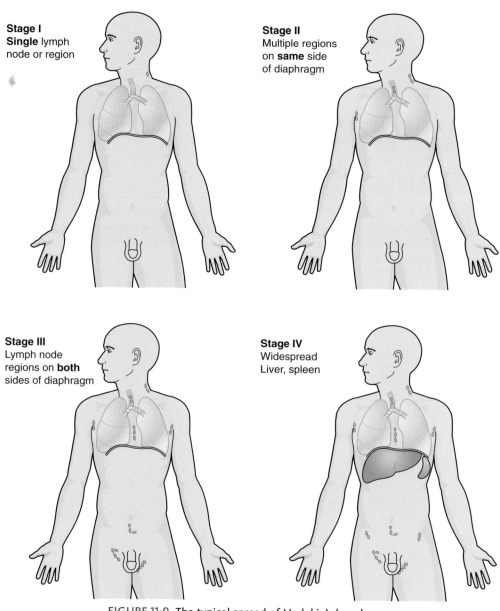

Stage I
Single lymph
node or region

Stage II
Multiple regions
on **same** side
of diaphragm

Stage III
Lymph node
regions on **both**
sides of diaphragm

Stage IV
Widespread
Liver, spleen

FIGURE 11-9 The typical spread of Hodgkin's lymphoma.

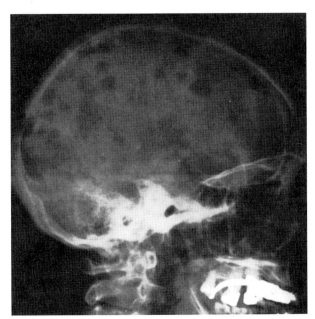

FIGURE 11-10 Multiple myeloma of the skull. Radiograph shows punched-out bone lesions filled with soft tumor. *(From Kumar V, Abbas AK, Fausto M: Robbins and Cotran Pathologic Basis of Disease, ed 7, Philadelphia, 2005, Saunders.)*

Multiple Myeloma or Plasma Cell Myeloma

▨ *Pathophysiology*

Multiple myeloma is a neoplastic disease of unknown etiology occurring in older adults and involving the plasma cells (mature B lymphocytes involved in production of antibodies). An increased number of malignant plasma cells replace the bone marrow and erode the bone (Fig. 11-10). Blood cell production is impaired, as well as production of antibodies. Multiple tumors with bone destruction develop in the vertebrae, ribs, pelvis, and skull. Pathologic or spontaneous fractures at weakened sites in the bone are common. Hypercalcemia develops as bone is broken down. The tumor cells can spread throughout the body, into lymph nodes and infiltrating many organs. Extensive testing is required for the diagnosis.

▨ *Signs and Symptoms*

The onset is usually insidious and the malignancy well advanced before diagnosis.
- Frequent infections may be the initial sign related to impaired production of antibodies.
- Pain, related to bone involvement, is common and is present at rest.
- Pathologic fractures may occur as bone is weakened.
- Anemia and bleeding tendencies are common because blood cell production is affected.
- Kidney function, particularly the tubules, is affected, leading to proteinuria and kidney failure.

▨ *Treatment*

Chemotherapy is used to encourage remission. Median survival is 3 years. Analgesics for bone pain and treatment for kidney impairment may be needed. Blood transfusions are required in the late stage.

THINK ABOUT 11-2
a. Explain why infections occur frequently in patients with lymphomas.
b. State the prognosis for a person with a stage I and stage IV Hodgkin's lymphoma and explain your reasoning.

Lymphedema

Lymphedema is a condition in which the tissues in the extremities swell due to an obstruction of the lymphatic vessels and the subsequent accumulation of lymph.

▨ *Etiology*

The most common form of the disorder is congenital and may involve not only the vessels, but the lymph nodes as well. It is most often seen in women between the ages of 15 and 25 years. This condition can also be caused by blockage of the lymph vessels by infestation of parasitic worms. This specific form of lymphedema results in a condition called elephantiasis, which is addressed as a separate disorder.

▨ *Signs and Symptoms*

The extremities swell as the lymph accumulates. The swelling may initially be soft, but as the condition progresses, the extremity affected may become firm, painful, and unresponsive to treatment.

Chronic lymphedema may lead to frequent infections, resulting in high fever and chills

▨ *Treatment*

Treatments include:
- Diuretics to reduce the swelling
- Strict bed rest
- Massage of the affected area
- Elevation of the affected extremity

If the edema is severe, infection has set in, or the patient's mobility has been severely impaired, surgical removal of the affected tissue and surrounding fascia may be required. Other surgical options, such as the implanting of a drainage shunt to drain lymph from the superficial to the deep lymphatic circulation, are also possible solutions.

Elephantiasis (Filariasis)

This is a type of lymphedema caused primarily by an infestation and blockage of the lymph vessels of the

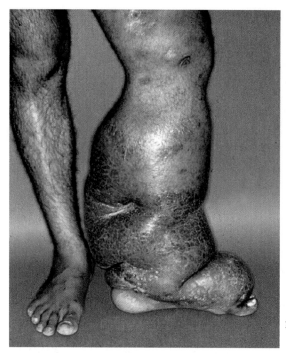

FIGURE 11-11 Elephantiasis. Prolonged infestation of the lymphatic system by *Filaria* worms produces so much swelling (lymphedema) that the affected limbs begin to resemble those of an elephant. *(From Goldstein B, editor:* Practical Dermatology, *ed 2, St. Louis, 1997, Mosby.)*

extremities by a parasitic worm called filaria. There is also relatively rare, nonfilarial form of elephantiasis found primarily in Africa and caused by chemicals from volcanic ash.

■ *Etiology*

The parasitic worms infest the small lymph vessels blocking lymph flow and resulting in significant swelling of the affected extremity. In severe cases the swelling can be so pronounced that the extremity may resemble an elephant's limb, giving this disorder its name (Fig. 11-11).

The nonfilarial elephantiasis is caused by chemicals entering the body through cuts on the feet. The chemicals in the ash irritate the lymph vessels causing swelling, which in turn blocks the lymph vessels, causing excessive swelling of the affected area.

There are other situations that can lead to this condition such as protozoal infection, birth defects in lymphatic vessels, repeated streptococcal infections, and the removal of cancerous lymph nodes.

■ *Signs and Symptoms*

Manifestations of this disorder include:
- Extreme swelling of the legs, breasts, or genitalia
- Thickening of the subcutaneous tissue
- Frequent infections
- Skin ulcerations
- Fever

■ *Diagnosis and Treatment*

Positive diagnosis of lymphatic filariasis is by the detection and identification of the parasitic worms in the blood. Urine can also reveal the presence of the parasites as well as examination of hydrocele fluid.

The primary treatment for lymphatic filariasis is a medication regimen to kill the parasite. In elephantiasis cases resulting in massive enlargement of the legs and resultant ulceration, surgery to perform a fluid shunting procedure may be necessary.

Castleman Disease

Castleman disease is a rare illness that involves the overgrowth of lymphoid tissue. Although this disease is characterized by overgrowth of lymphatic cells, it is not considered a cancer, but is associated with a higher risk of lymphoma.

■ *Pathophysiology and Etiology*

Also known as giant lymph node hyperplasia and angiofollicular lymph node hyperplasia, this disease is classified as a lymphoproliferative disorder. There are two types of Castleman disease: unicentric, which affects only a single lymph node, and multicentric, which affects multiple lymph nodes and tissue and may lead to a severe weakening of the immune system.

■ *Signs and Symptoms*

In the unicentric form of the disease, manifestations include:
- Difficulty breathing or eating due to fullness or pressure in the chest or abdomen
- A large lump in the neck, armpit, or groin
- Unexplained weight loss and anorexia
- Persistent cough

In the multicentric form of the disease, manifestations include:
- Fever and night sweats
- Nausea and vomiting leading to a loss of appetite and resulting in weight loss
- Weakness and overall fatigue
- Enlarged spleen, liver and/or peripheral lymph nodes in the neck, groin, or armpits
- Numbness or weakness in the hands and feet due to nerve damage

■ *Diagnosis*

A number of tests can be used to diagnosis the disease, which include:
- Physical examination of the lymph nodes
- Blood and urine tests for anemia, which can be associated with the disease
- Imaging techniques such as x-ray, computed tomography scans, or magnetic resonance imaging to detect the presence and number of any enlarged lymph

nodes as well as the enlargement of organs such as the spleen or liver
- Lymph node biopsy

Treatment

The type of Castleman disease a patient has will determine the specific treatment.

For the unicentric form of the disease, surgical removal of the diseased and enlarged lymph node is the preferred method of treatment. In those cases in which surgical removal of the node may not be possible due to its location, medication such as corticosteroids or radiation treatment may be used to shrink or destroy the node.

For the multicentric form of the disease, the treatment is generally more difficult. Surgical removal of the affected nodes is not practical because the number of nodes involved; however, the removal of an enlarged spleen can ease symptoms in some cases. The primary treatment is the use of medications to target the affected nodes or organs. These medications such as corticosteroids, monoclonal antibodies, antiviral drugs, immune modulators, and some anticancer drugs are being used with varying results.

THINK ABOUT 11-3

Why might the absence of a parasitic nematode in the blood not be a definitive proof that a patient is not suffering from elephantiasis?

CASE STUDY A

Hodgkin's Disease

J.R., age 32 years, noticed a lump on the side of his neck a few months ago. The lump is relatively large, painless, and not tender to the touch. A few days ago he experienced some difficulty swallowing as if there was something putting pressure on his esophagus. He has also noticed unexplained weight loss, fever, night sweats, and general fatigue over the last few weeks. A visit to his physician produced lab results showing a marked decrease in the lymphocyte count as well as the presence of a giant cell in the tissue of a biopsied lymph node, subsequently confirmed as a Reed-Sternberg cell. The lab results confirmed Hodgkin's lymphoma.

1. Describe the pathophysiology of Hodgkin's lymphoma.
2. Outline the conditions of the disease at each of the four stages as defined by the Ann Arbor staging system.
3. List some of the differences between Hodgkin's and non-Hodgkin's lymphoma.
4. List the treatment methods currently available to treat this disease.

CHAPTER SUMMARY

Lymph and the associated vessels, structures, and organs function to return excess interstitial fluid and protein to the blood, to filter and destroy unwanted material from the body fluids, and to initiate an immune response.

- Lymphatic vessels originate as microscopic capillaries that are in direct contact with tissue cells and the interstitial fluid surrounding the cells.
- Lymph nodes containing many lymphocytes and macrophages are situated along all lymphatic and blood vessels, ensuring constant filtration and surveillance of body fluids.
- The spleen has many functions: defense, hematopoiesis, and red blood cell and platelet destruction, as well as serving as a reservoir for blood.
- The thymus gland plays a critical role as part of the immunity mechanism against infections.
- Lymphomas are malignant neoplasms involving lymphocyte proliferation in the lymph nodes.
- In Hodgkin's lymphoma, the T lymphocytes appear to be defective, and the lymphocyte count is decreased.
- Non-Hodgkin's lymphoma is similar to Hodgkin's lymphoma; however, about 80% of the cases involve B lymphocytes, which is not the case in Hodgkin's lymphoma.
- Multiple myeloma is a neoplastic disease of unknown etiology occurring in older adults and involving the plasma cells (mature B lymphocytes involved in production of antibodies).
- Lymphedema is a condition in which the tissues in the extremities swell due to an obstruction of the lymphatic vessels and the subsequent accumulation of lymph.
- Castleman disease is a rare illness that involves the overgrowth of lymphoid tissue; however, it is not considered a cancer.

STUDY QUESTIONS

1. Describe the functions of the lymph nodes, the thymus gland, the tonsils, and the spleen.
2. Trace the basic path of the lymphatic circulation.
3. Compare and contrast Hodgkin's and non-Hodgkin's lymphomas based on pathophysiology, signs and symptoms, diagnosis, and treatments.

4. What are the two forms of Castleman disease and what characteristic(s) distinguish(es) one from another?

ADDITIONAL RESOURCES

Kumar V, Abbas AK, Fausto M: *Robbins and Cotran Pathologic Basis of Disease*, ed 8, Philadelphia, 2007, Saunders.

Patton KT, Thibodeau GA: *Anatomy and Physiology*, ed 7, St. Louis, 2010, Mosby.

Web Sites

http://www.mayoclinic.com *Mayo Clinic*
http://www.lls.org/ *The Leukemia & Lymphoma Society*
http://www.emedicinehealth.com *e medicine health*
www.cancer.org *American Cancer Society*

CHAPTER 12

Cardiovascular System Disorders

CHAPTER OUTLINE

Review of the Cardiovascular System
Heart
Blood Pressure
Heart Disorders
Diagnostic Tests for Cardiovascular
Function
General Treatment Measures for
Cardiac Disorders
Coronary Artery Disease or Ischemic
Heart Disease or Acute Coronary
Syndrome

Cardiac Dysrhythmias
(Arrhythmias)
Congestive Heart Failure
Young Children with Congestive Heart
Failure
Congenital Heart Defects
Inflammation and Infection in the
Heart
Vascular Disorders
Arterial Disorders
Venous Disorders

Shock
Case Studies
Chapter Summary
Study Questions
Additional Resources

LEARNING OBJECTIVES

After studying this chapter, the student is expected to:

1. Describe the common diagnostic tests for cardiovascular function.
2. Describe the dietary and lifestyle changes, and the common drug groups used, in the treatment of cardiovascular disease.
3. Explain the role of cholesterol and lipoproteins in the development of atheromas.
4. Explain the significance of metabolic syndrome in the development of cardiovascular disease.
5. State the factors predisposing to atherosclerosis.
6. Compare angina and myocardial infarction.
7. Describe the common arrhythmias and cardiac arrest.
8. Discuss the causes of congestive heart failure and the effects of left-sided and right-sided failure.

9. Explain the changes in blood flow and their effects in common congenital heart defects.
10. Discuss the development of rheumatic fever and rheumatic heart disease.
11. Describe the etiology and pathophysiology of infectious endocarditis and pericarditis.
12. Explain the development and possible effects of essential hypertension.
13. Compare the arterial peripheral vascular diseases atherosclerosis and aneurysms.
14. Describe the development and effects of the venous disorders varicose veins, phlebothrombosis, and thrombophlebitis.
15. Discuss the types of shock and the initial and progressive effects of shock on the body.

KEY TERMS

adrenergic	baroreceptors	electrodes	orthopnea
anastomoses	bradycardia	endarterectomy	sulcus
angioplasty	cardiomegaly	hemoptysis	syncope
auscultation	depolarization	microcirculation	synergistic
autoregulation	ectopic	murmurs	tachycardia

Review of the Cardiovascular System

Heart

Anatomy

The heart functions as the pump for the circulating blood in both the pulmonary and systemic circulations. The path of a specific component of the blood, such as a red blood cell, through the heart and circulation is illustrated in Figure 12-1.

The heart is located in the *mediastinum* between the lungs and is enclosed in the double-walled *pericardial sac* (see Fig. 12-29). The outer fibrous pericardium

anchors the heart to the diaphragm. The visceral pericardium, also called the epicardium, consists of a serous membrane that provides a small amount of lubricating fluid within the pericardial cavity between the two pericardial membranes to facilitate heart movements. The middle layer of the heart is the myocardium, composed of specialized cardiac muscle cells that contract rhythmically and forcefully to pump blood throughout the organs. The left ventricular wall is thicker because it must eject blood into the extensive systemic circulation. The inner layer of the heart is the *endocardium*, which also forms the four heart valves that separate the chambers of the heart and ensure *one-way flow* of blood.

The atrioventricular (AV) valves separate the atria from the ventricles; they comprise, on the right side, the tricuspid valve with three leaflets or cusps, and on the left side, the mitral or bicuspid valve with two leaflets. The semilunar valves, each with three cusps, include the aortic and pulmonary valves located at the exits to the large arteries from the ventricles. The *septum* separates the left and right sides of the heart.

Conduction System

Impulses to initiate cardiac contractions are conducted along specialized myocardial (cardiac muscle) fibers. No nerves are present within the cardiac muscle. The unique characteristics of cardiac muscle include the presence of intercalated disks at the junctions between fibers. These disks contain desmosomes, connections to prevent muscle cells from separating during contraction; and gap junctions, which permit ions to pass from cell to cell, facilitating rapid transmission of impulses. These specialized structures ensure that all muscle fibers of the two atria normally contract together, followed shortly by the two ventricles. This coordinated effort results in a rhythmic and efficient filling and emptying of the atria and ventricles that has sufficient force to sustain the flow of blood through the body.

The pathway for impulses in the cardiac conduction system is as follows:

- All cardiac muscle cells can initiate impulses, but normally the conduction pathway originates at the sinoatrial (SA) node, often called the *pacemaker*, located in the wall of the right atrium.
- The SA node automatically generates impulses at the basic rate, called the *sinus rhythm* (approximately 70 beats per minute), but this can be altered by autonomic nervous system fibers that innervate the SA node and by circulating hormones such as epinephrine.
- From the SA node, impulses then spread through the atrial conduction pathways, resulting in contraction of both atria.
- The impulses then arrive at the AV node, located in the floor of the right atrium near the septum. This is

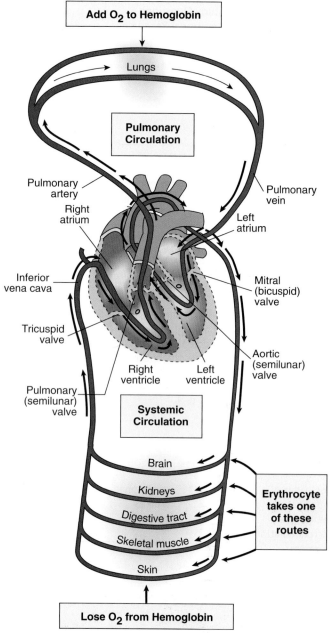

FIGURE 12-1 Path of erythrocyte in the circulation.

the only anatomical connection between the atrial and ventricular portions of the conduction system.

- There is a slight delay in conduction at the AV node to allow for complete ventricular filling; then the impulses continue into the ventricle through the AV bundle (Bundle of His), the right and left bundle branches, and the terminal Purkinje network of fibers, stimulating the simultaneous contraction of the two ventricles.

Conduction of impulses produces a change in electrical activity that can be picked up by electrodes attached to the skin at various points on the body surface, producing the *electrocardiogram (ECG)* (see Fig. 12-2). The atrial contraction is represented by the depolarization in the P wave, and the ventricular contraction is shown by the large wave of depolarization in the ventricles (QRS). This wave masks the effect of atrial repolarization, but the third wave (T wave) represents the repolarization of the ventricles, or recovery phase. Abnormal variations in the ECG known as *arrhythmias* or *dysrhythmias* may indicate acute problems, such as an infarction, or systemic problems, such as electrolyte imbalances (for example, potassium deficiency [see Fig. 2-8]).

Control of the Heart

Heart rate and force of contraction are controlled by the *cardiac control center* in the medulla of the brain. The baroreceptors in the walls of the aorta and internal carotid arteries detect changes in blood pressure and the cardiac center then responds through stimulation of the sympathetic nervous system (SNS) or the parasympathetic nervous system to alter the rate and force of cardiac contractions as required. Sympathetic innervation increases heart rate (tachycardia) and contractility, whereas parasympathetic stimulation by the vagus nerve slows the heart rate (bradycardia). The sympathetic or beta$_1$-adrenergic receptors in the heart (see Chapter 14) are an important site of action for some drugs, such as beta-blockers. Because beta-blockers fit the receptors and prevent normal SNS stimulation, they are used to block any increases in rate and force of contractions after the heart has been damaged.

Factors that increase heart rate include:
- Elevated body temperature, such as in fever
- Increased environmental temperatures, especially if humidity is high
- Exertion or exercise, notably when beginning, followed by a leveling off
- Smoking even one cigarette
- Stress response
- Pregnancy
- Pain

Any stimulation of the SNS, as with stress, increases the secretion of epinephrine, which in turn stimulates beta-receptors and increases both the heart rate and contractility.

[handwritten note: < 60 = bradycardia, >100 = tachycardia]

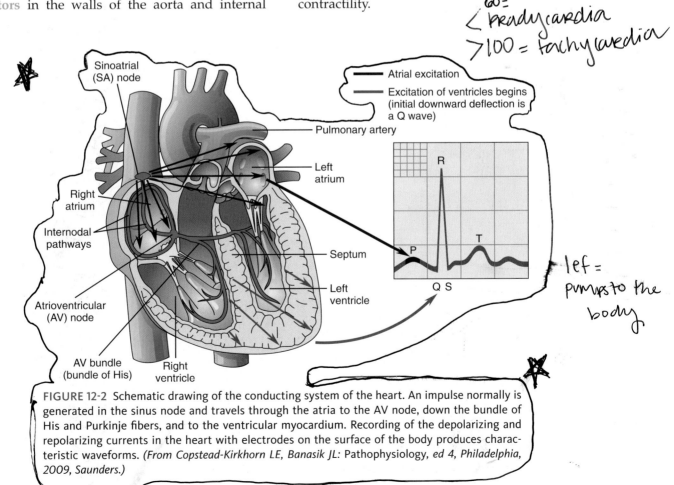

[handwritten note: lef = pumps to the body]

FIGURE 12-2 Schematic drawing of the conducting system of the heart. An impulse normally is generated in the sinus node and travels through the atria to the AV node, down the bundle of His and Purkinje fibers, and to the ventricular myocardium. Recording of the depolarizing and repolarizing currents in the heart with electrodes on the surface of the body produces characteristic waveforms. *(From Copstead-Kirkhorn LE, Banasik JL:* Pathophysiology, *ed 4, Philadelphia, 2009, Saunders.)*

THINK ABOUT   12-1

a. Where is the mitral valve located? Describe the direction and type of blood (oxygenated or nonoxygenated) that flows through this valve.
b. List two functions of the AV node.
c. Describe the control of heart rate during and after exercise.

Coronary Circulation

Cardiac muscle requires a constant supply of oxygen and nutrients to conduct impulses and contract efficiently, but it has very little storage capacity for oxygen.

The distribution of the major blood vessels in the coronary circulation is:

1. Two major arteries, the right and left coronary arteries, branch off the aorta immediately above the aortic valve (Fig. 12-3).
2. The left coronary artery soon divides into the *left anterior descending* or *interventricular artery*, which follows the anterior interventricular sulcus or groove downward over the surface of the heart, and the *left circumflex artery*, which circles the exterior of the heart in the left atrioventricular sulcus.
3. Similarly, the *right coronary artery* follows the right atrioventricular sulcus on the posterior surface of the heart and branches into the right marginal artery and the posterior interventricular artery, and then descends in the posterior interventricular groove

toward the apex of the heart, where it comes close to the terminal point of the left anterior descending artery.

The passage of arteries over the surface of the heart in these grooves is helpful because it permits surgical replacement of obstructed arteries with "bypasses"—using sections of other veins or arteries (see Fig. 12-13 for a diagram of a bypass).

4. Many small branches extend inward from these large arteries to supply the myocardium and endocardium. Blood flow through the myocardium is greatest during diastole or relaxation and is reduced during systole or contraction as the contracting muscle compresses the arteries. Thus, very rapid or prolonged contractions can reduce the blood supply to the cardiac muscle cells.

Anastomoses, or direct connections, exist between small branches of the left and right coronary arteries near the apex, as well as in other areas in which branches are nearby (see Fig. 12-3). These junctions have the potential to open up and provide another source of blood to an area. *Collateral* circulation (alternative source of blood and nutrients) is important if an artery becomes obstructed. When obstruction develops gradually, more capillaries from nearby arteries tend to enlarge or extend into adjacent tissues to meet the metabolic needs of the cells. Regular aerobic exercise contributes to cardiovascular fitness by stimulating the development of collateral channels.

Any interference with blood flow will affect heart function, depending on the specific area supplied by

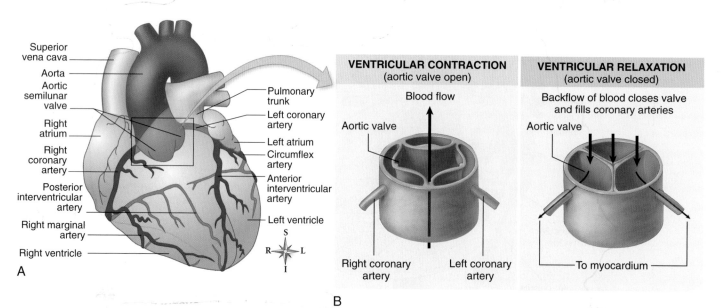

FIGURE 12-3 **Coronary arteries. A,** Diagram showing the major coronary arteries (anterior view). Clinicians often refer to the interventricular arteries as *descending* arteries. Thus a cardiologist would refer to the *anterior descending artery* and an anatomist would refer to the same vessel as the *anterior interventricular artery*. **B,** The unusual placement of the coronary artery opening behind the leaflets of the aortic valve allows the coronary arteries to fill during ventricular relaxation. *(From Patton KT, Thibodeau GA: Anatomy & Physiology, ed 8, St. Louis, 2013, Mosby.)*

that artery. Generally, the right coronary artery supplies the right side of the heart and the inferior portion of the left ventricle, as well as the posterior interventricular septum. The left anterior descending artery brings blood to the anterior wall of the ventricles, the anterior septum, and the bundle branches, and the circumflex artery nourishes the left atrium and the lateral and posterior walls of the left ventricle. The source of blood for the SA node depends on the specific position of the arteries, which varies in individuals. The SA node is supplied by the right coronary artery in slightly more than half the population and by the left circumflex artery in the remainder. The AV node is nourished primarily by the right coronary artery. This information implies that blockage of the right coronary artery is more likely to result in conduction disturbances of the AV node (resulting in dysrhythmias), whereas interference with the blood supply to the left coronary artery will most likely impair the pumping capability of the left ventricle (potentially leading to congestive heart failure).

The course of the coronary or cardiac veins generally parallels that of the arteries, with the majority of the blood returning to the coronary sinus and emptying directly into the right atrium.

APPLY YOUR KNOWLEDGE 12-1

Predict three basic ways that cardiac function could be impaired.

Cardiac Cycle

The cardiac cycle refers to the alternating sequence of *diastole*, the relaxation phase of cardiac activity, and *systole*, or cardiac contraction, which is coordinated by the conduction system for maximum efficiency (see Fig. 12-4).

1. The cycle begins with the two atria relaxed and filling with blood (from the inferior and superior venae cavae into the right atrium, and from the pulmonary veins into the left atrium).
2. The AV valves open as the pressure of blood in the atria increases and the ventricles are relaxed.

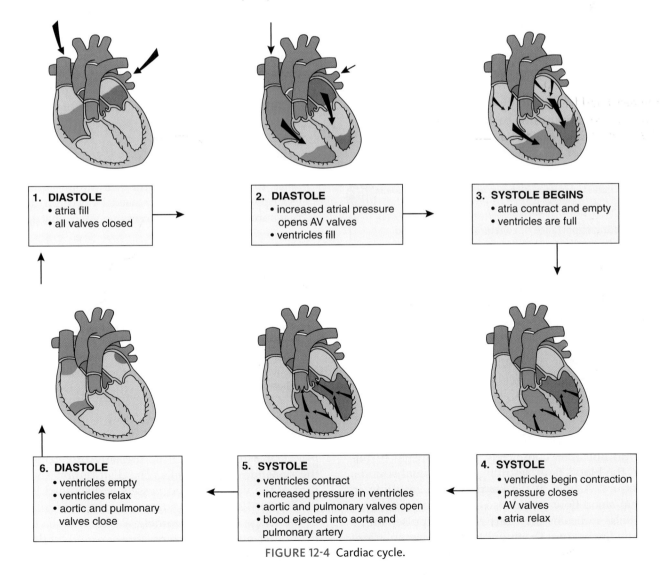

1. DIASTOLE
- atria fill
- all valves closed

2. DIASTOLE
- increased atrial pressure opens AV valves
- ventricles fill

3. SYSTOLE BEGINS
- atria contract and empty
- ventricles are full

6. DIASTOLE
- ventricles empty
- ventricles relax
- aortic and pulmonary valves close

5. SYSTOLE
- ventricles contract
- increased pressure in ventricles
- aortic and pulmonary valves open
- blood ejected into aorta and pulmonary artery

4. SYSTOLE
- ventricles begin contraction
- pressure closes AV valves
- atria relax

FIGURE 12-4 Cardiac cycle.

3. Blood flows into the ventricles, almost emptying the atria.
4. The conduction system stimulates the atrial muscle to contract, forcing any remaining blood into the ventricles.
5. The atria relax.
6. The two ventricles begin to contract, and pressure increases in the ventricles.
7. The AV valves close.
8. For a brief moment, all valves are closed, the ventricular myocardium continues to contract, building up pressure in this isovolumetric phase (no change in blood volume in the ventricles).
9. Then the increasing pressure opens the semilunar valves; blood is forced into the pulmonary artery and aorta. Note that the muscle contraction must be strong enough to overcome the opposing pressure in the artery to force the valve open. This is significant, particularly in the left ventricle, in which the pressure must be greater than the diastolic pressure in the aorta. Because the pulmonary circulation is a low-pressure system, the right ventricle does not have to exert as much pressure to pump blood into the pulmonary circulation.
10. At the end of the cycle, the atria have begun to fill again, the ventricles relax, the aortic and pulmonary valves close to prevent backflow of blood, and the cycle repeats.

The same volume of blood is pumped from the right and left sides of the heart during each cycle. This is important to ensure that blood flow through the systemic and pulmonary circulations is consistently balanced.

THINK ABOUT 12-2

a. Discuss the importance of collateral circulation and explain how collateral circulation can be maximized.
b. Why is there a pause after the atrial contraction and before the ventricular contraction?
c. Predict the outcome if more blood is pumped into the pulmonary circulation than into the systemic circulation during each cardiac cycle.

The *heart sounds,* "lubb-dupp," which can be heard with a stethoscope, result from vibrations due to closure of the valves. Closure of the AV valves at the beginning of ventricular systole causes a long, low "lubb" sound, followed by a "dupp" sound as the semilunar valves close with ventricular diastole. Defective valves that leak or do not open completely cause unusual turbulence in the blood flow, resulting in abnormal sounds, or murmurs. A hole in the heart septum resulting in abnormal blood flow would also cause a heart murmur.

The *pulse* indicates the heart rate. The pulse can be felt by the fingers (not the thumb) placed over an artery that passes over bone or firm tissue, most commonly at the wrist (Fig. 12-5). During ventricular systole, the surge of blood expands the arteries. The characteristics of the pulse, such as weakness or irregularity in a peripheral pulse (e.g., the radial pulse in the wrist), often indicate a problem. The *apical* pulse refers to the rate measured at the heart itself. A *pulse deficit* is a difference in rate between the apical pulse and the radial pulse.

Cardiac function can be measured in a number of ways.

- *Cardiac output* is the volume of blood ejected by a ventricle in one minute and depends on heart rate and *stroke volume,* the volume pumped from one ventricle in one contraction) (Fig. 12-6). This means that at rest, the heart pumps into the system an amount equal to the total blood volume in the body every minute, which is a remarkable feat. When necessary, the normal heart can increase its usual output by four or five times the minimum volume.
- *Stroke volume* varies with sympathetic stimulation and venous return. When an increased amount of blood returns to the heart, as during exercise, the heart is stretched more and the force of the contraction normally increases proportionately. During exercise, stress, or infection, cardiac output increases considerably.
- *Cardiac reserve* refers to the ability of the heart to increase output in response to increased demand.
- *Preload* refers to the mechanical state of the heart at the end of diastole with the ventricles at their maximum volume.
- *Afterload* is the force required to eject blood from the ventricles and is determined by the *peripheral resistance* to the opening of the semilunar valves. For example, afterload is increased by a high diastolic pressure resulting from excessive vasoconstriction.

THINK ABOUT 12-3

a. What information does the ECG provide about heart function?
b. Describe the function of the areas of the heart usually supplied by the left coronary artery.
c. Describe the effect if the atria were to contract at the same time as the ventricles, or if the ventricles contracted slightly before the atria.

Blood Pressure

Blood pressure refers to the pressure of blood against the systemic arterial walls. The distribution and structure of the various blood vessels is discussed in detail in Chapter 10. In adults a normal pressure is commonly in the range of 120/70 mmHg at rest. *Systolic pressure,* the higher number, is the pressure exerted by the blood when ejected from the left ventricle. *Diastolic pressure,*

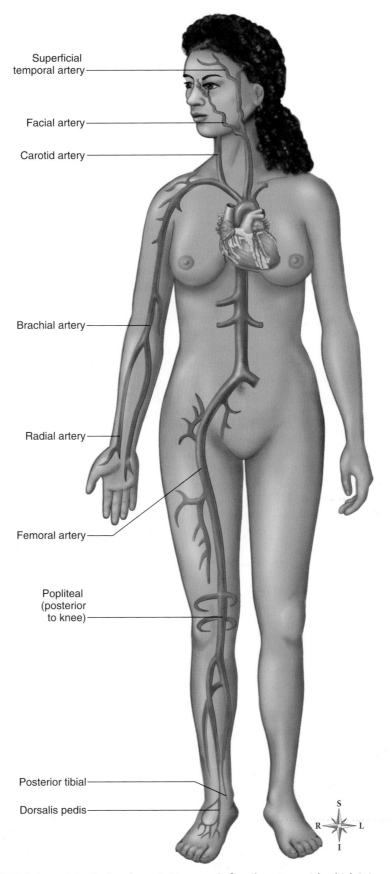

FIGURE 12-5 Pulse points. Each pulse point is named after the artery with which it is associated. (Some arteries in the figure have been enlarged to clarify the location of pulse points.) *(From Patton KT, Thibodeau GA:* Anatomy & Physiology, *ed 8, St. Louis, 2013, Mosby.)*

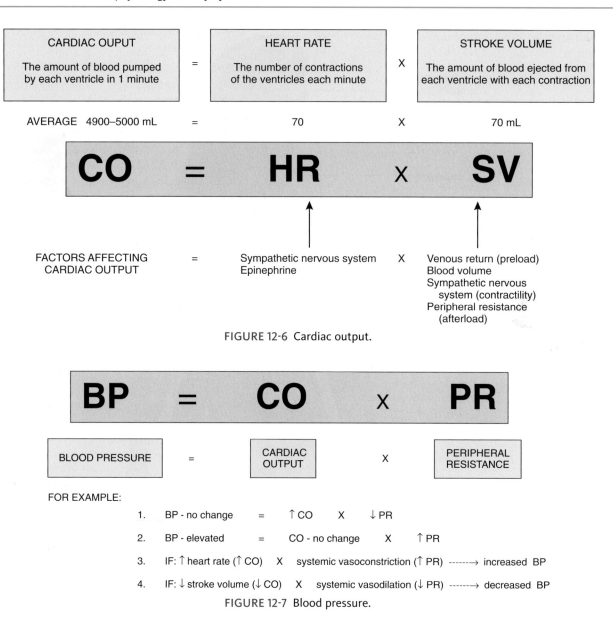

FIGURE 12-6 Cardiac output.

FIGURE 12-7 Blood pressure.

the lower value, is the pressure that is sustained when the ventricles are relaxed. The brachial artery in the arm is used to measure blood pressure with a sphygmomanometer and an inflatable blood pressure cuff. *Pulse pressure* is the difference between the systolic and diastolic pressures.

Blood pressure depends on cardiac output and peripheral resistance (Fig. 12-7). Specific variables include blood volume and viscosity, venous return, the rate and force of heart contractions, and the elasticity of the arteries. *Peripheral resistance* is the force opposing blood flow, or the amount of friction with the vessel walls encountered by the blood. Decreasing the diameter (or lumen) of the blood vessel increases the resistance to blood flow. Normally peripheral resistance can be altered by the systemic constriction or dilation of the arterioles. Systemic or widespread vasoconstriction occurs in response to sympathetic stimulation and increases blood pressure. Systemic or general vasodilation that leads to decreased blood pressure results from reduced SNS stimulation. (There is *no parasympathetic* nervous system innervation in the blood vessels.) Any obstruction in the blood vessel also increases resistance. Local vasoconstriction or dilation does *not* affect the overall systemic blood pressure.

Changes in blood pressure are detected by the baroreceptors and relayed to the vasomotor control center in the medulla, which adjusts the distribution of blood to maintain normal blood pressure. For example, when one rises from a supine position, blood pressure drops momentarily owing to gravitational forces until the reflex vasoconstriction mechanism in the body ensures that more blood flows to the brain.

Blood pressure is elevated by increased SNS stimulation in two ways:

1. SNS and epinephrine act at the beta$_1$-adrenergic receptors in the heart to increase both the rate and force of contraction.

2. SNS, epinephrine, and norepinephrine increase vasoconstriction by stimulating the alpha$_1$-receptors in the arterioles of the skin and viscera. This reduces the capacity of the system and increases venous return.

Other hormones also contribute to the control of blood pressure:

- Antidiuretic hormone (ADH) increases water reabsorption through the kidney, thus increasing blood volume. Antidiuretic hormone, also known as vasopressin, also causes vasoconstriction.
- Aldosterone increases blood volume by increasing reabsorption of sodium ions and water.
- The renin-angiotensin-aldosterone system in the kidneys is an important control and compensation mechanism that is initiated when there is any decrease in renal blood flow. This stimulates the release of renin, which in turn activates angiotensin (vasoconstrictor) and stimulates aldosterone secretion (see Chapter 18). Angiotensin II is a powerful vasoconstrictor.

THINK ABOUT 12-4

a. Explain four factors that can increase blood pressure.
b. List the compensatory mechanisms (in the correct sequence) that can help return the blood pressure to normal levels following a slight drop such as standing up too rapidly.
c. List three ways that systemic circulation could be impaired.
d. Describe the effect of a hot compress on the tissues to which it is applied.
e. How does vasoconstriction in the skin and viscera result in increased venous return to the heart?

Heart Disorders

Heart disease is ranked as a major cause of morbidity and mortality in North America. Common heart diseases include congenital heart defects, hypertensive heart disease, angina and heart attacks, cardiac arrhythmias, and congestive heart failure. There is increasing emphasis on routine preventive measures for all individuals, with a focus on factors such as a healthy diet, regular exercise, moderation in alcohol intake, cessation of smoking, safe sexual practices, immunizations, monitoring body weight and blood pressure, and basic screening tests for cholesterol levels and the presence of cancer.

Diagnostic Tests for Cardiovascular Function

Because many of the same tests are used in the diagnosis and monitoring of a variety of cardiovascular disorders, a few of the basic tests are summarized here.

- An ECG is useful in the initial diagnosis and monitoring of arrhythmias, myocardial infarction, infection, and pericarditis (see Fig. 12-17). It is a noninvasive procedure and can illustrate the conduction activity of the heart as well as the effects of systemic abnormalities such as serum electrolyte imbalance. A portable *Holter monitor* may be worn by an individual to record ECG changes while he or she pursues daily activities. A log of activities is usually maintained to match with the changes in ECG. A normal baseline ECG recording is recommended for everyone; it can be used for comparison if cardiovascular disease ever develops.
- Valvular abnormalities or abnormal shunts of blood cause *murmurs* that may be detected by auscultation of heart sounds by means of a stethoscope. A recording of heart sounds may be made with a phonocardiograph. In *echocardiography,* ultrasound, or reflected sound waves, is used to record the image of the heart and valve movements (see Fig. 12-25). These tests provide useful information regarding valvular abnormalities, congenital defects, and changes in heart structure or function.
- *Exercise stress tests* (bicycle, step, or treadmill) are useful in assessing general cardiovascular function and in checking for exercise-induced problems such as arrhythmias. They may be used in fitness clubs before setting up an individualized exercise program or by insurance companies in the evaluation of an individual's health risks, as well as in cardiac rehabilitation programs following heart attacks or cardiovascular surgery.
- *Chest x-ray films* can be used to show the shape and size of the heart, as well as any evidence of pulmonary congestion associated with heart failure.
- *Nuclear imaging* with radioactive substances such as thallium assesses the size of an infarct in the heart, the extent of myocardial perfusion, and the function of the ventricles. *Tomographic studies,* which illustrate various levels of a tissue mass may be used when available. *Nuclear medicine studies* can identify dead or damaged areas of myocardial tissues and may be used to assess the extent of myocardial damage after a myocardial infarction.
- *SPECT* is a specialized CAT scan that accurately assesses cardiac ischemia at rest. Therapeutic intervention is not possible during this procedure. (Compare with coronary angiography below.)
- *Cardiac catheterization,* passing a catheter through an appropriate blood vessel, usually a large vein in the leg, into the ventricle, may also be utilized to visualize the inside of the heart, measure pressures, and assess valve and heart function. Determination of *central venous pressure* and *pulmonary capillary wedge pressure,* which indicate blood flow to and from the heart, can be made with a catheter. After contrast dye is injected into the ventricle, fluoroscopy can

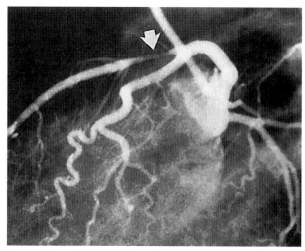

FIGURE 12-8 Coronary angiography shows stenosis (*arrow*) of left anterior descending coronary artery. *(From Braunwald E: Heart Disease: A Textbook of Cardiovascular Medicine, ed 4, Philadelphia, 1992, Saunders.)*

monitor blood movement continuously and check for abnormalities. There is some risk with this procedure, but it has proved beneficial in many instances.

- Blood flow in the coronary arteries can be visualized with coronary *angiography* (Fig. 12-8). Current research using very tiny ultrasound instruments within the vessels has proved more effective in diagnosing obstructions. Obstructions can be assessed and then treated with the basic catheterization procedure, with injected thrombolytic agents or laser therapy to break down clots, or balloon angioplasty to open a narrow coronary artery mechanically.

- *Troponin Blood test* is used to measure the levels of blood proteins called troponins. These proteins are released when cardiac muscle has been damaged. The more damage to the heart, the higher the levels of the troponins. Very high levels of the proteins are an indication that a heart attack has occurred.

- Blood flow in the peripheral vessels can be assessed with *Doppler* studies, in which essentially a microphone that records the sounds of blood flow or obstruction is placed over the blood vessel.

- *Blood tests* are used to assess serum triglyceride and cholesterol levels and the levels of sodium, potassium, calcium, and other electrolytes. Hemoglobin, hematocrit, blood cell counts, and the differential count for white cells are also routine aspects of blood tests.

- *Arterial blood gas determination* is essential in patients with shock or myocardial infarction, to check the current oxygen level and acid-base balance.

Other specific tests are mentioned under the appropriate topic and in Ready Reference 5 at the back of the book. More specialized tests may be necessary.

General Treatment Measures for Cardiac Disorders

Because some treatment measures apply to many disorders, a number of common therapies are covered here. Additional specific treatment modalities are mentioned with the disorder to which they apply.

1. Dietary modifications usually include reducing total fat intake and intake of saturated (hydrogenated or animal) fat as well as "trans" fats, which are commercially hydrogenated plant oils used to stabilize convenience foods. General weight reduction may be recommended for some persons. Salt (sodium) intake is decreased as well in order to reduce blood pressure. The American Heart Association has current dietary guidelines.

2. A regular exercise program is suggested to improve overall cardiovascular function and circulation to all areas of the body. Exercise assists in lowering serum lipid levels, increasing high-density lipoprotein (HDL) levels, and reducing stress levels, which in turn lessen peripheral resistance and blood pressure.

3. Cessation of cigarette smoking decreases the risk of coronary disease. Smoking appears to increase vasoconstriction and the heart rate, thus increasing the workload on the heart. Smoking increases platelet adhesion and the risk of thrombus (clot) formation, as well as increasing serum lipid levels. Also, carbon monoxide, a product of smoking, displaces oxygen from hemoglobin. In a compromised patient, this decrease in oxygen can be dangerous.

4. Drug therapy is an important component in the maintenance of cardiac patients. Many individuals take several drugs. Common medications include:
   - *Vasodilators,* such as nitroglycerin or long-acting isosorbide, reduce peripheral resistance systemically and therefore the workload for the heart and also act as coronary vasodilators. These actions provide a better balance of oxygen supply and demand in the heart muscle. Vasodilators may cause a decrease in blood pressure, resulting in dizziness or syncope and a flushed face. A person should sit quietly for a few minutes after taking nitroglycerin sublingually.
   - *Beta-blockers* such as metoprolol or atenolol are used to treat hypertension and dysrhythmias, as well as to reduce the number of angina attacks. These drugs block the beta$_1$-adrenergic receptors in the heart and prevent the SNS from increasing heart activity.
   - *Calcium channel blockers,* which block the movement of calcium ions into the cardiac and smooth muscle fiber, make up another group of effective cardiovascular drugs. Members of the group may be used as agents to decrease cardiac contractility, as an antidysrhythmic particularly for excessive atrial activity, or as an antihypertensive and

vasodilator. They also serve a prophylactic purpose for angina. Some drugs such as diltiazem are more selective for the myocardium and reduce both conduction and contractility. Verapamil slows the heart rate by depressing the action of the SA and AV nodes, preventing tachycardia and fibrillation. Others, like nifedipine, are more effective as peripheral vasodilators. Amlodipine (Norvasc) has been useful in lowering blood pressure. Note that these drugs do not affect skeletal muscle contraction because more calcium is stored in skeletal muscle cells.

- *Digoxin,* a cardiac glycoside, has been used for many years as a treatment for heart failure and as an antiarrhythmic drug for atrial dysrhythmias. It slows conduction of impulses and heart rate. Digoxin improves the efficiency of the heart because it also is inotropic, increasing the contractility of the heart. The contractions are less frequent but stronger. Because the effective dose is close to the toxic dose, patients must be observed for signs of toxicity, and blood levels of the drug must be checked periodically.

- *Antihypertensive drugs* may be used to lower blood pressure to more normal levels. There are a number of groups in this category, including the adrenergic or sympathetic-blocking agents, the calcium blockers, the diuretics, the angiotensin-converting enzyme (ACE) inhibitors, and the angiotensin II receptor blocking agents. Combinations of drugs from various classifications are frequently prescribed to effectively lower blood pressure. Some of these drugs do cause orthostatic hypotension, a drop in blood pressure accompanied by dizziness, when arising from a recumbent position. These drugs may be used for treatment of essential hypertension or congestive heart failure or after myocardial infarction. Calcium blockers and beta-adrenergic blockers were discussed previously.

- *Adrenergic-blocking drugs* may act on the SNS centrally (brain), may block peripheral (arteriolar) alpha$_1$-adrenergic receptors, or may act as direct vasodilators.

- *Angiotensin-converting enzyme inhibitors* (ACE inhibitors) are currently preferred in the treatment of many patients with hypertension and congestive heart failure (CHF). They act by blocking the conversion of angiotensin I to angiotensin II (stimulated by the release of renin from the kidney). These drugs, such as enalapril (Vasotec), ramipril (Altace), captopril (Capoten) and perindopril (Coversyl), reduce both peripheral resistance (vasoconstriction) and aldosterone secretion (thus decreasing sodium and water retention). The result is a decrease in preload and afterload. Angiotensin II receptor blocking agents such as losartan (Cozaar) and irbesartan (Avapro) prevent angiotensin acting on blood vessels, and thus lower blood pressure. They do not appear to have side effects.

- *Diuretics* remove excess sodium and water from the body through the kidneys by blocking the reabsorption of sodium or water (see Chapter 18). Patients often refer to them as "water pills." They are useful drugs in the treatment of high blood pressure and congestive heart failure because they increase urine output, reducing blood volume and edema. Examples are hydrochlorothiazide, a mild diuretic, and furosemide, a more potent drug. These diuretics may also remove excessive potassium from the body, requiring supplements to prevent hypokalemia. Spironolactone is an example of a "potassium-sparing" diuretic.

- *Anticoagulants* or "blood thinners" may be used to reduce the risk of blood clot formation in coronary or systemic arteries or on damaged or prosthetic heart valves. In many cases, a small daily dose of aspirin (ASA) is recommended to decrease platelet adhesion. Oral anticoagulants such as warfarin (Coumadin) may be taken by individuals in high-risk groups. These drugs block the coagulation process (see Fig. 10-9). Individuals must be cautious about taking other medication, including nonprescription drugs, drinking alcohol, and making dietary changes, and avoid potentially traumatic activities. It is essential to monitor clotting ability, measuring prothrombin time or activated partial thromboplastin time closely in these patients to prevent hemorrhage and to observe patients for increased bleeding tendencies (see blood clotting in Chapter 10).

- *Cholesterol or lipid-lowering* drugs are prescribed when diet and exercise are ineffective in reducing blood levels. These drugs, referred to as the "statins" include simvastatin (Zocor) and atorvastatin (Lipitor). They reduce low-density lipoprotein (LDL) and cholesterol content of the blood by blocking synthesis in the liver. Current investigations are assessing their ability to lower C-reactive protein levels, which has a role in the inflammation associated with atheroma formation.

Table 12-1 provides a summary of common cardiovascular drugs. A drug index may be found in Ready Reference 8 at the back of the book.

Coronary Artery Disease or Ischemic Heart Disease or Acute Coronary Syndrome

Sometimes called coronary heart disease, coronary artery disease includes angina pectoris or temporary cardiac ischemia and myocardial infarction or heart attack. Myocardial infarction results in damage to part of the heart muscle because of obstruction in a coronary

TABLE 12-1   Selected Cardiovascular Drugs

Name	Use	Action	Adverse Effects
Nitroglycerin	Angina attacks and prophylaxis	Reduces cardiac workload, peripheral and coronary vasodilator	Dizziness, headache
Metoprolol (Lopressor)	Hypertension, angina, antiarrhythmic	Blocks beta-adrenergic receptors, slows heart rate	Dizziness, fatigue
Nifedipine (Adalat)	Angina, hypertension, peripheral vasodilator, antiarrhythmic	Calcium blockers, vasodilator	Dizziness, fainting, headache
Digoxin (Lanoxin)	Congestive heart failure and atrial arrhythmias	Slows conduction through AV node and increases force of contraction (cardiotonic) to increase efficiency	Nausea, fatigue, headache, weakness
Enalapril (Vasotec)	Hypertension	ACE inhibitor—blocks formation of angiotensin II and aldosterone	Headache, dizziness, hypotension
Furosemide (Lasix) hypertension	Edema with CHF, hypertension	Diuretic—increases excretion of water and sodium	Nausea, diarrhea, dizziness
Simvastatin (Zocor)	Hypercholesteremia (CHD)	Decreases cholesterol and LDL	Digestive discomfort
Warfarin (Coumadin)	Prophylaxis and treatment of thromboemboli	Anticoagulant—interferes with vitamin K in synthesis of clotting	Excessive bleeding (antidote: vitamin K)
ASA (aspirin)	Prophylaxis of thromboemboli	Prevents platelet adhesion, anti-inflammatory	Gastric irritation, allergy

CHD, Coronary heart disease; CHF, congestive heart failure; LDL, low-density lipoprotein.

artery. The basic problem is insufficient oxygen for the needs of the heart muscle.

A common cause of disability and death, coronary artery disease may ultimately lead to heart failure, serious dysrhythmias, or sudden death. It is the leading cause of death in men and women in the United States, causing approximately 385,000 deaths each year. Statistics for 2009 reveal that one in four deaths are the result of some form of heart disease, and the incidence for new or repeated heart attacks is 935,000 Americans. It is estimated that 13.2 million live with coronary artery disease in the United States. An additional 6 million are currently diagnosed with congestive heart failure (there is some overlap within these figures). The CDC reported that in 2008, high blood pressure was listed as a factor in 348,000 deaths and affects 68 million Americans. Males tend to develop heart disease at an earlier age than women, but women tend to have more complications likely due to later diagnosis. The current statistics show a decrease in numbers of individuals being diagnosed with heart disease, which many attribute to prevention awareness programs.

Arteriosclerosis and Atherosclerosis

■ Pathophysiology

Arteriosclerosis can be used as a general term for all types of arterial changes. It is best applied to degenerative changes in the small arteries and arterioles, commonly occurring in individuals over age 50 and those with diabetes. Elasticity is lost, the walls become thick and hard, and the lumen gradually narrows and may become obstructed. This leads to diffuse ischemia and necrosis in various tissues, such as the kidneys, brain, or heart.

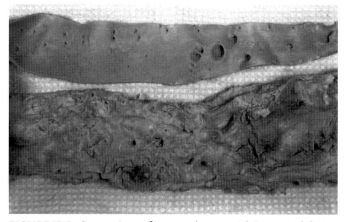

FIGURE 12-9 Comparison of a normal aorta with its smooth lining and patent openings into branching arteries *(top)* with an atherosclerotic aorta *(bottom)*. Note the rough surface and blocked openings to branches. *(Courtesy of Paul Emmerson and Seneca College of Applied Arts and Technology, Toronto, Canada.)*

Atherosclerosis is differentiated by the presence of *atheromas*, plaques consisting of lipids, cells, fibrin, and cell debris, often with attached thrombi, which form inside the walls of large arteries. Note in Figure 12-9 how the unaffected artery is smooth, and the openings to branch arteries are clearly defined. By comparison, the atherosclerotic artery has a very rough, elevated surface, with loose pieces of plaque and thrombus, and the openings to branching arteries are blocked. Atheromas form primarily in the large arteries, such as the aorta and iliac arteries, the coronary arteries, and the carotid arteries, particularly at points of bifurcation,

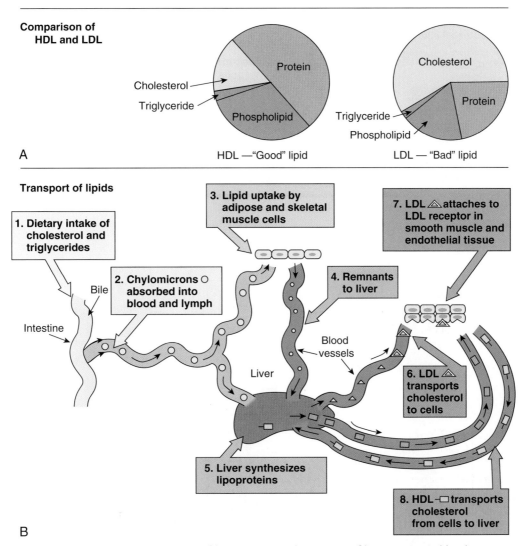

Comparison of HDL and LDL

Cholesterol

Protein

Triglyceride

Phospholipid

Cholesterol

Protein

Triglyceride

Phospholipid

A   HDL —"Good" lipid   LDL — "Bad" lipid

Transport of lipids

3. Lipid uptake by adipose and skeletal muscle cells

1. Dietary intake of cholesterol and triglycerides

7. LDL △ attaches to LDL receptor in smooth muscle and endothelial tissue

Bile

2. Chylomicrons ○ absorbed into blood and lymph

4. Remnants to liver

Intestine

Blood vessels

Liver

6. LDL △ transports cholesterol to cells

5. Liver synthesizes lipoproteins

8. HDL ▭ transports cholesterol from cells to liver

B

FIGURE 12-10 Composition of lipoproteins and transport of lipoproteins in blood.

where turbulent blood flow may encourage the development of atheromas.

Lipids or fats, which are usually transported in various combinations with proteins (lipoproteins), play a key role in this process (Fig. 12-10). Lipids, including cholesterol and triglycerides, are essential elements in the body and are synthesized in the liver; therefore they can never be totally eliminated from the body.

Analysis of serum lipids includes assessment of all the subgroups (total cholesterol, triglycerides, low-density lipoproteins, and high-density lipoproteins) because the proportions indicate the risk factor for the individual. The serum lipids of particular importance follow:

- Low-density lipoprotein, which has a *high* lipid content and transports cholesterol from the liver *to* cells, is the dangerous component of elevated serum levels of lipids and cholesterol. It is a major factor contributing to atheroma formation. Also, LDL binds to receptors, for example on the membranes of vascular smooth muscle cells and enters them; it is

considered the "bad" lipoprotein that promotes atheroma formation.

- High-density lipoprotein is the "good" lipoprotein; it has a *low* lipid content and is used to transport cholesterol *away* from the peripheral cells to the liver, where it undergoes catabolism and excretion.

The process appears to begin with endothelial injury in the artery, often at a very young age. Endothelial injury causes inflammation in the area, leading to elevated C-reactive protein (CRP) levels. White blood cells, particularly monocytes and macrophages, and lipids accumulate in the intima, or inner lining, of the artery and in the media, or muscle layer. Smooth muscle cells proliferate or multiply (Fig. 12-11). Thus, a plaque forms and inflammation persists. Platelets adhere to the rough, damaged surface of the arterial wall, forming a thrombus and partial obstruction of the artery.

Lipids continue to build up at the site of arterial injury, along with fibrous tissue. Platelets adhere and release prostaglandins, which precipitate inflammation and vasospasm. This draws more platelets to aggregate

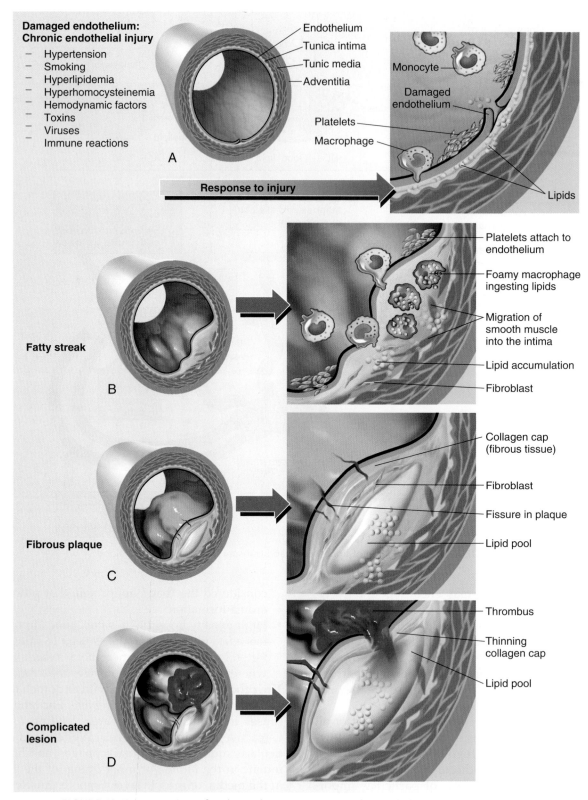

Damaged endothelium:
Chronic endothelial injury

- Hypertension
- Smoking
- Hyperlipidemia
- Hyperhomocysteinemia
- Hemodynamic factors
- Toxins
- Viruses
- Immune reactions

Endothelium
Tunica intima
Tunic media
Adventitia
Monocyte
Damaged endothelium
Platelets
Macrophage
Lipids

A

Response to injury

Platelets attach to endothelium
Foamy macrophage ingesting lipids
Migration of smooth muscle into the intima
Lipid accumulation
Fibroblast

Fatty streak

B

Collagen cap (fibrous tissue)
Fibroblast
Fissure in plaque
Lipid pool

Fibrous plaque

C

Thrombus
Thinning collagen cap
Lipid pool

Complicated lesion

D

FIGURE 12-11 Progression of artherosclerosis. **A,** Damaged endothelium. **B,** Diagram of fatty streak and lipid core formation. **C,** Diagram of fibrous plaque. **D,** Diagram of completed lesion; thrombus is red; collagen is blue. Plaque is complicated by red thrombus deposition. *(From McCance KL, et al: Pathophysiology, ed 6, St. Louis, 2010, Mosby.)*

at the site, enlarging the thrombus. Arterial flow becomes more turbulent, again promoting thrombus formation. A vicious cycle persists. Blood flow progressively decreases as the lumen narrows. At some point, the plaque may ulcerate and break open. This may precipitate more inflammation or a thrombus may form at this site, resulting in total obstruction in a very short time. This may be the precipitating factor for myocardial infarction.

The atheroma also damages the arterial wall, weakening the structure and decreasing its elasticity. In time, atheromas may calcify, causing further rigidity of the wall. This process may lead to aneurysm, a bulge in the arterial wall (see Fig. 12-34), or to rupture and hemorrhage of the vessel.

Initially the atheroma manifests as a yellowish fatty streak on the wall. It becomes progressively larger, eventually becoming a large, firm projecting mass with an irregular surface on which a thrombus easily forms. As the atheroma increases in size and the coronary arteries are partially obstructed, angina (temporary myocardial ischemia) may occur; a total obstruction leads to myocardial infarction. Atheromas are also a common cause of strokes, renal damage, and peripheral vascular disease, which affects the legs and feet (Fig. 12-12).

■ *Etiology*

The cause of atherosclerosis appears to be multifactorial, and some of the factors are synergistic, enhancing the total effect. There are two groups of risk factors for atherosclerosis, one group that can be modified to some extent and one that cannot.

The factors that cannot be changed (nonmodifiable) include:

- Age, with atherosclerosis more common after age 40 years, particularly in men
- Gender, that is, women are protected by higher HDL levels until after menopause, when estrogen levels decrease.
- Genetic or familial factors seem to have a strong influence on serum lipid levels, metabolism, and cell receptors for lipids; some conditions are inherited, such as familial hypercholesterolemia, but family lifestyle factors may also have a role.
- The other group of predisposing factors are *modifiable*. These include factors such as:
  - Obesity or diets high in cholesterol and animal fat, which elevate serum lipid levels, especially LDL. The significant increase in obesity in children is of great concern with regards to a relative increase in cardiovascular disease in the coming years. The Centers for Disease Control and Prevention estimate that more than12.5 million children and adolescents under age 19 in the United States are obese and at risk of metabolic syndrome. Data collected in the United States for 2011 also indicated that 35.7% of adult men and women were clinically obese. Obesity is the primary indicator of *metabolic syndrome*, which is directly linked with the development of coronary artery disease in adulthood (see Chapter 23).
  - Cigarette smoking. The risk associated with smoking is directly related to the number of packs of cigarettes smoked per day. Smoking decreases

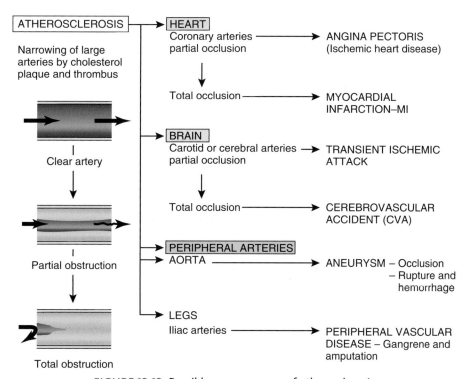

FIGURE 12-12 Possible consequences of atherosclerosis.

HDL, increases LDL, promotes platelet adhesion, and increases fibrinogen and clot formation as well as vasoconstriction.

- Sedentary lifestyle, which predisposes to sluggish blood flow and obesity. Exercise also reduces blood pressure and stress level and increases HDL while lowering LDL and cholesterol. Increasing numbers of children and adults report declining levels of physical activity.
- The presence of diabetes mellitus. In individuals with diabetes, especially those whose disease is not well controlled, serum lipid levels are increased and there is a tendency toward endothelial degeneration. The substantial increase in incidence and earlier onset in recent years of type 2 diabetes has increased the incidence of cardiovascular disease.
- Poorly controlled hypertension, which causes endothelial damage
- Combination of some oral contraceptives and smoking
- The combination of high blood cholesterol and high blood pressure in an individual has been shown to increase the risk of atherosclerosis and coronary artery disease significantly.

■ Diagnostic Tests

Serum lipid levels, including those of LDL and HDL, should be checked to identify the patient's risk and monitor the efficacy of treatment. Serum levels of high-sensitivity CRP indicate the presence of inflammation, indicating increased risk. However, CRP may be elevated due to other chronic inflammatory disease. Low CRP levels appear to indicate a low risk of developing cardiovascular disease. Exercise stress testing can be used for screening or to assess the degree of obstruction in arteries. Nuclear medicine studies can be used to determine the degree of tissue perfusion, the presence of collateral circulation, and the degree of local cell metabolism. To minimize risk and promote early diagnosis and treatment, the acceptable range for test results may be modified or lowered as new evidence becomes available.

APPLY YOUR KNOWLEDGE 12-2

Research is continuing to investigate the role of microbial infections in the damage of blood vessels. What are some portals of entry or potential sources from which bacteria may gain entry into the circulatory system and reach vessels such as the coronary arteries? What measures could be taken to prevent these types of infections and subsequent vessel damage?

■ Treatment

1. Losing weight and maintaining weight at healthy levels reduces the onset of metabolic syndrome as well as hypertension and atherosclerosis. Waist measurements below 35 in/87.5 cm in females and below 40 in/100 cm in males are considered healthy benchmarks.
2. Lowering serum cholesterol and LDL levels by substituting nonhydrogenated vegetable oils for trans fats and saturated fats has been well promoted as an effective means of slowing the progress of atherosclerosis. Vegetable oils containing linolenic acid and fish oils and other foods containing Omega 3 fatty acids are considered particularly useful. High dietary fiber intake also appears to decrease LDL levels. General weight reduction decreases the workload on the heart. Lipid-reducing (cholesterol or LDL) drugs such as probucol, clofibrate, and lovastatin may help in resistant cases. These measures may slow the progress of previously formed lesions and also prevent new ones.
3. Sodium intake should be minimized as well to control hypertension.
4. Control of primary disorders such as diabetes or hypertension is important.
5. Cease smoking.
6. Exercise appropriate for age and health status will promote collateral circulation and reduce LDL levels.
7. If thrombus formation is a concern, oral anticoagulant therapy may be required; this may include a small daily dose of ASA or warfarin (Coumadin).
8. When atheromas are advanced, surgical intervention (percutaneous transluminal coronary angioplasty may be required to reduce obstruction by means of invasive procedures requiring cardiac catheterization. The catheter contains an inflatable balloon that flattens the atheroma. Newer techniques use laser angioplasty, a laser beam, and fiberoptic technology with a catheter. The high-energy laser causes the obstruction to disintegrate into microscopic particles that are removed by macrophages. There appears to be less risk of recurrence with this method. Stents, small tube-like structures, may be inserted into arteries after angioplasty, to maintain an opening. Surgery such as coronary artery bypass grafting (CABG) to reroute blood flow around the obstruction, using veins or the left internal mammary artery for a graft, appears to have an improved long-term prognosis (Fig. 12-13). A graft can also be placed around an obstructed aorta. Less invasive means of CABG are currently being used in some patients.

THINK ABOUT 12-5

a. Explain three ways of reducing the risk of atherosclerosis.
b. Give three common locations of atheromas.
c. Describe two ways in which an artery can become totally obstructed.

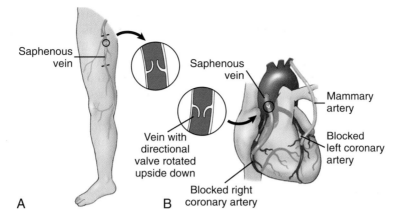

FIGURE 12-13 Coronary artery bypass graft (CABG) surgery. *(From Shiland BJ: Medical Terminology and Anatomy for ICD-10 Coding. St. Louis, 2012, Mosby.)*

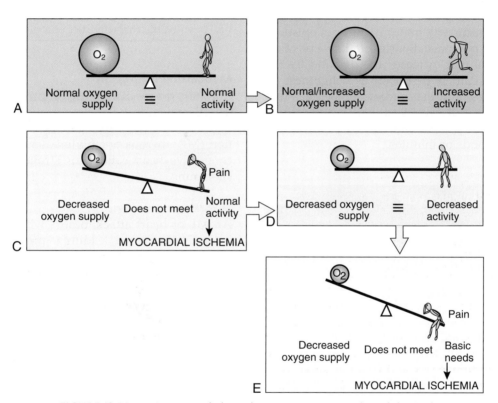

FIGURE 12-14 Angina—an imbalance between oxygen supply and demand.

Angina Pectoris

▪ *Pathophysiology*

Angina, or chest pain, occurs when there is a deficit of oxygen to the heart muscle. This can occur when the blood or oxygen supply to the myocardium is impaired, when the heart is working harder than usual and needs more oxygen, or when a combination of these factors is present (Fig. 12-14). Usually the heart can adapt its blood supply to its own needs by vasodilation (auto-regulation) unless the vessel walls are damaged or cannot relax. The reduced blood supply may be due to partial obstruction by atherosclerosis or spasm in the coronary arteries. When the supply and demand for oxygen are marginally balanced, an increase in cardiac demand with any physical or emotional exertion can cause a relative deficit of oxygen to the myocardium.

Chest pain may occur in a variety of patterns: classic or exertional angina; variant angina, in which vasospasm occurs at rest; and unstable angina, a more serious form. Unstable angina refers to prolonged pain at rest and of recent onset, perhaps the result of a break in an atheroma. This may precede a myocardial infarction. Most commonly, an episode of anginal pain occurs when the demand for oxygen increases suddenly, with exertion. In most cases, no permanent damage to the myocardium results from angina unless the episodes are frequent, prolonged, and severe.

■ *Etiology*

Insufficient myocardial blood supply is associated with atherosclerosis, arteriosclerosis, vasospasm (a localized contraction of arteriolar smooth muscle), and myocardial hypertrophy, in which the heart has outgrown its blood supply. Severe anemias and respiratory disease can also cause an oxygen deficit. Increased demands for oxygen can arise in circumstances such as tachycardia associated with hyperthyroidism or the increased force of contractions associated with hypertension.

Precipitating factors of angina attacks are related to activities that increase the demands on the heart, such as running upstairs, getting angry, respiratory infection with fever, exposure to weather extremes or pollution, or eating a large meal.

■ *Signs and Symptoms*

Angina occurs as recurrent, intermittent brief episodes of substernal chest pain, usually triggered by a physical or emotional stress that increases the demand by the heart for oxygen. Pain is described as a tightness or pressure in the chest and may radiate to the neck and left arm. Often pallor, diaphoresis (excessive sweating), and nausea are also present. Attacks vary in severity and last a few seconds or minutes.

EMERGENCY TREATMENT FOR ANGINA ATTACK

1. Let patient rest, stop activity.
2. Seat patient in an upright position.
3. Administer nitroglycerin sublingually (preferably patient's own supply).
4. Check pulse and respiration.
5. Administer oxygen if necessary.
6. For a patient known to have angina, the American Heart Association recommends that a second dose of nitroglycerin be given if pain persists more than 5 minutes. After three doses within a 10-minute period and no pain relief, the pain should be treated as a heart attack. Call for assistance and emergency medical intervention.
7. For a patient without a history of angina, emergency medical aid should be sought after 2 minutes without pain relief.

■ *Treatment*

Anginal pain is usually quickly relieved by rest and the administration of coronary vasodilators, such as nitroglycerin. The drug may relieve vasospasm in the coronary arteries but primarily acts to reduce systemic resistance, thus decreasing the demand for oxygen. Many patients carry nitroglycerin (in the correct dosage) with them at all times to be administered sublingually in an emergency (the tablet is not swallowed but dissolves under the tongue and enters the blood directly for instant effect). If chest pain persists following treatment, it is important to seek hospital care because the pain may indicate the presence of a myocardial infarction.

It is important to determine the history of angina and the factors predisposing to attacks to minimize their frequency and severity. The avoidance of sudden physical exertion, especially in cold or hot weather, marked fatigue, or strong emotional incidents, is recommended. Antianxiety and stress reduction techniques may be necessary in certain situations. Some clients use nitroglycerin in the form of a topical ointment, a skin patch, a nasal spray, or oral tablets (isosorbide) on a regular basis to reduce the number of attacks.

THINK ABOUT   12-6

a. Describe the characteristics of anginal pain.

Myocardial Infarction

Coronary heart disease is the primary cause of death in US males and females as well as a major cause of disability. For those who survive a myocardial infarction (MI), there is notably greater risk of a second MI, congestive heart failure, or stroke occurring within a short time.

■ *Pathophysiology*

An MI, or heart attack, occurs when a coronary artery is totally obstructed, leading to prolonged ischemia and cell death, or infarction, of the heart wall (Fig. 12-15A,B). The most common cause is atherosclerosis, usually with thrombus attached (see previous discussion under Coronary Artery Disease).

Infarction may develop in three ways:
1. The thrombus may build up to obstruct the artery.
2. Vasospasm may occur in the presence of a partial occlusion by an atheroma leading to total obstruction.
3. Part of the thrombus may break away, forming an embolus or emboli that flow(s) through the coronary artery until lodging in a smaller branch, blocking that vessel (see Fig. 12-11). Most infarctions are transmural; that is, all three layers of the heart are involved. The majority involve the critical left ventricle. The size and location of the infarct determine the severity of the damage.

At the point of obstruction the heart tissue becomes necrotic, and an area of injury, inflammation, and ischemia develops around the necrotic zone (see Fig. 12-15A). With cell destruction, specific enzymes are released from the myocardium into tissue fluid and blood; these enzymes appear in the blood and are diagnostic. The functions of myocardial contractility and conduction are lost quickly as oxygen supplies are depleted. If the blood supply can be restored in the first 20 to 30 minutes,

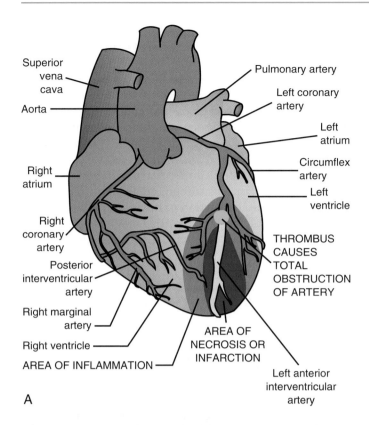

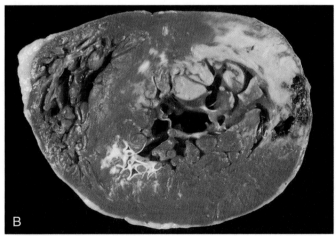

FIGURE 12-15 **A,** Damage caused by myocardial infarction. **B,** Acute myocardial infarct of the posterolateral left ventricle, shown by lack of stain in the necrotic area. Note the dark area on the right indicating hemorrhage and ventricular rupture. The white area on the lower left indicates an old infarct. *(From Kumar V, Abbas AK, Fausto M: Robbins and Cotran Pathologic Basis of Disease, ed 7, Philadelphia, 2005, Saunders.)*

irreversible damage may be prevented. After 48 hours, the inflammation begins to subside. If sufficient blood supply has been maintained in the outer area of inflammation, function can resume. On the other hand, if treatment has not been instituted quickly or is not effective, the area of infarction may increase. Because the myocardial fibers do not regenerate, the area of necrosis is gradually replaced by fibrous (nonfunctional) tissue,

beginning around the seventh day. It may take 6 to 8 weeks to form a scar, depending on the size of the infarcted area.

The presence of collateral circulation may reduce the size of the infarct (see Review of the Normal Cardiovascular System earlier in this chapter). The effectiveness of collateral circulation depends on the location of the obstruction, the presence or absence of anastomoses, and whether collateral circulation was established before infarction in response to the gradual development of a partial occlusion. Also, if the atheroma has developed gradually, there may have been several warning episodes of chest pain with exertion. If the infarction results from an embolus, there is no opportunity for collateral channels to develop, and therefore the infarcted area will usually be larger. Cardiac demand during the attack will also determine the effectiveness of collateral circulation.

> **WARNING SIGNS OF HEART ATTACK**
>
> (These signs may be intermittent initially.)
> 1. Feeling of pressure, heaviness, or burning in the chest, especially with increased activity
> 2. Sudden shortness of breath, sweating, weakness, fatigue
> 3. Nausea, indigestion
> 4. Anxiety and fear

■ Signs and Symptoms

It is important to seek a diagnosis and medical care as soon as these signs occur to prevent permanent heart damage or death. If thrombolytic therapy is administered within 20 minutes of the onset, blood flow can be restored, and no permanent damage occurs in the heart. Many paramedic teams can now administer fibrinolytic drugs, saving many lives. Automated external defibrillators (AEDs) may be found in many public buildings to be used in event of cardiac arrest.

As a myocardial infarction develops, the following manifestations become more evident:

* Pain: Sudden substernal chest pain that radiates to the left arm, shoulder, jaw, or neck is the hallmark of myocardial infarction. The pain is usually described as severe, steady, and crushing, and no relief occurs with rest or vasodilators. In some cases, pain is not present (*silent* myocardial infarction) or is interpreted as gastric discomfort. Women often report a milder pain, more like indigestion.
* Pallor and diaphoresis, nausea, dizziness and weakness, and dyspnea
* Marked anxiety and fear
* Hypotension: Hypotension is common, and the pulse is rapid and weak as cardiac output decreases and shock develops.
* Low-grade fever

■ Diagnostic Tests

1. Typical changes occur in the ECG during the course of a myocardial infarction, which confirm the diagnosis and assist in monitoring progress.
2. Serum enzymes and isoenzymes released from necrotic cells also follow a typical pattern, with elevations of lactic dehydrogenase (LDH-1), aspartate aminotransferase (AST, formerly SGOT), and creatine phosphokinase with M and B subunits (CK-MB or CPK-2) (Fig. 12-16). The particular isoenzymes, LDH-1 and CK-MB, are more specific for heart tissue.
3. Serum levels of myosin and cardiac troponin are elevated a few hours after MI, providing for an earlier confirmation. A rise in cardiac troponin levels is considered most specific for myocardial tissue damage.
4. Serum electrolyte levels, particularly potassium and sodium, may be abnormal.
5. Leukocytosis and an elevated CRP and erythrocyte sedimentation rate are common, signifying inflammation. There is evidence that high blood levels of CRP indicate a more marked inflammatory response, with plaques more inclined to rupture, thrombus to form, and ultimately a more severe heart attack.
6. Arterial blood gas measurements will be altered particularly if shock is pronounced.
7. Pulmonary artery pressure measurements are also helpful in determining ventricular function.

■ Complications

The following are common occurrences immediately following the infarction and also at a later time:

- Sudden death shortly after myocardial infarction occurs frequently (in about 25% of patients), usually owing to ventricular arrhythmias and fibrillation (see next section, Cardiac Dysrhythmias). This is the major cause of death in the first hour after an MI. One type of dysrhythmia, heart block, may occur when the conduction fibers in the infarcted area can no longer function. Second, an area of necrosis and inflammation outside the conduction pathway may stimulate additional spontaneous impulses at an ectopic site, causing, for example, *premature ventricular contractions* (PVCs) that lead to ventricular tachycardia and/or ventricular fibrillation. In some cases, dysrhythmias occur later as inflammation spreads to the conduction pathways, leading to heart block. Conduction irregularities may also be precipitated by hypoxia, by increased potassium released from necrotic cells, acidosis, and drug toxicities.
- Cocaine users may suffer fatal heart attacks, even at a young age, because cocaine interferes with cardiac conduction as well as causing vasospasm and occlusion.
- *Cardiogenic shock* may develop if the pumping capability of the left ventricle is markedly impaired. This greatly reduces cardiac output, leading to significant hypoxia (see the topic of shock later in this chapter).
- *Congestive heart failure* is a common occurrence when the contractility of the ventricle is reduced and stroke volume declines. This may occur a few days after the MI or much later as activity is resumed. (CHF is covered later in this chapter.)

Less frequent complications include:

- *Rupture* of the necrotic heart tissue, particularly in patients with a ventricular aneurysm or those with significant hypertension. This usually develops 3 to 7 days after the MI when the necrotic tissue is breaking down.
- *Thromboembolism* may result from a thrombus that develops over the infarcted surface inside the heart *(mural thrombus)* and eventually breaks off. If originating in the left side of the heart, the embolus will travel to the brain or elsewhere in the body, whereas if the source is the right ventricle, the result will be a pulmonary embolus. (A thrombus may form in the deep leg veins due to immobility and poor circulation and also cause a pulmonary embolus [see Chapter 13].)

■ Treatment

As mentioned, paramedics in many areas are equipped to provide immediate life-saving treatment. Keeping the patient calm, oxygen therapy, and analgesics such as morphine for pain relief are the usual treatment modalities. Anticoagulants such as heparin or warfarin may be used, or the newer thrombolytic agents, including streptokinase, urokinase, or tissue plasminogen activator, may be administered immediately to reduce the clot in the first hours. Depending on the individual circumstances, medication to reduce dysrhythmias, defibrillation, or a pacemaker (which may be temporary) may be

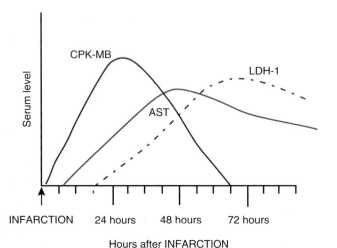

FIGURE 12-16 Serum enzymes and isoenzyme levels with myocardial infarction. *AST*, aspartate aminotransferase; *CPK-MB*, creatine phosphokinase containing M and B subunits; *LDH-1*, lactate dehydrogenase.

required. Drugs, such as digoxin, support the heart function. Specific measures may be required if shock or congestive heart failure develops. Bypass surgery may be performed. Other specific drugs are mentioned in the general treatment section.

Cardiac rehabilitation programs that offer individualized plans for regular exercise, dietary modifications, and stress reduction are useful following recovery. A schedule for the resumption of normal activities, such as climbing stairs, returning to work, and resuming sexual activities, can be established. Appropriate medications to treat any predisposing condition, as well as those to minimize the effects of the MI, are prescribed. Frequently a low dose of ASA is recommended to reduce the risk of further thrombi. The American Heart Association has organized a hospital-based program "Get With The Guidelines" to provide optimum treatment to all patients and promote patient compliance after discharge, thus improving outcomes.

The prognosis depends on the site and size of the infarct, the presence of collateral circulation, and the time elapsed before treatment. The mortality in the first year is 30% to 40% and results from complications or recurrences.

THINK ABOUT 12-7

a. Compare the causes of the chest pain that occurs with angina to that which occurs with myocardial infarction.

b. Explain why an embolus may cause a larger infarction than an atheroma with thrombus.

c. List the tests that confirm a diagnosis of myocardial infarction.

d. Explain why part of the myocardium is nonfunctional following myocardial infarction.

e. Suggest several treatment measures that may minimize the area of infarction. Why is time a critical element in treatment of MI?

Cardiac Dysrhythmias (Arrhythmias)

Deviations from normal cardiac rate or rhythm may result from damage to the heart's conduction system or systemic causes such as electrolyte abnormalities (see Chapter 2 for the effects of potassium imbalance), fever, hypoxia, stress, infection, or drug toxicity. Interference with the conduction system may result from inflammation or scar tissue associated with rheumatic fever or myocardial infarction. The ECG provides a method of monitoring the conduction system and detecting abnormalities (see Fig. 12-16). Holter monitors record the ECG over a prolonged period as a patient follows normal daily activities.

Dysrhythmias reduce the efficiency of the heart's pumping cycle. A slight increase in heart rate increases cardiac output, but a very rapid heart rate prevents adequate filling during diastole, reducing cardiac output, and a very slow rate also reduces output to the tissues, including the brain and the heart itself. Irregular contractions are inefficient because they interfere with the normal filling and emptying cycle. Among the many types of abnormal conduction patterns that exist, only a few examples are considered here.

Sinus Node Abnormalities

The SA node is the pacemaker for the heart, and its rate can be altered.

- *Bradycardia* refers to a regular but slow heart rate, less than 60 beats per minute; it often results from vagal nerve or parasympathetic nervous system stimulation. An exception occurs in athletes at rest, who may have a slow heart rate because they are conditioned to produce a large stroke volume.
- Tachycardia is a regular rapid heart rate, 100 to 160 beats per minute (Fig. 12-17). This may be a normal response to sympathetic stimulation, exercise, fever, or stress, or it may be compensation for decreased blood volume.
- *Sick sinus syndrome* is a heart condition marked by alternating bradycardia and tachycardia and often requires a mechanical pacemaker.

Atrial Conduction Abnormalities

Atrial conduction abnormalities are the most common dysrhythmias, (i.e., clinical abnormalities of heart conduction). Hospital admissions for paroxysmal atrial fibrillation have increased by 66% primarily due to aging of the population and an increase in the prevalence of coronary heart disease.

Premature atrial contractions or *beats* (PAC/PAB) are extra contractions or *ectopic* beats of the atria that usually arise from a focus of irritable atrial muscle cells outside the conduction pathway. They tend to interfere with the timing of the next beat. Ectopic beats may also develop from *re-entry* of an impulse that has been delayed in damaged tissue and then completes a circuit to re-excite the same area before the next regular stimulus arrives. Sometimes people feel *palpitations*, which are rapid or irregular heart contractions that often arise from excessive caffeine intake, smoking, or stress.

Atrial *flutter* refers to an atrial heart rate of 160 to 350 beats per minute, and atrial *fibrillation* is a rate over 350 beats per minute. With flutter, the AV node delays conduction, and therefore the ventricular rate is slower. A pulse deficit may occur because a reduced stroke volume is not felt at the radial pulse. Atrial fibrillation causes pooling of blood in the atria and is treated with anticoagulant medications to prevent clotting and potential cerebrovascular accident (stroke). Ventricular filling is not totally dependent on atrial contraction, and therefore these atrial arrhythmias are not always symptomatic unless they spread to the ventricular conduction pathways.

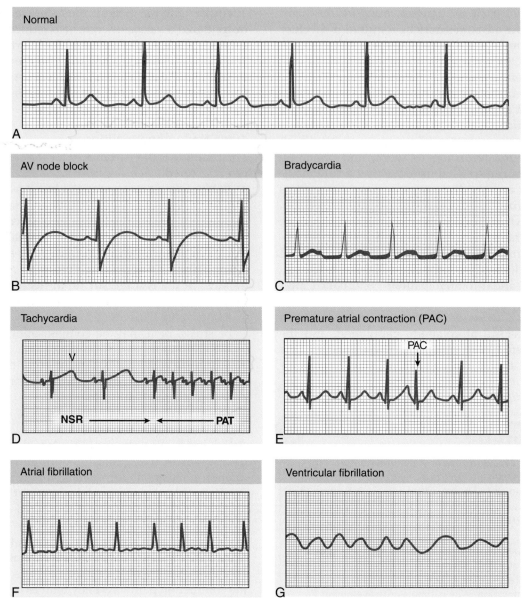

FIGURE 12-17 ECG strip chart recordings. **A,** Normal ECG. **B,** AV node block. Very slow ventricular contraction (25 to 45 beats/min at rest); P waves widely separated from peaks of QRS complexes. **C,** Bradycardia. Slow heart rhythm (less than 60 beats/min); no disruption of normal rhythm pattern. **D,** Tachycardia. Rapid heart rhythm (greater than 100 beats/min); no disruption of normal rhythm pattern. *NSR,* Normal sinus rhythm; *PAT,* paroxysmal (sudden) atrial tachycardia. **E,** Premature atrial contraction (PAC). Unexpected, early P wave that differs from normal P waves; PR interval may be shorter or longer than normal; normal QRS complex; more than 6 PACs per minute may precede atrial fibrillation. **F,** Atrial fibrillation. Irregular, rapid atrial depolarizations; P wave rapid (greater than 300/min) with irregular QRS complexes (150 to 170 beats/min). **G,** Ventricular fibrillation. Complete disruption of normal heart rhythm. *(From Patton KT, Thibodeau GA:* Anatomy & Physiology, *ed 8, St. Louis, 2013, Mosby.)*

Atrioventricular Node Abnormalities—Heart Blocks

Heart block occurs when conduction is excessively delayed or stopped at the AV node or bundle of His.
    Partial blocks may be:
1. First-degree, in which the conduction delay prolongs the PR interval, the time between the atrial and ventricular contractions

2. Second-degree, in which a longer delay leads periodically to a missed ventricular contraction
3. *Total,* or third-degree, blocks occur when there is no transmission of impulses from the atria to the ventricles. The ventricles contract spontaneously at a slow rate of 30 to 45 beats per minute, totally independent of the atrial contraction, which continues

normally (see Fig. 12-17C). In this case, cardiac output is greatly reduced, sometimes to the point of fainting (syncope), causing a *Stokes-Adams* attack or cardiac arrest.

Ventricular Conduction Abnormalities

1. *Bundle branch block* refers to interference with conduction in one of the bundle branches. This usually does not alter cardiac output but does appear on the ECG as a wide QRS wave.
2. Ventricular *tachycardia* is likely to reduce cardiac output because the filling time is reduced and the force of contraction is reduced.
3. In ventricular *fibrillation* the muscle fibers contract independently and rapidly (uncoordinated quivering) and therefore are ineffective in ejecting blood (see Fig. 12-17D). The lack of cardiac output causes severe hypoxia in the myocardium, and contraction ceases.
4. *Premature ventricular contractions (PVCs)* are additional beats arising from a ventricular muscle cell or ectopic pacemaker. Occasional PVCs do not interfere with heart function, but increasing frequency, multiple ectopic sites, or paired beats are of concern because ventricular fibrillation can develop from these, leading to cardiac arrest.

A summary of these abnormalities may be found in Table 12-2.

Treatment of Cardiac Dysrhythmias

The cause of the dysrhythmia should be determined and treated. Easily correctable problems include those caused by drugs, such as digitalis toxicity, bradycardia due to beta-blockers, or potassium imbalance related to some diuretics. In these examples a change in dosage or drug may eliminate the dysrhythmia.

Antiarrhythmic drugs are effective in many cases of heart damage. Beta$_1$-adrenergic blockers and calcium channel blockers are discussed earlier in this chapter. Atrial dysrhythmias often respond to digoxin, which slows AV node conduction and strengthens the contraction, thus increasing efficiency.

Sinoatrial nodal problems or total heart block requires a pacemaker, either a temporary attachment or a device that is permanently implanted in the chest; such a device provides electrical stimulation through electrodes directly to the heart muscle (Fig. 12-18). Pacemakers may stimulate a heart contraction only as needed or take over total control of the heart rate. Caution is required with the use of some electronic equipment when certain types of pacemakers are in place. Serious life-threatening dysrhythmias may require the use of defibrillators and cardioversion devices that transmit an electric shock to the heart to interrupt the disorganized electrical activity that occurs with fibrillation, for example, and then

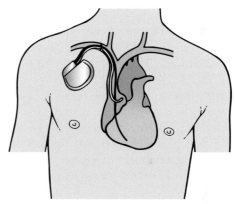

FIGURE 12-18 Permanent pacemaker implanted in the chest. *(From deWit S, Kumagai C: Medical-Surgical Nursing: Concepts and Practice, Philadelphia, 2013, Saunders.)*

TABLE 12-2 Cardiac Dysrhythmias

Name	Conduction change	Effect
Bradycardia	Rate regular, slower than 60/minute	Stroke volume increased Possibly reduced cardiac output
Tachycardia	Rate regular, fast, 100-160/minute	Possibly reduced cardiac output
Atrial flutter	Rate 160-350/min	Less filling time Often reduced cardiac output
Fibrillation	Rate over 300/min; uncoordinated muscle contractions	No filling, no output—cardiac standstill
Premature ventricular contractions	Additional ectopic beats	May induce fibrillation
Bundle Branch Block	Delayed conduction in one bundle branch, wide QRS wave	No effect
Heart Block 1° (partial)	Delays conduction in A-V node, prolongs PR interval	No effect
Heart Block 2° (partial)	Delays conduction in A-V node, gradually increasing PR until one contraction missed	Periodic decrease in output
Total Heart Block	No conduction in A-V node, ventricles slowly contract independent of atrial contraction	Marked decrease in output, causing syncope

allows the SA node to take control again, returning the heart to sinus rhythm. These devices may be external or implanted internally. Newer devices have electronic memory, which can be downloaded to assess cardiac function and efficiency of the device.

THINK ABOUT   12-8

a. Compare PVCs, atrial flutter, atrial fibrillation, and total heart block.
b. Using one type of dysrhythmia as an example, explain how cardiac output may be reduced.
c. Explain the absence of peripheral pulses in ventricular fibrillation.

Cardiac Arrest or Standstill (Asystole)

Cardiac arrest is the cessation of all activity in the heart. There is no conduction of impulses, and the ECG shows a flat line. Lack of contractions means that no cardiac output occurs, thus depriving the brain and heart itself of oxygen. Loss of consciousness takes place immediately, and respiration ceases. There is no pulse at any site, including the apical and carotid sites (see Fig. 12-17).

Arrest may occur for many reasons; for example, excessive vagal nerve stimulation may slow the heart, drug toxicity may occur, or there may be insufficient oxygen to maintain the heart tissue due to severe shock or ventricular fibrillation. In order to resuscitate a person, blood flow to the heart and brain must be maintained.

EMERGENCY TREATMENT FOR CARDIAC ARREST

1. Call for emergency medical help and begin CPR.
2. Commence use of an automatic electrical defibrillator if one is available. (These are located in public buildings and marked with a red symbol showing an electrical flash through a heart. The letters AED appear on the cover [Fig. 12-19].)
3. Continue CPR if no AED device is available or if instructed to do so by the device.

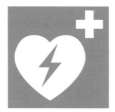

FIGURE 12-19 The universal AED symbol indicates presence and location of automatic electrical defibrillator. Symbol may be red or green in color.

Congestive Heart Failure

▪ *Pathophysiology*

Congestive heart failure occurs when the heart is unable to pump sufficient blood to meet the metabolic needs of the body. Usually CHF occurs as a complication of another condition. It may present as an acute episode but usually is a chronic condition. It may result from a problem in the heart itself, such as infarction or a valve defect; it may arise from increased demands on the heart, such as those imposed by hypertension or lung disease; or it may involve a combination of factors. Depending on the cause, one side of the heart usually fails first, followed by the other side. For example, an infarction in the left ventricle or essential hypertension (high blood pressure) affects the left ventricle first, whereas pulmonary valve stenosis or pulmonary disease affects the right ventricle first. It is helpful in the early stages to refer to this problem as left-sided CHF or right-sided CHF.

Initially various compensation mechanisms maintain cardiac output (Fig. 12-20, top part). Unfortunately, these mechanisms often aggravate the condition instead of providing assistance:

- The reduced blood flow into the systemic circulation and thus the kidneys leads to increased renin and aldosterone secretion. The resulting vasoconstriction (increased afterload) and increased blood volume (increased preload) add to the heart's workload.
- The SNS response also increases heart rate and peripheral resistance. Increased heart rate may decrease the efficiency of the heart and impede filling, as well as increasing work for the heart.
- The chambers of the heart tend to dilate (enlarge), and the cardiac muscle becomes hypertrophied (cardiomegaly), with the wall of the ventricle becoming thicker. This process demands increased blood supply to the myocardium itself, and eventually some myocardial cells die, to be replaced with fibrous tissue.

There are two basic effects when the heart cannot maintain its pumping capability:

1. *Cardiac output or stroke volume decreases,* resulting in less blood reaching the various organs and tissues, a "forward" effect. This leads to decreased cell function, creating fatigue and lethargy. Mild acidosis develops, which is compensated for by increased respirations (see Chapter 2). Because the affected ventricle cannot pump its load adequately, the return of blood to that side of the heart is also impaired.
2. *"Backup" congestion develops* in the circulation behind the affected ventricle (Fig. 12-21). The output from the ventricle is *less* than the inflow of blood.

For example, if the left ventricle cannot pump all of its blood into the systemic circulation, the normal volume of blood returning from the lungs cannot enter the left side of the heart. This eventually causes congestion in the pulmonary circulation, increased capillary

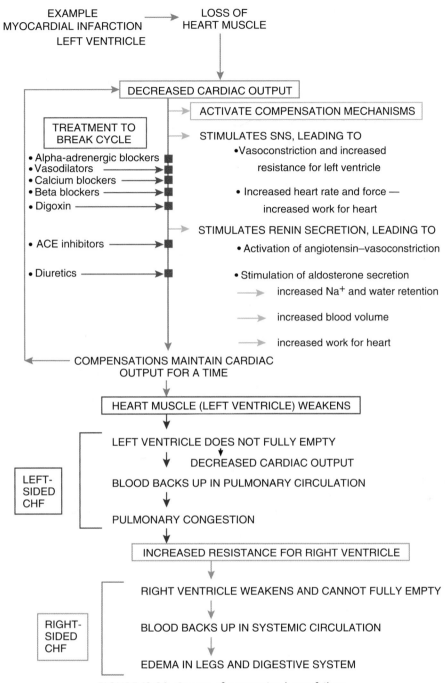

FIGURE 12-20 Course of congestive heart failure.

pressure, and possible pulmonary edema, in which fluid is forced into the alveoli. This situation is termed left-sided CHF.

In right-sided CHF, the right ventricle cannot maintain its output, so less blood proceeds to the left side of the heart and the systemic circulation (forward effect). The backup effect, or congestion, is apparent in the systemic circulation, as shown by increased blood volume and congestion in the legs and feet and eventually also in the portal circulation (liver and digestive tract) and neck veins. Right- and left-sided cardiac failures are compared in Table 12-3.

■ Etiology

Infarction that impairs the pumping ability or efficiency of the conducting system, valvular changes, or congenital heart defects may cause failure of the affected side. Presently coronary artery disease is the leading cause of CHF. Increased demands on the heart cause heart failure that may take various forms, depending on the ventricle most adversely affected. For example, essential hypertension increases diastolic blood pressure, requiring the left ventricle to contract with more force to open the aortic valve and eject blood into the aorta. The left ventricle hypertrophies and eventually

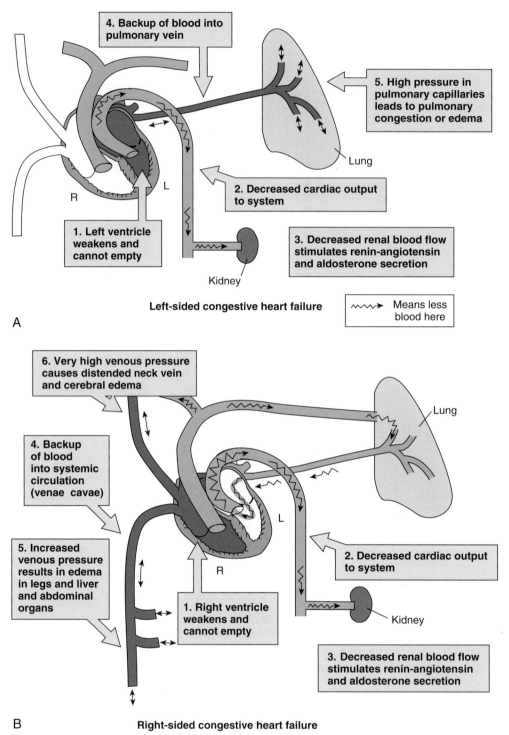

FIGURE 12-21 Effects of congestive heart failure.

fails (Fig. 12-22A). Pulmonary disease, which damages the lung capillaries and increases pulmonary resistance, increases the workload for the right ventricle; the muscle hypertrophies and eventually fails. Right-sided CHF due to pulmonary disease is often referred to as *cor pulmonale* (see Fig. 12-22B and further discussion in Chapter 13).

■ *Signs and symptoms*

The signs and symptoms become more marked as the condition progresses. Drugs may be controlling the severity of the manifestations, but there is an increased risk of sudden death from CHF.

1. With failure of either side, the *forward* effects are similar: decreased blood supply to the tissues and

TABLE 12-3   **Congestive Heart Failure**

	Left-Sided CHF	Right-Sided CHF
Causes	Infarction of left ventricle, aortic valve stenosis, hypertension, hyperthyroidism	Infarction of right ventricle, pulmonary valve stenosis, pulmonary disease (cor pulmonale)
Basic Effects	Decreased cardiac output, pulmonary congestion	Decreased cardiac output, systemic congestion, and edema of legs and abdomen
Signs and Symptoms		
Forward effects (decreased output)	Fatigue, weakness, dyspnea, exercise intolerance, cold intolerance	Fatigue, weakness, dyspnea, exercise intolerance, cold intolerance
Compensations	Tachycardia and pallor, secondary polycythemia, daytime oliguria	Tachycardia and pallor, secondary polycythemia, daytime oliguria
Backup effects	Orthopnea, cough producing white or pink-tinged phlegm, shortness of breath, paroxysmal nocturnal dyspnea, hemoptysis, rales	Dependent edema in feet, hepatomegaly and splenomegaly, ascites, distended neck veins, headache, flushed face

CHF, Congestive Heart Failure.

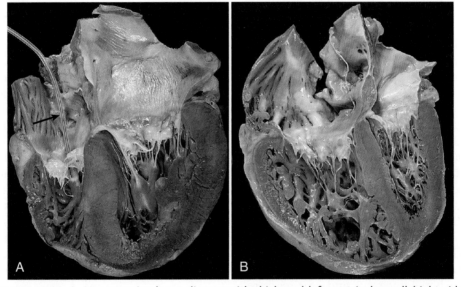

FIGURE 12-22 **A,** Hypertensive heart disease with thickened left ventricular wall (right side). Arrow indicates incidental pacemaker in the right ventricle. **B,** Chronic cor pulmonale showing dilated and enlarged right ventricle with thickened wall (left side). *(From Kumar V, Abbas AK, Fausto M:* Robbins and Cotran Pathologic Basis of Disease, *ed 7, Philadelphia, 2005, Saunders.)*

general hypoxia. Fatigue and weakness, dyspnea (breathlessness), and shortness of breath, especially with exertion, exercise intolerance, cold intolerance, and dizziness occur.

2. *Compensation* mechanisms are indicated by tachycardia, pallor, and daytime oliguria.

3. The *backup* effects of *left-sided* failure are related to pulmonary congestion and include:
   - Dyspnea and orthopnea, or difficulty in breathing when lying down, develop as increased fluid accumulates in the lungs in the recumbent position.
   - Cough is commonly associated with the fluid irritating the respiratory passages. The lungs become

a dependent area when the body is recumbent. In this position as well, excess interstitial fluid returns to the blood, reducing edema but increasing blood volume and pooled fluid in the lungs.
   - *Paroxysmal nocturnal dyspnea* indicates the presence of *acute pulmonary edema.* This usually develops during sleep, when the increased blood volume in the lungs leads to increased fluid in the alveoli and interferes with oxygen diffusion and lung expansion. The individual awakes in a panic, struggling for air and coughing, sometimes producing a frothy, blood-stained sputum (hemoptysis) if capillaries have ruptured with the pressure.

Rusty-colored sputum may be present with recurrent pulmonary edema, indicating the presence of hemosiderin-containing macrophages in the lungs. Rales (bubbly sounds of fluid in the lungs) and a rapid, weak pulse, together with cool, moist skin, are usually present. Sleeping with the upper body elevated may prevent this complication. Excess fluid in the lungs frequently leads to infections such as pneumonia.

4. Signs of *right-sided* failure and *systemic backup* include:
   • Dependent edema in the feet or legs or areas such as buttocks
   • Hepatomegaly and splenomegaly, and eventually digestive disturbances as the wall of the digestive tract becomes edematous
   • *Ascites,* a complication that occurs when fluid accumulates in the peritoneal cavity, leading to marked abdominal distention; hepatomegaly and ascites may impair respiration if upward pressure on the diaphragm impairs lung expansion
   • Acute right-sided failure, indicated by increased pressure in the superior vena cava, resulting in flushed face, distended neck veins, headache, and visual disturbances; this condition requires prompt treatment to prevent brain damage due to reduced perfusion of brain tissue.

Young Children with Congestive Heart Failure

Infants and young children manifest heart failure somewhat differently than adults. Heart failure is often secondary to congenital heart disease (see next section, Congenital Heart Defects). Feeding difficulties are often the first sign, with failure of the child to gain weight or meet developmental guidelines. Sleep periods are short because the baby falls asleep while feeding and is irritable when awake. There may be a cough, rapid grunting respirations, flared nostrils, and wheezing. With right-sided failure, hepatomegaly and ascites are common. Often a third heart sound is present (gallop rhythm).

■ *Diagnostic Tests*

Radiographs show cardiomegaly and the presence or absence of fluid in the lungs. Cardiac catheterization can be used to monitor the hemodynamics or pressures in the circulation. Arterial blood gases are used to measure hypoxia.

■ *Treatment*

The underlying problem should be treated if possible. Reducing the workload on the heart by avoiding excessive fatigue, stress, and sudden exertion is important in preventing acute episodes. Prophylactic measures such as influenza vaccine are important in preventing respiratory infections and added stress on the heart. Other common treatment measures have been outlined earlier in this chapter. Maintaining an appropriate diet with a low sodium intake, low cholesterol, adequate protein and iron, and sufficient fluids is essential. Antianxiety drugs or sedatives may be useful. Depending on the underlying problem, cardiac support is provided by drugs previously mentioned. Medications such as ACE inhibitors can reduce renin secretion and vasoconstriction, digoxin improves cardiac efficiency, antihypertensives and vasodilators reduce blood pressure, and diuretics decrease sodium and water accumulations. Because patients often take a number of medications on a long-term basis, it is important to check all of them for effectiveness, cumulative toxicities, and interactions.

> **THINK ABOUT   12-9**
>
> a. Explain how cor pulmonale may develop.
> b. Explain two causes of left-sided heart failure, one related to the heart and one systemic.
> c. How should a patient with left-sided heart failure be positioned in a reclining chair or bed for treatment?

Congenital Heart Defects

Cardiac *anomalies* are structural defects in the heart that develop during the first 8 weeks of embryonic life. A structure such as a valve may be altered or missing. Several specific examples are described following this introduction. It is estimated that in the United States, 8 of every 1000 infants (approximately 40,000 babies) per year are born with heart defects, the majority of which are mild. Heart defects are the major cause of death in the first year of life. Mortality rates have dropped considerably with improvements in surgical procedures. Both genetic and environmental factors contribute to the occurrence of congenital heart defects and these defects often occur with other developmental problems.

■ *Pathophysiology*

Congenital heart disease may include valvular defects that interfere with the normal flow of blood (Fig. 12-23), septal defects that allow mixing of oxygenated blood from the pulmonary circulation with unoxygenated blood from the systemic circulation, shunts or abnormalities in position or shape of the large vessels (aorta and pulmonary artery), or combinations of these (Fig. 12-24). Selected examples follow. Most defects can be detected by the presence of heart murmurs. All significant defects result in a decreased oxygen supply to the tissues unless adequate compensations are available. If untreated, the child may develop heart failure.

Many variations and degrees of severity are possible with these defects, but if the basic cardiac cycle is understood, the effects of a change in blood flow in each situation can be predicted. Different methods of classifying the defects are possible, using either the type of defect

NORMAL VALVE

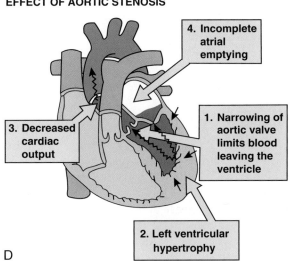

A Blood flows freely forward   No backflow of blood

STENOSIS

B Less blood flows through   No backflow of blood
    narrowed opening

INCOMPETENT VALVE

C Blood flows freely forward   Blood regurgitates
                                  backward through
                                  "leaky" valve

EFFECT OF AORTIC STENOSIS

4. Incomplete atrial emptying

3. Decreased cardiac output

1. Narrowing of aortic valve limits blood leaving the ventricle

2. Left ventricular hypertrophy

D

FIGURE 12-23 Effects of heart valve defects.

or the presence of cyanosis, a bluish color in the lips and oral mucosa.

When an abnormal communication permits mixing of blood, the fluid always flows from a high-pressure area to a low-pressure area, and flow occurs only in one direction. For example, a left-to-right shunt means that blood from the left side of the heart is recycled to the right side and to the lungs, resulting in an increased volume in the pulmonary circulation, a decreased cardiac output, and an inefficient system. On the other hand, a right-to-left shunt means that unoxygenated blood from the right side of the heart bypasses the lungs directly and enters the left side of the heart. The direction and amount of the abnormal blood flow determine the effects on the individual.

Acyanotic conditions are disorders in which systemic blood flow consists of oxygenated blood, although the amount may be reduced. In cyanotic disorders, venous blood mixes with arterial blood, permitting significant

amounts of unoxygenated hemoglobin in the blood to bypass the lungs and enter the systemic circulation. The high proportion of unoxygenated blood produces a bluish color (characteristic of cyanosis) in the skin and mucous membranes, particularly the lips and nails. Death occurs in infancy in some severe cases, but many anomalies can be treated successfully shortly after birth.

■ *Etiology*
Most defects appear to be multifactorial and reflect a combination of genetic and environmental influences. These defects are often associated with chromosomal abnormalities, such as Down syndrome. Environmental factors include viral infections such as rubella, maternal alcoholism (fetal alcohol syndrome), and maternal diabetes.

■ *Compensation Mechanisms*
Through a sympathetic response, the heart increases its rate and force of contraction in an effort to increase cardiac output. This response increases the oxygen demand in the heart, restricts coronary perfusion, and increases peripheral resistance. The heart dilates and becomes hypertrophied. However, this response is ineffective because of the defect in the heart itself. Respiratory rate increases if the oxygen deficit results in acidosis due to increased lactic acid in the body, but oxygen levels must drop considerably before this factor influences the respiratory rate (see Chapter 13). Secondary polycythemia develops with chronic hypoxia as erythropoietin secretion increases as compensation.

■ *Signs and Symptoms*
Small defects are asymptomatic other than the presence of a heart murmur. Large defects lead to:
- Pallor and cyanosis
- Tachycardia, with a very rapid sleeping pulse and frequently a pulse deficit
- Dyspnea on exertion and tachypnea, in which the signs of heart failure are often present
- A squatting position, often seen in toddlers and older children, that appears to modify blood flow and be more comfortable for them
- Clubbed fingers (thick, bulbous fingertips) developed in time
- A marked intolerance for exercise and exposure to cold weather
- Delayed growth and development

■ *Diagnostic Tests*
Congenital defects, particularly severe ones, may be diagnosed at birth, but others may not be detected for some time. Many techniques and modalities, both invasive and noninvasive, can be used. Cardiomegaly can be observed on radiography. Examination techniques include diagnostic imaging, cardiac catheterization, echocardiograms, and ECG.

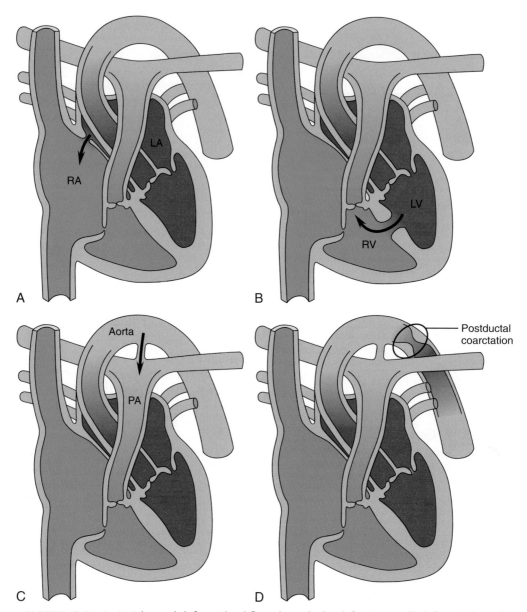

FIGURE 12-24 **A,** Atrial septal defect. Blood flow through the defect is usually left to right and produces an acyanotic shunt. **B,** Ventricular septal defect. Blood flow through the defect is usually left to right and produces an acyanotic shunt. **C,** Patent ductus arteriosus. Blood flow through the ductus is usually from the aorta to the pulmonary artery and produces an acyanotic shut. **D,** Coarction of the aorta. The arterial narrowing can produce a weaker pulse in lower extremities.

■ *Treatment*

Surgical repair is often needed to close abnormal openings or to replace valves or parts of vessels. Palliative surgery may take place immediately and then is followed up several years later by additional surgery. The timing of surgery depends on the individual situation, the severity of the defect, the ability of the individual to withstand surgery, and the impact of surgery on growth. In some cases, septal defects close spontaneously with time. Supportive measures and drug therapy are similar to those used for CHF. Prophylactic antimicrobial therapy may be administered before certain invasive procedures to prevent bacterial endocarditis (see Endocarditis in this chapter).

Ventricular Septal Defect

Ventricular septal defect (VSD) is the most common congenital heart defect and is commonly called a "hole in the heart." It is an opening in the interventricular septum, which may vary in size and location. (Septal defects may also occur in the atrial septum when the foramen ovale fails to close after birth.) Small defects do not affect cardiac function significantly but increase the risk of infective endocarditis.

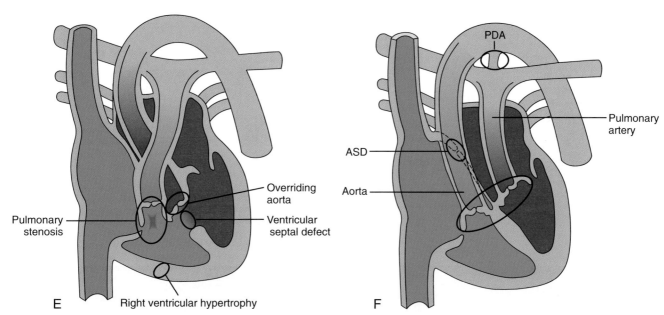

FIGURE 12-24, cont'd **E**, Tetralogy of Fallot showing the four characteristic abnormalities: pulmonary stenosis, ventricular septal defect, overriding aorta, and right ventricular hypertrophy. Tetralogy of Fallot is a cyanotic defect. **F**, Transposition of the great arteries. Two separate circulations are formed, which is incompatible with lilfe unless mixing blood occurs through other defects. *(From Copstead LE, Banisik J: Pathophysiology, ed 5, St. Louis, 2013, Saunders.)*

Large openings permit a *left-to-right* shunt of blood (see Fig. 12-24*A*). Blood can flow in *only one direction,* from the *high-pressure area* to the *low-pressure area.* In this case, the *left* ventricle is the high-pressure area, and therefore blood flows through the septal defect from the left ventricle to the right ventricle. The effect of this altered flow is that less blood leaves the left ventricle, reducing stroke volume and cardiac output to the systemic circulation. More blood enters the pulmonary circulation, some of which is already oxygenated; this reduces the efficiency of the system and in time overloads and irreversibly damages the pulmonary blood vessels, causing pulmonary hypertension. This complication, which may occur in untreated VSD, would lead to an abnormally high pressure in the right ventricle and a reversal of the shunt to a right-to-left shunt, leading to cyanosis.

THINK ABOUT 12-10

a. Describe the altered blood flow in the presence of an atrial septal defect. Include the direction of flow and the type of blood present in each circulation.

b. Patent ductus arteriosus results when the ductus arteriosus, a vessel between the aorta and the pulmonary artery that is present during fetal development, fails to close after birth. Using your knowledge of normal anatomy, trace the abnormal pattern of blood flow, including the rationale for it. Would a heart murmur be present?

Valvular Defects

Malformations most commonly affect the aortic and pulmonary valves. Valve problems may be classified as *stenosis,* or narrowing of a valve, which restricts the forward flow of blood, or valvular *incompetence,* which is a failure of a valve to close completely, allowing blood to regurgitate or leak backward (see Fig. 12-23). Mitral valve *prolapse* is a common occurrence; it refers to abnormally enlarged and floppy valve leaflets that balloon backward with pressure or to posterior displacement of the cusp, which permits regurgitation of blood. An effect similar to stenosis arises from abnormalities of the large vessels near the heart; for example, in coarctation (constriction) of the aorta.

Valvular defects reduce the efficiency of the heart "pump" and reduce stroke volume. If the opening is narrow, as in pulmonary stenosis, the myocardium must contract with more force to push the blood through (see Fig. 12-23 B and 12-24*B*). In time, that heart chamber will hypertrophy and may eventually fail. If a valve leaks and blood regurgitates backward, the heart must also increase its efforts to maintain cardiac output.

Mitral stenosis and its effects are demonstrated in an echocardiogram in Figure 12-25. Part *B* shows the normal valves and heart wall. In comparison, part *C* illustrates the thickened mitral valve leaflets and the narrow opening into the left ventricle. The left atrium is enlarged from the backup pressure and the increased workload has produced the thickened atrial wall.

Surgical replacement by mechanical, animal (porcine) or tissue engineered valves is often done (Fig. 12-26).

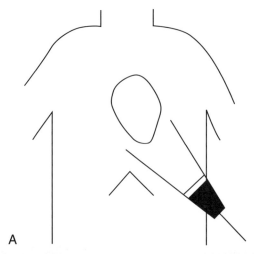

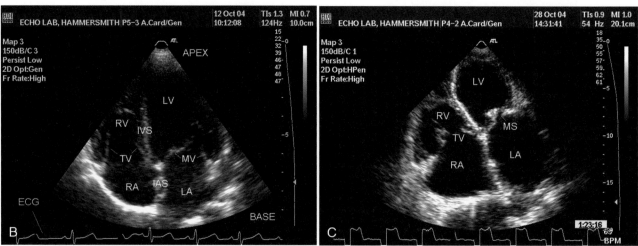

FIGURE 12-25 Echocardiograph showing mitral stenosis. *LA*, Left atrium; *LV*, left ventricle; *MS*, mitral stenosis; *MV*, mitral valve; *RA*, right atrium; *RV*, right ventricle; *TV*, tricuspid valve. **A**, Position of the transducer at the apical window. **B**, A 2-D image of a normal heart from the apical window, showing the four chambers and atrioventricular valves. An ECG is taken at the same time. **C**, The heart of a patient with mitral stenosis, indicated by thickening of the mitral valve leaflets, hypertrophy of the atrial wall, and enlargement of the atrial chambers. Note the change in the ECG indicating the cardiac phase affected by the abnormality. *(Courtesy of Helen Armstrong-Brown and Dr. P. Nihoyannopolous, Hammersmith Hospital, London, England.)*

These prosthetic valves may last up to 10 years, but are susceptible to thrombus formation, requiring patients to take daily ASA (see Fig. 12-26*B*). Also, infectious endocarditis is a risk, so prophylactic antimicrobial drugs are suggested before any procedure that might cause bacteremia.

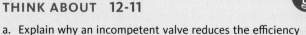

THINK ABOUT 12-11

a. Explain why an incompetent valve reduces the efficiency of the heart contraction.
b. Would symptomatic mitral valve prolapse cause a cyanotic or an acyanotic condition? Explain your reasoning.

Tetralogy of Fallot

Tetralogy of Fallot is the most common cyanotic congenital heart condition. It is more complex and more serious than the others described so far because it includes four (Greek *tetra*) abnormalities and is a cyanotic disorder (infants are sometimes called "blue babies"). The four defects are pulmonary valve stenosis, VSD, dextroposition of the aorta (to the right over the VSD), and right ventricular hypertrophy (see Fig. 12-24*C*). This combination alters pressures within the heart and therefore alters blood flow.

The pulmonary valve stenosis restricts outflow from the right ventricle, leading to right ventricular hypertrophy and high pressure in the right ventricle. This pressure, now higher than the pressure in the left ventricle, leads to a right-to-left shunt of blood through the VSD. The flow of unoxygenated blood from the right ventricle directly into the systemic circulation is promoted by the position of the aorta, over the septum or VSD. The end result is that the pulmonary circulation

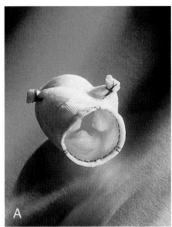

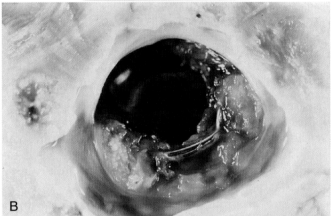

FIGURE 12-26 **A**, Porcine (pig) heart valve used to replace defective human valve. *(From deWit S, Kumagai C: Medical-Surgical Nursing: Concepts and Practice, Philadelphia, 2013, Saunders.)* **B**, Thrombosis obstructs mechanical prosthetic heart valve. *(From Kumar V, Abbas AK, Fausto M: Robbins and Cotran Pathologic Basis of Disease, ed 7, Philadelphia, 2005, Saunders.)*

receives a small amount of unoxygenated blood from the right ventricle, and the systemic circulation receives a larger amount of blood consisting of mixed oxygenated and unoxygenated blood. The oxygen deficit is great; hence, there are marked systemic effects and cyanosis.

THINK ABOUT 12-12

a. List the four defects present in the tetralogy of Fallot and state the effect each has on blood flow.
b. Describe the altered path of blood flow.
c. How does cyanosis occur with the altered blood flow?
d. Describe three signs of CHF in infants.

Inflammation and Infection in the Heart

Rheumatic Fever and Rheumatic Heart Disease

■ *Pathophysiology*

Rheumatic fever is an acute systemic inflammatory condition that appears to result from an abnormal immune

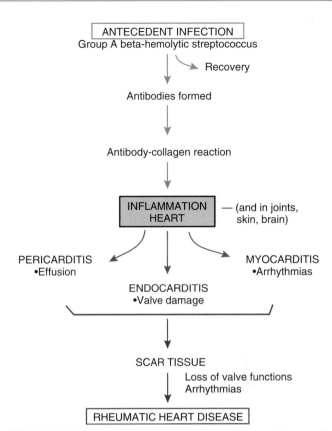

FIGURE 12-27 Development of rheumatic fever and rheumatic heart disease.

reaction occurring a few weeks after an untreated infection, usually caused by certain strains of group A beta-hemolytic *Streptococcus* (see Figs. 6-1*A* and 6-2*B*). The inflammation involves the heart and other parts such as joints and skin. It usually occurs in children 5 to 15 years of age. Although rheumatic fever occurs less frequently now in many areas, it remains a threat because new strains of *Streptococcus,* the cause of the antecedent infection, continue to appear. Also the long-term effects, seen as rheumatic heart disease, may be complicated by infective endocarditis and heart failure in older adults.

The antecedent or preceding infection commonly appears as an upper respiratory infection, tonsillitis, pharyngitis, or strep throat (awareness of the risk of rheumatic fever has led to increased use of rapid tests to quickly identify and treat a strep infection). Antibodies to the streptococcus organisms form as usual and then react with connective tissue (collagen) in the skin, joints, brain, and heart, causing inflammation (Fig. 12-27). The heart is the only site where scar tissue occurs, causing rheumatic heart disease.

During the acute stage, the inflammation in the heart may involve one or more layers of the heart:

• Pericarditis, inflammation of the outer layer, may include effusion (excessive fluid accumulation), which impairs filling.

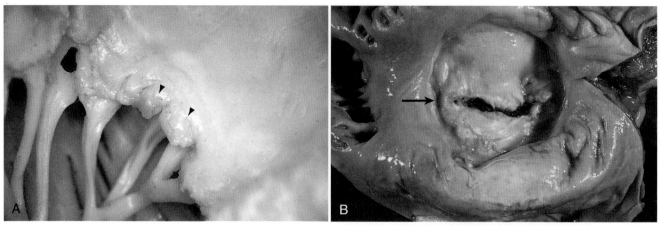

FIGURE 12-28 Rheumatic heart disease. **A,** Acute rheumatic mitral valvulitis superimposed on rheumatic heart disease (note thick cords). Verrucae *(arrows)* are visible along the edge of mitral valve leaflet. **B,** Mitral stenosis with fibrous thickening and distortion of valve leaflets. Arrow marks commissural fusion. *(From Kumar V, Abbas AK, Fausto M:* Robbins and Cotran Pathologic Basis of Disease, *ed 7, Philadelphia, 2005, Saunders.)*

- Myocarditis, in which the inflammation develops as localized lesions in the heart muscle, called Aschoff bodies, may interfere with conduction.
- Endocarditis, the most common problem, affects the valves, which become edematous, and *verrucae* form. Verrucae are rows of small, wartlike vegetations along the outer edge of the valve cusps (Fig. 12-28A). The mitral valve is affected most frequently. The inflammation disrupts the flow of blood and the effectiveness of the left ventricle. Eventually, the valve may be scarred, leading to stenosis if the cusps fuse together or to incompetence if fibrous tissue shrinks, or to a combination of these, ending in rheumatic heart disease (see Fig. 12-28B). In some cases the chordae tendineae are involved in the inflammatory reaction, and fibrosis ensues, leading to shortened chordae and malfunctioning valve. Recurrent inflammation is likely to cause more damage to the valves and increase risk for infective endocarditis.

Other sites of inflammation in patients with rheumatic fever include the:

- Large joints, particularly in the legs, which may be involved with synovitis in a migratory polyarthritis (often multiple joints affected)
- Skin, which may show a nonpruritic rash known as erythema marginatum (red macules or papules that enlarge and have white centers)
- Wrists, elbows, knees, or ankles, where small, nontender subcutaneous nodules usually form on the extensor surfaces
- Basal nuclei in the brain (more frequently in girls) causing involuntary jerky movements of the face, arms, and legs (Sydenham's chorea or Saint Vitus' dance)

Not all signs and symptoms occur in a single individual. Diagnosis is based on the presence of several of the preceding criteria including general signs of inflammatory disease, as well as high levels of antistreptolysin O antibodies and a history of prior streptococcal infection.

Rheumatic heart disease develops years later in some individuals, when scarred valves or arrhythmias compromise heart function. Congestive heart failure may occur in either the acute or chronic stage.

Signs and Symptoms

The general indications of a systemic inflammation are usually present in acute rheumatic fever:

- low-grade fever
- Leukocytosis
- Malaise
- Anorexia, and fatigue
- Tachycardia, even at rest, is common.
- Heart murmurs indicate the site of inflammation.
- Epistaxis and abdominal pain may be present. Acute heart failure may develop from the dysrhythmias or severe valve distortion. Recovery often requires a prolonged period of rest and treatment.

Diagnostic Tests

Elevated serum antibody levels remain after the infection has been eradicated (antistreptolysin O titer). Leukocytosis and anemia are common. Heart function tests, as previously mentioned, may be required. Characteristic ECG changes develop.

Treatment

Antibacterial agents such as penicillin V may be administered to eradicate any residual infection and prevent additional infection. Penicillin may be continued for some time to prevent recurrences, depending on previous attacks and the time lapse, the risk of infection, and the presence of cardiac damage. Any future streptococcal infection should be promptly treated. Anti-inflammatory agents such as ASA or corticosteroids (prednisone) may be given. Specific treatment is required for dysrhythmias or heart failure, as previously described.

Potential complications, such as heart failure resulting from severe valve damage, are similar to those mentioned earlier under congenital heart defects. Valve replacement may be necessary (see Fig. 12-26). The prognosis depends on the severity of heart damage and prevention of recurrences.

When valve damage has occurred, precautionary measures such as prophylactic penicillin prior to invasive procedures or dental treatment marked by significant bleeding are recommended to prevent bacteremia and infective endocarditis (see section on Infective Endocarditis).

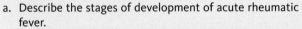

THINK ABOUT 12-13

a. Describe the stages of development of acute rheumatic fever.

b. Explain how valvular damage due to rheumatic fever may be asymptomatic until increased exercise or pregnancy occurs.

Infective Endocarditis

■ *Pathophysiology*

Infective endocarditis, formerly called bacterial endocarditis, occurs in two forms: the subacute type, in which defective heart valves are invaded by organisms of low virulence, such as *Streptococcus viridans* (part of the normal flora of the mouth); and the acute type, in which normal heart valves are attacked by highly virulent organisms, such as *Staphylococcus aureus*, which tend to cause severe tissue damage and may be difficult to treat successfully. It is now recognized that many different types of organisms can cause infective endocarditis, and it is important to identify and treat the specific organism promptly.

The basic effects are the same, regardless of the causative organism. Microorganisms in the general circulation attach to the endocardium and invade the heart valves, causing inflammation and formation of vegetations on the cusps. Vegetations are large, fragile masses made up of fibrin strands, platelets and other blood cells, and microbes. In the acute stage, these may interfere with the opening and closing of the valves. Pieces may break away, forming infective or septic emboli that then cause infarction and infection in other tissues. This process causes additional destruction and scarring of the valve and the chordae tendineae.

■ *Etiology*

A combination of factors predisposes to infection: the presence of abnormal tissue in the heart, the presence of microbes in the blood, and reduced host defenses.

Abnormal valves associated with many predisposing conditions increase the risk of subacute infective endocarditis. These conditions include congenital defects, rheumatic fever, mitral prolapse, and artificial or replacement valves. Persons with septal defects, catheters, or other artificial implants are also susceptible to infection.

Some individuals should be premedicated with penicillin or another antibacterial drug before any instrumentation or invasive procedure such as scaling of the teeth, in which a transient bacteremia could occur. Specific recommendations have been issued by the American Heart Association and American Dental Association regarding the conditions and procedures under which prophylactic medication should be given, the recommended drugs, and dosing. Medical conditions are classified with regard to the degree of risk for endocarditis. The drug of choice for prophylaxis is amoxicillin taken 1 hour before the procedure; the alternative in cases of allergy to penicillin is clindamycin or cephalexin.

Abscesses or other sources of infection should be treated promptly. Intravenous drug users have an increased incidence of acute endocarditis. Anyone in whom the immune system is suppressed, such as those taking corticosteroids or those with acquired immunodeficiency syndrome, is vulnerable. Endocarditis, both bacterial and fungal, is also a risk with open heart surgery.

THINK ABOUT 12-14

Explain why a tooth extraction or scaling procedure could pose a special danger to an individual with an altered heart valve.

■ *Signs and Symptoms*

Various new heart murmurs are the common indicator, as well as other signs of impaired heart function. Initially it may be difficult to detect any change in the heart murmur from the predisposing condition, but the increasing impairment soon affects the sounds. Transesophageal echocardiogram may also be used to reveal the presence of vegetations. Subacute infective endocarditis is frequently insidious in onset, manifesting only as an intermittent low-grade fever or fatigue. Anorexia, splenomegaly, and Osler's nodes (painful red nodules on the fingers) are often present. Septic emboli from the vegetations that cause vascular occlusion or infection and abscesses in other areas of the body, will result in additional manifestations depending on the location of the secondary problem. The release of bacteria into the blood may lead to intermittent increased fever. Congestive heart failure develops in severe cases.

Acute endocarditis has a sudden, marked onset, with spiking fever, chills, and drowsiness. Heart valves are badly damaged causing severe impairment of heart function. As in the subacute form, septic emboli may cause infarctions or abscesses in organs, resulting in appropriate signs related to location.

■ *Treatment*

Following a blood culture/rapid test to identify the causative agent, antimicrobial drugs are given, usually for a minimum of 4 weeks, to eradicate the infection completely. Other medication to support heart function is usually required.

THINK ABOUT 12-15

Describe the possible destination of an embolus from the mitral valve.

Pericarditis

■ *Pathophysiology*

Pericarditis may be acute or chronic and is usually secondary to another condition in either the heart or the surrounding structures. Pericarditis can be classified by cause or by the type of exudate associated with the inflammation. Acute pericarditis may involve a simple inflammation of the pericardium, in which the rough, swollen surfaces cause chest pain and a friction rub (a grating sound heard on the chest with a stethoscope). In some cases, an *effusion* may develop, with a large volume of fluid accumulating in the pericardial sac (Fig. 12-29). This fluid may be serous as with inflammation, may be fibrinous and purulent as with infection, or may contain blood (hemopericardium) as with trauma or cancer.

Small volumes of fluid in the pericardium have little effect on heart function, but a large amount of fluid that accumulates rapidly may compress the heart and impair its expansion and filling, thus decreasing cardiac output (*cardiac tamponade*). The right side (low-pressure side) of the heart is affected first, causing increased pressure in

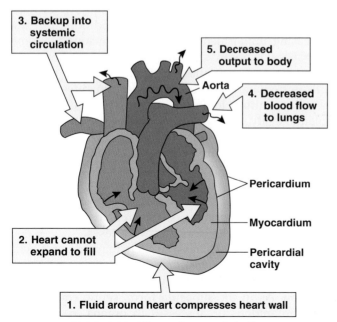

3. Backup into systemic circulation

5. Decreased output to body

Aorta

4. Decreased blood flow to lungs

Pericardium

Myocardium

2. Heart cannot expand to fill

Pericardial cavity

1. Fluid around heart compresses heart wall

FIGURE 12-29 Effects of pericardial effusion

the systemic veins and, if acute, distended neck veins. If fluid accumulates slowly, the heart adjusts, and a very large amount can build up before signs appear. A radiograph would show the enlargement of the heart.

Chronic pericarditis results in formation of adhesions between the pericardial membranes which may become constrictive, causing the pericardium to become a tight fibrous enclosure, thus limiting movement of the heart.

■ *Etiology*

Acute pericarditis may be secondary to open heart surgery, myocardial infarction, rheumatic fever, systemic lupus erythematosus, cancer, renal failure, trauma, or viral infection. The fibrous tissue of chronic pericarditis often results from tuberculosis or radiation to the mediastinum. Inflammation or infection may develop from adjacent structures, for example, pleurisy or pneumonia in the lungs. Effusion may be secondary to hypoproteinemia resulting from liver or kidney disease.

■ *Signs and Symptoms*

Signs vary with the underlying problem and its effects on the pericardium. Tachycardia is present, and chest pain, dyspnea, and cough are common signs. Electrocardiogram changes and a friction rub may be present.

Effusion and cardiac tamponade lead to distended neck veins, faint heart sounds, and pulsus paradoxus, in which systolic pressure drops 10 mmHg during inspiration.

Chronic pericarditis causes fatigue, weakness, and abdominal discomfort owing to systemic venous congestion.

■ *Treatment*

First, the primary problem must be treated successfully. Fluid may be aspirated from the cavity (paracentesis) and analyzed to determine the cause. If effusion is severe, immediate aspiration of the excess fluid may be required to prevent tamponade and shock.

THINK ABOUT 12-16

Explain the process by which a large volume of fluid in the pericardial cavity decreases cardiac output.

Vascular Disorders

Arterial Disorders

Hypertension

■ *Pathophysiology*

Hypertension, or high blood pressure, in both its primary and secondary forms is a very common problem. Recent estimates indicate one in three adults has high blood pressure. Within this group, one third are undiagnosed, and some are not controlled. Men are more likely to have high blood pressure than women until age 55; after menopause the proportion of women exceeds that of men. Another third of the adult population are considered to have *prehypertension*, with blood pressure in the high normal range and not currently prescribed medication. African Americans have a higher prevalence of hypertension; the onset is earlier and the average blood pressure is higher. Because of the insidious onset and mild signs, hypertension is often undiagnosed until complications arise and has been called the "silent killer." However, it is hoped that the availability of self-testing machines and other screening programs will aid in an early diagnosis. Compliance with treatment measures may not occur until the problem is severe enough to interfere with function.

Hypertension is classified in three major categories:

1. Primary or *essential* hypertension is idiopathic and is the form discussed in this section.
2. *Secondary* hypertension results from renal (e.g., nephrosclerosis) or endocrine (e.g., hyperaldosteronism) disease, or pheochromocytoma, a benign tumor of the adrenal medulla or SNS chain of ganglia. In this type of hypertension, the underlying problem must be treated to reduce the blood pressure.
3. *Malignant* or *resistant* hypertension, the third type, is an uncontrollable when treated with three or more drugs, severe, and rapidly progressive form with many complications. Diastolic pressure is very high. Sometimes hypertension is classified as systolic or diastolic, depending on the measurement that is elevated. For example, elderly persons with loss of elasticity in the arteries frequently have a high systolic pressure and low diastolic value.

Essential hypertension develops when the blood pressure is consistently above 140/90. This figure may be adjusted for the individual's age. The diastolic pressure is important because it indicates the degree of peripheral resistance and the increased workload of the left ventricle. The condition may be mild, moderate, or severe.

In essential hypertension there is an increase in arteriolar vasoconstriction, which is attributed variously to increased susceptibility to stimuli or increased stimulation or perhaps a combination of factors. A very slight decrease in the diameter of the arterioles causes a major increase in peripheral resistance, reduces the capacity of the system, and increases the diastolic pressure or afterload substantially. Frequently, vasoconstriction leads to decreased blood flow through the kidneys, leading to increased renin, angiotensin, and aldosterone secretion. These substances increase vasoconstriction and blood volume, further increasing blood pressure (Fig. 12-30). If this cycle is not broken, blood pressure can continue to increase.

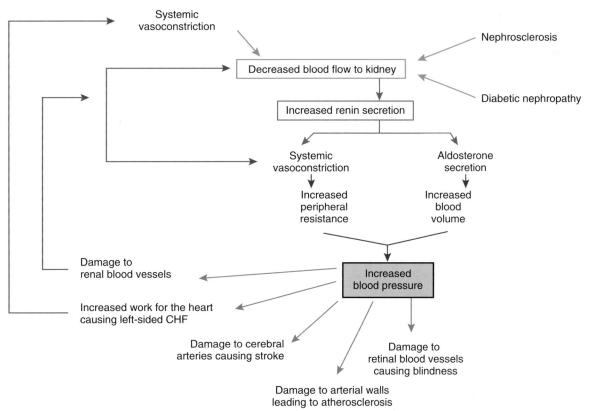

FIGURE 12-30 Development of hypertension

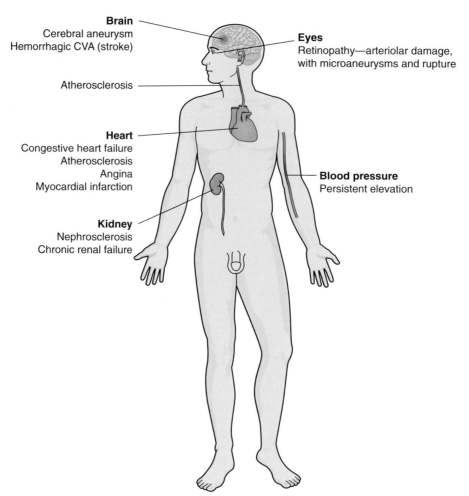

Brain
Cerebral aneurysm
Hemorrhagic CVA (stroke)

Eyes
Retinopathy—arteriolar damage,
with microaneurysms and rupture

Atherosclerosis

Heart
Congestive heart failure
Atherosclerosis
Angina
Myocardial infarction

Blood pressure
Persistent elevation

Kidney
Nephrosclerosis
Chronic renal failure

FIGURE 12-31 Effects of uncontrolled hypertension

Over a long period of time, the increased blood pressure causes damage to the arterial walls. They become hard and thick *(sclerotic)*, narrowing the lumen. The wall may dilate or tear, forming an aneurysm, or encourage atheroma formation. Blood supply to the involved area is reduced, leading to ischemia and necrosis with loss of function. In many cases, the progressive changes are asymptomatic until well advanced.

The areas most frequently damaged by elevated pressure are the kidneys, brain, and retina. One area that is easily checked through the pupil of the eye is the retina, where the blood vessels can easily be observed for sclerotic changes and rupture (Fig. 12-31). The end result of poorly controlled hypertension can be chronic renal failure, stroke due to hemorrhage, loss of vision, or congestive heart failure. Lifespan may be considerably shorter, particularly in men, when hypertension is not controlled.

■ Etiology

Even in idiopathic hypertension, the form discussed here, many factors appear to predispose to the condition. The incidence increases with age, although hypertension does occur in children. Men are affected more frequently and more severely, but the incidence in women increases after middle age. Genetic factors are reflected by the fact that African Americans have a higher incidence than do Caucasians and experience a more severe form of hypertension. There are also familial trends, but these reflect lifestyle characteristics as well as heredity.

Other factors implicated in the development of essential hypertension include high sodium intake, excessive alcohol intake (small amounts of alcohol appear to decrease blood pressure), obesity, and prolonged or recurrent stress.

■ Signs and Symptoms

Hypertension is frequently asymptomatic in the early stages, and the initial signs are often vague and nonspecific. They include:
* Fatigue
* Malaise
* Morning headache
* Consistently elevated blood pressure under various conditions is the key sign of hypertension. The

complications are also asymptomatic until they are well advanced.

■ *Treatment*

Essential hypertension is usually treated in a sequence of steps, beginning with lifestyle changes, as needed, to reduce salt intake, reduce body weight and stress, and generally increase cardiovascular fitness.

The recommendations and drugs selected are individualized. Mild diuretics such as the thiazide diuretics, which also have an antihypertensive action, are suggested for the next stage. Physicians recommend ACE inhibiters for many as the initial treatment. Subsequently, one or more drugs may be added to the regimen until blood pressure is reduced. Combinations of drugs with different actions are quite effective, and the adverse effects are minimal. The choice of drug also depends on the individual situation. For example, a patient with a high serum sodium level needs a stronger diuretic, such as furosemide, and a patient with high renin levels may take an ACE inhibitor. Other antihypertensive agents block the sympathetic stimulation in various ways: alpha$_1$-blockers causing vasodilation, calcium blockers reducing heart action and peripheral resistance, and beta-blockers reducing heart action and sometimes renin release (see Table 12-1).

Patient compliance can be difficult when no obvious signs of illness are present. However it is important to continue to follow all the physician's recommendations to prevent unseen damage and complications. Unfortunately, some of the drugs do have significant side effects, such as nausea, erectile dysfunction, and orthostatic hypotension. Orthostatic hypotension results from the lack of reflex vasoconstriction when rising from a supine position causing a decrease in blood flow to the brain. This results in dizziness and fainting and can result in falls. Rising slowly to a standing position and using support will decrease the risk of falls. Diuretics may cause increased urinary frequency in the morning and generalized weakness. Beta-blockers may prevent the heart rate from increasing with exercise. This interference with normal responses can lead to misinterpretation of the results of exercise stress testing.

Prognosis depends on treating any underlying problems and maintaining constant control of blood pressure to prevent complications.

THINK ABOUT 12-17

a. State the cause of elevated blood pressure in essential hypertension.
b. Describe the long-term effects of uncontrolled hypertension.
c. Explain why orthostatic (postural) hypotension may occur with vasodilator drugs.
d. Explain how compensation by the renin-angiotensin pathway aggravates hypertension.

Peripheral Vascular Disease and Atherosclerosis

■ *Pathophysiology*

Peripheral vascular disease refers to any abnormality in the arteries or veins outside the heart. The cause, development, and effects of atheromas have been discussed previously in this chapter (see Figs. 12-8 to 12-11). The most common sites of atheromas in the peripheral circulation are the abdominal aorta and the femoral and iliac arteries (see Fig. 10-1), where partial occlusions may impair both muscle activity and sensory function in the legs. Total occlusions may result from a thrombus obstructing the lumen or breaking off (an embolus) and eventually obstructing a smaller artery. Loss of blood supply in a limb leads to necrosis, ulcers, and gangrene, which is a bacterial infection of necrotic tissue.

■ *Signs and Symptoms*

• Increasing fatigue and weakness in the legs develop as blood flow decreases.
• *Intermittent claudication,* or leg pain associated with exercise due to muscle ischemia, is a key indicator. Initially pain subsides with rest. As the obstruction advances, pain becomes more severe and may be present at rest, particularly in the distal areas such as the feet and toes.
• Sensory impairment may also be noted as paresthesias, or tingling, burning, and numbness.
• Peripheral pulses distal to the occlusion (e.g., the popliteal and pedal pulses) become weak or absent (see Fig. 12-4).
• The appearance of the skin of the feet and legs changes, with marked pallor or cyanosis becoming evident when the legs are elevated and rubor or redness when they are dangling. The skin is dry and hairless, the toenails are thick and hard, and poorly perfused areas in the legs or feet feel cold.

■ *Diagnostic Tests*

Blood flow can be assessed by Doppler studies (ultrasonography) and arteriography. Plethysmography measures the size of limbs and blood volume in organs or tissues.

■ *Treatment*

Treatment has several aspects, including slowing the progress of atherosclerosis, maintaining circulation in the leg, and treating complications.
• Reduction of serum cholesterol levels is recommended.
• Thrombus formation can be reduced by platelet inhibitors or anticoagulant medications.
• Cessation of smoking, which causes increased platelet adhesion, is highly recommended.
• An exercise program can be helpful in preserving existing circulation.
• Maintaining a dependent position for the legs can improve arterial perfusion.

- Peripheral vasodilators such as calcium blockers may be helpful because they may enhance the collateral circulation.
- Surgical procedures to restore blood flow include bypass grafts using a vein or synthetic material, angioplasty to reduce plaques, or endarterectomy (removal of the intima and obstructive material).
- Care should be taken to avoid any skin trauma, and regular examination of the feet is important to avoid pressure from shoes, especially if there is sensory impairment. Specially fitted shoes may be required.
- Gangrenous ulcers can be treated with antibiotics and débridement of dead tissue.
- Amputation of a gangrenous toe or foot is often required to prevent spread of the infection into the systemic circulation and to relieve the severe pain of ischemia. In many cases, multiple amputations are required, beginning with a toe, then a foot, lower leg, and so on. Vascular disease is the primary reason for amputation. Healing is very slow because of the poor blood supply, and a prosthesis may be difficult to fit and maintain unless circulation can be improved.

THINK ABOUT   12-18

a. What is the cause of weak peripheral pulses when the iliac artery is blocked?
b. Why should the feet be carefully inspected on a daily basis in arterial PVD?
c. How does gangrene develop in arterial PVDs and why may healing following amputation to treat gangrene be reduced?

Aortic Aneurysms

■ *Pathophysiology*

An aneurysm is a localized dilatation and weakening of an arterial wall. The most common location is either the abdominal or thoracic aorta. The aneurysm may take different shapes: a saccular shape is a bulging wall on one side, whereas a *fusiform* shape is a circumferential dilatation along a section of artery (Fig. 12-32). *Dissecting* aneurysms develop when there is a tear in the intima, allowing blood to flow along the length of the vessel between the layers of the arterial wall. Aneurysms also occur in the cerebral circulation and are discussed in Chapter 14.

The aneurysm develops from a defect in the medial layer, often associated with turbulent blood flow at the site, from a bifurcation, or from an atheroma. Trauma such as a motor vehicle accident may result in tearing of tissues. Syphilis may also damage the tissues in the arterial wall. Over time the dilatation enlarges, particularly if hypertension develops. Frequently, a thrombus forms in the dilated area, obstructing branching arteries

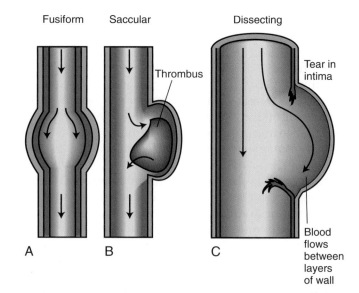

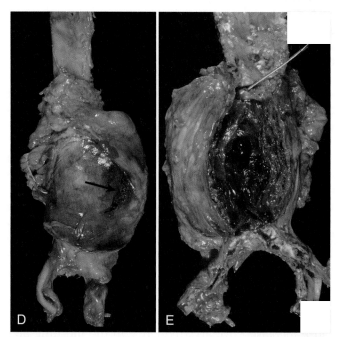

FIGURE 12-32 A-C, Types of aortic aneurysms. **D,** External view of abdominal aortic aneurysm with arrow marking rupture. **E,** Open view with probe marking rupture. Note thin bulging wall of aneurysm and lumen filled with thrombus. (*D and E from Kumar V, Abbas AK, Fausto M: Robbins and Cotran Pathologic Basis of Disease, ed 7, Philadelphia, 2005, Saunders.*)

such as the renal arteries, or becoming a source of embolus. Many aneurysms eventually rupture, causing massive hemorrhage (see Fig. 12-32E).

■ *Etiology*

Common causes are atherosclerosis, trauma (particularly car accidents), syphilis and other infections, as well as congenital defects. Hypertension is present in half the patients diagnosed with aortic aneurysms.

■ Signs and Symptoms

Aneurysms are frequently asymptomatic for a long period of time until they become very large or rupture. Abdominal aneurysms are sometimes detected as palpable pulsating masses with bruits (abnormal sounds). In certain locations, earlier diagnosis may be achieved if a large aneurysm compresses the nearby structures, causing signs such as dysphagia from pressure on the esophagus or pain if a spinal nerve is compressed.

Rupture occasionally leads to moderate bleeding but most often causes severe hemorrhage and death. Signs include severe pain and indications of shock. A dissecting aneurysm causes obstruction of the aorta and its branches as the intima peels back and blood flow is diverted between the layers. The dissection tends to progress down the aorta and sometimes back toward the heart as well. Dissection causes severe pain, loss of pulses, and organ dysfunction, as normal blood flow is lost. Many dissecting aneurysms ultimately rupture.

■ Diagnostic Tests

Radiography, ultrasound, CT scans, or MRI confirm the problem.

■ Treatment

Pending surgery, it is of critical importance to maintain blood pressure at a normal level, preventing sudden elevations due to exertion, stress, coughing, or constipation. In some cases, small tears may occur before a major rupture; these need immediate surgical repair. Surgical repair with resection and replacement with a synthetic graft can prevent rupture.

Venous Disorders

Varicose Veins

■ Pathophysiology

Varicosities are irregular dilated and tortuous areas of the superficial or deep veins (see Fig. 10-2). The most common location is the legs, but varicosities are also found in the esophagus (esophageal varices) and the rectum (hemorrhoids).

Varicose veins in the legs may develop from a defect or weakness in the vein walls or in the valves (Fig. 12-33). Long periods of standing during which the pressure within the vein is greatly elevated can also lead to varicosities. Superficial veins lack the muscle support of the deep veins. If a section of vein wall is weak, eventually the excessive hydrostatic pressure of blood under the influence of gravity causes the wall to stretch or dilate. The weight of blood then damages the valve below, leading to backflow of blood into the section distal to the starting point. If the basic problem is a defective valve, reflux of blood into the section of vein distal to the valve occurs, the overload distending and

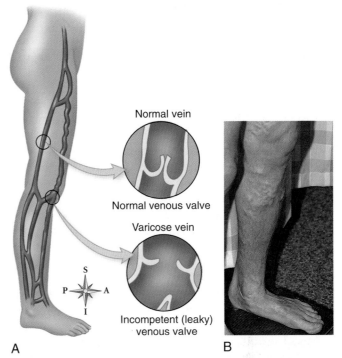

FIGURE 12-33 Varicose veins. **A,** Veins near the surface of the body—especially in the legs—may bulge and cause venous valves to leak. **B,** Photograph showing varicose veins on the surface of the leg. (**A,** *From Patton KT, Thibodeau GA:* Anatomy & Physiology, *ed 8, St. Louis, 2013, Mosby.* **B,** *From Kumar V, Abbas A, Fausto N:* Robbins and Cotran Pathologic Basis of Disease, *ed 7, Philadelphia, 2005, Saunders.*)

stretching the walls. The continued back pressure of blood in the leg veins leads to progressive damage down the vein. Some blood may be diverted into other veins, such as blood flowing from the deep veins through connecting veins into the superficial veins, further extending the damage. Varicosities can predispose to thrombus formation in the presence of other contributing factors such as immobility.

■ Etiology

A familial tendency to varicose veins is probably related to an inherent weakness in the vein walls. The superficial leg veins are frequently involved because there is less muscle support for these veins. Valves may be damaged by trauma, intravenous administration of fluids, or thrombophlebitis. Many factors can increase pressure in the leg veins, such as standing for long periods of time, crossing the legs, wearing tight clothing, or pregnancy.

■ Signs and Symptoms

Superficial varicosities on the legs appear as irregular, purplish, bulging structures. There may be edema in the feet as the venous return is reduced. Fatigue and aching are common as the increased interstitial fluid interferes with arterial flow and nutrient supply (see Chapter 2).

Increased interstitial fluid or edema also leads to a shiny, pigmented, and hairless skin, and varicose ulcers may develop as arterial blood flow continues to diminish leading to skin break down. Healing is slow because of impaired blood flow.

■ Treatment

Treatment is directed toward keeping the legs elevated and using support stockings to encourage venous return and relieve discomfort. Restrictive clothing and crossing the legs should be avoided. When standing or sitting for long periods, intermittent voluntary muscle contractions or position changes are helpful. For more severe varicosities, sclerosing agents that obliterate the veins or surgical vein stripping may be tried, rerouting the blood to functional veins.

THINK ABOUT 12-19

a. Compare the ideal position in a chair for a client with arterial obstruction with that for a client with varicose veins.

b. Explain how leg ulcers may develop in people with varicose veins.

Thrombophlebitis and Phlebothrombosis
■ Pathophysiology

The terms *thrombophlebitis* and *phlebothrombosis,* as well as *phlebitis* and *thromboembolic disease* are often used interchangeably. It can be difficult to differentiate the two conditions, but sometimes there is a significant difference in the predisposing factors, early signs, and risks of emboli.

Thrombophlebitis refers to the development of a thrombus in a vein in which inflammation is present. The platelets adhere to the inflamed site, and a thrombus develops. In phlebothrombosis, a thrombus forms spontaneously in a vein without prior inflammation, although inflammation may develop secondarily in response to thrombosis. The clot is less firmly attached in this case, and its development is asymptomatic or silent.

Several factors usually predispose to thrombus development:

- The first group of factors involves stasis of blood or sluggish blood flow, which is often present in people who are immobile or where blood flow is constricted by clothing or other devices.
- Endothelial injury, which may have arisen from trauma, chemical injury, intravenous injection, or inflammation, is another factor.
- The third factor involves increased blood coagulability, which may result from dehydration, cancer, pregnancy, or increased platelet adhesion.

The critical problem is that venous thrombosis may lead to pulmonary embolism (see Chapter 13). A piece of thrombus (often the tail) breaks off, usually because of some activity, and flows in the venous blood returning to the heart. The first smaller blood vessels along the route are those of the lungs, where the clot lodges, obstructing the pulmonary circulation and causing both respiratory and cardiovascular complications. Sudden chest pain and shock are indicators of pulmonary embolus.

THINK ABOUT 12-20

Based on predisposing factors, explain why the elderly, immobile or extremely obese individuals often experience thrombophlebitis or phlebothrombosis.

■ Signs and Symptoms

Often thrombus formation is unnoticed until a pulmonary embolus occurs, with severe chest pain and shock. Thrombophlebitis in the superficial veins may present with aching or burning and tenderness in the affected leg. The leg may be warm and red in the area of the inflamed vein. A thrombus in the deep veins may cause aching pain, tenderness, and edema in the affected leg as the blood pools distal to the obstructing thrombus. A positive Homans' sign (pain in the calf muscle when the foot is dorsiflexed) is common, but not always reliable. Systemic signs such as fever, malaise, and leukocytosis may be present.

■ Treatment

Preventive measures, such as exercise, elevating the legs, and minimizing the effects of primary conditions, are important. Depending on the particular situation, compression or elastic stockings as well as exercise may be needed to reduce stasis. Anticoagulant therapy, including heparin, fibrinolytic therapy, and surgical interventions such as thrombectomy, may be used to reduce or remove the clot and prevent embolization.

Shock

Shock or hypotension results from a decreased *circulating* blood volume, leading to decreased *tissue perfusion* and general hypoxia. In most cases, cardiac output is low. There are several methods of classifying shock. Shock is most easily classified by the cause, which also indicates the basic pathophysiology and treatment (Table 12-4).

Shock may be caused by a loss of circulating blood volume (hypovolemic shock), inability of the heart to pump the blood through the circulation (cardiogenic shock), and its subcategory, interference with blood flow through the heart (obstructive shock), or changes

TABLE 12-4	Types of Shock	
Type	Mechanism	Specific Causes
Hypovolemic	Loss of blood or plasma	Hemorrhage, burns, dehydration, peritonitis, pancreatitis
Cardiogenic	Decreased pumping capability of the heart	Myocardial infarction of left ventricle, cardiac arrhythmia, pulmonary embolus, cardiac tamponade
Vasogenic (neurogenic or distributive)	Vasodilation owing to loss of sympathetic and vasomotor tone	Pain and fear, spinal cord injury, hypoglycemia (insulin shock)
Anaphylactic	Systemic vasodilation and increased permeability owing to severe allergic reaction	Insect stings, drugs, nuts, shellfish
Septic (endotoxic)	Vasodilation owing to severe infection, often with gram-negative bacteria	Virulent microorganisms (gram-negative bacteria) or multiple infections

in peripheral resistance leading to pooling of blood in the periphery (distributive, vasogenic, neurogenic, septic, or anaphylactic shock).

■ *Pathophysiology*

Blood pressure is determined by blood volume, heart contraction, and peripheral resistance. When one of these factors fails, blood pressure drops (Fig. 12-34). When blood volume is decreased, it is difficult to maintain pressure within the distribution system. If the force of the pump declines, blood flow slows, and venous return is reduced. The third factor, peripheral resistance, is altered by general vasodilation, which increases the capacity of the vascular system, leading to a lower pressure within the system and sluggish flow.

In patients with shock there is usually less cardiac output, and blood flow through the microcirculation is decreased, leading to reduced oxygen and nutrients for the cells. Less oxygen results in *anaerobic* metabolism and increased lactic acid production.

Compensation mechanisms are initiated as soon as blood pressure decreases:

- The SNS and adrenal medulla are stimulated to increase the heart rate, the force of contractions, and systemic vasoconstriction.
- Renin is secreted to activate angiotensin, a vasoconstrictor, and aldosterone to increase blood volume.
- Increased secretion of ADH also promotes reabsorption of water from the kidneys to increase blood volume and acts as a vasoconstrictor.

- Glucocorticoids are secreted that help stabilize the vascular system.
- Acidosis stimulates respirations, increasing oxygen supplies and reducing carbon dioxide levels.

Note: Organs which are the source of the problem cannot compensate for the problem. Thus cardiogenic shock cannot be compensated for by increased cardiac output.

If shock is prolonged, cell metabolism is diminished, and cell wastes are not removed, leading to lower pH, or *acidosis,* which impairs cell enzyme function. Acidosis also tends to cause vasodilation and relaxes precapillary sphincters first, contributing further to the pooling of blood in the periphery and decreasing venous return to the heart (Fig. 12-35).

If shock is not reversed quickly, it becomes even more difficult to reverse because the compensations and effects of shock tend to aggravate the problem. Vasoconstriction reduces arterial blood flow into tissues and organs, causing ischemia and eventually necrosis. Thrombi form in the microcirculation, further reducing venous return and cardiac output. Fluid shifts from the blood to the interstitial fluid as more cytokines are released from damaged cells. Organs and tissues can no longer function or undergo mitosis. Eventually the cells degenerate and die. When organ damage occurs, shock may be irreversible. Of concern is the occurrence of multiple organ failure after the patient appears stabilized.

Decompensation causes complications of shock, such as:

- Acute renal failure owing to tubular necrosis
- Shock lung, or acute respiratory distress syndrome (ARDS), due to pooling of blood and alveolar damage
- Hepatic failure due to cell necrosis
- Paralytic ileus, and stress or hemorrhagic ulcers
- Infection or septicemia from digestive tract ischemia or from the primary problem; septic shock, primarily endotoxic shock, has a much higher mortality rate because the toxins cause depressed myocardial function and acute respiratory distress syndrome (ARDS) and activate the coagulation process
- Disseminated intravascular coagulation (DIC) as the clotting process is initiated
- Depression of cardiac function by the oxygen deficit, acidosis and hyperkalemia, and myocardial depressant factor released from the ischemic pancreas; eventually cardiac arrhythmias and ischemia develop, perhaps resulting in cardiac arrest
- With multiorgan failure, shock becomes irreversible and death ensues

■ *Etiology*

Shock has a multitude of causes. A few are mentioned here.

1. *Hypovolemic shock* results from loss of blood or loss of plasma from the circulating blood. In patients with

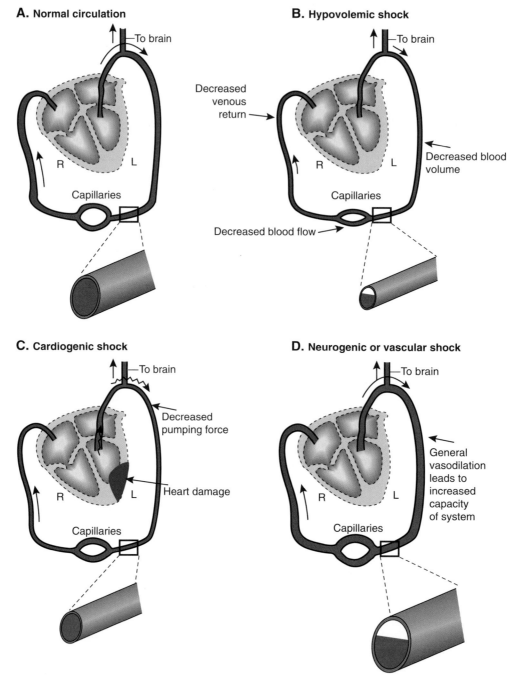

A. Normal circulation

To brain

R   L

Capillaries

B. Hypovolemic shock

To brain

Decreased venous return

Decreased blood volume

R   L

Capillaries

Decreased blood flow

C. Cardiogenic shock

To brain

Decreased pumping force

R   L

Heart damage

Capillaries

D. Neurogenic or vascular shock

To brain

General vasodilation leads to increased capacity of system

R   L

Capillaries

FIGURE 12-34 Causes of shock.

burns (see Chapter 5) the inflammatory response leads to edema with shift of fluid and protein from the blood into surrounding tissues and continued loss from the burn wound area due to loss of skin. Peritonitis (see Chapter 17) causes hypovolemia when infection and inflammation in the peritoneal membranes cause a fluid shift out of the blood into another compartment, the peritoneal space, a condition termed "third-spacing." Dehydration can reduce the circulating blood volume and blood pressure.

2. *Cardiogenic shock* is associated with cardiac impairment, such as acute infarction of the left ventricle,

or arrhythmias. A subcategory, *obstructive shock*, is caused by cardiac tamponade or a pulmonary embolus that blocks blood flow through the heart.

3. The causes of *vasogenic shock* (it may be called *distributive shock*, since the blood has been relocated within the system because of vasodilation) may be classified in a variety of ways:

• *Neurogenic* or *vasogenic shock* may develop from pain, fear, drugs, or loss of SNS stimuli with spinal cord injury. Metabolic dysfunction, such as hypoglycemia or insulin shock (see Chapter 16) or severe acidosis, may lead to this type of shock.

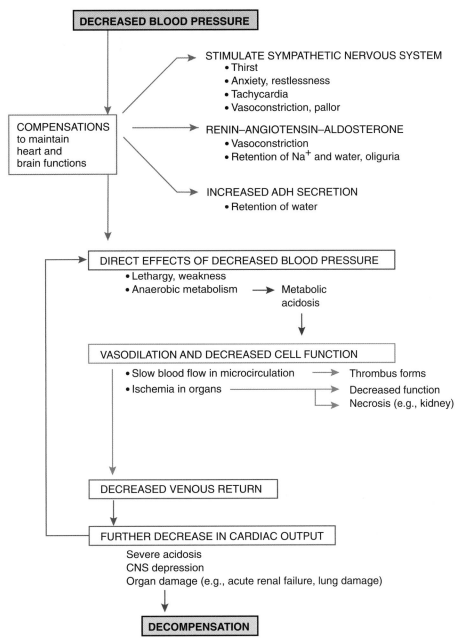

FIGURE 12-35 Progress of shock.

- *Anaphylactic shock* results from rapid general vasodilation due to the release of large amounts of histamine in a severe allergic reaction (see Chapter 7).
4. *Septic shock* may develop in persons with severe infection, particularly infections with gram-negative endotoxins, such as *Escherichia coli, Klebsiella pneumoniae,* and *Pseudomonas.* Initial circulatory changes vary with the causative organism, but eventually systemic vasodilation develops. In some cases, the organism affects the heart as well.

◼ Signs and Symptoms
Often missed, the first signs of shock are thirst and agitation or restlessness because the SNS is quickly stimulated

by hypotension. This is followed by the characteristic signs of compensation: cool, moist, pale skin; tachycardia; and oliguria (Fig. 12-36). Vasoconstriction shunts blood from the viscera and skin to the vital areas.

In cases of septic shock, the patient may experience "warm shock" with fever; warm, dry, flushed skin; rapid, strong pulse; and hyperventilation, evidence of infection.

Then the direct effects of a decrease in blood pressure and blood flow become manifest by lethargy, weakness, dizziness, and a weak, thready pulse. Initially hypoxemia and respiratory alkalosis are present as respirations increase. Acidosis or low serum pH due to anaerobic metabolism is compensated for by increased respirations (see Chapter 2). As shock progresses, metabolic acidosis

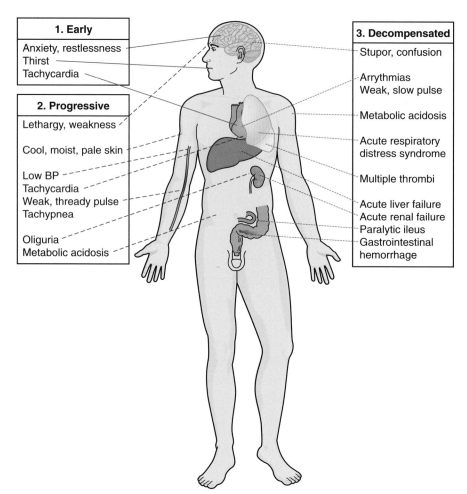

1. Early

Anxiety, restlessness
Thirst
Tachycardia

2. Progressive

Lethargy, weakness

Cool, moist, pale skin

Low BP
Tachycardia
Weak, thready pulse
Tachypnea

Oliguria
Metabolic acidosis

3. Decompensated

Stupor, confusion

Arrythmias
Weak, slow pulse

Metabolic acidosis

Acute respiratory
distress syndrome

Multiple thrombi

Acute liver failure
Acute renal failure
Paralytic ileus
Gastrointestinal
hemorrhage

FIGURE 12-36 General effects of shock.

dominates. Manifestations of shock with rationale are summarized in Table 12-5.

If shock is prolonged, the body's responsiveness decreases as oxygen supplies dwindle and wastes accumulate in the body. Compensated metabolic acidosis progresses to decompensated acidosis when serum pH drops below 7.35 (see Chapter 2). Decompensated acidosis leads to central nervous system depression, reduced of cell metabolism and diminished effectiveness of medications. Acute renal failure, indicated by increasing serum urea and creatinine due to tubular ischemia and necrosis, is a common occurrence in decompensated shock.

When shock is severe and prolonged, monitoring may include the use of arterial catheters to assess blood pressure, ventricular filling, and cardiac output. Constant monitoring of arterial blood gases is essential to maintain acid-base balance.

■ *Treatment*

The Emergency Treatment box that follows lists the treatment for shock.

EMERGENCY TREATMENT FOR SHOCK

1. Place patient in supine position.
2. Cover and keep warm.
3. Call for assistance.
4. Administer oxygen if possible.
5. Determine underlying cause and treat if possible, such as using an EpiPen for anaphylaxis or applying pressure for bleeding.

The primary problem must be treated as quickly as possible to prevent decompensation. In patients with hypovolemic shock, whole blood, plasma or fluid with electrolytes and bicarbonate is required. When the cause is anaphylaxis, antihistamines and corticosteroids are given as well. Antimicrobials and glucocorticoids are necessary with septic shock. The oxygen supply should be maximized. The use of vasoconstrictors and vasodilators depends on the specific situation. Epinephrine acts both to reinforce heart action and constrict blood vessels. Dopamine and dobutamine increase heart

TABLE 12-5	Manifestations of Shock	
	Manifestations	Rationale
Early signs	Anxiety and restlessness	Hypotension stimulates SNS
Compensation	Tachycardia	SNS response stimulates heart
	Cool, pale, moist skin	Peripheral vasoconstriction
	Oliguria	Renal vasoconstriction and renin mechanism
	Thirst	Osmoreceptors stimulated
	Rapid respirations	Anaerobic metabolism increases lactic acid secretion, which leads to increased respiratory rate
Progressive	Lethargy, weakness, faintness	Decreased blood flow and cardiac output
	Metabolic acidosis secretion.	Anaerobic metabolism increases lactic acid
		Decreased renal excretion of acids and production of bicarbonate owing to decreased glomerular filtration rate

SNS, Sympathetic nervous system.

function and, in low doses, dilate renal blood vessels, which may prevent acute renal failure.

The prognosis is good in the early stages. However, the mortality rate increases as decompensated shock develops in conjunction with renal failure, ARDS, or DIC.

THINK ABOUT 12-21

a. List and explain the signs indicating that compensation is occurring in patients with shock.
b. Explain two reasons why acidosis develops in shock.
c. State the expected changes in the arterial blood gas measurements with rationale for compensated acidosis with shock (see Chapter 2).
d. Explain several reasons why shock tends to become progressively more serious.
e. Explain why septic shock could be referred to as "warm shock."

CASE STUDY A

Myocardial Infarction

Ms. X., aged 55 years, has been complaining of severe fatigue and "indigestion." Her son is quite concerned and decides to take her to the emergency department. On arrival she appears very anxious, and her facial skin is cool and clammy; her blood pressure is 90/60, and the pulse is around 90, weak, and irregular. She is given oxygen, an intravenous line is opened, and leads for ECG are attached. Blood is taken for determination of serum enzymes and electrolytes. Tentative diagnosis is myocardial infarction involving the left ventricle. Her son provides information that indicates Ms. X is a long-time smoker, has a stressful job as a high school teacher, is recently separated after 20 years of marriage, and is fearful of losing the family home. She has also seemed to be more fatigued and stopped going to the gym about 18 months ago. She has begun to rely on "fast foods" like pizza and fried chicken and cooks infrequently. Her

father had died of a heart attack at age 50. She had also noticed more fatigue and intermittent leg pain when walking or climbing stairs at work. Generalized atherosclerosis is suspected.

1. List the high-risk factors for atherosclerosis in this patient's history.
2. Describe how atherosclerosis causes myocardial infarction.
3. It is suspected that the indigestion reported in the history was really angina. Explain how this pain may have occurred.
4. Explain each of the admitting signs.
5. What is "atypical" in Ms. X's symptoms? How does this affect treatment and prognosis?
6. What information do serum enzyme and electrolyte levels provide?
7. What purpose does the ECG serve?
    It is determined that Ms. X. has a large infarct in the anterior left ventricle.
8. Ms. X. is showing increasing PVCs on the ECG. State the cause and describe the effect if these continue to increase in frequency.
9. On day 6 after admission Ms. X is preparing to go home with her son and they receive instructions on lifestyle modifications that are desirable if Ms. X is to avoid another MI. What measures should be included in such a discussion?
    Ms. X's condition becomes less stable and she remains in the hospital. On the seventh day following admission, she is found unconscious on the floor of her bathroom. Her pulse is weak and elevated, and her skin is moist with pallor evident. Her BP is 50 systolic. A diagnosis of cardiogenic shock is made and resuscitation efforts are started.
10. Explain why Ms. X. has experienced cardiogenic shock at this time.
11. Describe the effects of cardiogenic shock on the organs of the body.
12. What problems will occur if decompensated shock occurs? How is compensation limited in this situation?
13. Ms. X dies shortly later. What is the cause of death in this case?

CASE STUDY B

Essential Hypertension

Ms. J., aged 48 years, has essential hypertension, diagnosed 4 years ago. She has not been taking her medication during the past 6 months because she has been feeling fine. Now she has a new job and has been too busy to enjoy her usual swimming and golf. She has decided to have a checkup because she is feeling tired and dyspneic and has had several bouts of dizziness, blurred vision, and epistaxis (nosebleeds) lately. On examination, her blood pressure is found to be 190/120, some rales are present in the lungs, and the retinas of her eyes show some sclerosis and several arteriolar ruptures. The physician orders rest and medication to lower the blood pressure, as well as an appointment with a nutritionist and urinary tests to check kidney function.

1. Describe the pathophysiology of essential hypertension.
2. Explain the possible problems associated with the high diastolic pressure.
3. Explain the significance of the retinal changes.
4. The doctor suspects mild congestive heart failure. Explain how this can develop from hypertension.
5. Give two other possible signs of CHF.
6. List two medications that are helpful in treating hypertension and describe their actions.

CHAPTER SUMMARY

Heart function may be impaired by conduction system abnormalities, interference with the blood supply to the myocardium, or structural abnormalities. Arterial and venous disorders usually affect cardiac function as well. Multiple long-term factors usually predispose to heart dysfunction. Treatment of cardiovascular disorders frequently involves dietary changes, exercise programs, and cessation of cigarette smoking, as well as drug therapy and possibly surgery.

- Arteriosclerosis refers to degeneration of small arteries with loss of elasticity; development of thick, hard walls and narrow lumens causing ischemia; and possibly local necrosis.
- In atherosclerosis, large arteries such as the aorta and the coronary and carotid arteries are obstructed by cholesterol plaques and thrombi. Obstructions may be partial or complete, and emboli are common. Factors such as genetic conditions, high cholesterol diet, elevated serum LDL levels, and elevated blood pressure predispose patients to development of atheromas.
- Angina pectoris attacks are precipitated when the demand for oxygen by the myocardium exceeds the supply. Chest pain is relieved by intake of the vasodilator nitroglycerin and decreasing demands on the heart.
- MI results from total obstruction in a coronary artery, resulting in tissue necrosis and loss of function. Continuing chest pain, hypotension, and typical changes in the ECG are diagnostic. Arrhythmias are a common cause of death shortly after infarction occurs.
- Cardiac arrhythmias may result from MI or systemic abnormalities such as electrolyte imbalance, infection, or drug toxicity. Arrhythmias include abnormally slow or rapid heart rates, intermittent additional heart contractions (extrasystoles), or missed contractions (heart blocks).
- Depending on the cause, congestive heart failure may develop first in either the right or the left side of the heart, causing systemic backup and congestion or pulmonary congestion, respectively. In either case, cardiac output to the body is reduced, causing general fatigue and weakness, and stimulating the renin-angiotensin mechanism.
- Congenital heart defects consist of a variety of single or multiple developmental abnormalities in the heart. These structural abnormalities may involve the heart valves, such as mitral stenosis; the septae, such as ventricular septal defect; or the proximal great vessels. The primary outcome is decreased oxygen to all cells in the body.
- Cyanotic defects such as the tetralogy of Fallot refer to congenital defects where blood leaving the left ventricle consists of mixed oxygenated and unoxygenated blood, thereby delivering only small amounts of oxygen to all parts of the body.
- Rheumatic fever is a systemic inflammatory condition caused by an abnormal immune response to certain strains of hemolytic streptococcus. Inflammation causes scar tissue on heart valves and in the myocardium, leading to rheumatic heart disease.
- Infectious endocarditis causes destruction and permanent damage to heart valves and chordae tendineae. Individuals with heart defects or damage should take prophylactic antibacterial drugs before invasive procedures in which bacteremia is a threat.
- When pericarditis leads to a large volume of fluid accumulating in the pericardial cavity, filling of the heart is restricted, and cardiac output is reduced.
- Essential or primary hypertension is idiopathic and marked by a persistent elevation of blood pressure above 140/90, related to increased systemic vasoconstriction. It is frequently asymptomatic, but if not monitored and controlled may cause permanent damage to the kidneys, brain, and retinas as well as possible congestive heart failure.
- Atherosclerosis in the abdominal aorta or iliac arteries may cause ischemia in the feet and legs, resulting in fatigue, intermittent claudication, sensory impairment, ulcers, and possibly gangrene and amputation.
- Aortic aneurysms are frequently asymptomatic until they are very large or rupture occurs.

- Varicose veins in the legs tend to be progressive. They cause fatigue, swelling, and possible ulcers in the skin.
- Pulmonary emboli are a greater risk with phlebothrombosis, usually a silent problem, than with thrombophlebitis, in which inflammation is more apparent.
- Circulatory shock may result from decreased blood volume, impaired cardiac function with reduced output, or generalized vasodilation, any of which reduce blood flow and available oxygen in the microcirculation. Compensation mechanisms include the sympathetic nervous system; renin mechanism; increased secretion of ADH, aldosterone, and cortisol; and increased respirations. Decompensated shock develops with complications such as organ failure or infection.

STUDY QUESTIONS

1. Name three mechanisms that can increase cardiac output.
2. Explain the effect on blood flow of mitral valve incompetence.
3. Explain the importance/function for each of the following:
   a. High elastic fiber content in the aorta
   b. Smooth muscle in the arterioles
   c. Extensive capillaries in the liver and lungs
   d. Valves in the leg veins
4. Differentiate angina from myocardial infarction with regard to its cause and the characteristics of pain associated with it.
5. If you had a client with persistent chest pain following rest and administration of nitroglycerin, what action would you take?
6. Explain why vasodilator drugs are of limited value in arterial disease.
7. List and explain briefly three possible causes of cardiac dysrhythmias.
8. Differentiate heart blocks from PVCs with regard to causes and effects on heart action.
9. Describe the stages in the development of an atheroma in an artery
10. Why would you recommend avoidance of prolonged stress for a patient with congenital heart disease?
11. Explain how aortic stenosis may develop following rheumatic fever.
12. For which conditions could secondary polycythemia develop as compensation: VSD, CHF, chronic lung disease, aplastic anemia, multiple myeloma?
13. Explain why untreated essential hypertension is dangerous.
14. Define and explain the term *intermittent claudication*.
15. Describe three early signs of shock and the rationale for each.
16. Explain how neurogenic and hypovolemic shock may occur with major burns.
17. List four types of congenital heart defects and briefly describe each.

ADDITIONAL RESOURCES

Applegate EJ: *The Anatomy and Physiology Learning System Textbook*, ed 3, Philadelphia, 2006, Saunders.

Copstead L, Banasik J: *Pathophysiology*, ed 4, St. Louis, 2010, Saunders.

Kumar V, Abbas AK, Fausto N, Mitchell RN: *Robbins Basic Pathology*, ed 8, Philadelphia, 2007, Saunders.

McCance K, Huether S, Brashers V, Rote N: *Pathophysiology: The Biologic Basis for Disease in Adults and Children*, ed 6, St. Louis, 2010, Mosby.

Mosby's Drug Consult 2006. St. Louis, 2006, Mosby.

Mosby's Medical, Nursing & Allied Health Dictionary, ed 8, St. Louis, 2009, Mosby.

Patton K, Thibodeau G: *Anatomy & Physiology*, ed 7, St. Louis, 2010, Mosby.

Phibbs B: *The Human Heart: A Basic Guide to Heart Disease*, ed 2, Philadelphia, 2007, Lippincott Williams & Wilkins.

Web Sites

http://www.pbs.org/wgbh/nova/heart

http://www.acc.org *American College of Cardiology*

http://www.ada.org *American Dental Association*

http://www.americanheart.org *American Heart Association*

http://www.nhlbi.nih.gov *National Heart, Lung, and Blood Institute, National Institutes of Health*

http://www.webmd.com *Web MD*

http://www.cdc.gov *Centers for Disease Control and Prevention*

http://www.mayoclinic.com *Mayo Clinic*

CHAPTER 13

Respiratory System Disorders

CHAPTER OUTLINE

Review of Structures of the Respiratory System
Purpose and General Organization
Structures in the Respiratory System
The Upper Respiratory Tract
The Lower Respiratory Tract
Ventilation
The Process of Inspiration and Expiration
Pulmonary Volumes
Control of Ventilation
Gas Exchange
Factors Affecting Diffusion of Gases
Transport of Oxygen and Carbon Dioxide
Diagnostic Tests
General Manifestations of Respiratory Disease
Common Treatment Measures for Respiratory Disorders
Infectious Diseases
Upper Respiratory Tract Infections

Common Cold (Infectious Rhinitis)
Sinusitis (Laryngotracheobronchitis)
Epiglottitis
Influenza (Flu)
Scarlet Fever
Lower Respiratory Tract Infections
Bronchiolitis (RSV Infection)
Pneumonia
Severe Acute Respiratory Syndrome
Tuberculosis
Histoplasmosis
Anthrax
Obstructive Lung Diseases
Cystic Fibrosis
Lung Cancer
Aspiration
Obstructive Sleep Apnea
Asthma
Chronic Obstructive Pulmonary Disease
Emphysema

Chronic Bronchitis
Bronchiectasis
Restrictive Lung Disorders
Pneumoconioses
Vascular Disorders
Pulmonary Edema
Pulmonary Embolus
Expansion Disorders
Atelectasis
Pleural Effusion
Pneumothorax
Flail Chest
Infant Respiratory Distress Syndrome
Adult or Acute Respiratory Distress Syndrome
Acute Respiratory Failure
Case Studies
Chapter Summary
Study Questions
Additional Resources

LEARNING OBJECTIVES

After studying this chapter, the student is expected to:

1. Describe the common upper respiratory tract infections.
2. Explain how secondary bacterial infections occur in the respiratory tract.
3. Compare the different types of pneumonia.
4. Differentiate the effects of primary from secondary tuberculosis.
5. Describe the pathophysiology and complications of cystic fibrosis.
6. Describe the etiology and pathophysiology of bronchogenic carcinoma.
7. Describe the possible outcomes of aspiration.
8. Compare the types of asthma and describe the pathophysiology and manifestations of an acute attack.
9. Compare emphysema and chronic bronchitis.
10. Explain how bronchiectasis develops as a secondary problem and also its manifestations.
11. Describe the causes of pulmonary edema and explain how it affects oxygen levels.

12. Compare the effects of small, moderate, and large-sized pulmonary emboli.
13. Describe the causes of atelectasis and the resulting effects on ventilation and oxygen levels.
14. Explain the effects of pleural effusion on ventilation.
15. Compare the types of pneumothorax.
16. Explain how a flail chest injury affects ventilation, oxygen levels, and circulation.
17. Describe the pathophysiology and signs of infant respiratory distress syndrome.
18. Describe the possible causes of adult respiratory distress syndrome and the pathophysiology.
19. Describe the etiology and changes in blood gases with acute respiratory failure.
20. Explain the cause of sleep apnea and describe the effects and complications of this disorder.

KEY TERMS

apnea	empyema	paroxysmal nocturnal dyspnea	steatorrhea
bifurcation	eupnea	proteases	stridor
bronchodilation	expectorant	pulsus paradoxus	surface tension
caseation	hemoptysis	rales	wheezing
clubbing	hypercapnia	rhonchi	
cohesion	hypoxemia	sputum	

Review of Structures of the Respiratory System

Purpose and General Organization

The respiratory system provides the mechanisms for transporting oxygen from the air into the blood and for removing carbon dioxide from the blood. Oxygen is essential for cell metabolism, and the respiratory system is the only means of acquiring oxygen. Carbon dioxide is a waste material resulting from cell metabolism, and it influences the acid-base balance in body fluids.

The respiratory system consists of two anatomic areas. The *upper respiratory* tract is made up of the passageways that conduct air between the atmosphere and the lungs, and the *lower respiratory* tract consists of the trachea, bronchial tree, and the lungs, where gas exchange takes place. In addition, the pulmonary circulation, the muscles required for ventilation, and the nervous system, which plays a role in controlling respiratory function, are integral to the function of the respiratory system.

Structures in the Respiratory System

The Upper Respiratory Tract

When air is inhaled into the respiratory system, it first enters the nasal passages, passing over the conchae or turbinates, where it is warmed and moistened by the highly vascular mucosa. Foreign material is filtered out by the mucous secretions and hairs before the air enters the delicate lung tissue. Opening off the nasal cavity through small canals are four pairs of paranasal sinuses, which are small cavities in the skull bones (Fig. 13-1). The presence of the hollow sinuses reduces the weight of the facial bones and adds resonance to the voice. They are named according to the bones in which they are located—the frontal, ethmoid, sphenoid, and maxillary sinuses.

The sinuses are lined by a continuation of the respiratory mucosa. The *respiratory mucosa* consists of pseudostratified ciliated columnar epithelium, which includes mucus-secreting goblet cells. The resultant mucous blanket "traps" foreign particles, and the cilia "sweep" the mucus and debris up and out of the

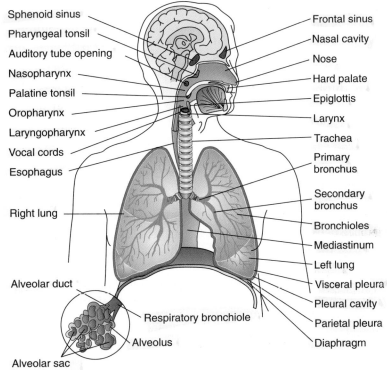

FIGURE 13-1 Anatomy of the respiratory system.

respiratory tract. This process is referred to as "ciliary escalator." Excessive amounts of mucus or particles stimulate a sneeze or a cough, which assists in expelling unwanted material away from the lungs. Smoking impairs the function of the cilia, and the irritation caused by smoke leads to replacement of ciliated epithelium by squamous cells, thereby removing this protective mechanism.

The airflow continues through the *nasopharynx and larynx* into the trachea. On the posterior wall of the nasopharynx are located the *pharyngeal tonsils* or adenoids, which consist of lymphoid tissue, another defense against the inhalation of foreign material. If these tonsils become enlarged owing to infection, they can obstruct the flow of air through the nasopharynx, leading to mouth breathing. When air passes through the mouth directly into the respiratory tract, it is not warmed, moistened, and filtered properly before it reaches the delicate lung tissue. The tissues of the mouth become dry and irritated, and there is a risk of increased dental caries as normal salivary cleansing function is lost. The *palatine tonsils*, popularly called the tonsils, are lymphoid tissue located in the posterior portion of the oral cavity (see Fig. 17-2 in Chapter 17). Also opening off the nasopharynx are the two *auditory* (eustachian) tubes, which connect to the middle ear cavities. The continuation of the respiratory mucosa into the sinuses and middle ear creates a predisposition to the spread of infection from the upper respiratory tract. The upper respiratory tract has a *resident flora*, whereas the lungs are sterile, containing no microorganisms.

The *pharynx*, where the nasopharynx joins the oropharynx, serves as a common passage for air and food and descends to the point of separation of the esophagus and trachea. When infection is present, the inflammation and swelling in the area causes sore throat and painful swallowing. In the airway, the cartilaginous *epiglottis* protects the opening into the larynx, or voice box, by flipping up or down during swallowing or ventilation.

The *larynx* consists of various cartilages and their associated muscles. The largest is the thyroid cartilage, which forms the "Adam's apple," a structure that may protrude in the anterior neck area. There are two pairs of vocal cords, which are infoldings of the mucous membrane: the upper, or "false," pair, and the lower pair, comprising the *true vocal cords*. The *glottis* refers to the true vocal cords and the space between them. When air is expired through the larynx, the true vocal cords vibrate, producing the sound of the voice. Other structures affect the characteristics of this sound, including the mouth, tongue, pharynx, and sinuses. The vocal cords, when approximated, prevent food from entering the trachea and lungs.

As inspired air is tracked downward through the larynx, it flows into the *trachea*, or windpipe. The wall of the trachea contains 16 to 20 hyaline cartilage rings,

fibroelastic tissue, and smooth muscle tissue. The trachea is flexible enough to allow bending and elongation. The cartilage rings prevent the collapse of the trachea and keep the airway open even with the pressure changes. The posterior wall of the trachea is not rigid, thus allowing the esophagus to expand as swallowed food moves through it.

THINK ABOUT 13-1

a. Name and locate the lymphoid structures in the upper respiratory tract.
b. Describe the structure and function of the paranasal sinuses.
c. Describe how inhaled air may be altered as it passes through the nasal passages and pharynx.
d. Explain how allergens such as pollen affect the upper respiratory tract.

The Lower Respiratory Tract

At the lower end of the trachea, inhaled air proceeds into the right or left primary *bronchus*. The right bronchus is larger and straighter and therefore is the more likely destination for any aspirated material. The point at which the bronchus enters the lung is the hilum. Each major or primary bronchus then branches into many smaller (secondary) bronchi and then into bronchioles, forming an inverted bronchial "tree." As the bronchi become smaller, the cartilaginous rings are replaced by irregular plates of cartilage. As the bronchi divide into bronchioles, supportive cartilage is no longer present. The smooth muscle contracts or relaxes to adjust the diameter of the bronchioles. Bronchodilation results when sympathetic stimulation relaxes the smooth muscle, dilating or enlarging the bronchioles. Many elastic fibers are present in the lung tissue, enabling the expansion and recoil of the lungs during ventilation. The respiratory mucosa thins and changes from pseudostratified columnar to simple columnar and then to simple cuboidal epithelium in the terminal and respiratory bronchioles.

Air in the bronchioles then flows into the *alveolar ducts* and *alveoli*, or air sacs, which resemble a cluster of grapes. The alveoli are formed by a single layer of simple squamous epithelial tissue, which promotes the diffusion of gases into the blood, the end-point for inspired air (see Fig. 13-5). The respiratory membrane is the combined alveolar and capillary wall, a very thin membrane, through which gas exchange takes place. There are millions of alveoli, and the capillaries of the pulmonary circulation are in close contact, providing a very large surface area for the diffusion of gases. The alveoli contain macrophages (alveolar macrophages), whose function is to remove any foreign material that penetrates to this level. However some substances can escape any action by macrophages.

The inside surfaces of the alveoli are coated with a very small amount of fluid containing *surfactant*, produced by specialized cells in the alveolar wall. Surfactant has a detergent action that reduces surface tension of the alveolar fluid (the tendency for fluid to reduce its surface area by forming droplets), facilitating inspiration and preventing total collapse of the alveoli during expiration. When inspiration is complete, the process of expiration reverses airflow in the passageways, forcing air out of the alveoli and up the bronchi, trachea, and nose.

The *lungs* are cone-shaped structures positioned on either side of the heart. The *mediastinum* is the region in the center of the chest, which contains the heart, the major blood vessels, the esophagus, and the trachea. The dome-shaped muscular diaphragm forms the inferior boundary. The right lung is divided into three lobes and the left lung into two lobes because of the position of the heart, and each lobe is then divided into segments. The lung tissue (lungs, bronchi, and pleurae) is nourished by the bronchial arteries, which branch from the thoracic aorta.

Each lung is covered by its own double-walled sac, the *pleural membrane*. The *visceral pleura* is attached to the outer surface of the lung and then doubles back to form the *parietal pleura*, which lines the inside of the thoracic cavity, adhering to the chest wall and the diaphragm. The visceral pleura lies closely against the parietal pleura, separated only by very small amounts of fluid in the pleural cavity or space, which is considered only a *potential* space. The slightly negative pressure (less than atmospheric pressure) in the pleural cavity also assists in holding the pleura in close approximation and promoting lung expansion. The pleural fluid provides lubrication during respiratory movements and a force that provides cohesion, or "sticking together" (high surface tension), between the two pleural layers during inspiration.

The *thorax*, consisting of ribs, vertebrae, and sternum (breastbone) provides a rigid protective wall for the lungs. The upper seven pairs of ribs (true ribs) articulate with the vertebrae and are attached to the sternum by costal (hyaline) cartilage. The next three pairs of ribs are "false" ribs, which are connected to the costal cartilage of the seventh rib, not directly to the sternum. The last two ribs (also false), the eleventh and twelfth pairs, are attached only to vertebrae and are therefore called floating ribs. Between the ribs are located the external and internal intercostal muscles, which move the thoracic structures during ventilation.

APPLY YOUR KNOWLEDGE 13-1

Predict three ways by which ventilation or gas exchange could be impaired.

Ventilation

The Process of Inspiration and Expiration

Airflow during inspiration and expiration depends on a *pressure* gradient, with air always moving from a *high pressure* area to a *low pressure* area (flow is *one way* only!). If atmospheric pressure is higher than air pressure inside the lungs, air will move from the atmosphere into the lungs (inspiration). For expiration to occur, pressure must be higher in the lungs than in the atmosphere. These pressure changes in the lungs result from alterations in the size of the thoracic cavity. *As the size of the thoracic cavity decreases, the pressure inside the cavity increases* (Boyle's law).

A sequence of events is responsible for the change in size of the thorax and the changes in airflow with inspiration and expiration:

1. Normal *quiet inspiration* begins with contraction of the diaphragm (the primary muscle of inspiration) and the external intercostal muscles.
2. The diaphragm flattens and descends, increasing the length of the thoracic cavity (Fig. 13-2).
3. The external intercostal muscles raise the ribs and sternum up and outward, increasing the transverse and anteroposterior diameters of the thorax.
4. The increased size of the thoracic cavity results in decreased pressure in the pleural cavity and in the alveoli and airways.
5. As the ribs and diaphragm move, the attached parietal pleura pulls the adhering visceral pleura and lungs along with it.
6. As the visceral pleura moves outward, the elastic lungs expand with it, resulting in a decrease in air pressure inside the lungs.
7. At this point, atmospheric pressure is greater than intra-alveolar pressure, so air flows from the atmosphere down the airways into the alveoli.. Note that the thorax and lungs must expand *before* more air can enter the lungs; it is not the air entering the lungs that makes them expand. Breathing requires physical effort and cellular energy.
8. During *normal expiration* the diaphragm and external intercostal muscles relax, leading to a decrease in thoracic size.
9. This decrease, combined with the natural elastic recoil of the alveoli, results in increased intra-alveolar pressure (greater than atmospheric pressure).
10. Therefore air flows out of the alveoli into the atmosphere. Quiet expiration is a *passive* process and does not require cellular energy.

Forced inspiration or expiration requires additional energy and muscular activity. In forced inspiration the sternocleidomastoid, scalene, pectoralis minor, and serratus muscles contract to increase the elevation of the ribs and sternum. During forceful expiration the abdominal muscles contract to increase upward pressure on

Resting

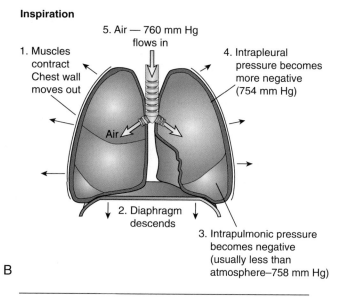

A

Inspiration

B

Expiration

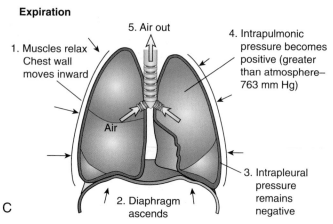

C

FIGURE 13-2 Ventilation: Changes in pressure with inspiration and expiration.

the diaphragm, and the intercostal muscles contract, pulling the ribs and sternum down and inward.

Compliance is the term used to refer to the ability of the lungs to expand. Compliance depends largely on the elasticity of the tissues, but can also be affected by other factors, such as alveolar surface tension and the shape, size, and flexibility of the thorax.

Changes in ventilation occur during pregnancy (see Chapter 22) and with aging (see Chapter 24).

THINK ABOUT 13-2

a. Describe the purpose of: (1) surfactant, (2) the ribs, (3) the respiratory membrane, (4) the diaphragm, (5) alveolar macrophages, and (6) the bronchial artery.
b. Describe the sequence of events that takes place during inspiration.
c. Explain the oxygen demands of quiet respiration versus forced respirations.
d. Explain why frequent forced expirations are fatiguing.

Pulmonary Volumes

Pulmonary volumes are a measure of ventilatory capacity in that they measure the air moving in and out of the lungs with normal or forced inspiration and expiration (Fig. 13-3). Pulmonary volumes can change with disease processes and are helpful in monitoring a patient's progress or response to treatment. For example, impaired expiration can cause an increase in residual volume and therefore increased carbon dioxide levels in body fluids. Some of the basic volumes are summarized in Table 13-1.

- *Residual volume* is the volume of air remaining in the lungs after maximum expiration. This air continues to provide gas exchange and maintains partial inflation of the lungs.
- *Vital capacity* is another important measure that represents the maximal amount of air that can be moved in and out of the lungs. It can be altered by lung disease, size of the thorax, amount of blood in the lungs, or body position.
- *Dead space* refers to the passageways or areas where gas exchange cannot take place. This is the space first filled by newly inspired air. More effort is required to open and fill the alveoli for gas exchange. Anatomic dead space includes areas such as the bronchi and bronchioles. Dead space can be increased by obstruction in the passageways or collapse of alveoli.

Control of Ventilation

The primary control centers for breathing are located in the medulla and the pons. The inspiratory center in the medulla controls the basic rhythm by stimulating the phrenic nerves to the diaphragm and the intercostal nerves to the external intercostal muscles. These stimuli occur spontaneously in a rhythmic fashion, each lasting about 2 seconds. The expiratory center in the medulla appears to function primarily when forced expiration is required because normal quiet expiration is a cessation of activity following each inspiration. Additional centers

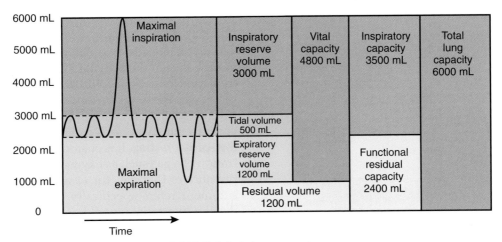

FIGURE 13-3 Pulmonary volumes.

TABLE 13-1	Pulmonary Volumes	
Name	Volume	Meaning
Tidal volume (TV)	500 mL	Amount of air entering lungs with each normal breath
Residual volume (RV)	1200 mL	Amount of air remaining in the lungs after forced expiration
Inspiratory reserve (IRV)	3000 mL	Maximal amount of air that can be inhaled in excess of normal quiet inspiration
Expiratory reserve (ERV)	1100 mL	Maximal volume of air expired following a passive expiration
Vital capacity (VC)	4600 mL	Maximal amount of air expired following a maximal inspiration
Total lung capacity (TLC)	5800 mL	Total volume of air in the lungs after maximal inspiration

in the pons play a role in coordinating inspiration, expiration, and the intervals for each.

The rate and depth of breathing set by the medullary center can be modified by a number of factors. Any depression of central nervous system activity, for example, by drugs (such as morphine), can lead to slow, shallow breathing. Other factors include activity of the hypothalamus, perhaps in response to emotions; or the stretch receptors in the lungs or the Hering-Breuer reflex, which prevents excessive lung expansion; or voluntary control, as required when singing. However, voluntary control is limited by the levels of carbon dioxide in the blood. When the concentration or partial pressure of carbon dioxide ($Paco_2$) in the blood rises, breathing resumes automatically. For this reason, a child who intentionally holds his or her breath will eventually have to breathe spontaneously.

Chemical factors are most important in respiratory control. Chemoreceptors sense changes in the levels of carbon dioxide, hydrogen ions, and oxygen in blood or cerebrospinal fluid (Fig. 13-4).

- The *central* chemoreceptors in the medulla respond quickly to slight elevations in Pco_2 (from a normal 40 to 43 mmHg) or to a decrease in pH (increased H^+) of the cerebrospinal fluid.
- The *peripheral* chemoreceptors, located in the carotid bodies at the bifurcation of the common carotid arteries and in the aortic body in the aortic arch, are sensitive to decreased oxygen levels in arterial blood as well as to low pH.

Normal oxygen levels provide a substantial reserve of oxygen in the venous blood. *A marked decrease in oxygen* (from approximately 105 to 60 mmHg) is necessary before the chemoreceptors respond to hypoxemia. This control mechanism can be important when individuals with chronic lung disease adapt to a sustained elevation in PCO_2 and move to a *hypoxic drive*. Such individuals are dependent on low oxygen levels rather than the normal slight elevation in carbon dioxide to stimulate inspiration. Therefore it is important for these patients always to remain slightly hypoxic and not be given excessive amounts of oxygen at any time.

THINK ABOUT 13-3

a. Name the major stimulus for inspiration.
b. How do elevated carbon dioxide levels alter serum pH and respiratory pattern?
c. State the normal serum pH and describe how compensation for decreased serum pH due to a respiratory impairment is achieved.
d. Describe how acidosis affects the central nervous system and give two physiologic signs of this condition.
e. Predict the effects on ventilation and carbon dioxide levels if a patient with chronic hypercapnia is given a large amount of 100% oxygen.

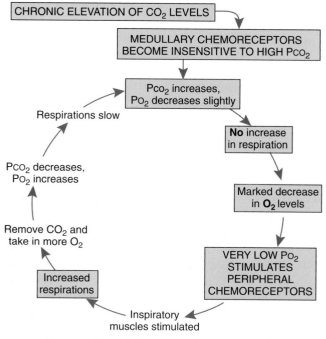

A. NORMAL CYCLE

B. HYPOXIC DRIVE WITH CHRONIC ELEVATED Pco$_2$ LEVELS (e.g., emphysema)

FIGURE 13-4 Respiratory control and hypoxic drive.

When carbon dioxide levels in the blood increase (**hypercapnia**), the gas easily diffuses into the cerebrospinal fluid, lowering pH and stimulating the respiratory center, resulting in an increased rate and depth of respirations (hyperventilation). Hypercapnia causes respiratory acidosis, and acidosis depresses the nervous system. Hypocapnia, or low Pco$_2$, may be caused by hyperventilation after excessive amounts of carbon dioxide have been expired. Hypocapnia causes respiratory alkalosis. To review the conditions of respiratory acidosis and alkalosis and the role of arterial blood gases, refer to Chapter 2.

Gas Exchange

Gas exchange, or external respiration, is the flow of gases between the alveolar air and the blood in the pulmonary circulation. Diffusion of oxygen and carbon dioxide in the lungs depends on the relative concentrations or partial pressures of the gases, and movement of each gas always occurs from a high-pressure area to a low-pressure area. It is customary to refer to the concentration of a gas such as oxygen in a mixture as the partial pressure of that gas, for example, Po$_2$. When the measurement refers specifically to the partial pressure of oxygen in arterial blood, it is expressed as Pao$_2$.

Each gas in a mixture moves or diffuses according to its own partial pressure gradient and independent of other gases (Dalton's law). For example, oxygen diffuses from alveolar air, an area with a high concentration of oxygen, to the blood in the pulmonary capillary, which has a low concentration of oxygen, until the concentrations become equal (Fig. 13-5). Meanwhile, carbon dioxide diffuses out of the pulmonary capillary into the alveolar air depending on its relative concentrations. Atmospheric air contains oxygen, carbon dioxide, nitrogen, and water. Because the air is not totally expired from the alveoli during expiration and has been humidified during its passage into the lungs, alveolar air has different concentrations of gases than either atmospheric air or blood. The residual air in the alveoli allows continuing gas exchange between expiration and inspiration because blood continually flows through the pulmonary circulation.

The pulmonary circulation is composed of the pulmonary arteries, which bring venous blood (dark blue-red in color) from the right ventricle of the heart to be oxygenated; the pulmonary capillaries, in which diffusion or gas exchange occurs; and the pulmonary veins, which return the oxygenated blood (bright red) to the left atrium of the heart. The oxygenated blood moves from the left ventricle of the heart, which pumps the blood into the aorta, and the systemic circulation starts.

APPLY YOUR KNOWLEDGE 13-2

1. Predict specific changes in structure or function that would likely decrease oxygen levels in the body.
2. Predict specific changes in structure or function that would likely increase carbon dioxide levels in the body.

Factors Affecting Diffusion of Gases

In addition to the partial pressure gradient, diffusion can be altered by other factors such as the thickness of the respiratory membrane. When fluid accumulates in the alveoli or interstitial tissue, diffusion, particularly of oxygen, is greatly impaired. Normally the pressure in the pulmonary circulation is very low, reducing the risk

A. Pulmonary capillaries around alveolus

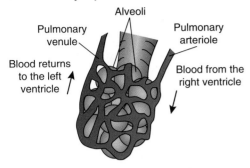

B. Cross-section of an alveolus

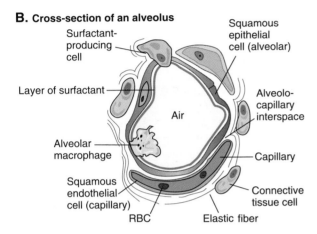

C. Diffusion of gases

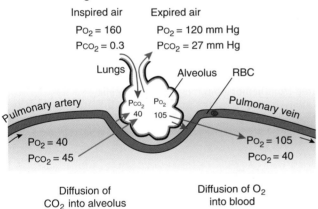

FIGURE 13-5 The alveolus and diffusion of gases.

the alveoli is obstructed or the capillaries are damaged, the involved surface area becomes nonfunctional.

This imbalance is measured by the ventilation-perfusion ratio ($\dot{V}a/\dot{Q}$). An autoregulatory mechanism in the lungs can adjust ventilation and blood flow in an attempt to produce a good match. For example, if P_{O_2} is low because of poor ventilation in an area, vasoconstriction occurs in the pulmonary arterioles, shunting the blood to other areas of the lungs where ventilation may be better. If airflow is good, the pulmonary arterioles dilate to maximize gas exchange.

THINK ABOUT 13-4

a. Explain why oxygen diffuses from alveolar air into the blood.
b. Name the blood vessels bringing blood into the pulmonary circulation, and describe the blood in these vessels.
c. Describe the effect of a thickened respiratory membrane on blood levels of oxygen and carbon dioxide. Which gas is affected more?
d. Death by drowning can occur in either of two ways, by the airways filling with water (more common), or a reflex laryngospasm (strong muscle contraction of the larynx closing it). Explain how each mechanism causes death.

Transport of Oxygen and Carbon Dioxide

Only about 1% of total oxygen is dissolved in plasma because oxygen is relatively insoluble in water. This factor also limits the ease with which oxygen can diffuse. The *dissolved* form of the gas is that which diffuses from the alveolar air into the blood in the pulmonary capillaries and also diffuses into the interstitial fluid and the cells during the process of internal respiration. Most oxygen is transported reversibly bound to hemoglobin by the iron molecules and is called oxyhemoglobin (see Fig. 10-16*A* for a diagram of hemoglobin and attachments). When all four heme molecules in hemoglobin have taken up oxygen, the hemoglobin is termed *fully saturated* (measurement expressed as Sa_{O_2}).

As oxygen diffuses out of the blood into the interstitial fluid and the cells, hemoglobin releases oxygen to replace it, so dissolved oxygen is always available in the plasma, ready to diffuse into the cells. The rate at which hemoglobin binds or releases oxygen depends on factors such as P_{O_2} (the partial pressure of dissolved oxygen), P_{CO_2} temperature, and plasma pH (Fig. 13-6). Normally approximately 25% of the bound oxygen is released to the cells for metabolism during an erythrocyte's trip through the systemic circulation, leaving 75% of the hemoglobin in the venous blood still saturated with oxygen. This provides a good safety margin of oxygen that is available to meet increased cell demands.

Carbon dioxide, a waste product from cell metabolism, is transported in several forms. Approximately 7% is dissolved in the plasma and can easily diffuse across

of excessive fluid in the interstitial space and alveoli. The presence of extra fluid may also impede blood flow through the pulmonary capillaries and increase surface tension in the alveoli, restricting expansion of the lung.

Other major factors in gas exchange are the total surface area available for diffusion and the thickness of the alveolar membranes. The alveoli are the only structures that provide such a surface area, and both ventilation and perfusion must be adequate for diffusion to occur (see Fig. 13-20). If part of the alveolar wall is destroyed, as in emphysema, or fibrosis occurs in the lungs, the surface area is greatly reduced. If airflow into

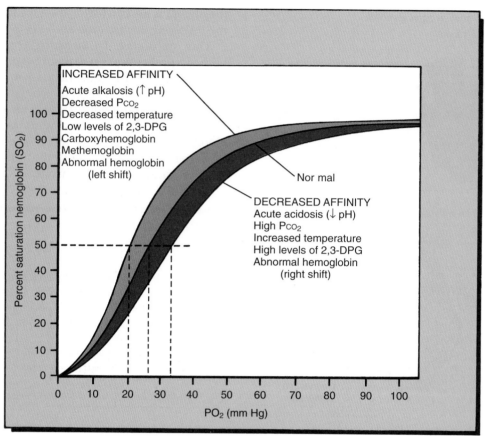

FIGURE 13-6 Oxyhemoglobin dissociation curve. This graph illustrates the factors affecting the bond between oxygen and hemoglobin. The steep slope of the curve on the left represents the rapid dissociation of oxygen from hemoglobin as blood circulates through the tissues. This oxygen diffuses into the cells. The flat portion of the curve at the top of the graph illustrates the binding of oxygen with hemoglobin in the lungs. The lighter colored section above the line marked "normal" shows the effect of increased affinity, when more oxygen is bound to hemoglobin, termed a shift to the left. The darker area below the normal line shows a shift to the right, the condition in which more oxygen that is dissociated from hemoglobin moves into the cells. *(From Lane EE, Walker JF: Clinical Arterial Blood Gas Analysis, St. Louis, 1987, Mosby.)*

membranes. Roughly 20% is loosely and reversibly bound to hemoglobin, attached to an amino group on the globin portion (not the heme). This is termed carbaminoglobin. The majority of carbon dioxide resulting from cell metabolism diffuses into the red blood cells (RBCs), where, under the influence of the enzyme carbonic anhydrase, it transitions very briefly as carbonic acid, then is immediately converted into bicarbonate ions (see the following equation). These bicarbonate ions can then diffuse back into the plasma to function in the buffer pair (see Chapter 2).

$$CO_2 + H_2O \longleftrightarrow H_2CO_3 \longleftrightarrow H^+ + HCO_3^-$$

carbon dioxide + water $\leftarrow \rightarrow$ carbonic acid $\leftarrow \rightarrow$ hydrogen ions + bicarbonate ions

(in presence of enzyme, carbonic anhydrase)

A ratio of 20 parts bicarbonate ion to 1 part carbonic acid maintains blood pH at 7.35. Thus, carbon dioxide plays a major role in control of blood pH through this buffer system.

Diagnostic Tests

Common tests include:
- Spirometry-pulmonary function testing (PFT) is used to test pulmonary volumes, measuring volume and airflow times.
- Arterial blood gas determinations are used to check oxygen, carbon dioxide, and bicarbonate levels as well as serum pH.
- Oximeters measure O_2 saturation.
- Exercise tolerance testing is useful in patients with chronic pulmonary disease for diagnosis and monitoring of the patient's progress.
- Radiography may be helpful in evaluating tumors or infections such as pneumonia or tuberculosis.
- Bronchoscopy may be used in performing a biopsy or in checking for the site of a lesion or bleeding.
- Culture and sensitivity tests on exudates from the upper respiratory tract or sputum specimens can

identify pathogens and assist in determining the appropriate therapy.

General Manifestations of Respiratory Disease

1. *Sneezing* is a reflex response to irritation in the upper respiratory tract and assists in removing the irritant. It is associated with inflammation or foreign material in the nasal passages.
2. *Coughing* may result from irritation caused by a nasal discharge dripping into the oropharynx, or from inflammation or foreign material in the lower respiratory tract, or from inhaled irritants such as tobacco smoke. An occasional cough is considered a normal event in a healthy person, but a persistent cough may be evidence of a respiratory disease or chronic irritation. Aspiration of food or fluid may cause a spasm of coughing.

   The *cough reflex* is controlled by a center in the medulla and consists of coordinated actions that inspire air and then close the glottis and vocal cords. This is followed by forceful expiration in which the glottis is opened and the unwanted material is blown upward and out of the mouth. In some cases, the product of a cough is swallowed. The effectiveness of the cough depends on the strength of the muscle action during both inspiration and expiration.

   A constant dry or unproductive cough is fatiguing because it interferes with sleep, and the respiratory muscles are used excessively. In such cases, a cough-suppressant medication (e.g., codeine or dextromethorphan) may be used at night. A productive cough usually occurs when secretions or inflammatory exudate accumulate in the lungs, and removal of such fluids from the airways is beneficial. Excess secretions may become infected and tend to obstruct the airways. It is helpful in such cases to increase fluid intake to keep the secretions thin and easy to remove. An expectorant medication (e.g., guaifenesin) or the use of a humidifier also may assist in removing secretions. Thick or sticky mucus is particularly difficult to raise from the lungs, especially in elderly or debilitated patients.

3. *Sputum* or mucoid discharge from the respiratory tract may have significant characteristics depending on the abnormality causing it. Normal secretions are relatively thin, clear, and colorless or cream color.
   a. Yellowish-green, cloudy, thick mucus is often an indication of a bacterial infection.
   b. Rusty or dark-colored sputum is usually a sign of pneumococcal pneumonia.
   c. Very large amounts of purulent (contains pus) sputum with a foul odor may be associated with bronchiectasis.
   d. Thick, tenacious (sticky) mucus may occur in patients with asthma or cystic fibrosis. Blood-tinged secretions may result from a chronic cough and irritation that causes rupture of superficial capillaries, but it may also be a sign of a tumor or tuberculosis.
   e. Hemoptysis is blood-tinged (bright red) frothy sputum that is usually associated with pulmonary edema. It is important not to confuse hemoptysis with hematemesis, which is vomitus containing blood and is usually granular and dark in color (coffee-grounds vomitus).
4. *Breathing patterns* and characteristics may be altered with respiratory disease (Fig. 13-7). The normal rate

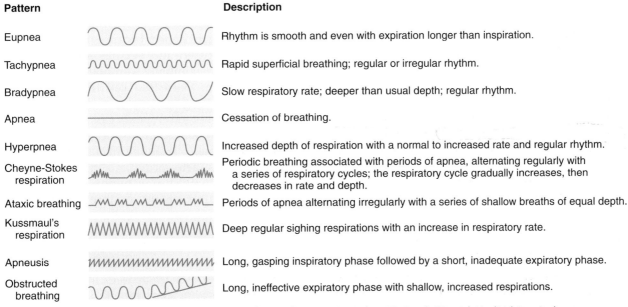

Pattern		Description
Eupnea		Rhythm is smooth and even with expiration longer than inspiration.
Tachypnea		Rapid superficial breathing; regular or irregular rhythm.
Bradypnea		Slow respiratory rate; deeper than usual depth; regular rhythm.
Apnea		Cessation of breathing.
Hyperpnea		Increased depth of respiration with a normal to increased rate and regular rhythm.
Cheyne-Stokes respiration		Periodic breathing associated with periods of apnea, alternating regularly with a series of respiratory cycles; the respiratory cycle gradually increases, then decreases in rate and depth.
Ataxic breathing		Periods of apnea alternating irregularly with a series of shallow breaths of equal depth.
Kussmaul's respiration		Deep regular sighing respirations with an increase in respiratory rate.
Apneusis		Long, gasping inspiratory phase followed by a short, inadequate expiratory phase.
Obstructed breathing		Long, ineffective expiratory phase with shallow, increased respirations.

FIGURE 13-7 Respiratory patterns. *(From Phipps WJ, Monahan FD, Sands JK, et al:* Medical-Surgical Nursing: Health and Illness Perspectives, *ed 7, St. Louis, 2003, Mosby.)*

(eupnea) is 10 to 18 inspirations per minute, and the normal pattern is regular and effortless. Changes in the rate, rhythm, depth, and effort of ventilation are significant.

a. Kussmaul respirations, deep rapid respirations or "air hunger," are typical of a state of acidosis or may follow strenuous exercise.

b. Labored respirations or prolonged inspiration or expiration times are often associated with obstruction of the airways.

c. Wheezing or whistling sounds indicate obstruction in the small airways.

d. Stridor, a high-pitched crowing noise, usually indicates upper airway obstruction.

5. Breath sounds may be abnormal or absent in respiratory disorders. Rales and rhonchi are abnormal sounds resulting from air mixing with excessive secretions in the lungs.

a. Rales are light bubbly or crackling sounds associated with serous secretions.

b. Rhonchi are deeper and harsher sounds resulting from thicker mucus.

c. Absence of breath sounds indicates nonaeration or collapse of a lung (atelectasis).

6. Dyspnea is a subjective feeling of discomfort that occurs when a person feels unable to inhale enough air. It may be manifested as breathlessness or shortness of breath, either with exertion or at rest.

a. Severe dyspnea may be accompanied by flaring of the nostrils (nares), use of the accessory respiratory muscles, or retraction (pulling in) of the muscles between or above the ribs. For example, intercostal retractions between the ribs are visible to the observer.

b. Orthopnea is dyspnea that occurs when a person is lying down. Pulmonary congestion develops as more blood pools in the lungs when the person lies down and also as the abdominal contents push upward against the lungs. Raising the upper part of the body with pillows often facilitates breathing in persons with respiratory or cardiovascular disorders.

c. Paroxysmal nocturnal dyspnea is a sudden acute type of dyspnea common in patients with left-sided congestive heart failure. During sleep the body fluid is redistributed, leading to pulmonary edema, and the individual wakes up gasping for air and coughing (see Chapter 12).

7. Cyanosis is the bluish coloring of the skin and mucous membranes that results from large amounts of unoxygenated hemoglobin in the blood. It may develop in peripheral areas as a result of exertion or be more generalized. This may occur in patients with cardiovascular conditions as well as respiratory disease, and its presence must be considered in conjunction with other data. Cyanosis is not a reliable early indicator of hypoxia.

8. Pleural pain results from inflammation or infection of the parietal pleura. It is a cyclic pain that increases as the inflamed membrane is stretched with inspiration or coughing.

9. Friction rub may be heard, a soft sound produced as the rough membranes move against each other. Pleural inflammation may be caused by lobar pneumonia or lung infarction.

10. Clubbed fingers and sometimes toes result from chronic hypoxia associated with respiratory or cardiovascular diseases. Clubbing is a painless, firm, fibrotic enlargement at the end of the digit.

11. Changes in arterial blood gases (ABGs): Hypoxemia refers to inadequate oxygen in the blood (Pao_2). Hypoxia, or inadequate oxygen supply to the cells, may have many causes:

a. A deficit of RBCs or hemoglobin levels that are too low for adequate oxygen transport

b. Circulatory impairment, which may lead to decreased cardiac output from the heart to the lungs or the systemic circulation

c. Excessive release of oxygen from RBCs if circulation is sluggish through the system or is partially obstructed by vascular disease

d. Impaired respiratory function, including inadequate ventilation, inhalation of oxygen-deficient air, or impaired diffusion

e. Carbon monoxide poisoning, in which carbon monoxide binds tightly and preferentially to heme, displacing oxygen. Unfortunately, carbon monoxide does not cause obvious signs of hypoxia (rather a bright red coloring of the skin and mucosa with headache and drowsiness) or affect ventilation, but it can be fatal very quickly and quietly.

Hypoxia affects cell metabolism, reducing cell function and leading to anaerobic metabolism and the development of metabolic acidosis. The brain is most susceptible to an oxygen deficit because it has little storage capacity for oxygen and yet has a constant demand. Cerebral hypoxia initially stimulates the sympathetic nervous system. Decreased cell function is indicated by fatigue, lethargy or stupor, and muscle weakness. Extreme or prolonged hypoxia can result in cell death.

Compensation mechanisms for hypoxia due to respiratory impairment include increased cardiovascular activity such as tachycardia and increased blood pressure. In people with chronic hypoxia due to respiratory or circulatory impairment, erythropoietin secretion is increased, stimulating the bone marrow to produce additional red blood cells (secondary polycythemia).

Acid-base imbalance may develop from respiratory disorders (see Chapter 2). Respiratory acidosis due to excess carbon dioxide (increased carbonic acid) is more common and results from impaired expiration. Arterial blood gases in this situation indicate high Pco_2 and low serum pH. Respiratory alkalosis occurs when the respiratory rate is increased, usually because of acute anxiety or excessive intake of aspirin.

THINK ABOUT 13-5

a. Define the terms sputum, rales, orthopnea, and hemoptysis.

b. Differentiate a productive cough from an unproductive cough by general cause, signs, and possible complications.

c. List the signs indicating a possible obstruction in the airways.

Common Treatment Measures for Respiratory Disorders

A number of treatment modalities are recommended for many respiratory diseases. A few examples are summarized in Table 13-2.

Infectious Diseases

Upper Respiratory Tract Infections

Common Cold (Infectious Rhinitis)

The common cold is caused by a viral infection of the upper respiratory tract. The most common pathogen is a rhinovirus, but it may also be an adenovirus, parainfluenza virus, or coronavirus. There are more than 200 possible causative organisms, so it is difficult for an individual to develop sufficient immunity to avoid all colds. Children do acquire more colds than adults, usually as a brief, self-limiting infection, unless a secondary bacterial infection develops. The common cold is spread through respiratory droplets, which either are directly inhaled or are spread by secretions on hands or contaminated objects such as facial tissue. The infection is highly contagious because the virus is shed in large numbers from the infected nasal mucosa during the first few days of the infection and can survive for several hours outside the body.

Initially the mucous membranes of the nose and pharynx are red and swollen, with increased secretions. The signs of a cold include nasal congestion and copious watery discharge (rhinorrhea, sneezing, and sometimes watery eyes). Mouth breathing is common, and a change in the tone of voice is noticeable. There may be sore throat, headache, slight fever, and malaise. Cough may develop from the irritation of the secretions dripping into the pharynx. Sometimes the feeling of stuffiness and irritation persists as the secretions become more viscous for a few days after the acute period has passed. The infection and inflammation may spread to cause pharyngitis, laryngitis, or acute bronchitis.

Treatment is symptomatic, consisting of acetaminophen for fever and headache and decongestants (vasoconstrictors) to reduce the edema and congestion in the respiratory passages. A cold is a self-limiting infection. Antihistamines reduce secretions but may cause excessive drying of tissues and cough. Humidifiers aid in keeping the secretions liquid and easily drained. The role of vitamin C in prevention and therapy remains controversial. Antibiotics do not cure viral infections and are usually reserved for secondary bacterial infections such as sinusitis, otitis media (see Chapter 15), or tracheitis, or for prophylactic use in high-risk patients (such as those with chronic illnesses). Proper handwashing and disposal of tissues as well as avoidance of crowded areas reduce the risk of transmission to others.

Secondary bacterial infections, for example, pharyngitis or "strep throat," are usually caused by streptococcus invading inflamed and necrotic mucous membranes (Fig. 13-8). A purulent exudate forms and systemic signs such as fever develop. These bacteria should be identified by culture and treated quickly with antimicrobial drugs to reduce the risk of rheumatic fever or acute glomerulonephritis arising from group A beta-hemolytic *Streptococcus pneumoniae.*

Sinusitis

Sinusitis is usually a bacterial infection secondary to a cold or an allergy that has obstructed the drainage of one or more of the paranasal sinuses into the nasal cavity (see Fig. 13-1). Common causative organisms include pneumococci, streptococci, or *Haemophilus influenzae.* As the exudate accumulates, pressure builds up inside the sinus cavity, causing severe pain in the facial bone. The pain may be confused with headache (ethmoid sinus) or toothache (maxillary sinus). Other signs, such as nasal congestion, fever, or sore throat, may already be present. Diagnosis may be confirmed by radiograph or transillumination. Decongestants and analgesics are recommended until the sinuses are draining well, and a course of antibiotics is often required to eradicate the infection totally.

Laryngotracheobronchitis (Croup)

Laryngotracheobronchitis is a common viral infection, particularly in children between 1 and 2 years of age, although adults may also contract laryngitis, tracheitis, or bronchitis. Common causative organisms are parainfluenza viruses and adenoviruses (Table 13-3). The infection begins as an upper respiratory condition with nasal congestion and cough. In the young child, the larynx and subglottic area become inflamed with swelling and exudate, leading to obstruction and a characteristic barking cough (croup), hoarse voice, and inspiratory stridor. The condition often becomes more severe at night. Cool, moisturized air from a humidifier or shower or croup tent often relieves the obstruction. The infection is usually self-limited, and full recovery occurs in several days. In some children with allergic tendencies,

TABLE 13-2   Basic Therapies for Respiratory Disorders

Treatment	Effect	Example
Avoid inhaling irritants and maintain good ventilation	Reduce inflammation and infection	Cigarette smoke Industrial pollutants
Current immunizations	Prevent infection	Influenza and pneumonia vaccines
Humidify air	Moist mucosa resists damage Thin and remove secretions	Cool-air humidifiers Croup tents
Moderate exercise	Improves lung function and circulation	Walking, swimming
Breathing and coughing	Improve lung expansion and remove secretions	Techniques appropriate for specific condition (e.g., pursed-lip breathing)
Chest physiotherapy	Remove thick secretions and reduce Infections	Clapping, postural drainage
Oxygen	Improve oxygen supply to all body cells	Nasal cannula, face mask or mechanical ventilation
Drugs		
Decongestants	Vasoconstriction in nasal mucosa, reduce edema	phenylpropanolamine, pseudoephedrine
Expectorants	Thin respiratory secretions for easier removal	guaifenesin
Antitussives	Reduce cough reflex	codeine, dextromethorphan (DM),
Antihistamines	Block H1 receptors to reduce allergic response	diphenhydramine, loratadine
Analgesics	Reduce pain	acetaminophen, codeine
Antimicrobials	Prophylaxis and treatment of infection (sputum culture and sensitivity)	Antibacterial—penicillin Antiviral—amantadine, zanamivir Antitubercular—isoniazid rifampin
Bronchodilators	Stimulate beta-2 adrenergic receptors to open bronchioles	theophylline (oral) salbutamol (inhaler)
Glucocorticoids	Anti-inflammatory, antiallergenic	beclomethasone (inhaler) prednisone (oral)
Surgical Interventions		
Thoracentesis	Removal of excess fluid from pleural cavity, prevent atelectasis	Pleurisy, cancer
Tracheotomy	Incision into the trachea below the larynx to permit air intake	Emergency obstructed airway (e.g., aspiration, edema)
Surgery	Remove tumor, abscess or damaged tissue	Resection, lobectomy

TABLE 13-3   General Comparison of Respiratory Infections in Children

	Laryngotracheobronchitis	Epiglottitis	Bronchiolitis
Age group	3 months to 3 years	3-7 years	2-12 months
Cause	Virus	*Haemophilus influenzae*	Virus—RSV
Pathology	Inflammation of mucosa of larynx and trachea obstructs airway	Supraglottic inflammation and swelling of epiglottis obstructs airway	Inflammation of mucosa of bronchioles obstructs small passages
Onset	Gradual	Rapid	Gradual
Signs	Hoarse, barking cough Inspiratory stridor Restlessness	Drooling, dysphagia High fever, appears ill Rapid respirations and pulse Tripod position	Increasing dyspnea Paroxysmal cough, wheezing Chest retractions Flared nares

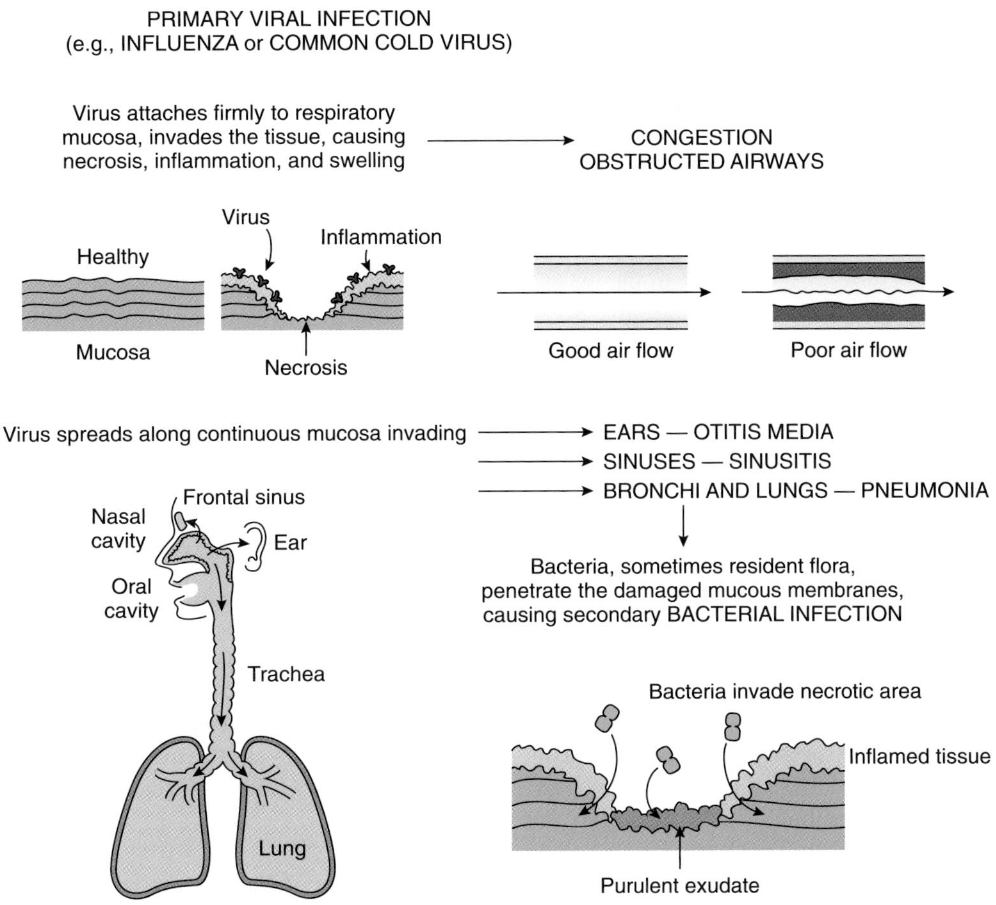

PRIMARY VIRAL INFECTION
(e.g., INFLUENZA or COMMON COLD VIRUS)

Virus attaches firmly to respiratory
mucosa, invades the tissue, causing ———————→ CONGESTION
necrosis, inflammation, and swelling   OBSTRUCTED AIRWAYS

Virus
Healthy   Inflammation

Mucosa   Good air flow   Poor air flow
        Necrosis

Virus spreads along continuous mucosa invading ——————→ EARS — OTITIS MEDIA
                                                ——————→ SINUSES — SINUSITIS
                                                ——————→ BRONCHI AND LUNGS — PNEUMONIA

Frontal sinus
Nasal   Bacteria, sometimes resident flora,
cavity   Ear   penetrate the damaged mucous membranes,
Oral   causing secondary BACTERIAL INFECTION
cavity

                                         Bacteria invade necrotic area
Trachea

                                                              Inflamed tissue

Lung

                                         Purulent exudate

FIGURE 13-8   Complications of viral respiratory infection.

smooth muscle spasm may exacerbate the obstruction, requiring additional medical treatment.

Epiglottitis

Epiglottitis is an acute infection usually caused by the bacterial organism, *H. influenzae* type B. It is common in children in the 3- to 7-year-old group, although the incidence has been increasing in adults. The infection causes swelling of the larynx, supraglottic area, and epiglottis, which appears as a round, red ball obstructing the airway. Onset is rapid, fever and sore throat develop, and the child refuses to swallow. Drooling of saliva is apparent, and inspiratory stridor is heard. The child appears anxious and pale and assumes a sitting position (tripod position) with the mouth open, struggling to breathe. Caution is required during laryngeal examination to prevent reflex spasm and total obstruction of the airway. Treatment consists of oxygen and antimicrobial therapy, with intubation or tracheotomy if necessary.

Influenza (Flu)

Influenza is a viral infection that may affect both the upper and the lower respiratory tracts. As indicated in the discussion of this topic at the end of Chapter 6 (influenza is presented as an example of infection), there are three groups of the influenza virus—type A, the most

prevalent pathogen, and types B and C. These viruses mutate constantly, preventing effective immune defense for prolonged time periods.

Flu differs from a common cold in that it usually has a sudden, acute onset with fever, marked fatigue, and aching pains in the body. It may also cause a viral pneumonia. Similarly to the common cold, a mild case of influenza can be complicated by secondary problems such as bacterial pneumonia. Most deaths during flu epidemics result from pneumonia.

Treatment is symptomatic and supportive unless bacterial infection occurs. Antiviral drugs, such as amantadine (Symmetrel, Endantadine), zanamivir (Relenza inhaler), or oseltamivir (Tamiflu) taken by adults in the first 2 days, may reduce the symptoms and duration as well as reduce the risk of infecting others. These drugs are useful in the control of flu outbreaks in hospitals or nursing homes. The incubation period for the virus is 1 to 4 days, with an average of 2, but the individual can pass the virus on a day before symptoms develop and for up to 5 days after.

Prevention of influenza by vaccination is highly recommended for all individuals. If flu does develop following immunization, it is a mild infection. A period of 2 to 3 weeks after vaccination is required before immunity develops.

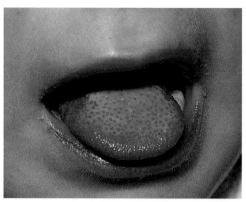

FIGURE 13-9 Scarlet fever. "Strawberry" tongue with its prominent papillae. *(From Zitelli BJ, Davis HW: Atlas of pediatric physical Diagnosis, ed 4. St. Louis, 2002, Mosby.)*

Scarlet Fever

An upper respiratory infection caused by group A β-hemolytic streptococcus (*Streptococcus pyogenes*). Incubation period is generally 1 to 2 days. Symptoms usually begin with a fever and sore throat; chills, vomiting, abdominal pain, and malaise may occur as well. The typical "strawberry" tongue (Fig. 13-9) is caused by the exotoxin produced by the bacteria. A fine rash on the chest, neck, groin, and thighs are characteristic also. Once a serious childhood disease, upper respiratory infection is now generally treatable with antibiotics.

THINK ABOUT   13-6

a. Compare the signs of the common cold, sinusitis, influenza, and epiglottitis.
b. Explain why secondary bacterial infections may commonly follow viral infections in the respiratory tract of elderly clients.
c. Explain why frequent handwashing may reduce the transmission of influenza.
d. Explain why antibacterial drugs are not effective against virus infections (see Chapter 6).
e. Describe how antiviral agents act against infection.

Lower Respiratory Tract Infections

Bronchiolitis (Respiratory Syncytial Virus Infection)

Bronchiolitis is a common infection in young children 2 to 12 months of age and is caused by the respiratory syncytial virus (RSV), a myxovirus. It is transmitted directly by oral droplet and occurs more frequently in the winter months. Predisposing factors include a familial history of asthma and the presence of cigarette smoke. Bronchiolitis varies in severity. The virus causes necrosis and inflammation in the small bronchi and

bronchioles, with edema, increased secretions, and reflex bronchospasm leading to obstruction of the small airways. Signs include wheezing and dyspnea; rapid, shallow respirations; cough; rales; chest retractions; fever; and malaise. There may be areas of hyperinflation with air trapping due to partial obstruction (see Fig. 13-19C) or areas of atelectasis or nonaeration resulting from total obstruction (see Fig. 13-24). Treatment is supportive and symptomatic, with monitoring of blood gases in severe cases to ensure that oxygen levels are adequate. Respiratory syncytial virus-immunoglobulin serum or palivizumab, an RSV monoclonal antibody, may be administered to reduce the severity of infection, particularly in premature infants.

Pneumonia

Pneumonia may develop as a primary acute infection in the lungs or it may be secondary to another respiratory or systemic condition in which tissue resistance is reduced. Pneumonia is a risk following any aspiration or inflammation in the lung, when fluids pool or defense mechanisms such as cilia are reduced. In most cases the organisms enter the lungs directly, by inhalation (virus), resident bacteria spreading along the mucosa, or aspiration in secretions. Occasionally the infection is blood-borne.

Classification of the Pneumonias

Numerous methods are available for classifying pneumonias. Categories may be based on the causative agent, anatomic location of the infection, pathophysiologic changes, or epidemiologic data.

For example, the causative agent may be a virus, bacterium, or fungus. Pneumonia may involve multiple microbes following aspiration. Usually lobar pneumonia is bacterial, the most common agent being a pneumococcus, but other causative organisms include *Staphylococcus aureus* and *Legionella* (Legionnaire's disease). Severe pneumococcal pneumonia is less common now because antibacterial medications are quickly administered, but it remains a major threat to those with chronic disease. A vaccine that provides protection against the seven most common agents of pneumonia is available for those with chronic respiratory or cardiovascular disease as well as clients greater than 65 years of age. Re-immunization does not appear to be necessary, but may be done without risk. In immune-suppressed individuals, other organisms such as *Candida* (fungus) or *Pneumocystis carinii* may cause pneumonia.

Anatomic distribution of lesions may be diffuse and patchy throughout both lungs or *lobar*, meaning consolidated in one lobe (Fig. 13-10). In some pneumonias, such as viral, pathophysiologic changes occur primarily in the interstitial tissue or alveolar septae. In other types, such as pneumococcal, the alveoli are inflamed and filled with exudate, resulting in a solid mass in a lobe.

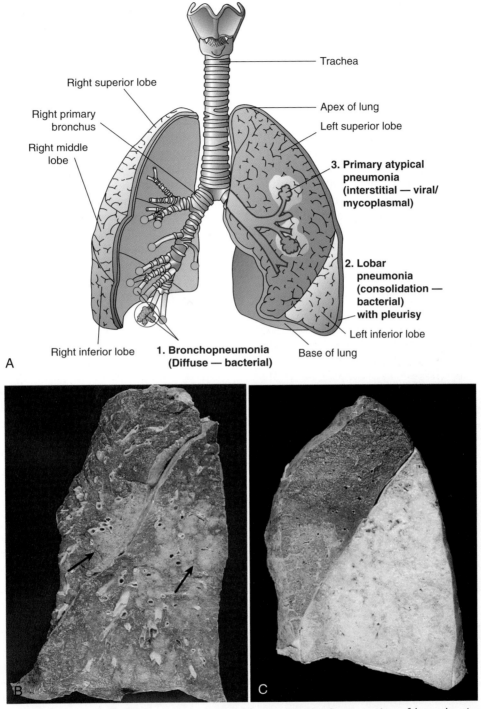

Right superior lobe

Right primary bronchus

Right middle lobe

Trachea

Apex of lung

Left superior lobe

3. Primary atypical pneumonia (interstitial — viral/ mycoplasmal)

2. Lobar pneumonia (consolidation — bacterial) with pleurisy

Left inferior lobe

Base of lung

Right inferior lobe

1. Bronchopneumonia (Diffuse — bacterial)

A

B

C

FIGURE 13-10 A, Types of pneumonia. **B,** Bronchopneumonia. Gross section of lung showing patches of consolidation (*arrows*). **C,** Lobar pneumonia. Lower lobe is uniformly consolidated (*light color*). (***B** and **C** from Kumar V, Abbas AK, Fausto M:* Robbins and Cotran Pathologic Basis of Disease, *ed 7, Philadelphia, 2005, Saunders.*)

Epidemiologic categories refer to *nosocomial* (hospital-acquired) pneumonia, which affects those with less resistance, the elderly, the debilitated, the malnourished, or the immune suppressed. In these cases, infection often results from gram-negative organisms such as *Klebsiella pneumoniae* or *Pseudomonas aeruginosa.*

Community-acquired pneumonia may be viral or bacterial. It can affect healthy persons, such as following influenza, as well as persons with underlying cardiovascular or respiratory disease. Aspiration pneumonia may be nosocomial or community acquired. It frequently involves aspiration of vomitus, which is irritating to tissues, or nasopharyngeal secretions. Mixed bacteria are usually isolated from the resultant infection. When periodontal disease is marked, aspiration pneumonia results from infection by gram-negative microbes.

A brief comparison of common types of pneumonia is found in Table 13-4.

Lobar Pneumonia

Lobar pneumonia (pneumococcal pneumonia) is usually caused by *Streptococcus pneumoniae* (pneumococcus), and the infection is localized in one or more lobes (Fig. 13-11). This microbe sometimes colonizes the nasopharynx without producing symptoms. The first stage in its development is *congestion*, in which inflammation and vascular congestion develop in the alveolar wall, and exudate forms in the alveoli. This change interferes greatly with oxygen diffusion. Next, neutrophils, RBCs, and fibrin accumulate in the alveolar exudate, forming a solid mass in the lobe, called *consolidation*. The

presence of these RBCs in the exudate produces the typical rusty sputum associated with lobar pneumonia. Eventually the RBCs break down, and as the infection resolves, macrophages break down the exudate to allow it to be expectorated or resorbed. Because a complete lobe is usually involved in the inflammatory process, the adjacent pleurae are frequently involved, producing pleuritic pain at the affected site (*pleurisy* or *pleuritis*). As well, infection may spread into the pleural cavity, causing empyema. If not resolved quickly, empyema can cause adhesions between the pleural membranes, restricting ventilation. Chest x-rays confirm the typical distribution of the infection, and a sputum culture identifies the organism.

The filling of the alveoli with exudate reduces the diffusion of gases, particularly oxygen, and decreases blood flow through the affected lobe. Hypoxia results and is more marked because the demand for oxygen increases with the higher metabolic rate associated with

TABLE 13-4   Types of Pneumonia

	Lobar Pneumonia	Bronchopneumonia	Interstitial Pneumonia (Primary Atypical Pneumonia, PAP)
Distribution	All of one or two lobes	Scattered small patches	Scattered small patches
Cause	*Streptococcus pneumoniae*	Multiple bacteria	Influenza virus *Mycoplasma*
Pathophysiology	Inflammation of alveolar wall and leakage of cells, fibrin, and fluid into alveoli causing consolidation Pleura may be inflamed	Inflammation and purulent exudate in alveoli often arising from prior pooled secretions or irritation	Interstitial inflammation around alveoli Necrosis of bronchial epithelium
Onset	Sudden and acute	Insidious	Variable
Signs	High fever and chills Productive cough with rusty sputum Rales progressing to absence of breath sounds in affected lobes	Mild fever Productive cough with yellow-green sputum Dyspnea	Variable fever, headache Aching muscles Nonproductive hacking cough

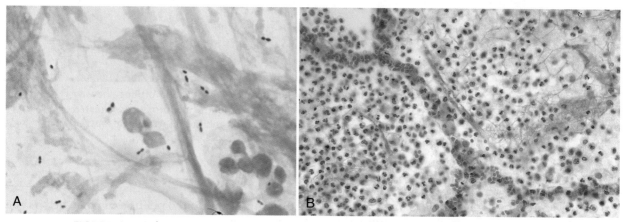

FIGURE 13-11   Lobar or streptococcal pneumonia. **A**, Respiratory secretions contain gram-positive diplococci suggesting *Streptococcus pneumonia*. *(From de la Maza LM, Pezzlo MT, Baron EJ:* Color Atlas of Diagnostic Microbiology, *St. Louis, 1999, Mosby.)* **B**, Pneumococcal pneumonia/alveoli filled with exudate containing neutrophils. *(From Kumar V, Abbas AK, Fausto M:* Robbins and Cotran Pathologic Basis of Disease, *ed 7, Philadelphia, 2005, Saunders.)*

the infection. The oxygen deficit also leads to metabolic acidosis. Dehydration may result from the high fever, hyperventilation, and inadequate fluid intake.

Typical manifestations of pneumococcal pneumonia include:

- Sudden onset
- Systemic signs of high fever with chills, marked fatigue, and leukocytosis
- Dyspnea, tachypnea, tachycardia
- Pleuritic pain with splinting or restriction of respiratory expansion on the affected side
- Rales, heard initially over the affected lobe, and then disappearing as consolidation occurs
- Productive cough, with the typical rusty-colored sputum
- Confusion and disorientation if infection is severe or several lobes are involved

Treatment involves the administration of antibacterial medications such as penicillin in combination with supportive measures such as fluids, drugs to reduce fever, and oxygen. Pneumococcal vaccine (considered a once-in-a-lifetime immunization) is recommended particularly for the elderly and those at risk because of other disease.

Bronchopneumonia

Bronchopneumonia occurs as a diffuse pattern of infection in both lungs, more often in the lower lobes. One or several species of microorganisms may cause the infection, beginning in the bronchial mucosa and spreading into the local alveoli. In many cases, pooled secretions in the lungs become infected by organisms draining from the upper passages, a hazard particularly in immobilized patients (hypostatic pneumonia). The inflammatory exudate forms in the alveoli, interfering with oxygen diffusion. Onset tends to be insidious, with moderate fever, cough, and rales. Congestion causes a productive cough with purulent sputum, usually yellow or green in color. Sputum culture and sensitivity tests indicate the appropriate choice of antibacterial treatment. Recovery usually occurs without residual lung damage.

Legionnaires' Disease

Legionnaires' disease is a pneumonia caused by a gram-negative bacteria, *Legionella pneumophila*. The microbe thrives in warm, moist environments, such as air conditioning systems and spas. It arises as a nosocomial infection in hospitals or other institutions, especially among those with other lung disease. It was unknown until a number of deaths occurred at a convention in 1976. The microbe has been difficult to identify because the organism is found inside pulmonary macrophages and requires a special culture medium. If untreated, the infection causes severe congestion and consolidation, with necrosis in the lung and possibly fatal consequences.

Primary Atypical Pneumonia

Primary atypical pneumonia (PAP) differs in both the causative organisms, often viral or mycoplasma, and the pathophysiology, which involves interstitial inflammation.

Mycoplasma pneumoniae is a very small bacterium that lacks a cell wall and can appear in varying shapes. It is found normally in the upper respiratory tract.

Mycoplasma pneumonia is common in older children and young adults. It is transmitted by aerosol but is not considered highly contagious. Frequent cough is a prominent sign. Mycoplasma responds to erythromycin or tetracycline therapy.

Viral pneumonia is often caused by influenza A or B, as well as adenoviruses and respiratory syncytial virus (RSV). The infection frequently begins insidiously, with inflammation in the mucosa of the upper respiratory tract, and then it descends to involve the lungs. These organisms produce inflammation that is diffuse and interstitial, with little exudate forming in the alveoli. Therefore, cough is unproductive, and rales are not pronounced. A radiograph may show some poorly defined patches of congestion. The infection varies greatly in severity, from mild cases that may not even be diagnosed to severe cases that may be complicated by secondary bacterial infection. The onset of primary atypical pneumonia is often vague, with nonproductive cough, hoarseness and sore throat, headache, mild fever, and malaise. The infection is usually self-limiting.

Chlamydial pneumonia, caused by the organism *Chlamydia pneumoniae*, is also considered a cause of PAP and pharyngitis. Infection is often mild, so sometimes it is not diagnosed.

Pneumocystis carinii *Pneumonia*

Pneumocystis carinii pneumonia (PCP), a type of atypical pneumonia, occurs as an opportunistic and often fatal infection in patients with acquired immunodeficiency syndrome (AIDS) (see Chapter 7). It also causes pneumonia in premature infants. This microbe was formerly classified as a protozoan, now it is considered a fungus (see Fig. 7-16A). It appears to be inhaled and attaches to alveolar cells, causing necrosis and diffuse interstitial inflammation. Then the alveoli fill with exudate and fungi, including the cystic form. Its onset is marked by difficulty breathing and a nonproductive cough. For AIDS patients with low CD4 T-cell counts, prophylactic drugs such as sulfamethoxazole-trimethoprim combination or pentamidine aerosol are recommended.

Severe Acute Respiratory Syndrome

Severe acute respiratory syndrome (SARS) is of importance because its advent triggered extensive global efforts to quickly identify this previously unknown microorganism and its mode of transmission, then to develop a system to contain and control the spread of such emerging infections. These guidelines could be implemented for other emerging infectious diseases. In October 2004, the World Health Organization (WHO) revised the guidelines for global surveillance and reporting of SARS and laboratory precautions. At that time, the last case of SARS had occurred in a laboratory worker in China in April 2004. The Centers for Disease Control and Prevention continues to focus on early detection of cases, and monitors and updates information about this and other emerging diseases.

Severe acute respiratory syndrome, an acute respiratory infection, was first diagnosed in China in 2002. It did not attract attention until February 2003, when China informed WHO about a new form of atypical pneumonia clustered in one province. Work began to identify the infectious agent and the genetic sequence of the virus was announced on April 14, 2003, confirming it as a previously unknown agent. (By contrast, the agent for Legionnaires' disease was not identified by researchers until 2 years after its first appearance.) By July 2003, in excess of 8000 cases and almost 800 deaths were reported in 29 countries around the world. The rapid spread and high morbidity and mortality rates prompted immediate cooperative action by epidemiologists and public health officials globally.

The causative microbe is a coronavirus, named SARS-CoV (SARS-associated coronavirus), an RNA virus that is transmitted by respiratory droplets during close contact. To date, a close exposure to existing cases has always been identified; casual contact has not been documented.

The incubation period is 2 to 7 days, average 4 to 6 days. The first stage presents as a flulike syndrome, with fever, headache, myalgia, chills, anorexia, and frequently diarrhea, lasting 3 to 7 days. Effects on the lungs are evident several days later, with a dry cough and marked dyspnea. Chest radiographs by day 7 indicate spreading patchy areas of interstitial congestion and hypoxia increases rapidly, with mechanical ventilation often required. Lymphopenia and thrombocytopenia are often present, as are increased C-reactive protein levels. Elevated liver enzymes were found in many cases and appeared to result from liver damage by the virus. A number of patients continue into a third stage with severe, sometimes fatal, respiratory distress.

Treatment included the antiviral ribavirin and the glucocorticoid methylprednisolone.

The case fatality rate is high, about 10%, increasing to greater than 50% in patients more than 60 years of age.

The lack of a rapid diagnostic test (antibodies are not present until 3 weeks after onset) and the nonspecific early manifestations of SARS combine to make immediate identification of the infection difficult.

Currently risk factors that may be monitored to prevent future outbreaks include:

- Travel to China, Hong Kong, and Taiwan or close contact with such a traveler

- The presence of a cluster of undiagnosed atypical pneumonia cases
- Employment involving close contact with the virus (nursing a patient or a laboratory worker handling the virus). During the epidemic in 2003 in Canada, a second wave of infection, among health care workers and visitors who were in direct contact with the first hospitalized SARS cases, occurred 4 weeks later. This confirmed the need for additional protective clothing for those in close contact with cases and tighter infection control measures within institutions. Patients were treated in specific institutions and those in contact with active cases were quarantined at home until shown to be clear of infection.

Tuberculosis

Once thought to be declining and well under control, tuberculosis (TB) is increasing globally, with many new cases each year in some areas of the world, particularly among AIDS patients in Africa. One to two percent of new cases are multiple drug resistant forms of the disease, which has complicated control of the infection and its spread within the community. Tuberculosis is a disease of poverty and crowding. Predicted new cases annually in the United States are dropping in many areas; but areas in which HIV infection and homelessness are high show rates closer to those of developing countries. Prevalence is difficult to estimate because of the large number of latent cases (many are undiagnosed). Ten percent of diagnosed infections will progress to active pulmonary TB. Two billion people worldwide are infected, and the death rate is 2000 deaths per year globally, with the highest mortality rates among those who are HIV positive.

■ *Pathophysiology*

Tuberculosis is an infection that is usually caused by *Mycobacterium tuberculosis* and primarily affects the lungs, but the pathogen may invade other organs as well. *Mycobacterium* is an acid-fast, aerobic, slow-growing bacillus that is somewhat resistant to drying and many disinfectants. The microbe can survive in dried sputum for weeks. They are destroyed by ultraviolet light, heat, alcohol, glutaraldehyde, and formaldehyde. The cell wall also appears to protect the organism from destruction by normal body defenses, so that the normal response by neutrophils (PMNs) to infection and production of purulent exudate does not occur.

There are two stages in the pathogenesis of tuberculosis—primary infection (TB infection) and secondary infection or reinfection (TB disease) (Fig. 13-12). *Primary infection* occurs when the microorganisms first enter the lungs, are engulfed by macrophages, and cause a local inflammatory reaction, usually on the periphery of the upper lobe. Some bacilli migrate to the lymph nodes, activating a type IV or cell-mediated

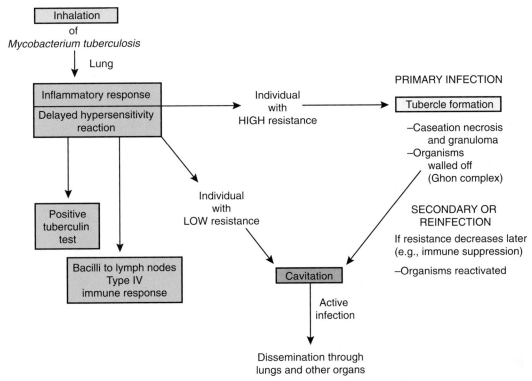

FIGURE 13-12 Development of tuberculosis.

hypersensitivity response (see Chapter 7). Lymphocytes and macrophages cluster together to form a granuloma at the site of inflammation. The granuloma contains the bacilli, some of which remain alive, forming a *tubercle*. In the center of the tubercle, caseation necrosis develops, forming a core of cheese-like material consisting of dead macrophages and necrotic tissue. A healthy person can resist this invasion, so these lesions remain very small and become walled off by fibrous tissue, eventually calcifying. These lesions in the lung and lymph nodes are referred to as Ghon complexes. When calcified, the tubercle may be visible on a chest radiograph. However, the bacilli may remain viable, in a dormant state inside the tubercle for years, and are therefore a potential danger. As long as the *individual's resistance* and immune responses remain high, the bacilli remain walled off within the tubercle. The individual has been exposed to the bacillus and infected but does *not* have active disease and is asymptomatic. By about 6 to 8 weeks the immune response is complete. This is considered primary or latent infection.

The hypersensitivity reaction first initiated by *M. tuberculosis* is the basis for the tuberculin test (e.g., Mantoux test), which is used to detect exposure to the bacillus. Several weeks after exposure, the person has become hypersensitive and will produce a positive skin reaction, a large area of induration (a hard, raised, red area), in response to administration of tuberculoprotein. A chest x-ray and sputum culture will determine whether active infection is present.

In people with *low resistance* for any reason, the primary infection may not be controlled but instead progress to active infection, spreading through the lungs and to other organs.

Miliary or *extrapulmonary* tuberculosis is a rapidly progressive form in which multiple granulomas affect large areas of the lungs and rapidly disseminate into the circulation and to other tissues, such as bone or kidney. This form of infection is more common in children and immunosuppressed adults. If the patient with extrapulmonary TB has no cough, she or he is not considered to have a contagious disease.

Secondary or *reinfection* tuberculosis is the stage of active infection. It often arises years after primary infection, when the bacilli, hidden in the tubercles, are reactivated, usually because of decreased host resistance. Occasionally there is a new invasion of microbes. As the organisms multiply, tissue destruction occurs, forming a large area of necrosis (Fig. 13-13*A*). *Cavitation* occurs, with formation of a large open area in the lung and erosion into the bronchi and blood vessels (Fig. 13-13*B*). Hemoptysis is common as blood vessels are eroded. With cavitation, spread of the organisms into other parts of the lung is promoted, and bacilli are present in the sputum, where they may be passed to others. Bacteria may be swallowed to infect the digestive tract. Infection may also spread into the pleural cavity, causing pleuritis and adhesions.

Patients with cough and positive sputum tests or x-ray showing cavitation are infectious, and proper

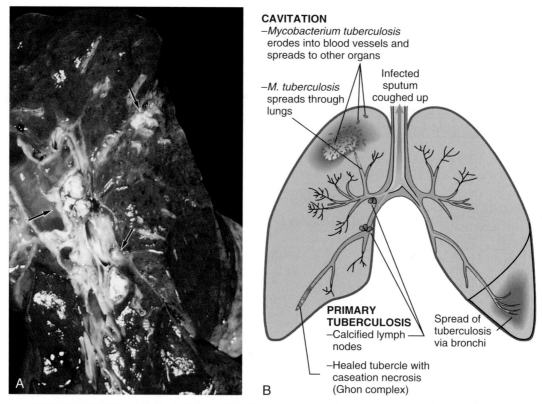

FIGURE 13-13 Tuberculosis. **A,** Primary TB, Ghon complex, in lower part of upper lobe. (*Top arrow shows gray-white area. Lower arrows show hilar lymph nodes with caseation.*) **B** Cavitation. (*From Kumar V, Abbas AK, Fausto M:* Robbins and Cotran Pathologic Basis of Disease, *ed 7, Philadelphia, 2005, Saunders.*)

respiratory hygiene measures must be followed. These include covering the mouth when coughing, wearing a mask when in contact with others, and avoidance of sustained close contact with others.

■ *Etiology*

Mycobacterium tuberculosis is transmitted by oral droplets released from a person with active infection that are inhaled into the lungs. In some countries in which milk is not pasteurized, tuberculosis may be caused by the related *Mycobacterium bovis*, which infects cows.

Tuberculosis occurs more frequently in persons living in crowded conditions or those whose resistance is lowered because of immunodeficiency, malnutrition, alcoholism, conditions of war, or chronic disease. There is probably a genetic susceptibility, and children are more easily infected than adults. Some factors leading to an increasing incidence in recent years are more frequent travel, an increased homeless population who are malnourished and frequently have other diseases, prevalence of the infection in patients with AIDS, and development of drug-resistant strains of the organism.

■ *Signs and Symptoms*

Primary tuberculosis is asymptomatic. The onset of secondary or active pulmonary tuberculosis is insidious.

Systemic signs often appear first, with vague manifestations such as anorexia, malaise, fatigue, and weight loss. Afternoon low-grade fever and night sweats develop. Cough is prolonged and becomes increasingly severe and, as cavitation develops, more productive. Sputum becomes purulent and often contains blood.

■ *Diagnostic Tests*

First exposure or primary infection is indicated by a positive tuberculin test result. This test is of no value (that is, it produces a false-positive result) if the person has previously received the bacillus Calmette-Guérin (BCG) vaccine for tuberculosis or has had a previous positive tuberculin test. Active infection can be confirmed by chest x-ray, acid-fast staining of sputum specimens, and sputum culture (a lengthy time required). A CT scan is more sensitive than the traditional x-ray in identifying TB lesions. Newer testing techniques involving the nucleic acid amplification (NAA) from microbial genetic material provide faster confirmation. Routine testing of health care providers is common practice and prophylactic medication may be required if the person shows a new positive tuberculin test in the absence of any other signs or symptoms of infection. Detailed protocols vary with the licensing bodies responsible for professional practice and the public health statutes.

Treatment

A person with active tuberculosis is now usually treated at home or in a general hospital. Long-term treatment with a combination of drugs is recommended, so as to totally eradicate the infecting microbes and reduce the risk of resistant bacteria. The length of treatment varies from 6 months to a year or longer depending on the situation. Drugs of choice include isoniazid (INH), rifampin, ethambutol, pyrazinamide, and streptomycin. Sputum culture usually is negative for tuberculosis organisms after 1 to 2 months of treatment, and the risk of transmission becomes much less. Patient compliance with the drug regimen for the entire time is essential to totally eradicate the infection and prevent the development of drug-resistant microbes. The WHO recommends a Directly Observed Therapy (DOT) regimen in all cases. The DOT program requires a health care worker to observe the administration of each drug dose in the treatment protocol. This approach requires government commitment to reduce the incidence of TB, adequate drugs, and adequate funding to administer them. Case finding of early active cases is also part of the protocol. Directly Observed Therapy is expensive in terms of human resources, but when used in highly endemic areas it has reduced TB infection rates significantly. Unfortunately, not all TB infected individuals accept the need for supervision, drug shortages are common, and funding for DOT may not be available; as a result cure rates remain low.

It is recommended that contacts of the patient be given prophylactic isoniazid for 1 year and receive tuberculin testing as well. The BCG vaccine is not widely used in North America because it is not considered sufficiently effective, particularly in adults, and its use prevents diagnosis by skin test. Because BCG immunization continues to be used in some countries, a health history should include this immunization. In North America all babies should be tested for TB on or before their first birthday unless symptoms and history suggest earlier testing.

THINK ABOUT 13-7

a. Compare the causative organism and two significant signs of lobar pneumonia with those of bronchopneumonia.
b. What factors predispose to bronchopneumonia in immobilized persons?
c. Describe and explain the significance of a tubercle and cavitation in the progress of TB infection.
d. Describe several specific precautions that could be taken by affected individuals or health professionals that would limit the spread of *M. tuberculosis*.

Histoplasmosis

Histoplasmosis, a fungal infection, is common in the midwestern United States, where the fungus *Histoplasma capsulatum* and its spores can be inhaled on dust particles. As well, histoplasmosis occurring as an opportunistic infection is common in persons with AIDS, in whom the fungus tends to disseminate or spread easily throughout the body. The fungus is found as a parasite inside macrophages.

The effects of histoplasmosis are similar to those of tuberculosis in that the first stage often involves asymptomatic, limited infection that may be followed by a second stage of active infection. This second stage involves granuloma formation and necrosis and consolidation in the lungs as well as possible spread to other organs. Signs include cough, marked fatigue, fever, and night sweats. A skin test can differentiate histoplasmosis from TB, and the organisms can be cultured to confirm the diagnosis. Current treatment consists of the antifungal agent amphotericin B (Fungizone).

Anthrax

Anthrax is a bacterial infection of the skin, respiratory tract or gastrointestinal tract of humans and cattle. Although rare in developed countries, it has recently gained attention as a biological weapon. The causative organism is a gram-positive bacillus that forms grayish white spores that can remain viable for long periods of time. Inhalation anthrax causes flulike symptoms following a usual incubation period of 1 to 7 days. Within 3 to 5 days severe acute respiratory distress occurs with mediastinal widening on x-ray and fever. Shock follows quickly due to the release of toxins, and case fatality rates were 45% in the 2001 illnesses as a result of exposure to anthrax spores in Washington, DC. Anthrax is treated with the antimicrobial ciprofloxacin (Cipro). If anthrax infection is suspected, the local medical officer of health and federal law enforcement agencies must be contacted. Strict respiratory barrier measures are required until the source of the infection is identified and removed.

Animal vaccines for protection against anthrax are in common use in North America and are effective in reducing infection. Vaccination of individuals is available and recommended for those who work with the organism in the laboratory, persons who work with animal hides imported from areas with a high incidence of animal anthrax, and military personnel. Pregnant women should *not* be immunized with anthrax vaccine.

Obstructive Lung Diseases

Cystic Fibrosis

Cystic fibrosis (CF) is a common inherited disorder in children. The incidence of CF differs with the ethnic community of the parents, and is 1 in 3419 live births to parents who are of white, European ancestry and 1 in 12,163 to parents who are of African ancestry in the

United States. In Canada the incidence rate is 1 in 3600 live births. The mean survival age in 2006 was 37 years. Many states include CF in newborn screening programs for early identification and prevention of infections.

■ *Pathophysiology*

Cystic fibrosis, sometimes called mucoviscidosis, is a genetic disorder. Several mutations to the CFTR gene have been identified and relate to a protein involved in chloride ion transport in the cell membrane. This defect in the exocrine glands causes abnormally thick secretions, such as tenacious mucus. The primary effects of cystic fibrosis are seen in the lungs and the pancreas, where the sticky mucus obstructs the passages; other tissues are affected less frequently. Usually several areas in the body are affected in an individual. The severity of the effects varies among individuals.

In the *lungs*, the mucus obstructs airflow in the bronchioles and small bronchi, causing air trapping or atelectasis with permanent damage to the bronchial walls (Fig. 13-14). Because stagnant mucus is an excellent medium for bacterial growth, infections are common and add to the progressive destruction of lung tissue. Organisms commonly causing infection in patients with cystic fibrosis include *P. aeruginosa* and *S. aureus*. Bronchiectasis and emphysematous changes are seen frequently as fibrosis and obstructions advance. Eventually respiratory failure or cor pulmonale (right-sided congestive heart failure) develops.

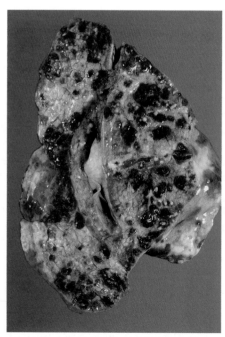

FIGURE 13-14 Lung from a patient with cystic fibrosis. The lung shows widespread bronchopneumonia with pus from dilated bronchi and bronchioles. *(From Cooke RA, Stewart B: Colour Atlas of Anatomical Pathology, ed 3, Sydney, 2004, Churchill Livingstone.)*

In the digestive tract, the first indication of abnormality may be *meconium ileus* in newborns, in which the small intestine of the neonate is blocked by mucus at birth, preventing the excretion of meconium shortly after birth (Fig. 13-15). In the *pancreas*, the ducts of the exocrine glands become blocked, leading to a deficit of pancreatic digestive enzymes in the intestine. Malabsorption and malnutrition result. Also, the obstruction and backup of secretions eventually cause damage to the pancreatic tissue, including the islets of Langerhans, resulting in diabetes mellitus in some individuals. The *bile ducts* of the liver may be blocked by viscid mucus, preventing bile from reaching the duodenum and interfering with digestion and absorption of fats and fat-soluble vitamins. Ultimately this abnormality also contributes to the general state of malabsorption, malnutrition, and dehydration. If obstruction is severe, the backup of bile behind the obstruction may cause inflammation and permanent damage to the liver in the form of biliary cirrhosis.

The *salivary glands* are often mildly affected, with secretions that are abnormally high in sodium chloride and mucus plugs that cause patchy fibrosis of the submaxillary and sublingual glands. The *sweat glands* are also affected, producing sweat that is very high in sodium chloride content. This is usually not a serious problem unless hot weather or strenuous exercise lead to excessive loss of electrolytes in the sweat. The *reproductive system* may be affected, with thick mucus obstructing the vas deferens in males or the cervix in females, leading to sterility or infertility. In some males the testes and ducts do not develop normally.

■ *Etiology*

The mutated CFTR gene for cystic fibrosis is located on the seventh chromosome, and the disease is transmitted as an autosomal recessive disorder (see Chapter 21). It is much more common in whites from northern Europe. Asymptomatic carriers form a high proportion of the population. When a family history of cystic fibrosis warrants testing, the defect can be diagnosed prenatally and in carriers with reliable results.

■ *Signs and Symptoms*

- Signs such as meconium ileus may appear at birth.
- Salty skin may be noticed by a mother when kissing a newborn with cystic fibrosis. This may lead to a *sweat test* and the diagnosis of cystic fibrosis. In some cases, the diagnosis may be delayed a few months or several years.
- The signs of malabsorption may become apparent during the first year of life, with steatorrhea (bulky, fatty, foul stools), abdominal distention, and failure to gain weight. These signs indicate a lack of the pancreatic enzymes and bile needed to digest food and absorb nutrients. Fats and the fat-soluble vitamins (vitamins A, D, E, and K) are affected

CYSTIC FIBROSIS—AN AUTOSOMAL RECESSIVE DISORDER

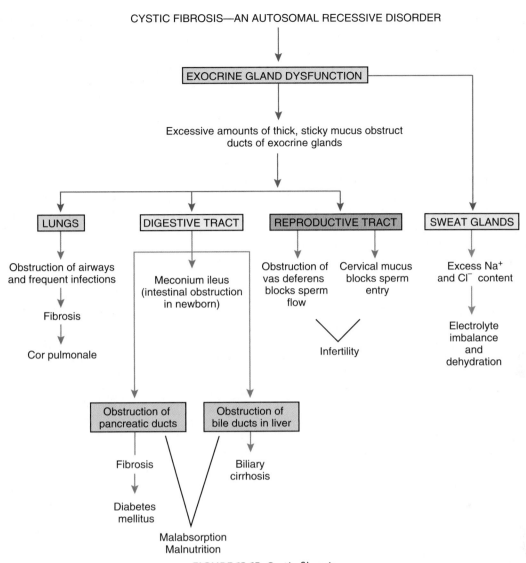

FIGURE 13-15 Cystic fibrosis.

initially, but in turn protein and carbohydrate deficits develop.

- Chronic cough and frequent respiratory infections indicate pulmonary involvement in the child. These tend to increase over time. As lung damage proceeds, hypoxia, fatigue, and exercise intolerance develop. The chest may be overinflated owing to air trapping, and rhonchi are audible.
- Failure to meet the normal growth milestones is common, usually because of chronic respiratory problems.

▣ *Diagnostic Tests*

Genetic testing can identify the CFTR mutations at birth or any time after birth. Sweat is analyzed for abnormal electrolyte content. This test may not be accurate until the infant is at least 2 to 3 weeks old. Stools may be checked for fat content and trypsin (pancreatic enzyme) content. Lung involvement can be assessed with x-rays, pulmonary function tests, and blood gas analysis.

▣ *Treatment*

Treatment of a child with cystic fibrosis requires a team or interdisciplinary approach because there is multisystemic involvement with numerous complications and implications for the child's growth and development.

Replacement therapy for pancreatic enzymes, for example, pancrelipase (Cotazym), and if necessary, bile salt replacement can be administered with meals and snacks to improve digestion and absorption and promote general health and resistance to infection. A well-balanced diet, with high protein, low fat, and vitamin supplements, is recommended, but the suggested total dietary intake is much greater than is usually recommended for a specific child or adult to allow for some malabsorption. It is important to avoid dehydration resulting from excessive losses in the sweat or stool because a fluid deficit may result in thicker and more tenacious respiratory mucus.

Intensive chest physiotherapy, including postural drainage, percussion, and coughing techniques, is a very time-consuming but necessary daily exercise to ensure removal of the tenacious mucus. The use of bronchodilators and humidifiers also promotes drainage. Regular moderate aerobic exercise is helpful in removing secretions and promoting general health.

Immediate aggressive treatment is required for infections and has extended the life span of patients. In patients with advanced lung disease, oxygen therapy as well as medication for congestive heart failure may be required (see Chapter 12).

With improved treatment, the life span of children with cystic fibrosis has been extended into adulthood. Respiratory failure is the usual cause of death. Heart-lung transplants have been performed in some individuals with cystic fibrosis (see Chapter 7). Research continues to repair the genetic mutation or alter its expression.

THINK ABOUT 13-8

a. Describe how cystic fibrosis affects the lungs and sweat glands.
b. Describe the potential complications of cystic fibrosis in the lungs and pancreas.
c. Explain the probability of cystic fibrosis occurring in a child when one parent is a carrier.

Lung Cancer

The lungs are a common site of both primary and secondary lung cancer. Benign lung tumors are rare. Lung cancer ranks as the third most common cancer in the United States. The incidence has declined slightly, but the mortality rate remains high. Estimates for 2008 indicate 215,000 individuals will be diagnosed in the United States with lung cancer and more than 162,000 patients with lung cancer in the United States will die. Incidence and mortality rates are similar in Canada. Women are more apt to develop lung cancer and die of it than are men. There is a higher incidence in black men than white men. Almost 90% of lung cancers are related to smoking. This has precipitated legislation in many areas to ban smoking in all public places.

Secondary metastatic cancer develops frequently in the lungs because the venous return and lymphatics bring tumor cells from many distant sites in the body to the heart and then into the pulmonary circulation, which provides the first small blood vessels and hospitable environment in which tumor cells can lodge (see Fig. 20-5).

■ *Pathophysiology*

Bronchogenic carcinoma, arising from the bronchial epithelium, is the most common type of malignant lung tumor (Fig. 13-16). A number of subgroups occur. Squamous cell carcinoma usually develops from the

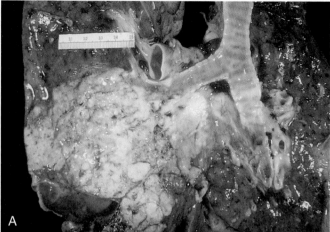

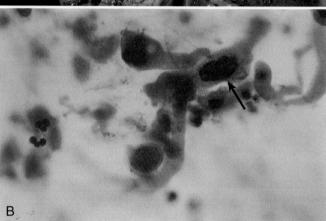

FIGURE 13-16 **A,** Bronchogenic carcinoma. The tumor, a squamous cell carcinoma, appears gray-white, infiltrating the lung tissue. **B,** Cytologic examination of a sputum specimen shows a squamous carcinoma cell with large nucleus (*arrow*). (***A** and **B** from Kumar V, Abbas AK, Fausto M: Robbins and Cotran Pathologic Basis of Disease, ed 7, Philadelphia, 2005, Saunders.)*

epithelial lining of a bronchus near the hilum and projects into the airway (see Fig. 20-3). Adenocarcinomas (from glands) and bronchoalveolar cell carcinomas are usually found on the periphery of the lung, making them less symptomatic and more difficult to detect in the early stages. The cells of adenocarcinomas may secrete mucin. Small cell or "oat cell" carcinomas are a rapidly growing type of lung cancer often located near a major bronchus in the central part of the lung. They tend to be invasive and metastasize very early in their development. Large cell carcinomas are usually found in the periphery and consist of undifferentiated large cells that have a rapid growth rate and metastasize early.

The first change in the lungs is usually metaplasia, a change in the epithelial tissue, associated with smoking or chronic irritation, which is reversible if the irritation ceases. The loss of normal protective, ciliated, pseudostratified epithelium leaves the lung tissue more vulnerable to irritants and inflammation from smoking. Various chemicals in cigarette smoke are carcinogenic and act as initiators and promoters. Dysplasia or carcinoma in situ then develops. These changes are difficult to detect. Lung cancer is staged at the time of diagnosis based on the tumor size-node involvement-metastases (TNM) classification (see Chapter 20). Stage I tumors are localized, whereas stage III lesions are disseminated. Common sites of metastases from the lungs include the brain, bone, and liver.

Tumors in the lungs have many effects:

- Obstruction of airflow by tumor growth into a bronchus causes abnormal breath sounds and dyspnea.
- Inflammation surrounding the tumor stimulates a cough and predisposes to secondary infection. Frequent infections may occur because secretions pool distal to the tumor.
- Pleural effusion, hemothorax, pneumothorax, or combination of these is common with tumors located on the lung periphery owing to inflammation or erosion of the pleural membrane.
- Paraneoplastic syndrome may accompany bronchogenic carcinoma when the tumor cell secretes hormones or hormone-like substances such as antidiuretic hormone (ADH) or adrenocorticotropic hormone (ACTH). The endocrine effects may complicate both diagnosis and treatment. This syndrome may include neuromuscular disturbances or hematologic disorders such as disseminated intravascular coagulation (DIC) (see Chapter 10).
- Tumors in the lungs also cause the usual systemic effects of cancer.

Etiology

The incidence of lung cancer continues to rise and is now very high in women as well as men. Cigarette smoking is the major factor in its development. "Secondhand smoke" in the environment has been implicated in a significant number of cases. The risk of developing cancer is higher in persons who begin smoking early, persist for many years, and are considered heavy smokers (i.e., they smoke more than a pack per day). Not all smokers develop lung cancer, and therefore there is probably a genetic factor involved that also influences the cellular changes (see Chapter 20). Tumors may develop in persons with chronic obstructive pulmonary disease (COPD), also associated with smoking (see Fig. 13-21C).

Occupational or industrial exposure to carcinogens such as silica, vinyl chloride, or asbestos is the other major cause of lung cancer, and the risk is greatly increased if a second factor such as cigarette smoking is also present in an occupationally exposed individual.

In addition to the direct carcinogenic effect, any irritant such as smoke leads to chronic inflammation and frequent infections in the respiratory tract, which in turn cause cellular changes. For example, in the mucosa, cigarette smoking causes a change from ciliated columnar epithelium to squamous cell epithelium. The alterations in the respiratory mucosa as it changes through metaplasia to dysplasia demonstrate the cell mutations caused by carcinogens and could perhaps lead to earlier diagnosis.

Signs and Symptoms

The onset of lung cancer is insidious because the early signs of cancer are often masked by signs of the predisposing factor, such as a "smoker's cough." In many cases, the cancer has already metastasized before diagnosis, and the signs of a metastatic tumor lead to diagnosis. There are four possible categories of signs of lung cancer: (1) those related to the direct effects of the tumor on the respiratory structures; (2) those representing the systemic effects of cancer; (3) those caused by associated paraneoplastic syndromes; and (4) those resulting from metastatic tumors at other sites.

1. Early signs related to respiratory involvement include:
   a. Persistent productive cough, dyspnea, and wheezing
   b. Detection on a chest x-ray taken when an individual develops pneumonia or other complications
   c. Hemoptysis, when tumors erode tissue
   d. Pleural involvement, which may lead to pleural effusion, pneumothorax, or hemothorax
   e. Chest pain, occurring with advanced tumors that involve the pleura or mediastinum
   f. Hoarseness (laryngeal nerve compression), facial or arm edema and headache (compression of the superior vena cava), dysphagia (compression of the esophagus), or atelectasis, caused by large tumors or involved lymph nodes
2. Systemic signs of lung cancer include weight loss, anemia, and fatigue.
3. Paraneoplastic syndrome is indicated by the signs of an endocrine disorder related to the specific hormone secreted.
4. Signs of metastases depend on the site. For example, metastatic bone cancer would be indicated on a bone scan and be manifested by bone pain or pathologic fracture.

Diagnostic Tests

There is no readily available screening test for lung cancer, although research continues to identify means to diagnose tumors before metastasis and spread. Specialized helical CT scans and MRI are more effective in early diagnosis than chest x-rays, which demonstrate later lesions and complications such as atelectasis or pleural effusion. Bronchoscopy provides secretions containing malignant cells from central lesions for definitive diagnosis, and biopsy may be required for less accessible lesions. Mediastinoscopy is useful to check lymph nodes, whereas bone scans are used to detect metastasis. These are useful in the staging process. Pulmonary function tests can clarify the effects of the tumor on airflow.

Treatment

Radiofrequency ablation (RFA) can be used to destroy single small tumors (see Chapter 20). Surgical resection or lobectomy may be performed on localized lesions. Chemotherapy and radiation may be used in conjunction with surgery or as palliative treatment, although many tumors are not responsive to such therapy. Photodynamic therapy (a chemical is injected and migrates to tumor cells, where it is activated by laser light and destroys the cancer cells) is sometimes effective. The prognosis is poor unless the tumor is in a very early stage of development.

Aspiration

Aspiration involves the passage of food or fluid, vomitus, drugs, or other foreign material into the trachea and lungs. The right lower lung is often the destination of aspirated material because anatomically the right branching bronchus tends to continue almost straight down, whereas the bronchus in the left lung branches at a sharper angle. Normally a cough removes such material from the upper tract, and the vocal cords and epiglottis prevent entry into the lower tract.

Pathophysiology

The characteristics of the aspirate determine the specific effects on respiratory function. For example, vomitus may contain solid objects as well as highly acidic gastric secretions, lipids, or alcohol. The common result is obstruction, whether the aspirate is a solid object causing obstruction directly or an irritating liquid causing inflammation and swelling. In addition, inflammation may interfere with gas exchange and predispose to pneumonia.

Some examples of the effects of aspirated solid objects follow:

- Solid objects lodge in a passageway and totally obstruct airflow at that point. The physical size of the object is one factor, which may be augmented by inflammation and swelling in the area. A small obstruction may be asymptomatic.
- A large object may occlude the trachea and block all airflow, a life-threatening situation. In such cases, no sound can be made to alert others to the problem, and consciousness is lost very quickly as oxygen supplies are depleted.
- Solid objects lodging in a bronchus lead to nonaeration and collapse of the area distal to the obstacle (see Fig. 13-24C).
- Sometimes solid objects create a ball-valve effect, in which air is able to pass down the tract on inspiration, but the passageway totally closes on

expiration, leading to a buildup of air distal to the obstruction.

- Foods such as dried beans may swell after aspiration and become more firmly lodged.
- Sharp pointed objects, such as bone fragments, also lodge in a passageway. Although it does not totally occlude the airway by itself, such an object traumatizes the mucosa, causing an acute inflammatory response that adds to the barrier. The inflammatory response may stimulate bronchoconstriction. Also, an object that straddles the airway will collect any other material entering the area, increasing the obstruction.
- Fatty or irritating solids such as peanuts also cause inflammation around the area, creating edema and further impeding airflow. If not removed, a granuloma or fibrous tissue develops around such material (Fig. 13-17).

When liquids are aspirated, the effects are somewhat different. Irritating liquids, particularly acids (vomitus), alcohol, or oils (milk), tend to disperse into several bronchi. These materials cause severe inflammation, leading to narrow airways and increased secretions, which make the lungs more difficult to expand. In some cases, the alveoli are involved in the inflammation, and gas diffusion is impaired. This type of inflammation may be called chemical or *aspiration pneumonia*; it predisposes to the development of infection later.

Other potential complications include:

- *Respiratory distress syndrome* may develop if inflammation is widespread.
- Pulmonary abscess may develop if microbes are in the aspirate.
- Certain materials such as solvents, if aspirated in large amounts, may be absorbed into the blood and cause systemic effects.

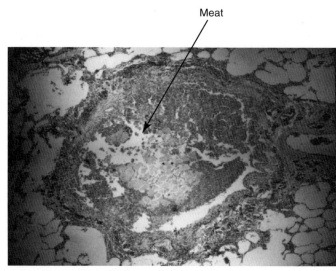

Meat

FIGURE 13-17 Photomicrograph of granuloma in the lung resulting from aspiration of meat in a patient with multiple sclerosis. *(Courtesy of R.W. Shaw, MD, North York General Hospital, Toronto, Ontario, Canada.)*

Etiology

Aspiration is a common problem in young children. When children are very young, they put most objects in their mouths. Children also tend to move about with objects in their mouths, thus increasing the risk of aspiration. *Smooth, round* objects are most dangerous. Common examples are chunks of hot dogs, candy, nuts, grapes, and raw carrots. Buttons or coins and balloons are frequent nonfood examples. Children may accidentally aspirate toxic fluids such as cleaning materials or lighter fluid. Some fluids, such as those containing hydrocarbons, for example, turpentine, have a low viscosity and a low surface tension and therefore tend to spread in a very thin film over a large area of the lung, causing extensive irritation and damage. Inhalation of substances such as baby powder can also cause inflammation in the delicate lung tissue.

Children with congenital anomalies such as a cleft palate or tracheoesophageal fistula are especially at risk for aspiration until surgical repair takes place (see Chapter 17).

Aspiration can occur under many different circumstances. It is often a complication in individuals of any age when the swallowing or gag reflex is depressed for any reason, for example, following anesthesia or stroke, or in patients with coma or neurologic damage. Vomitus may be aspirated postoperatively from the effects of anesthetics or drugs. Usually a patient is not allowed to eat or drink preoperatively to reduce the risk of aspiration, but emergency situations do not allow for this precaution.

Individuals who eat or drink or perhaps take medications when lying down also risk aspiration because the gravitational force is of no value in moving food quickly and completely down the esophagus. Residual liquid often remains in the mouth and oropharynx, to drip at a later time into the trachea.

Adults frequently aspirate food or fluid, especially when combining eating with talking at social events (sometimes called a *café coronary*). A chunk of meat is the common culprit, particularly if the food is not well chewed and alcohol intake has depressed protective reflexes. Because such food causes total obstruction, the person cannot speak, but may have time to gesture to the chest or neck before falling unconscious, and this could be interpreted as a heart attack or coronary. It is important to sweep the mouth for any object and carry out the Heimlich maneuver before commencing cardiopulmonary resuscitation.

Signs and Symptoms

Common manifestations:
- Coughing and choking with marked dyspnea are common.
- Stridor and hoarseness are characteristic of upper airway obstruction.

- Wheezing occurs with aspiration of liquids into the lungs.
- Tachycardia and tachypnea are responses to respiratory distress.
- Nasal flaring, chest retractions, and marked hypoxia occur in individuals with severe respiratory distress.
- As mentioned, total obstruction at the larynx or trachea prevents any sounds or cough from being produced. A person may reach for the chest or neck area. Cardiac or respiratory arrest quickly ensues.

Prevention and Treatment

Aspiration is easier to prevent than treat. Caregivers are advised to keep toys with small pieces away from toddlers; to not provide food that can choke the child. Adults should avoid talking or moving about when chewing and swallowing to reduce the risk. Avoid swallowing large chunks of food.

EMERGENCY TREATMENT FOR ASPIRATION

1. The Heimlich maneuver to dislodge the solid object is recommended (stand behind the victim with encircling arms, position a fist, thumb side against the abdomen, below the sternum, place the other hand over the fist and thrust forcefully inward and upward).
2. A foreign object may be ejected from an infant by back blows administered between the infant's shoulder blades, while the infant's body is supported over an arm or leg, head lower than the trunk.

Sometimes an individual can use a finger probe successfully to access an object at the back of the tongue. Instrumentation may be necessary in some cases to remove the offending object. In case of total obstruction, an emergency tracheotomy is necessary. Patients with widespread inflammation should be monitored for adult respiratory distress syndrome or pneumonia. Oxygen and supportive therapy may be required as well as prophylactic antibiotics.

THINK ABOUT 13-9

a. Describe the incidence of lung cancer.
b. Explain why: (1) wheezing, (2) hemoptysis, and (3) pleural effusion may occur in patients with lung cancer.
c. Explain the result of aspirating food and explain why the problem may be difficult to identify.
d. Explain why an infant should never be put to bed with a bottle.

Obstructive Sleep Apnea

Sleep apnea results when the pharyngeal tissues collapse during sleep leading to repeated and momentary cessation of breathing. Men are more often affected the women and the incidence increases with age and obesity (BMI >30). Sleep apnea is usually diagnosed when the sleeping partner notes loud snoring with intermittent gasps for air. Many cases go undiagnosed and untreated. Current estimates suggest that 3% to 5% of the adult population is affected. Complications are directly related to chronic hypoxia and fatigue and include type 2 diabetes, pulmonary hypertension, right-sided congestive heart failure, cerebrovascular accident, erectile dysfunction, depression, and daytime sleepiness. Operating a motor vehicle or other machinery is dangerous because the person tends to become sleepy and unaware of changes in the environment. It is recommended that patients avoid ingestion of sleeping pills or alcohol. Treatment involves the use of a continuous positive airway pump (CPAP) machine, which delivers humidified room air at a pressure that maintains an open airway. Patients using a CPAP machine during sleep prevent progression of complications and accidents owing to sleepiness. Oral appliances may reduce the collapse of the pharyngeal tissues in some cases. Devices are also available to prevent the patient sleeping in a supine position, which predisposes to apnea. In many jurisdictions, if the client refuses effective treatment, his or her driver's license will be revoked.

Asthma

Asthma is a disease that involves periodic episodes of severe but reversible bronchial obstruction in persons with hypersensitive or hyperresponsive airways. Frequent repeated attacks of acute asthma may lead to irreversible damage in the lungs and the development of chronic asthma (chronic obstructive lung disease). Acute attacks may continue to be superimposed on the chronic condition.

A significant rise in episodes of acute asthma requiring hospitalization in children has occurred during the past 20 years. In the age group 5 to 17 years, about 15 million persons have been diagnosed with asthma in the United States. It was reported that 4 million children under age 18 had an asthma attack during one 12-month period. The number of attacks peaks in school children in September, often associated with an increase in incidence of the common cold. As well, the incidence of asthma in the general population has greatly increased, and it appears that many additional cases have not been diagnosed; thus incidence rates are probably lower than the actual occurrence of the disease.

▪ *Pathophysiology*

Asthma may be classified in different ways. It may be acute or chronic, *acute* referring to a single episode, and *chronic* referring to the long-term condition. A recently developed system rates a case of asthma on a clinical scale ranging from mild and intermittent to severe and persistent. In the traditional method based on etiology and the presence of a hypersensitivity reaction, there are two basic types of asthma. The first is often called

extrinsic asthma and involves acute episodes triggered by a type I hypersensitivity reaction to an inhaled antigen (see Chapter 7). Frequently there is a familial history of other allergic conditions such as allergic rhinitis (hay fever) or eczema, and onset commonly occurs in children. Some patients are no longer subject to attacks after adolescence. The second type of asthma is *intrinsic* asthma, with onset during adulthood. In this disease other types of stimuli target hyper-responsive tissues in the airway, initiating the acute attack. These stimuli include respiratory infections, exposure to cold, exercise, drugs such as aspirin, stress, and inhalation of irritants such as cigarette smoke. Many patients have a combination of the two types.

All types of asthma exhibit the same pathophysiologic changes related to inflammation during an acute attack. The bronchi and bronchioles respond to the stimuli with three changes, inflammation of the mucosa with edema, contraction of smooth muscle (bronchoconstriction), and increased secretion of thick mucus in the passages (Fig. 13-18). These changes create obstructed airways, partially or totally, and interfere with airflow and oxygen supply.

In patients with extrinsic asthma, the antigen reacts with immunoglobulin E (IgE) on the previously sensitized mast cells in the respiratory mucosa, releasing histamine, kinins, prostaglandins, and other chemical mediators, which then cause inflammation, bronchospasm, edema, and increased mucus secretion. The reaction also stimulates branches of the vagus nerve, causing reflex bronchoconstriction.

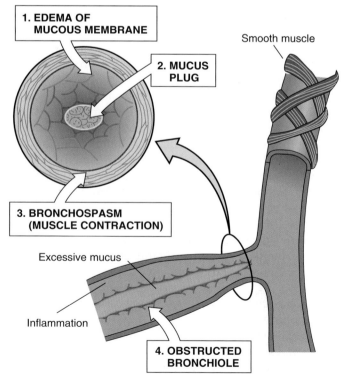

FIGURE 13-18 Asthma—acute episode.

In the second stage of the allergic response, which occurs a few hours later, the increased leukocytes, particularly eosinophils, release additional chemical mediators such as leukotrienes, resulting in prolonged inflammation, bronchoconstriction, and epithelial damage. Chemotactic factors and cytokines are released by mast cells and draw more white blood cells. The outcome is obstruction in the airways, partial and total, and marked hypoxia.

The precise mechanism whereby a similar response occurs in patients with intrinsic asthma has not been determined, but research suggests that chronic T lymphocyte activation possibly due to an internal antigen is the cause. The tissues are hyper-responsive, and an underlying chronic inflammation or imbalance in autonomic innervation to the tissues is also suspected.

Partial obstruction of the small bronchi and bronchioles results in *air trapping* and hyperinflation of the lungs (see Fig. 13-18C). Air passes into the areas distal to the obstruction and alveoli, but is only partially expired. Because expiration is a passive process, less force is available to move air out, and forced expiration often collapses the bronchial wall, creating a further barrier to expiratory airflow. Residual volume increases. As a result, it becomes more difficult to inspire fresh air or to cough effectively to remove the mucus. To understand hyperinflation of the lungs, take several breaths but exhale only partially after each inspiration. Consider how your lungs feel and the position of your ribs. Can you take a deep breath? Can you cough?

Total obstruction of the airway results when mucus plugs completely block the flow of air in the already narrowed passage. This leads to atelectasis or nonaeration of the tissue distal to the obstruction (see Fig. 13-24C). The air in the distal section diffuses out and is not replaced, resulting in collapse of that section of the lung. Both partial and total airway obstruction lead to marked hypoxia. Oxygen levels are further depleted by the increased demand for oxygen to supply increased muscle activity and the stress response as the individual fights for air. Both respiratory and metabolic acidosis result from severe respiratory impairment. Hypoxemia causes vasoconstriction in the pulmonary blood vessels, reducing blood flow through the lungs and increasing the workload of the right side of the heart.

Status asthmaticus is a persistent severe attack of asthma that does not respond to therapy. It is often related to inadequate medical treatment. It may be fatal owing to severe hypoxia and acidosis leading to cardiac arrhythmias or central nervous system depression.

Chronic asthma and chronic obstructive lung disease may develop from irreversible damage in the lungs when frequent and severe acute asthmatic attacks form a pattern. The bronchial walls become thickened, and fibrous tissue resulting from the frequent infections that follow attacks develops in atelectatic areas. Because it is impossible to remove all the tiny mucus plugs in the small passages, complications are common following frequent episodes of asthma.

■ *Etiology*
A family history of hay fever, asthma, and eczema is common. Viral upper respiratory infections frequently precipitate attacks. Contributing factors include an increase in sedentary lifestyles, with children remaining indoors, resulting in increased exposure to allergens amid poor ventilation. Increased air pollution has also been a factor.

■ *Signs and Symptoms*
Typical manifestations of an acute asthma attack include:
- Cough, marked dyspnea, a tight feeling in the chest, and agitation develop as airway obstruction increases. The patient is unable to talk.
- Wheezing is characteristic as air passes through the narrowed bronchioles.
- Breathing is rapid and labored, with use of accessory muscles and possible chest retractions.
- Thick and tenacious or sticky mucus is coughed up.
- Tachycardia occurs and perhaps pulsus paradoxus when the pulse differs on inspiration and expiration. Paradoxic pulse is observed when a blood pressure measurement is taken during an asthma attack. The sounds registering systolic pressure are heard first during expiration, and there is a gap of 10 mmHg or more before the sounds of both inspiration and expiration are heard.
- Hypoxia develops.
- Respiratory alkalosis develops initially because of hyperventilation.
- Respiratory acidosis develops in time due to air trapping, and marked fatigue causes decreased respiratory effort with weaker cough. This is aggravated by developing metabolic acidosis due to hypoxia (increased lactic acid) and from metabolic acid accumulating from increased metabolic activity and dehydration.
- Severe respiratory distress is evident. Hypoventilation leads to increasing hypoxemia and respiratory acidosis.
- Respiratory failure is indicated by decreasing responsiveness, cyanosis, and arterial blood gas measurements indicating a Pao_2 of less than 50 mmHg or a $Paco_2$ of greater than 50 mmHg.

■ *Treatment*
Minimizing the number and severity of acute attacks is necessary to prevent permanent lung damage, reduce the risk of infection, and prevent the development of emphysematous changes or chronic obstructive lung disease.
1. General measures include:
   a. Skin tests for allergic reactions are helpful in determining specific stimuli to be avoided.

b. Avoidance of common triggering factors, including airborne irritants or drugs such as aspirin, is recommended.

c. Good ventilation in the home, school, and workplace is helpful.

d. Regular swimming sessions are of great benefit, particularly to affected children, to strengthen chest muscles and improve cardiovascular fitness as well as reduce stress. Walking and swimming are recommended for adults.

e. It has been suggested that prophylactic medication be given as children return to school or at the first sign of a cold.

2. Measures for acute attacks include:

a. Controlled breathing techniques and a reduction in anxiety often lessen the severity and extent of the attack because a feeling of panic frequently aggravates the condition.

b. Many individuals carry inhalers so that they can self-administer a bronchodilator, usually a beta$_2$-adrenergic agent such as salbutamol (Ventolin). These more specific drugs, which have largely replaced isoproterenol and epinephrine, act on receptors to relax bronchial smooth muscle but have minimal effects on the heart. These inhalers, properly used, provide a measured dose of the medication and are most effective when used at the first indication of an attack. They may also be administered before exercise or exposure to a known stimulus.

c. Glucocorticoids such as beclomethasone (Beclovent) may be administered by inhalation also, but are more effective in reducing the second stage of inflammation in the airways. This type of drug may be useful when chronic inflammation develops.

3. Measures for status asthmaticus include:

a. Hospital care is essential when a patient does not respond to the bronchodilator.

4. Prophylaxis and treatment of chronic asthma includes:

a. Leukotriene receptor antagonists such as zafirlukast (Accolate) and montelukast (Singulair) block inflammatory responses in the presence of stimuli. Medication is taken orally on a regular basis to prevent attacks due to allergens, exercise, and aspirin. Leukotriene receptor antagonists are not effective in the treatment of acute attacks.

b. Cromolyn sodium is a prophylactic medication that is administered by inhalation on a regular daily basis. The drug inhibits release of chemical mediators from sensitized mast cells in the respiratory passages and decreases the number of eosinophils, thus reducing the hyperresponsiveness of the tissues. It is particularly useful for athletes and sports enthusiasts. It is of no value during an acute attack.

THINK ABOUT   13-10

a. Which structures in the lungs contain a higher percentage of smooth muscle?

b. Explain how obstruction develops in an asthmatic patient following exposure to an inhaled allergen.

c. Compare the effects of partial and total obstruction of the airways on ventilation and on oxygen levels in the blood.

d. Explain the timing and development of respiratory alkalosis, respiratory acidosis, and metabolic acidosis during an asthma attack.

Chronic Obstructive Pulmonary Disease

Chronic obstructive pulmonary disease (COPD), sometimes also called chronic obstructive lung disease (COLD), is a group of common chronic respiratory disorders that are characterized by progressive tissue degeneration and obstruction in the airways of the lungs. They are debilitating conditions that affect the individual's ability to work and function independently. Examples of these disorders are emphysema, chronic bronchitis, and chronic asthma. Their characteristics are compared in Table 13-5. In some patients, several primary diseases overlap; for example, asthma and bronchitis. Other conditions such as cystic fibrosis and bronchiectasis may lead to similar obstructive effects. In contrast, many occupational lung diseases, such as silicosis, asbestosis, and farmer's lung are classified as *restrictive lung diseases* because the irritant causes *interstitial* inflammation and fibrosis, resulting in loss of compliance, or "stiff lung."

Chronic obstructive pulmonary disease causes irreversible and progressive damage to the lungs. Eventually, respiratory failure may result because of severe hypoxia or hypercapnia. In many patients COPD leads to the development of *cor pulmonale*, right-sided congestive heart failure due to lung disease (see Chapter 12).

The prevalence of COPD is probably underestimated because many people are unaware they have it, particularly in the early stages when symptoms are minimal or masked by the primary problem. The percentage of females has greatly increased, as has the number of deaths. In 2002, there were 124,816 deaths in the United States. In 2005, the breakdown by disease showed approximately 4.1 million persons had emphysema, 9.5 million had chronic bronchitis, and 16 million had asthma in the United States. The CDC states that COPD is the fourth most common cause of mortality in the United States and WHO estimates that COPD will become the fourth cause of deaths globally by 2020; the current global mortality is 2.74 million.

TABLE 13-5 Chronic Obstructive Lung Disease

Disease Characteristic	Emphysema	Chronic Bronchitis	Asthma—Acute
Etiology	Smoking, genetic	Smoking, air pollution	Hypersensitivity type I, hyperresponsive tissue
Location	Alveoli	Bronchi	Small bronchi, bronchioles
Pathophysiology	Destruction of alveolar walls, loss of elasticity, impaired expiration, barrel chest, hyperinflation	Increased mucous glands and secretion, inflammation, and infection, obstruction	Inflammation, broncho-constriction, increased mucus produced, obstruction, repeat attacks lead to damage
Cough, dyspnea	Some coughing, marked dyspnea	Early, constant cough, some dyspnea	Cough and dyspnea, wheezing
Sputum	Little	Large amount, purulent	Thick, tenacious mucus
Cyanosis	No	Yes	Yes if status asthmaticus
Infections	Some	Frequent	Some
Cor pulmonale	Perhaps late	Common	Rare

Emphysema

■ *Pathophysiology*

The significant change in emphysema is the destruction of the alveolar walls and septae, which leads to large, permanently inflated alveolar air spaces (Fig. 13-19). Emphysema may be further classified by the specific location of the changes; for example, in the distal alveoli (panacinar) or bronchiolar (centrilobular) area.

Several factors contribute to the destruction of tissue in the alveoli. In some individuals there is a genetic deficiency of alpha$_1$-antitrypsin, a protein normally present in tissues and body fluids that inhibits the activity of proteases, which are destructive enzymes released by neutrophils during an inflammatory response. An example of a protease is elastase, which breaks down elastic fibers. This destructive process seems to be accelerated in persons with low alpha$_1$-antitrypsin levels. This genetic tendency is often found in individuals who develop emphysema relatively early in life. Cigarette smoking increases both the number of neutrophils in the alveoli and the release and activity of elastase, but decreases the effect of alpha$_1$-antitrypsin, thus greatly contributing to the breakdown of alveolar structures. Certain pathogenic bacteria present with infection also release proteases.

The changes in the lung tissue have many effects on lung function:

1. The breakdown of the alveolar wall results in:
   a. Loss of surface area for gas exchange
   b. Loss of pulmonary capillaries, affecting perfusion and the diffusion of gases
   c. Loss of elastic fibers, affecting the ability of the lung to recoil on expiration
   d. Altered ventilation-perfusion ratio as various changes occur in the alveoli (Fig. 13-20)
   e. Decreased support for other structures such as the small bronchi, which often leads to collapse of the walls and additional obstruction of airflow during expiration
2. Fibrosis and thickening of the bronchial walls have resulted from chronic irritation and the frequent infections associated with smoking and increased mucus production. These conditions lead to:
   a. Narrowed airways
   b. Weakened walls
   c. Interference with passive expiratory airflow
3. Progressive difficulty with expiration leads to:
   a. Air trapping (see Fig. 13-19C), and increased residual volume
   b. Overinflation of the lungs
   c. Fixation of the ribs in an inspiratory position, and an increased anterior-posterior diameter of the thorax (barrel chest)
   d. Diaphragm appears flattened on x-rays
4. With advanced emphysema, and significant loss of tissue:
   a. Adjacent damaged alveoli coalesce forming very large air spaces. Normally the uninflated lung appears to be a solid mass. With emphysema, the lung appears to have many large holes in it. Sometimes one can see through the scraps of remaining tissue from one side to the other. These air-filled spaces are called blebs or bullae (Fig. 13-21B).
   b. The tissue and pleural membrane surrounding large blebs near the surface of the lung may rupture, resulting in pneumothorax.
   c. Hypercapnia becomes marked.
   d. Hypoxic drive for inspiration develops as the patient's respiratory control adapts to a chronic elevation of carbon dioxide levels, and hypoxia becomes the driving force for respiration.

A. Normal Alveolus

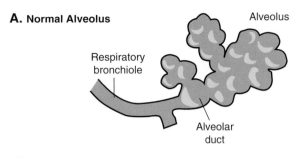

Alveolus

Respiratory bronchiole

Alveolar duct

B. Emphysema

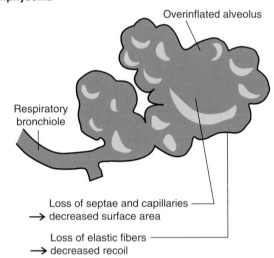

Overinflated alveolus

Respiratory bronchiole

Loss of septae and capillaries → decreased surface area

Loss of elastic fibers → decreased recoil

C. Air Trapping

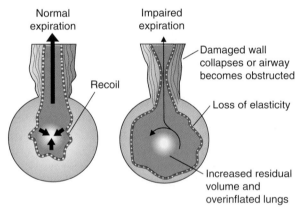

Normal expiration

Impaired expiration

Recoil

Damaged wall collapses or airway becomes obstructed

Loss of elasticity

Increased residual volume and overinflated lungs

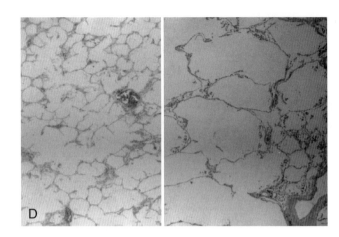

D

FIGURE 13-19 Emphysema. **A**, Normal alveolus. **B**, Emphysema. **C**, Air trapping. **D**, *Left*, Normal lung. *Right*, Large spaces characteristic of emphysema. *(Courtesy of R.W. Shaw, MD, North York General Hospital, Toronto, Ontario, Canada.)*

e. Infections develop frequently because secretions are more difficult to remove past obstructions, and airway defenses are impaired.

f. Pulmonary hypertension and cor pulmonale may develop in a late stage as the pulmonary blood vessels are destroyed and hypoxia causes pulmonary vasoconstriction. The increased pressure in the pulmonary circulation increases resistance to the right ventricle, and eventually the ventricle

fails. Many patients with respiratory disease manifest signs of heart failure (see Chapter 12).

■ *Etiology*

Cigarette smoking is implicated in most cases of emphysema. However, a genetic factor contributes to early development of the disease in nonsmokers. Exposure to other air pollutants also predisposes to emphysematous

A. Normal ventilation
and perfusion

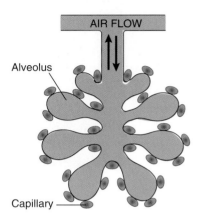

AIR FLOW

Alveolus

Capillary

B. Decreased ventilation

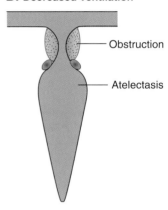

Obstruction

Atelectasis

C. Good ventilation –
Obstruction in pulmonary
circulation
⟶ Decreased perfusion

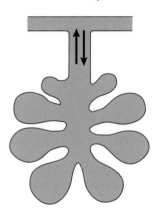

D. Destruction of alveolar wall
and capillaries ⟶ Decreased
ventilation and perfusion

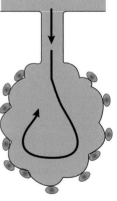

E. Inflammation impairs ventilation, perfusion,
and diffusion of O_2

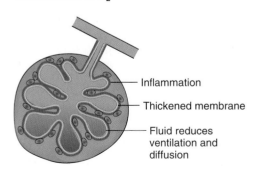

Inflammation

Thickened membrane

Fluid reduces
ventilation and
diffusion

FIGURE 13-20 Changes in ventilation and perfusion.

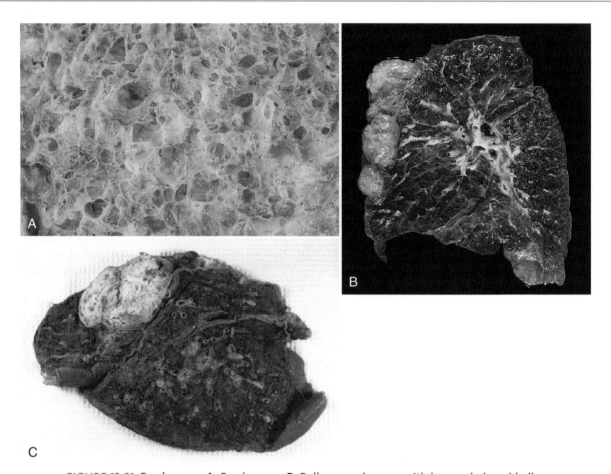

FIGURE 13-21 Emphysema. **A**, Emphysema. **B**, Bullous emphysema with large subpleural bullae (*left*). **C**, Emphysematous lung with tumor. (**A** *and* **B** *from Kumar V, Abbas AK, Fausto M: Robbins and Cotran Pathologic Basis of Disease, ed 7, Philadelphia, 2005, WB Saunders.* **C**, *Courtesy of Paul Emmerson and Seneca College of Applied Arts and Technology, Toronto, Ontario, Canada.*)

changes, which may develop in conjunction with other chronic lung disorders, such as cystic fibrosis and chronic bronchitis.

■ Signs and Symptoms
The onset of emphysema is insidious.
- Dyspnea occurs first on exertion and then progresses until it is marked even at rest.
- Hyperventilation with a prolonged expiratory phase, use of the accessory muscles, and hyperinflation leading to development of a "barrel chest" mark the ventilation difficulty. Typical posture is a sitting position, leaning forward (tripod position), to facilitate breathing. The chest is hyperresonant on percussion. Hyperventilation maintains adequate oxygen levels until later stages.
- Anorexia and fatigue contribute to weight loss.
- Clubbed fingers and secondary polycythemia may develop as compensations.

■ Diagnostic Tests
Chest x-rays and pulmonary function tests indicate the presence of increased residual volume and total lung capacity as well as decreased forced expiratory volume and vital capacity.

■ Treatment
Avoidance of respiratory irritants and sources of respiratory infections and cessation of smoking may slow the progress of emphysema.

Immunization against influenza and pneumonia is essential.

Pulmonary rehabilitation programs provide appropriate exercise and facilitate breathing. Patients can increase their endurance for walking and learn methods to optimize oxygen levels.

Learning appropriate breathing techniques such as pursed-lip breathing can maximize expiration and ventilation with less expenditure of energy.

Maintenance of adequate nutrition and hydration contributes to improved energy levels, resistance to infection, and general well-being.

Bronchodilators, antibiotics, and oxygen therapy may be necessary as the condition advances.

Lung reduction surgery has proved helpful, although recovery time is prolonged, and there is increased risk of complications. By removing part of the lung, air trapping can be reduced and expiration improved.

THINK ABOUT   13-11

a. Explain the factors that interfere with oxygenation of the blood in patients with emphysema.
b. Explain why expiration is significantly impaired in patients with emphysema.
c. Explain why heart failure may develop in patients with emphysema.
d. Describe and explain the preferred position for patient with COPD (e.g., one who is having dental treatment). Should the patient be relatively supine, upright, or otherwise positioned?

Chronic Bronchitis

■ *Pathophysiology*

Although there may be some overlap in the basic conditions comprising COPD, chronic bronchitis is differentiated by significant changes in the *bronchi* resulting from constant irritation from smoking or exposure to industrial pollution. The effects are irreversible and progressive.

Inflammation and obstruction, repeated infections, and chronic coughing characterize bronchitis as the following occur:

- The mucosa is inflamed and swollen.
- There is hypertrophy and hyperplasia of the mucous glands, and increased secretions are produced. The number of goblet cells is increased, and there is decreased ciliated epithelium.
- Chronic irritation and inflammation lead to fibrosis and thickening of the bronchial wall and further obstruction. Secretions pool distal to obstructions and are difficult to remove.
- Oxygen levels are low. During episodes of coughing cyanosis may be seen. Historically the characteristic manifestations of emphysema have been differentiated from those of chronic bronchitis by using the term "pink puffer" to summarize the dyspnea, hyperventilation, and overinflation that maintain oxygen levels in emphysema, compared with the typical clinical presentation of lower oxygen levels, cyanosis, and edema, the "blue bloater" of bronchitis.
- Severe dyspnea and fatigue interfere with nutrition, communication, and daily activities, leading to general debilitation.
- Pulmonary hypertension and cor pulmonale are common.

■ *Etiology*

Individuals with chronic bronchitis usually have a history of cigarette smoking or living in an urban or industrial area, particularly in geographic locations where smog is common. Heavy exposure to inhaled irritants leads to inflammation and frequent infections, initiating the cycle. In some cases, asthma is an associated condition.

■ *Signs and Symptoms*

Constant productive cough is the significant indicator of chronic bronchitis, as is tachypnea and shortness of breath. Frequently secretions are thick and purulent. Cough and rhonchi are usually more severe in the morning because the secretions have pooled during sleep. Airway obstruction leads to hypoxia and eventually to cyanosis as well as to hypercapnia. Secondary polycythemia, severe weight loss, and signs of cor pulmonale (systemic edema) often develop as the vascular damage and pulmonary hypertension progress.

■ *Treatment*

Reducing exposure to irritants and prompt treatment of infection slow the progress of the disease. The influenza and pneumonia vaccines provide useful prophylaxis, as will antimicrobials when appropriate. Use of expectorants, bronchodilators, and appropriate chest therapy, including postural drainage and percussion, assist in removing excessive mucus. Low-flow oxygen and nutritional supplements are helpful.

Bronchiectasis

Bronchiectasis is usually a secondary problem, rather than a primary one, that develops in patients with conditions such as cystic fibrosis or COPD. Some cases result from childhood infection, aspiration of foreign bodies, or a congenital weakness in the bronchial wall. Depending on the cause, the condition may be localized in one lobe, or more often it is diffuse in both lungs. The incidence in North America has decreased owing to effective use of antibiotics in treatment of the predisposing disorders.

■ *Pathophysiology*

Bronchiectasis is an irreversible abnormal dilation or widening, primarily of the medium-sized bronchi. These dilations may be saccular or elongated (fusiform). They arise from recurrent inflammation and infection in the airways. This leads to obstruction in the airways or a weakening of the muscle and elastic fibers in the bronchial wall, or a combination of these. Fibrous adhesions may pull the wall of a bronchus outward, dilating it.

In dilated or ballooning areas, large amounts of fluid constantly collect and become infected. Infecting organisms are usually mixed and include streptococci, staphylococci, pneumococci, and *H. influenzae*. These infections then cause loss of cilia and metaplasia in the epithelium, additional fibrosis, and progressive obstruction. The obstructions and loss of cilia interfere with the removal of the fluids, continuing the cycle of events.

■ Signs and Symptoms

The significant signs of bronchiectasis are chronic cough and production of copious amounts of purulent sputum (1 to 2 cups per day). Cough may be paroxysmal in the morning as the purulent sputum shifts in the lungs with changes in body position, stimulating the cough reflex. Other signs include rales and rhonchi in the lungs, foul breath, dyspnea, and hemoptysis. Systemic signs include weight loss, anemia, and fatigue.

■ Treatment

Antibiotics, bronchodilators, and chest physiotherapy as well as treatment of the primary condition reduce the severity of the infections and progressive damage to the lungs.

THINK ABOUT 13-12

a. Describe the conditions predisposing to chronic bronchitis and relate them to the pathologic changes occurring in the lungs.
b. Describe the factors contributing to recurrent infections in the lungs and relate them to your professional practice.
c. Explain why bronchiectasis tends to be progressive.
d. Prepare a chart comparing emphysema, cystic fibrosis, and bronchiectasis with regard to pathologic changes in the lungs, the significant signs that can be observed in a patient, and potential complications.

Restrictive Lung Disorders

The term *restrictive lung disorders* applies to a group of diseases in which lung expansion is impaired and total lung capacity is reduced. Some pulmonary diseases may be classified in several categories; that is, they have both obstructive and restrictive components.

Restrictive disorders include two groups, those in which an abnormality of the chest wall limits lung expansion and those in which lung disease impairs expansion. In the first group are included conditions such as kyphosis or scoliosis (affecting the thorax), poliomyelitis or amyotrophic lateral sclerosis or botulism (respiratory muscle paralysis), or muscular dystrophy (weak muscles).

The second group includes diseases affecting the tissues providing the supportive framework of the lungs, rather than airway obstruction or alveolar destruction. Idiopathic pulmonary fibrosis is an example of such a disease that appears to have an immune basis. This group also includes occupational diseases in which inhaled irritants cause chronic low-grade but damaging inflammation over a long period of time. Loss of elastic fibers and fibrosis in chronic conditions results in loss of compliance. Acute forms occur as pulmonary edema

TABLE 13-6	Pneumoconioses	
Disease	Agent	Occurrence
Coal workers disease or anthracosis	Coal dust	Coal mines
Silicosis	Silica	Stone-cutting, sand-blasting, mines
Asbestosis	Asbestos	Insulation, shipbuilding
Farmer's lung	Fungal spores	Hay

and adult respiratory distress syndrome (ARDS). A "stiff lung" and reduced compliance reduce total lung capacity.

Pneumoconioses

Pneumoconioses are chronic restrictive diseases resulting from long-term exposure to irritating particles such as asbestos (see Fig. 28-2). Table 13-6 lists some examples. Large particles are usually captured by nasal hairs and mucus or by cilia and mucus in the lower passages, and then removed. The normal defenses in the upper respiratory system cannot handle the overload of foreign material, especially small particles, with long-term occupational exposure such as in mining. Although there are minor variations in the effects, this discussion includes the general changes. More damage occurs when larger numbers of particles enter the lungs, the particles are very small, the material is more reactive with tissue, and exposure continues over a long time period. Very small particles can penetrate into alveolar ducts and sacs. Smoking cigarettes aggravates the condition.

■ Pathophysiology

Inflammation and fibrous tissue develops, with gradual destruction of connective tissue. Immune responses may add to the damage in the case of more reactive particles, such as silica. As fibrosis extends, the functional areas of the lungs, including alveoli, are lost. Inspiration becomes difficult as compliance is lost. The tissue changes are irreversible. Infections are common.

Asbestos fibers have two additional effects, frequently causing pleural fibrosis and greatly increasing the risk of lung cancer, particularly in cigarette smokers. The risk of cancer has raised public concern regarding the presence of asbestos insulation in schools and homes.

■ Signs and Symptoms

Onset is insidious, with dyspnea developing first. As the disease progresses, increasing effort is required for inspiration. Cough is common and may or may not be productive.

■ *Treatment*

Identifying and ending exposure to the damaging agent will slow the progression of the disease, as will prompt treatment of infection.

Vascular Disorders

Pulmonary Edema

■ *Pathophysiology*

Pulmonary edema refers to fluid collecting in the alveoli and interstitial area. Many conditions can lead to this development. This accumulation of fluid reduces the amount of oxygen diffusing into the blood and interferes with lung expansion, also reducing oxygenation of the blood.

Excess fluid in the alveolar tissue may develop when:
- Inflammation is present in the lungs, increasing capillary permeability.
- Plasma protein levels are low, decreasing plasma osmotic pressure.
- Pulmonary hypertension develops.

Normally pressure in the pulmonary capillaries is very low, and there is minimal fluid in the air passages and alveoli. When hydrostatic pressure in the pulmonary capillaries becomes high, for example with congestive heart failure (see Chapter 12), this leads to a shift of fluid out of the capillaries into the alveoli (see Chapter 2).

Excessive amounts of fluid in the interstitial areas and alveoli interfere with the diffusion of oxygen, causing severe hypoxemia, as well as with the action of surfactant, leading to difficulty in expanding the lungs, which ultimately collapse (Fig. 13-22). Capillaries may rupture, causing blood-streaked sputum.

■ *Etiology*

Pulmonary edema can result from many primary conditions. With left-sided congestive heart failure, backup of blood from the failing left ventricle causes high pressure in the pulmonary circulation. This may be a chronic or acute condition. Pulmonary edema also results from hypoproteinemia due to kidney or liver disease, in which serum albumin levels are low. Inflammation in the lungs with increased capillary permeability develops due to inhalation of toxic gases, or in association with tumors. Blocked lymphatic drainage due to tumors or fibrosis in the lungs may cause edema. Pulmonary hypertension may occur idiopathically or secondary to obstructive sleep apnea that is not treated.

■ *Signs and Symptoms*

Signs of mild pulmonary edema include cough, orthopnea, and rales. As congestion increases, hemoptysis often occurs. Sputum is frothy owing to air mixed with the secretions, and blood-tinged owing to ruptured capillaries in the lungs. Breathing becomes labored as it becomes more difficult to expand the lungs. The individual feels as if he or she is drowning. Hypoxemia increases, and cyanosis develops in the advanced stage. Acute congestive heart failure may cause such an episode, called paroxysmal nocturnal dyspnea, during a sleep period (see Chapter 12).

■ *Treatment*

The causative factors must be treated, and supportive care such as oxygen is offered. In severe cases positive-pressure mechanical ventilation may be necessary. There is an increased risk of pneumonia developing after an episode of pulmonary edema because of the residual secretions. Individuals with a tendency to pulmonary edema should be positioned with the upper body elevated.

Pulmonary Embolus

A pulmonary embolus is a blood clot or a mass of other material that obstructs the pulmonary artery or a branch of it, blocking the flow of blood through the lung tissue. Most pulmonary emboli are thrombi or blood clots originating from the deep leg veins (see Chapter 12). An embolus to the lungs travels from its source through larger and larger veins until it reaches the heart and pulmonary artery. It then lodges as soon as it reaches a smaller artery in the lungs through which it cannot pass.

Pulmonary embolus due to deep vein thrombosis (DVT) is a leading cause of death in hospitals. More than 600,000 people in United States have a pulmonary embolism each year, resulting in more than 60,000 deaths, usually within the first hour after symptoms develop.

■ *Pathophysiology*

The effects of a pulmonary embolus depend somewhat on the material, but largely on the size and therefore the location of the obstruction in the pulmonary circulation (Fig. 13-23). Because lung tissue is supplied with oxygen and nutrients by the separate bronchial circulation, infarction does not follow obstruction of the pulmonary circulation unless the general circulation is compromised or there is prior lung disease. Infarction usually involves a segment of the lung and the pleural membrane in the area.

Small pulmonary emboli are frequently "silent" or asymptomatic. However, multiple small emboli (a "shower") often have an effect equal to that of a larger embolus.

Emboli that block moderate-sized arteries usually cause respiratory impairment because fluid and blood fill the alveoli of the involved area. Reflex vasoconstriction often occurs in the area, further increasing the pressure in the blood vessels.

Large emboli (usually those involving more than 60% of the lung tissue) affect the cardiovascular system, causing right-sided heart failure and decreased cardiac

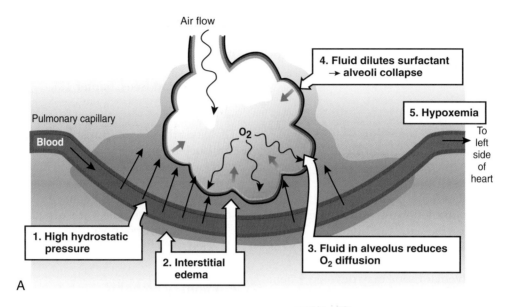

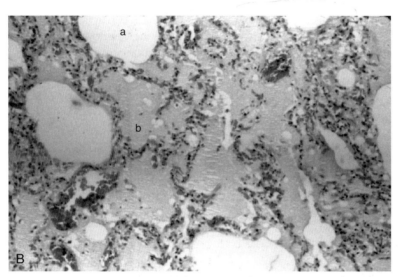

FIGURE 13-22 **A,** Pulmonary edema associated with congestive heart failure. **B,** Photomicrograph showing acute pulmonary edema due to congestive heart failure: *a,* alveolar air space; *b,* fluid-filled alveolus. *(Courtesy of R.W. Shaw, MD, North York General Hospital, Toronto, Ontario, Canada.)*

output (shock). Sudden death often results in these cases, which involve greatly increased resistance in the pulmonary arteries because of the embolus plus reflex vasoconstriction due to released chemical mediators such as serotonin and histamine. This resistance to the output from the right ventricle causes acute cor pulmonale. There is also much less blood returning from the lungs to the left ventricle and then to the systemic circulation (decreased cardiac output). This can be appreciated by visualizing a large embolus lying across the bifurcation of the pulmonary artery (a "saddle embolus") and totally blocking the flow of blood from the right ventricle into the lungs.

■ *Etiology*

Ninety percent of pulmonary emboli have originated from deep veins, primarily in the legs. Many travel from the deep veins of the legs as a result of phlebothrombosis or thrombophlebitis (see Chapter 12). Risk factors for these emboli include immobility, trauma or surgery to the legs, childbirth, congestive heart failure, dehydration, increased coagulability of the blood, and cancer. Sitting in a plane or car for a long time period can predispose to thromboembolus. Thrombi tend to break off with sudden muscle action or massage, trauma, or changes in blood flow. Postoperative risk can be reduced by early ambulation, constant mechanical movement of

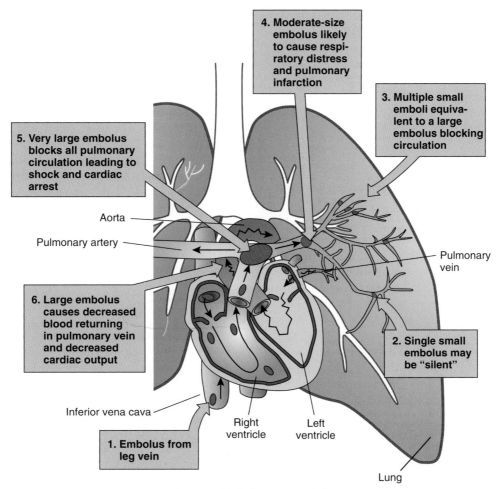

FIGURE 13-23 Pulmonary embolus.

the affected leg or use of thromboembolic deterrent stockings (TEDS).

Other types of pulmonary emboli include fat emboli from the bone marrow resulting from fracture of a large bone (e.g., the femur, particularly if poorly immobilized), vegetations resulting from endocarditis in the right side of the heart, amniotic fluid emboli from placental tears occurring during labor and delivery, tumor cell emboli that break away from a malignant mass, or air embolus injected into a vein.

■ Signs and Symptoms

With small emboli, a transient chest pain, cough, or dyspnea may occur. This is often unnoticed but can be significant because it may be a warning of more emboli developing. For larger emboli, chest pain that increases with coughing or deep breathing, tachypnea, and dyspnea develop suddenly. Later, hemoptysis and fever are present. Hypoxia stimulates a sympathetic response, with anxiety and restlessness, pallor, and tachycardia. Massive emboli cause severe crushing chest pain, low blood pressure, rapid weak pulse, and loss of consciousness. Fat emboli are distinguished by the development

of acute respiratory distress, a petechial rash on the trunk, and neurologic signs such as confusion and disorientation.

Diagnosis can be confirmed with x-ray, lung scan, MRI, or pulmonary angiography. The source of the embolus can be determined using Doppler ultrasound or venography.

■ Treatment

Assessment of risk factors in an individual situation and preventive measures are recommended. With prolonged bed rest, compression stockings are helpful. In some

THINK ABOUT 13-13

a. Explain three possible causes of pulmonary edema.
b. Explain which is more likely to occur with acute pulmonary edema—hypoxemia, hypercapnia, or both equally.
c. Explain how a pulmonary embolus can cause immediate death.

cases, a filter can be surgically inserted in the inferior vena cava to remove blood clots. The underlying cause of the embolus must be considered. In patients with pulmonary embolus due to thrombus, oxygen is administered and usually heparin or streptokinase (fibrinolytic agents) as well to prevent additional clots. Mechanical ventilation may be necessary, and in some cases an embolectomy is performed.

Expansion Disorders

Atelectasis

Atelectasis is the nonaeration or collapse of a lung or part of a lung leading to decreased gas exchange and hypoxia. It occurs as a complication of many primary conditions. Treatment depends on removing the underlying cause, whether obstruction or compression, before reinflating the lung.

■ *Pathophysiology*

When the alveoli become airless, they shrivel up as the natural elasticity of the tissues dominates. This process also interferes with blood flow through the lung. Both ventilation and perfusion are altered, and this in turn primarily affects oxygen diffusion. Unless a very large proportion of the lungs is affected, the increased respiratory rate can control carbon dioxide levels, because this gas diffuses easily.

If the lungs are not reinflated quickly, the lung tissue can become necrotic and infected, and permanent lung damage results.

■ *Etiology*

A variety of mechanisms can result in atelectasis (Fig. 13-24):

- *Obstructive* or *resorption* atelectasis develops when total obstruction of the airway due to mucus or tumor leads to diffusion into the tissue of air distal to the obstruction; this air is not replaced.
- *Compression* atelectasis results when a mass such as a tumor exerts pressure on a part of the lung and prevents air from entering that section of lung. Alternatively, when the pressure in the pleural cavity is increased, as with increased fluid or air, and the adhesion between the pleural membranes is destroyed, the lung cannot expand.
- Increased surface tension in the alveoli occurs with pulmonary edema or respiratory distress syndrome, preventing expansion of the lung.
- Fibrotic tissue in the lungs or pleura (sometimes called *contraction* atelectasis) may restrict expansion and lead to collapse.
- *Postoperative* atelectasis commonly occurs 24 to 72 hours after surgery, particularly abdominal surgery. A number of factors are implicated in this situation, including restricted ventilation due to pain or abdominal distention; slow, shallow respirations due to anesthetics and analgesics; increased secretions due to the supine position; and decreased cough effort.

■ *Signs and Symptoms*

Small areas of atelectasis are asymptomatic. Large areas cause dyspnea, increased heart and respiratory rates, and chest pain. Chest expansion may appear abnormal or asymmetric, depending on the cause of the atelectasis. For example, obstructive atelectasis leads to a potential low pressure "gap" or space on the affected side; therefore the mediastinum shifts toward it, and the other lung compensates by overinflating. The affected side often "lags" behind the unaffected side during ventilation. With compression atelectasis, the mediastinum may shift toward the other unaffected side.

Pleural Effusion

A pleural effusion is the presence of excessive fluid in the pleural cavity. Normally a very small amount of fluid is present to provide lubrication for the membranes. Effusions vary in type and mechanism according to the primary problem. Both lungs may be involved, but more often only one lung is affected because each lung is enclosed in a separate pleural membrane. The effects of effusion depend on the amount, type, and rate of accumulation of the fluid.

Pleurisy or *pleuritis* may precede or follow pleural effusion or occur independently. Pleurisy is a condition in which the pleural membranes are inflamed, swollen, and rough, often in association with lobar pneumonia.

■ *Pathophysiology*

Small amounts of fluid are drained from the pleural cavity by the lymphatics and have little effect on respiratory function. Large amounts of fluid first increase the pressure in the pleural cavity and then cause separation of the pleural membranes, preventing their cohesion during inspiration. These effects prevent expansion of the lung, leading to atelectasis, particularly when fluid accumulates rapidly (see Fig. 13-24A). A large amount of fluid causes atelectasis on the affected side and a shift of the mediastinal contents toward the unaffected lung, limiting its expansion also. A tracheal deviation indicates this shift. Venous return in the inferior vena cava and cardiac filling may be impaired because large effusions increase pressure in the mediastinum.

■ *Etiology*

Different types of fluid may collect in the pleural cavity. *Exudative* effusions are a response to inflammation, perhaps from a tumor, in which increased capillary permeability allows fluid containing protein and white blood cells to leak into the pleural cavity. *Transudates* are

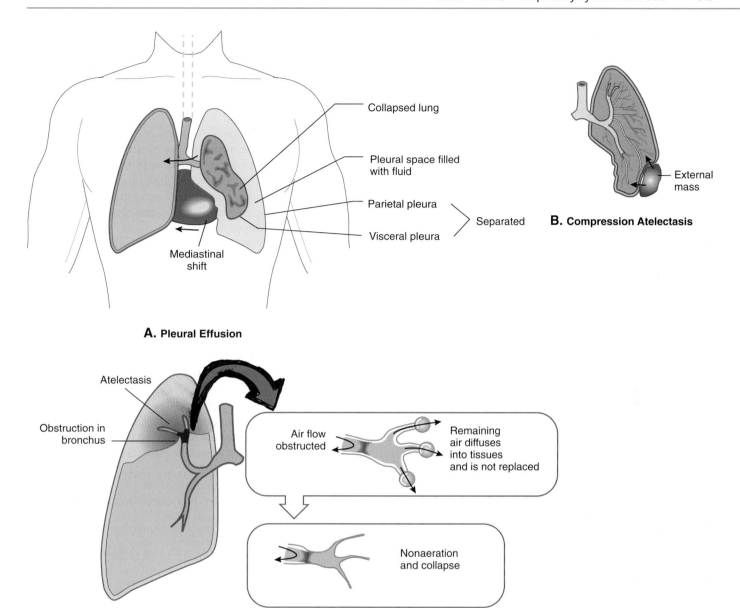

A. Pleural Effusion

B. Compression Atelectasis

C. Obstructive Atelectasis – Absorption Atelectasis

FIGURE 13-24 Atelectasis.

watery effusions, sometimes called *hydrothorax*, that result from increased hydrostatic pressure or decreased osmotic pressure in the blood vessels, leading to a shift of fluid out of the blood vessels into the potential space in the pleural cavity. These effusions may occur secondary to liver or kidney disease. *Hemothorax* is the term used when the fluid is blood resulting from trauma, cancer, or surgery. Empyema occurs when the fluid is purulent as a result of infection, often related to pneumonia.

■ *Signs and Symptoms*

The general signs of pleural effusion include dyspnea, chest pain, and increased respiratory and heart rates. Usually dullness to percussion and absence of breath sounds over the affected area are found because air no longer flows through the passages. Tracheal deviation and hypotension indicate a massive effusion that interferes with both respiratory and circulatory function.

Pleurisy is manifested by cyclic pleuritic pain and a friction rub heard on auscultation as the rough, swollen membranes move against each other during respiratory movements.

■ *Treatment*

Measures are required to remove the underlying cause and treat the respiratory impairment. The fluid may have to be analyzed to confirm the cause. Chest drainage tubes may be used to assist inflation. If a large quantity of fluid forms, thoracocentesis (needle aspiration) is required to remove the fluid and relieve the pressure.

> **THINK ABOUT   13-14**
>
> a. Compare the mechanisms involved in the development of atelectasis in a patient with cystic fibrosis and one with pleural effusion.
> b. Explain why a large pleural effusion may have more serious consequences than an obstruction in a major bronchus.
> c. Explain the signs of atelectasis.

Pneumothorax

Pneumothorax refers to air in the pleural cavity. The presence of air at atmospheric pressure in the pleural cavity and the separation of the pleural membranes by air prevent expansion of the lung, leading to atelectasis. When pneumothorax is caused by a malignant tumor or trauma, fluid or blood may also be present in the cavity. For example, with fluid in the more dependent area and air above it, the condition could be called *hydropneumothorax*. Chest x-rays can determine the type and extent of pneumothorax.

There are several different types of pneumothorax (Table 13-7):

* *Closed pneumothorax* occurs when air can enter the pleural cavity through an opening directly from the internal airways. There is no opening in the chest wall. This can be a simple or spontaneous pneumothorax or can be secondary to another disease.
* *Simple* or *spontaneous pneumothorax* occurs when a tear on the surface of the lung allows air to escape from inside the lung through a bronchus and the visceral pleura into the pleural cavity (Fig. 13-25A). As the lung tissue collapses, it seals off the leak. Simple pneumothorax often occurs in young men who have no prior lung disease but perhaps an idiopathic bleb or defect on the lung surface. Following collapse, the mediastinum can shift toward the affected lung, allowing the other lung to expand more.
* *Secondary pneumothorax* is associated with underlying respiratory disease resulting from rupture of an emphysematous bleb on the surface of the lung (see Fig. 13-21B) or erosion by a tumor or tubercular cavitation through the visceral pleura. Again, this condition lets inspired air pass into the pleural cavity.
* *Open pneumothorax* refers to atmospheric air entering the pleural cavity through an opening in the chest wall. This could result from trauma or surgery.
* *"Sucking wound"* is used to describe a *large* opening in the chest wall, in which the sound of air moving in and out makes a typical sucking sound (see Fig. 13-25B). Because larger quantities of air are moving in and out, there is a greater effect on respiratory and cardiovascular function.

In open pneumothorax, air enters the pleural cavity through the opening in the chest wall and parietal

TABLE 13-7	Types of Pneumothorax		
	Closed	**Open**	**Tension**
Cause	Spontaneous, idiopathic Ruptured emphysematous bleb	Puncture wound through chest wall	Open—puncture through thorax Closed—tear in lung surface Both with flap or one-way valve
Air entry	From inside lung through tear in visceral pleura	From outside body through opening in thorax and parietal pleura	Through the thorax or tear in lung surface
Effects	Atelectasis Leak seals as lung collapses	Atelectasis Air enters pleural cavity with each inspiration and leaves with each expiration	Atelectasis Air enters pleural cavity with each inspiration Flap closes with expiration, and air pressure increases in pleural cavity pressure
	One lung impaired	Unaffected lung compressed by mediastinal shift on inspiration	Unaffected lung increasingly compressed by mediastinal shift
	No additional cardiovascular effects	Mediastinal flutter impairs venous return to heart	Mediastinal shift reduces venous return to heart
Signs	All three types: Increased, labored respirations with dyspnea, tachycardia, pleural pain, and asymmetrical chest movements		
	Breath sounds absent	"Sucking" noise if large Tracheal swing Decreased blood pressure	Breath sounds absent on affected side Tracheal deviation to unaffected side Increasing respiratory distress Shock, distended neck veins, cyanosis
	Hypoxemia	Moderate hypoxemia	Severe hypoxemia

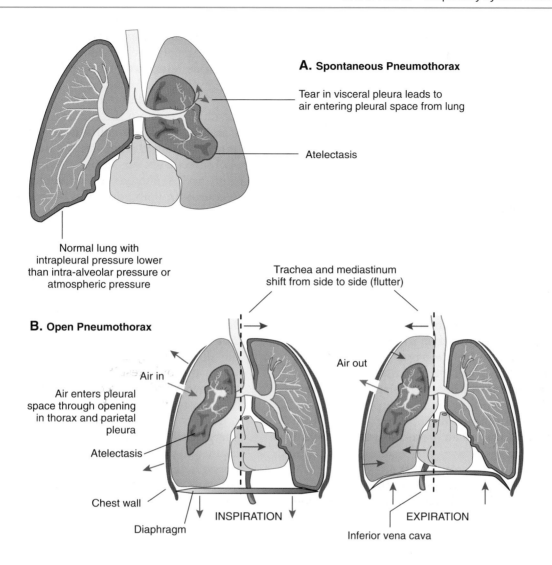

A. Spontaneous Pneumothorax

Tear in visceral pleura leads to
air entering pleural space from lung

Atelectasis

Normal lung with
intrapleural pressure lower
than intra-alveolar pressure or
atmospheric pressure

B. Open Pneumothorax

Trachea and mediastinum
shift from side to side (flutter)

Air in

Air enters pleural
space through opening
in thorax and parietal
pleura

Air out

Atelectasis

Chest wall

INSPIRATION

Diaphragm

EXPIRATION

Inferior vena cava

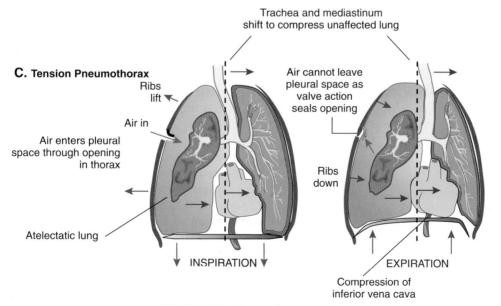

Trachea and mediastinum
shift to compress unaffected lung

C. Tension Pneumothorax

Ribs
lift

Air in

Air enters pleural
space through opening
in thorax

Air cannot leave
pleural space as
valve action
seals opening

Ribs
down

Atelectatic lung

INSPIRATION

EXPIRATION

Compression of
inferior vena cava

FIGURE 13-25 Types of pneumothorax.

pleura, causing immediate atelectasis on the affected side. Because more air enters the pleural cavity during inspiration, the mediastinum pushes against the unaffected lung, limiting its expansion. Subsequently, on expiration, as air is pushed out of the pleural cavity through the opening, the mediastinal contents shift back toward the affected side.

These abnormal movements occur as the pressure changes with rib movements on inspiration and expiration. This *mediastinal flutter* or "to-and-fro" motion impairs both ventilation in the unaffected lung and venous return through the inferior vena cava. (Recall that normal respiratory movements and pressure changes promote movement of venous blood upward to the heart.)

- *Tension pneumothorax* is the most serious form of pneumothorax (see Fig. 13-25C). This situation may result from an opening through the chest wall and parietal pleura (open pneumothorax) or from a tear in the lung tissue and visceral pleura (closed pneumothorax) that causes atelectasis. The particular pattern of damage creates a flap of tissue or a *one-way valve* effect, whereby the opening enlarges on inspiration, promoting airflow into the pleural cavity. However, on expiration, the opening is sealed off, preventing removal of air from the pleural cavity. Thus, with each inspiration this lesion leads to continual increases in the amount of air in the pleural cavity. Pressure increases on the affected side eventually push the mediastinal contents against the other lung, compressing the other lung and the inferior vena cava. Severe hypoxia and respiratory distress develop quickly and can become life threatening if the source of the valve effect and increasing intrapleural pressure is not treated.

■ *Signs and Symptoms*

The general signs of pneumothorax include those of atelectasis, dyspnea, cough, and chest pain. Breath sounds are reduced over the atelectatic area. Other signs related to chest movements, unequal expansion, and mediastinal shift vary with the type of pneumothorax.

> **EMERGENCY TREATMENT FOR PNEUMOTHORAX**
>
> 1. Transport to a hospital as soon as possible.
> 2. An open pneumothorax or sucking wound is covered with an occlusive dressing or covering to prevent the air moving in and out of the pleural cavity. The dressing should be checked to ensure that a tension pneumothorax has not developed.
> 3. Penetrating objects should not be removed from the chest wall until medical assistance is available.
> 4. If possible, tension pneumothorax should be converted to an open pneumothorax, by removing loose tissue or enlarging the opening.

Hypoxia develops and leads to a sympathetic response, including anxiety, tachycardia, and pallor. Interference with venous return leads to hypotension.

Flail Chest

Falls and car accidents cause most chest injuries. Flail chest results from fractures of the thorax, usually fractures of three to six ribs in two places or fracture of the sternum and a number of consecutive ribs. There is often contusion with edema and some bleeding in the lung tissue adjacent to the flail section. Atelectasis does not occur as a direct result of the trauma but may follow as a complication if a broken rib punctures the pleura.

Chest wall rigidity is lost, resulting in *paradoxical* (opposite) movement during inspiration and expiration (Fig. 13-26). A sequence of pressure changes follows affecting ventilation and oxygen levels.

During *inspiration* there is the usual decrease in pressure inside the lungs, then:

- The flail or broken section of ribs moves inward rather than outward as intrathoracic pressure is decreased.
- This inward movement of the ribs prevents expansion of the affected lung.
- A large flail section can compress the adjacent lung tissue, pushing the air out of that section and up the bronchus. Because air is flowing down the trachea and into the other lung, the "stale" air from the damaged lung crosses into the other lung, along with newly inspired air.

On *expiration*:

- The unstable flail section is pushed outward by the increasing intrathoracic pressure.
- If the flail section is large, the paradoxical movement of the ribs alters airflow during expiration.
- Air from the unaffected lung moves across into the affected lung as the outward movement of the ribs decreases pressure in the affected lung.

Mediastinal flutter occurs when the flail section is large. As the lungs shift back and forth, the mediastinum is pushed to and fro. The pressure changes and possible kinking of the inferior vena cava interferes with venous return to the heart and thus reduces cardiac output and oxygen supplies to the cells.

Hypoxia results from the limited expansion and decreased inspiratory volume of the flail lung, the shunting of stale air between lungs, which lowers the oxygen content of the air; and the decreased venous return.

> **EMERGENCY TREATMENT FOR FLAIL CHEST**
>
> The abnormal movement is obvious, and therefore first aid measures include stabilizing the flail section with a flat, heavy object, thus limiting the outward paradoxic movement of the thorax until surgical repair can be performed.

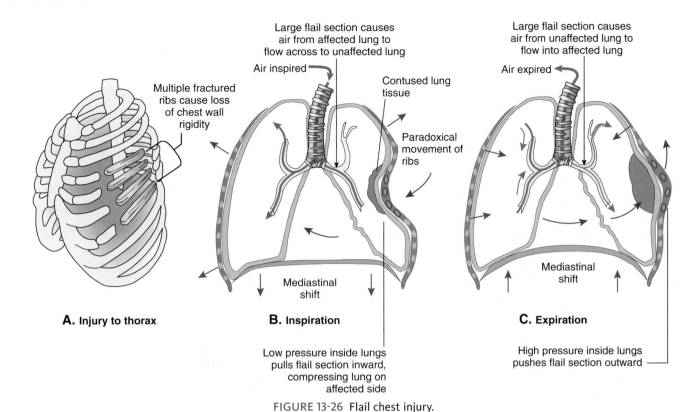

FIGURE 13-26 Flail chest injury.

A. Injury to thorax

Multiple fractured ribs cause loss of chest wall rigidity

B. Inspiration

Large flail section causes air from affected lung to flow across to unaffected lung

Air inspired

Contused lung tissue

Paradoxical movement of ribs

Mediastinal shift

Low pressure inside lungs pulls flail section inward, compressing lung on affected side

C. Expiration

Large flail section causes air from unaffected lung to flow into affected lung

Air expired

Mediastinal shift

High pressure inside lungs pushes flail section outward

THINK ABOUT   13-15

a. Describe two ways in which atmospheric air can enter the pleural cavity.

b. List in the proper sequence the changes in the structures and the pressures that occur during normal inspiration and inspiration with flail chest.

c. Prepare a chart comparing the cause and effects of closed pneumothorax, tension pneumothorax, and flail chest on ventilation and cardiovascular activity.

Infant Respiratory Distress Syndrome

Infant respiratory distress syndrome (IRDS) or neonatal respiratory distress syndrome (NRDS, or hyaline membrane disease) is a common cause of neonatal deaths, particularly in premature infants. With improved methods of testing for lung maturity, and more effective prenatal and postnatal therapy as well as supportive treatment, the mortality rate has decreased in the past decade. Some children have suffered developmental impairment, particularly those born late in the second trimester of pregnancy.

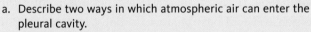 *Pathophysiology*

During the third trimester of fetal development, the alveolar surface area and lung vascularity greatly increase in preparation for independent lung function immediately after birth. Surfactant, which reduces surface tension in the alveoli and promotes expansion,

is first produced between 28 and 36 weeks of gestation, depending on the maturity of the individual lung. It has been shown that in utero stress hastens the maturation of lung tissue. Infant lung maturity can be assessed by measuring the surfactant level of the fetus with a test such as the lecithin-sphingomyelin (L/S) ratio in amniotic fluid, which is obtained by amniocentesis. Initially sphingomyelin is high, then it decreases and lecithin increases until the ratio represents adequate surfactant function at around 35 weeks of gestation.

Normally the first few inspirations after birth are difficult as the lungs are first inflated; then breathing becomes easier as residual air volume increases. Without adequate surfactant, each inspiration is very difficult because the lungs totally collapse during each expiration, thereby requiring use of the accessory muscles and much energy to totally reinflate the lungs. The poorly developed alveoli are difficult to inflate, and an inadequate blood and oxygen supply further deters the production of surfactant by alveolar cells (see Fig. 13-5). Diffuse atelectasis results, which decreases pulmonary blood flow and leads to reflex pulmonary vasoconstriction and severe hypoxia.

Poor lung perfusion and lack of surfactant lead to increased alveolar capillary permeability, with fluid and protein (fibrin) leaking into the interstitial area and alveoli, forming the hyaline membrane (Fig. 13-27). This further impairs lung expansion and decreases oxygen diffusion. Some of the surviving neonates experience brain damage due to severe hypoxia.

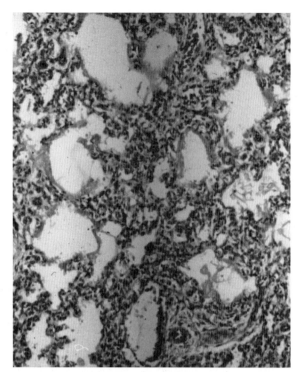

FIGURE 13-27 Infant respiratory distress syndrome. Photomicrograph of lung tissue with infant respiratory distress syndrome and atelectasis. Note the decreased number and size of air spaces. *(Courtesy of R.W. Shaw, MD, North York General Hospital, Toronto, Ontario, Canada.)*

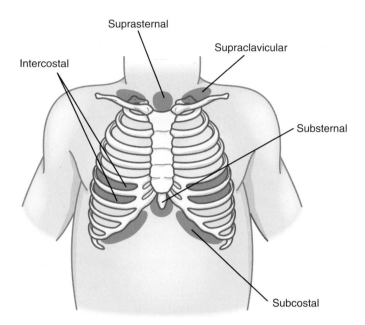

FIGURE 13-28 Retractions of the Infant Chest in IRDS. *(From McCance KL, et al: Pathophysiology: The Biologic Basis for Disease in Adults and Children, ed 6, St. Louis, 2010, Mosby.)*

A vicious cycle develops as acidosis develops from respiratory impairment and metabolic factors. The strenuous muscle activity needed to breathe requires more oxygen than is available, and this leads to anaerobic metabolism and increased lactic acid. In turn, acidosis causes pulmonary vasoconstriction and impairs cell metabolism, reducing the synthesis and secretion of surfactant.

■ Etiology

Infant respiratory distress syndrome is usually related to premature birth, but other factors are involved. It occurs more commonly in male children and following cesarean delivery. Infants born to diabetic mothers are predisposed to this syndrome.

■ Signs and Symptoms

Respiratory difficulty may be evident at birth or shortly after birth. Signs include a persistent respiratory rate of more than 60 breaths per minute, nasal flaring, subcostal and intercostal retractions, rales, and low body temperature. Chest retractions are quite marked in a neonate because of the soft chest wall (Fig. 13-28). As infant respiratory distress syndrome continues, respirations become more rapid and shallow, frothy sputum and expiratory grunt develop, blood pressure falls, and cyanosis and peripheral edema become evident. Signs of severe hypoxemia are decreased responsiveness, irregular respirations with periods of apnea, and decreased breath sounds.

■ Diagnostic Tests

Arterial blood gas analysis is helpful in monitoring both oxygen and acid-base balance. Initially, hypoxemia (low Pao_2) and metabolic acidosis (low serum HCO_3^-) are present. Respiratory acidosis (high Pco_2) develops as ventilation becomes more difficult. Chest x-rays indicate areas of congestion and atelectasis.

■ Treatment

Glucocorticoids given to women in premature labor appear to benefit the premature infant by speeding up the maturation process. Synthetic surfactant, colfosceril (Exosurf Neonatal), administered to the high-risk neonate both as prophylaxis immediately following birth and as necessary therapy, has greatly improved the prognosis. Ventilation using CPAP, oxygen therapy, and nitrous oxide drugs have improved outcomes but are not without risk. High concentrations of oxygen may cause pulmonary damage (bronchodysplasia) and retrolental fibroplasia causing permanent damage to the retina of the eye and loss of vision. Other systemic problems are often present in the premature infant and require specialized care.

Adult or Acute Respiratory Distress Syndrome

Adult or acute respiratory distress syndrome (ARDS) is also known as shock lung, wet lung, stiff lung, postperfusion lung, and a variety of other names related to specific causes. It is considered to be a restrictive lung disorder. A multitude of predisposing conditions such as systemic sepsis, prolonged shock, burns, aspiration, and smoke inhalation may cause ARDS. The onset of respiratory distress usually occurs 1 to 2 days after an injury or other precipitating event. In many cases, it is associated with multiple organ dysfunction or failure secondary to a severe insult to the body.

■ *Pathophysiology*

The basic changes in the lungs result from injury to the alveolar wall and capillary membrane, leading to release of chemical mediators, increased permeability of alveolar capillary membranes, increased fluid and protein in the interstitial area and alveoli, and damage to the surfactant-producing cells (Fig. 13-29). These events result in decreased diffusion of oxygen, reduced blood flow to the lungs, difficulty in expanding the lungs, and diffuse atelectasis. Reductions in tidal volume and vital capacity occur. Damage to lung tissue progresses as increased numbers of neutrophils migrate to the lungs,

releasing proteases and other mediators. Hyaline membranes form from protein-rich fluid in the alveoli, and platelet aggregation and microthrombi develop in the pulmonary circulation, causing stiffness and decreased compliance. If the patient survives, diffuse necrosis and fibrosis are apparent throughout the lungs.

Excess fluid in the lungs predisposes to pneumonia as a complication. Congestive heart failure may develop.

■ *Etiology*

Severe or prolonged shock may cause ARDS because of ischemic damage to the lung tissue. Inflammation in the lungs arises directly from such events as inhalation of toxic chemicals or smoke; excessive oxygen concentration in inspired air; severe viral infections in the lungs; toxins from systemic infection, particularly by gram-negative organisms; fat emboli; explosions; aspiration of highly acidic gastric contents; or lung trauma. Other causes include disseminated intravascular coagulation (see Chapter 10), cancer, acute pancreatitis, and uremia.

■ *Signs and Symptoms*

Early signs may be masked by the effects of the primary problem. Onset is usually marked by dyspnea, restlessness, rapid, shallow respirations, and increased heart rate. Arterial blood gas measurements indicate a significant decrease in Po_2. As lung congestion increases, the accessory muscles are used, rales can be heard, productive cough with frothy sputum may be evident, and cyanosis and lethargy with confusion develop. A combination of respiratory and metabolic acidosis evolves as diffusion is impaired and anaerobic metabolism is required.

■ *Treatment*

The underlying cause must be successfully treated, and supportive respiratory therapy such as oxygen therapy and mechanical ventilation must be maintained until the causative factors are removed and healing occurs. Administration of fluid may be limited to minimize alveolar edema, although this may be difficult in patients with multisystem failure. The prognosis is generally poor, with a case fatality rate of 30% to 40%, but depends on the underlying problem (with infection, the case fatality rate is 80% to 90%).

Acute Respiratory Failure

■ *Pathophysiology*

Acute respiratory failure (ARF) can be the end result of many pulmonary disorders. Respiratory failure is indicated when Pao_2 is less than 50 mmHg (severe hypoxemia) or $Paco_2$ is greater than 50 mmHg (hypercapnia) and serum pH is decreasing (<7.3). Normal values are approximately 80 to 100 mmHg for oxygen and 35 to 45 mmHg for carbon dioxide. The abnormal values

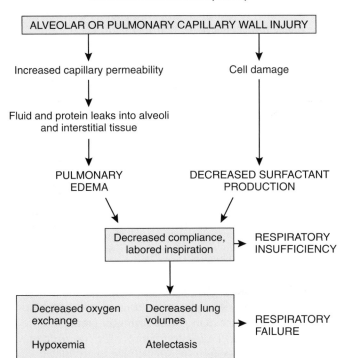

ADULT RESPIRATORY DISTRESS SYNDROME (ARDS)

ALVEOLAR OR PULMONARY CAPILLARY WALL INJURY

Increased capillary permeability

Cell damage

Fluid and protein leaks into alveoli and interstitial tissue

PULMONARY EDEMA

DECREASED SURFACTANT PRODUCTION

Decreased compliance, labored inspiration

RESPIRATORY INSUFFICIENCY

Decreased oxygen exchange

Decreased lung volumes

Hypoxemia

Atelectasis

RESPIRATORY FAILURE

CONFUSION AND DECREASED RESPONSIVENESS
SEVERE HYPOXEMIA
PROGRESSIVE METABOLIC AND RESPIRATORY ACIDOSIS
CARDIAC ARRHYTHMIAS
SHOCK

FIGURE 13-29 Adult respiratory distress syndrome.

mentioned are considered inadequate for the body's metabolic needs at rest. Oxygen is always a major concern because the lungs are the only source of oxygen for the body. The central nervous system, including the respiratory control center, is affected.

The precise figures used for these criteria may vary somewhat with the cause of the problem, but the significant factor is the trend or progressive changes in the values that occur over time. *Respiratory insufficiency* is the term applied to an interim state in which blood gases are abnormal but cell function can continue. Very low oxygen levels can be related to ventilation and perfusion abnormalities that arise for many reasons, sometimes from a combination of problems. A primary problem may be complicated by reflex pulmonary vasoconstriction due to hypoxia or acidosis, which further impairs lung perfusion and increases cardiac workload. The heart may be limited in its ability to compensate for reduced oxygen levels.

Acidosis of respiratory origin (elevated CO_2) may become decompensated because of failure in other systems, resulting in respiratory failure.

Respiratory arrest refers to cessation of respiratory activity and is quickly followed by cardiac arrest.

■ Etiology

Acute respiratory failure may result from acute or chronic disorders:

- Chronic conditions such as emphysema may lead to respiratory failure if the degenerative tissue changes progress to the point at which ventilation and gas exchange are minimal.
- A combination of a chronic with an acute disorder may lead to ARF. For example, ARF may develop in an earlier stage of emphysema or other chronic lung disease if it is complicated by pneumonia, or pneumothorax, or central nervous system depression caused by narcotics or other depressant drugs.
- Acute respiratory disorders such as chest trauma (flail chest or tension pneumothorax), pulmonary embolus, or acute asthma may lead to failure.
- Many neuromuscular diseases such as myasthenia gravis, amyotrophic lateral sclerosis (see Chapter 14), or muscular dystrophy (see Chapter 9) ultimately cause ARF.

■ Signs and Symptoms

The signs may be masked or altered by the primary problem. Manifestations include rapid, shallow, often labored respirations. General signs of hypoxia and hypercapnia include headache, tachycardia, lethargy, and confusion.

■ Treatment

As in many other situations, the primary problem must be resolved and supportive treatment given to maintain respiratory function.

THINK ABOUT 13-16

a. Compare the factors contributing to infant respiratory distress syndrome and ARDS.
b. Describe the basic pathophysiology of respiratory distress syndrome and its initial effect on arterial blood gases.
c. Using an example, explain how respiratory failure may develop and explain why this is life threatening.
d. Explain how severe hypoxia and hypercapnia affect the central nervous system.

CASE STUDY A

Influenza and Pneumonia

Mrs. A.H. has had an acute episode of influenza A, complicated by pneumococcal pneumonia. She lives in a seniors' apartment building, where a number of residents have had influenza in the past month.

1. State the cause of influenza and describe briefly how it affects the lungs.
2. Describe the normal mechanisms that defend against infection in the respiratory tract.
3. Explain why it can be expected that a number of residents in such a building would be affected by influenza.
4. What precautions could be taken by the residents to avoid the infection?
5. What precautions could you take in your particular profession to reduce the risk of respiratory infection for yourself, your colleagues, and your patients?
6. Explain why antibacterial drugs are not directly effective in cases of influenza. Why may they be prescribed?
7. Explain why Mrs. A.H. is predisposed to develop pneumonia.

Mrs. H. was admitted to the hospital after she developed severe chest pain and appeared confused to friends. Pneumococcal pneumonia was suspected.

8. Describe the appropriate diagnostic tests that would be used for Mrs. A.H. and give the rationale for each.
9. Mrs. A.H. indicates that the chest pain increases on inspiration or coughing. Explain the probable cause of this chest pain and her confusion.
10. Describe how other signs and symptoms would probably change as pneumonia develops and give the reason for each (include the relevant respiratory and systemic signs).
11. Predict the values of arterial blood gases in Mrs. A.H. in the early stage of pneumococcal pneumonia and in the advanced stage if two lobes are involved. (Use general descriptions such as increased slightly or greatly, not specific figures.)
12. Explain how Mrs. A.H. can compensate to maintain a normal serum pH.
13. List several reasons why Mrs. A.H. may become dehydrated.
14. Explain several ways in which dehydration could complicate Mrs. A.H.'s status.
15. Describe several treatment measures that would be helpful in this case.

CASE STUDY B

Acute Asthma

Eight-year-old B.J. has had asthma for 2 years since he had acute bronchitis. He was tested for allergies and demonstrated marked responses to a number of animals, pollens, and molds. B.J. also has a history of asthma related to exposure to very cold weather.

1. Describe the pathophysiology of an acute asthma attack in B.J. following exposure to cats.
2. Describe the early signs of an acute asthma attack and relate each of these to the changes taking place in the lungs.
3. If you were updating a medical and drug history for B.J., list several significant questions that should be asked.
4. Describe what precautions you would take if you were treating or dealing with B.J. and include your reasons. Describe your actions if B.J. had an attack while he was with you.
5. State and explain the effects of a prolonged asthma attack.
6. Explain the factors contributing to severe hypoxia and acidosis in a prolonged attack.
7. Define status asthmaticus.
8. Explain why B.J. is likely to have frequent respiratory infections.
9. Suggest several measures that B.J. can take to reduce anxiety and perhaps the risk of an asthma attack.
10. Explain how a beta$_2$-adrenergic agent is helpful in treating asthma and how it is usually administered.

CASE STUDY C

Emphysema

Mr. C.Y., age 71, has had significant emphysema for 6 years. He has reduced his cigarette smoking since mild congestive heart failure was diagnosed (right-sided heart failure; refer to Chapter 12). He has been admitted to the hospital with a suspected closed pneumothorax and respiratory failure.

1. Describe the pathophysiologic changes in the lungs with emphysema, and explain how these affect oxygen and carbon dioxide levels in the blood.
2. Explain the possible role of smoking in Mr. C.Y.'s case and its general effects on respiratory function (consider effects on cardiovascular function also).
3. What significant characteristics related to emphysema and heart failure would you expect to observe in Mr. C.Y.?
4. Explain how a pneumothorax has probably occurred in the presence of emphysema.
5. Explain how a pneumothorax has precipitated respiratory failure, using the effects on lung function and gas exchange in your answer. Include the criteria for respiratory failure.
6. Explain why caution must be exercised in administering oxygen to Mr. C.Y.
7. Mr. C.Y. is resting quietly. Suggest three complications of immobility that could develop in Mr. C.Y. and one preventive measure that could be taken for each.

8. Explain how congestive heart failure develops from emphysema.
9. Describe respiratory therapy that might be helpful to Mr. C.Y.
   With aggressive treatment, Mr. C.Y. recovered and returned home.
10. Suggest some reasons why Mr. C.Y. may not receive adequate nutrition and hydration at home.
11. Suggest other support measures that would be useful in this case.

CASE STUDY D

Cystic Fibrosis

M.T., age 5 years, has cystic fibrosis, which was diagnosed following an intestinal obstruction after birth (meconium ileus). M.T. has frequent lung infections despite daily respiratory therapy. She is given pancrelipase with her meals and snacks to facilitate digestion and absorption. At a recent checkup, M.T. was found to be shorter and under the weight range for her age.

1. M.T.'s parents would like to have another child. What is the probability that a future child would have cystic fibrosis? (Hint: What is the genetic status of each parent?)
2. Describe the basic pathophysiology of cystic fibrosis and briefly describe the various effects in the body.
3. Explain the possible effects on airflow of mucus obstructions in the lungs.
4. Explain why M.T. has frequent infections.
5. M.T.'s parents are arranging a dental appointment for her. Describe any possible limitations in arranging the appointment and list what precautions should be taken when she arrives for the appointment.
6. State several criteria that would be helpful in maintaining adequate nutrition for M.T.
7. If M.T. does not take pancrelipase regularly, she has steatorrhea (frequent loose, fatty stools). Explain why this occurs and how it might affect her respiratory function if prolonged.
8. Using your basic knowledge of physiology, describe the possible effects on M.T. if she fails to digest and absorb adequate amounts of protein, calcium, vitamin D, vitamin K, and iron.
9. Explain why M.T. is likely to develop bronchiectasis at a later time, and describe the significant signs of its development.
10. Explain why M.T. may have a fluid-electrolyte imbalance if she has a high fever with a lung infection.

CHAPTER SUMMARY

Because the respiratory system is the sole source of oxygen for cell metabolism, respiratory impairment has widespread effects in the body. Respiratory and/or metabolic acidosis often accompany hypoxia. Respiratory disorders may result from airway obstructions, alveolar damage, reduced lung expansion, or interference with pulmonary blood flow.

- Characteristic breathing patterns, type of cough, and sputum, as well as other manifestations, are helpful in diagnosing the cause of the disorder. For example, a cough producing purulent sputum is typical of bacterial infection, and wheezing indicates airway obstruction.
- Viruses cause both upper and lower respiratory tract infections, including the common cold, laryngotracheobronchitis (croup), influenza, bronchiolitis, and primary atypical pneumonia.
- Pneumonia impairs oxygen diffusion when exudate fills the alveoli or interstitial tissue in the lungs. Pneumonia may be classified in several ways, including primary or secondary, by etiology or type of causative microbe, or by the anatomical distribution of the infection in the lung.
- Severe acute respiratory syndrome is an acute respiratory infection caused by a previously unknown virus. The recent epidemic stimulated a global effort to identify the causative microbe and contain the infection.
- The incidence of tuberculosis is increasing in individuals with low host resistance. The number of drug-resistant bacteria has risen as well. The hypersensitivity reaction developing with primary infection and tubercle formation is the basis of the tuberculin (Mantoux) test. Infection can be spread when active infection or cavitation occurs in the lungs.
- Cystic fibrosis is an inherited disorder (recessive gene) affecting the exocrine glands, particularly the mucous glands of the lungs. The pancreas, liver, and sweat glands are also involved. Airway obstructions and frequent lung infections cause permanent damage to the lungs.
- Exposure to cigarette smoke and industrial carcinogens are predisposing factors to lung cancer. Prognosis is poor because early diagnosis is rare, and many types of tumors resist chemotherapy or radiation. The lungs are also a common site for secondary tumors.
- Aspiration of solids or liquids may cause inflammation, laceration, or direct obstruction of airways.
- Obstructive sleep apnea occurs when pharyngeal tissues collapse on expiration during sleep, leading to intermittent periods of apnea.
- The pathophysiology of acute asthma is based on airway obstruction related to bronchoconstriction, inflammation and edema, and production of excessive thick mucus. Obstruction leads to severe respiratory distress and hypoxia. Status asthmaticus is a potential complication.
- Emphysema (COPD) is characterized by loss of elasticity and destruction of alveolar walls, septae, and capillaries, leading to overinflation of the lungs and hypercapnia as well as hypoxia.
- Chronic bronchitis is associated with constant irritation in the airways and frequent infections, leading to fibrosis. Cor pulmonale is a common complication.
- Restrictive disorders include those with chest wall dysfunction, such as kyphosis or respiratory muscle paralysis, and those disorders causing pulmonary fibrosis and loss of compliance, such as occupational pneumoconioses (silicosis).
- Pulmonary edema refers to increased fluid in the alveoli reducing oxygen diffusion and lung expansion.
- Most pulmonary emboli arise from thrombi in leg veins. Moderate-sized emboli cause respiratory impairment; large emboli interfere with cardiovascular function. Fat emboli cause ARDS.
- Atelectasis may affect part or all of a lung. Causes include airway obstruction, decreased ventilation, compression of the lung, or increased surface tension in the alveoli.
- A large open pneumothorax impairs ventilation and circulation (venous return) due to mediastinal flutter. Flail chest injury causes paradoxic motion and decreases oxygen concentration in the alveolar air as well as impeding venous return.
- Respiratory distress syndrome occurs in newborn infants, IRDS associated with prematurity, and also in adults whose lungs are damaged by ischemia or inhalation of toxic materials. Lung expansion is reduced and oxygen diffusion impaired by fluid in the lungs.
- Acute respiratory failure applies to a marked deficit of oxygen, a great increase in carbon dioxide, or a combination of these. It may occur with acute conditions (tension pneumothorax), chronic disorders (emphysema), or chronic diseases complicated by a secondary acute problem (cystic fibrosis plus pneumonia).

STUDY QUESTIONS

1. Explain the purpose of the specialized cells in the respiratory mucosa.
2. a. Describe the function of the external intercostal muscles.
   b. Describe the mechanism of and the energy required for quiet expiration and for forced expiration.
3. a. Describe the location of the chemoreceptors that respond to elevated carbon dioxide levels and those that respond to low oxygen levels.
   b. Which gas creates the primary respiratory drive under normal circumstances?
4. State and explain the effect of increased carbon dioxide levels on serum pH.

5. a. Describe how carbon dioxide is transported in the blood.
   b. Name a gas that can displace oxygen from hemoglobin.
6. What physiologic compensations are available for chronic hypoxia due to respiratory impairment and for chronic hypercapnia?
7. Explain how respiratory infection can cause serious respiratory obstruction in a young child and include examples.
8. a. Name the organisms that commonly cause primary atypical pneumonia.
   b. Compare the pathophysiologic changes in viral and pneumococcal pneumonia.
9. a. Explain the significance and limitations of a positive tuberculin test.
   b. Explain the conditions under which tuberculosis may be contagious.
   c. What measures can be taken by health professionals to minimize the spread of infection?
10. a. Why has anthrax become an infectious disease of concern?
    b. How can illness from inhalation anthrax be prevented?
11. What is the primary cause of obstructive sleep apnea and how does it affect oxygen levels in the body?
12. a. Explain how obstruction develops with chronic bronchitis.
    b. Explain how acute asthma causes air trapping or atelectasis.
    c. How does hypoxia and respiratory alkalosis develop in the early stages of an asthma attack?
    d. Explain why serum pH is lowered when an asthma attack persists.
13. a. Explain why the anteroposterior diameter of the chest is increased in a patient with emphysema.
    b. Explain why hypercapnia may be a major problem in patients with emphysema.
    c. Explain how each of the following develops in patients with emphysema: (1) cor pulmonale, (2) secondary polycythemia.
14. a. Define meconium ileus.
    b. Describe the effects of cystic fibrosis on the lungs and the liver.
    c. Explain several ways whereby permanent damage can occur in the lungs and in the pancreas.
15. a. Explain why the lung is a common site for secondary cancer.
    b. State two systemic signs or symptoms of cancer, two local respiratory signs, and two signs related to paraneoplastic syndrome.

c. Explain why the prognosis for lung cancer is poor (include three factors).
16. a. List three factors predisposing to aspiration.
    b. Describe the potential effects of aspirating vomitus.
17. a. Describe the factors predisposing to atelectasis following abdominal surgery.
    b. Describe the signs of atelectasis.
18. a. Explain why pulmonary edema causes severe hypoxia.
    b. Trace the path of a pulmonary embolus resulting from thrombophlebitis.
    c. Compare the effects on respiration of a very small embolus and a very large one.
19. a. Describe the effects of a large open pneumothorax on respiratory function and on cardiovascular function.
    b. Explain how covering an open pneumothorax improves oxygen levels.
    c. Explain a possible cause of increased respiratory distress following the covering of an open pneumothorax.
20. a. Explain how paradoxic motion develops with a flail chest injury and how it causes hypoxemia.
    b. Explain why atelectasis does not occur directly with a flail chest injury.
21. a. Compare the causes of infant and adult respiratory distress syndromes.
    b. Describe the signs of infant respiratory distress.
    c. Describe the criteria for a diagnosis of respiratory failure.
22. Respiratory problems frequently occur in patients with burns, particularly those with facial burns or who were injured in enclosed spaces such as a car or small room (see Chapter 2). Apply your knowledge to explain how each of the following affects respiratory function in a burn patient and the end result:
    a. Inhaling carbon monoxide
    b. Inhaling very hot air with irritant particles and gases
    c. A deep burn covering the chest and back
23. The "bends" or decompression sickness is a form of air embolism. When scuba or deep sea divers are under higher pressure, more nitrogen gas dissolves in the blood and tissue fluids. Usually a slow ascent to the surface (lower pressure) allows the gas to be gradually dissipated and exhaled. If a diver rises to the surface too rapidly, the gas comes out of solution, forming bubbles or gas emboli in the circulation. Explain why ischemia and pain may occur in various tissues such as muscle, joints, or the heart.

ADDITIONAL RESOURCES

Greenwood D, Slack RCB, Peutherer JF: *Medical Microbiology,* ed 17, Edinburgh, 2007, Churchill Livingstone.

Heymann DL: *Control of Communicable Disease Manual,* ed 18, 2004, American Public Health Association.

Heart & Lung: The Journal of Acute and Critical Care.

Kumar V, Abbas AK, Fausto M: *Robbins and Cotran Pathologic Basis of Disease,* ed 8, Philadelphia, 2007, Saunders.

Ware LB, et al: The acute respiratory distress syndrome. *N Engl J Med* 342:1334, 2000.

Web Sites

http://www.cancer.gov *National Cancer Institute, U.S. National Institutes of Health*

http://www.cdc.gov/cancer/lung *Cancer prevention and control (Centers for Disease Control and Prevention)*

http://www.cdc.gov/flu *Information on influenza (Centers for Disease Control and Prevention)*

http://www.cdc.gov/sars/index.html *Information on severe acute respiratory syndrome (SARS) (Centers for Disease Control and Prevention)*

http://www.niaid.nih.gov *National Institute of Allergy and Infectious Diseases*

http://www.nhlbi.nih.gov *National Heart, Lung and Blood Institute, National Institutes of Health*

http://www.nlhep.org *National Lung Health Education Program*

http://www.who.int *World Health Organization*

Nervous System Disorders

CHAPTER OUTLINE

LEARNING OBJECTIVES

After studying this chapter, the student is expected to:

1. Relate the focal effect of a lesion to the specific area of damage in the brain.
2. Describe the possible effects of increased intracranial pressure on level of consciousness, motor and sensory functions, vital signs, vision, and language.
3. Explain the effects of herniation.
4. Compare the effects of brain tumors in different areas of the brain.
5. Compare transient ischemic attacks (TIAs) to cerebrovascular accidents (CVAs).
6. Explain how cerebral aneurysms develop, their effects, and possible complications.

7. Describe the cause, pathophysiology, and manifestations of bacterial meningitis.
8. Explain how a brain abscess may cause focal and general effects.
9. Differentiate the types of hematomas and describe the effect of a hematoma on the brain.
10. Explain how seizures may be related to infection or injury.
11. Describe how various types of spinal cord injury may occur.
12. Explain how the effects of spinal cord injury depend on the location of the damage.
13. Compare the signs of spinal shock with the permanent effects of spinal cord injury.

KEY TERMS

afferent	coma	hyperreflexia	prodromal
amnesia	contralateral	infratentorial	ptosis
anencephaly	disorientation	ipsilateral	retina
anomalies	efferent	labile	scotoma
aphasia	fissure	nuchal rigidity	spastic
athetoid	flaccid	paralysis	stupor
atresia	flaccid	paresis	sulcus, sulci
aura	foramina	paresthesia	supratentorial
bifurcation	fulminant	photophobia	sutures
choreiform	ganglion	postictal	tetraplegia
clonic	gyri	precursor	tonic
cognitive	hyperreflexia	pressoreceptors	transillumination

Review of Nervous System Anatomy and Physiology

The nervous system consists of the central and peripheral nervous system.

- Central nervous system—brain and spinal cord
- Peripheral nervous system—cranial and spinal nerves; ganglia; sensory neurons, neuromuscular junctions

Brain

The brain is the communication and control center of the body. It receives, processes, and evaluates many kinds of input; decides on the response or action to be taken; and then initiates the response. Responses include both involuntary activity that is required to maintain homeostasis in the body (regulated by the autonomic nervous system) and voluntary actions (controlled by the somatic nervous system). With both reflex and voluntary activities, the individual is often not aware of the amount and diversity of input received or the integration or assessment of that input, but knows only of the response (Fig. 14-1).

Protection for the Brain

The brain is protected by the rigid bone of the skull, the three membranes or meninges, and the cerebrospinal fluid (CSF). The cranial and facial bones are connected by sutures, which are relatively immovable joints consisting of fibrous tissue. If pressure inside the skull increases in infants before the sutures fuse or ossify, the cranial bones may separate, causing the head to enlarge. The skull contains a number of cavities, or fossae, as well as foramina (openings) and canals through which nerves and blood vessels pass. The largest opening, the foramen magnum, is located in the occipital bone at the base of the skull, where the spinal cord emerges.

Meninges

The meninges consist of three continuous connective tissue membranes covering the brain and spinal cord.

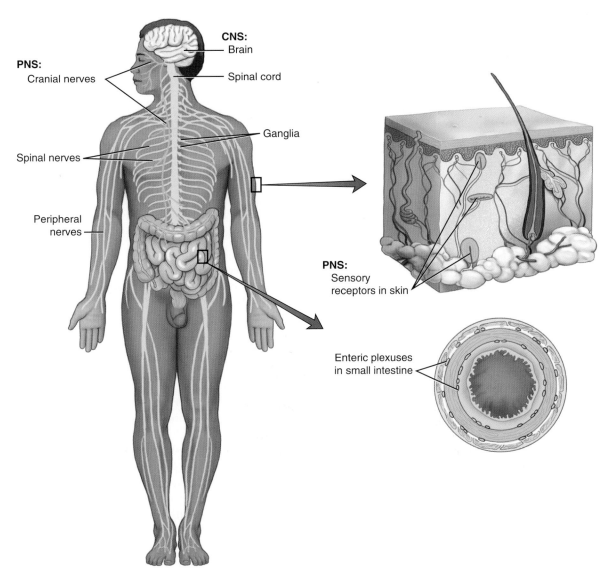

PNS:
Cranial nerves

CNS:
Brain

Spinal cord

Ganglia

Spinal nerves

Peripheral
nerves

PNS:
Sensory
receptors in skin

Enteric plexuses
in small intestine

FIGURE 14-1 Overview of the Nervous System The nervous system is divided into two components: the central nervous system composed of the brain and the spinal cord, and the peripheral nervous system containing the cranial and spinal nerves, ganglia, and sensory receptors. *(From VanMeter K, Hubert R:* Microbiology for the Healthcare Professional, *St. Louis, 2010, Elsevier.)*

The meninges and the contents of the spaces between the layers are as follows:
- The *dura mater*, the outer layer, is a tough, fibrous, double-layered membrane that separates at specific points to form the dural sinuses, which collect *venous* blood and CSF for return to the general circulation
- The *subdural space*, lying beneath the dura, is a *potential space* (i.e., normally empty, this space could fill with blood after an injury).
- The *arachnoid (arachnoid mater)*, a loose, weblike covering, is the middle layer.
- The *subarachnoid space*, which contains the *CSF* and the cerebral arteries and veins, lies beneath the arachnoid.

- *Arachnoid villi* are projections of arachnoid into the dural sinuses at several places around the brain, through which CSF can be absorbed into the venous blood.
- The *pia mater*, a delicate connective tissue that adheres closely to all convolutions on the surface of the brain, is the inner layer. Many small blood vessels are found in the pia mater (Fig. 14-2).

Cerebrospinal Fluid
The cerebrospinal fluid (CSF) provides a cushion for the brain and spinal cord. Similar to plasma in appearance, it is a clear, almost colorless liquid, but it differs from plasma in the concentrations of electrolytes,

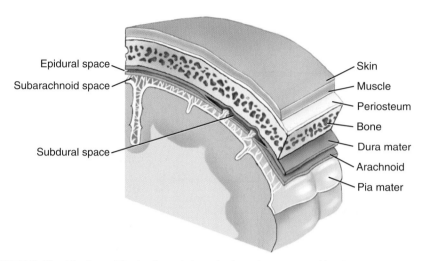

FIGURE 14-2 **The Meninges** The brain and the spinal cord are covered by three protective membranes, collectively called *meninges*. The outermost membrane is the dura mater, the middle layer is the arachnoid, and the innermost membrane is the pia mater. *(From VanMeter K, Hubert R: Microbiology for the Healthcare Professional, St. Louis, 2010, Elsevier.)*

TABLE 14-1	Characteristics of Normal Cerebrospinal Fluid
Appearance	Clear and colorless
Pressure	9-14 mmHg or 150 mm H$_2$O
Red blood cells	None
White blood cells	Occasional
Protein	15-45 mg/dL
Glucose	45-75 mg/dL
Sodium	140 mEq/L
Potassium	3 mEq/L
Specific gravity	1.007
pH	7.32-7.35
Volume in the system at one time	125-150 mL
Volume formed in 24 hours	500-800 mL

glucose, and protein (Table 14-1), which remain relatively *constant*. A change in the characteristics of the CSF is a useful diagnostic tool (see Fig. 14-11). For example, the presence of significant numbers of erythrocytes in CSF indicates bleeding in the central nervous system.

Cerebrospinal fluid is formed constantly in the choroid plexuses in the ventricles and then flows into the subarachnoid space, where it circulates around the brain and spinal cord and eventually passes through the arachnoid villi, returning into the venous blood. To maintain a relatively constant pressure within the skull (intracranial pressure), it is important for equal amounts of CSF to be produced and reabsorbed at the same rate.

Blood-Brain Barrier and Blood-Cerebrospinal Fluid Barrier

The blood-brain barrier is a protective mechanism provided primarily by relatively impermeable capillaries in the brain. The endothelial cells of the capillaries are tightly joined together by tight junctions rather than possessing pores. This barrier limits the passage of potentially damaging materials into the brain and controls the delicate but essential balance of electrolytes, glucose, and proteins in the brain. There is a similar blood-CSF barrier at the choroid plexus to control the constituents of CSF. The blood-brain barrier is poorly developed in neonates, and therefore substances such as bilirubin (see Chapter 22) or other toxic materials can pass easily into the infant's brain, causing damage. When fully developed, the blood-brain barrier can be a disadvantage, because it does not allow the passage of many essential drugs into the brain (i.e., certain antibiotics and anticancer drugs). Lipid-soluble substances, including alcohol, pass freely into the brain.

THINK ABOUT 14-1

a. List, in order, the brain coverings and spaces with their contents, from the brain tissue outward.
b. Explain the effect of the production of more CSF than can be reabsorbed.

Functional Areas
Cerebral Hemispheres

The cerebral hemispheres make up the largest and most obvious portions of the brain. The outer surface is covered by elevations, or gyri (sing., gyrus), that are

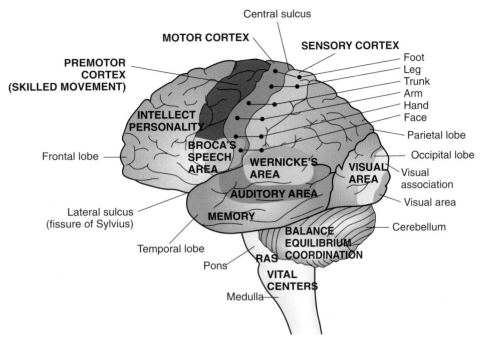

FIGURE 14-3 Functional areas of the brain showing the *left* side of the cerebral hemispheres.

separated by grooves, or sulci (sing., sulcus). The longitudinal fissure separates the left and right hemispheres. The corpus callosum consists of nerve fibers connecting the left and right hemisphere for the purpose of communication between the two hemispheres.

Each hemisphere is divided into four major lobes, each of which has specific functions (Fig. 14-3). Complex functions, such as language and memory, involve many areas of the brain. Each hemisphere is concerned with voluntary movement and sensory function in the opposite (contralateral) side of the body, and these areas of the cortex have been well mapped. In Figure 14-3, note the large number of nerve cells required to innervate the face compared with the amount of cortex allocated to the trunk. The cells of the motor cortex of the frontal lobe initiate specific voluntary movements, and these cells are often referred to as upper motor neurons (UMNs). Their axons form the corticospinal tracts in the spinal cord. Because the crossover of most of these tracts occurs in the medulla, damage to the motor cortex in the left frontal lobe adjacent to the longitudinal fissure (on top of the head) results in paralysis or paresis of the muscles of the right leg.

Each special sensory area of the cortex has an *association area* surrounding the primary cortex, in which the sensory input is recognized and interpreted. For example, the occipital lobe contains the primary visual cortex, which receives the stimuli from the eye, and the surrounding association cortex identifies the object seen. If the primary cortex is damaged, the person is blind, but if the association area is damaged, the person can see an object but cannot comprehend its significance.

The right and left hemispheres are generally similar in structure but not necessarily in function (Table 14-2). The term *dominant hemisphere* refers to the side of the brain that controls *language*, which in most people is the left hemisphere. There are two special areas involved in language skills. *Broca's area* is considered the motor or expressive speech area, in which the output of words, both verbal and written, is coordinated in an appropriate and understandable way. This area is located at the base of the premotor area of the left frontal lobe. *Wernicke's area* is the integration center that comprehends language received, both spoken and written. This area is located in the posterior temporal lobe and has connecting fibers to the prefrontal, visual, and auditory areas. The left hemisphere also appears to be responsible for mathematical, problem-solving, and logical reasoning abilities. The right hemisphere has greater influence on artistic abilities, creativity, spatial relationships, and emotional and behavioral characteristics.

The *prefrontal cortex* lies anterior to the motor and premotor cortex and recent research indicates that it functions in coordinating complex cognitive behavior as well as providing components for expression of personality. It plays a very significant role in social relationships and impulse control.

The *basal nuclei* (previously called the basal ganglia) are clusters of cell bodies or gray matter located deep among the tracts of the cerebral hemispheres. These are part of the *extrapyramidal system* (EPS) of motor control, which controls and coordinates skeletal muscle activity, preventing excessive movements and initiating accessory and often involuntary actions, such

TABLE 14-2 **Major Functional Areas of the Brain**

Area	Function
Frontal lobe	
Prefrontal area (left cortex)	Intellectual function and personality
Premotor cortex	Skilled movements
Motor cortex	Voluntary movements
Broca's area (left cortex)	Speech (expression)
Parietal lobe	
Somatosensory area	Sensation (e.g., touch, pain)
Occipital lobe	
Visual cortex	Vision
Temporal lobe	
Auditory cortex	Hearing
Olfactory cortex	Smell
Wernicke's area (left cortex)	Comprehension of speech
	Memory
Cerebellum	Body balance and position, coordinated movement
Medulla oblongata	Control and coordination centers for respiration and cardiovascular activity
	Swallow reflex center, vomiting reflex, cough reflex
	Nuclei of five cranial nerves
Hypothalamus	Autonomic nervous system
	Link with endocrine system
	Control of body temperature, fluid balance
	Centers for thirst, hunger
Thalamus	Sensory sorting and relay center
Basal nuclei	Coordination and control of body movement
Reticular activating System	Arousal or awareness
Limbic system	Emotional responses

as arm-swinging when walking. Two additional nuclei located in the midbrain, the substantia nigra and the red nucleus, are also connected to the basal nuclei and the EPS.

The *limbic system* consists of many nuclei and connecting fibers in the cerebral hemispheres that encircle the superior part of the brain stem. The limbic system is responsible for emotional reactions or feelings, and for this purpose, it has many connections to all areas of the brain. Part of the hypothalamus is involved with the limbic system. The hypothalamus provides the link for the autonomic responses, such as altered blood pressure or nausea, which occur when one experiences fear, excitement, or an unpleasant sight or odor. Any

cognitive (intellectual) decision arising from the higher cortical centers may be accompanied by an emotional aspect mediated through the limbic system.

Diencephalon

The diencephalon is the central portion of the brain. It is surrounded by the hemispheres and contains the thalamus, the hypothalamus, and the epithalamus. The *thalamus* consists of many nerve cell bodies, the major function of which is to serve as a sorting and relay station for incoming sensory impulses. From the thalamus, connecting fibers transmit impulses to the cerebral cortex and other appropriate areas of the brain. The *hypothalamus* has a key role in maintaining homeostasis in the body, controlling the autonomic nervous system and much of the endocrine system through the hypophysis, or pituitary gland. It is responsible for the regulation of body temperature, intake of food and fluid, and the regulation of sleep cycles. The hypothalamus is also the key to the stress response and plays major roles in emotional responses through the limbic system and in biologic behaviors, such as the sex drive (libido).

Brain Stem

The inferior portion of the brain, called the brain stem, is the connecting link to the spinal cord. The *pons* is composed of bundles of afferent (incoming) and efferent (outgoing) fibers. Several nuclei of cranial nerves are also located in the pons. The *medulla oblongata* contains the vital control centers that regulate respiratory and cardiovascular function and the coordinating centers that govern the cough reflex, swallowing, and vomiting. The medulla is the location of the nuclei of several cranial nerves. It is distinguished by two longitudinal ridges on the ventral surface, termed the pyramids, marking the site of crossover (decussation) of the majority of fibers of the corticospinal (pyramidal) tracts, which results in the contralateral control of muscle function.

The *reticular formation* is a network of nuclei and neurons scattered throughout the brain stem that has connections to many parts of the brain. The *reticular-activating system (RAS)* is part of this formation and determines the degree of arousal or awareness of the cerebral cortex. In other words, these neurons decide which of the incoming sensory impulses the brain ignores and which it notices. Many drugs can affect the activity of the RAS, thus increasing or decreasing the input to the brain.

Cerebellum

The cerebellum is located dorsal to the pons and medulla, below the occipital lobe. It functions to coordinate movement and maintain posture and equilibrium by continuously assessing and adjusting to input from the pyramidal system, the proprioceptors in joints and muscles, the visual pathways, and the vestibular pathways from the inner ear.

THINK ABOUT 14-2

a. Describe the specific location and function of each of the following: the prefrontal cortex, somatosensory area, the RAS, Wernicke's area, the basal nuclei, and the visual association area.

b. Describe white matter—what it is and what its function is—and give an example.

c. Predict the effects of brain damage in the prefrontal cortex, left frontal lobe, the cerebellum, or the hypothalamus.

Blood Supply to the Brain

Blood is supplied to the brain by the internal carotid arteries and the vertebral arteries. Each *internal carotid artery* is a branch of a common carotid artery (right or left) and includes the carotid sinus, which is the location of the pressoreceptors, or baroreceptors, that signal changes in blood pressure and the chemoreceptors that monitor variations in blood pH and oxygen levels.

At the base of the brain, each internal carotid artery divides into an anterior and middle cerebral artery (see Fig. 14-14).

- The *anterior cerebral artery* supplies the frontal lobe.
- The *middle cerebral artery* supplies the lateral part of the cerebral hemispheres, primarily the temporal and parietal lobes, which comprise a high proportion of the brain tissue.

Posteriorly, the *vertebral arteries* join to form:

- The *basilar artery,* which supplies branches to the brain stem and cerebellum as it ascends.

At the base of the brain, the basilar artery divides into:

- The right and left *posterior cerebral arteries,* which supply blood to the occipital lobes.
- The anterior, middle, and posterior cerebral arteries follow a course over the surface of each hemisphere, with many branches penetrating into the brain substance (see Fig. 14-13*A*).

Anastomoses between these major arteries at the base of the brain are provided by the:

- *Anterior communicating artery* between the anterior cerebral arteries
- *Posterior communicating arteries* between the middle cerebral and posterior cerebral arteries
- This arrangement forms the *circle of Willis* and provides an alternative source of blood when the internal carotid or vertebral artery is obstructed. This circle of arteries surrounds the pituitary gland and optic chiasm.

Blood flow in the cerebral arteries is relatively constant because the brain cells constantly use oxygen and glucose (essential nutrients for neurons) and have little storage capacity. *Autoregulation* is a mechanism by which increased carbon dioxide levels or decreased pH in the blood, or decreased blood pressure, in an area of the brain results in immediate local vasodilation. The pressoreceptors (baroreceptors) and chemoreceptors protect the brain from damage related to abnormal blood pressure or pH levels in the systemic flow.

As mentioned, venous blood from the brain collects in the dural sinuses and then drains into the right and left internal jugular veins, to be returned to the heart.

Cranial Nerves

There are 12 pairs of cranial nerves. They originate from the brain stem and pass through the foramina in the skull to serve structures in the head and neck, including the eyes and ears. The vagus nerve (cranial nerve X) serves a more extensive area, branching to innervate many of the viscera. A cranial nerve may consist of motor fibers only (with associated sensory fibers from proprioceptors in the skeletal muscles) or of sensory fibers only, or it may be a mixed nerve, containing both motor and sensory fibers (Table 14-3). Four cranial nerves (III, VII, IX, X) include parasympathetic fibers.

THINK ABOUT 14-3

a. Explain the function of the circle of Willis.

b. Describe the effect of an obstruction in the right anterior cerebral artery.

c. Explain how a lack of glucose or oxygen will affect brain function.

d. What are the different types of fibers and the functions of cranial nerves II, III, and IX? Describe the effects of damage to each.

Spinal Cord

Spinal Cord

The spinal cord is protected by the bony vertebral column, the meninges, and the CSF. The cord is continuous with the medulla oblongata and ends at the level of the first lumbar vertebra. Beyond this extends a bundle of nerve roots known as the cauda equina. This arrangement is significant because there is little risk of damaging the cord when a needle is inserted into the subarachnoid space below the first lumbar level (usually in the space between L3 and L4) to obtain a sample of CSF (see Fig. 14-11).

The spinal cord consists of the white matter (outer region) containing the spinal cord tracts, composed of myelinated fibers, and the gray matter (inner region) containing the nerve cell bodies, dendrites, and nonmyelinated axons. Within the gray matter three distinct areas can be identified:

- Ventral horn
  - Contain motor neurons and their axons leave via the ventral root

TABLE 14-3   Major Components of Cranial Nerves

Number	Name	Type of Fibers	Function
I	Olfactory	Sensory	Special sensory—smell
II	Optic	Sensory	Special sensory—vision
III	Oculomotor	Motor	Eye movements
			Four extrinsic eye muscles
			Upper eyelid—levator palpebrae muscle
		PNS	Iris—pupillary constrictor muscle
			Ciliary muscle—accommodation
IV	Trochlear	Motor	Eye movements—superior oblique eye muscle
V	Trigeminal	Sensory	General sensory—eye, nose, face and oral cavity, teeth
		Motor	Muscles of mastication with sensory proprioceptive fibers; speech
VI	Abducens	Motor	Eye movements—lateral rectus eye muscle
VII	Facial	Sensory	Special sensory—taste, anterior two-thirds of tongue
		Motor	Muscles of facial expression
			Scalp muscles
		PNS	Lacrimal gland, nasal mucosa, salivary glands (sublingual and submandibular)
VIII	Vestibulocochlear	Sensory	Special sensory—hearing and balance (inner ear)
IX	Glossopharyngeal	Sensory	Special sensory—taste, posterior one-third of tongue
			General sensory—pharynx and soft palate (gag reflex)
			Sensory—carotid sinus for baroreceptors and chemoreceptors
		Motor	Pharyngeal muscles—swallowing
		PNS	Salivary gland (parotid)
X	Vagus	Sensory	Special sensory—taste, pharynx, posterior tongue
			General sensory—external ear and diaphragm
			Visceral sensory—viscera in thoracic and abdominal cavities
		Motor	Pharynx and soft palate—swallowing and speech
		PNS	Heart and lungs; smooth muscle and glands of digestive system
XI	Spinal accessory	Motor	Voluntary muscles of palate, pharynx, and larynx
			Head movements—sternocleidomastoid and trapezius muscles
XII	Hypoglossal	Motor	Muscles of tongue

PNS, parasympathetic nervous system.

- Dorsal horn
  - Contain interneurons receiving information from sensory neurons of the dorsal root ganglia
- Lateral horns
  - Contain visceral motor neurons

The white matter is composed of afferent (sensory) and efferent (motor) fibers that are organized into tracts and communicating fibers that run between the two sides of the spinal cord. Each tract is assigned a unique position in the white matter; a cross-section of the cord would illustrate the "map" of tracts (Fig. 14-4B). The name of the tract is based on its source and destination, and the fibers in it transmit one type of impulse. For example, the lateral spinothalamic tract is made up of *ascending* fibers that conduct pain or temperature *sensations*, which are relayed from spinal nerves and receptors on the opposite side of the body, to the thalamus.

The *descending* tracts are of two types. The *pyramidal*, or corticospinal, tracts conduct impulses concerned with voluntary movement from the motor cortex (*upper motor neurons*) to the *lower motor neurons* in the anterior horn at the appropriate level of the spinal cord. Most of these tracts cross in the medulla. The *extrapyramidal* tracts carry impulses that modify and coordinate voluntary movement and maintain posture. Lower motor neurons may receive both stimulatory and inhibitory input from upper motor neurons and from interneurons in the spinal cord. The sum of the input determines what activity occurs in the spinal nerves and skeletal muscles.

Spinal Nerves

Thirty-one pairs of spinal nerves emerge from the spinal cord, carrying motor and sensory fibers to and from the

THE SPINAL CORD   CROSS-SECTION OF THE SPINAL CORD SHOWING TRACTS

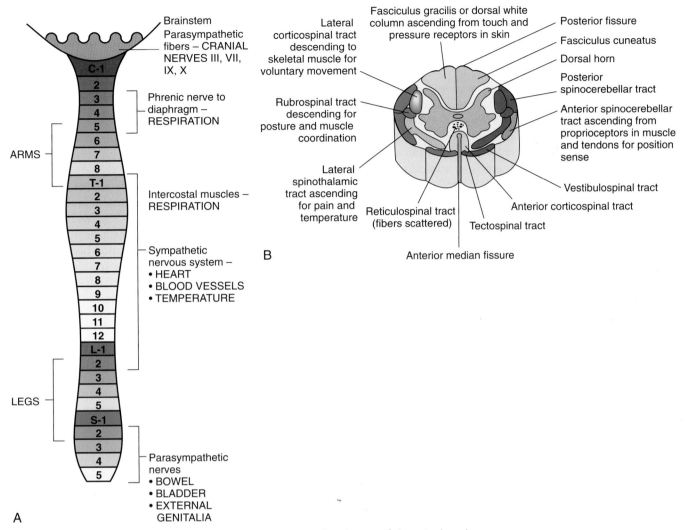

FIGURE 14-4 Functional areas of the spinal cord.

organs and tissues of the body. They are named by the location in the vertebral column where they emerge (see Fig. 14-4) and are numbered within each section. For example, there are eight pairs of *cervical nerves*, numbered *C1 to C8*. Each spinal nerve is connected to the spinal cord by two short roots. The ventral, or anterior, root is made up of efferent or motor fibers from the lower motor neurons in the anterior horn. The dorsal, or posterior, root consists of afferent or sensory fibers from the dorsal root ganglion (a collection of nerve cell bodies in the peripheral nervous system), where sensory fibers from peripheral receptors have already synapsed.

The area of sensory innervation of the skin by a specific spinal nerve is called a *dermatome*, and these can be drawn on a "map" of the body surface (see Fig. 14-22). Assessment of sensory awareness using the dermatome map can be a useful tool in determining the level of damage to the spinal cord.

Four *plexuses* are located where fibers from several spinal nerves branch and then reform in different combinations to become specific peripheral nerves: the cervical, brachial, lumbar, and sacral. This networking means that the phrenic nerve, for example, consists of fibers from spinal nerves C3 to C5, and the sciatic nerve contains fibers from spinal nerves L4 to L5 and S1 to S3. Also, the fibers in each spinal nerve can be distributed in several peripheral nerves. This dispersal pattern can minimize the effects on a muscle's contraction of damage to one spinal cord segment.

Reflexes

Reflexes are automatic, rapid, involuntary responses to a stimulus. A simple reflex involves a sensory stimulus from a receptor that is conducted along an afferent nerve fiber, a synapse in the spinal cord, and an efferent impulse that is conducted along a peripheral nerve to elicit the response. Touching a hot object with the hand thus results in an immediate movement of the hand away from the object. At the same time, connecting neurons or interneurons transmit the sensory information up to the brain to initiate an assessment and further action if required. Many reflexes that control visceral activities or posture take place continuously, *without* the individual's awareness. In addition, each individual has *acquired*, or learned, reflexes, such as those developed when learning to ride a bicycle. Certain basic reflexes, such as the patellar, or knee-jerk reflex, or oculocephalic (doll's head eye response) reflex are useful in diagnosis. Absent, weak, or abnormal responses may indicate the presence of a neurologic problem and sometimes can show the location of spinal cord damage.

THINK ABOUT   14-4

a. At which level of the spine would a lumbar puncture occur, and why?
b. Describe the general location of the cervical spinal nerves.
c. Describe a dermatome and its purpose.
d. Describe the path of nerve impulses involved in the withdrawal reflex that occurs when one pricks a finger on a sharp pin. Name each element in the reflex arc and state its function.

Neurons and Conduction of Impulses

Neurons

Neurons, or nerve cells, are highly specialized, nonmitotic cells that conduct impulses throughout the central nervous system (CNS) and the peripheral nervous system. They require glucose and oxygen for metabolism. There are many variations in the specific structural characteristics of each neuron, depending on its function. The cell body has a variable number of processes, or extensions, depending on the type of neuron involved. These processes make up nerves and tracts. The dendrite is the receptor site, which conducts impulses toward the cell body. The cell body contains the nucleus. The axon conducts impulses away from the cell body toward an effector site or connecting neuron, where it can release neurotransmitter chemicals at its terminal point.

Many nerve fibers are covered by a myelin sheath, which insulates the fiber and speeds up the rate of conduction. The myelin sheath, which wraps many layers of its plasma membrane around the axon, is formed by Schwann cells in the peripheral nervous system and by oligodendrocytes in the central nervous system. The interruptions in the myelin sheath are called the nodes of Ranvier.

The neurons are supported and protected by large numbers of *glial (neuroglial) cells*. Astroglia or astrocytes provide a link between neurons and capillaries for physical and probably metabolic support, as well

as contributing to the blood-brain barrier. Oligodendrocytes provide myelin for axons in the CNS. Microglia have phagocytic activity. Ependymal cells line the ventricles and neural tube cavity and form part of the choroid plexus. Researchers are investigating specific roles that glial cells may play in areas such as synapses and intercellular communication, as well as neuronal metabolism.

Regeneration of Neurons

Neurons cannot undergo cell division. If the cell body is damaged, the neuron dies. In the peripheral nervous system, axons may be able to regenerate if the cell body is viable. After damage to the axon occurs, the section distal to the injury degenerates because it lacks nutrients and is removed by macrophages and Schwann cells. The Schwann cells then attempt to form a new tube at the end of the remaining axon. The cell body becomes larger and synthesizes additional proteins for the growth of the replacement axon. The new growth does not always occur appropriately or make its original connections, because the surrounding tissue may interfere. Much of spinal cord research is focused on reducing damage to neurons immediately after injury and facilitating functional reconnections.

Conduction of Impulses

A stimulus increases the permeability of the neuronal membrane, allowing sodium ions to flow inside the cell, thus *depolarizing* it and generating an action potential when threshold is reached. The change to a positive electrical charge inside the membrane results in increased permeability of the adjacent area, and the impulse moves along the membrane. Recovery, or *repolarization*, occurs as potassium ions move outward; the normal permeability of the membrane is restored, and the sodium-potassium pump returns the sodium and potassium ions to their normal locations (see Fig. 2-5). In myelinated fibers, this action potential is generated only at the nodes of Ranvier, and therefore the impulse can "skip" along rapidly (saltatory conduction). Generally the larger axons conduct impulses more rapidly than smaller ones. The synapse provides the connection between two or more neurons or a neuron and an effector site. Complex "electrical circuits" exist in the nervous system, with multiple synapses on each neuron. The electrical activity of the brain can be monitored by attaching electrodes to the scalp and measuring the brain waves by means of an electroencephalogram (EEG).

APPLY YOUR KNOWLEDGE   14-1

Predict five possible points of dysfunction and explain how each might occur and the effects to be expected.

Synapses and Chemical Neurotransmitters

A chemical synapse involves the release of neurotransmitters from vesicles in the synaptic buds of the axons (Fig. 14-5). These transmitters may stimulate or inhibit the postsynaptic neuron. A typical synapse consists of the terminal axon of the presynaptic neuron, containing the vesicles with neurotransmitter (synaptic vesicles), and the receptor site on the membrane of the postsynaptic neuron. The axon and the receptor site are separated by the synaptic cleft. When the action potential reaches the axon terminal, the neurotransmitter is released from the vesicles and diffuses across the cleft to act on the receptor in the postsynaptic membrane, creating a postsynaptic potential. Receptors are specific for each neurotransmitter. Neurotransmitters are then either inactivated by specific enzymes or taken up by the presynaptic axon to prevent continued stimulation. Because there are usually many impulses from a variety of neurons arriving at one postsynaptic neuron, that neuron can process the input and then transmit the net result of the information to the next receptor site.

There are many neurotransmitters in the body; a few examples follow:

- Acetylcholine (ACh) is present at neuromuscular junctions and in the autonomic nervous system, the peripheral nervous system, and, less commonly, the CNS.
- Catecholamines, including norepinephrine, epinephrine, and dopamine, are present in the brain.
- Norepinephrine is a neurotransmitter in the sympathetic nervous system (SNS).
- Both norepinephrine and epinephrine, when released from the adrenal medulla in response to SNS stimulation, circulate in the blood and interstitial fluid, ultimately diffusing into the synaptic cleft and stimulating the appropriate receptors in the SNS.
  - Serotonin involved in mood, emotions, and sleep
  - Histamine involved in emotions, regulation of body temperature, and water balance
  - Gamma-aminobutyric acid (GABA), most common inhibitory neurotransmitter in the brain
  - Glycine, most common inhibitory neurotransmitter in the spinal cord

The roles of many neurotransmitters in mental illness and other pathologies are being studied intensively. For example, norepinephrine and dopamine are excitatory, and thus low levels may be linked to depression. The enkephalins and beta-endorphins are of interest because they can block the conduction of pain impulses in the spinal cord and brain (see Chapter 4). Many drugs have been developed that can mimic the effects of natural chemical neurotransmitters by stimulating specific receptors and promoting similar effects (see Chapter 3). Other drugs are designed to bind to certain receptors but not stimulate them. These drugs block the action of normal neurotransmitters, inhibiting the activity initiated by them. Drugs can also affect neurotransmission, by either inhibiting the enzymes that normally inactivate transmitters or interfering with the uptake of neurotransmitters into the axons for recycling.

THINK ABOUT 14-5

a. If postsynaptic membrane permeability is increased, is the neuron more easily stimulated or less excitable?

b. Explain the effect of the myelin sheath and the nodes of Ranvier on the conduction of impulses.

c. Briefly describe, in the correct sequence, the events that occur in synaptic transmission.

d. Explain how and why surface receptors on neurons are specific for certain neurotransmitters?

Autonomic Nervous System

The autonomic nervous system (ANS) incorporates the sympathetic and parasympathetic nervous systems. These systems generally have antagonistic effects, thereby providing a fine balance that aids in maintaining homeostasis in the body (Table 14-4).

The autonomic system provides motor and sensory innervation to smooth muscle, cardiac muscle, and glands. Although the individual is largely unaware of this involuntary activity, it is integrated with somatic activity by the higher brain centers. The neural pathways in the motor fibers of the autonomic system differ from somatic nerves because each involves two neurons and a ganglion. The *preganglionic* fiber is located in the brain or spinal cord (see Fig. 14-5). This axon then synapses with the second neuron in the *ganglion* outside the CNS, and the *postganglionic* fiber continues to the effector organ or tissue.

Sympathetic Nervous System

The sympathetic nervous system (SNS), or thoracolumbar nervous system, increases the general level of activity in the body, increasing cardiovascular, respiratory, and neurologic functions. The SNS is necessary for the fight-or-flight, or stress, response and is augmented by the increased secretions of the adrenal medulla in response to SNS stimuli.

The preganglionic fibers of the sympathetic nerves arise from the thoracic and the first two lumbar segments of the spinal cord. The ganglia are located in two *chains* or trunks, one on either side of the spinal cord. In the ganglia, preganglionic fibers synapse with postganglionic fibers or connecting fibers to other ganglia in the chain.

Neurotransmitters

A. Neuromuscular junction

3. Excess neurotransmitter taken up by neuron or destroyed by enzyme

Synaptic cleft

Receptor in skeletal muscle

Impulse

Nerve

Impulse

1. Vesicle releases neurotransmitter

2. Neurotransmitter stimulates receptor

Spinal cord

Acetylcholine

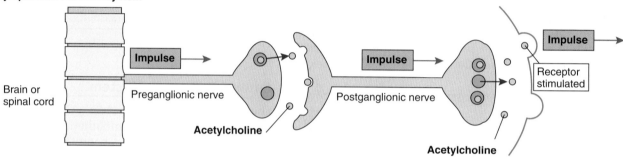

B. Parasympathetic nervous system

Brain or spinal cord

Impulse

Preganglionic nerve

Acetylcholine

Postganglionic nerve

Impulse

Receptor stimulated

Acetylcholine

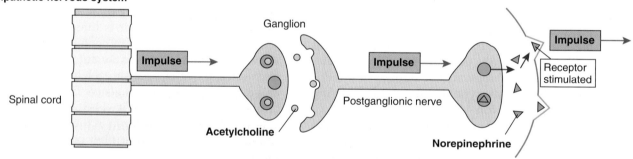

C. Sympathetic nervous system

Ganglion

Spinal cord

Impulse

Acetylcholine

Postganglionic nerve

Impulse

Receptor stimulated

Norepinephrine

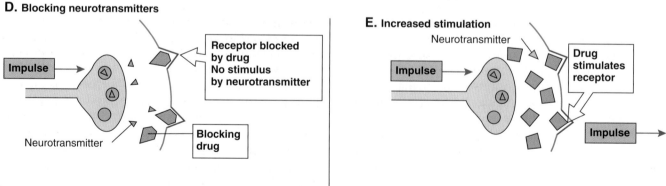

D. Blocking neurotransmitters

Impulse

Receptor blocked by drug
No stimulus by neurotransmitter

Neurotransmitter

Blocking drug

E. Increased stimulation

Neurotransmitter

Impulse

Drug stimulates receptor

Impulse

FIGURE 14-5 Neurotransmitters at the synapse.

TABLE 14-4 Effect of Stimulation of the Autonomic Nervous System

Area	SNS Receptor	Sympathetic	Parasympathetic
Cardiovascular System			
Heart blood vessels	β-1 (beta-1)	Increases rate and force of contractions	Decreases rate and contractility
Skin, mucosa, viscera	α-1 (alpha-1)	Vasoconstriction	No innervation
Skeletal muscle	β-2	Vasodilation	No innervation
Adrenal medulla		Secretion of epinephrine and norepinephrine	No innervation
Respiratory system	β-2	Bronchodilation (smooth muscle)	Bronchoconstriction
Eye	α-1	Pupil dilation (radial muscle)	Pupil constriction (sphincter or circular muscle)
Sweat glands	α-1	Increased secretion	
Digestive system	α-2		
Secretions		Decreased	Increased
Peristalsis		Decreased	Increased
Sphincters	α-1	Constricts	Relaxes
Urinary system			
Sphincters of bladder	α-1	Constricts	Relaxes
Renin	β-1	Increased secretion	
Male genitalia	α-1	Ejaculation	Erection

SNS, sympathetic nervous system.

The neurotransmitters and receptors are important in the autonomic nervous system because they are closely linked to drug actions. The neurotransmitter released by preganglionic fibers at the ganglion is acetylcholine; hence these fibers are termed *cholinergic* fibers. Most SNS postganglionic fibers release *norepinephrine*, also called *adrenaline* (*adrenergic* fibers). The postganglionic fibers to sweat glands and blood vessels in skeletal muscle are cholinergic.

Several types of *adrenergic receptors* in the tissues respond to norepinephrine and epinephrine. Norepinephrine acts primarily on *alpha* (α) receptors, and epinephrine acts on both alpha and *beta* (β) receptors. (See Table 14-4 for a summary of the major sites of the receptors and the effects of stimulation.) An organ or tissue may have more than one type of receptor, but one type is usually present in greater numbers and exerts the dominant effect. It is possible that other specific types of receptors will be discovered in the future.

Drugs may be used to stimulate these receptors or to prevent stimulation (see Fig. 14-5D,E). For example, beta₁-adrenergic receptors (sympathetic receptors) are located in the cardiac muscle. With SNS stimulation, epinephrine stimulates these receptors, resulting in an increased heart rate and force of contraction. In a patient with a damaged heart, drugs such as beta-adrenergic blocking agents (commonly called beta-blockers) may be used to block these receptors, thus preventing the stimulation and the resulting excessive heart activity. A patient may, in contrast, require a drug that can stimulate the beta receptors to improve heart function (a beta-adrenergic drug). The best drugs are specific for one type of receptor in one organ or tissue and do not alter function in other areas of the body; that is, the more specific the drug action is, the milder the adverse effects of the drug.

Parasympathetic Nervous System

The parasympathetic nervous system (PNS), or craniosacral nervous system, dominates the digestive system and aids in the recovery of the body after sympathetic activity. There are two locations of PNS preganglionic fibers—cranial nerves III, VII, IX, and X at the brain stem level and the sacral spinal nerves. The vagus nerve (cranial nerve X) provides extensive innervation to the heart and digestive tract. In the PNS, the ganglia are scattered and located close to the target organ, and the neurotransmitter at both preganglionic and postganglionic synapses is ACh.

There are two types of cholinergic receptors: nicotinic and muscarinic. Nicotinic receptors are always stimulated by ACh and are located in all postganglionic cholinergic neurons in the PNS and SNS. Muscarinic receptors are located in all effector cells and may be stimulated or inhibited by ACh, depending on the organ. Similar to the pharmacologic effects of drugs in the SNS, cholinergic blocking agents reduce PNS activity, whereas cholinergic or anticholinesterase agents (which prevent the enzyme cholinesterase from breaking down ACh) increase PNS activity.

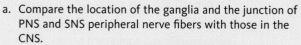

THINK ABOUT   14-6

a. Compare the location of the ganglia and the junction of PNS and SNS peripheral nerve fibers with those in the CNS.

b. Explain how the PNS and SNS affect cardiovascular activity and blood pressure.

c. List the synapses in which ACh is the neurotransmitter.

d. Which part of the autonomic nervous system promotes digestion and absorption? How does this occur?

e. Briefly describe the action and effect of a drug classified as an alpha-1 adrenergic blocking agent.

f. Briefly describe where a cholinergic drug acts and how it affects the postsynaptic receptors. Give two examples of its possible effects on function.

General Effects of Neurologic Dysfunction

The effects of neurologic damage from different causes have many similarities, because specific areas of the brain and spinal cord have established functions. Therefore damage to a certain area from a tumor or head injury, for example, can result in the same neurologic loss and signs. Also, the effects of increased pressure within the CNS are basically similar, regardless of the cause. To facilitate study and prevent repetition, these common effects are discussed in this section and are then referred to in the subsequent sections on specific disorders. Some unique variations in the effects of damage to the nervous system do occur, given the diversity of pathologic conditions and the possible combinations of effects.

Local (Focal) Effects

Local effects are signs related to the specific area of the brain or spinal cord in which the lesion is located (see Fig. 14-3). Examples include paresis or paralysis of the right arm that results from damage to a section of the left frontal lobe and loss of vision that results from damage to the occipital lobe. With an expanding lesion, such as a growing tumor or hemorrhage, additional impairment is noted as the adjacent areas become involved.

Supratentorial and Infratentorial Lesions

Supratentorial lesions occur in the cerebral hemispheres above the tentorium cerebelli. A lesion in this location leads to a specific dysfunction in a discrete area, perhaps numbness in a hand. The lesion must become very large before it affects consciousness. An infratentorial lesion is located in the brain stem, or below the tentorium. A relatively small lesion in this location may affect many motor and sensory fibers, resulting in widespread impairment, because the nerves are bundled together

when passing through the brain stem. Also, respiratory and circulatory function and the level of consciousness may be impaired by a small lesion in this area.

Left and Right Hemispheres

Certain effects of brain damage are unique to the left or right hemisphere. These occur in addition to focal effects. In most individuals, damage to the left hemisphere leads to loss of logical thinking ability, analytical skills, other intellectual abilities, and communication skills. Right-sided brain damage impairs appreciation of music and art and causes behavioral problems. Spatial orientation and recognition of relationships may be deficient, resulting in interference with mobility and "neglect" of the contralateral side of the body (which is not recognized as "self"). For a further explanation of the role of the right and left hemisphere, please consult your physiology text.

Level of Consciousness

Normally a person is totally aware of surrounding activities and incoming stimuli and oriented to time, place, and people; the person can respond quickly and appropriately to questions, commands, or events. An individual may exert various levels of attention on different aspects of the immediate environment. The cerebral cortex and the RAS in the brain stem determine the level of consciousness. Information must be processed in the association areas of the cortex before one is conscious of the information.

One of the early changes noted in those with acute brain disorders is a decreasing level of consciousness or responsiveness. Usually extensive supratentorial lesions must be present in the cerebral hemispheres to cause loss of consciousness, whereas relatively small lesions in the brain stem (infratentorial lesions) can affect the reticular activating system (RAS). Space-occupying masses in the cerebellum can also compress the brain stem and RAS. In addition to CNS lesions, many systemic disorders, such as acidosis or hypoglycemia, can depress the CNS, reducing the level of consciousness.

Various levels of reduced consciousness may present as lethargy, confusion, disorientation, memory loss, unresponsiveness to verbal stimuli, or difficulty in arousal. Standard categories, in tools such as the *Glasgow Coma Scale*, provide consistency in the medical assessment (Table 14-5). The most serious level is loss of consciousness or coma, in which the affected person does not respond to painful or verbal stimuli and the body is motionless, although some reflexes are present. The terminal stage, deep coma, is marked by a loss of all reflexes, fixed and dilated pupils, and slow and irregular pulse and respirations.

A *vegetative state* is a loss of awareness and mental capabilities, resulting from diffuse brain damage,

TABLE 14-5 Glasgow Coma Scale and Use in Assessment

Criteria	Maximum	Example—0700Hours	Example—0900Hours	Example—1100Hours
Eye opening				
Spontaneous	4			
Response to speech	3	×	×	
Response to pain	2			
None	1			×
Motor response				
Obeys commands	6	×		
Localizes pain	5		×	
Normal flexion (to pain)	4			
Abnormal flexion (decorticate)	3			
Abnormal extension (decerebrate)	2			
None (flaccid)	2			×
Verbal response				
Oriented to time and place	5			
Confused	4	×		
Inappropriate words	3		×	
Incomprehensible	2			
None	1			×
Score	15 (good, normal)	13	11	4

although brain stem function continues, supporting respiratory, cardiovascular, and autonomic functions. There appears to be a sleep-wake cycle (eyes are open or closed), but the person is unresponsive to external stimuli. Some individuals may in time recover consciousness but often survive with significant neurologic impairment.

Locked-in syndrome refers to a condition in which an individual with brain damage is aware and capable of thinking but is paralyzed and cannot communicate. Some individuals can move their eyes in a "yes" or "no" response.

A diagnosis of *brain death* is often required to terminate medical intervention, because individuals can be maintained artificially on cardiopulmonary support systems. The criteria for brain death include:
- Cessation of brain function, including function of the cortex and the brain stem (e.g., a flat or inactive EEG)
- Absence of brain stem reflexes or responses
- Absence of spontaneous respirations when ventilator assistance is withdrawn
- Establishment of the certainty of irreversible brain damage by confirmation of the cause of the dysfunction

Drug overdose or hypothermia can cause loss of brain activity temporarily; thus, a longer time period and additional testing are required before brain death can be confirmed in these cases.

Motor Dysfunction

Damage to the upper motor neurons in the posterior zone of the frontal lobe of cerebral cortex or to the corticospinal tracts in the brain interferes with voluntary movements, causing weakness or paralysis on the opposite (contralateral) side of the body. This contralateral effect is determined by the crossover of the corticospinal tracts in the medulla. The area affected, such as a leg or arm, depends on the specific site of damage. Muscle tone and reflexes may be increased (hyperreflexia) because the intact spinal cord continues to conduct impulses with no moderating or inhibiting influences sent from the brain (spastic paralysis). This frequently leads to immobility resulting in contractures in the affected limbs.

Damage to the lower motor neurons in the anterior horns of the spinal cord causes weakness or paralysis on the same side of the body, at and below the level of damage. In the area of damage, the muscles are usually flaccid (absence of tone), and reflexes are absent (flaccid paralysis). If the cord distal to the damage is intact, some reflexes in that area may be present and hyperactive (hyperreflexia). Lower motor neurons are also located in the nuclei of *cranial nerves* in the brain stem, and similarly, ipsilateral weakness or flaccid paralysis may result from damage to any cranial nerves containing motor fibers (see Table 14-3).

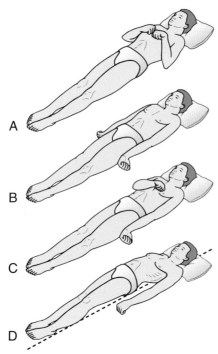

FIGURE 14-6 Decorticate and Decerebrate Posturing A, Decorticate response. Flexion of arms, wrists, and fingers with adduction in upper extremities. Extension, internal rotation, and plantar flexion in lower extremities. **B**, Decerebrate response. All four extremities in rigid extension, with hyperpronation of forearms and plantar flexion of feet. **C**, Decorticate response on right side of body and decerebrate response on left side of body. **D**, Opisthotonic posturing. *(From Lewis SM, Heitkemper MM, Dirksen SR: Medical-Surgical Nursing, ed 6, St. Louis, 2004, Mosby).*

Two involuntary motor responses that occur in persons with severe brain trauma include *decorticate* and *decerebrate* posturing (Fig. 14-6). Decorticate responses include rigid flexion in the upper limbs, with adducted arms and internal rotation of the hands; the lower limbs are extended. This response may occur in persons with severe damage in the cerebral hemispheres. Decerebrate responses occur in persons with brain stem lesions and CNS depression caused by systemic effects. Both the upper and lower limbs are extended, as is the head, and the body is arched.

Sensory Deficits

Sensory loss may involve touch, pain, temperature, and position and the special senses of vision, hearing, taste, and smell. The somatosensory cortex in the parietal lobe (see Fig. 14-3), which receives and localizes basic sensory input from the body, is mapped to correspond to receptors in the skin and skeletal muscles of various body regions. The specific site of damage determines the deficit. Mapping of the dermatomes (see Fig. 14-22) assists in the evaluation of spinal cord lesions. Damage to the cranial nerves or their nuclei or to the assigned area of the brain may interfere with vision or other special senses.

Visual Loss: Hemianopia

Because of the unique anatomy of the visual pathway, loss of the visual field depends on the site of damage in the visual pathway (Fig. 14-7). (See Chapter 15 for review of the structure of the eye.) At the optic chiasm, the fibers in each optic nerve come together and then divide. If the optic chiasm is totally destroyed, vision is lost in both eyes. Partial loss can result in a variety of effects, depending on the particular fibers damaged. Fibers from the medial (inner) half of each retina (cells receive visual stimuli) cross over to the other hemisphere, whereas fibers from the lateral or outer half of the retina remain on the same side. Thus, the optic tract coursing from the optic chiasm to the occipital lobe on one side includes fibers from half of each eye. If the optic tract or occipital lobe is damaged, vision is lost from the medial half of one eye and the lateral half of the other eye; this is called *homonymous hemianopia*. The overall effect is loss of the visual field on the side opposite to that of the damage. In other words, damage to the left occipital lobe means loss of the right visual field because the left half of both retinas receives light waves from the right side of the visual field. If you were caring for this patient, it would be best to stand on the patient's left side.

Other types of visual loss may occur depending on the point of damage in the visual pathway. Partial loss of vision may lead to inability to coordinate input from right and left visual fields. This may lead to diplopia or double vision as well as loss of depth perception and hand to eye coordination.

Language Disorders

Aphasia refers to an inability to comprehend or to express language. There are many types of aphasia; the main types are expressive, receptive, and global (Table 14-6). Variations and combinations may occur in individual cases. Dysphasia refers to partial impairment, which is more common, but the term *aphasia* is frequently used to refer to both partial and total loss of communicating ability.
- *Expressive*, or *motor*, *aphasia* results in an impaired ability to speak or write fluently or appropriately. Such a person may be unable to find any intelligible words or construct a meaningful sentence. This type of aphasia occurs when Broca's area in the dominant (usually the left lobe) frontal lobe, inferior motor cortex, is damaged (see Fig. 14-3).
- *Receptive*, or *sensory*, *aphasia* is an inability to read or understand the spoken word. This category does not include hearing or visual impairment. The source of the problem is the inability to process information in

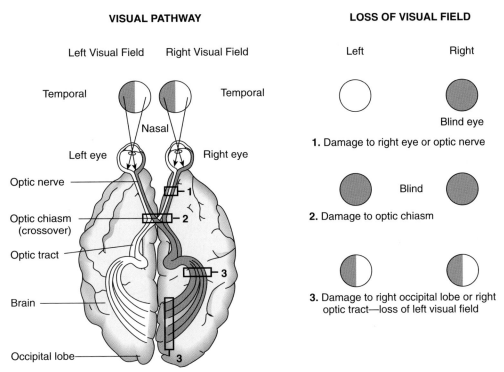

FIGURE 14-7 The visual pathway.

TABLE 14-6	Aphasia	
Type	Site of Damage	Effect
Expressive (motor)	Broca's area Left frontal lobe	Cannot speak or write fluently or appropriately
Receptive (sensory)	Wernicke's area Left temporal lobe, prefrontal	Unable to understand written or spoken language
Global	Broca's and Wernicke's areas and connecting fibers	Cannot express self or comprehend others' language

the brain. The individual may be capable of fluent speech, but frequently it is meaningless. Damage to Wernicke's area in the left temporal lobe results in receptive aphasia.

- *Global aphasia* commonly describes a combination of expressive and receptive aphasia that results from major damage to the brain, including Broca's area, Wernicke's area, and many communicating fibers throughout the brain.

Aphasia may also be described as *fluent* or *nonfluent*; in fluent aphasia the pace of speech is relatively normal but contains made-up words and sentences that do not make sense. Fluent aphasia is associated with damage to Wernicke's area. Nonfluent aphasia is slow and labored speech with short phrases; often small words are omitted. It is associated with damage to Broca's area.

Other types of language disorders include the following:

- *Dysarthria*, in which words cannot be articulated clearly, is a motor dysfunction that usually results from cranial nerve damage or muscle impairment.
- *Agraphia* is impaired writing ability.
- *Alexia* is impaired reading ability.
- *Agnosia* is loss of recognition or association. For example, visual agnosia indicates an inability to recognize objects.

Thorough testing is required before a specific diagnosis can be made of any of these disorders.

THINK ABOUT 14-7

a. Compare normal function and coma, using two characteristics of these levels of consciousness.
b. Describe two possible areas of CNS damage that might cause flaccid paralysis.
c. Describe the effects on motor function of damage to the lateral surface of the frontal lobe.
d. Describe the characteristics of expressive aphasia, and state the usual location of the damage.

Seizures

Seizures or convulsions are caused by spontaneous excessive discharge of neurons in the brain. This state may be precipitated by inflammation, hypoxia, or bleeding in the brain. Often the seizure is focal or is related to the particular site of the irritation, but it may become generalized. Frequently the seizure is manifested by involuntary repetitive movements or abnormal sensations.

Increased Intracranial Pressure

The skull contains brain tissue, blood, and CSF. The volume of each of these normally remains relatively constant, thus maintaining a normal pressure inside the cranial cavity. Temporary fluctuations in blood flow and blood pressure may occur with activities such as coughing or bending over. The fluids, blood and CSF, are not compressible. Because the brain is encased in the rigid, nonexpandable skull, any increase in fluid, such as blood or inflammatory exudate, or any additional mass, such as a tumor, causes an increase in pressure in the brain. The result is that less arterial blood can enter the "high pressure" area in the brain, and eventually the brain tissue itself is compressed. Both of these effects decrease the function of the neurons, both locally and generally. Eventually brain tissue dies. The pressure increases at the site of the problem initially but gradually is dispersed throughout the CNS by means of the continuous flow of CSF and blood, leading to widespread loss of function. Changes in intracranial pressure (ICP) can be monitored directly by instruments placed in the ventricles (an invasive procedure) or indirectly by methods such as radiologic examinations or assessment of the level of consciousness and vital signs.

Increased ICP is common in many neurologic problems, including brain hemorrhage, trauma, cerebral edema, infection, tumors, or accumulation of excessive amounts of CSF (Fig. 14-8). All of these problems create the same general set of manifestations, which are summarized in Table 14-7.

Early Signs

When ICP increases, the body initially attempts to compensate for it by shifting more CSF to the spinal cavity, for example, and increasing venous return from the brain. These compensation mechanisms are effective for only a short time. The resulting hypoxia triggers arterial vasodilation in the brain through local autoregulatory reflexes, in an attempt to improve the blood supply to the brain. However, this adds to the fluid volume inside the skull and is also effective for only a short time. Because of these compensatory mechanisms, ICP is often significantly elevated before signs become apparent.

If the cause of the increased pressure has not been removed, the *first* indication of increased ICP is usually a *decreasing level of consciousness* or decreased responsiveness (lethargy). Additional early indications of increased ICP include the following:

- *Severe headache* occurs from stretching of the dura and walls of large blood vessels.

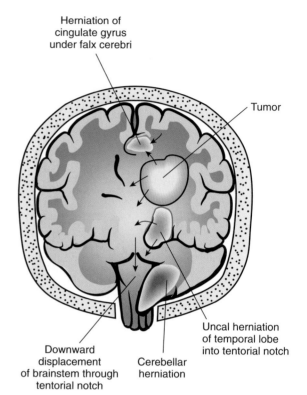

FIGURE 14-8 Increased intracranial pressure and possible herniations.

TABLE 14-7	Effects of Increased Intracranial Pressure
General Signs	**Rationale**
Decreasing level of consciousness	Pressure on RAS (brain stem) or cerebral cortex
Headache	Stretching or distortion of meninges or walls of large blood vessels
Vomiting	Pressure on emetic center in medulla
Vital Signs	
Increasing blood pressure with increasing pulse pressure	Cushing's reflex; response to cerebral ischemia causes systemic vasoconstriction
Slow heart rate	Response to increasing blood pressure
Signs Affecting Vision	
Papilledema	Increased pressure of CSF causes swelling around the optic disc
Pupil, fixed and dilated	Pressure on cranial nerve III (oculomotor)

CSF, cerebrospinal fluid; RAS, reticular activating system.

- *Vomiting*—often projectile vomiting that is not associated with food intake—is the result of pressure stimulating the emetic center in the medulla.
- *Papilledema* may be present, caused by increased ICP and swelling of the optic disc (Fig. 14-9).

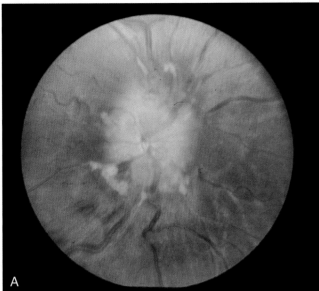

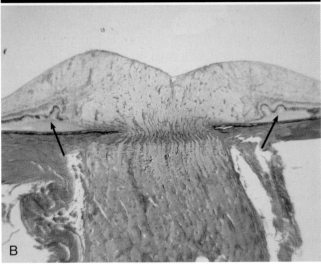

FIGURE 14-9 **A,** Papilledema. **B,** Papilledema showing displacement and folding of the retina (*arrows*) as well as edema and congestion of the optic nerve head. (*A, Courtesy John W. Payne, MD, The Wilmer Ophthalmological Institute, The Johns Hopkins University and Hospital, Baltimore, MD, from Seidel HM, Ball JW, Dains JE, et al: Mosby's Guide to Physical Examination, ed 5, St. Louis, 2003, Mosby; B, From Cotran RS, Kumar V, Collins T: Robbins Pathologic Basis of Disease, ed 6, Philadelphia, 1999, Saunders.*)

Papilledema can be observed by looking through the pupil of the eye at the retina, where the optic disc provides a "window" into the brain (see Fig. 15-1). The optic nerve (cranial nerve II) is essentially a projection of brain tissue that is surrounded by CSF and meninges and enters the eye at the optic disc, where it reflects the effects of increased ICP in the brain. These early manifestations continue to increase in severity as long as ICP continues to rise.

Vital Signs

If ICP continues to build, a sequence of events occurs in an effort to supply critical oxygen to the brain, as follows:

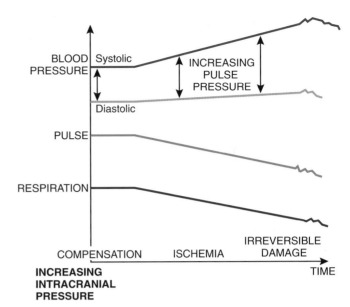

FIGURE 14-10 Vital signs with increased intracranial pressure.

1. Cerebral ischemia develops, which stimulates a powerful response (Cushing's reflex) from the vasomotor centers in an attempt to increase the arterial blood supply to the brain.
2. Systemic vasoconstriction occurs to increase systemic blood pressure and force more blood into the brain to relieve the ischemia.
3. Baroreceptors in the carotid arteries respond to the increased blood pressure by slowing the heart rate.
4. Chemoreceptors respond to the low carbon dioxide levels that accompany the accelerated systemic circulation by reducing the respiratory rate.
5. As improved cerebral circulation relieves ischemia, the reflex vasoconstriction momentarily ceases. However, the increasing ICP causes ischemia to recur in a very short time, and the cycle is repeated.

In other words, the brain responds to ischemia by one mechanism, whereas feedback control for blood pressure uses other mechanisms to protect the rest of the body, resulting in a conflict of interests.

As ICP continues to rise, so does systemic blood pressure (Fig. 14-10). An increasing *pulse pressure* (the difference between systolic and diastolic pressures) is significant in people with ICP. The widening gap in pulse pressure results from the slow heart rate and the intermittent but rapid on-off cycle of Cushing's reflex controlling systemic vasoconstriction.

Eventually severe ischemia and neuronal death prevent any circulatory control, and the blood pressure drops. Pressure and ischemia also destroy respiratory controls. Various abnormal respiratory patterns develop, such as Cheyne-Stokes respirations, with alternating apnea and periods of increasing and decreasing respirations, depending on the site of the lesion (see Fig. 13-7).

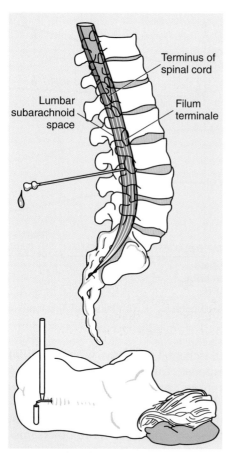

FIGURE 14-11 **Lumbar Puncture** Cerebrospinal fluid is obtained by inserting a needle into the subarachnoid space in the lumbar region. *(From Mahon CR, Manuselis G: Textbook of Diagnostic Microbiology, ed 2, Philadelphia, 2000, Saunders.)*

Visual Signs

In addition to papilledema and specific reflex changes, several other significant indicators of increasing ICP are seen in the eyes. Pressure on the oculomotor nerve (cranial nerve III) affects the size and response of the pupils. Usually one pupil ipsilateral to the lesion becomes fixed (unresponsive to light) and dilated as the PNS fibers in the affected oculomotor nerve become nonfunctional. With an additional pressure increase, both pupils become fixed and dilated ("blown").

Other signs of increased ICP may include ptosis, or "droopy eyelid," which is another effect of pressure on cranial nerve III because innervation to the muscle of the upper eyelid is impaired, and abnormal or excessive eye movements, such as nystagmus.

Changes in Cerebrospinal Fluid

A specimen may be procured with a lumbar puncture by inserting a fine needle between the vertebrae at L3-4, into the subarachnoid space, and withdrawing a small sample of CSF (Fig. 14-11). A manometer may be attached to the syringe to measure pressure. The pressure of CSF is elevated (above 20 mmHg) in patients with increased ICP.

The composition of the fluid may vary with the cause of the problem (see Table 14-1). The CSF may be pinkish in color and contain erythrocytes, suggesting hemorrhage. A cloudy, yellowish fluid that contains numerous WBCs may indicate infection, whereas abnormal protein levels in the CSF may indicate a neoplasm.

Herniation

When a mass, such as a blood clot or tumor, becomes large enough, it may displace brain tissue, leading to herniation. There are several different types of herniation (see Fig. 14-8). In transtentorial (central) herniation, the cerebral hemispheres, diencephalon, and midbrain are displaced downward. The resulting pressure affects the flow of blood and CSF, the RAS, and respiration. Uncal (uncinate) herniation occurs when the uncus of the temporal lobe is displaced downward past the tentorium cerebelli, creating pressure on the third cranial nerve, the posterior cerebral artery, and the RAS. Cerebellar, or tonsillar (infratentorial), herniation develops when the cerebellar tonsils are pushed downward through the foramen magnum, which compresses the brain stem and vital centers and causes death.

THINK ABOUT 14-8

a. List the early signs of increased ICP.
b. Explain why headache occurs with an increase in ICP.
c. Describe the usual changes in vital signs that result from increased ICP in early and later stages.
d. Explain why a lesion in the brain stem is more critical than one in the cerebral hemisphere.

Diagnostic Tests

Computed tomographic (CT) scans, magnetic resonance imaging (MRI), cerebral angiography, Doppler ultrasound (for assessing patency of the carotid and intracerebral vessels), and EEG provide useful information. A radionuclide such as technetium may be added to track perfusion in CNS. Lumbar puncture is used to check pressure and analyze the CSF for altered components.

Clinical assessment routinely includes tools such as the assessment of normal reflexes and the Glasgow coma scale to assess the level of consciousness.

Acute Neurologic Problems

Neurologic disorders have been divided into acute problems and chronic problems. Although some overlap occurs, there are major differences in onset, course, and management of the two groups.

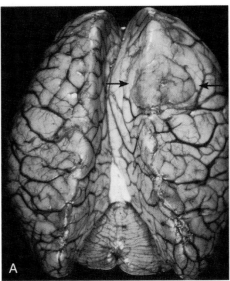
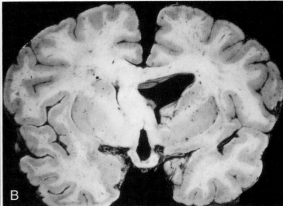

FIGURE 14-12 **Brain Tumor A**, Astrocytoma in right frontal lobe has expanded the gyri (arrows indicate flattening). **B**, Expanded white area in left hemisphere distorts brain structures. *(From Kumar V, Abbas AK, Fausto M: Robbins and Cotran Pathologic Basis of Disease, ed 7, Philadelphia, 2005, Saunders.)*

Brain Tumors

Tumors serve as a good example of space-occupying lesions that cause increased ICP because of space constraints within the rigid skull, and localized dysfunction related to their location. Therefore benign tumors as well as malignant tumors can be life threatening, unless they are in an accessible superficial location where they can be removed. Gliomas form the largest category of primary malignant tumors. They arise from one of the glial cells, the parenchymal cells in the CNS (see Fig. 20-13 for CT scan of a brain tumor). This group of tumors is further classified according to the cell of derivation (e.g., astrocytomas are the most common) and the location of the tumor. In addition, tumors may develop in the meninges (meningioma) or pituitary gland (adenoma, see Chapter 16), causing similar neurologic effects that result from pressure on the brain. Primary malignant tumors rarely metastasize outside the CNS, but multiple tumors may be present within the CNS. Secondary brain tumors are quite common, usually metastasizing from breast or lung tumors, and they cause effects similar to those of primary brain tumors.

The combined incidence rate for brain cancer in children and adults is 22,000 in 2008 with 13,000 deaths. Case fatality rates with this cancer are relatively high. Brain cancer is responsible for greater than 2% of cancer deaths. Diagnosis is made by MRI, with a stereotactic biopsy providing confirmation.

■ *Pathophysiology*

Primary malignant brain tumors, particularly astrocytomas, do not usually have well-defined margins but are invasive and have irregular projections into adjacent tissue that are difficult to totally remove (see Fig. 14-12). There is usually an area of inflammation around the tumor, adding to the pressure. In some cases, obstruction of the flow of CSF or of the venous sinuses increases ICP. As the mass expands, it compresses and distorts the tissue around it, eventually resulting in herniation. A relatively small tumor in the brain stem or cerebellum can compress the medulla within a short time. However, tumors in the cerebral hemispheres, particularly in "silent" areas (without obvious function), may grow quite large before their effects are noticeable.

■ *Etiology*

Brain stem and cerebellar tumors are common in young children, and research into the cause of these tumors continues, particularly with regard to prenatal parental exposure to carcinogens and embryonic development. Tumors occur in adults most often in mid-life. Adults are affected more frequently by tumors in the cerebral hemispheres; predisposing factors have not been established.

■ *Signs and Symptoms*

The specific site of the tumor determines the focal signs. If the tumor grows rapidly, signs of increased ICP develop quickly, often beginning with morning headaches. Over time, these headaches increase in severity and frequency. Vomiting occurs. Lethargy and irritability may develop, along with personality and behavioral changes. In some cases, focal or generalized seizures are the first sign, as the tumor irritates the surrounding tissue. Brain stem or cerebellar tumors may affect several cranial nerves, possibly causing unilateral facial paralysis or visual problems. Unlike other forms of cancer, brain tumors do not cause the usual systemic signs of malignancy because they do not metastasize outside the CNS, and they will cause death before they are large enough to cause general effects.

Pituitary adenomas in the brain usually cause endocrinologic signs, depending on the type of excess secretion (see Chapter 16). Headaches and visual signs may result from increased ICP, and compression of the adjacent optic chiasm, nerves, or tracts, resulting in visual disturbances, is common.

■ Treatment

Surgery is the treatment of choice, if the tumor is reasonably accessible. Chemotherapy is often accompanied by radiation, and the prognosis for many types of tumors is improving as new drugs are developed. Some targeted drugs are being used to reduce blood flow to the tumor. It continues to be difficult to deliver drugs to CNS tumors because of the blood-brain barrier. In some cases, surgery and radiation may cause substantial damage to normal tissue in the CNS.

THINK ABOUT 14-9

a. Explain the specific signs of dysfunction that would be expected in a young child with a cerebellar tumor.

b. Choose a possible tumor site in one cerebral hemisphere and list the signs (focal and general) that would be expected as the tumor grows.

c. Explain why a tumor in the cerebral hemisphere may grow quite large before any signs appear, but a brain stem tumor causes signs in the early stages.

d. Explain why the general signs of cancer, such as weight loss and anemia, do not develop with brain tumors.

e. Explain why the brain is a common site of metastatic cancer from the lung.

Vascular Disorders

Vascular disorders may be hemorrhagic or ischemic in origin. Interference with blood supply to a specific area of the brain results in local damage and manifestations depending on the particular cerebral artery involved. If the deficit results from hemorrhage, the additional effects of increased intracranial pressure will cause local ischemia and generalized symptoms. Global cerebral ischemia, which may develop secondary to severe shock or cardiac arrest, occurs when impaired perfusion of the entire brain results in loss of function and generalized cerebral edema. In mild cases, confusion and neurologic dysfunction develop temporarily, followed by recovery with no permanent damage. If severe or prolonged ischemia occurs, significant diffuse necrosis or infarction

results in deep coma. If death does not result, a vegetative state may ensue.

Transient Ischemic Attacks

A transient ischemic attack (TIA) results from a temporary localized reduction of blood flow in the brain. Recovery occurs within 24 hours. Transient ischemic attacks may occur singly or in a series.

■ Pathophysiology

A TIA may be caused by partial occlusion of an artery, caused by atherosclerosis, or from a small embolus, a vascular spasm, or local loss of autoregulation. Transient ischemic attacks are advantageous if they serve as a warning and lead to early diagnosis and treatment of a problem before the occurrence of a cerebrovascular accident (CVA, or stroke). The brain must have a constant source of glucose and oxygen or suffer permanent damage. Not all strokes are preceded by TIAs.

■ Signs and Symptoms

The manifestations of TIA are directly related to the location of the ischemia. The patient remains conscious. Intermittent short episodes of impaired function, such as muscle weakness in an arm or leg, visual disturbances, or numbness and paresthesia in the face, may occur. Transient aphasia or confusion may develop. The attack may last a few minutes or longer but rarely lasts more than 1 to 2 hours, and then the signs disappear. Repeated attacks are frequently a warning of the development of obstruction related to atherosclerosis.

Such attacks should be investigated immediately and treatment instituted, depending on the cause, to prevent permanent brain damage.

Cerebrovascular Accidents (Stroke)

It is estimated that in United States, someone has a stroke every 45 seconds. Of the approximate 700,000 strokes experienced annually, about 500,000 are first strokes and 200,000 are recurrent attacks. Cerebrovascular accidents (CVAs) account for more than 1 out of 15 deaths (about 160,000 per year). Incidence increases with age, most occurring in people who are over 65 years old. Strokes are considered a major cause of disability.

■ Pathophysiology

A CVA (stroke) is an infarction of brain tissue that results from lack of blood. Tissue necrosis may be an outcome of total occlusion of a cerebral blood vessel by atheroma or embolus, which causes ischemia, or may be the consequence of a ruptured cerebral vessel, which causes hemorrhage and increased intracranial pressure (see Fig. 14-13). Five minutes (or less) of ischemia causes irreversible nerve cell damage. A central area of necrosis develops, surrounded by an area of inflammation, and

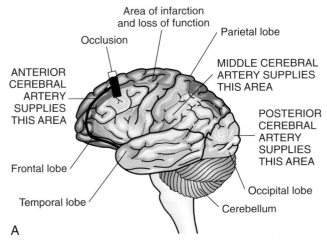

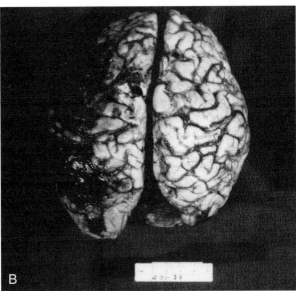

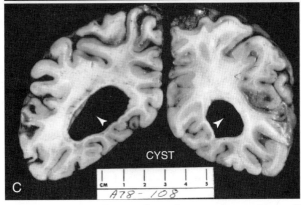

FIGURE 14-13 **A**, Effects of cerebrovascular accident (CVA). **B**, External superior surface of the brain showing acute hemorrhagic infarction. Note blood vessels on surface of brain. **C**, Cut surface of brain showing cyst from healed infarction. *(Courtesy of R.W. Shaw, MD, North York General Hospital, Toronto, Ontario, Canada.)*

function in this area is lost immediately. The tissue liquefies, leaving a cavity in the brain.

The development and effects of a stroke vary with the cause. There are three common categories (Table 14-8), described as follows:

- Occlusion of an artery by an atheroma is the most common cause of CVA. (*Atherosclerosis* is discussed in Chapter 12.) Atheromas often develop in the large arteries, such as the carotid arteries. This condition causes gradual narrowing of the arterial lumen by plaque and thrombus, leading to possible TIAs and eventually infarction.

- A sudden obstruction caused by an *embolus* lodging in a cerebral artery is the second type of stroke. Thrombi may break off of an atheroma, or mural thrombi may form inside the heart after a myocardial infarction and then break away. Emboli can also result from other materials, such as tumors, air, or infection (e.g., endocarditis).

- Intracerebral *hemorrhage*, usually caused by rupture of a cerebral artery in a patient with severe hypertension (see Chapter 12), is the third class of stroke. Hemorrhagic strokes are frequently more severe and destructive than other CVAs, because they affect large portions of the brain (see Fig. 14-13*B*). Because of the greater increase in ICP with hemorrhage, the effects are evident in both hemispheres and are complicated by the secondary effects of bleeding, in addition to the disrupted blood supply. The presence of free blood in interstitial areas affects the cell membranes and can lead to significant secondary damage as vasospasm, electrolyte imbalances, acidosis, and cellular edema develop.

An MRI can determine the cause of the stroke or illustrate other possible causes of the dysfunction.

Cerebral edema and an increasing area of infarction in the first 48 to 72 hours tend to increase the neurologic deficits. As the inflammation subsides, neurologic function increases. The inflammation and pressure in the brain must be minimized as quickly as possible and therapy instituted to dissolve thrombi and maintain adequate perfusion to limit the area of permanent damage. Collateral circulation may have already developed in areas gradually affected by atherosclerosis (see Chapter 12). Because neurons do not regenerate, an area of residual scar tissue and often cysts remains, with a permanent loss of neurons in that area (see Fig. 14-13*C*). In many cases, because specific functions result from integrated output from many areas, it is possible with intensive therapy for a person who has experienced a stroke to develop new neural pathways in the brain or to relearn a task, thus recovering some lost function.

Complications are common. These include recurrent CVA; secondary problems related to immobility such as pneumonia, aspiration, and constipation; or contractures related to paralysis.

TABLE 14-8	**Types of Cerebrovascular Accidents**		
	Thrombus	Embolus	Hemorrhage
Predisposing condition	Atherosclerosis in cerebral artery	Atherosclerosis (carotid artery) or systemic source (e.g., heart)	Hypertension—arteriosclerosis
Onset	Gradual—may be preceded by transient ischemic attacks Often occurs often at rest	Sudden	Sudden—often occurs with activity
Increased ICP	Minimal	Minimal	Present; often high
Effects	Localized—may be less permanent damage if collateral circulation has been established	Localized unless multiple emboli are present	Widespread and severe—often fatal

■ *Etiology*

Risk factors for stroke include diabetes, hypertension, systemic lupus erythematosus, elevated cholesterol levels, hyperlipidemia, atherosclerosis, a history of TIAs, increasing age, obstructive sleep apnea, and heart disease. The risk factors for atherosclerosis (see Chapter 12) apply similarly to CVA. The combination of oral contraceptives and cigarette smoking has been well documented as an etiologic factor. Emboli may arise from atheromas in the large arteries, such as the carotids, or from cardiac disorders of the left ventricle, such as acute myocardial infarction, atrial fibrillation, or endocarditis or from an implant such as a prosthetic valve. Severe or long-term hypertension and arteriosclerosis in the elderly increase the risk of intracerebral hemorrhage.

> **WARNING SIGNS OF STROKE (CVA, OR BRAIN ATTACK)**
>
> 1. Sudden transient weakness, numbness, or tingling in the face, an arm or leg, or on one side of the body
> 2. Temporary loss of speech, failure to comprehend, or confusion
> 3. Sudden loss of vision
> 4. Sudden severe headache
> 5. Unusual dizziness or unsteadiness
>   Immediate medical treatment may prevent permanent brain damage.

■ *Signs and Symptoms*

The National Institutes of Health has developed a diagnostic *stroke scale* that is designed to assist with rapid diagnosis of a cerebral vascular accident in an emergency situation. The stroke scale includes commands to determine capacity for speech, level of consciousness, motor abilities, and assessment of eye movements. The scale also identifies areas of damage based on resulting dysfunction.

Signs and symptoms depend on the location of the obstruction, the size of the artery involved, and the functional area affected (see Figs. 14-13*A* and 14-3). The presence of collateral circulation may diminish the size of the affected area. There are "silent" areas of the brain,

in which dysfunction resulting from small infarctions is not obvious. Obstruction of small arteries may not lead to obvious signs until several small infarctions have occurred. In some cases, the effects of a stroke develop slowly over a period of hours (termed *evolving stroke*).

Initially flaccid paralysis is present; spastic paralysis develops several weeks later, as the nervous system recovers from the initial insult. Generally the functional deficits increase during the first 48 hours as inflammation develops at the site and then subside as some neurons around the infarcted area recover.

Occlusion of large arteries, such as the internal carotid artery or the middle cerebral artery, or a hemorrhage may cause severe, widespread effects, including coma, loss of consciousness, or death, almost immediately. Hemorrhagic strokes usually begin suddenly with a blinding headache and increasingly severe neurologic deficits.

Specific local signs depend on the area affected. For example, occlusion of an anterior cerebral artery affects the frontal lobe. Common signs include contralateral muscle weakness or paralysis, sensory loss in the leg, confusion, loss of problem-solving skills, and personality changes.

The middle cerebral artery supplies a large portion of the cerebral hemisphere; therefore, lack of blood supply to this artery leads to contralateral paralysis and sensory loss, primarily of the upper body and arm. Aphasia occurs when the dominant hemisphere of the brain is affected, whereas spatial relationships may be more severely impaired if the right side is damaged.

Because the posterior cerebral artery supplies the occipital lobe, visual loss is likely if it is occluded.

> **EMERGENCY FIRST AID FOR STROKE (CVA, OR BRAIN ATTACK)**
>
> 1. Call 911 immediately and state the person has the symptoms of a stroke.
> 2. The patient should be transported to hospital as quickly as possible with a record of common drugs used and medical conditions being treated.
> 3. Time between onset of the stroke and treatment is directly related to the severity of the damage to the brain. Minutes count!

■ *Treatment*

Rapid treatment with "clot-busting agents," such as tissue plasminogen activator (tPA) (see Chapter 12), has reduced the effects of CVA in some individuals, but initial screening to rule out hemorrhage or other contraindications for anticoagulant drugs is essential. Surgical intervention may be possible to relieve carotid artery obstruction.

Glucocorticoids may reduce cerebral edema. Supportive treatment to maximize cerebral circulation and oxygen supply is usually initiated. Assisting the patient's return to a sitting or standing position as soon as the vital signs are stable helps to maintain muscle tone and minimize perceptual deficits.

A team approach to care, including occupational and physical therapists and speech-language pathologists, encourages recovery and minimizes complications in patients in whom many basic functions are impaired. Speech, mobility, swallowing, and other functions may be affected in one individual. Correct positioning, frequent changes of position, and passive exercises to prevent muscle atrophy, contractures, and skin breakdown are required (see Chapter 25).

Rehabilitation programs should be instituted as soon as possible.

The underlying problem (hypertension, atherosclerosis, or thrombus) requires treatment to prevent recurrences. The prognosis varies considerably, depending on the underlying causative factors, the artery affected, and the general health status of the individual.

Approximately 20% of stroke patients die within the first few days. Complete recovery is rare. However, the sooner improvement and rehabilitation therapy begin, the more optimistic the prognosis can be. Newer therapies such as constraint induced therapy, which stimulates the use of the weaker side of the body, can be effective many years after the occurrence of a CVA. Ongoing assessment and rehabilitation are of value to any client who has experienced a CVA.

Cerebral Aneurysms
■ *Pathophysiology*

An aneurysm is a localized dilation in an artery. Cerebral aneurysms are frequently multiple and usually occur at the points of bifurcation on the circle of Willis (Fig. 14-14). These "berry" aneurysms develop where

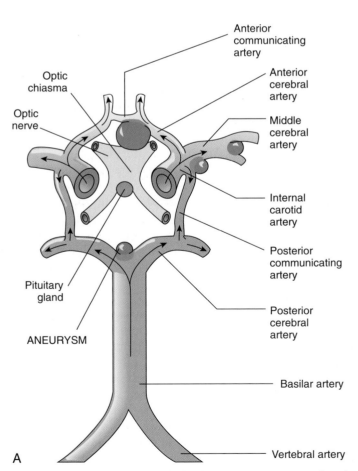
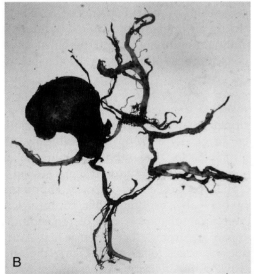

FIGURE 14-14 **A,** Cerebral aneurysm. **B,** Dissected circle of Willis showing a large cerebral aneurysm. *(From Kumar V, Abbas AK, Fausto M: Robbins and Cotran Pathologic Basis of Disease, ed 7, Philadelphia, 2005, Saunders.)*

there is a weakness in the arterial wall where branching occurs. The force of blood at this point leads to bulging in the wall, which is often aggravated by hypertension. Initially the aneurysms are small and *asymptomatic*, but they tend to enlarge over years, until compression of the nearby structures (e.g., a cranial nerve) causes clinical signs or rupture occurs.

Rupture often results from a sudden increase in blood pressure during exertion, and bleeding occurs into the subarachnoid space (the location of the circle of Willis) and the CSF. This rupture may be a small leak or a massive tear. Blood is irritating to the meninges and causes an inflammatory response and irritation of the nerve roots passing through the meninges. This free blood also causes *vasospasm* in the cerebral arteries, further reducing perfusion and leading to additional ischemia. Hemorrhage from the ruptured vessel causes increased ICP and its associated signs. No focal signs are present because the additional blood is dispersed through the system. Subarachnoid hemorrhages may be classified according to their clinical effects.

■ Signs and Symptoms

The enlarging aneurysm may cause pressure on the surrounding structures, such as the optic chiasm or the cranial nerves, leading to loss of the visual fields (see Figs. 14-7 and 14-14) or other visual disturbances. The mass may also result in headache as tension increases on the blood vessel wall and meninges.

A small leak is likely to cause headache, photophobia (increased sensitivity of the eyes to light), and intermittent periods of dysfunction, such as confusion, slurred speech, or weakness. Nuchal rigidity, or a stiff, extended neck, often develops because the escaped blood irritates the spinal nerve roots and causes muscle contractions in the neck.

A massive rupture or subarachnoid hemorrhage is manifested by an immediate, severe, "blinding" headache, vomiting, photophobia, and, perhaps, seizures or loss of consciousness. Death may occur shortly after rupture.

■ Treatment

An aneurysm that is diagnosed *before* rupture can be treated surgically as soon as possible by clipping or tying it off. In the interim, while the patient is waiting for surgery, sudden increases in blood pressure must be prevented. Surgical clipping of the aneurysm may also be done after rupture. Unfortunately, there is a substantial risk of rebleeding at the site of repair or from other aneurysms. Additional therapeutic measures focus on reducing the effects of increased ICP and cerebral vasospasm. Approximately 35% of patients die with the initial rupture, and an additional 15% die of a second rupture within several weeks.

> **THINK ABOUT 14-10**
>
> a. Differentiate a TIA from a CVA with regard to the cause of each and the effects of each on function.
> b. Describe the three causes of CVAs and the characteristic onset of signs with each.
> c. Describe several factors that influence the degree of functional recovery that is attained after a CVA.
> d. List common signs of an expanding aneurysm and of a bleeding aneurysm.
> e. Why does a headache occur with a subarachnoid hemorrhage?
> f. Explain why skin breakdown or ulcers may occur in a person who has had a stroke and list the common sites of these problems.

Infections

Meningitis

Meningitis is an infection, usually of bacterial origin, in the meninges of the CNS. Many microbes can infect the CNS and all age groups are susceptible. Early diagnosis and treatment is essential to prevent deficits or death.

■ Pathophysiology

Microorganisms reach the brain via the blood, by extension from nearby tissue, or by direct access through wounds. Microbes such as meningococcus can bind to nasopharyngeal cells in an individual, cross the mucosal barrier, attach to the choroid plexus, and enter CSF.

Because the membranes are continuous around the CNS and CSF flows in the subarachnoid space, infection spreads rapidly through the coverings of the brain. Focal signs are absent because there is no localized mass of infection. The inflammatory response to the infection leads to increased ICP, and the pia and arachnoid layers become edematous. The common bacterial infections lead to a purulent exudate that covers the surface of the brain and fills the sulci, causing the surface to appear flat. The exudate is present in the CSF, and the blood vessels on the surface of the brain appear dilated (Fig. 14-15*D*).

■ Etiology

Different age groups are susceptible to different organisms that cause meningitis. In some categories, vaccines have reduced the risk of meningitis:

- In children and young adults, *Neisseria meningitidis*, or *meningococcus*, which is the classic meningitis pathogen, is frequently carried in the nasopharynx of asymptomatic carriers. It is spread by respiratory droplets. Epidemics are common in schools or institutions where close contact between the children is likely to spread the organism. Any close contacts of affected persons should be given prophylactic treatment. This type of meningitis occurs more frequently in late winter and early spring.

- In neonates, *Escherichia coli* is the most common causative organism; this form of meningitis is usually seen in conjunction with a neural tube defect, premature rupture of the amniotic membranes, or a difficult delivery.
- In young children, meningitis results most often from bacterial infections caused by *Haemophilus influenzae* and occurs more often in the autumn or winter.
- In elderly persons and young children, *Streptococcus pneumoniae* is a major cause of meningitis.

In any age group, meningitis may be secondary to other infections, such as sinusitis or otitis, or it may result from an abscess located where the infection can spread through the bone to the meninges (e.g., an abscessed tooth). Any form of head trauma or surgery can result in meningitis from a variety of microorganisms. Aseptic or viral meningitis results from an infection, such as mumps or measles.

■ *Signs and Symptoms*

Sudden onset of meningitis is common, with severe headache, back pain, photophobia, and nuchal rigidity (a hyperextended, stiff neck). These signs result from meningeal irritation. Two other clinical signs of meningeal irritation include *Kernig's sign* (resistance to leg extension when lying with the hip flexed) and *Brudzinski's sign* (neck flexion causes flexion of hip and knee). Vomiting, irritability, and lethargy progressing to stupor or seizures are common early indicators of increased ICP. Fever and chills with leukocytosis indicate infection.

Meningococcal infections result in a rose colored petechial rash or extensive ecchymoses over the body (see Fig. 14-15*B*). Different signs, including feeding problems, irritability, lethargy, a typical high-pitched cry, and bulging fontanelles, occur in the newborn.

Potential complications include hydrocephalus, if CSF flow is blocked by pus or adhesions, and cranial nerve damage. In some cases, damage to the cerebral cortex may occur, resulting in mental retardation, seizures, or motor impairment.

In fulminant (rapidly progressive, severe) cases caused by highly virulent organisms, frequently meningococcal, disseminated intravascular coagulation (see Chapter 10) develops, with associated hemorrhage of the adrenal glands, or meningococcal septicemia may directly cause adrenal hemorrhage (Waterhouse-Friderichsen syndrome) (see Fig. 14-15*C*). These cases usually result in vascular collapse or shock and death.

■ *Diagnostic Tests*

Examination of CSF, obtained by lumbar puncture, confirms the diagnosis. If meningitis is present, the CSF pressure is elevated; it will appear cloudy and usually contains an increased number of leukocytes. The causative organism in the CSF or blood must be identified to ensure adequate and effective treatment.

■ *Treatment*

Aggressive antimicrobial therapy (e.g., ampicillin) is required, along with specific treatment measures for ICP and seizures as needed. Glucocorticoids reduce cerebral inflammation and edema. With prompt diagnosis and treatment, the majority of patients survive. The mortality rate in neonatal meningitis is high, and there is some risk of permanent brain damage in young children. Between 10% and 20% of patients with meningitis are estimated to have some neurologic deficits as sequelae.

Vaccines are available as a preventive measure for some types of meningococcal, *S. pneumoniae* and *H. influenzae* meningitis, especially when outbreaks occur. Carriers should be identified in institutional epidemics, and contacts should be notified and treated. Vaccination may be undertaken as a preventive measure when cases occur in institutions such as schools.

Brain Abscess

An abscess is a localized infection, frequently occurring in the frontal or temporal lobes (see Fig. 14-16). There is usually necrosis of brain tissue and a surrounding area of edema. A medical history may be helpful in making the diagnosis. Abscesses usually result from the spread of organisms from ear, throat, lung, or sinus infections; multiple septic emboli from acute bacterial endocarditis; or directly from a site of injury or surgery. Common organisms are staphylococci, streptococci, and pneumococci.

The onset of a brain abscess tends to be insidious. Focal signs indicating neurologic deficits and increasing ICP develop. Both surgical drainage and antimicrobial therapy are required. The mortality rate is around 10%.

Encephalitis

Encephalitis is considered an infection of the parenchymal or connective tissue in the brain and cord, particularly the basal ganglia, although various viruses demonstrate an affinity for particular types of cells. The infection may include the meninges. Necrosis and inflammation develop in the brain tissue, often resulting in some permanent damage. Early signs of infection include severe headache, stiff neck, lethargy, vomiting, seizures, and fever.

Encephalitis is usually of viral origin but may be related to other organisms. In some cases, there may be considerable delay before signs appear. A few examples of specific diseases follow.

Western equine encephalitis is an arboviral infection spread by mosquitoes, which occurs more frequently in the summer months and is common in young children.

St. Louis encephalitis is found throughout the United States and affects older persons more seriously than younger ones.

West Nile fever is a form of encephalitis that originated in the northeastern United States but has now spread to

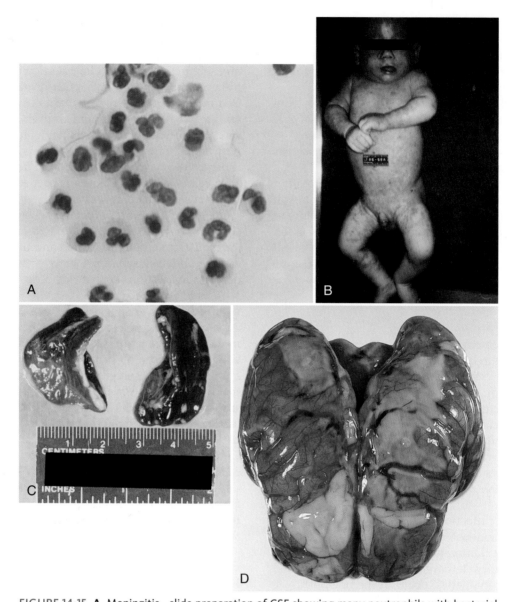

FIGURE 14-15 **A,** Meningitis—slide preparation of CSF showing many neutrophils with bacterial meningitis. **B,** Petechial rash associated with meningococcemia. **C,** Hemorrhage (dark areas) in the adrenal glands with Waterhouse-Friderichsen syndrome. **D,** Meningitis due to coliform microorganisms. The meninges are reddened from vascular congestion. Thick, greenish pus fills the subarachnoid space over both hemispheres. (*A from Stevens ML:* Fundamentals of Clinical Hematology, *Philadelphia, 1997, Saunders; **B** and **C** from Mahon CR, Manuselis G:* Textbook of Diagnostic Microbiology, *ed 2, Philadelphia, 2000, Saunders; **D** from Cooke RA, Stewart B:* Colour Atlas of Anatomical Pathology, *ed 3, Sydney, 2004, Churchill Livingstone.)*

a number of states across the country and into Canada. It is caused by a flavivirus, spread by mosquitoes, with certain birds as an intermediate host. The focus for control has been to track the spread and reduce the risk of mosquito bites in affected areas. The infection initially causes flulike symptoms with low-grade fever and headache, sometimes followed by confusion and tremors.

Neuroborreliosis (Lyme disease) is caused by a spirochete, *Borrelia burgdorferi,* transmitted by tick bites in summertime. The site of the tick bite is red with a pale center, gradually increasing in size to form the unique marker lesion, a "bull's eye" that may become quite large and persist for some time. The microbes then disseminate through the circulation, causing first, sore throat, dry cough, fever, and headache, followed by cardiac arrhythmias and neurologic abnormalities (e.g., facial nerve paralysis) related to meningoencephalitis. Last, pain and swelling may develop in large joints, sometimes progressing to chronic arthritis. The effects may persist for months. Prolonged therapy with antimicrobials such as doxycycline is prescribed.

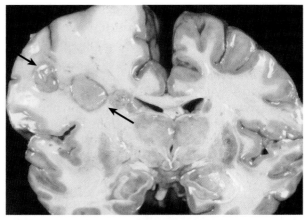

FIGURE 14-16 **Brain—Frontal Abscess** Infection causes central liquefactive necrosis and surrounding edema. *(From Kumar V, Abbas AK, Fausto M: Robbins and Cotran Pathologic Basis of Disease, ed 7, Philadelphia, 2005, Saunders.)*

Herpes simplex encephalitis occurs occasionally and is dangerous, arising from the spread of herpes simplex virus type 1 (HSV-1) from the trigeminal nerve ganglion. This virus causes extensive necrosis and hemorrhage in the brain, often involving the frontal and temporal lobes. Early treatment with an antiviral drug, such as acyclovir, may control the infection. Otherwise, treatment is supportive.

THINK ABOUT 14-11

a. List the signs of developing meningitis.
b. Describe the changes that occur in the CSF with meningitis.
c. What are the causes of death in meningococcal infection?
d. Why does an abscess cause focal signs, whereas meningitis does not?

Other Infections

Many other microorganisms specifically target the central and/or peripheral nervous systems. Brief descriptions of several of the diseases they cause are given here.

Rabies (hydrophobia) is caused by a virus that is transmitted by the bite of a rabid animal. The virus travels along peripheral nerves to the CNS, where it causes severe inflammation and necrosis, particularly in the brain stem and basal ganglia. The incubation period (often 1 to 3 months) depends on the distance between the bite and access to the CNS. Onset is marked by headache and fever; nervous hyperirritability, including sensitivity to touch; and seizures. The virus also travels to the salivary glands. Difficulty swallowing, caused by muscle spasm, and foaming at the mouth are typical. Respiratory failure causes death. Immediate cleansing

of the bite area and prophylactic immunization are necessary treatments.

Tetanus (lockjaw) is caused by *Clostridium tetani*, a spore-forming bacillus. The spores survive for years in soil. The vegetative form is an anaerobe, thriving deep in tissues, for example, in a puncture wound. The exotoxin enters the nervous system, causing tonic muscle spasms. Symptoms of infection include jaw stiffness, difficulty swallowing, stiff neck, headache, skeletal muscle spasm, and eventually respiratory failure. The mortality rate is 50%. Immunizations are advised, with boosters as needed or after injury.

Poliomyelitis (infantile paralysis) is now rare in North America because of immunization but still occurs in other parts of the world. An immunization program is underway to combat an epidemic occurring in West and Central Africa, where large numbers of young children have been infected and threatened with paralysis in large numbers. The goal of the World Health Organization (WHO) is worldwide eradication through immunization. The polio virus is highly contagious through direct contact or oral droplet. It reproduces in lymphoid tissue in the oropharynx and digestive tract, and then enters the blood and, eventually, the CNS. The virus attacks the motor neurons of the spinal cord and medulla, causing minor flulike effects in many cases, but paralysis and respiratory failure in other cases, depending on the level of the destruction. Symptoms include fever, headache, and vomiting, followed by the typical stiff neck, pain, and flaccid paralysis.

Other microorganisms, such as *Candida albicans* or *Toxoplasma gondii*, may cause infection in the brain, most often in immune-suppressed individuals.

Infection-Related Syndromes
Herpes Zoster (Shingles)

Herpes zoster or shingles is caused by varicella-zoster virus (VZV) in adults. It is seen years after the primary infection of varicella or chickenpox, which usually occurs in childhood.

Shingles usually affects *one cranial nerve* or *one dermatome*, a cutaneous area innervated by a spinal nerve (see Fig. 14-22 for dermatomes) on *one* side of the body. Pain, paresthesia, and a vesicular rash develop in a line, unilaterally. This may occur on the face (e.g., following the trigeminal nerve) or along the path of a lumbar nerve from the spine extending around one side in the hip area. The lesions persist for several weeks and then clear in the majority of cases.

In some cases, particularly in older individuals, neuralgia or pain continues after the lesions disappear. In patients with immune deficiencies, the lesions tend to spread locally. Visual impairment has resulted from involvement of the ophthalmic division of the trigeminal nerve. Antiviral medications such as acyclovir or vidarabine have provided some relief from symptoms. A new shingles vaccine, Zostrix, is available for those 60 years of age or older. It prevents initial and recurrent outbreaks as well as reducing postherpetic nerve pain.

Postpolio Syndrome

Postpolio syndrome (PPS) has been occurring 10 to 40 years after recovery from the original infection, with progressive and debilitating fatigue, weakness, pain, and muscle atrophy. It is estimated that 25% to 50% of individuals infected with polio will develop PPS. Symptoms have developed in individuals who, as young children in the 1950s and earlier, were diagnosed with mild forms as well as paralytic forms of polio, and in those who were misdiagnosed at the time, but are now considered to have been infected. The more severe the original infection was, the more severe the effects of PPS. The syndrome does not appear to be a recurrence of latent infection, but the precise basis for the neuronal damage has not been determined. It appears that surviving motor neurons have now degenerated and died, possibly because they developed new additional axon branches to serve muscle cells as compensation for damage, but could not maintain them.

Reye's Syndrome

■ Pathophysiology

The cause of Reye's syndrome has not yet been fully determined, but it is linked to a viral infection, such as influenza, in young children that have been treated with aspirin (ASA). Depending on the particular virus, signs appear 3 to 5 days after the onset of the viral infection. The number of cases has decreased with awareness of this potential danger, and acetaminophen is now used to treat fever in children.

The major pathologic changes occur in the brain and the liver. A noninflammatory cerebral edema develops, leading to increased ICP. Brain function is severely impaired by cerebral edema and the effects of high ammonia levels in serum related to liver dysfunction.

The liver enlarges, develops fatty changes in the tissue, and progresses to acute failure. Jaundice is not present, but serum levels of liver enzymes are elevated. The resultant metabolic abnormalities include hypoglycemia and increased lactic acid in the blood and body fluids, which also contribute to acute encephalopathy. In some cases, the kidneys are also affected by fatty degenerative changes, leading to increases in serum urea and creatinine levels.

■ Signs and Symptoms

Manifestations vary in severity. Encephalopathy initially causes lethargy, headache, and vomiting, which are quickly followed by disorientation, hyperreflexia, hyperventilation, seizures, stupor, or coma.

■ Treatment

There is no immediate cure. Treatment is supportive and symptomatic, managing the metabolic imbalances and cerebral edema. The mortality rate is high if diagnosis and treatment are not initiated quickly. Average mortality is 30% and neurologic damage is possible.

Guillain-Barré Syndrome

Guillain-Barré syndrome is also known as postinfectious polyneuritis, acute idiopathic polyneuropathy, and acute infectious polyradiculoneuritis. The syndrome is an inflammatory condition of the peripheral nervous system.

■ Pathophysiology

The precise cause of Guillain-Barré is unknown, but evidence indicates that an abnormal immune response, perhaps an autoimmune response, precipitated by a preceding viral infection or immunization, may be responsible. Local inflammation, accompanied by accumulated lymphocytes, demyelination, and axon destruction, occurs. These changes cause impaired nerve conduction, particularly in the efferent (motor) fibers, although afferent (sensory) and autonomic fibers may also be involved. If the cell body remains alive through the acute period, the axon can regenerate. Initially the inflammatory and degenerative processes affect the peripheral nerves in the legs; then the inflammation ascends to involve the spinal nerves to the trunk and neck and frequently includes the cranial nerves as well. The critical period develops when the ascending paralysis involves the diaphragm and respiratory muscles. Recovery is usually spontaneous with the manifestations diminishing in reverse order; that is, motor function is regained first in the upper body and then gradually improves in the trunk and the lower extremities.

■ Signs and Symptoms

Progressive muscle weakness and areflexia, beginning in the legs, lead to an ascending flaccid paralysis, which may be accompanied by paresthesia, or pain and general muscle aching. As paralysis advances upward, vision and speech may be impaired. This process may occur rapidly over a few hours or several days. If swallowing and respiration are affected, a life-threatening situation develops. Many patients sustain autonomic nervous system impairment, manifested as cardiac arrhythmias, labile (fluctuating) blood pressure, or loss of sweating capability.

■ Treatment

Treatment is primarily supportive, and a ventilator is required in many cases. The use of immunoglobulin therapy or plasmapheresis, in which IgG is separated and removed from the patient's blood, in the early stage may shorten the acute period of the disease in some patients and hasten recovery. Physiotherapy, occupational therapy, and respiratory therapy throughout the recovery period are essential to maximize restoration of function. About 30% of patients experience some degree of residual weakness.

Brain Injuries

Brain injuries may involve skull fractures, hemorrhage and edema, or direct injury to brain tissue. An injury may be mild, causing only bruising of the tissue, or it can be severe and life-threatening, causing destruction of brain tissue and massive swelling of the brain. The skull protects the brain but can also destroy it by means of bone fragments that penetrate or compress the brain tissue and by its inability to expand to relieve pressure.

Types of Head Injuries

Various terms are used to classify and describe brain trauma, in some cases with overlap, as follows:

- *Concussion, also termed mild traumatic brain injury (MTBI)* is a reversible interference with brain function, usually resulting from a mild blow to the head, which causes sudden excessive movement of the brain, disrupting neurologic function and leading to loss of consciousness. Amnesia, or memory loss, and headaches may follow a concussion, but recovery with no permanent damage usually occurs within 24 hours. Recurrent concussions have been shown to cause progressive and permanent brain damage; thus at-risk individuals may need to change activities to prevent further damage.
- *Contusion* is a bruising of brain tissue with rupture of small blood vessels and edema that usually results from a blunt blow to the head. The possibility of residual damage depends on the force of the blow and the degree of tissue injury.
- *Closed* head injury occurs when the skull is not fractured in the injury, but the brain tissue is injured and blood vessels may be ruptured by the force exerted against the skull (Fig. 14-17). Extensive damage may occur when the head is rotated with considerable force.
- *Open* head injuries are those involving fractures or penetration of the brain by missiles or sharp objects.
- *Linear* fractures are simple cracks in the bone.
- *Comminuted* fractures consist of several fracture lines but may not be complicated.
- *Compound* fractures involve trauma in which the brain tissue is exposed to the environment and is likely to be severely damaged because bone fragments may penetrate the tissue and the risk of infection is high.
- *Depressed* skull fractures involve displacement of a piece of bone below the level of the skull, thereby compressing the brain tissue. With this type of fracture, the blood supply to the area is often impaired, and considerable pressure is exerted on the brain.

- *Basilar* fractures occur at the base of the skull and are often accompanied by leaking of CSF through the ears or nose. These fractures may occur when the forehead hits a car windshield with considerable force. Cranial nerve damage and dark discoloration around the eyes are common.
- *Contrecoup* injury occurs when an area of the brain contralateral to the site of direct damage is injured as the brain bounces off the skull. This injury may be secondary to acceleration or deceleration injuries, in which the skull and brain hit a solid object, which causes the brain to rebound against the opposite side of the skull, usually causing minor damage.

■ *Pathophysiology*

Primary brain injuries are direct injuries, such as lacerations or crushing of the neurons, glial cells, and blood vessels of the brain.

Secondary injuries result from the additional effects of cerebral edema, hemorrhage, hematoma, cerebral vasospasm, infection, and ischemia related to systemic factors.

Primary injuries may involve a laceration or compression of brain tissue by a piece of bone or foreign object or rupture or compression of the cerebral blood vessels. Because the brain is not held tightly in place, the application of unusual force may rotate or shift it inside the skull. The brain tissue may be damaged by the rough and irregular inner surface of the skull or by the movement of the lobes of the brain against each other (shearing injury).

Any trauma to the brain tissue causes loss of function in the part of the body controlled by that specific area of the brain. Cell damage and bleeding lead to inflammation and vasospasm around the site of the injury, increased ICP and further general ischemia and dysfunction (Fig. 14-18). After the bleeding and inflammation subside, some recovery of the neurons in the area surrounding the direct damage may occur. The central area of damage undergoes necrosis and is replaced by scar tissue or a cyst.

Secondary brain damage is caused by the development of additional injurious factors. A *hematoma* is a collection of blood in the tissue that develops from ruptured blood vessels, either immediately after the injury or after some delay (Fig. 14-19). Hematoma may also develop after surgery.

Hematomas and hemorrhages are classified by their location in relation to the meninges, as follows:

- *Epidural* (extradural) *hematoma* results from bleeding between the dura and the skull, usually caused by tearing of the middle meningeal artery in the temporal region. Signs of trouble usually arise within a few hours of injury, when the person loses consciousness after a brief period of responsiveness.
- *Subdural hematoma* develops between the dura and the arachnoid (Fig. 14-20). Frequently there is a small

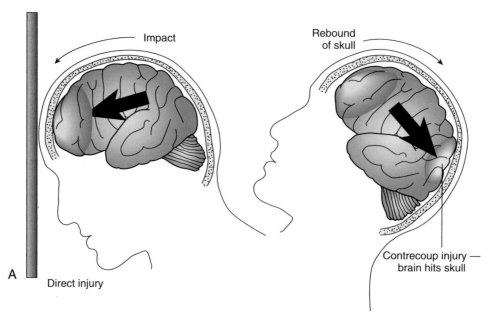

Closed Injury — Direct and Contrecoup Injury

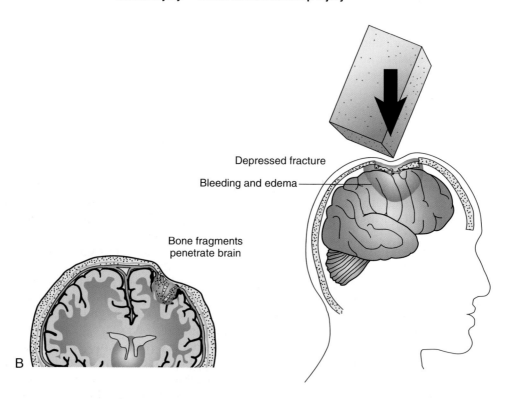

Open Injury

FIGURE 14-17 Types of head injury—closed and open.

tear in a vein, which causes blood to accumulate slowly. A hematoma may be acute (signs present in about 24 hours) or subacute (increasing ICP develops over a week or so). A chronic subdural hematoma may occur in an elderly person, in whom brain atrophy allows more space for a hematoma to develop. Also, a tear in the arachnoid can allow CSF to leak into the subdural space (hygroma), creating additional pressure.

- *Subarachnoid* hemorrhage occurs in the space between the arachnoid and pia and is associated with traumatic bleeding from the blood vessels at the base of the brain. Because the blood mixes with circulating CSF, a localized hematoma cannot form.

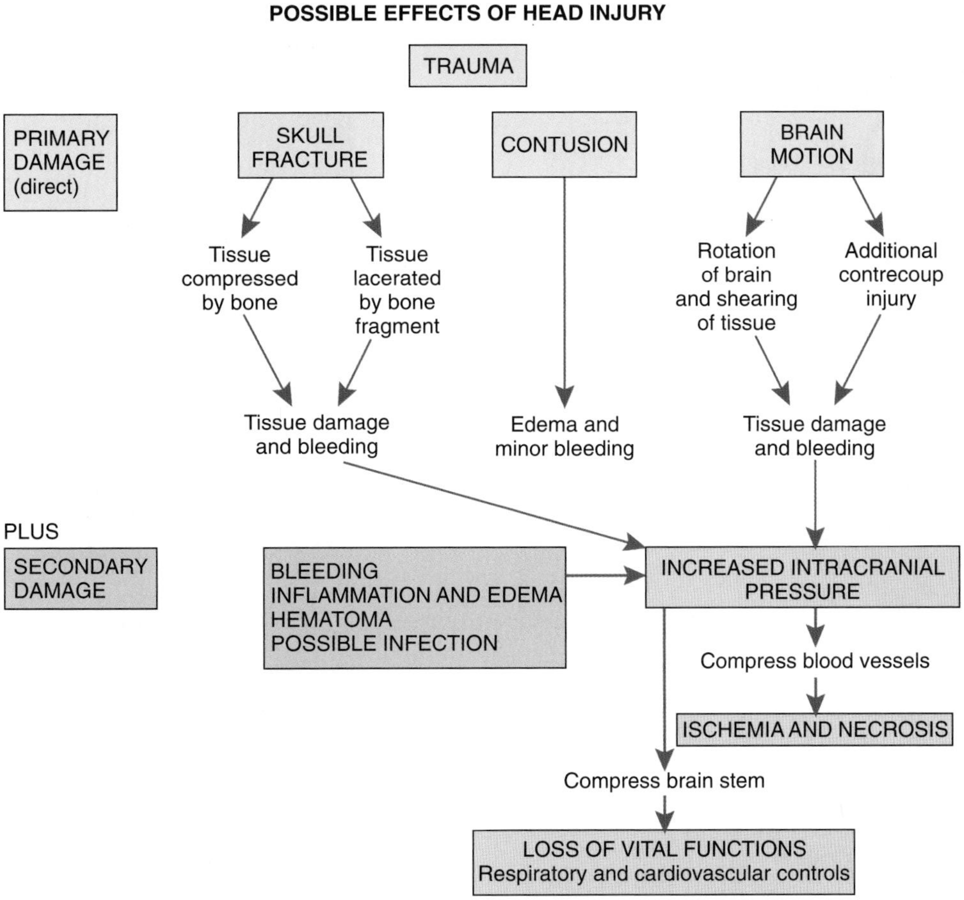

POSSIBLE EFFECTS OF HEAD INJURY

FIGURE 14-18 Possible effects of head injury.

- *Intracerebral hematoma* results from contusions or shearing injuries and may develop several days after injury.

In all types of hematomas, the bleeding leads to local pressure on adjacent tissue and a general increase in ICP. Blood may be partially coagulated, forming a solid mass. When the blood accumulates slowly, the blood cells undergo hemolysis. The fluid in this area of cell breakdown exerts osmotic pressure, drawing more and more water into the area, increasing the size and pressure of the mass, and raising the ICP. Herniation may result from an untreated mass. Any bleeding in the brain may precipitate cerebral vasoconstriction (vasospasm), leading to further ischemia and more damage to the neurons.

Other factors that may cause secondary brain damage include infection, which is usually a significant risk in persons with open head injuries, and hypoxia, which is related to systemic injury or shock. Respiratory or cardiovascular impairment may cause additional ischemia in the brain.

■ *Etiology*
The majority of head injuries occur in young adults as a result of sports injuries and accidents involving cars

or motorcycles. In many of these accidents, excessive alcohol intake is a contributing factor. Unfortunately, a high blood alcohol level can impede neurologic assessment by masking the signs of injury. Alcohol, because of its dehydrating effects, tends to delay the onset of cerebral edema and elevation of ICP, but there may be a greater increase in ICP at a later time. Other systemic injuries, such as a chest injury or shock, can have the same effect.

Falls are a common cause of head injury in any age group, but more often in elderly persons. Boxers and other athletes engaged in contact sports are at risk for repeated head injury. Infants, when violently shaken, can experience severe damage to the brain and brain stem as the head swings. Other injuries may involve objects that fall on the head or a blow to the head.

■ *Signs and Symptoms*
The person with a head injury manifests the characteristic focal signs and the general signs of increased ICP. In addition, one or more of the following may develop:
1. Seizures, which are often focal but may be generalized, occur because of the irritating quality of blood.
2. Cranial nerve impairment may occur, particularly in persons who have sustained basilar fractures.

TYPES OF HEMATOMAS AND THE MENINGES

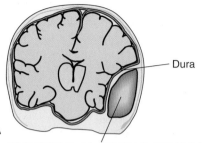

A

EXTRADURAL OR EPIDURAL HEMATOMA
Blood fills space between
dura and bone

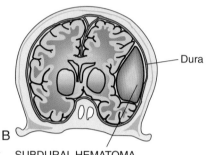

B

SUBDURAL HEMATOMA
Blood fills space between dura
and arachnoid

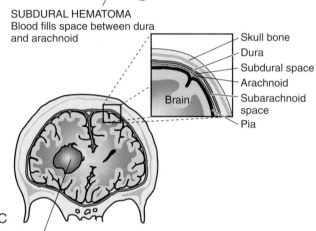

C

INTRACEREBRAL HEMATOMA

FIGURE 14-19 Types of hematomas.

3. Otorrhea or rhinorrhea (leaking of CSF from the ear or nose, respectively) occurs with fractures and tearing of the meninges, which allows fluid to pass out of the subarachnoid space. This type of trauma provides microbes with an entry point into the brain.
4. Otorrhagia is blood leaking from the ear through a fracture site with torn vessels and meninges.
5. Fever may be a sign of hypothalamic impairment or of cranial or systemic infection.
6. Stress ulcers may develop from increased gastric secretions.

If the individual is unconscious for a prolonged period of time, other problems may develop. Immobility may cause complications such as pneumonia or decubitus ulcers (see Chapter 25).

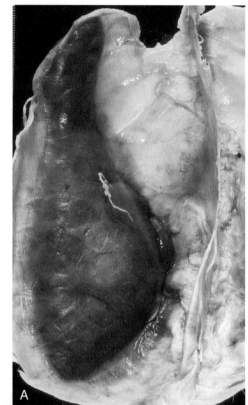

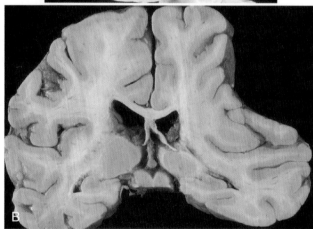

FIGURE 14-20 **A**, Large organizing subdural hematoma attached to the dura. **B**, Coronal section of the brain showing compression of the brain tissue under the hematoma. *(From Kumar V, Abbas AK, Fausto M: Robbins and Cotran Pathologic Basis of Disease, ed 7, Philadelphia, 2005, Saunders.)*

■ *Treatment*

Computed tomographic (CT) and MRI scans are useful in determining the extent of brain injury. Glucocorticoid agents, which decrease edema, and antibiotic agents, which reduce the risk of infection, are helpful. Surgery may be necessary to reduce ICP. Blood products and oxygen may be administered to protect the remaining brain tissue. Any other injuries must be treated promptly, particularly if they interfere with respiration or circulation.

Individuals with brain injuries may be examined and discharged from the hospital if no brain damage is apparent. The person's family or friends are usually asked to continue to perform a simplified head injury assessment for the next day or so to detect delayed hematoma formation. This routine involves awakening the person periodically to check the level of consciousness (i.e., response to questions and orientation to time, place, and people), checking for reactive pupils, and watching for vomiting or any change in movement, sensation, or behavior. Headache, irritability, and fatigue are often present for a few days in persons with minor injuries.

The prognosis for recovery from a brain injury is better now because of improved surgical techniques, monitoring devices, supportive rehabilitation and drug therapies. Physiotherapy is used to increase mobility. Occupational therapy addresses motor, visual and cognitive activity, whereas speech and language therapy address communication. There may be permanent residual damage in specific areas of the brain, resulting in motor or sensory deficits that may cause disability. Seizures, focal or generalized, are common sequelae because of the increased irritability of tissue around the scar. Often, general fatigue, frequent headaches, and memory loss are present for some time after recovery.

THINK ABOUT 14-12

a. Differentiate an open head injury from a closed head injury in terms of appearance and effects.

b. Describe the location, common source, and time of development of a subdural hematoma.

c. Describe three significant signs of an injury to the right occipital lobe, including one specific focal sign and two general signs.

Spinal Cord Injury

Approximately 11,000 Americans experience spinal cord injuries each year and 200,000 Americans live with ongoing disability due to spinal cord injury. Injury to the spinal cord usually results from fracture or dislocation of the vertebrae, which compresses, stretches, or tears the spinal cord (Fig. 14-21). The supporting ligaments and the intervertebral disc may be damaged also. Most injuries occur in areas of the spine that provide more mobility but less support (i.e., C1 to C7 and T12 to L2) (see Fig. 14-4). A few common types of injuries are described as follows:

- Cervical spine injuries may result from hyperextension or hyperflexion of the neck, with possible fracture. Usually damage to the disc and ligaments occurs, leading to dislocation, loss of alignment of the vertebrae, and compression or stretching of the spinal cord.

- Dislocation of any vertebra may crush or compress the spinal cord and compromise the blood supply.

- Compression fractures cause injury to the spinal cord when great force is applied to the top of the skull or to the feet and is transmitted up or down the spine. Diving into an empty pool, jumping from a height and landing on the feet, or an object falling on a standing person's head may cause this injury. The shattered bone is compressed and protrudes, exerting pressure horizontally against the cord. The sharp edges of bone fragments may lacerate or tear nerve fibers and blood vessels.

- Spinal cord damage also may result directly from penetration injuries, such as stab or bullet wounds.

Vertebral fractures may be classified as simple (single line break), compression (crushed or shattered bone in multiple fragments), wedge (a displaced angular section of bone), or dislocation (a vertebra forced out of its normal position).

Because spinal cord injuries are often unstable, immediate appropriate immobilization is essential to prevent secondary damage.

■ *Pathophysiology*

Damage to the spinal cord may be temporary or permanent. Nerves in the spinal cord do not undergo mitosis but axonal regrowth may occur. Laceration of nerve tissue by bone fragments usually results in permanent loss of conduction in the affected nerve tracts. Complete transection (severing) or crushing of the cord causes irreversible loss of all sensory and motor functions at and below the level of injury. Partial transection or crushing injuries may allow recovery of some function.

Bruising is reversible damage when mild edema and minor bleeding temporarily impair conduction of nerve impulses. Any compression of the cord must be relieved quickly to maintain adequate blood supply. Prolonged ischemia and necrosis lead to permanent damage. As with any trauma, bleeding and inflammation develop locally, creating additional pressure and further interfering with blood flow. Edema and hemorrhage extend for several segments above and below the level of injury. In addition, damaged tissue releases mediators such as norepinephrine, serotonin, and histamine in the area. These mediators cause vasoconstriction, leading to additional local ischemia and possible necrosis. Destructive enzymes are released as well, causing more inflammation and necrosis.

Initially the loss of function may appear to be extensive because of this additional compression, but as the edema subsides, there may be partial recovery of function. Regular assessment of movement and sensory response using the dermatome map (Fig. 14-22) can determine the degree of damage or recovery in the spinal cord. When injury occurs in the *cervical* region, the inflammation may extend upward to the level of C3

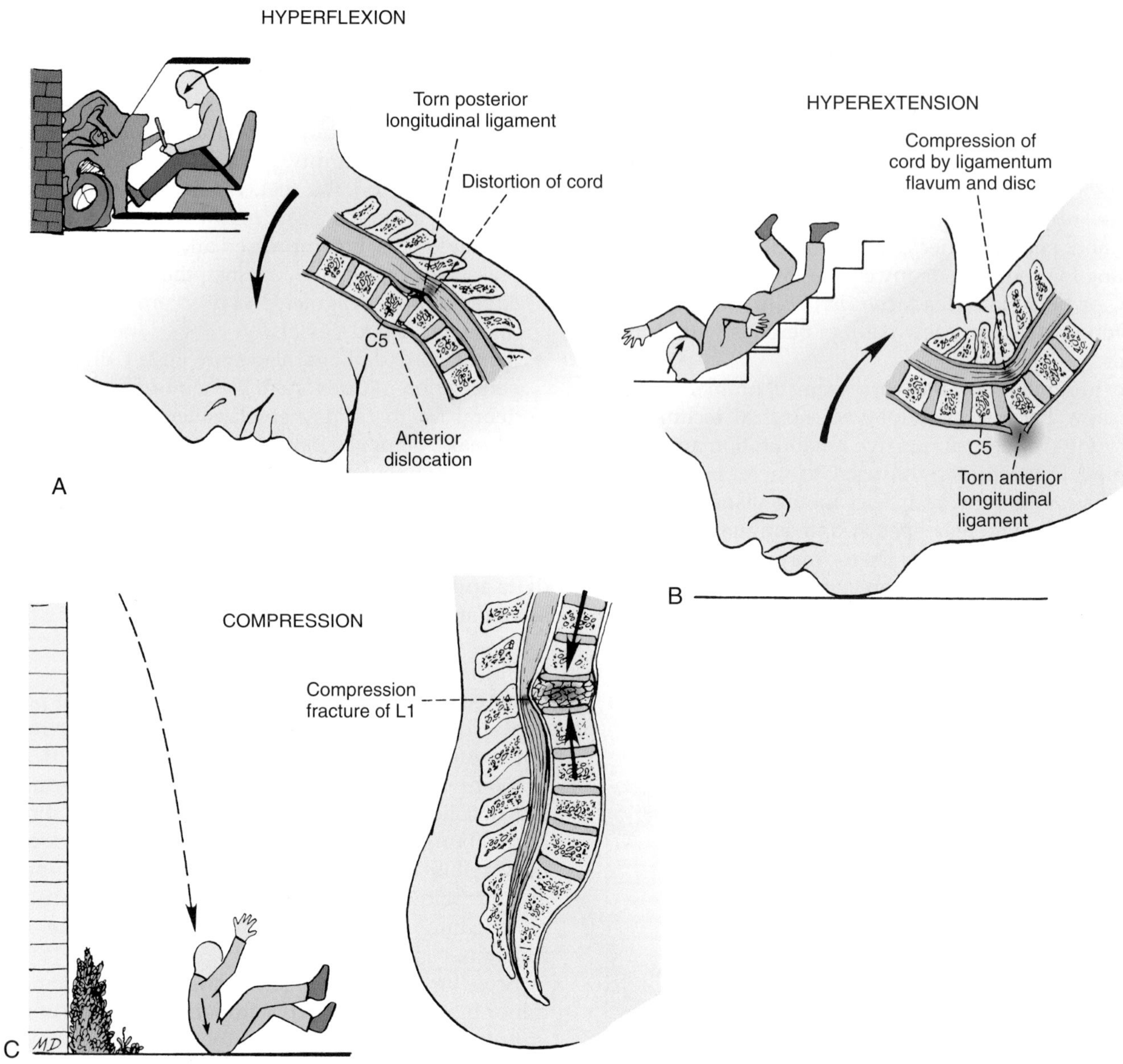

HYPERFLEXION

HYPEREXTENSION

COMPRESSION

FIGURE 14-21 Types of spinal cord injuries. *(From Copstead LC:* Perspectives on Pathophysiology, *Philadelphia, 1995, Saunders.)*

to C5, interfering with *phrenic nerve* innervation to the diaphragm and therefore affecting respiration. Ventilatory assistance may be required.

In the initial period after the injury, conduction of impulses ceases in the nerve tracts and in the gray matter, a period known as *spinal shock* (which is a form of neurogenic shock). The extent of the injury, the amount of resultant bleeding, and the need for surgical intervention determine the rate and degree of recovery. The inflammation gradually subsides, damaged tissue is removed by phagocytes, and scar tissue begins to form. During this period, reflex activity resumes in the spinal cord below the level of injury, and any undamaged tracts continue to conduct impulses through the level of damage (Fig. 14-23).

■ *Etiology*

Most spinal cord injuries occur in young men and around 50% result from motorcycle or automobile accidents. The second most common cause is sports (e.g., diving, football). The other major cause of injury is falls, which elderly persons often experience. The average age for persons with SCI has increased over the past few years and now is 38 years.

■ *Signs and Symptoms*

There are two stages in the post-traumatic period, the early stage of spinal shock and increasing impairment, followed by recovery and recognition of the extent of functional loss. During the initial period of *spinal shock*, all neurologic activity ceases at, below, and slightly

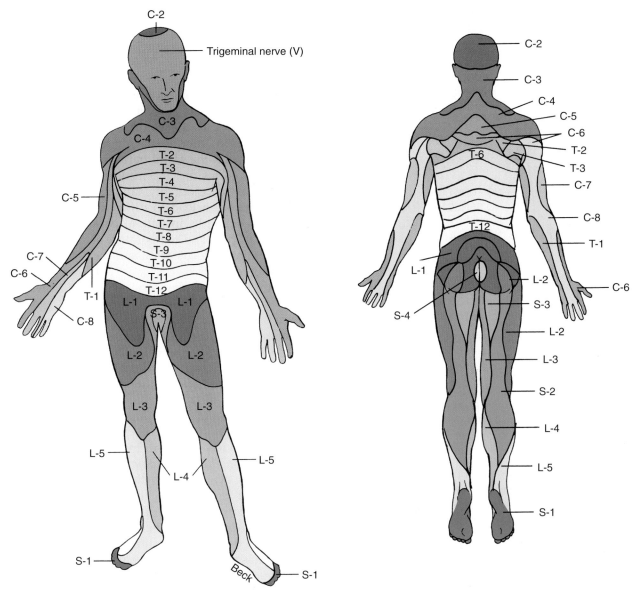

FIGURE 14-22 Dermatomes. *(From Thibodeau GA: Anatomy and Physiology, St. Louis, 1987, Mosby.)*

above the level of injury (see Fig. 14-23). No reflexes are present, including the skeletal muscle, sensory, and autonomic systems (bladder and bowel function). This condition may persist for days or weeks. During the period of spinal shock, signs include flaccid paralysis and sensory loss at and below the injured area, an absence of all reflex responses, and loss of central control of autonomic function. In patients with cervical injury, this includes loss of control of vasomotor tone, blood pressure, diaphoresis and body temperature, and bowel and bladder emptying. Blood pressure is low and labile. Urinary retention and paralytic ileus are present.

Recovery from spinal shock is indicated by the gradual return of reflex activity below the level of injury. No impulses, including reflexes, can pass through the specific area of damaged neurons. In most cases, *hyperreflexia* develops, because the normal inhibitory, or

"dampening," impulses cannot reach the cord levels below the injury. Following recovery from spinal shock and the return of reflexes, spastic paralysis, sensory deficits, and reflex or neurogenic bladder and bowel function (urinary incontinence and reflex defecation) are present below the level of damage.

Gradually the extent of permanent damage is revealed. For example, a check of the dermatome response can assess sensory function. Voluntary motor activity and sensory impulses are blocked at the level of damage. The specific effects of permanent damage depend on the level at which the spinal cord trauma occurred (see Figs. 14-4 and 14-23). For example, cervical injuries affect motor and sensory function in the arms, trunk, and legs; respiratory function; SNS function (T1 to L2); and sacral parasympathetic fibers. In patients with cervical injuries, respiratory function may

**DURING SPINAL SHOCK (PERIOD
IMMEDIATELY FOLLOWING INJURY)**

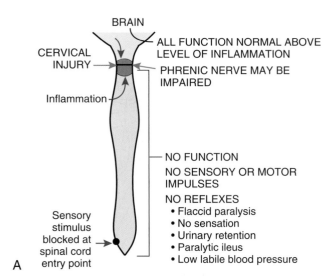

A

**OVERVIEW OF PERMANENT EFFECTS –
POSTSPINAL SHOCK**

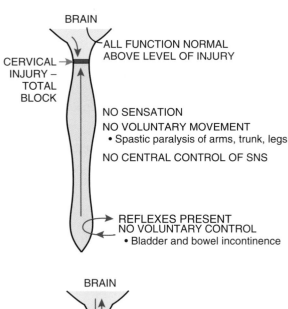

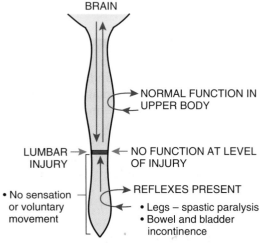

B

FIGURE 14-23 Effects of spinal cord damage.

continue to be a matter of concern owing to phrenic nerve impairment and the loss of intercostal muscle innervation. Blood pressure and body temperature may be labile, because central control of vasomotor tone and diaphoresis is lacking.

Paralysis of all four extremities is termed *tetraplegia (quadriplegia)*, whereas *paraplegia* refers to paralysis of the lower part of the trunk and legs. Trauma in the lumbar region interferes with function in the lower extremities and the sacral parasympathetic nerves.

Many injuries are incomplete, and the permanent effects vary considerably among individuals. Partial cord injuries can lead to different patterns of impairment, for example, ipsilateral paralysis and contralateral loss of pain and temperature sensation, depending on the point of decussation and the location of the specific injured tracts.

With injury of the cervical spine, stimulation of the sympathetic system may result in *autonomic dysreflexia* (Fig. 14-24). This is a potentially serious complication caused by a sensory stimulus that triggers a massive sympathetic reflex response that cannot be controlled from the brain. The trigger may be any noxious stimulus in the body, but most frequently is a distended bladder or decubitus ulcer. A sensory stimulus to the SNS below the level of injury can stimulate the entire chain of SNS ganglia, leading to excessive vasoconstriction, with a sudden increase in blood pressure, severe headache, and visual impairment. Bradycardia accompanies this syndrome as the baroreceptors sense the high blood pressure and respond through the vagus nerve by slowing the heart rate. Note that the excessive vasoconstriction cannot be reduced through the cardiovascular control center. Immediate resolution of this problem is necessary to prevent a stroke or heart failure. This means finding and removing the cause of the stimulus and administering medication to lower blood pressure.

Complications are common after spinal cord injury because of immobility and loss of function (see Chapter 25). Contractures may develop from muscle spasms and decubitus ulcers are common; respiratory and urinary infections are frequent.

Sexual function and reproductive capacity are likely to be affected. The sensory and psychological components of the sexual response are usually blocked by the injury. Men may have neurogenic reflex erections. Penetration depends on sustaining this reflex, which can be difficult. Many men, particularly those with high-level cord injuries, are infertile, because sperm production in the testes is impaired. Women usually resume menstrual cycles once they have recovered from the acute trauma period, and they can bear children. Close monitoring of the pregnancy is necessary, and vaginal delivery may be difficult. With counseling and supportive mates, many individuals with spinal cord injury can develop or maintain sexual relationships.

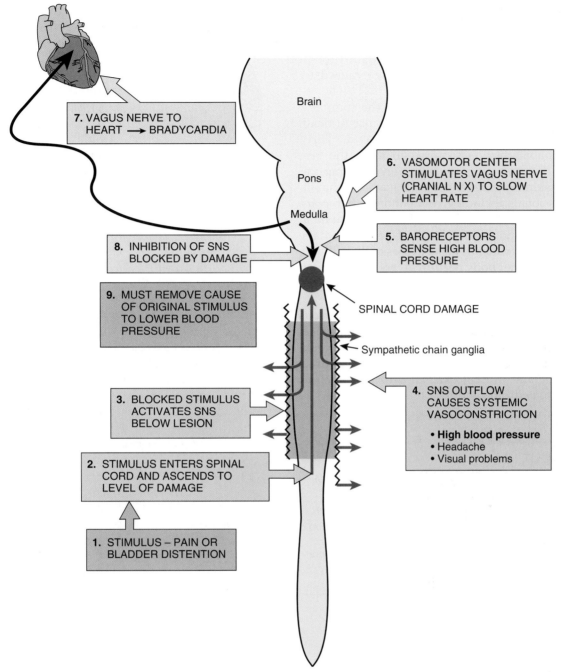

7. VAGUS NERVE TO HEART ⟶ BRADYCARDIA

Brain

Pons

Medulla

6. VASOMOTOR CENTER STIMULATES VAGUS NERVE (CRANIAL N X) TO SLOW HEART RATE

8. INHIBITION OF SNS BLOCKED BY DAMAGE

5. BARORECEPTORS SENSE HIGH BLOOD PRESSURE

9. MUST REMOVE CAUSE OF ORIGINAL STIMULUS TO LOWER BLOOD PRESSURE

SPINAL CORD DAMAGE

Sympathetic chain ganglia

3. BLOCKED STIMULUS ACTIVATES SNS BELOW LESION

4. SNS OUTFLOW CAUSES SYSTEMIC VASOCONSTRICTION
- **High blood pressure**
- Headache
- Visual problems

2. STIMULUS ENTERS SPINAL CORD AND ASCENDS TO LEVEL OF DAMAGE

1. STIMULUS – PAIN OR BLADDER DISTENTION

FIGURE 14-24 Autonomic dysreflexia following spinal cord damage.

■ *Treatment*

Assessment of damage is usually carried out using the American Spinal Injury Association (ASIA)* criteria:
- A = Complete: No motor or sensory function is preserved in the sacral segments S4-S5
- B = Incomplete: Sensory but not motor function is preserved below the neurologic level and includes the sacral segments S4-S5

- C = Incomplete: Motor function is preserved below the neurologic level, and more than half of key muscles below the neurologic level have a muscle grade less than 3
- D = Incomplete: Motor function is preserved below the neurologic level, and at least half of key muscles below the neurologic level have a muscle grade of 3 or more
- E = Normal: Motor and sensory function are normal.

Treatment and rehabilitation begin at the time of the injury. Care must be taken to immobilize the spine, maintain breathing, and prevent shock. In the hospital,

*From American Spinal Injury Association: International Standards for Neurological Classification of Spinal Cord Injury, reprint Chicago, IL.

traction or surgery may be required to relieve pressure and repair tissues. Glucocorticoids such as methylprednisolone may be administered to reduce edema and stabilize the vascular system. Other injuries require prompt treatment to minimize secondary damage caused by decreased oxygen or circulation.

Ongoing care is necessary to prevent the complications related to immobility. The leading cause of death now is pneumonia, rather than renal failure. Early, extensive rehabilitation is required to learn the best ways to use the remaining function, prevent complications, and maximize independence. A team of rehabilitation professionals including occupational therapists, physiotherapists, respiratory therapists (for lesions at C4 and above), and psychotherapists can assist the patient with performance of the activities of daily living, ventilation, and other body needs. Advances in technology have provided myriad assistive devices, which can be tailored to the patient's individual needs.

With improved treatment and rehabilitation, persons with SCI are living much longer, adding the complications of aging to those of SCI. These include skin breakdown, respiratory problems, digestive and urinary tract complications, and musculoskeletal problems such as carpal tunnel syndrome and torn rotator cuff.

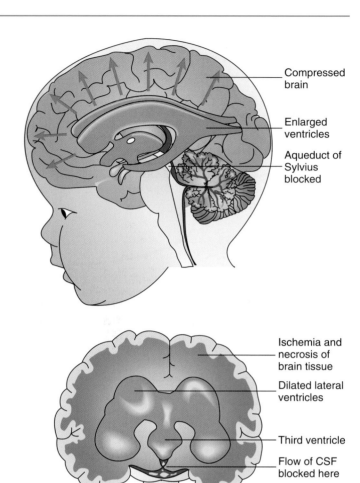

FIGURE 14-25 Hydrocephalus.

> ## THINK ABOUT 14-13
> a. Compare the immediate and permanent effects on motor function of a lumbar spinal cord injury.
> b. Explain why micturition may not occur immediately after an injury (urinary retention), but urinary incontinence may develop later.
> c. Explain several reasons why a cervical injury is much more serious than a lumbar injury.
> d. Explain the cause of spinal shock and its effects.

Congenital Neurologic Disorders

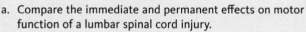

Down syndrome is discussed in Chapter 21.

Hydrocephalus

▓ *Pathophysiology*

Hydrocephalus is a condition in which excess cerebrospinal fluid (CSF) accumulates within the skull, compressing the brain tissue and blood vessels. The condition is sometimes called "water on the brain." Because the cranial sutures have not yet closed, the infant's head enlarges beyond the normal size as the amount of fluid increases. Excess CSF accumulates because more is produced than is absorbed, often because of obstruction to the flow at some point. In the majority of cases, production of CSF is normal, but there is a reduction in the amount reabsorbed. Most cases are apparent shortly after birth, but some may not be diagnosed until later in childhood.

There are two types of hydrocephalus. *Noncommunicating* or *obstructive hydrocephalus* occurs in babies when the flow of CSF through the ventricular system is blocked, usually at the aqueduct of Sylvius or the foramen magnum (Fig. 14-25). This condition usually results from a fetal developmental abnormality, such as stenosis or a neural tube defect. In many neonates, an associated myelomeningocele or Arnold-Chiari malformation is present. The obstruction leads to increased back pressure of fluid in the ventricles of the brain, which gradually dilates or enlarges the ventricles and compresses the blood vessels and brain tissue.

In the second type, *communicating hydrocephalus*, the absorption of CSF through the subarachnoid villi is impaired, resulting in increased pressure of CSF in the system. In neonates, the skull can expand to some degree in the early stages of hydrocephalus to relieve the pressure, but if the condition is not treated quickly, the brain tissue is permanently damaged.

In older children and adults, intracranial pressure (ICP) increases more rapidly than in neonates, because the fused sutures of the skull prevent expansion to accommodate the increased volume of CSF. The amount of brain damage that results depends on the rate at which pressure increases and the time that elapses before relief occurs. Other factors that increase the risk of damage may also be present in a particular patient. Brain damage may result in major physical disability and intellectual impairment because all areas of the brain are affected.

■ *Etiology*

Developmental abnormalities are the most frequent cause of hydrocephalus, particularly stenosis or atresia (the absence of a canal or opening) at the connecting channels between the ventricles or a thickened arachnoid membrane.

Obstruction may also develop at any age from tumors, infection, or scar tissue. Meningitis can cause obstructive hydrocephalus during the acute infection or lead to fibrosis in the meninges, impairing absorption.

■ *Signs and Symptoms*

The signs of increasing CSF depend on the age of the patient. In the *neonate* or young *infant*, in whom the sutures have not yet closed, the head can enlarge and the fontanels bulge in the early stages of hydrocephalus. Recording head size is a standard procedure after birth and often is done during routine examinations. With the currently brief periods of hospitalization after childbirth, this measurement may not be taken, but it can provide a basic reference point if a problem is suspected.

In the patient with hydrocephalus, scalp veins appear dilated and the eyes show the "sunset sign," in which the white sclera is visible above the colored pupil. Pupil response to light is sluggish. The infant is lethargic but irritable and difficult to feed. A high-pitched or shrill cry often occurs when the infant is moved or picked up. The condition must be diagnosed and treated as soon as possible to minimize brain damage. In older children and adults, the head cannot enlarge and the classical signs of increased ICP develop as the volume of CSF expands. These may include decreased memory, difficulty in coordination, and impaired balance. Often urinary incontinence is present. Depending on the underlying cause, other manifestations may be present.

■ *Diagnostic Tests*

A computed tomography (CT) or magnetic resonance imaging (MRI) scan can locate the obstruction or abnormal flow and determine the size of the ventricles.

■ *Treatment*

Surgery is usually performed to remove an obstruction or provide a shunt for CSF from the ventricle into the peritoneal cavity or other extracranial site, such as the right atrium of the heart. A shunt must be replaced as the child grows. Shunts are vulnerable to blockage or infection and thus require continued close monitoring to prevent further brain damage.

> **THINK ABOUT 14-14**
> a. Differentiate between communicating and noncommunicating hydrocephalus.
> b. Explain the effects of ventricular dilation.
> c. Explain why there are no focal signs of hydrocephalus in neonates.

Spina Bifida

Spina bifida refers to a group of neural tube defects that are congenital anomalies of varying severity. They are a common developmental defect, myelomeningocele occurring in an estimated 1500 to 2000 of the 4 million live births per year in the United States. The incidence rate varies in different countries, with the incidence in Canada being slightly higher than that in the United States.

■ *Pathophysiology*

The neural tube develops during the fourth week of gestation, beginning in the cervical area and progressing toward the lumbar area. The basic problem in spina bifida is failure of the posterior spinous processes on the vertebrae to fuse, which may permit the meninges and spinal cord to herniate, resulting in neurologic impairment. Any number of vertebrae can be involved, and the lumbar area is the most common location.

Three types of spina bifida are common (Fig. 14-26*A*):
- *Spina bifida occulta* develops when the spinous processes do not fuse, but herniation of the spinal cord and meninges does not occur. The defect may not be visible, although often a dimple or a tuft of hair is present on the skin over the site. The defect may be diagnosed by means of routine x-ray examination or when mild neurologic signs manifest owing to tension on the cord during a growth period.
- *Meningocele* is the same bony defect, but herniation of the meninges occurs through the defect, and the meninges and CSF form a sac on the surface. Transillumination confirms the absence of nerve tissue in the sac. Neurologic impairment is usually not present, although infection or rupture of the sac may lead to neurologic damage.
- *Myelomeningocele* is the most serious form of spina bifida. Herniation of the spinal cord and nerves along with the meninges and CSF occurs, resulting in considerable neurologic impairment (see Fig. 14-26*C*). The location and extent of the herniation determine how much function is lost. This defect is often seen in conjunction with hydrocephalus.

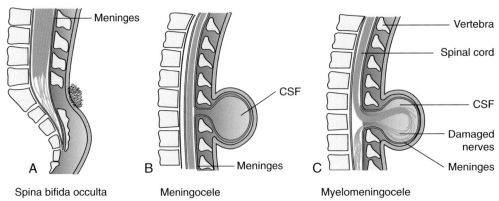

FIGURE 14-26 Spina bifida.

■ Diagnostic Tests

Alpha-fetoprotein (AFP) that has leaked from the defect results in an elevated level in maternal blood in a specimen obtained at 16 to 18 weeks' gestation. Amniocentesis detects the presence of AFP that has leaked into the amniotic fluid surrounding the fetus. The presence of spina bifida can be diagnosed prenatally by ultrasound.

■ Etiology

Spina bifida appears to have a multifactorial basis, with a combination of genetic and environmental factors contributing to its development. There is a high familial incidence of spina bifida and associated defects, such as anencephaly (absence of the cerebral hemispheres and superior cranial vault).

Environmental factors include exposure to radiation, gestational diabetes, and deficits of vitamin A or folic acid. Folic acid supplements are recommended before conception and for the first 6 weeks of pregnancy as a preventive measure. Research has shown that such supplementation reduces the incidence rate of the disorder.

■ Signs and Symptoms

Meningocele and myelomeningocele are visible as a protruding sac over the spine. In myelomeningocele, the extent of the neurologic deficit depends on the level of the defect (see Fig. 14-4) and the status of the nerve tissue; sensory and motor function at and below the level of the herniation is impaired. Some degree of muscle weakness or paralysis is present. Bladder and bowel control is usually impaired. Depending on the level of damage and the availability of reflex and sphincter control, there may be fecal and urinary incontinence.

■ Treatment

Some surgical repair of spina bifida has been done successfully in utero before birth.

Controversy continues about the timing of the surgical repair of the sac if done postnatally—whether it should take place immediately or be delayed. Rupture and infection are potential complications when repair is delayed. The decision regarding surgery also depends on the presence of other anomalies (abnormal structures) that may be present in the infant. After repair, ongoing assistance and occupational and physical therapy are required to manage the neurologic deficits. Local community services and the Spina Bifida Association, which has many local chapters, provide continuing support for the parents and the child.

Cerebral Palsy

Cerebral palsy (CP) is a group of disorders marked by some degree of motor impairment, caused by genetic mutations, abnormal fetal formation of functional brain areas, infection, or brain damage in the perinatal period. In addition, damage usually occurs in other areas of the brain, resulting in a clinical presentation that is highly variable, depending on the specific areas affected and the severity of the trauma. The damage may occur before, during, or shortly after birth and is nonprogressive. It is estimated that there are about 500,000 individuals with CP in the United States, with approximately 10,000 children developing CP each year. With improved treatment, rehabilitation, and education, many individuals with CP live into adulthood.

■ Pathophysiology

Pathologically, the brain tissue is altered by malformation, mechanical trauma, hypoxia, hemorrhage, hypoglycemia, hyperbilirubinemia, infection, or some other factor, resulting in necrosis. In some cases, generalized necrosis and atrophy of brain tissue have occurred, whereas in other cases only one or two localized areas of the brain are affected. Although all children have some degree of altered mobility, which provides the basis for classifying cerebral palsy, an assortment of other problems is present in individual cases.

■ Etiology

Single or multiple factors may be implicated in the development of cerebral palsy. Hypoxia or ischemia is the major cause of brain damage; it may occur prenatally, perinatally, or postnatally. Hypoxia may be caused by placental complications or a difficult delivery or by vascular occlusion, hemorrhage, aspiration, or respiratory impairment in the premature infant. High bilirubin levels, resulting from problems such as prematurity or Rh blood incompatibility may cause *kernicterus,* in which accumulated bilirubin crosses the blood-brain barrier and damages the neurons. Other causes of cerebral palsy include infection or metabolic abnormalities, such as hypoglycemia, in either the mother or the child.

■ Signs and Symptoms

In some cases the effects are evident at birth, whereas in others the delay in motor development or abnormal muscle tone does not become apparent for several months. Persistence of early reflexes, such as the Moro reflex, may indicate cerebral palsy.

Cerebral palsy is classified either on the basis of area affected (e.g., quadriplegia or diplegia) or on the basis of the motor disability that results (Table 14-9). Three major groups of motor disability have been identified:

- The first and largest group includes those with *spastic paralysis,* which results from damage to the pyramidal tracts (diplegia) or the motor cortex (hemiparesis), or from general cortical damage (quadriparesis). As the name indicates, this form is characterized by hyperreflexia (excessive reflex response). For example, crossed legs are apparent when the child is held up or a child with some mobility walks with a typical scissors gait (i.e., on the toes and with crossed legs).
- The second group is *dyskinetic* disease, which results from damage to the extrapyramidal tract, basal nuclei, or cranial nerves. This form of cerebral palsy is manifested by athetoid or choreiform involuntary

movements and loss of coordination with fine movements.
- The third group, *ataxic* cerebral palsy, commonly develops from damage to the cerebellum and manifests as loss of balance and coordination.
- Spasticity is manifested by increased muscle tone or resistance to passive movement, with excessive reflex responses. Unilateral use of the hands or feet and asymmetric body movements are indications of abnormality. Writhing movements or facial grimaces may indicate athetoid cerebral palsy. Feeding difficulties and constant tongue thrusting are signs of motor dysfunction and may interfere with nutrition and growth. The position of the child's limbs when resting or when held up is often unusual (e.g., scissors position of the legs).

In addition to the motor deficit, cerebral palsy may be accompanied by many other problems, which depend on the other areas of brain damage. A few common areas of dysfunction are:

- Intellectual function
- Communication and speech
- Seizures
- Visual problems

With regard to cognitive function, one third of persons with cerebral palsy are considered to have normal intelligence, one third are mildly impaired, and one third are severely cognitively disabled.

Communication and speech development are difficult because of motor disability, possible impaired mentation, and visual or hearing deficits. A number of children have learning disabilities and behavioral problems, such as attention deficit disorder, spatial disorientation, and hyperactivity.

Seizures, primarily of the generalized tonic-clonic type, are common. Visual problems, such as astigmatism and strabismus, occur frequently.

■ Treatment

Because each infant has a unique set of problems, individualized and immediate therapy is necessary. Early stimulation programs with a team of health professionals are helpful in encouraging motor skills, coordination, and intellectual development. Assessment and therapy by speech and language pathologists can assist parents in dealing with feeding and swallowing problems, positioning the child correctly, reducing the effects of tongue thrusting, and encouraging communication.

Physical therapy is essential to maximize physical development. Regular exercise therapy and use of devices such as braces can improve mobility and reduce deformities. A program called MEDEK (CME) is a therapeutic exercise program offered by trained professionals to some infants and young children with developmental problems involving skeletal muscle, particularly hypotonia. This is a strenuous program of repetitive exercises designed to promote strength, mobility, and

TABLE 14-9	**Cerebral Palsy**		
Type	Percentage of Cases	Area of Damage	Effects
Spastic	65%-75%	Motor cortex or pyramidal tracts	Paralysis Hyperreflexia and increased muscle tone
Dyskinetic	20%-25%	Basal nuclei or extrapyramidal tracts	Loss of motor control and coordination Athetoid or choreiform movements
Ataxic	5%	Cerebellum	Gait disturbance Loss of balance
Mixed	13%	All of above	Some of each of above

independence. No devices or machines are used. The program may be offered in private clinics or combined with traditional therapies, which are required for older children. Family members can be trained to provide regular exercise and thus reduce the incidence of complications.

Occupational therapy works with the child to maximize hand function, teach the use of adaptive devices, and facilitate the development of skills associated with normal development and academic work, as well as providing adaptive devices to maximize mobility and independence.

Specialists in early education for developmentally handicapped children can work with the child and the family to develop and maximize motor skills, eye-hand coordination, and reflex responses. As the child develops, simple exercises can be instituted to help in learning to recognize familiar objects or sounds, associating cause with effect, and identifying likes and dislikes. Appropriate medication to control seizures prevents complications.

Hearing and vision require monitoring in the early stages, and some form of communication must be developed as soon as possible. Many new devices and techniques are now available to promote communication. Technologic advances, including computers, provide aids for many different problems and enable many individuals to live more independently and develop individual interests and skills. In many areas, children with cerebral palsy are being integrated into mainstream classes in schools and other activities.

THINK ABOUT 14-15

a. Compare Down syndrome (see Chapter 21) and cerebral palsy with regard to cause and effects on motor and cognitive abilities.
b. Describe the factors that could interfere with communication in a child with cerebral palsy.
c. Discuss how technology may provide accommodation for communication deficits.

Seizure Disorders

Seizures result from uncontrolled, excessive discharge of neurons in the brain. The activity may be localized or generalized. They have many possible causes. Seizure disorders are characterized by recurrent seizures, sometimes called convulsions. It is estimated that 3 to 6 million affected individuals exist in the United States. The onset occurs before age 20 in 75% of cases. *Epilepsy* is the old term for recurrent seizures, rarely used today because of the stigma once attached to the term.

Seizure disorders are classified by their location in the brain and their clinical features, including characteristic EEG patterns during and between seizures. The

---

BOX 14-1 Classification of Seizures

I. Partial seizures (focal)
  a. Simple
    1. Motor (includes jacksonian)
    2. Sensory (e.g., visual, auditory)
    3. Autonomic
    4. Psychic
  b. Complex (impaired consciousness)
    1. Temporal lobe or psychomotor
  c. Partial leading to generalized seizures
II. Generalized (both hemispheres affected with loss of consciousness)
  a. Tonic-clonic (grand mal)
  b. Absence (petit mal)
  c. Myoclonic
  d. Infantile spasms
  e. Atonic (akinetic)
  f. Lennox-Gastaut syndrome (febrile seizures)
III. Unclassified

---

international classification of seizures is summarized in Box 14-1, a commonly accepted classification that incorporates current terminology and divides seizures into two basic categories, generalized and partial.

Generalized seizures have multiple foci or origins in the deep structures of both cerebral hemispheres and the brain stem and cause loss of consciousness, whereas *partial seizures* have a single or focal origin, often in the cerebral cortex, and may or may not involve altered consciousness. However, partial seizures may progress to generalized seizures.

Seizures may be primary (idiopathic) or secondary (acquired) with an identified cause, such as posttraumatic syndrome. Seizures can be categorized on other grounds because they may result from an abnormality in the brain or from systemic causes, such as hypoglycemia or withdrawal from certain drugs. They may be a temporary problem, such as febrile seizures in an infant, or they may be chronic and frequent. An individual can have more than one type of seizure. For example, absence seizures, which are common in children, may decrease or be replaced by tonic-clonic or psychomotor seizures. Common types of seizures are described in the section on signs and symptoms.

■ *Pathophysiology*

A seizure results from a sudden, spontaneous, uncontrolled depolarization of neurons, which causes abnormal motor or sensory activity and possibly loss of consciousness. The neurons in the epileptogenic focus are hyperexcitable and have a lowered threshold for stimulation. Any physiologic change, such as alkalosis or other sensory stimulus—for example, flashing lights—can easily activate the "irritable" neurons. These focal cells stimulate the surrounding normal cells, spreading the activity. There are various theories about the specific mechanism for seizure activity, including altered permeability of the neuronal membrane, reduced inhibitory control of neurons, or a transmitter imbalance.

Each seizure lasts for a few seconds or minutes, and the excessive activity of the neurons then ceases *spontaneously.* The altered pattern of electrical activity, or brain waves, during a seizure can be demonstrated on an EEG, indicating the type of seizure and its focus. Also, observation and description of the seizure by bystanders, particularly its initial effects, is useful in identifying the origin or focus of the seizure.

Complications may arise from generalized tonic-clonic (grand mal) seizures that are severe and frequent. Injuries may occur during a seizure.

Recurrent or continuous seizures without recovery of consciousness are termed *status epilepticus.* This condition may lead to serious consequences if it is not treated promptly. Respiration is impaired during a generalized tonic-clonic seizure and skeletal muscle activity is intense; the combination of these events in status epilepticus can lead to severe hypoxia, hypoglycemia, acidosis, and decreased blood pressure, potentially resulting in brain damage.

■ *Etiology*

Many seizure disorders are idiopathic. To date, four genes have been identified as having a role in seizure disorders. Familial incidence is more evident in young children.

Children with congenital disorders, such as cerebral palsy, may have seizures resulting from the brain damage. Acquired seizures that occur after head injury or infection are more common now because improved treatment of these primary conditions has led to a higher survival rate. A seizure may be initiated by a tumor, infection, or hemorrhage in the brain, or by a high fever in an infant or young child (febrile seizure). Some systemic disorders, such as renal failure or hypoglycemia, may precipitate a seizure in an individual who has no previous history of seizures. Sudden withdrawal from sedatives or alcohol can precipitate seizures as well as drugs such as cocaine.

Precipitating factors, or triggers, of an individual seizure may include physical stimuli, such as loud noises or bright lights, or biochemical stimuli, such as stress, excessive premenstrual fluid retention, hypoglycemia, change in medication, or hyperventilation (alkalosis). Awareness and avoidance of the potential precipitating factors in an individual can reduce the frequency of seizures. The medical history should be updated frequently to note changes in precipitating factors and the type of seizure.

■ *Signs and Symptoms*

■ *Generalized Seizures. Absence (petit mal) seizures* are generalized seizures that are more common in children

than adults, beginning about age 5. The seizure lasts for 5 to 10 seconds and may occur many times during the day. There is a brief loss of awareness and sometimes transient facial movements, such as twitches of the eyelids or lip smacking. Usually the child simply stares into space for a moment and then resumes the activity previously pursued. No memory of the episode is retained.

Tonic-clonic (grand mal) seizures are generalized seizures that may occur spontaneously or after simple seizures. There is a pattern for this type of seizure, which usually ends spontaneously:

- Prodromal signs occur in some individuals, such as nausea, irritability, depression, or muscle twitching some hours before the seizure.
- An aura, such as a peculiar visual or auditory sensation, immediately precedes the loss of consciousness in many persons.
- Loss of consciousness occurs, and the individual falls to the floor.
- Strong tonic muscle contraction, resulting briefly in flexion, is followed by extension of the limbs and rigidity in the trunk (ictal phase).
- A cry escapes as the abdominal and thoracic muscles contract, forcing air out of the lungs. The jaws are clenched tightly, and respiration ceases.
- The clonic stage follows, in which the muscles alternately contract and relax, resulting in a series of forceful jerky movements that involve the entire body. Increased salivation (foaming at the mouth) and bowel and bladder incontinence may occur.
- Contractions gradually subside spontaneously in several minutes; the body is limp and consciousness slowly returns.
- The person is confused and fatigued, with aching muscles, and falls into a deep sleep in this postictal period.

EMERGENCY TREATMENT FOR SEIZURES

1. If possible, clear a space and gently place the person on the floor, positioning him or her on the side, cushioning the head, and loosening neckwear.
2. Move potentially harmful objects away from the patient.
3. Do not force a specific position or unduly restrain the person, which can cause injury.
4. Do not put anything in the person's mouth.
5. When the seizure ends, offer reassurance and check breathing and patient orientation to surroundings.
6. If the seizure continues or immediately repeats, seek medical assistance.

The prodromal indications and occasionally the aura may be remembered by the person but not the entire seizure (amnesia). Hypoxia is common at this time because of interference with respiration during the seizure and because some airway obstruction may be present, owing to excess saliva or tongue position. Also, the contracting muscles present an increased demand for oxygen during the seizure. Increased levels of lactic acid and carbon dioxide in the body fluids contribute to acidosis. Recurrent tonic-clonic seizures without full return to consciousness are termed *status epilepticus* and carry an increased risk of complications.

■ *Partial Seizures.* Simple partial or focal seizures arise from an epileptogenic focus, often related to a single area of damage in the cortex. They are manifested by repeated motor activity, such as jerking or turning the head or eye aside, jerky movements of a leg, or by a sensation such as tingling that begins in one area and may spread. Auditory or visual experiences, such as ringing in the ears or a sensation of light, may occur if the focus is in the related area. Memory and consciousness remain, although awareness is reduced. A *jacksonian seizure* is a focal motor seizure in which the clonic contractions begin in a specific area and spread progressively; for example, the contractions "march" up the arm and then to the face.

Children and adults may have complex partial, temporal lobe, or psychomotor seizures. They usually arise from the temporal lobe, but may involve the limbic system or frontal lobe. Sometimes an aura is present, such as the perception of an odd odor. The seizure itself consists of bizarre behavior, perhaps repetitive and purposeful but *inappropriate*; for example, waving or clapping the hands. Frequently visual or auditory hallucinations or feelings of déjà vu (perceiving strange surroundings as familiar) occur. The person is unresponsive to people or activities during the seizure, and afterward he or she is amnesic and drowsy.

■ Diagnostic Tests
A detailed medical history and description of the seizure is required. An EEG will determine the type and location of the seizure. An MRI can detect any structural abnormality in the brain.

■ Treatment
Any primary cause should be treated, and the specific factors that precipitate seizures should be identified and avoided.

Anticonvulsant drugs, such as phenytoin (Dilantin), are prescribed to raise the threshold for neuronal stimulation and prevent seizures. A choice of anticonvulsant drugs is available to treat different types of seizures and for optimum control in an individual patient. In many cases, anticonvulsant drugs are combined with sedatives, such as phenobarbital, to allow a reduction in the dosage and side effects of the drugs, while simultaneously decreasing the occurrence of seizures. Phenobarbital increases liver enzyme activity, and therefore may affect the dosage of other medications. Phenytoin may cause gingival hyperplasia (Fig. 14-27), which can cause

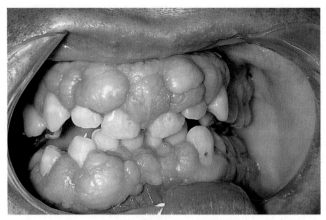

FIGURE 14-27   An example of gingival hyperplasia associated with the medication phenytoin (Dilantin) used to treat seizures. Compare with normal gingiva in Figure 20-7A. *(Courtesy of Evie Jesin, RRDH, BSe, George Brown College of Applied Arts and Technology, Toronto, Ontario, Canada.)*

difficulty in maintaining good oral hygiene and create a cosmetic problem for the patient. Many anticonvulsant drugs reduce leukocyte counts, thus predisposing the patient to infection. Several drugs reduce blood-clotting capability. It is essential to continue medication as prescribed at set intervals and without omissions, because sudden withdrawal can cause more severe seizures or status epilepticus, with its risk of brain damage.

Once a seizure begins it cannot be stopped. Single episodes require no additional medical treatment unless the individual continues to be disoriented. Prolonged or recurrent seizures (status epilepticus) are life threatening and require hospital treatment with medications such as intravenous diazepam, oxygen, and fluids.

During pregnancy, some women have an increased number of seizures. There is an increase in the incidence of congenital abnormalities in children born to mothers with seizure disorders; this is probably related to drug therapy.

> **THINK ABOUT 14-16**
>
> a. Describe how a seizure develops in the brain tissue.
> b. Differentiate a partial seizure from a general seizure and give an example of each.
> c. Describe factors that should be avoided if a patient has a history of seizures.
> d. List the sequence of events in a generalized tonic-clonic seizure.

Chronic Degenerative Disorders

Multiple Sclerosis

Multiple sclerosis (MS) involves a progressive demyelination of the neurons of the brain, spinal cord, and

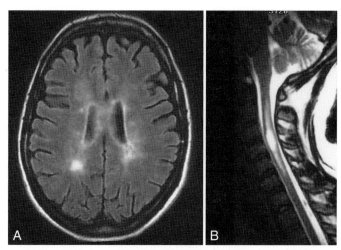

FIGURE 14-28 **A,** Typical white matter changes around the ventricles shown on MRI in multiple sclerosis. **B,** Change in the spinal cord in multiple sclerosis. *(From Perkin GD:* Mosby's Color Atlas and Text of Neurology, *ed 2, London, 2002, Mosby.)*

cranial nerves. There are a number of types of MS with considerable variation in the effects, severity, and progression in any one individual. Multiple sclerosis is characterized by remissions and exacerbations, but nevertheless is marked by progressive degeneration. Estimated incidence runs from 30 to 100 per 100,000 persons. It is the second most common cause of disability in the United States; motor vehicle accidents are the first.

Pathophysiology

Loss of myelin interferes with the conduction of impulses in the affected fibers. It affects all types of nerve fibers—motor, sensory, and autonomic—and occurs in diffuse patches throughout the nervous system (Fig. 14-28). Recent research has shown that cognitive function can be impaired in the client with MS, particularly with respect to attention to tasks and memory.

The earliest lesion occurs as an inflammatory response as cells that normally do not enter the brain or spinal cord do so and attack neurons, with loss of myelin in the white matter of the brain or spinal cord. Recent research has identified a protein in the body's blood clotting mechanism as a potential trigger of the immune response. Later larger areas of inflammation and demyelination, termed *plaques,* become visible, frequently beside the lateral ventricles in the brain, in the brain stem, and in the optic nerves.

Initially the area of plaque appears pinkish and edematous, but then it becomes gray and firm. Each plaque varies in size, and several may coalesce into a single patch. The initial inflammation may subside, and neural function may return to normal for a short time, until another exacerbation occurs. In time neural degeneration becomes irreversible, and function is lost permanently. With each recurrence, additional areas of the central nervous system (CNS) are involved. Multiple

sclerosis varies in severity, occurring in mild and slowly progressive patterns in some individuals and in rapidly progressive forms in others.

Etiology

The onset of symptoms usually occurs in individuals between ages 20 and 40, with a peak at 30 years. The disease is more common in women by a 2:1 ratio. The cause is unknown, although many researchers believe it is an autoimmune disorder. However it may be even more complex in its origins. Multiple sclerosis appears to have genetic, immunologic, and environmental components. Multiple sclerosis occurs more frequently in people of European descent, and there is an increased risk for close relatives of affected individuals. The environmental factors have not yet been determined, although it is thought that climate may play a role because the disease is more common in temperate zones (northern United States and Canada) and in individuals who grow up in temperate climates. However there are exceptions to this factor, where MS occurs in warm climates. Viral infection and an abnormal immune response have also been suspected.

Signs and Symptoms

The manifestations of MS are determined by the areas that are demyelinated in each individual (Fig. 14-29). Blurred vision is a common early sign. Initially weakness in the legs often occurs, resulting from plaques on the corticospinal tract. If the cranial nerves are affected, diplopia (double vision), scotoma (a spot in the visual field), or dysarthria (poor articulation) may occur. Paresthesias, areas of numbness, burning, or tingling develop if the sensory nerve fibers are damaged. As the number of plaques increases with each exacerbation, progressive weakness and paralysis extending to the upper limbs, loss of coordination, and bladder, bowel, and sexual dysfunction occur. Chronic fatigue is common. Sensory deficits include paresthesias and loss of position sense in the upper body, face, and legs. The clinical picture and mode of progression vary greatly among individuals. Later in the course of the disease, depression or euphoria may develop. Complications related to immobility, such as respiratory infection, decubitus ulcers, and contractures, are common as the disease progresses.

Diagnostic Tests

There is no definitive test for multiple sclerosis, and a long delay may precede the diagnosis. A history of exacerbations and remissions, involvement of multiple focal areas, progression, and absence of other neurologic diagnostic criteria are often the basis for an initial diagnosis of MS. Magnetic resonance imaging studies are best for diagnosis and monitoring and are able to detect multiple CNS lesions. Often patients have elevated protein, gamma globulin, and lymphocytes levels in the CSF.

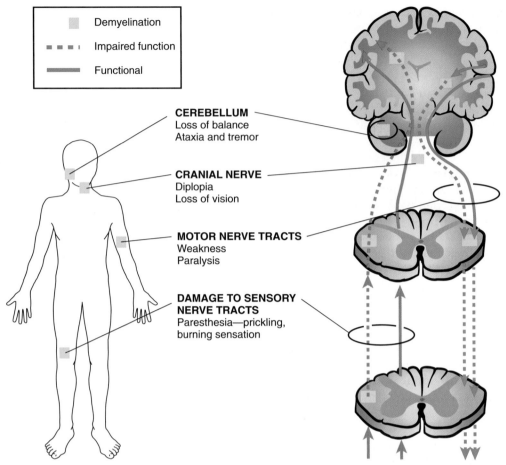

FIGURE 14-29 Multiple sclerosis—distribution of lesions.

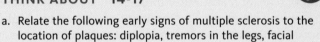

▓ *Treatment*

No specific treatment is available at this time, although new measures are always being investigated. Interferon beta-1b (Betaseron) appears to reduce the frequency and severity of exacerbations through its effects on the immune system. Glucocorticoid agents may help to control acute signs during exacerbations. Drugs to target the abnormal clotting proteins in the brain are being developed. Additional drugs may be prescribed as muscle relaxants or for other complications. The number of exacerbations can be reduced by avoiding excessive fatigue, stress, injury, or infection.

Therapy includes physical therapy and exercise to maintain mobility. Occupational therapy is essential in assessing the need for and provision of adaptive devices to simplify work and reduce fatigue. Special problems, such as constipation or incontinence, require individual attention. Communication and interest must be maintained by addressing issues such as visual impairment or speech disorders early in the course of the disease. Early intervention by a speech and language pathologist can maximize communication and assist with some feeding problems. As with any disabling condition, rehabilitation and psychosocial support are essential in maximizing function.

THINK ABOUT 14-17

a. Relate the following early signs of multiple sclerosis to the location of plaques: diplopia, tremors in the legs, facial weakness.

b. Relate the frequency of exacerbations to the progress of the disease.

Parkinson's Disease (Paralysis Agitans)

Parkinson's disease is a progressive degenerative disorder, affecting motor function through loss of extrapyramidal activity. It is estimated that 5000 individuals develop Parkinson's disease each year and that between 500,000 and 1.5 million Americans have Parkinson's disease.

▓ *Pathophysiology*

In Parkinson's disease, dysfunction of the *extrapyramidal motor system* occurs because of progressive degenerative changes in the basal nuclei, principally in the *substantia nigra*. In this condition, a decreased number of neurons in the substantia nigra secrete dopamine, an inhibitory neurotransmitter, leading to an imbalance between excitation and inhibition in the basal nuclei. The excess stimulation affects movement and posture by increasing muscle tone and activity, leading to resting tremors, muscular rigidity, difficulty in initiating movement, and postural instability. Many patients with Parkinson's disease have a reduced number of cortical neurons, which is characteristic of dementia. Diagnosis depends on the physical manifestations and clinical history.

■ Etiology

Primary or idiopathic Parkinson's disease usually develops after age 60 and occurs in both men and women. Several genes have been identified in cases of familial Parkinson's disease, but a common focus of research is the possible damaging effects of viruses or toxins on cells. Recent research has focused on the mitochondrial changes in cells from patients with Parkinson's disease; these changes suggest periods of significant oxidative stress leading to the accumulation of free radicals within the cells.

Secondary Parkinsonism may follow encephalitis, trauma, or vascular disease. Drug-induced Parkinson's disease is linked particularly to use of the phenothiazines (e.g., chlorpromazine). The effects may be reversible or diminished when the drug is discontinued.

■ Signs and Symptoms

Early signs include fatigue, muscle weakness, muscle aching, decreased flexibility, and less spontaneous change in facial expression. More obvious signs are tremors in the hands at rest and a repetitive "pill-rolling" motion of the hands. Tremors cease with voluntary movement and during sleep. As the disease advances, tremors affect the hands and feet, the face, tongue, and lips. Further motor impairment, increased muscle rigidity, difficulty in initiating movement, slow movements (bradykinesia), and a lack of associated involuntary movement occurs; for example, loss of arm-swinging when walking or spontaneous postural adjustments when sitting. The characteristic standing posture is stooped, leaning forward with the head and neck flexed (Fig. 14-30). Festination, or a propulsive gait (short, shuffling steps with increasing acceleration), occurs as postural reflexes are impaired, leading to falls. Complex activities, such as getting up out of a chair, become slow and difficult.

Other functions are affected as the voice becomes low and devoid of inflection (the person speaks in a quiet monotone) and dysarthria develops. Chewing and swallowing become difficult, prolonging eating time and causing recurrent drooling. The face of the patient resembles a mask, and blinking of the eyelids is reduced, resulting in a blank, staring face. Autonomic dysfunction is manifested in the later stages by urinary retention, constipation, and orthostatic hypotension. As orthostatic hypotension develops, the threat of falls increases. Urinary tract and respiratory infections are

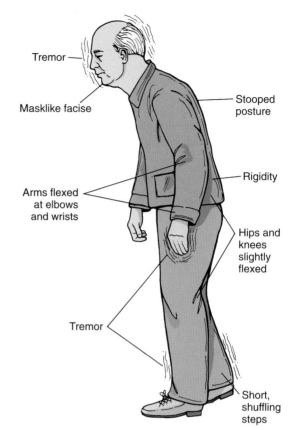

FIGURE 14-30 Parkinson's disease. *(From Monahan FD, Drake T, Neighbors M:* Nursing Care of Adults, *Philadelphia, 1994, Saunders.)*

common complications. Dementia develops late in the course of the disease in 20% of affected persons.

■ Treatment

Dopamine replacement therapy has been used to reduce motor impairment. Levodopa (l-dopa), a precursor of dopamine, is administered because dopamine itself does not cross the blood-brain barrier. Selegiline (Eldepryl), a drug that blocks the breakdown of l-dopa in the brain, has resulted in improvement for some individuals. Anticholinergic drugs are also helpful. Several drugs are under investigation, as are new surgical procedures and transplants of fetal dopamine-producing cells or adult stem cells. Drug treatment may also include the use of antidepressant drugs to deal with the depression that often develops as the disease progresses.

Swallowing and speech impairments require early attention from a speech and language pathologist to maintain function as long as possible. Physical therapy is helpful in maintaining general mobility. Exercise that promotes the use of the arms and forceful movements are helpful. Occupational therapists work to improve balance, coordination, and safe use of adaptive devices.

Constant monitoring and immediate treatment of respiratory and urinary tract infections can reduce the risk of damage to the organs involved.

THINK ABOUT 14-18

a. Describe the pathophysiology of Parkinson's disease.
b. Describe three common manifestations that can be observed in a person with Parkinson's disease.
c. Explain why adequate nutrition and hydration may be difficult to maintain in a person with Parkinson's disease.
d. If adequate nutrition and hydration are not maintained, what potential complications may ensue?

Amyotrophic Lateral Sclerosis

The name of this disease, amyotrophic lateral sclerosis (ALS), is indicative of the pathology: amyotrophic means "muscle wasting" and sclerosis refers to the degenerative "hardening" of the lateral corticospinal tracts. The cause has not been identified, although a number of genes on various chromosomes have been linked to the disease. Ten percent of cases are considered familial. Most cases are random and do not reflect any ethnic trends in incidence. The disease is invariably fatal over time.

The disease, also called Lou Gehrig's disease, primarily affects individuals between the ages of 40 and 60, particularly men. The prevalence is 6 to 8 per 100,000. Although the disease is not common, it has attracted public attention because there is no means of preventing the continuous and rapid decline of motor and respiratory function, whereas cognitive function remains intact. Amyotrophic lateral sclerosis has been the focus of debate by the public and legislative and medical groups regarding ethical issues surrounding euthanasia for patients with such diseases.

Pathophysiology

Amyotrophic lateral sclerosis is a progressive degenerative disease affecting both upper motor neurons in the cerebral cortex and lower motor neurons in the brain stem and spinal cord. There is no indication of inflammation around the nerves. Recent studies have shown that supportive glial cells called *astrocytes* secrete a neurotoxin leading to the death of motor neurons. The loss of upper motor neurons leads to spastic paralysis and hyperreflexia; damage to lower motor neurons results in flaccid paralysis, with decreased muscle tone and reflexes. Sensory neurons, cognitive function, and cranial nerves III, IV, and VI to the eye muscles are not affected. The loss of neurons occurs in a diffuse and asymmetric pattern but proceeds without remission. Progressive muscle weakness eventually affects respiratory function. Although a specific diagnostic test has not been available to confirm the presence of the disease, many tests are required to eliminate other possible diagnoses. At present, a new test for specific biomarkers in CSF is under evaluation. Nerve conduction velocity tests and tests of muscle response to electrical stimulation are also used to evaluate the patient's myoneural function.

Signs and Symptoms

Initially in most cases, the upper extremities, particularly the hands, manifest weakness and muscle atrophy, with loss of fine motor coordination commencing with the distal fibers. Stumbling and falls are common. Muscle cramps or twitching may result from an imbalance of antagonistic muscles. The weakness and paralysis progress throughout the body. Dysarthria develops as the cranial nerves controlling speech are lost. Eventually swallowing and respiration are impaired, and a ventilator is required.

Treatment

At this time, no specific treatment is available to slow the degenerative process. Stem cell therapy is under investigation. A new drug, Rilutek (riluzole) has been developed to slow further damage to neurons; this can assist with maintaining swallowing and ventilation reflexes. A well-balanced program of moderate exercise and rest is helpful. Electronic communication devices are recommended for use relatively early in the course of the disease. A team approach to care can minimize the complications of immobility, sustain function as long as possible, and support the family. The team includes a respiratory therapist, nutritionist, speech pathologist, occupational therapist, physical therapist, psychologist, and social worker. In most cases respiratory failure occurs in 2 to 5 years, although some individuals survive for a longer period.

Myasthenia Gravis

Myasthenia gravis is an autoimmune disorder that impairs the receptors for acetylcholine (ACh) at the neuromuscular junction. The specific cause is not known, although many patients have thymus disorders, such as hyperplasia or benign tumors. Women are more frequently affected than men, and the age of onset is between ages 20 and 30 for women and greater than age 50 for men.

Pathophysiology

In myasthenia gravis, IgG autoantibodies to ACh receptors form, blocking and ultimately destroying the receptor site, thus preventing any further stimulation of the muscle. This change leads to skeletal muscle weakness and rapid fatigue of the affected muscles. The facial and ocular muscles are usually affected initially, followed by the arm and trunk muscles.

Diagnostic Tests

Several tests are available, including electromyography, to test for muscle fatigue, and an assay of serum antibodies. One test uses edrophonium chloride (Tensilon), a short-acting anticholinesterase inhibitor, to prolong the action of ACh at the myoneural junction, resulting in a short period of increased skeletal muscle function.

Signs and Symptoms

Muscle weakness is noticeable in the face and eyes, and fatigue develops quickly when the muscles are being used. Diplopia and ptosis impair vision, and speech becomes a nasal monotone. Spontaneous facial expressions are lost, and the face appears to droop with sadness. Attempts to smile may result in what appears to be a snarl. Chewing and swallowing become difficult as the weakness progresses and the risk of aspiration increases. The head droops as the neck muscles become involved. As the arms become weaker, it is difficult for the person to comb hair, brush teeth, or prepare and eat food. Muscle fatigue becomes more marked as the day progresses. Upper respiratory infections occur frequently and tend to be prolonged, because it becomes more difficult to remove secretions. *Myasthenic crisis*, which may occur when there is added stress—such as infection, trauma, or alcohol intake—involves an increase in weakness and fatigue, and respiratory impairment may develop.

Treatment

Anticholinesterase agents, such as pyridostigmine (Mestinon) or neostigmine (Prostigmin), may be used to temporarily improve neuromuscular transmission. These agents prolong the action of ACh at the neuromuscular junction and facilitate eating and swallowing. Glucocorticoids such as prednisone are effective in suppressing the immune system. Plasmapheresis, a process that removes antibodies from the blood, may help temporarily. Thymectomy may be helpful in reducing symptoms if hyperplasia or an adenoma is present. The long-term prognosis is increasing generalized weakness with eventual weakness of respiratory muscles.

> **THINK ABOUT 14-19**
>
> a. Explain why a person with myasthenia gravis might prefer a soft diet. List several potential complications of a continued soft diet.
> b. Describe how oral hygiene might be affected by myasthenia gravis.
> c. Compare the pathophysiology, significant early signs or symptoms, and course of amyotrophic lateral sclerosis, myasthenia gravis, multiple sclerosis, and Guillain-Barré syndrome

Huntington Disease

Huntington disease (HD), or Huntington's chorea, is an inherited disorder that does not manifest until midlife. Maternal inheritance delays onset longer than inheritance from fathers. It has a prevalence of 5 per 100,000

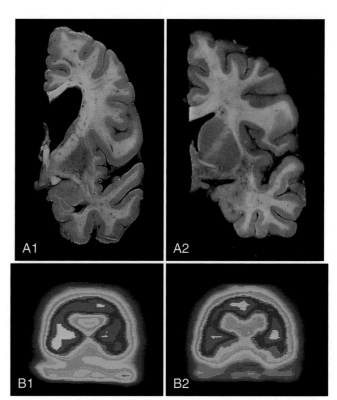

FIGURE 14-31 Huntington's Disease A, Coronal section of the brain shows a dilated lateral ventricle with caudate and lentiform atrophy on the left compared with a normal brain on the right. **B,** Reduced caudate blood flow shown on the left, compared to normal blood flow on the right, shown in single photon emission CT scan. *(From Perkin GD: Mosby's Color Atlas and Text of Neurology, ed 2, St. Louis, 2002, Mosby.)*

people and affects all ethnic groups. It is estimated that 15,000 people have HD in the United States and greater than 150,000 individuals face a 50% chance of inheriting the disorder.

Pathophysiology

Progressive atrophy of the brain occurs, with degeneration of neurons, particularly in the basal ganglia and the frontal cortex. The ventricles are dilated (Fig. 14-31). There is depletion of gamma-aminobutyric acid (GABA), an inhibitory neurotransmitter in the basal nuclei and substantia nigra. Levels of ACh in the brain also appear to be reduced.

Etiology

This condition is inherited as an autosomal-dominant trait (about a 50% probability of having an affected child) and is carried on chromosome 4. Until recently there were no diagnostic tests available to identify affected individuals before the onset of symptoms; therefore children with a high risk of inheritance were once born to affected parents before the disease was diagnosed in the parents. This combination of factors increased the incidence of the disorder. That trend is changing because testing and genetic counseling are available. However, in one in three newly diagnosed cases there is no record of family members with the disorder.

Signs and Symptoms

At the onset, mood swings and personality changes develop, as well as restlessness and choreiform (rapid, jerky) movements in the arms and face. There may also be early indications of intellectual impairment, such as difficulty learning new information, loss of problem-solving skills, poor judgment, inability to concentrate, and memory lapses. With progressive degeneration, rigidity and akinesia develop, making any movement difficult. Personality changes, moodiness, and behavioral disturbances become more marked as dementia progresses.

Diagnostic Tests

The presence of the defective gene can be detected by DNA analysis.

Treatment

No therapy is available to slow the progress of the disease. Symptomatic therapy, such as physiotherapy or tetrabenazine, a new drug approved in 2008, may reduce the choreiform movements and maintain mobility for a longer time. Other drugs may be used to treat behavior changes. In later stages the patient with HD requires significant supportive care for physical needs.

Dementia

There are many formal definitions of dementia, based on the following characteristics. It is a progressive chronic disease, in which cortical function is decreased, impairing cognitive skills such as language and innumeracy, logical thinking and judgment, ability to learn new information, as well as motor coordination. Loss of memory affects primarily short-term or recent memory, but includes confusion about the events in long-term memory. Memory loss is often progressive, leading to long-term as well as short-term memory loss. Behavioral and personality changes are usually present. These changes lead to inability to work and perform activities of daily living.

Tests are available for a behavioral assessment and to distinguish between "normal forgetfulness" and memory loss related to dementia. For example, forgetful people can remember when clues are available, handle finances, and function independently. In a person with dementia, recall does not occur after being given clues, the day cannot be identified, calculations are difficult, and reminders are needed for meals and hygiene.

There are many causes of dementia, including vascular disease (e.g., arteriosclerosis), infections, toxins, and genetic disorders. Alzheimer's disease accounts for more than 50% of those affected with dementia with vascular causes of dementia in second place.

Alzheimer's Disease

Approximately 10% of the population greater than 65 years of age has Alzheimer's disease (AD), and this increases to over 25% in the age group greater than 85 years. Females are affected more than males. It is estimated that between 4.5 and 5.4 million Americans are affected by AD.

In Alzheimer's disease there is a progressive loss of intellectual function that eventually interferes with work, relationships, and personal hygiene. Personality changes, lack of initiative, and repetitive behavior and impairments in judgment, abstract thinking, and problem-solving abilities are characteristic of the disease.

Pathophysiology

Typical changes in Alzheimer's disease include progressive cortical atrophy, which leads to dilated ventricles, and widening of the sulci (Fig. 14-32). Neurofibrillary tangles in the neurons and senile plaques are found in large numbers in the affected parts of the brain. The plaques, which disrupt neural conduction, contain fragments from beta-amyloid precursor protein (βAPP); the role of this protein is a focus of research. Some neurofibrils and plaques have been found in the brains of elderly people whose cognitive function is not impaired, and therefore it appears that the numbers and distribution of the plaques are the significant factors. A deficit of the neurotransmitter ACh also occurs in the affected brain.

No definitive diagnostic tests are available; the diagnosis is based on observations and ruling out other possible causes. Progressive tests of memory are very helpful in making a probable diagnosis of AD. Some cases of dementia have been labeled Alzheimer's disease, and then later classified as another form of dementia.

Etiology

The specific cause is unknown.

At least four defective genes located on different chromosomes have been associated with AD. Three gene mutations on chromosomes 1, 14, and 21 are inherited as autosomal dominant traits resulting in early onset AD. The genetic factor is also supported by the high incidence in older persons with Down syndrome (trisomy 21). One form of late onset AD has been linked to a mutation on chromosome 19. Other forms of Alzheimer's disease appear to be multifactorial in origin. The National Institute on Aging has launched major research investigations into genetic and other suspected factors, including exposure to metals, viruses, and metabolic syndrome.

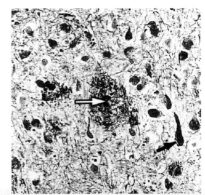

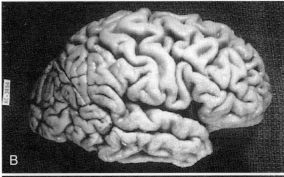

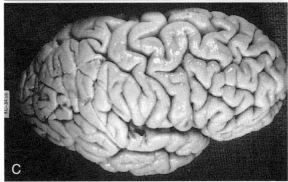

FIGURE 14-32 **Pathologic Changes in Alzheimer's Disease A**, A mature plaque with central amyloid core (*white arrow*) next to a neurofibrillary tangle (*black arrow*). **B**, Alzheimer's disease: brain is smaller with narrower gyri and wider sulci, particularly in frontal and temporal lobes. **C**, Comparable normal brain. *(From Damjanov I, Linder J: Anderson's Pathology, ed 10, St. Louis, 1996, Mosby.)*

▓ *Signs and Symptoms*

There is less emphasis on differentiating the pathophysiology and signs of early versus late-onset disease. Several research projects are, however, focused on defining the signs at the time of onset and through the stages to determine the pattern of neurologic damage.

Onset tends to be insidious. The course may extend over 10 to 20 years:

- In the early stage, gradual loss of memory and lack of concentration become apparent. Ability to learn new information and to reason is impaired and behavioral changes, such as irritability, hostility, and mood swings, are common.
- Cognitive function, memory, and language skills continue to decline. Problem solving, mathematical

ability, and judgment are poor. Apathy, indifference, and confusion become more marked. Managing the activities of daily living becomes difficult, affecting meal preparation, dressing, and personal hygiene. Wandering is common and the person may become confused and lost, even in familiar territory.

- In the late stage, the person does not recognize his or her family, lacks awareness or interest in the environment, is incontinent, and is unable to function in any way. Degenerative changes may gradually interfere with motor function.

▓ *Treatment*

Although no specific treatment is available to reverse the effects of AD, occupational therapy is important in assessment and provision of adaptive devices to provide for a safe environment as long as is possible. Specific problems, such as depression or anxiety, are treated symptomatically. Many drugs are contraindicated because they add to mental confusion. Anticholinesterase drugs, such as donepezil (Aricept), have led to some temporary improvement resulting from improved cholinergic transmission.

Moderate stimulation, perhaps in a daycare setting, is helpful, while maintaining a daily routine and exercise program is also advisable. A team approach to care is helpful in prolonging independence and supporting the family. Social workers, occupational therapists, psychologists, and speech therapists can provide direction and assistance. A daily routine and secure surroundings facilitate compliance with care. Often the primary caregiver is included in such therapy programs. Survival ranges up to 20 years, with an average of 7 years.

THINK ABOUT 14-20

a. List the early signs of Alzheimer's disease.
b. Describe three ways that AD can interfere with activities of daily living.
c. Compare the effects of AD, HD, ALS, and Parkinson's disease.

Other Forms of Dementia

Vascular Dementia

Vascular dementia is a form of dementia that is caused by cerebrovascular disease and frequently is a result of multiple small brain infarctions. It is common in persons older than age 70, particularly those with hypertension. Onset is insidious, with memory loss, apathy, and inability to manage daily routines. Progression may be in stages that are connected to the infarctions and loss of brain tissue. Other neurologic impairment is common.

Creutzfeldt-Jakob Disease

Creutzfeldt-Jakob disease (CJD) is a rare, but rapidly progressive, form of dementia caused by infection by a prion, an altered infectious protein particle (PrP) with a preference for nervous tissue. The infecting protein appears to alter normal host PrP or the coding gene for protein shape. Often the origin of the infection is not identified. Some cases show a familial incidence (defect in human prion protein gene) and some have been iatrogenic, including sources such as surgery, corneal transplants, or other invasive procedures. Most are sporadic. Creutzfeldt-Jakob disease is more common in older individuals.

Creutzfeldt-Jakob disease has a very long incubation period after its introduction into the brain, where more abnormal prions are produced. This is followed by rapid destruction of neurons, formation of plaques and vacuoles (empty spaces) in the neurons (spongiform encephalopathy). Early indicators are memory loss, behavioral changes, motor dysfunction, and progressive dementia. An EEG and MRI study aids the diagnosis. The course is 6 to 12 months. No treatment is available at this time.

The prions resist common methods of sterilization and disinfection. A link has been established between bovine spongiform encephalopathy (BSE, or mad cow disease) and a variant form of CJD (vCJD), with transmission by infected beef.

AIDS Dementia

Dementia is common in the later stages of AIDS (see Chapter 7). The virus itself invades brain tissue and may be exacerbated by other infections, including those of *Candida* or *Toxoplasma* species, and by tumors, such as lymphomas. Gradual loss of memory and cognitive ability and impaired motor function (e.g., ataxia, weakness, and abnormal reflexes) are typical.

In children with congenital HIV infection, the brain is frequently affected, causing mental retardation and delayed motor development.

Mental Disorders

Mental illness is classified using the *Diagnostic and Statistical Manual of Mental Disorders (DSM)*, published by the American Psychiatric Association. Mental health problems involve significant dysfunction in the areas of behavior or personality that interferes with the person's ability to function. Biochemical and structural abnormalities in the brain appear to contribute to these pathologies. Many disorders have a genetic component. Stressors may play a role in the development of the illness. Psychotic illness includes the more serious disorders, such as schizophrenia, delusional disorders, and some affective or mood disorders. Many patients with psychotic disorders receive large doses of drugs with obvious side effects. Other common mental disorders include anxiety and panic disorders, which are less severe but nevertheless disruptive. This section provides a brief introduction to the pathophysiology of several common mental disorders. Further information can be obtained from texts focusing on mental health.

Schizophrenia

■ *Pathophysiology*

Schizophrenia affects approximately 1.3% of the population and includes a variety of syndromes, which present differently in each individual. Although the etiology and pathogenesis have not been fully determined, some common changes do occur in the brains of schizophrenic patients, including reduced gray matter in the temporal lobes, enlarged third and lateral ventricles, abnormal cells in the hippocampus (part of the limbic system), excessive dopamine secretion, and decreased blood flow to the frontal lobes. Some of these changes appear to be linked to the neurologic manifestations seen in schizophrenic patients, such as abnormal eye movements (staring or periodic jerky eye movements).

■ *Etiology*

Theories about the cause of schizophrenia focus on a genetic predisposition along with brain damage in the fetus caused by perinatal complications or viral infection in the mother during pregnancy. Twin studies show a high concordance in both monozygotic and dizygotic twins pointing to a genetic component. Onset of schizophrenia usually occurs between ages 15 and 25 in men and 25 and 35 in women. Stressful events appear to initiate the onset and recurrences.

■ *Signs and Symptoms*

Symptoms may be grouped as positive (e.g., delusions, bizarre behavior) or negative (e.g., flat emotions, decreased speech). Both the excesses and the deficits may appear in one patient. Subtypes are based on the predominant characteristics.

Generally disorganized thought processes are the basic problem. Communication is often impaired by inadequate language skills, including lack of appropriate association of thoughts, meaningless repetition of words or thoughts, or development of new words without accepted meanings (neologisms). Delusions or false beliefs and ideas are persistent. Delusions may include a belief in persecution by others or ideas of grandeur or power over others. Problem-solving ability is impaired, and the attention span is brief. Hallucinations or abnormal sensory perceptions are common. The patient may withdraw socially from people and show little emotion but also may experience mood swings and become anxious. Often self-care is neglected.

■ *Treatment*

Drugs are the major therapeutic modality, often in conjunction with psychotherapy and psychosocial rehabilitation. The antipsychotic drugs (major tranquilizers or neuroleptics), chlorpromazine (Thorazine), fluphenazine (Prolixin, Moditen), haloperidol (Haldol), and clozapine (Clozaril), act by decreasing dopamine activity in the brain. These drugs frequently cause side effects related to excessive extrapyramidal activity (or parkinsonian signs). Dystonia and tardive dyskinesia cause involuntary muscle spasms in the face, neck, arms, or legs. Tardive dyskinesia may present as chewing or grimacing, repetitive jerky or writhing movements of the limbs, tremors, or a shuffling gait. With prolonged use and high doses of these drugs, tardive dyskinesia may be irreversible. Some of these side effects may be reduced by anti-Parkinson agents (anticholinergics), but these drugs also have adverse effects, such as blurred vision and dry mouth.

Depression

Depression is classified as a mood disorder, of which there are several subgroups. Major depression, or unipolar disorder, is endogenous, and a precise diagnosis is based on biologic factors or personal characteristics. Etiologic factors include genetic, developmental, and psychosocial stressors. Bipolar disorder involves alternating periods of depression and mania. Depression may also occur as an exogenous or reactive episode, a response to a life event, or secondarily to many systemic disorders, including cancer, diabetes, heart failure, and systemic lupus erythematosus. Depression is a common problem, and many patients with milder forms may be misdiagnosed and not receive treatment.

■ *Pathophysiology*

Depression is classified as an affective or mood disorder on the basis of characteristic disorganized emotions. It results from decreased activity by the excitatory neurotransmitters, norepinephrine and serotonin, in the brain. The exact mechanism has not yet been established, but twin studies do suggest a genetic component. The depressed client often has a history of major psychosocial trauma, which may contribute to the development of the disorder.

■ *Signs and Symptoms*

Depression is indicated by a prolonged period of profound sadness marked by hopelessness and an inability to find pleasure in any activity. Lack of energy and loss of self-esteem and motivation interfere with daily activity. Some individuals may be irritable and agitated. The individual has difficulty in concentrating and solving problems. Sleep disorders, such as insomnia or, occasionally, excessive sleep, usually accompany depression. Loss of appetite and libido (sex drive) are common. The degree to which the individual is affected varies over time and between individuals. In some cases

disability results as the individual is unable to meet the demands of daily life.

■ *Treatment*

Antidepressant drugs that increase norepinephrine activity are effective in treating many cases of depression. There is concern about the increased risk of suicide in children and adolescents taking antidepressant medications without concurrent psychiatric counselling.

A group of drugs in common use, the selective serotonin reuptake inhibitors (SSRIs), including fluoxetine (Prozac), have fewer cardiovascular side effects than drugs that block norepinephrine uptake. They prolong the activity at serotonin receptors, with antidepressant and anxiolytic effects. A new class, called serotonin-norepinephrine reuptake inhibitors (SNRIs) (e.g., venlafaxine [Effexor]), may be more selective in receptor action and have fewer side effects.

The tricyclic antidepressants (TCAs), such as amitriptyline (Elavil), block the reuptake of the neurotransmitters, particularly norepinephrine, into the presynaptic neuron. These mechanisms allow the stimulation by excitatory neurotransmitters to continue in the brain.

Monoamine oxidase (MAO) inhibitors, such as tranylcypromine (Parnate), block the destruction of norepinephrine and serotonin by the enzyme MAO at the synapse. Monoamine oxidase inhibitors cause many interactions involving certain foods and other drugs that may result in a hypertensive crisis (marked increase in high blood pressure). Foods to be avoided include tyramine-containing substances, such as chocolate, aged cheese, beer, and red wine. Monoamine oxidase inhibitors are not taken with SNRIs or SSRIs due to dangerous synergistic effects.

Another treatment of severe depression involves electroconvulsive therapy (ECT, shock treatments), which increases norepinephrine activity, but may result in some memory loss.

Panic Disorder

Panic attacks are common but do not necessarily lead to panic disorder. *Panic attack* refers to a sudden brief episode of discomfort and anxiety. Panic disorder, an anxiety disorder, develops when panic attacks are frequent or prolonged. These attacks occur in situations that most individuals would not find threatening.

■ *Pathophysiology*

A genetic factor has been implicated. An increased discharge of neurons may occur in the temporal lobes. Biochemical abnormalities involving the neurotransmitters norepinephrine, serotonin, and GABA may also be involved. Patients are fearful of having another panic attack, leading to increased irritability of the limbic system.

■ *Signs and Symptoms*

Repeated episodes of intense fear without provocation, which may last for minutes or hours, characterize this disorder. Palpitations or tachycardia, hyperventilation, sweating, sensations of choking or smothering, and nausea accompany the feeling of terror. Patients who anticipate attacks may develop a fear of open spaces (agoraphobia) or a fear of being in a place where no help is available and may refuse to leave their homes.

■ *Treatment*

Treatment consists of psychotherapy combined with drug therapy, usually antianxiety agents, such as alprazolam (Xanax) or diazepam (Valium). Antianxiety agents or minor tranquilizers, such as the benzodiazepines, potentiate the activity of GABA, an inhibitory neurotransmitter. Large doses may be necessary, which can cause drowsiness and ataxia. These drugs have a wide safety margin when used appropriately. In some patients, antidepressants may be prescribed.

THINK ABOUT   14-21

a. Compare three signs of schizophrenia with three signs of depression.

b. Explain how antipsychotic drugs act to reduce signs of mental illness.

c. Describe common signs of extrapyramidal side effects of antipsychotic drugs.

d. Describe a panic attack.

Spinal Cord Disorder

Herniated Intervertebral Disc

■ *Pathophysiology*

The vertebrae are separated by cartilaginous discs, which act as cushions and provide some flexibility to the spinal column. Herniation involves protrusion of the nucleus pulposus, the inner gelatinous component of the intervertebral disc, through a tear in the annulus fibrosus, the tough outer covering of the disc (Fig. 14-33). Such protrusions into the extradural space, usually laterally exert pressure on the spinal nerve root or spinal cord at the site, interfering with nerve conduction. The tear in the capsule may occur suddenly or develop gradually. Depending on which site is involved, sensory, motor, or autonomic function can be impaired. The most common location is the lumbosacral discs, at L4 to L5 or L5 to S1. Some herniations involve cervical discs between C5 and C7. If pressure on the nerve tissue or blood supply is prolonged and severe, permanent damage to the nerve may result.

■ *Etiology*

A person may be predisposed to herniation because of degenerative changes in the intervertebral disc,

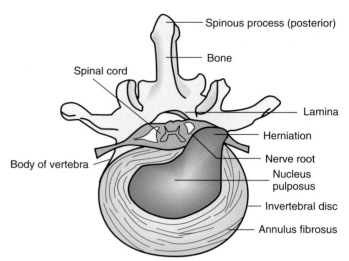

FIGURE 14-33 Herniated intervertebral disc.

resulting from age or metabolic changes. The herniation usually is caused by trauma or poor body mechanics, leading to excessive stress on the muscles, for example, by improper lifting or transfer of patients. Trauma accounts for about 50% of herniations.

■ *Signs and Symptoms*

Signs depend on the location and extent of the protrusion (see Figs. 14-4 and 14-23). In most cases, the effects are unilateral; however, large protrusions may cause bilateral effects. Because of pressure on the sensory nerve fibers in the dorsal root, lumbosacral herniations cause pain in the lower back, radiating down the posterior aspect of one or both legs (sciatic nerve pain). Actions such as coughing or straight leg-raising usually aggravate the pain. Paresthesia or numbness and tingling may occur. If the nerve compression is extensive, muscle weakness develops. Interference with micturition (bladder emptying) may develop.

Similarly a herniated disc in the cervical region causes pain in the neck and shoulder that radiates down the arm. Sensory impairment, reduced neck movement, and weakness may accompany the pain. The pressure may lead to skeletal muscle spasm in the neck or back, further increasing the pain.

■ *Diagnostic Tests*

Myelography with contrast dye, CT scans, and MRI confirm the herniation.

■ *Treatment*

Conservative treatment, including bed rest; application of heat, ice, or traction; or drugs, such as analgesics, anti-inflammatory agents, and skeletal muscle relaxants, are the initial approach. Back education programs are helpful in establishing appropriate positions for rest and activity. It is important to note that the pressure on the disks is highest in the sitting position. Physiotherapy and an appropriate program of exercise are usually undertaken. An occupational therapist can recommend appropriate modifications to daily life and workplace activities. Surgery may be considered in selected cases of unremitting chronic back pain and includes laminectomy or diskectomy. Spinal fusion is required if several vertebrae are involved creating added instability.

THINK ABOUT 14-22

Explain how a herniated intervertebral disc causes pain in the leg.

CASE STUDY A

Brain Tumor

Mr. A.H., age 44, had a generalized tonic-clonic seizure unexpectedly at work. He had no history of seizures, trauma, infection, or other illness. Investigation revealed a tumor in the right parietal lobe. This was removed surgically, although the diffuse nature of the malignant mass prevented its complete elimination. Follow-up radiation treatment was recommended.

1. Describe briefly several diagnostic tests that would be of value in this case.
2. Explain the basis of this seizure activity, and describe how it might be controlled.
3. Describe each stage, in sequence, of a generalized tonic-clonic seizure.

After surgery, Mr. A.H. demonstrated considerable weakness and sensory loss on his left side.

4. Match each of these effects with the functional areas of the brain that control them.

A few days after surgery, Mr. A.H. developed a bacterial infection at the operative site.

5. Explain why this infection is likely to increase motor and sensory deficits.

The infection was eradicated quickly with treatment, but the tumor did not respond to radiation and chemotherapy. As a result, several tumors in the brain grew relatively large during the next 2 months.

6. The cancer treatments caused severe anemia, nausea, and vomiting. Explain how these side effects could cause other complications for Mr. A.H.; describe these complications clearly.
7. Suggest several types of therapy or assistance that would be helpful to Mr. A.H. during this period. (Extend this question to focus on your specialty area, when possible.)

Mr. A.H. developed severe headaches and diplopia and became increasingly lethargic, and his seizures increased in frequency despite anticonvulsant medication. He was given medication to reduce the frequency of vomiting.

8. Explain the specific rationale for each of his manifestations.

As the tumors increased in size Mr. A.H.'s vital signs indicated increased pulse pressure.

9. Explain the cause of each of this sign.
10. Describe the changes that are likely to occur as coma develops in Mr. A.H.

CASE STUDY B

Spinal Cord Injury

B.L., age 17, has a compression fracture at C5 to C6, a result of diving from a bridge into a river and hitting a submerged rock. Fortunately a companion who had first aid training as a lifeguard rescued her and tried to minimize any secondary damage. In the emergency department, B.L. could not move her limbs or sense touch and lacked reflexes in her limbs.

1. Explain why caution is needed when handling a person with possible spinal cord injury.
2. Describe a compression fracture and how it can affect neurologic function.
3. Explain why reflexes are absent in B.L. at this early stage. What type of paralysis is present?
4. Explain why and how B.L.'s respiratory function may be impaired at any time.
5. Explain why the full extent of permanent damage cannot be estimated in this initial period.

Surgery was performed to relieve pressure and stabilize the fracture site.

6. Describe several additional factors that may result in secondary damage to the spinal cord.
7. Explain the anticipated effect in the immediate period of this injury on B.L.'s blood pressure and bladder function.

Several weeks later, routine examination indicated that some spinal cord reflexes were returning in the lower extremities.

8. Explain the significance of the returning reflexes.
9. Explain why each of the following complications could develop in B.L. and state the early signs for each:
    a. pneumonia
    b. decubitus ulcer
    c. muscle atrophy
    d. contracture
10. Briefly describe how the risk for each of the above complications could be minimized.

Gradually more reflexes returned. Some muscle tone and movement of the shoulder and upper arm became apparent, but no other function returned.

11. Explain how the dermatomes can assist in detecting functional areas.
12. Describe the change to be expected in bowel and bladder function as reflexes return.

One day, B.L. suddenly developed a severe headache and blurred vision. Her blood pressure was 210/120 mmHg and her pulse was 62 beats per minute.

13. What has probably caused this effect, and what action needs to be taken?
14. Suggest the specific components for a rehabilitation program for B.L. Expand your comments in areas of particular concern to you.

CASE STUDY C

Increased Intracranial Pressure

R.T. is a 16-year-old girl who has just received her driver's license. She has taken several friends to a "bush party" at a classmate's farm where beer and liquor were available. She leaves the party at 2:00 AM after having several drinks. Her friends tease her as she attempts to put on her seat belt and one calls her a sissy. She begins driving home without a seat belt. Her car drifts across the median and is involved in a head-on collision. Her most serious problem appears to be severe brain injury following ejection from the car. She is transported to the area trauma center, where treatment begins immediately.

1. Examination indicates papilledema in the right eye, a subdural hematoma in the temporal region, loss of consciousness and decreased responsiveness to painful stimuli. Explain how each symptom or sign is related to increased intracranial pressure.
2. Describe a subdural hematoma, its location, and how it developed and caused ICP.
3. R.T. develops bilaterally dilated pupils and a CT scan shows ventricular shift. What are the implications of these findings?
4. Surgery is performed to reduce the pressure in her cranium and R.T. recovers but requires rehabilitation for several deficits, including problems with hearing and memory as well as comprehension of speech. How will these deficits affect her academic work? Which regions of the cortex have been damaged?

One year after the accident, R.T. returns to high school and with the aid of a special education program for with head injuries, she graduates.

CASE STUDY D

Multiple Sclerosis

W.H., a woman, age 36, has received a diagnosis of multiple sclerosis. She has lost part of her left visual field and has weakness in her left leg. W.H.'s mother had multiple sclerosis.

1. State the factors in the history and the diagnostic tests that would indicate multiple sclerosis as a diagnosis.
2. Describe the pathophysiology of multiple sclerosis.
3. State the possible locations of the lesions that have caused visual and motor deficits.
4. Describe the typical course of multiple sclerosis that W.H. can expect in future.
5. Suggest several measures that can be used to minimize exacerbations.
6. Explain why adequate nutrition and hydration are important in patients with chronic neurologic conditions, including specific potential complications that may be avoided.
7. Explain why a program of moderate activity is important for W.H.

CASE STUDY E

Alzheimer's Disease

D.N. developed Alzheimer's disease at age 50. Early signs were vague and included occasional errors in judgment and increased criticism of others, noted only in retrospect. Several years later, following several episodes of extreme anger, a diagnosis of

Alzheimer's disease was made. At this time, it was suspected that his father had also had AD, but had died from an unrelated cause before a diagnosis could be made.

1. Why is a diagnosis difficult in the early stage of AD?
2. Could there be a familial factor?
3. Describe the pathologic changes that occur in the brain with AD.

The neurologist prescribed galantamine (Reminyl), an anticholinesterase inhibitor and regular attendance at a group center offering appropriate activities.

4. How would this drug be useful in treating AD?

The degeneration progressed rapidly over the next 2 years. The maximum dose of galantamine is no longer effective. He is confused about any change and not capable of performing simple activities. Communication is impaired, including that with family members.

5. Describe what might be expected in the final stage of AD.

CHAPTER SUMMARY

The brain and spinal cord are mapped in specific areas related to functions. Damage to a certain area results in a precise dysfunction and manifestations (focal signs) regardless of the exact cause. Damage to the right side of the brain (motor or sensory cortex) affects the contralateral side of the body. Loss of consciousness occurs when the RAS is depressed or large areas of the cerebral cortex are damaged. Aphasia, the inability to communicate, may be expressive, receptive, or a combination, and is often related to damage in Broca's area or Wernicke's area in the dominant hemisphere (left). Regeneration or replacement of neurons does not occur in the CNS.

Increased Intracranial Pressure

- The manifestations of *ICP* are common to all types of lesions in the brain and include a decreasing level of consciousness; headache; vomiting; increasing pulse pressure; papilledema; fixed, dilated pupil; and increasing CSF pressure.
- *Brain tumors*, both benign and malignant, cause focal effects and increased ICP, and are often life threatening.

Vascular Problems

- *Transient ischemic attacks* are caused by temporary reductions in blood supply, causing brief impairment of speech or motor function. They may serve as a warning of impending obstruction of blood flow.
- *Cerebrovascular accident* may result from atheroma, embolus, or hemorrhage causing total loss of blood supply to an area of the brain and subsequent infarction. Cerebral edema adds to the neurologic deficit during the first 48 hours. The presence of collateral circulation or immediate clot dissolution may minimize permanent damage.

- *Cerebral aneurysm* is frequently asymptomatic and undiagnosed until it is very large or rupture occurs.

Infections

- *Meningitis* is frequently caused by meningococcus, often carried in the upper respiratory tract, but a variety of other microbes may cause infection depending on the individual circumstances. Inflammation and swelling of the meninges leads to increased ICP, but no focal signs are present. Typical signs are severe headache, nuchal rigidity, photophobia, lethargy, and vomiting.

Injuries

- *Brain injury* may be mild with only transient dysfunction (e.g., concussion) or very serious with extensive damage to brain tissue (e.g., compound skull fracture). Inflammation and bleeding will create increased ICP and focal signs will reflect both the primary site and contrecoup injury. Secondary brain damage may be caused by hematoma formation, infection, or ischemia due to shock or other systemic factors.
- *Spinal cord injury* may result from a dislocation or fracture of a vertebra related to flexion, hyperextension, compression, or penetration injury. Additional neurologic damage is caused by hemorrhage, inflammation, or vasospasm. Immediately after the injury, a period of spinal shock develops in which reflexes and all functions cease at and below the level of injury. Following this period, reflexes return below the level of injury, and other functions may return, depending on the extent of spinal cord damage and the level of the injury. Cervical injury is particularly dangerous because of the risk of respiratory failure related to phrenic nerve dysfunction.

Congenital Neurologic Disorders

- *Hydrocephalus* occurs in the neonate when excessive amounts of cerebrospinal fluid force separation of the cranial bones, enlargement of the head, and compression of brain tissue. A shunt may be used to reroute CSF to prevent continued damage.
- *Spina bifida* involves a number of developmental neural tube defects. In *myelomeningocele*, the most serious form, the spinal cord and nerves as well as meninges and CSF herniate through the vertebral defect, resulting in neurologic dysfunction at and below that level of the spinal cord.
- *Cerebral palsy* refers to a group of disorders resulting from brain damage during fetal development or in the neonate, all of which involve a motor disability. A variety of other abnormalities (e.g., seizures or cognitive impairment) is present in each child depending on the areas of the brain that are damaged.

- *Seizure disorders* consist of a diversity of conditions caused by intermittent episodes of excessive uncontrolled neuronal discharge in the brain. Generalized seizures of the tonic-clonic type (grand mal) follow a typical pattern of initial aura, loss of consciousness, tonic muscle contraction, a cry, clonic muscle contraction, cessation, and postictal recovery.

Chronic Degenerative Diseases

- *Multiple sclerosis* is marked by progressive loss of myelin from nerves in the CNS, resulting in a loss of motor, sensory, and autonomic functions. The clinical effects vary with the individual, depending on the specific areas affected and the number of exacerbations.
- *Parkinson's disease* involves a deficit of dopamine caused by degenerative changes in the basal nuclei. Extrapyramidal dysfunction leads to tremors, muscular rigidity, and loss of the commonly associated involuntary movements such as arm swinging.
- *Amyotrophic lateral sclerosis* is a disorder marked by degeneration of upper and lower motor neurons, hence by progressive wasting of skeletal muscle, whereas other functions such as intellect persist.
- *Huntington's disease* is unusual because the effect of the autosomal dominant trait is not evident until midlife. Atrophy of the brain and decreased neurotransmitters cause choreiform movements and progressive cognitive impairment.
- *Alzheimer's disease* is a form of dementia or progressive loss of intellectual function and personality changes. Cortical atrophy and other pathologic changes in the neurons disrupt conduction, and in time all functions deteriorate.

Mental Disorders

- *Schizophrenia* is linked to specific chemical and physical abnormalities in the brain, resulting in disorganized thought processes, delusions, or decreased responsiveness.
- *Depression* encompasses a number of mood disorders linked to deficits of excitatory neurotransmitters. It may also develop secondary to a number of systemic disorders.
- *Panic disorder* is diagnosed when panic attacks, periods of intense fear and anxiety, occur at frequent intervals and persist. Chemical imbalance is considered to be the underlying cause.

Spinal Cord

- *Herniated intervertebral disc* is a common problem in older individuals or in cases of spinal trauma or undue stress. A tear occurs in the annulus fibrosis, allowing the inner nucleus pulposus to protrude and exert pressure on the spinal nerve or root, causing pain and weakness.

STUDY QUESTIONS

1. a. List the contents of the subdural space, subarachnoid space, and dura mater.
   b. Describe the specific location and list the functions of each of the following: auditory association area, prefrontal area, Broca's area, cerebellum, RAS.
   c. Using Table 14-2, Table 14-3, or Figure 14-3, describe the effects of damage to each area of the brain.

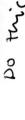

2. Draw a simple line diagram of the circle of Willis at the base of the brain by doing the following:
   a. Draw a line to show the division between the two hemispheres and label the top "frontal" and the bottom "occipital."
   b. In the lower half of the drawing, show the basilar artery dividing into two posterior cerebral arteries, and extend each down and to the side to the occipital lobes.
   c. Midway on the line and on either side of it, draw a circle showing each carotid artery.
   d. Draw two branches from each carotid: one extending upward toward the frontal lobe, and one outward and away from your central line.
   e. Label the arteries you have drawn.
   f. Add the communicating arteries to complete the circle, and label them.

3. a. Explain why the circle of Willis is important in the cerebral circulation.
   b. Predict the effects of obstruction of the left middle cerebral artery.
   c. Explain why a constant supply of oxygen and glucose to the brain is necessary.

4. a. Describe the characteristics of a spinal cord tract, using an example.
   b. Differentiate an upper motor neuron from a lower motor neuron by location and function.
   c. Describe a nerve plexus and how it affects nerve distribution.
   d. Describe an acquired reflex and include an example.

5. Compare the location and three basic effects of the SNS and the PNS.

6. a. Describe how the effects of deep coma differ from normal consciousness.
   b. Describe the sites of damage that would cause left-sided hemiplegia, receptive aphasia, and loss of hearing.

7. a. Describe the visual signs of increased ICP.
   b. State the rationale for headache with increased ICP.
   c. Describe what changes occur in vital signs (i.e., blood pressure, pulse, respiration) with rising ICP.

8. a. State the common signs and symptoms of a frontal lobe tumor.
   b. Predict the initial and progressive signs of a tumor growing in the left parietal lobe.
   c. Compare the effects of similar-sized tumors in the occipital lobe and the brain stem.
   d. Explain why there are general signs of increasing pressure in a person with a brain tumor.

9. a. Compare the pathophysiology and effects of TIAs and CVAs.
   b. Compare the origins and extent of damage in the three categories of CVAs.
   c. Describe several important factors in minimizing permanent damage from a CVA.

10. a. List several causative organisms of meningitis and the age groups primarily affected by each.
    b. Describe the significant signs of brain infection, including signs of meningitis and brain abscess and general signs of infection.

11. a. Compare open and closed head injuries, including a description of each, their effects, and their potential complications.
    b. Describe the location, usual cause, and basic effect of an epidural hematoma.

12. a. Describe two ways in which the spinal cord can be damaged in a fall.
    b. Explain why it is difficult to predict the degree of permanent damage to the spinal cord during the first few days.
    c. Describe the usual effects of transection of the spinal cord at C4-C5, immediately after injury and after recovery from spinal shock. Explain why there is a difference in the effects over time.
    d. Describe the cause and effect of autonomic dysreflexia. How are the signs different from those of a stress response?

13. a. Compare the pathophysiology of communicating and noncommunicating hydrocephalus.
    b. Explain why hydrocephalus occurs in adults.

14. Compare myelomeningocele with cerebral palsy in terms of etiology and effects on motor function and communication.

15. a. Describe the sequence of events in a generalized tonic-clonic seizure.
    b. Define status epilepticus.
    c. Explain why a focal seizure may occur in a person with a head injury.

16. Compare the pathophysiology and early signs of multiple sclerosis and Parkinson's disease.

17. Describe the changes occurring in the brain with Alzheimer's disease and compare its early effects on function with the later effects.
18. Compare depression and panic disorder in regard to:
    a. Classification
    b. Two significant signs or symptoms
    c. Recommended drug therapy
19. Describe the factors leading to herniation of the intervertebral disc.
20. Explain why pain is a common indicator of herniated intervertebral disc.

ADDITIONAL RESOURCES

Applegate E: *The Anatomy and Physiology Learning System Textbook*, ed 3, Philadelphia, 2006, Saunders.

Chabner DE: *The Language of Medicine*, ed 8, St. Louis, 2007, Saunders.

Kumar V, Abbas AK, Fausto M: *Robbins and Cotran Pathologic Basis of Disease*, ed 8, Philadelphia, 2007, Saunders.

Perkin GD: *Mosby's Color Atlas and Text of Neurology*, ed 3, St. Louis, 2009, Mosby.

Web Sites

http://www.aan.com/ *American Academy of Neurology*

http://www.aapmr.org/condtreat/injuries/sciadvance.htm *American Academy of Physical Medicine and Rehabilitation-Information on SCI*

http://www.mayoclinic.com *Mayo Clinic*

http://www.ninds.nih.gov *National Institute of Neurologic Disorders and Stroke*

http://stroke.ninds.nih.gov/resources/ *Know Stroke: Know the Signs. Act in Time (National Institutes of Health, National Institute of Neurological Disorders and Stroke)*

http://www.alsa.org *Amyotrophic Lateral Sclerosis Association*

http://www.asbah.org *Association for Spina Bifida and Hydrocephalus, with many links*

http://www.cdc.gov/ncidod/diseases/ *National Center for Infectious Diseases*

http://www.msaa.com *Multiple Sclerosis Association of America*

http://www.nlm.nih.gov/medlineplus/multiplesclerosis.html *Medline Plus—Research on multiple sclerosis*

http://www.ninds.nih.gov *National Institute of Neurological Disorders and Stroke*

http://www.neurosurgery.org *American Association of Neurological Surgeons and Congress of Neurological Surgeons*

http://www.wfnals.org *World Federation*

CHAPTER 15

Disorders of the Eyes, Ears and Other Sensory Organs

CHAPTER OUTLINE

LEARNING OBJECTIVES

After studying this chapter, the student is expected to:

1. Define sensory receptors and classify them by location and stimuli.
2. Describe the common structural defects impairing vision: hyperopia, presbyopia, myopia, astigmatism, amblyopia, and nystagmus.
3. Describe common infections in the eye and their possible effects on vision.
4. Explain how intraocular pressure may become elevated and how it may affect vision.
5. Compare the signs of chronic glaucoma, acute glaucoma, cataract, macular degeneration, and detached retina. Include the rationale for each.
6. Describe how the retina may become detached and the possible effects on vision.
7. Describe the types of hearing loss with an example of each.
8. Describe otitis media and its cause, pathophysiology, and signs.
9. Describe the pathophysiology and signs of otosclerosis and of Ménière's syndrome.
10. Explain how permanent hearing loss is caused by acute otitis media, chronic otitis media, Ménière's syndrome, and damage to the auditory area of the brain.

KEY TERMS

diplopia	photophobia	refraction	visceroceptors
exteroceptors	proprioceptors	tinnitus	visual acuity
ototoxic	ptosis	trachoma	

Sensory Receptors

Sensory receptors/sense organs are classified into two categories: general senses and special senses. Special senses include the eye and the ear.

Sensory receptors can be classified by their location

- Exteroceptors
  - Located close to the body surface and are sometimes referred to as cutaneous receptors. Examples include receptors for touch, pressure, temperature, and pain.
- Visceroceptors (interoceptors)
  - Located internally and provide information about the environment around the viscera.
- Proprioceptors
  - Provide information about body movement, orientation, and muscle stretch. Proprioceptors are of the referred to as *muscle sense.*

Sensory receptors are classified by their stimuli:

- Mechanoreceptors
  - Stimulated by a mechanical force: touch, pressure, equilibrium, hearing
- Chemoreceptors
  - Activated by a change in chemical concentration
- Taste, smell
- Thermoreceptors
  - Stimulated by a change in temperature
- Warm and cold receptors
- Photoreceptors
  - Respond to light stimuli
- Nociceptors
  - Respond to any tissue damage, the sensation produced is pain
- Osmoreceptors
  - Specialized receptors concentrated in the hypothalamus. They recognize changes in the osmotic pressure of body fluids.

The Eye

Review of Structure and Function

Visual information is received from light rays that pass through the transparent cornea and then through the lens, which focuses the image on the receptor cells of the retina, the rods and cones. These visual stimuli are conducted by the optic nerves to the occipital lobe of the brain for interpretation and processing before they are sent to other appropriate areas of the brain.

Protection for the Eye

The eye is well protected in the bony *orbit* of the skull. The eyelids (*palpebrae*) and eyelashes deflect foreign material in the air away from the eyes and protect the eye from excessive sunlight and drying. The levator palpebrae superior, the muscle of the upper eyelid, is controlled by the oculomotor nerve (cranial nerve III). The eyelids are lined with a thin mucous membrane, the *conjunctiva*, which continues over the sclera of the eye.

The continual secretion of *tears* washes away particles, microbes, and irritating substances. This watery secretion contains *lysozyme*, an antibacterial enzyme. The tears form in the *lacrimal gland* located on the superior lateral area of the orbit. They flow across the eye and drain into the lacrimal canals in the medial corner of the eye and then into the nasal cavity through the nasolacrimal duct. The tears keep the external tissues of the eye moist and healthy.

The Eyeball

Six skeletal muscles (*extrinsic muscles*) control the movement of the eyeball in the bony orbit. They originate on the orbit and insert onto the sclerae on the outside of the eyeball. There are four straight (rectus) muscles and two angled (oblique) muscles, which are coordinated to move and rotate the eye and are under the control of cranial nerves III, IV, and VI.

The eyeball consists of a spherical three-layered wall filled with fluid (Fig. 15-1):

- The anterior portion of the three layers differs from the posterior section because these tissues must permit the passage of light rays.
- The outer layer is a tough fibrous coat, the posterior portion of which is the sclera and the anterior portion the cornea. The *sclera* is visible as the "white" of the eye, and the *cornea* is a transparent bulging portion through which light rays pass and are refracted. (If you look at another person's eye from the side, you can observe the curve of the cornea.) The cornea does not contain blood vessels, but is nourished by the fluids around it and by oxygen diffusing from the atmosphere. This source of oxygen is a concern for individuals wearing contact lenses for long periods of time.
- The middle layer of the eye, or *uvea*, is made up of the *choroid*, a dark, vascular layer adjacent to the sclera in the posterior portion of the eye. The dark color absorbs the light, preventing reflection of light within the orbit. The numerous blood vessels in the choroid supply nutrients to the outer layers of the retina.

In the anterior part of the eye, the choroid develops into the ciliary body and iris. The *ciliary body* consists of the *ciliary muscle*, which controls the shape of the lens to focus the image of near and distant objects accurately and clearly on the retina, and the *ciliary processes*, which secrete aqueous humor, the fluid in the anterior cavity of the eye.

The *iris* is a circular structure surrounding the *pupil*, an opening through which light rays pass into the interior of the eye. The iris is pigmented and gives the eye its distinctive brown or blue tone. The iris contains two muscles that control the size of the pupil. The *circular*, or sphincter, muscle contracts in response to parasympathetic stimuli or excessive light on the retina, resulting in a constricted or small pupil. Parasympathetic nervous system fibers reach the iris from cranial nerve III. Under sympathetic nervous system control, the *radial* muscles of the iris, when contracted, cause the pupil to dilate or open. This function is easier to remember if it is associated with the stress (GAS, see Chapter 26) or fight-or-flight response, in which sympathetic stimulation leads to pupil dilation and improved vision, especially in dim light.

The *lens* is a *transparent* biconvex structure made up of an elastic capsule surrounding an orderly alignment of fibers. There are no blood vessels or nerves to interfere with the transparency, nor are there organelles in the cells. However the lack of organelles limits repair in these cells. Nutrients are provided from the aqueous humor. Together with the cornea, the lens provides refractive power for the light entering the eye. Current

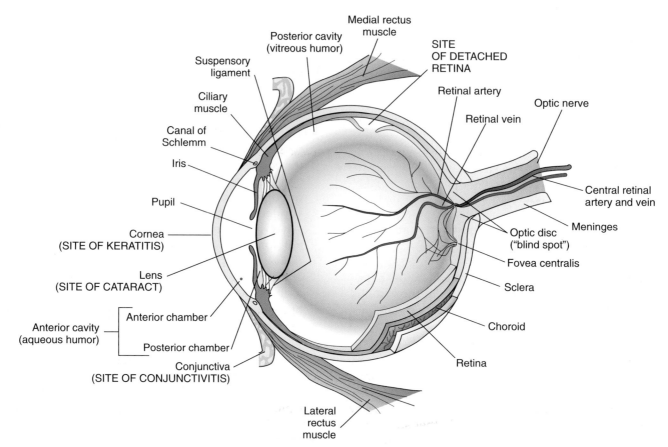

FIGURE 15-1 Structure of the eye.

interest relates to the mechanism by which these cells have lost the organelles and become transparent.

The *suspensory ligament* connects the lens to the ciliary body. The shape of the lens is altered as the contraction of the ciliary muscle alters tension on the suspensory ligament. This adjustment in lens curvature, or *accommodation*, bends the light rays (refraction) entering the eye sufficiently to focus a sharp image on the retina.

• The inner layer of the wall of the eye is the *retina*. This multilayered coat is present only in the posterior two thirds of the eye because light rays passing through the lens cannot bend enough to reach the retina if it is present in the anterior part of the eye. The retina consists of a pigmented layer and several layers of neurons. In the center of the posterior retina is the macula lutea, a yellowish area containing a depression called the *fovea centralis*, which is an area containing many cones that provides the most acute vision. The innermost layers of the retina consist of the rods and cones, which are light-sensitive *photoreceptor* nerve cells. *Rods* are specialized for dim light (for night vision), and *cones* are color sensitive. The light energy is absorbed by the rods and cones and converted into electrical energy in the neurons. Three types of cones, red, green, and blue, determine color perception. *Color blindness* is common in males and results from a deficit of one type of cone owing to an abnormal gene on the X chromosome (sex-linked recessive gene) (see Chapter 21).

Fluids in the Eye

The eye is divided into two cavities by the lens and ciliary body:

• The *posterior cavity* is the space between the lens and the retina, and it contains the transparent, jellylike *vitreous humor*. This material is formed during embryonic development and holds the retina approximated against the choroid to ensure diffusion of nutrients as well as to maintain the shape and size of the eyeball. Sometimes "floaters" may pass through a person's visual field, small specks or shadows that move about and eventually settle to the inferior portion of the eye. These are strands that form in the vitreous humor, more often with aging.

• The *anterior cavity* between the cornea and the lens is further divided into the *anterior chamber*, extending from the cornea to the iris, and the *posterior chamber*, between the iris and the lens. The chambers are connected through the pupil.

The anterior cavity is filled with *aqueous humor*, which is continuously secreted by the ciliary processes into the posterior chamber. It flows through the pupil into the anterior chamber and drains into the reticular network and canal of Schlemm (see Fig. 15-4). This canal encircles the eye at the junction of the cornea and iris and returns the fluid to the blood. To maintain normal intraocular pressure inside the eye (normal range 12 to 20 mmHg, average 15 mmHg), the amount of aqueous humor formed should equal the amount reabsorbed. Normal pressure maintains the shape of the eye. The aqueous humor supplies nutrients to the lens and cornea, which lack blood vessels.

The Visual Pathway

To review the physiology of vision, light rays from an object pass through the cornea, where they are refracted, and then through the aqueous humor and pupil. The curvature of the lens is adjusted to refract the light rays so that they converge on the retina, providing a sharp image of the object. The light continues through the transparent aqueous humor to the retina, where the photoreceptor neurons, the rods and cones, are stimulated. The light energy is converted into an electrical stimulus, which is transmitted by the optic nerve to the occipital lobe of the brain, where the image is identified and integrated with other information. The double image projected from different angles by the two eyes provides a wider visual field, and the central overlap of visual fields provides depth perception.

The nerve impulses from the ganglion cells of the retina converge in the fibers of the *optic nerve* (cranial nerve II), which leaves the eye at the *optic disc* in the posterior portion of the eye. The central retinal artery and vein, which supply the retina and other structures, also pass through the optic disc. There are no rods or cones at the optic disc, forming the "blind spot."

Because the optic nerve is essentially a projection of brain tissue surrounded by cerebrospinal fluid and meninges, it reflects pressure in the brain (see Chapter 14). Assessment of the eye can often provide useful information about other problems in the body, such as hypertension or vascular changes as a result of diabetes.

The optic nerves carry visual stimuli to the *occipital lobes* of the brain (see Fig. 14-1). At the optic chiasm, half of the fibers from each optic nerve cross to pass to the occipital lobe in the opposite hemisphere (see Fig. 14-7). Therefore the left occipital lobe receives images from the right visual field. Damage to the left occipital lobe results in loss of the right visual field.

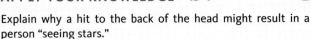

APPLY YOUR KNOWLEDGE 15-1

Explain why a hit to the back of the head might result in a person "seeing stars."

Diagnostic Tests

Basic tests include the following:
- The Snellen chart or similar eye charts, consisting of lines of progressively smaller letters and numbers, measure visual acuity.
- Visual field tests are used to check central and peripheral vision.
- Tonometry assesses intraocular pressure by checking the resistance of the cornea.
- An ophthalmoscope can be used to examine the interior structures.
- Gonioscopy measures the angle of the anterior chamber.
- Muscle function and coordination can also be tested.

Many other sophisticated tests are available for specific disorders. *Neurologic damage* to the visual pathway is covered in Chapter 14. *Retinopathies* are discussed in Chapter 12 under hypertension, and in Chapter 16 under diabetes mellitus.

Structural Defects

Structural defects interfere with the focusing of a clear image on the retina:
- *Myopia*, nearsightedness, occurs when the image is focused in front of the lens, perhaps because the eyeball is too long (Fig. 15-2).
- *Hyperopia*, or farsightedness, develops if the eyeball is too short and the image is focused behind the retina. In cases of myopia and hyperopia, the blurred image can be corrected with a lens, such as a concave lens for myopia, which refocuses the image on the retina.
- *Presbyopia* refers to farsightedness associated with aging, when the loss of elasticity reduces accommodation.
- *Astigmatism* develops from an irregular curvature in the cornea or lens.
- *Strabismus* (squint or cross-eye) results from a deviation of one eye, resulting in double vision (diplopia). Strabismus may be caused by a weak or hypertonic muscle, a short muscle, or a neurologic defect. In young children, strabismus must be treated immediately to prevent the development of *amblyopia*, the suppression by the brain of the visual image from the affected eye.
- *Nystagmus* is an involuntary abnormal movement of one or both eyes. It may be a back-and-forth rhythmic motion, jerky movement, or circular motion. This abnormality may result from neurologic causes, from

THINK ABOUT 15-1

a. Explain why one may have a "runny nose" when crying.
b. Describe the outer layer of the eye, naming and locating the parts and describing the function of each.
c. List the parts of the eye that do not contain blood vessels and explain how they are nourished.
e. Explain the effect of sudden fear or anger on the size of the pupil.
f. List the functions of the oculomotor nerve.
g. Describe the location and function of the photoreceptor cells.
h. Describe the type of impulses carried by the optic nerve.

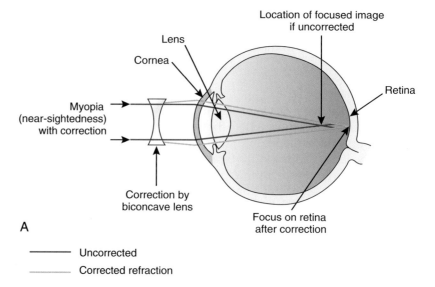

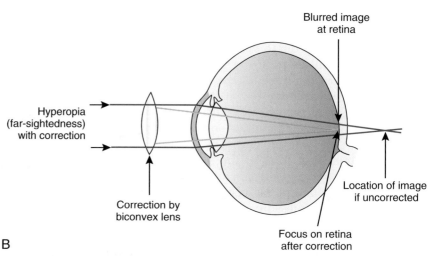

FIGURE 15-2 Refraction defects in the eye.

inner ear or cerebellar disturbances, or from drug toxicity.

- *Diplopia* (double vision) or paralysis of the upper eyelid (ptosis) may be caused by trauma to the cranial nerves, resulting in paralysis of the extraocular muscles.

Infections and Trauma

A *stye* (hordeolum) is an infection involving a hair follicle on the eyelid, usually by staphylococci. A swollen, red mass forms on the eyelid, which is uncomfortable when blinking.

Conjunctivitis

Conjunctivitis is a superficial inflammation or infection involving the conjunctiva lining the eyelids and covering the sclera. Allergens, bacteria, viruses, or irritating chemicals in the air are a frequent cause of inflammation, resulting in redness, itching, and excessive tearing with a watery discharge.

Organisms such as *Staphylococcus aureus* cause the highly contagious "pinkeye," which occurs frequently in children. The sclera of the eye and eyelid appears red, and there is a purulent discharge. Pinkeye is spread by the fingers or contaminated towels. Antibiotic treatment is required to reduce contagion and prevent damage to the cornea.

Contact lenses are a frequent source of infection in the eye, both conjunctivitis and keratitis (Fig. 15-3B,C). Other sources are contaminated medication or makeup. Medications or eye makeup should not be used past the expiry date or instructions. The infectious agent could be one of a variety of microorganisms.

Chlamydia trachomatis and gonorrhea cause infection in the reproductive tract (sexually transmitted disease, or STD) and may infect the eyes of newborns, who are routinely given medication after birth to prevent this infection. *Neisseria gonorrhoeae* is frequently transferred to the eyes by self-inoculation, causing conjunctivitis (see Fig. 15-3A). Redness and very heavy discharge running out of the eyes are typical.

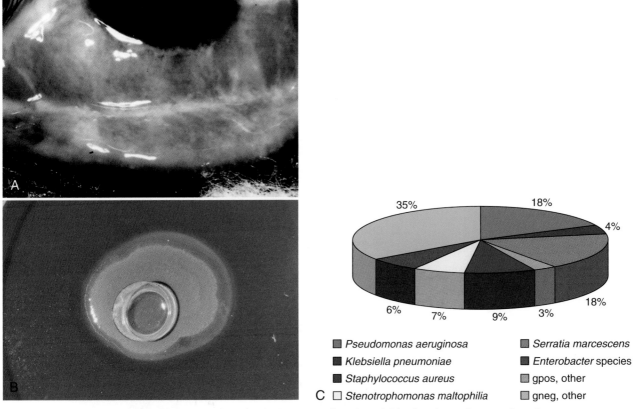

FIGURE 15-3 Infections in the eye. **A,** Gonococcal conjunctivitis showing redness and copious discharge in the eye caused by *Neisseria gonorrhoeae.* **B,** Growth of *Pseudomonas aeruginosa* surrounds the soft contact lens of a patient with ulcerative keratitis. **C,** Recent trends in bacteria recovered from contact lenses and solutions. gneg, gram-negative; *gpos,* gram-positive. *(From Mahon CR, Manuselis G:* Textbook of Diagnostic Microbiology, *ed 2, Philadelphia, 2000, Saunders.)*

Trachoma

Trachoma is an eye infection caused by *Chlamydia trachomatis* that causes follicles to develop on the inner surface of the eyelids. It occurs in situations in which there is not adequate water to wash the face and eyes or flies carry the organism to the eyes. Although common in children, it can occur in any age group. If not effectively treated with antibiotic ointments, the eyelids become scarred and the lashes turn inward to abrade the cornea. Globally, trachoma is the most common cause of vision loss, but it is also easily treated and prevented. The patient reports a "scratchy" eye and no exudate is normally present. Everting the upper eyelid shows the characteristic pearl-like follicles.

Keratitis

Severe pain and photophobia (sensitivity to light) develop when the cornea is infected or irritated because it has numerous pain receptors (trigeminal nerve-cranial nerve V). Herpes simplex virus is a cause of corneal inflammation and ulceration. The virus may be transferred from a herpes lesion around the mouth by the fingers, or in a dental office, by spray of contaminated saliva. With keratitis there is increased risk of ulceration eroding the cornea and scar tissue interfering with

vision. Corneal involvement is best treated by an ophthalmologist.

Trauma to the cornea also increases risk of visual loss. The cornea is finely structured to provide a transparent pathway for light. Abrasions may develop from foreign bodies caught under the eyelid, a damaged contact lens, or objects directly scratching the cornea. Abrasions can be seen using a fluorescein stain in the eye. Penetration injuries may cause damage to the internal structures or loss of the vitreous humor.

The eye is susceptible to damage from chemicals, splashes, or fumes. Prompt and prolonged flooding of the eye with cool running water is important. It may be necessary to hold the eye open to accomplish the flushing. Preventive measures such as wearing protective glasses, avoiding touching the eyes, and cleaning contact lenses appropriately can greatly reduce the risks of trauma to the eye.

Glaucoma

Pathophysiology

Glaucoma results from increased intraocular pressure caused by an excessive accumulation of aqueous humor. *Narrow-angle* glaucoma occurs when the angle between

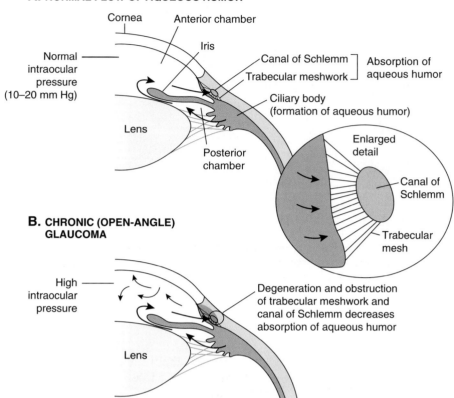

A. NORMAL FLOW OF AQUEOUS HUMOR

B. CHRONIC (OPEN-ANGLE) GLAUCOMA

FIGURE 15-4 Glaucoma.

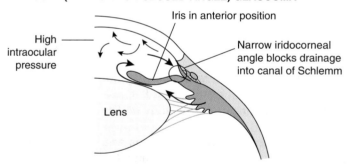

C. ACUTE (NARROW- OR CLOSED-ANGLE) GLAUCOMA

the cornea and the iris in the anterior chamber is decreased by factors such as an abnormal anterior insertion of the iris. With aging, the lens enlarges, pushing the iris more forward and to the side. This anatomic position may block the outflow of aqueous humor when the pupil is dilated and the thickened iris fills the narrow angle (Fig. 15-4). Pressure inside the eyeball can increase significantly within an hour of pupil dilation, blocking drainage of fluid. This leads to *acute* glaucoma, in which there is a sudden marked increase in intraocular pressure.

Chronic glaucoma, sometimes referred to as *wide-angle* or *open-angle* glaucoma, is a common degenerative disorder in older persons, affecting 1% to 2% of the population in the United States. The trabecular network and canal of Schlemm become obstructed, and the outflow of aqueous humor gradually diminishes. Intraocular pressure increases slowly and usually asymptomatically. The increased pressure compresses the blood flow to the retinal cells, causing ischemia and damage to the retinal cells. The anterior portion of the retina is affected first, including the receptor cells for peripheral vision. If pressure inside the eyeball continues to increase, more of the retina and the optic nerve will be damaged. When observed through the pupil, the optic disc appears eroded or "cupped" as the optic nerve fibers are compressed (Fig. 15-5). Damage to the retina and optic nerve is irreversible, and eventually blindness results.

■ *Etiology*

Chronic glaucoma develops frequently in older individuals, usually beginning after age 50. Narrow-angle

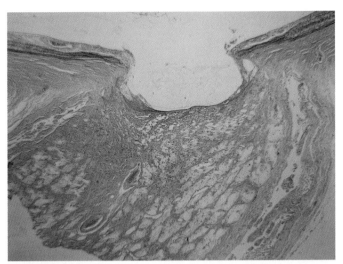

FIGURE 15-5 Glaucomatous cup: loss of nerve fibers leads to excavation of the optic disc. *(From Cotran RS, Kumar V, Collins T: Robbins Pathologic Basis of Disease, ed 6, Philadelphia, 1999, Saunders.)*

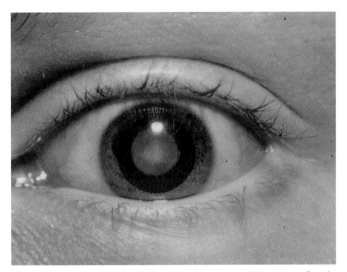

FIGURE 15-6 Appearance of eye with cataract. *(Courtesy of Ophthalmic Photography at the University of Michigan W.K. Kellogg Eye Center, Ann Arbor, from Black JM, Hawks JH: Medical-Surgical Nursing: Management for Positive Outcomes, ed 7, Philadelphia, 2005, Saunders.)*

glaucoma may be caused by a developmental abnormality, aging, or scar tissue in the eye from trauma or infection. Congenital glaucoma occurs as an inherited disorder of several types, both recessive and dominant.

▩ Signs and Symptoms

Chronic glaucoma has an insidious onset. Increased intraocular pressure is the initial indicator of chronic glaucoma. Routine screening tests are recommended as individuals age because increased intraocular pressure is often the only sign. Loss of peripheral vision may not be noticed initially except by a screening test because individuals automatically adjust the direction of the eyes to focus on an object.

As pressure increases over time, corneal edema and altered light refraction lead to blurred vision and the appearance of "halos" around lights. Mild eye discomfort develops as the corneal pain receptors are stimulated by the increased pressure.

In individuals with narrow-angle glaucoma, acute episodes of glaucoma may be triggered by pupil dilation resulting from adrenergic drugs such as those used for colds or hay fever (vasoconstrictors or decongestants, which may cause pupil dilation), by stress, or by prolonged periods in darkened rooms. As intraocular pressure rises rapidly, eye pain, nausea, and headache develop, vision is blurred, and the cornea appears bulging and cloudy. The pupil is dilated and unresponsive to light. This situation requires prompt treatment to prevent permanent damage.

▩ Treatment

Chronic glaucoma is treated by regular administration of eye drops to reduce secretion of aqueous humor (e.g., timolol or betaxolol, beta-adrenergic blocking agents) or to constrict the pupil (e.g., pilocarpine, a miotic or cholinergic agent). Some drugs also reduce the intraocular pressure through inhibition of carbonic anhydrase. Drug interactions and side effects should be carefully checked with any new medication that is prescribed. It is essential to maintain treatment, administering the medication on a regular basis, to control intraocular pressure and minimize the risk of retinal damage. If the condition is unresponsive to drugs, laser trabeculoplasty or trabeculectomy may be required to deepen the anterior chamber and thus increase the drainage of aqueous humor.

Acute glaucoma (narrow-angle), if severe, may require surgery, such as removal of part of the iris, to open a passageway for drainage into the canal of Schlemm (iridectomy). Laser iridotomy is a popular noninvasive procedure.

Cataracts

A cataract occurs when the normally clear lens becomes cloudy and interferes with light transmission (Fig. 15-6). The size, site, and density of the opacity/cloudiness vary among individuals and may differ in one individual's two eyes. The changes may be caused by degeneration related to aging or metabolic abnormalities such as diabetes. Excessive exposure to sunlight may be a factor. Congenital cataracts are usually a result of maternal infection due to rubella or toxoplasmosis. Traumatic cataracts are the result of blows to the eye, which imprint iris pigment on the lens. These injuries are often associated with sports activities in which eye protection is not used.

Blurred vision that progresses over the visual field and becomes darker with time is the only indicator. The rate at which impairment develops varies considerably, and a cataract in one eye may advance more quickly than one in the other eye. When severe enough to interfere with the person's ability to function or work, the damaged lens can be removed and replaced by an artificial intraocular lens. Tests are essential to assess retinal function, intraocular pressure, and the possible presence of other lesions such as tumors before surgery.

Cataract surgery is usually day surgery, and the patient is quickly ambulatory. The degenerated material inside the lens is broken up by phacoemulsification and removed by suction, and the intraocular lens placed in position to replace the natural lens that was removed. Peripheral iridectomy may be included to prevent post-operative glaucoma.

Detached Retina

A detached retina is an acute problem that occurs when the retina tears away from the underlying choroid because of marked myopia, degeneration with aging, or scar tissue that creates tension on the retina. The tear allows vitreous humor to flow behind the loose retinal portion (see Fig. 15-1). As increased vitreous humor continues to seep behind the retina, an increasing portion of the retina is lifted away from the choroid. The retinal cells cease to function as they are deprived of nutrients diffusing from the blood vessels of the choroid. This loss of function results in an area of blackness in the visual field. If separation continues, the retina is deprived of its source of nutrients in the choroid and dies.

There is *no pain* related to the tear, but initially the patient may see light or dark floating spots in the visual field, resulting from blood or exudate leaking from the tear. Then a darkened or blind area develops, which increases in size with time. Typically, this event has been described as a "dark curtain" drawn across the visual field.

Surgical intervention such as scleral buckling or laser therapy is required as soon as possible to close any holes and reattach the retina in its proper position against the choroid to restore the source of nutrients to the retinal cells before irreversible damage occurs. Retinal detachment may recur and requires immediate attention to prevent vision loss.

Macular Degeneration

Age-related macular degeneration (AMD) is a common cause of visual loss in older persons. It appears to arise from a combination of genetic factors and environmental exposure (e.g., ultraviolet rays and drugs). A similar condition found in younger persons has a stronger genetic basis.

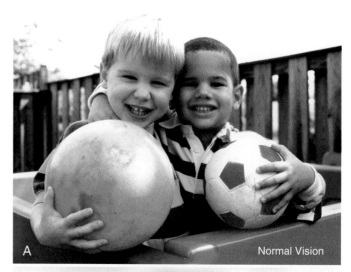

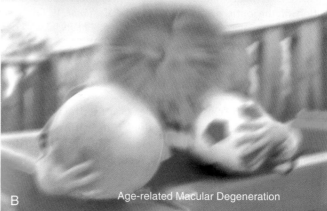

FIGURE 15-7 **A,** Normal vision. **B,** Age-related macular degeneration. *(From National Eye Institute, National Institutes of Health.)*

Degeneration occurs at the fovea centralis in the macula lutea, with its high density of cones, at the central point of the retina. There are two types of degeneration: in the more common type, the *dry* or atrophic AMD, deposits form in retinal cells gradually destroying them; in the *wet* or exudative form, neovascularization occurs, with the formation of abnormal, leaky blood vessels, rapidly destroying the retina. In both types, nutrients can no longer pass from the choroids to the retina.

Central vision with high acuity first becomes blurred, and then is lost. There is no treatment to reverse the effects. Depth perception is also affected. There is no pain. Peripheral vision is not affected (Fig. 15-7).

Visual field tests and angiography assist diagnosis. Photodynamic therapy (photosensitive drug plus laser) may help seal off neovasculature in some persons with the wet type. The new drug, pegaptanib (Macugen) may slow vascular growth in cases of the wet type. For the dry type of AMD, nutrition is assessed to ensure that vitamin, mineral, and antioxidant intake are sufficient. A high-dose formulation of antioxidants and zinc has been shown to reduce the risk of advanced AMD and its associated vision loss.

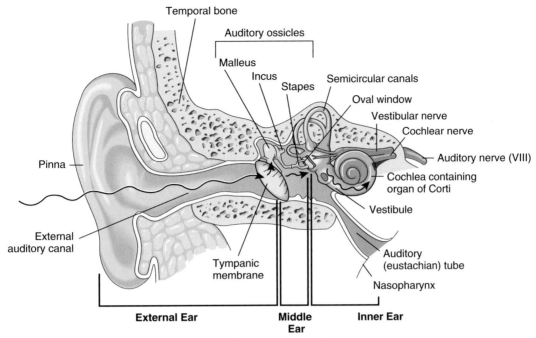

FIGURE 15-8 Structure of the ear.

THINK ABOUT   15-2

a. Explain why infection or trauma involving the cornea is more serious than that involving the conjunctiva.
b. Describe the characteristic signs of cataract development.
c. Compare wide-angle and narrow-angle glaucoma, including the pathophysiology and signs of each.
d. Explain the cause of blindness with cataract, acute glaucoma, detached retina, and damage to the optic chiasm.
e. Describe the two types of macular degeneration and current treatments.

The Ear

Review of Structure and Function

Parts of the Ear

The ear is divided into three anatomic sections, the external ear, the middle ear, and the inner ear (Fig. 15-8):

- The *external* ear consists of the *pinna*, or visible flap on the side of the head, and the *external auditory meatus* or canal. This canal passes through the temporal bone to the *tympanic membrane* or eardrum, which marks the separation between the external and middle ear.
- The *middle* ear consists of the *tympanic cavity*, a hollow area in the bone, which contains three tiny bones, the malleus, incus, and stapes, which compose the ossicles. The malleus is adjacent to the tympanic membrane, and the stapes fits against the oval window, a membrane connecting the middle ear and the inner ear.

The middle ear cavity opens into the *auditory* or eustachian tube, which connects to the nasopharynx. This tube equalizes pressure in the middle ear with pressure in the external ear canal. This equalization is important if atmospheric pressure changes suddenly, as when an airplane takes off. Chewing or swallowing helps to equalize the pressure on either side of the tympanic membrane. The middle ear cavity is also continuous with the *mastoid air cells* in the mastoid process of the temporal bone around the ear.

A *continuous mucous membrane* lines the middle ear cavity, the mastoid cells, the auditory tube, and the respiratory tract. This is significant because it provides a path for direct spread of infection through these structures.

- The *inner* ear is called the *labyrinth*. It is composed of two parts, the cochlea and the semicircular canals, joined by a vestibule. These structures consist of a bony labyrinth filled with a fluid, perilymph, inside of which is a membranous labyrinth filled with endolymph. The cochlea contains a complex arrangement of membranes surrounding the *organ of Corti,* where specialized hair cells (nerve receptors) provide stimuli to the sensory neurons for hearing. These neurons form the cochlear branch of the auditory nerve (cranial nerve VIII), which conducts impulses to the temporal lobe for reception and interpretation of sound. Some fibers from each ear cross to the auditory cortex in the opposite hemisphere, and some fibers remain on the same side, meaning that each auditory area receives some sound from each ear.

Pathway for Sound

Hearing begins with sound waves in the air. The height of a wave determines the loudness of the sound, and the number of sound waves per time period, or frequency, determines the pitch (high or low):

1. Sound waves enter the external ear canal and strike the tympanic membrane, causing it to vibrate.
2. Vibration of the tympanic membrane causes the malleus to vibrate, and then the incus and the stapes.
3. The motion of the stapes against the oval window initiates movement of the perilymph and endolymph in the cochlea.
4. These "water waves" stimulate movement of the membranes and hair cells in the organ of Corti, which converts the stimulus into a nerve impulse.
5. The nerve impulses are conducted to the auditory area in the temporal lobe of the brain, where the sound is received and interpreted.

The Semicircular Canals

The semicircular canals in the inner ear include three structures, each at right angles to the other two; the sense of balance and equilibrium is focused in the crista ampullaris, located in the ampulla of each semicircular canal and in the macula in the vestibule. These contain the receptor hair cells, which can be stimulated by motion of the endolymph fluid in response to head movements or position changes. Because of the arrangement of the canals, movement in any direction can be detected.

Any stimulus is conducted by the vestibular branch of the auditory nerve to the medulla oblongata and other parts of the brain. Many additional connections to the cerebellum, to incoming proprioceptive impulses (joints, muscles, and tendons), and to visual stimuli are required for the coordination of righting reflexes to maintain body position. Vestibular damage causes *vertigo*, a sense of rotation of self or the environment.

Hearing Loss

Hearing loss is of two basic types, conduction deafness and sensorineural deafness (sometimes sensorineural is broken down into sensory and neural deafness). Tests comparing conduction by air through the external canal and conduction through the mastoid bone can assist in differentiating the type of deafness.

Conduction deafness occurs when sound is blocked in the external ear or middle ear. For example:

- An accumulation of wax or a foreign object in the external ear canal can block sound waves.
- Scar tissue or adhesions may impair the function of the tympanic membrane or ossicles.
- *Sensorineural* impairment develops with damage to the organ of Corti or the auditory nerve. For example:
- Infection, particularly viral infection, including rubella, influenza, and herpes, can lead to deafness.
- Head trauma or neurologic disorders can affect the auditory nerve or temporal lobe.
- Ototoxic drugs such as the antibiotics streptomycin, neomycin, and vancomycin, the analgesics aspirin

and ibuprofen, the diuretic furosemide, and some antineoplastic agents have caused temporary or permanent hearing loss. The early sign of toxicity is often tinnitus, a ringing or buzzing in the ears.

- Sudden, very loud sounds or prolonged exposure to loud noise can damage the delicate hair cells because of the force exerted by excessive movement in response to the sound. This damage may be an occupational hazard, or it may be associated with loud music.
- *Presbycusis* is the sensorineural loss that occurs in elderly people owing to a reduced number of hair cells or receptor cells or other degeneration in the cochlea.
- *Congenital* deafness may be inherited or may result from infection or trauma during pregnancy or delivery. Most deaf infants are born to hearing parents. Early diagnosis and treatment are essential for development of the child. Hearing impairment in young children often interferes with speech and social development, as well as other interactions with persons and with learning ability.

In many areas, newborns are screened for hearing deficits. Additional tests can determine the source of the deficit. Audiologists and otolaryngologists may be consulted to determine the optimum therapy. Regular therapy with a speech-language pathologist is helpful. Lip reading and sign language (American Sign Language, ASL) may be learned. Many assistive devices are now available to improve communication skills.

Hearing aids may be used if appropriate for the individual hearing deficit. Various types of hearing aids to amplify sound are available to improve hearing capacity.

Cochlear implants have been in existence for some years. They are used successfully in some cases of sensorineural loss in very young congenitally deaf children or in adults, following appropriate screening by the medical team. With an implant, any sound is picked up by an external microphone and bypasses many structures in the ear to stimulate the auditory nerve (Fig. 15-9). The auditory area of the brain then interprets this input. The mechanism can be used when the receptor cells in the cochlea are not functioning, but the auditory nerve is intact. In very young children with profound hearing loss, the developing brain usually quickly adapts to the stimuli from the cochlear implant. Working with speech and language pathologists, they are able to develop normal speech and language skills in a short time. Adults who formerly could hear and speak also are able to match the "old" sounds to the new stimuli. However, deaf children greater than age 7 have had little success with this prosthesis. Controversy exists as to the need for cochlear implant therapy. Some parents who are deaf, deafened, or hard of hearing and have children who are hearing impaired do not consider deafness to be a disability; therefore they do not consider cochlear implants a necessary or valuable

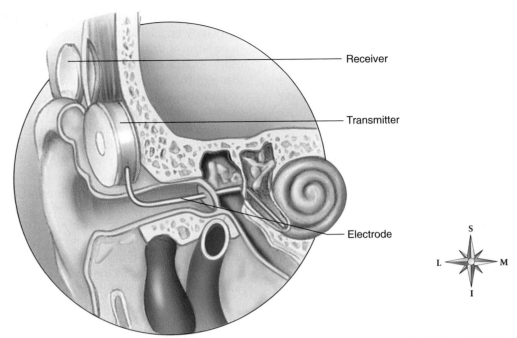

FIGURE 15-9 Cochlear implant. *(From Patton KT, Thibodeau GA: Anatomy & Physiology, ed 8, St. Louis, 2013, Mosby.)*

treatment option for their children. If a cochlear implant is chosen for treatment, it is preferable to use an implant at an early age if it is to be successful.

THINK ABOUT 15-3

a. Describe the location of the middle ear, including its boundaries, and the openings from it. Describe the structures in the middle ear and their function.

b. Compare the advantages and disadvantages of the auditory tube and its relationship to the middle ear.

c. Describe the location of the auditory nerve receptors and trace the connection to the brain.

d. Predict the effect on hearing capacity of damage to: (1) the cochlea in the right ear; (2) the left auditory nerve; and (3) the left temporal lobe.

e. Which parts of the hearing pathway can a cochlear implant replace?

f. Explain why a cochlear implant may not be successful in older children who are deaf.

Ear Infections

Otitis Media

Otitis media is an inflammation or infection of the middle ear cavity.

▪ *Pathophysiology*

Exudate builds up in the cavity, causing pressure on the tympanic membrane and interfering with the movement of the membrane and the ossicles. Usually the auditory tube is obstructed by inflammation, preventing drainage of the fluid into the nasopharynx. Enlarged adenoids may compress the tube. The middle ear cavity is encased in rigid bone, and therefore increasing pressure eventually causes rupture of the tympanic membrane.

Prolonged infection is likely to produce scar tissue and adhesions, leading to permanent conductive hearing loss. Chronic infection may lead to mastoiditis, infection involving the mastoid cells of the temporal bone.

▪ *Etiology*

The mucosa of the middle ear cavity may become inflamed because of allergies or infection that spreads along the continuous mucosa from the nasopharynx and respiratory structures. This happens more easily in infants and young children because the auditory canal is shorter and wider and forms more of a right angle to the nasopharynx, thereby facilitating drainage of respiratory secretions into the auditory tube. Also, infants tend to spend more time in a recumbent position, and feeding in a supine position encourages reflux of fluid into the ear.

Otitis media occurs more frequently in the winter months when there is an increase in upper respiratory infections. Common bacterial causes include *Haemophilus influenzae*, particularly in young children, and pneumococci, beta-hemolytic streptococci, and staphylococci. Viral infection may also lead to otitis media, which is frequently complicated by a secondary bacterial infection. Bacterial infections result in a purulent discharge.

Signs and Symptoms

Occasionally otitis media is asymptomatic. More often there is severe pain or earache (otalgia) related to the pressure on the tympanic membrane and the nerve receptors in the cavity. The tympanic membrane appears red and bulging (Fig. 15-10). An infant or young child tends to rub or pull at the ear to express distress. Mild hearing loss or a feeling of fullness is common. Signs of infection, such as fever and nausea, may be present. Rupture of the tympanic membrane results in a purulent discharge from the external ear canal, accompanied by relief of pain.

Treatment

The use of antibacterials to routinely treat otitis media has recently been questioned by American and Canadian medical associations. Although antibacterials are needed in recurrent otitis media, some physicians treat initial infections for at least 48 hours with ibuprofen (Advil) or acetaminophen (Tylenol) to reduce discomfort. The child is then reassessed, and if the condition has not resolved, antibacterials are administered. Decongestants may be useful in reducing the edema and obstruction in the auditory tube. Young children with recurrent otitis media may require insertion of drainage tubes through the tympanic membrane temporarily to relieve congestion. A person with an ear infection should use caution if he is planning to use air transportation because the pressures inside and outside the ear must be equalized to prevent additional damage (barotrauma). Chewing gum or swallowing during rapid ascent or descent may help. Scar tissue on the tympanic membrane or an open tear may follow infection and impair hearing. Recurrent infection may cause adhesions or damage to the ossicles. In these cases, surgery may be necessary to restore a functional tympanic membrane and ossicles (e.g., tympanoplasty) or treat chronic mastoiditis (e.g., mastoidectomy). Mastoiditis is less common now with antimicrobial treatment of ear infections.

Cholesteatoma, a cystlike mass, may develop with chronic otitis media and the accompanying ruptured tympanic membrane. Epithelial cells collect and become infected, forming a mass in the middle ear cavity that eventually erodes the ossicles and surrounding bone, impairing hearing. Surgical intervention is required.

Treatment of otitis media in the toddler or infant is essential if proper speech patterns are to develop. Children with a history of otitis media and delayed or impaired speech should be assessed by a speech therapist or speech pathologist as well as an audiologist.

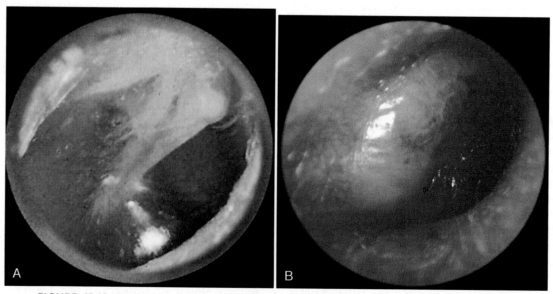

FIGURE 15-10 **A**, Normal tympanic membrane. **B**, Tympanic membrane with otitis media. (***A**, Courtesy Richard A. Buckingham, Clinical Professor, Otolaryngology, Abraham Lincoln School of Medicine, University of Illinois, Chicago, from Seidel HM, Ball JW, Dains JE, et al: Mosby's Guide to Physical Examination, ed 5, St. Louis, 2003, Mosby. **B**, Courtesy Michael Hawke, MD, from Zitelli BJ, Davis HD: Atlas of Pediatric Physical Diagnosis, ed 4, St. Louis, 2002, Mosby.)*

Otitis Externa

Otitis externa, sometimes called swimmer's ear, is an infection of the external auditory canal and pinna. It is usually of bacterial origin but occasionally is fungal. It may be associated with swimming, irritation or the introduction of organisms when cleaning the ear, or frequent use of earphones or earplugs. Pain, purulent discharge, and a hearing deficit are common signs of otitis externa. Otitis externa can be differentiated from otitis media because pain is usually increased with movement of the pinna.

Chronic Disorders of the Ear

Otosclerosis

Otosclerosis involves an imbalance in bone formation and resorption. With development of excess bone in the middle ear cavity, the stapes becomes fixed to the oval window, blocking conduction of sound into the cochlea. Otosclerosis appears to develop from a genetic factor, primarily in young adult females. Surgical removal of the stapes (stapedectomy) and replacement by a prosthesis restores hearing. If laser surgery is used in an early stage, the stapes may be freed and no prosthesis is required.

Ménière's Syndrome

Ménière's syndrome is an inner ear or labyrinth disorder beginning in adults 30 to 50 years of age. Usually it affects one ear. Excessive endolymph develops intermittently, stretching the membranes and interfering with the function of the hair cells in the cochlea and vestibule. Rupture of the labyrinth membrane may allow perilymph to mix with endolymph, increasing volume and causing an attack. The increased fluid may also be of vascular origin. Each attack may last minutes or hours and causes severe vertigo, tinnitus (excess noise like a roaring motor or ringing), and unilateral hearing loss. Vertigo, a sensation of whirling and weakness, is often accompanied by loss of balance and falls, nausea and sweating, inability to focus, and nystagmus. There is a feeling of pressure in the ear. Repeated occurrences lead to permanent damage to the hair cells, with permanent loss of hearing and vertigo.

The acute episodes occur over several months, followed by a brief period of relief, and then the cycle repeats. Stress is a predisposing factor, as are other conditions that affect blood flow. Changes in barometric pressure may precipitate an attack. Improvement occurs with stress reduction; avoidance of smoking, alcohol, and caffeine; observance of a low-sodium diet; and use of a mild diuretic.

Diagnostic tests include the balance test, electronystagmography (ENG), the fluid test, electrocholeography (ECOG), and magnetic resonance imaging to rule out a tumor or other abnormal structure.

Treatment of attacks consists of drugs such as dimenhydrinate, diazepam, or antihistamines. Home exercise programs have assisted in reducing the individual's sensitivity to motion. In severe cases surgery may be helpful to provide a shunt, remove excess endolymph, or resect the vestibular nerve.

> **THINK ABOUT 15-4**
> a. Explain why infants and young children are predisposed to otitis media.
> b. Explain why earache is often severe in persons with acute otitis media.
> c. Explain two ways in which permanent hearing loss may develop with ear infections.
> d. Differentiate conductive hearing loss from sensorineural loss and give an example of each.
> e. Explain why Ménière's syndrome causes both hearing loss and vertigo.

CASE STUDY A

Glaucoma

Mr. A., age 72, has been treated for chronic glaucoma for 6 years. He has lost some peripheral vision but does not feel seriously impaired. There is one incident in his history 2 years ago when he decided to discontinue his eye drops for a month because he was comfortable and there was no change in his vision. He developed some eye discomfort and blurred vision. Examination confirmed elevated intraocular pressure (IOP) but little additional permanent damage. Since then an increased strength of eye drops was ordered to control IOP.

1. Describe the pathophysiologic change in chronic glaucoma.
2. Why is there decreased peripheral vision?
3. Explain the reason for eye discomfort and blurred vision with increased IOP.

   Mr. A. consulted his doctor about a dark area in his field of vision. It developed suddenly, although he had noticed a few dark floaters recently. He has no pain or discomfort, but the dark area is increasing in size. A detached retina in the right eye is diagnosed.
4. Explain the cause of the: (1) floaters, and (2) dark area in the visual field.
5. Why is it essential to reattach the retina immediately?

CASE STUDY B

Ménière's Syndrome

Mrs K., age 42, had several episodes of vertigo with nausea and temporary loss of hearing. She also has essential hypertension, controlled by medication. Following tests to rule out other possible causes, Ménière's syndrome was diagnosed.

1. Explain how the attacks of vertigo are caused.
2. How might hypertension aggravate the attacks?

3. List three therapeutic measures that may reduce the severity of attacks.

     The attacks continue, although less frequently. She now has lost considerable hearing in the right ear and has difficulty maintaining balance on stairs and on heights.

4. Explain why there is permanent loss of hearing and loss of balance.

     Mrs. K. had surgery on the right ear, which has reduced the attacks of vertigo, but deafness in the right ear continues.

CASE STUDY C

Congenital Deafness in a Young Child

O.R. was diagnosed when 2 weeks old with severe-to-profound sensorineural hearing loss. Pregnancy and delivery were normal and O.R. was healthy at birth, with no evidence of other congenital problems. There was no family history of deafness.

1. Explain the meaning of sensorineural hearing loss.
2. Explain several ways in which profound deafness could affect a child's growth and development.

     His parents began classes in American Sign Language (ASL). English and Hindi were spoken in the home. Over a period of time, three types of behind-the-ear hearing aids were tried on O.R., all without success. Other options to assist O.R. were explored. Following assessment, O.R. was deemed a good candidate (good health and cognitive ability) and received a cochlear implant at age 18 months.

3. How does a cochlear implant differ from the normal hearing process?
4. How is the child's brain promoting the development of verbal skills?

     He received speech and language therapy and was soon responding to sounds and voices. In several months he was using some words in English and Hindi as well as continuing with ASL. By age 3 he was able to put several words together, although his words were not always clear. His verbal skills continue to develop and he is now able to attend a preschool program.

5. Why is family interest and support necessary for successful development of communication skills?
6. What impact might O.R.'s exposure to three languages have on the development of his communication skills?

CHAPTER SUMMARY

Sensory organs can be classified into general senses and special senses.

The eye and ear are special senses, complex structures, providing a major proportion of the body's sensory functions. These organs are vulnerable to damage from trauma, infection, and degenerative processes. Loss of vision or hearing can cause significant changes in lifestyle, employment opportunities, and relationships.

The Eye

- *Inflammation* may be caused by allergens, irritants, trauma, or microorganisms. *Keratitis* is more serious than *conjunctivitis*, because it involves the transparent cornea and therefore raises the potential for permanent visual loss. Keratitis is indicated by severe pain and photophobia.
- *Glaucoma* is characterized by increased intraocular pressure resulting from an excessive amount of aqueous humor in the anterior cavity. The common type, chronic wide-angle glaucoma, is a degenerative condition that causes retinal damage and loss of peripheral vision. If pressure is not controlled, the optic nerve is damaged.
- A *cataract* is a degenerative process with increasing opacity of the lens of the eye, resulting in blurred vision.
- A *detached retina* requires immediate treatment to prevent permanent visual loss, because the retinal cells are deprived of nutrients.
- *Macular degeneration* is manifested by loss of visual acuity and central vision in older persons.

The Ear

- *Hearing loss* may be categorized as conduction deafness when the cause is located in the external or middle ear, or as sensorineural deafness when the inner ear (organ of Corti) or the auditory nerve is damaged.
- *Otitis media* is inflammation or infection of the middle ear, frequently secondary to allergies or upper respiratory infections. Permanent hearing loss may result if the tympanic membrane or ossicles are damaged.
- *Otosclerosis* involves excessive bone formation fixing the stapes to the oval window, blocking sound conduction.
- *Ménière's syndrome* is characterized by episodes of increasing endolymph in the inner ear, impairing both hearing and equilibrium. Ultimately permanent damage to the nerve receptor cells occurs.

STUDY QUESTIONS

1. Describe the classification of senses by their sensory input.
2. Describe the function of each of the following structures in the eye: sclera, cornea, lens, choroid, and ciliary process.
3. Compare the signs of chronic glaucoma, acute glaucoma, cataract, detached retina, and macular degeneration.
4. Describe the progress of a sound wave until it is identified in the brain.

5. Describe two ways in which otitis media can impair hearing permanently.

6. Explain why Ménière's syndrome affects balance and hearing.

ADDITIONAL RESOURCES

Guyton AC, Hall JE: *Textbook of Medical Physiology*, ed 11, Philadelphia, 2005, Saunders.

Thibodeau G, Patton K: *Anatomy and Physiology*, ed 7, St. Louis, 2009, Mosby.

Web Sites

http://www.agbell.org *Alexander Graham Bell Association for the Deaf and Hard of Hearing*

http://www.asha.org *American Speech-Language-Hearing Association*

http://www.deafchildren.org *American Society for Deaf Children*

http://www.nad.org *National Association of the Deaf*

http://www.nei.nih.gov/health/glaucoma/glaucoma_ facts.asp *National Eye Institute-Glaucoma*

http://www.nidcd.nih.gov *National Institute on Deafness and other Communication Disorders*

Endocrine System Disorders

CHAPTER OUTLINE

LEARNING OBJECTIVES

After studying this chapter, the student is expected to:

1. Explain the homeostasis of hormones.
2. Name the endocrine glands and the hormones they secrete.
3. Describe the function of each hormone discussed.
4. Differentiate the action of steroid and nonsteroid hormones on the target cell.
5. Explain the relationship between metabolic syndrome and diabetes mellitus.
6. Differentiate Type 1 and Type 2 diabetes mellitus.
7. Compare the causes and development of hypoglycemia and hyperglycemia.
8. Describe the common degenerative effects of diabetes mellitus.
9. Explain the relationship between parathyroid hormone and calcium and their changes with various disorders.
10. Describe the possible effects of a pituitary tumor.
11. Compare the effects of an excess and a deficit of growth hormone in a child and an adult.
12. List the causes and effects of diabetes insipidus and inappropriate ADH syndrome.
13. Describe the causes of goiter.
14. Explain the effects of an excess and a deficit of thyroid hormones.
15. List the possible causes of Cushing's syndrome.
16. Compare the effects of Cushing's and Addison's diseases.

KEY TERMS

anabolic	glucosuria	ketones	neuropathy
catabolism	hyperglycemia	ketonuria	polydipsia
ectopic	hypoglycemia	macroangiopathy	polyphagia
endemic	iatrogenic	microangiopathy	polyuria
gluconeogenesis	ketoacidosis	negative feedback	tropic

Review of the Endocrine System

The major endocrine glands are scattered throughout the body and include the hypothalamus, pituitary gland (hypophysis), pineal gland, the two adrenal glands, the thyroid gland, the four parathyroid glands, the endocrine portion of the pancreas, the gonads, and the thymus (Fig. 16-1). Also, local hormones are secreted in the digestive tract, which regulates its secretions and motility. These hormones are discussed in Chapter 17. Endocrine glands secrete hormones directly into the blood, in contrast to exocrine glands that secrete into a duct, such as mucus, serous glands, or pancreatic digestive enzymes.

Hormones are chemical messengers that may be classified by action, source, or chemical structure. For example, several hormones affect blood glucose levels, including insulin, glucagon, epinephrine, cortisol, and growth hormone.

- Classification by source
  - Hypothalamus
    - Releasing and inhibiting hormones
    - Antidiuretic hormone (ADH—vasopressin)

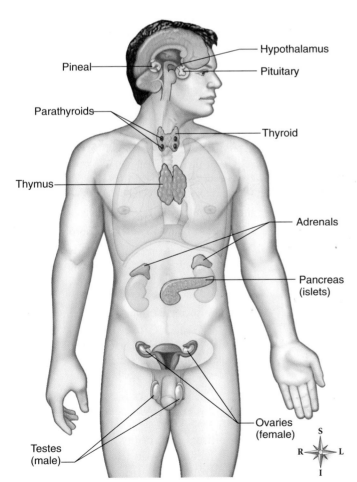

FIGURE 16-1 Locations of some major endocrine glands. *(From Patton KT, Thibodeau GA: Anatomy & Physiology, ed 8, St. Louis, 2013, Mosby.)*

- Oxytocin
  - Both ADH and oxytocin are produced in the hypothalamus, and transported to the neurohypophysis (posterior pituitary) where they are stored and released upon the appropriate stimulus.
- Pituitary
  - Growth hormone (GH)
  - Prolactin
  - FSH—follicle stimulating hormone
  - LH—luteinizing hormone
  - TSH—thyroid stimulating hormone
  - ACTH—adrenocorticotropic hormone
- Thymus
  - Thymosin and thymopoietin
- Thyroid
  - Thyroid hormone
  - Calcitonin
- Parathyroid glands
  - Parathyroid hormone
- Adrenal cortex
  - Mineralocorticoids
  - Glucocorticoids
  - Gonadocorticoids
- Adrenal medulla
  - Epinephrine and norepinephrine
- Pancreas
  - Insulin
  - Glucagon
  - Somatostatin
- Pineal gland
  - Melatonin
- Ovaries
  - Estrogen
  - Progesterone
- Testis
  - Testosterone
- Classification by chemical structure
  - Steroid
    - Steroids are lipids, they enter the cell and nucleus and act directly in the nucleus to engage in transcription (messenger RNA)
  - Nonsteroid
    - Need a second messenger system to finally activate the formation of mRNA

Following release from an endocrine gland, the hormones circulate to target cells in other glands or tissues. After acting on specific receptors on or in the target cells, the hormones are metabolized or inactivated by the target tissues or the liver and excreted by the kidneys to prevent excessive amounts from accumulating in the body over a period of time. Table 16-1 provides a brief review of major hormones, their sources, and primary effects.

The release of hormones from glands is most frequently controlled by a negative feedback mechanism (Fig. 16-2). For example, as levels of glucose increase,

TABLE 16-1 **Sources of Major Hormones and Primary Effects**

Hormone	Source	Primary Effects
Hypothalamic-releasing hormones	Hypothalamus	Stimuli to anterior pituitary to release specific hormone
Hypothalamic-inhibiting hormones	Hypothalamus	Decrease release of specific hormone by anterior pituitary
Growth hormone (GH, somatotropin)	Pituitary—anterior lobe (adenohypophysis)	Stimulates protein synthesis
Adrenocorticotropic hormone (ACTH)	Adenohypophysis	Stimulates adrenal cortex to secrete primarily cortisol
Thyroid-stimulating hormone (TSH)	Adenohypophysis	Stimulates thyroid gland
Follicle-stimulating hormone (FSH)	Adenohypophysis	Women: stimulates growth of ovarian follicles and estrogen secretion; men: stimulates sperm production
Luteinizing hormone (LH)	Adenohypophysis	Women: stimulates maturation of ovum and ovulation; men: stimulates secretion of testosterone
Prolactin (PRL)	Adenohypophysis	Stimulates breast milk production during lactation
Antidiuretic hormone (ADH, or vasopressin)	Pituitary- posterior lobe (neurohypophysis)	Increases reabsorption of water in kidney
Oxytocin (OT)	Neurohypophysis	Stimulates contraction of uterus after delivery Stimulates ejection of breast milk during lactation
Insulin	Pancreas—beta cells of islets of Langerhans	Transport of glucose and other substances into cells Lowers blood glucose level
Glucagon	Pancreas—alpha cells	Glycogenolysis in liver Increases blood glucose level
Parathyroid hormone (PTH)	Parathyroid gland	Increases blood calcium level by stimulating bone demineralization and increasing absorption of Ca^{++} in the digestive tract and kidneys
Calcitonin	Thyroid gland	Decreases release of calcium from the bone to lower blood calcium level
Thyroxine (T_4) and triiodothyronine (T_3)	Thyroid gland	Increases metabolic rate in all cells
Aldosterone	Adrenal cortex	Increases sodium and water reabsorption in the kidney
Cortisol	Adrenal cortex	Anti-inflammatory and decreases immune response Catabolic effect on tissues; stress response
Norepinephrine	Adrenal medulla	General vasoconstriction
Epinephrine	Adrenal medulla	Stress response Visceral and cutaneous vasoconstriction Vasodilation in skeletal muscle Increases rate and force of heart contraction Bronchodilation

the secretion of insulin increases. When glucose levels decrease, insulin secretion decreases.

The endocrine and nervous systems work together to regulate metabolic activities. The hypothalamus and pituitary gland comprise a complex control system for some hormones. The hypothalamus initially secretes releasing or inhibiting hormones; for example, thyrotropin-releasing factor acts on the pituitary gland to secrete thyroid-stimulating hormone (TSH). When determining the cause of a hormonal deficit or excess, it is necessary to check pituitary hormone levels as well as those of the target gland. For example, a deficit of

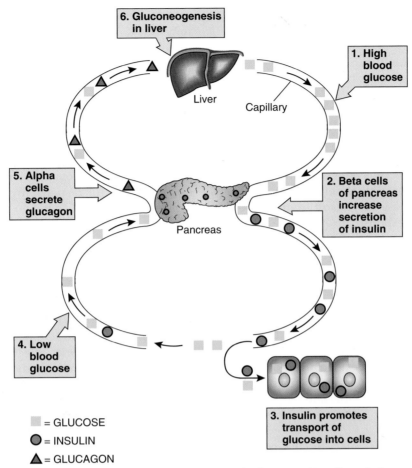

6. Gluconeogenesis in liver

1. High blood glucose

Liver

Capillary

5. Alpha cells secrete glucagon

2. Beta cells of pancreas increase secretion of insulin

Pancreas

4. Low blood glucose

3. Insulin promotes transport of glucose into cells

■ = GLUCOSE

● = INSULIN

▲ = GLUCAGON

FIGURE 16-2 Negative feedback mechanism with glucose and insulin and glucagon.

thyroxine could result from a pituitary problem (decreased secretion of TSH) or a problem in the thyroid gland. In the latter case, blood levels of TSH would be high, whereas thyroxine levels would be low (see Fig. 16-13 for the thyroid hormone feedback system).

In some cases, secretion is controlled by more than one mechanism (e.g., aldosterone is regulated by renin secretion and serum levels of Na^+ and K^+).

To assist in maintaining a well-controlled blood level of a substance such as calcium, a balance of several hormones, such as parathyroid hormone and calcitonin, is required. These are *antagonistic* hormones and have opposing actions on serum calcium. The blood level of glucose is critical to nervous system function and fluid balance; therefore, as mentioned, it is controlled by a number of hormones.

Another variable affecting hormone levels in the body is the rate or timing of secretion. Some hormones, such as thyroid hormone, are maintained at fairly constant levels, whereas others are released in large amounts intermittently as the demand occurs. Some hormones, such as estrogen, follow a cyclic pattern in women. Adrenocorticotropic hormone (ACTH) and cortisol are secreted in a diurnal pattern, the highest levels occurring in the morning and the lowest levels at night. If an

individual's sleep pattern changes, the hormonal secretion changes with it. However, any acute stress leads to the sympathetic nervous system overriding this pattern, resulting in a great outflow of ACTH and cortisol.

THINK ABOUT 16-1

a. State and explain the effect of a high-carbohydrate meal on insulin secretion.
b. Explain why it is beneficial for more than one hormone to control certain activities (e.g., blood pressure).
c. Construct a feedback chart for the glucocorticoids (hydrocortisone).
d. Describe the effect on the natural secretion of hormone from the pituitary gland and the adrenal gland when large amounts of glucocorticoids are administered.

Endocrine Disorders

There are essentially two categories of endocrine problems: an excessive amount of hormone and a deficit of hormone. The manifestations of hormonal disorders reflect the actions of the hormone. Frequently endocrine disorders cause distinctive changes in the individual's physical appearance, which may be helpful in diagnosis.

The most common cause of endocrine disorders is the development of a benign tumor, or *adenoma*. Adenomas may be secretory, causing excess hormone, or they may have a destructive effect on the gland, causing a hormonal deficit. In the case of an adenoma in the pituitary gland, located in the bony sella turcica on the inferior surface of the brain, this will cause increased intracranial pressure and neurologic effects.

In some cases, the target cells are resistant or insensitive to the hormone, thus creating the effect of a hormone deficit. This lack of response may result from a genetic defect, an autoimmune response, or excessive demand on the target cells. An example of this receptor insensitivity to insulin may be seen in Type 2 diabetes mellitus.

Other causes of hormonal imbalances include congenital defects in the glands, hyperplasia or infection in the glands, abnormal immune reactions, and vascular problems.

Not all hormones are covered in this chapter. However, if the normal effects of a hormone are known, it is possible to predict the effects of an excess or a deficit. Diagnostic tests and treatment follow similar patterns.

■ Diagnostic Tests

Levels of tropic hormones secreted by the pituitary gland, as well as the levels of hormones secreted by the target gland, must be evaluated to determine the source of an endocrine disorder. In some patients, an excessive amount of hormone may arise from an ectopic (outside) source, such as a bronchogenic cancer, rather than from a gland. In such cases, the levels of tropic hormones are low.

Blood tests are commonly used to check serum hormone levels, frequently making use of radioimmunoassay methods or, more recently, immunochemical methods (enzyme-multiplied immunoassay technique or chemoluminescence). The effectiveness of a hormone can be measured; for example, blood glucose or blood calcium levels may reflect the activity of the respective hormones. Twenty-four-hour *urine tests* are helpful for ascertaining daily levels of hormones or their metabolites rather than using a random level taken at a specific moment. *Stimulation* or *suppression tests* can be performed to confirm the hyperfunction or hypofunction of a gland.

Scans, ultrasound, and *magnetic resonance imaging* are also helpful for checking the location and type of lesion that may be present. *Biopsy* is essential to eliminate the possibility of malignancy.

■ Treatment

Treatment depends on the cause of the problem. Hormone deficits may be treated with replacement therapy; for example, insulin to treat diabetes mellitus.

Adenomas causing excessive secretions may be removed surgically or by radiation therapy. Removal may be essential when pressure from the mass causes additional problems. For example, pituitary tumors cause pressure inside the skull, compressing brain tissue.

Insulin and Diabetes Mellitus

Diabetes mellitus is caused by a relative deficit of insulin secretion from the beta cells in the islets of Langerhans or by the lack of response by cells to insulin (insulin resistance). To simplify the text, *insulin deficit* is used to cover both decreased secretion of the hormone and insulin resistance.

Insulin is an anabolic hormone (building up or synthesis of complex substances from simple molecules). Deficient insulin results in abnormal carbohydrate, protein, and fat metabolism because the transport of glucose and amino acids into cells is impaired, as well as the synthesis of protein and glycogen. In turn, these metabolic abnormalities affect lipid metabolism. Many tissues and organs in the body are adversely affected by diabetes.

Some types of cells are not affected *directly* by the deficit of insulin. Insulin is not required for the transport of glucose into brain cells. This is fortunate, because neurons require glucose constantly as an energy source. In the digestive tract, insulin is not required for glucose absorption. *Exercising* skeletal muscle can utilize glucose without proportionate amounts of insulin. This can be significant because excessive exercise can deplete blood glucose and result in hypoglycemia. Conversely, exercise is helpful in controlling blood glucose levels in the presence of an insulin deficit.

Type 1 and Type 2 Diabetes

There are two basic types of diabetes, Types 1 and 2 (Table 16-2). The classification system has been revised to better reflect the pathology. *Type 1,* formerly insulin-dependent diabetes mellitus, type I, or juvenile diabetes, is the more severe form. It occurs more frequently in children and adolescents, but can develop at any age. Although there is a genetic factor in the development of the disease, the insulin deficit results from destruction of the pancreatic beta cells in an autoimmune reaction, resulting in an absolute deficit of insulin in the body and therefore requiring replacement therapy. The amount of insulin required is equivalent to the metabolic needs of the body based on dietary intake and metabolic activity. Acute complications such as hypoglycemia or ketoacidosis are more likely to occur in this group. About 1 in every 400 to 500 children has Type 1 diabetes; Type 1 diabetes occurs in approximately 10% of all individuals diagnosed with diabetes. It is a major factor predisposing to strokes (cerebrovascular accident), heart attacks

TABLE 16-2	General Comparison of Type 1 and Type 2 Diabetes	
	Type 1	**Type 2**
Age at onset	Children and adults	Older but also younger adults
Onset	Acute	Insidious
Etiology	Autoimmune destruction	Familial, lifestyle and environmental factors, obesity
	Family history	
Body weight	Thin	Obese
Plasma insulin level	Very low	Decreased or normal
Treatment	Insulin replacement	Diet and exercise or oral hypoglycemic agents or insulin replacement
Occurrence of hypoglycemia or ketoacidosis	Frequent	Less common

(myocardial infarction, peripheral vascular disease and amputation, kidney failure, and blindness.

Type 2 diabetes, formerly referred to as non–insulin-dependent diabetes mellitus, Type II, or mature-onset diabetes, is based on decreased effectiveness of insulin or a relative deficit of insulin. This abnormality may involve decreased pancreatic beta cell production of insulin, increased resistance by body cells to insulin, increased production of glucose by the liver, or a combination of these factors.

This form of diabetes may be controlled by adjusting the need for insulin by:
• Regulating dietary intake
• Increase use of glucose, such as with exercise
• Reducing insulin resistance
• Stimulating the beta cells of the pancreas to produce more insulin

Type 2 is a milder form of diabetes, often developing gradually in older adults, the majority of whom are overweight. However, there has been an increased incidence in adolescents and younger adults who are identified with *metabolic syndrome*, a complex of several pathophysiologic conditions marked by obesity, cardiovascular changes, and significant insulin resistance due to increased adipose tissue (see Chapter 23). Individuals with metabolic syndrome often have developed vascular or other chronic complications before diagnosis. A major concern at this time is the rapid climb in incidence of Type 2 diabetes, with prevalence now estimated at about 9% (18 million) of the population greater than 20 years of age. With increasing obesity seen in the population, it is anticipated that future incidence will increase significantly. Also, it is thought that there may be one

undiagnosed case for every two to three diagnosed cases. Prevalence of Type 2 diabetes increases with age, with approximately half the cases found in persons greater than 55 years of age. There is a higher prevalence in African Americans, Hispanic Americans, and Native Americans.

Gestational diabetes may develop during pregnancy and disappear after delivery of the child (see Chapter 22). Approximately 5% to 10% of women who have gestational diabetes develop Type 2 diabetes some years later. A number of other types of diabetes and glucose intolerance vary in cause and severity. The following discussion focuses on Types 1 and 2.

A number of other types of diabetes are recognized and include:
• Prediabetes—an early manifestation of Type 2 diabetes
• Latent autoimmune diabetes in adults—a slow onset Type 1 autoimmune diabetes
• Maturity onset diabetes of the young—a rare form caused by a mutation in an autosomal dominant gene
• Diabetes insipidus—diabetes not related to blood sugar levels, but an insensitivity of the kidneys to ADH

■ *Pathophysiology*
An insulin deficit leads to the following sequence of events.

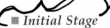

■ *Initial Stage*
1. Insulin deficit results in decreased transportation and use of glucose in many cells of the body.
2. Blood glucose levels rise (hyperglycemia).
3. Excess glucose spills into the urine (glucosuria) as the level of glucose in the filtrate exceeds the capacity of the renal tubular transport limits to reabsorb it.
4. Glucose in the urine exerts osmotic pressure in the filtrate, resulting in a large volume of urine to be excreted (polyuria), with the loss of fluid and electrolytes (e.g., sodium and potassium) from the body tissues.
5. Fluid loss through the urine and high blood glucose levels draw water from the cells, resulting in dehydration (see Chapter 2).
6. Dehydration causes thirst (polydipsia).
7. Lack of nutrients entering the cells stimulates appetite (polyphagia).

THINK ABOUT 16-2

List the signs, including rationale for each, of developing diabetes.

■ *Progressive Effects.* If the insulin deficit is severe or prolonged, the process continues to develop, resulting in additional consequences, ultimately, diabetic

ketoacidosis. This occurs more frequently in persons with Type 1 diabetes.

8. Lack of glucose in cells results in catabolism of fats and proteins, leading to excessive amounts of fatty acids and their metabolites, known as ketones or ketoacids, in the blood.

Ketones consist of acetone and two organic acids—beta-hydroxybutyric acid and acetoacetic acid. Because the liver and other cells are limited in the amount of lipids, fatty acids, or ketones they can process completely within a given time, excessive amounts of ketones in the blood cause ketoacidosis.

The ketoacids bind with bicarbonate buffer in the blood, leading to decreased serum bicarbonate and eventually to a decrease in the pH of body fluids. (Note that ketones can also accumulate in people on starvation diets.)

9. Ketoacids are excreted in the urine (ketonuria). Some diabetic patients test their urine for ketones.

10. However, as dehydration develops, the glomerular filtration rate in the kidney is decreased, and excretion of acids becomes more limited, resulting in *decompensated metabolic acidosis,* which has life-threatening potential (diabetic ketoacidosis [DKA] or diabetic coma).

THINK ABOUT 16-3

In people with diabetes mellitus Type 1, explain the reason for: (a) ketoacidosis, and (b) ketonuria.

Signs and Symptoms

As Type 2 diabetes develops weight gain or increased abdominal girth is common, whereas in Type 1 weight loss is common. As blood glucose rises in the early stage, fluid loss is significant. Polyuria is indicated by urinary frequency, which is often noticed by the patient at night (nocturia) with the excretion of large volumes of urine. Thirst and dry mouth occur in response to fluid loss. Fatigue and lethargy develop. Weight loss may follow. Appetite is increased. Typically, the three Ps—polyuria, polydipsia, and polyphagia—herald the onset of diabetes. If the insulin deficit continues, the patient progresses to the stage of diabetic ketoacidosis.

Diagnostic Tests

Fasting blood glucose level, the glucose tolerance test, and the glycosylated hemoglobin (HbA_1c) test are used to screen people with clinical and subclinical diabetes. There is less emphasis now on the "prediabetic stage" because tissue and organ damage appear to commence at an early stage. At present, a fasting blood sugar equal to or greater than 126 mg/dL, taken on more than one occasion, confirms a diagnosis of diabetes.

The test for HbA_{1c} is used to monitor long-term control (8 to 12 weeks) of blood glucose levels. The test should be repeated every 3 months. The acceptable level for HbA_{1c} has been lowered to 7%, and is likely to be lowered again to 6% (normal), so as to reduce the serious long-term effects of hyperglycemia.

Patients with diabetes can monitor themselves at home by taking a sample of capillary blood from a finger and checking it with a portable monitoring machine (glucometer). When performed regularly, this self-monitoring test helps reduce the fluctuations in blood glucose levels and therefore the risk of complications. Urine tests for ketones are helpful for those who are predisposed to ketoacidosis. Arterial blood gas analysis is required if ketoacidosis develops. Serum electrolytes may be checked as well.

Treatment

Maintenance of normal blood glucose levels is important to minimize the complications of diabetes mellitus, both acute and chronic. Glucose intake must be balanced with use. Treatment measures depend on the severity of the insulin deficit and may change over time. There are essentially three levels of control:

1. Diet and exercise
2. Oral medication to increase insulin secretion or reduce insulin resistance
3. Insulin replacement

Diet. Therapy is based on maintaining optimum body weight (weight reduction may be necessary) as well as control of blood glucose levels. This is important for persons with both types of diabetes. Recommended diets include more complex carbohydrates with a low glycemic index in contrast to simple sugars, which have a high glycemic index and elevate blood glucose rapidly; adequate protein; as well as maintaining low cholesterol and low lipid levels. Increased fiber with meals appears to reduce surges in blood sugar associated with food intake.

The total amount of food intake, as well as the distribution of the constituents, is important. Food intake must match available insulin and metabolic needs, including activity level. Various methods of meal planning are available from the diabetic associations and local diabetic clinics to ensure that the patient ingests a good balance of the various nutrients and provide information on the exchange of food components without disruption of goals. Nutritionists can be consulted on an individual basis in many diabetic clinics.

THINK ABOUT 16-4

How would omission of a meal affect blood glucose levels and insulin balance?

■ *Exercise.* A regular moderate exercise program is very beneficial to the diabetic. Exercise can increase the uptake of glucose by muscles substantially without an increase in insulin use. It also assists in weight control, reduces stress, and improves cardiovascular fitness.

There is a risk that hypoglycemia may develop with exercise, particularly strenuous or prolonged exercise. The increased use of glucose by skeletal muscle, plus the increased absorption of insulin from the injection site, may lower blood glucose levels precipitously. Increasing carbohydrate intake by eating a snack to compensate for exercise can decrease this risk.

■ *Oral Medications.* Antidiabetic agents or oral hypoglycemic drugs such as glyburide (Diaβeta®) and repaglinide (Prandin) are useful in the treatment of Type 2 diabetes when diet and exercise alone are not effective. These drugs stimulate the beta cells of the pancreas to increase insulin release. Drugs such as metformin (Glucophage) act to reduce insulin resistance and to reduce hepatic glucose production. The newer drugs (rosiglitazone/Avandia) increase tissue sensitivity to insulin, but they do have some side effects.

Frequently a combination of diet, exercise, and oral hypoglycemic drugs is effective in treating mild forms of diabetes.

■ *Insulin Replacement.* Insulin can be used for replacement therapy. It must be injected subcutaneously because it is a protein that is destroyed in the digestive tract if taken orally. Continuous infusions via a small pump are favored by some diabetics and may provide better control.

The primary form of insulin used now is a biosynthetic form of insulin, identical to human insulin (Humulin), synthesized by bacteria using recombinant DNA techniques. Insulin is standardized in units for subcutaneous administration and is produced in three forms: rapid-onset, short-acting (regular) insulin; intermediate-acting (Lente) insulin; and slow-onset, long-acting (protamine zinc or Ultralente) insulin. Newer insulins on the market have a very rapid onset, 15 minutes, or last for 24 hours, in an attempt to provide better control of serum levels. Any transition from one type of insulin to another must be carefully monitored by a physician. Blood glucose levels should be checked at more frequent intervals during any changes.

The type of insulin used and its effective period can be important factors in predicting periods of potential hypoglycemia in individual patients, and food intake can be timed to coincide with peak insulin levels, thus avoiding hypoglycemia. Each patient has an individualized schedule of insulin administration. Injection sites must be rotated to minimize skin damage. Insulin types may be mixed for administration, and several injections may be required in 1 day.

Insulin dosage may also require adjustment under special circumstances such as infection with high fever or vomiting, or at the time of surgery. Continuous control of blood glucose levels minimizes the risk of potential complications for the patient. Improved self-monitoring devices are helpful. Small, computerized recording and data bank devices have improved the compliance of young adults.

■ *Complications*

Many factors can lead to fluctuations in serum glucose levels and subsequent changes in cell metabolism throughout the body. These changes may result from variations in diet or physical activity, the presence of infections, or alcohol use. Complications may be acute (e.g., hypoglycemia) or chronic. Long-term complications such as vascular disease result from degenerative changes in the tissues. Stable blood glucose levels reduce the risk of complications.

■ *Acute Complications.*

Hypoglycemia (Insulin Shock). Hypoglycemia is precipitated by an excess of insulin, which causes a deficit of glucose in the blood (Fig. 16-3). It usually occurs in patients with Type 1 diabetes, often quite suddenly, following strenuous exercise, an error in dosage, vomiting, or skipping a meal after taking insulin. Many individuals are able to recognize their own response.

The lack of glucose quickly affects the nervous system, because neurons cannot use fats or protein as an energy source. The manifestations of hypoglycemia are related directly to the low blood glucose levels, not to the high insulin levels.

- One group of signs is related to *impaired neurologic function* resulting from the lack of glucose. These signs include poor concentration, slurred speech, lack of coordination, and staggering gait. Persons with hypoglycemia are sometimes assumed to be intoxicated with alcohol.
- The second group of signs is related to the hypoglycemic state stimulating the *sympathetic nervous system*, resulting in increased pulse; pale, moist skin; anxiety; and tremors. If hypoglycemia remains untreated, loss of consciousness, seizures, and death will follow.

Treatment consists of immediate administration of a concentrated carbohydrate, such as sweetened fruit juice or candy. If the person is unconscious, glucose or glucagon may be given parenterally (usually intravenously).

Hypoglycemia can be life threatening or can cause brain damage if it is not treated promptly. It is wise to verify that patients who have come for other treatments have eaten and taken the appropriate medications before the appointment to minimize the risk of a hypoglycemic episode during the appointment. Appointments should be scheduled so that meals are not unduly delayed or missed.

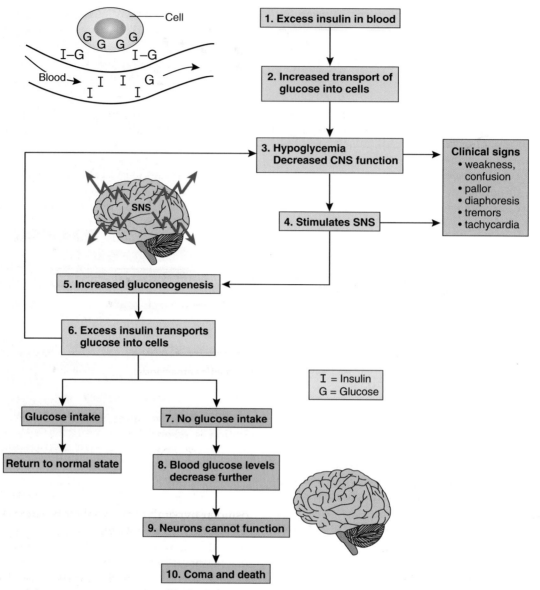

FIGURE 16-3 Hypoglycemic shock (insulin shock).

EMERGENCY TREATMENT FOR HYPOGLYCEMIC SHOCK

1. If conscious, immediately give sweet fruit juice (liquids are absorbed more quickly), honey, candy, or sugar.
2. If unconscious, give nothing by mouth. Intravenous glucose 50% is required.
3. Note: Diabetic ketoacidosis (diabetic coma or hyperglycemia) also causes loss of consciousness. The emergency treatment is insulin, fluid, and sodium bicarbonate. Assessment should be done to differentiate the cause.

Diabetic Ketoacidosis. As indicated earlier, DKA results from insufficient insulin, which leads to high blood glucose levels and mobilization of lipids. It is more common in Type 1 patients. Ketoacidosis usually develops over a few days and may be initiated by an infection or stress, which increases the demand for insulin in the body. It may also result from an error in dosage or overindulgence in food or alcohol (Fig. 16-4).

The signs and symptoms of diabetic ketoacidosis are related to dehydration, metabolic acidosis, and electrolyte imbalances (Table 16-3).

- Signs of dehydration include thirst; dry, rough oral mucosa; and a warm, dry skin. The pulse is rapid but weak and thready, and the blood pressure is low as the vascular volume decreases. Oliguria (decreased urine output) indicates that compensation mechanisms to conserve fluid in the body are taking place.
- Ketoacidosis leads to rapid, deep respirations (Kussmaul's respirations) and acetone breath (a sweet, fruity smell). Lethargy and decreased responsiveness indicate depression of the central nervous system owing to acidosis and decreased blood flow.

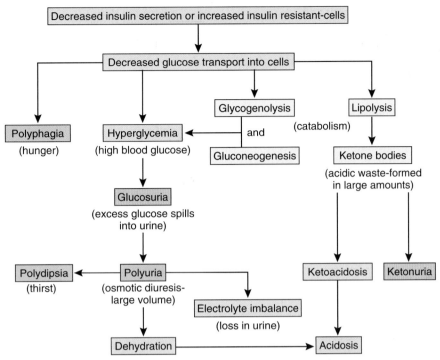

FIGURE 16-4 Development of diabetic ketoacidosis.

- Metabolic acidosis develops as ketoacids bind with bicarbonate ions in the buffer, leading to decreased serum bicarbonate levels and decreased serum pH (see Chapter 2). As dehydration progresses, renal compensation is reduced, acidosis becomes decompensated, and serum pH falls, resulting in loss of consciousness.
- Electrolyte imbalances include imbalances of sodium, potassium, and chloride. Signs include primarily abdominal cramps, nausea, and vomiting, as well as lethargy and weakness. Actual serum values of electrolytes may be misleading because the proportion of water lost can affect the serum level even though the electrolytes were lost in the urine. Serum sodium is often low, but the potassium concentration may be elevated because of acidosis (see Chapter 2). If the condition remains untreated, central nervous system depression develops owing to the acidosis and dehydration, leading to coma.

Treatment of diabetic ketoacidosis involves administration of insulin as well as replacement of fluid and electrolytes. Serum potassium levels may decrease when insulin is administered because insulin promotes transport of potassium into cells. Bicarbonate administration is essential to reverse the acidosis, as well as specific treatment to resolve the causative factor of the diabetic ketoacidosis episode.

Hyperosmolar Hyperglycemic Nonketotic Coma. Hyperosmolar hyperglycemic nonketotic coma develops more frequently in patients with Type 2 diabetes. Often the patient is an older person with an infection or one who has overindulged in carbohydrates, thereby using more insulin than anticipated. In these cases, hyperglycemia and dehydration develop because of the relative insulin deficit, but sufficient insulin is available to prevent ketoacidosis. Therefore, the condition may be difficult to diagnose initially. Severe cellular dehydration results in neurologic deficits, muscle weakness, difficulties with speech, and abnormal reflexes.

THINK ABOUT 16-6

Compare the characteristics of the urine and the effects on pulse and respiration of hypoglycemia, diabetic ketoacidosis, and hyperosmolar hyperglycemic nonketotic coma.

■ *Chronic Complications.* Degenerative changes occur in many tissues with both types of diabetes, particularly when blood glucose levels are poorly controlled. The insulin deficit and glucose excess cause a number of alterations in metabolic pathways involving carbohydrates, lipids, and proteins.

THINK ABOUT 16-5

a. Describe three signs that would help differentiate someone with hypoglycemia from someone with diabetic ketoacidosis.

b. Describe and explain the loss of consciousness that occurs with: (1) hypoglycemia, and (2) diabetic ketoacidosis.

TABLE 16-3   Progressive Effects of an Insulin Deficit (Diabetic Ketoacidosis)

Signs	Rationale
EARLY SIGNS	
Hyperglycemia	*Lack of Insulin*
Hunger (polyphagia)	Compensation for cell starvation
Glucosuria	Glucose in filtrate exceeds tubule transport
Polyuria	Osmotic diuresis due to glucosuria
Thirst (polydipsia)	Response to water loss
Weakness and weight loss	Loss of fluid and lack of glucose to cells
PROGRESSIVE SIGNS	
Increasing hyperglycemia	Gluconeogenesis owing to response by epinephrine, cortisol, and glucagon
Dehydration	*Polyuria*
Skin warm and dry; decreased turgor	Decreased interstitial fluid
Oral mucosa rough and dry	Decreased interstitial fluid
Eyeballs sunken and soft	Decreased interstitial fluid
Decreased blood pressure	Decreased blood volume
Pulse—rapid, thready	Compensation—sympathetic nervous system
Lethargy, weakness, confusion	Decreased oxygen and glucose to the brain resulting from hypovolemia. Also, acidosis and electrolyte imbalance
Ketoacidosis	*Catabolism of Fats And Protein*
Serum bicarbonate and serum pH low	Compensation for acidosis
Rapid, deep respirations (air hunger or Kussmaul's respirations)	Compensation for acidosis
Acetone breath—sweet, fruity odor	Acetone expired
Ketonuria	Ketoacids excreted in urine
Nausea, vomiting, weakness	Loss of Na^+, K^+, Cl^- in urine and ketonemia
LATE SIGNS	
Coma	Central nervous system depression owing to acidosis and dehydration

TABLE 16-4   Vascular Problems with Diabetes

Macroangiopathy

• Myocardial infarction (heart attack) • Cerebrovascular accident (stroke) • Peripheral vascular disease (ischemia, gangrene, and amputation affecting the legs)	Atherosclerosis in large arteries related to hyperlipidemia, hypertension, and degenerative changes in the intimal layer of the arterial wall

Microangiopathy

• Kidneys
  Diabetic nephropathy
  Chronic renal failure
	Thickening of the capillary basement membrane, leading to occlusion or rupture

• Eyes Retinopathy	Microaneurysms, neovascularization, and fibrosis Leads to blindness

• Nervous system
  Neuropathy in the central nervous system and peripheral nerves
  Decreased function of sensory, motor, and autonomic nervous system fibers
	Note—In addition to ischemia, there is also a metabolic abnormality that causes degeneration of myelin and deficit of *myo*-inositol, essential in the conduction of nerve impulses.

Vascular Problems. Changes occur in both the small and large arteries because of degeneration related to the metabolic abnormalities associated with diabetes (Table 16-4). Microangiopathy, in which the capillary basement membrane becomes thick and hard, causes obstruction or rupture of capillaries and small arteries, and results in tissue necrosis and loss of function. *Retinopathy* is a leading cause of blindness (Fig. 16-5). Retinal changes can be observed through the pupil of the eye. Diabetic *nephropathy*, or vascular degeneration in the kidney glomeruli, eventually leads to chronic renal failure (Fig. 16-6). It is responsible for 40% of patients in end-stage renal failure.

Macroangiopathy, like atherosclerosis, affects the large arteries (see Chapter 12), thus leading to a high incidence of heart attacks, strokes, and peripheral vascular disease in diabetics. Obstruction of the arteries in the legs frequently results in ulcers on the feet and legs that are slow to heal (Fig. 16-7). Ulcers are aggravated when peripheral neuropathy is present, reducing pain sensation. Peripheral vascular disease also causes intermittent claudication (pain with walking), which greatly impairs mobility. Decreased blood flow predisposes to frequent infection and gangrenous ulcers. In some cases, vascular problems necessitate amputation if gangrene develops. New surgical techniques allow for less invasive, less traumatic surgery to remove vascular obstructions, using angioscopic bypass surgery. This is very helpful to diabetics, who tend to have delayed healing.

Neuropathy. Peripheral neuropathy is a common problem for diabetics. This leads to impaired sensation,

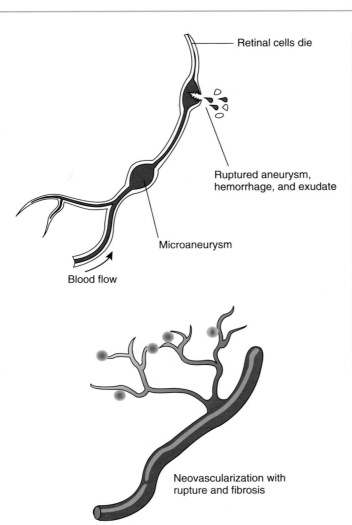

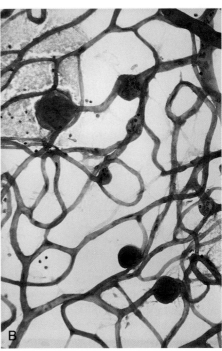

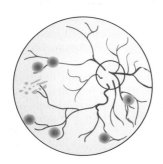

A   Retina with aneurysms and exudate

FIGURE 16-5 **A,** Diabetic retinopathy in the eye. **B,** Retina from a case of advanced diabetic microangiopathy showing several aneurysms. *(From Cotran RS, Kumar V, Collins T: Robbins Pathologic Basis of Disease, ed 6, Philadelphia, 1999, Saunders.)*

numbness, tingling, weakness, and muscle wasting. It results from ischemia and altered metabolic processes. Degenerative changes occur in both unmyelinated and myelinated nerve fibers. The risks of tissue trauma and infection are greatly increased when vascular impairment and sensory impairment coexist.

Autonomic nerve degeneration develops as well, leading to bladder incontinence, impotence, and diarrhea. Impaired vasomotor reflexes may cause dizziness when a person stands up.

Infections. Infections are more common and tend to be more severe in diabetics, probably because of the vascular impairment, which decreases tissue resistance, the delay in healing because of insulin deficit, and the increased glucose levels in body fluids that support

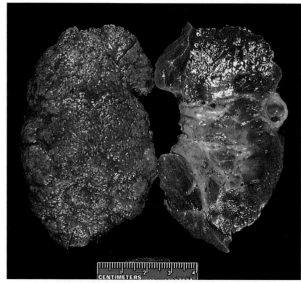

FIGURE 16-6 Diabetic nephrosclerosis in bisected kidney. (*Left*) Fine scarring on the outer surface of the kidney appears granular. (*Right*) Interior of the kidney shows thin cortex and several depressions, the result of pyelonephritis. (*From Kumar V, Abbas AK, Fausto M:* Robbins and Cotran Pathologic Basis of Disease, *ed 7, Philadelphia, 2005, Saunders.*)

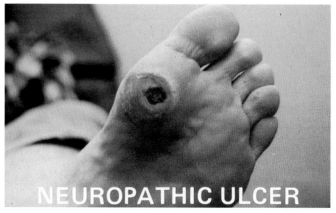

FIGURE 16-7 Classic neuropathic diabetic foot ulcer. Note ulceration in the callus is well circumscribed. The lesion is painless. (*From the Michigan Diabetes Research and Training Center, University of Michigan, Ann Arbor.*)

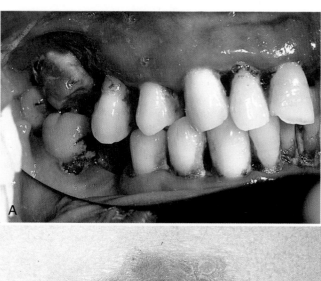

A

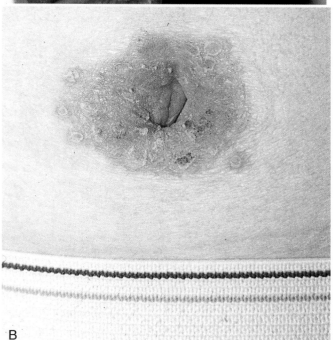

B

FIGURE 16-8 A, Periodontal disease in a diabetic-note the inflammation and infection.
(*Courtesy of Evie Jesin, RRDH, BSc, George Brown College of Applied Arts and Technology, Toronto, Ontario, Canada.*)
B, Candidiasis in the right axilla with satellite pustules. (*From Stone DR, Gorbach SL:* Atlas of Infectious Diseases, *Philadelphia, 2000, Saunders.*)

infection. Wound healing is slow, predisposing to infection in case of trauma or surgery. Diabetics are also susceptible to tuberculosis, which is increasing in incidence.

Infections in the feet and legs tend to persist because of vascular impairment, and healing is slow, contributing to a high incidence of gangrene and resultant amputation.

Fungal infections such as *Candida* occur frequently and persist on the skin in body folds (see Fig. 16-8), in the oral cavity (see Fig. 17-5*B*), and vagina. The urinary tract is a common site of infection, particularly if bladder function is compromised, and predisposes the patient to cystitis and pyelonephritis. Periodontal disease (infection in the tissues around the teeth) (see Fig. 16-8) and dental caries (infection and decay in teeth) are much more common in diabetics.

THINK ABOUT 16-7

a. Describe all the factors that may lead to a persistent infected foot ulcer in patients with diabetes.
b. Suggest several precautions for foot care that should be taken to prevent foot ulceration.

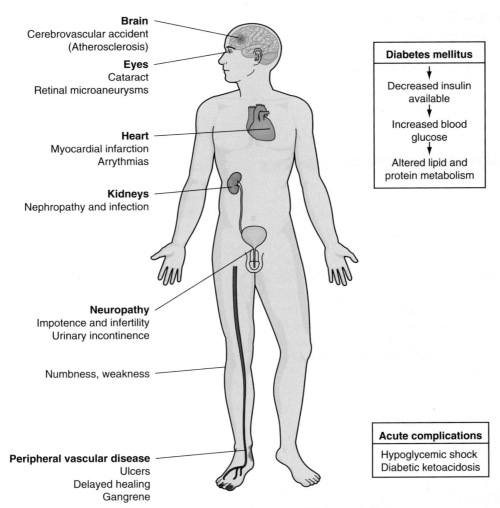

Brain
Cerebrovascular accident
(Atherosclerosis)

Eyes
Cataract
Retinal microaneurysms

Heart
Myocardial infarction
Arrythmias

Kidneys
Nephropathy and infection

Neuropathy
Impotence and infertility
Urinary incontinence

Numbness, weakness

Peripheral vascular disease
Ulcers
Delayed healing
Gangrene

Diabetes mellitus
↓
Decreased insulin
available
↓
Increased blood
glucose
↓
Altered lipid and
protein metabolism

Acute complications
Hypoglycemic shock
Diabetic ketoacidosis

FIGURE 16-9 Potential complications of diabetes mellitus.

Cataracts. Clouding of the lens of the eye is another degenerative process related to the abnormal metabolism of glucose, and it results in accumulated sorbitol and water in the lens, destroying the transparency. Cataracts may eventually lead to blindness and should be removed when they impair visual function (see Chapter 15).

A summary of complications of diabetes may be found in Figure 16-9.

Pregnancy. Complications for both the mother and the fetus may occur during pregnancy. Maternal diabetes may become more severe, control is more difficult with the continual hormonal and metabolic changes, and there is an increased incidence of spontaneous abortions and abnormalities in infants born to diabetic mothers.

APPLY YOUR KNOWLEDGE 16-1

Explain why research efforts into pancreatic beta cell transplants are being strongly supported.

The newborn infant is usually larger than average in size and predisposed to complications. Good prenatal care decreases these risks.

Parathyroid Hormone and Calcium

Hypoparathyroidism may be caused by a congenital lack of the four parathyroid glands, following surgery or radiation in the neck region, or as a result of autoimmune disease. Hypoparathyroidism leads to *hypocalcemia*, or low serum calcium levels.

Hypocalcemia affects nerve and muscle function in different ways. Low serum calcium levels result in *weak cardiac muscle* contractions but also increase the *excitability of nerves*, leading to spontaneous contraction of skeletal muscle. This causes muscle twitching and spasms, commonly known as tetany, which is usually observed first in the face and hands. Hypocalcemia does not weaken skeletal muscle contractions because sufficient calcium is stored in skeletal muscle cells. Cardiac muscle cells, on the other hand, do not have large stores of calcium but rely instead on calcium from the blood for contraction.

Hyperparathyroidism may be caused by an adenoma, hyperplasia, or secondary to renal failure. It causes *hypercalcemia*, or high serum calcium levels. Hypercalcemia leads to forceful cardiac contractions (see Table 2-7 for signs of calcium imbalance). The most serious effects of hyperparathyroidism occur in the bone tissue. Increased parathyroid hormone (PTH) causes calcium to leave the bone, leading to osteoporosis, weakening the bone so that it fractures easily (see Chapter 9). Hypercalcemia also increases predisposition to kidney stones (see Chapter 18).

Calcium metabolism may be modified by other factors, such as the presence of vitamin D and serum phosphate levels. Therefore, calcium imbalance may not be caused by hormone disorders. Serum levels of PTH and calcium may vary depending on the specific cause of the problem. For instance, in patients who are immobile or have bone cancer, *hypercalcemia* may be present along with a *low* level of PTH (Fig. 16-10). In patients with severe renal disease, there is decreased activation of vitamin D in the kidneys (see Chapter 18). Vitamin D is essential for calcium absorption and metabolism. Renal failure also leads to retention of phosphate ion and hyperphosphatemia. Because calcium and phosphate have a reciprocal relationship, hypocalcemia results. In this case, hypocalcemia leads to *high* levels of PTH. Therefore, any changes in the bone, kidneys, or digestive tract are significant in determining the cause of calcium imbalance, as are serum levels of calcium, phosphate, and PTH.

A comparison of the common effects of parathyroid imbalances is found in Figure 16-11. Treatment of parathyroid disorders depends on the cause. Any underlying disorder should be treated. Chronic hypoparathyroidism may be treated with calcium and vitamin D. Parathyroidectomy may be required for hyperparathyroidism.

THINK ABOUT   16-8

a. Describe three ways in which increased secretion of PTH can increase blood levels of calcium.
b. Describe the effect of increased calcitonin secretion on blood calcium levels.
c. Explain how malabsorption of calcium from the intestine would affect serum calcium and serum PTH.
d. Compare the effects of hypocalcemia on cardiac and skeletal muscle and explain the rationale for each.

Pituitary Hormones

As mentioned, it is important to determine the source of the imbalance in hormones controlled by the pituitary, whether it is in the pituitary gland, the hypothalamus, or the target gland (see Fig. 16-2).

Benign adenomas are the most common cause of pituitary disorders. They lead to two groups of manifestations in the patient:

- The effect of the mass as it enlarges and causes pressure in the skull (increased intracranial pressure, see Chapter 14). Signs of pressure on brain tissues include increasing headaches, seizures, and drowsiness. Visual defects such as hemianopsia are common because of pressure on the adjacent optic chiasm.
- The effect of the tumor on hormone secretion. The hormonal effects of the adenoma depend on which specific cells in the pituitary are involved and their location. For example, growth hormone is produced in cells in the anterior wings of the gland, whereas prolactin-producing cells are scattered throughout the gland. The tumor cells may secrete an excessive amount of a particular hormone (e.g., somatotropic cells secrete GH). Or the excess hormone could be ACTH or prolactin. Sometimes more than one hormone is secreted. In some cases, the adenoma may destroy an area of pituitary cells, causing a deficit of a particular hormone (e.g., decreased ACTH and therefore decreased adrenal cortex activity).

With some tumors, *hemorrhage* or *infarction* can occur, causing a sudden increase in intracranial pressure and destroying part of the pituitary (pituitary apoplexy). Untreated adenomas eventually destroy all types of cells, resulting in panhypopituitarism.

Pituitary adenomas make up more than 10% of intracranial tumors. They occur primarily in persons 30 to 50 years of age. Tumors are usually removed by surgery or radiation therapy. Replacement of one or more hormones is necessary after this therapy or any time that deficits develop.

Vascular thrombosis and infarction associated with obstetric delivery or other cardiovascular disorders damages the pituitary, causing hypopituitarism. Hypothalamic disorders include tumors or infection.

Growth Hormone

Dwarfism, or short stature, may be caused by a number of factors, one of which is a deficit of growth hormone (GH, somatotropin) or somatotropin-releasing hormone (Fig. 16-12). In some cases of pituitary adenomas, other types of pituitary cells are also affected, resulting in multiple deficits. Usually the pituitary dwarf has normal intelligence, normal body proportions, and some delay in skeletal maturation and puberty. Replacement therapy for GH deficiency in a child before closure of the epiphyses is available.

Gigantism, or tall stature, results from excess GH before puberty and fusion of the epiphyses.

Acromegaly refers to the effects of excess GH secretion in the adult, usually by an adenoma. The bones become broader and heavier, and the soft tissues grow, resulting in enlarged hands and feet, a thicker skull, and changes

NORMAL CONTROL AND FEEDBACK OF CALCIUM

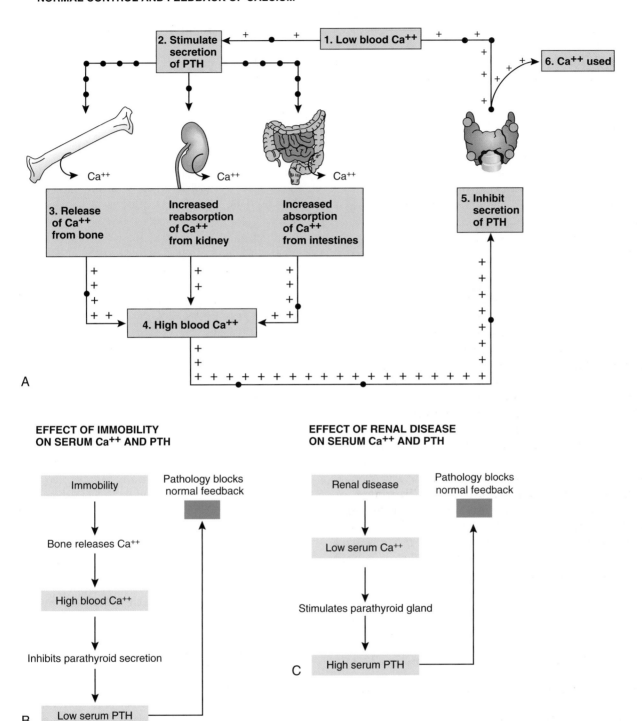

FIGURE 16-10 Calcium and PTH relationships. •, PTH; +, Ca⁺⁺.

in the facial features (see Fig. 16-12*B*). Thickening of the skull bones may compress nerves and blood vessels passing through the foramina. Overgrowth of bones and cartilage may lead to carpal tunnel syndrome (pain and weakness at the wrist and hand) or arthritis. A protruding mandible or jaw (prognathia, see Fig. 16-12*C*) and a large tongue (macroglossia) are common. Initially the patient notices a need for a larger shoe or glove size. In addition, GH affects glucose metabolism and the effectiveness of insulin, resulting eventually in diabetes. Hypertension and cardiovascular disease also develop with untreated acromegaly.

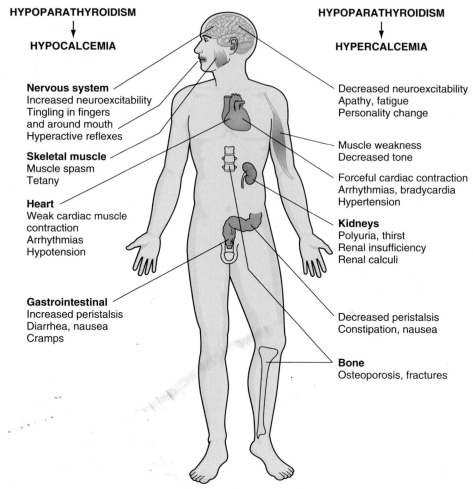

HYPOPARATHYROIDISM
↓
HYPOCALCEMIA

Nervous system
Increased neuroexcitability
Tingling in fingers
and around mouth
Hyperactive reflexes

Skeletal muscle
Muscle spasm
Tetany

Heart
Weak cardiac muscle
contraction
Arrhythmias
Hypotension

Gastrointestinal
Increased peristalsis
Diarrhea, nausea
Cramps

HYPOPARATHYROIDISM
↓
HYPERCALCEMIA

Decreased neuroexcitability
Apathy, fatigue
Personality change

Muscle weakness
Decreased tone

Forceful cardiac contraction
Arrhythmias, bradycardia
Hypertension

Kidneys
Polyuria, thirst
Renal insufficiency
Renal calculi

Decreased peristalsis
Constipation, nausea

Bone
Osteoporosis, fractures

FIGURE 16-11 Common effects of parathyroid hormone imbalances.

THINK ABOUT 16-9

a. Explain why longitudinal bone growth cannot occur in patients with acromegaly.
b. Compare dwarfism, gigantism, and acromegaly, including abnormal hormone secretion, age affected, and effect of hormonal change.

Antidiuretic Hormone (Vasopressin)

Diabetes Insipidus

Diabetes insipidus results from a deficit of ADH. This deficit may originate in the neurohypophysis. Head injury or surgery may cause a temporary condition. In some cases, the condition is considered to be nephrogenic, when the renal tubules do not respond to the hormone. The latter may be genetic or linked to electrolyte imbalance or drugs. The clinical manifestations include polyuria with large volumes of dilute urine and thirst, eventually causing severe dehydration. (Note that glucose is not present in the urine with diabetes insipidus as it is in cases of diabetes mellitus.) Replacement therapy for ADH is available.

Inappropriate Antidiuretic Hormone Syndrome

Inappropriate ADH syndrome, also called *syndrome of inappropriate ADH,* is due to excess ADH, which causes retention of fluid. In some cases, the additional ADH is temporary, triggered by stress, or may be secreted by an ectopic source (e.g., a bronchogenic carcinoma). The signs are related to severe hyponatremia, which causes mental confusion and irritability. Diuretics and sodium supplements are used to correct the problem, as well as investigating any underlying cause.

Thyroid Disorders

The two thyroid hormones, thyroxine and triiodothyronine, are secreted by the thyroid gland in response to hypothalamic-pituitary secretion of thyroid-stimulating hormone (Fig. 16-13). Disorders may result from pituitary or thyroid gland dysfunction.

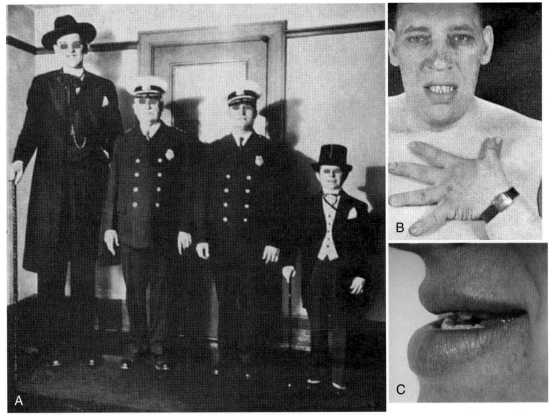

FIGURE 16-12 Effects of growth hormone. **A**, Comparison of (from left to right) gigantism, normal, and dwarfism. *(From Thibodeau GA:* Anatomy and Physiology. *St. Louis, 1987, Mosby. Courtesy of Dr. Edmund Beard, Cleveland, Ohio.)* **B**, The patient's hands and face show clinical signs of acromegaly. *(From Jarvis C:* Physical examination and health assessment, *Philadelphia, 1992, Saunders.)* **C**, Acromegaly. Excessive secretion of growth hormone in the adult caused characteristic malocclusion of the teeth resulting from the overgrowth of the mandible. *(From Cooke RA, Stewart B:* Colour Atlas of Anatomical Pathology, *ed 3, Sydney, 2004, Churchill Livingstone.)*

Goiter

Goiter refers to an enlargement of the thyroid gland, which is often visible on the anterior neck. Goiters are caused by various hypothyroid and hyperthyroid conditions. A goiter can become very large, compressing the esophagus and interfering with swallowing, or it can cause pressure on the trachea. It can also be of cosmetic concern (Fig. 16-14*A*).

Endemic goiter may affect large groups of people in a specific geographical area. It is a hypothyroid condition that occurs in regions where there are low iodine levels in the soil and food (e.g., mountainous areas or around the Great Lakes). Normally iodine is "trapped" by the thyroid gland and used to synthesize triiodothyronine (T_3) and thyroxine (T_4) (see Fig. 16-14*B*). This dietary deficiency leads to low T_3 and T_4 (thyroid hormone) production and a compensatory increase in TSH from the pituitary, producing hyperplasia and hypertrophy in the thyroid gland (see Fig. 16-14*C*). The use of iodized salt has solved this problem to a large extent.

Goitrogens are foods that contain elements that block synthesis of T_3 and T_4 but increase TSH secretion. Thyroid-stimulating hormone causes hyperplasia of the gland and can promote goiter formation when such substances are ingested in large quantities. These foods include cabbage, turnips, and other related vegetables. Lithium and fluoride may also be goitrogenic.

Toxic goiter is a hyperthyroid condition resulting from hyperactivity of the thyroid gland, perhaps due to excessive stimulation by TSH, which produces a large nodular gland.

Hyperthyroidism (Graves' Disease)

There are various forms of hyperthyroidism, with increased T_3 and T_4 secretion. Graves' disease provides an example.

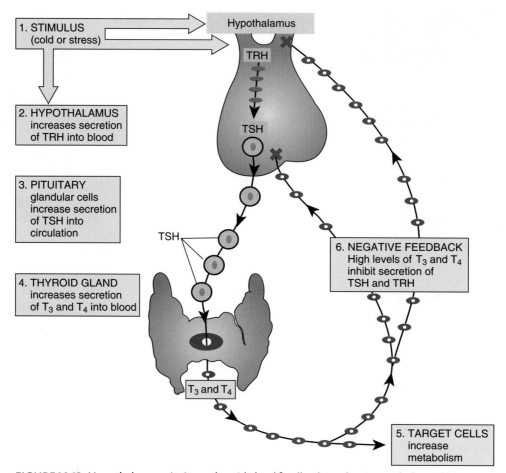

1. STIMULUS (cold or stress)

2. HYPOTHALAMUS increases secretion of TRH into blood

3. PITUITARY glandular cells increase secretion of TSH into circulation

4. THYROID GLAND increases secretion of T_3 and T_4 into blood

Hypothalamus

TRH

TSH

TSH

TSH

T_3 and T_4

6. NEGATIVE FEEDBACK High levels of T_3 and T_4 inhibit secretion of TSH and TRH

5. TARGET CELLS increase metabolism

FIGURE 16-13 Hypothalamus-pituitary-thyroid gland feedback mechanism with thyroid hormone.

Graves' disease occurs more frequently in women over 30 years of age and is related to an autoimmune factor. It is manifested by the signs of hypermetabolism, toxic goiter, and exophthalmos (Table 16-5). Increased stimulation of the sympathetic nervous system magnifies the metabolic effects.

Exophthalmos is evident by the presence of protruding, staring eyes and decreased blink and eye movements (Fig. 16-15). It results from increased tissue mass in the orbit pushing the eyeball forward and from increased sympathetic stimulation affecting the eyelids. If untreated, visual impairment may result from optic nerve damage or corneal ulceration.

Thyrotoxic crisis, or thyroid storm, is an acute situation in a patient with uncontrolled hyperthyroidism, usually precipitated by infection or surgery. It is life threatening because of the resulting hyperthermia, tachycardia, and heart failure and delirium.

Graves' disease is treated by a course of radioactive iodine, surgical removal of the thyroid gland, or the use of antithyroid drugs. Following treatment, there is a risk that patients may develop hypothyroidism or hypoparathyroidism.

TABLE 16-5   **General Comparison of Hypothyroidism and Hyperthyroidism**

	Hypothyroidism	Hyperthyroidism
Serum levels of T_3 and T_4	Low	High
Metabolic rate	Low	High
Goiter	Present with endemic goiter	Present with Graves' disease
Skin	Pale, cool, with edema	Flushed and warm
Temperature tolerance	Cold intolerance	Heat intolerance
Eyes	No changes	Exophthalmos with Graves' disease
Cardiovascular	Bradycardia, enlarged heart	Tachycardia, increased blood pressure
Nervous system	Lethargic, slow intellectual functions	Restless, nervous, tremors
Body weight	Some weight increase with decreased appetite	Thin, but increased appetite

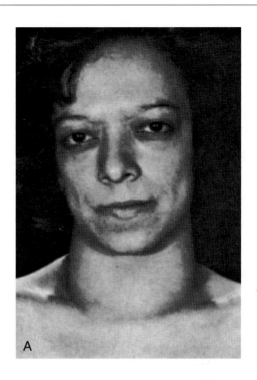

B. STRUCTURE OF THYROID HORMONES

Four iodine atoms

Three iodine atoms

THYROXINE (T₄)   TRIIODOTHYRONINE (T₃)

C. GOITER DEVELOPMENT

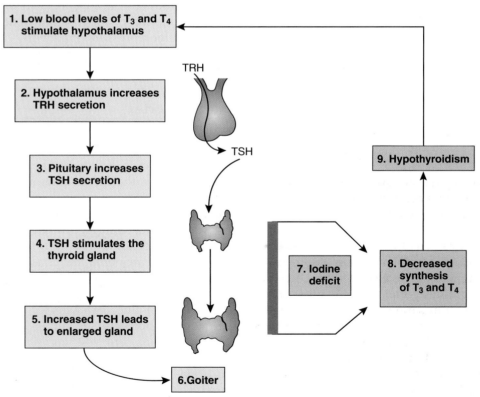

FIGURE 16-14 Endemic goiter and hypothyroidism. (**A,** *from Wilson JD, Foster DW:* Williams Textbook of Endocrinology, *ed 8, Philadelphia, 1992, Saunders.)*

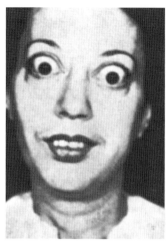

FIGURE 16-15 Hyperthyroidism showing exophthalmos. *(From Wilson JD, Foster DW: Williams Textbook of Endocrinology, ed 8, Philadelphia, 1992, Saunders.)*

Hypothyroidism

Mild hypothyroidism is very common and is easily treated by replacement doses of thyroid hormone. Signs of hypothyroidism are listed in Table 16-5.

Severe hypothyroidism occurs in several forms:
- *Hashimoto's thyroiditis,* a destructive autoimmune disorder
- *Myxedema,* severe hypothyroidism in adults ("myxedema" refers to the nonpitting edema manifested as facial puffiness and a thick tongue); myxedema coma refers to acute hypothyroidism resulting in hypotension, hypoglycemia, hypothermia, and loss of consciousness, a life-threatening complication occurring in undiagnosed or untreated elderly patients.
- *Cretinism,* untreated congenital hypothyroidism, may be related to iodine deficiency during pregnancy or may be a developmental defect. The thyroid gland may be nonfunctional or absent. Neonatal screening is standard in many areas of the country; it leads to early treatment and prevents the mental retardation that accompanies early hypothyroidism. Lack of treatment results in severe impairment of all aspects of growth and development because thyroid hormone affects the metabolism of all cells. For example, the child may have difficulty feeding, delayed tooth eruption, malocclusion, and a large protruding tongue, demonstrating stunted skeletal growth and *extreme* lethargy.

Diagnostic Tests

Current tests for thyroid disorders include checks of blood levels of T_4 and T_3, as well as serum TSH levels, and the uptake of radioactive iodine (T_3 uptake test).

Scans may be used to search for the presence of tumor nodules. Antibody assays may also be required to confirm a specific diagnosis.

THINK ABOUT 16-10
a. Why do weight loss and insomnia occur with hyperthyroidism?
b. Why are cold intolerance and bradycardia common with hypothyroidism?
c. What is a goiter and how may it develop?

Adrenal Glands

Adrenal Medulla

Pheochromocytoma is a benign tumor of the adrenal medulla that secretes epinephrine, norepinephrine, and sometimes other substances. Occasionally there are multiple tumors, or the tumor originates in the sympathetic ganglia. It may be bilateral or unilateral.

It is a relatively rare tumor, but it is one of the "curable" causes of hypertension if it is diagnosed. The signs it produces—headache, heart palpitations, sweating, and intermittent or constant anxiety—are related to elevated blood pressure. Frequently catecholamines are released intermittently, causing sudden hypertension and severe headache.

Adrenal Cortex

Cushing's Syndrome

Cushing's syndrome is caused by an excessive amount of glucocorticoids (e.g., hydrocortisone or cortisol). The mechanism for the excess amount of hormone and the effect on related hormones depends on the cause. Excess glucocorticoids may result from:
- Adrenal adenoma (Fig. 16-16)
- Pituitary adenoma (Fig. 16-17) or Cushing's disease
- An *ectopic* carcinoma that causes paraneoplastic syndrome (see Fig. 16-17C; see Chapter 20)
- Iatrogenic conditions, such as administration of large amounts of glucocorticoids for many chronic inflammatory conditions (see Fig. 16-17D; see Chapter 5)

Glucocorticoids are *essential for the stress response* and *essential for life.* They perform many important functions in the body. But in excess amounts, they produce many unfortunate effects. This is the reason why prolonged treatment with these drugs is not recommended.

Typical changes associated with Cushing's syndrome include:
- Characteristic change in the person's *appearance;* a moon face (round and puffy) and a heavy trunk with

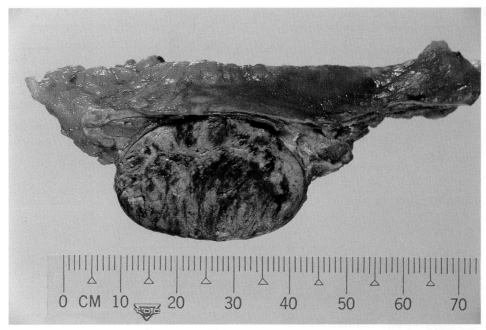

FIGURE 16-16 Cushing's syndrome. Adrenal cortical adenoma. Removal of the tumor cured the condition. *(From Cooke RA, Stewart B:* Colour Atlas of Anatomical Pathology, *ed 3, Sydney, 2004, Churchill Livingstone.)*

fat at the back of the neck (buffalo hump) and wasting of muscle in the limbs (Fig. 16-18)

- Fragile *skin* that may have red streaks as well as increased hair growth (hirsutism)
- *Catabolic* effects such as osteoporosis and decreased protein synthesis, which delays healing
- Metabolic changes include increased gluconeogenesis and insulin resistance, which may lead to glucose intolerance; this may result in diabetes mellitus or exacerbate an existing diabetic state
- Retention of sodium and water (mineral corticoid effect), leading to hypertension, edema, and possible hyperkalemia
- Suppression of the immune response and the inflammatory response with atrophy of the lymphoid tissue, predisposing the client to *infection*
- Stimulation of erythrocyte production
- Emotional lability and euphoria

Two concerns for health care professionals are:

1. The risk of infection in the patient with Cushing's syndrome and need for precautions; infection may be local or systemic (e.g., tuberculosis)
2. A *decreased stress response* in a patient with iatrogenic Cushing's syndrome because of the atrophy of the adrenal cortex; therefore the doses of medication may have to be increased before and during a stressful event. Similarly dosage must be *gradually reduced* over a period of time to permit resumption of normal secretory function by the gland

Treatment depends on the underlying cause.

THINK ABOUT 16-11

a. Explain how diagnostic tests could distinguish a pituitary Cushing's syndrome from an adrenal Cushing's syndrome.
b. List the catabolic effects of excess glucocorticoids.

Addison's Disease

Addison's disease refers to a deficiency of adrenocortical secretions, the glucocorticoids, mineralocorticoids, and androgens. An autoimmune reaction is the common cause. The gland may be destroyed by hemorrhage with meningococcal infection, or by viral, tubercular, or histoplasmosis infections. Destructive tumors may also cause hypoactivity.

The major effects of these hormonal deficits include decreased blood glucose levels, poor stress response, fatigue, weight loss, and frequent infections. Low serum sodium concentration, decreased blood volume, and hypotension, accompanied by high potassium levels, result from the mineralocorticoid (aldosterone) deficit and lead to cardiac arrhythmias and failure. Other manifestations include decreased body hair due to lack of androgens and hyperpigmentation in the extremities, skin creases, buccal mucosa, and tongue, because of increased ACTH resulting from low cortisol secretion.

A comparison of Cushing's syndrome and Addison's disease is found in Table 16-6.

Replacement therapy with the necessary hormones controls the diseases. Increased doses may be required in times of stress.

A. PITUITARY TUMOR
(increased serum ACTH and cortisol)

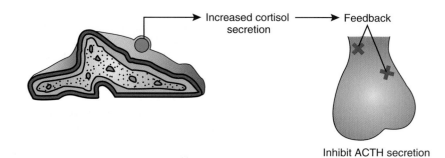

B. ADRENAL CORTEX TUMOR
(increased serum cortisol, decreased ACTH)

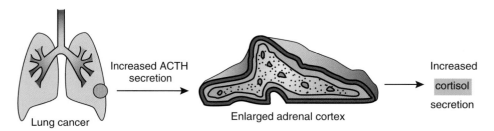

C. PARANEOPLASTIC SYNDROME
(increased serum ACTH and cortisol)

D. IATROGENIC
(increased serum cortisol, decreased ACTH)

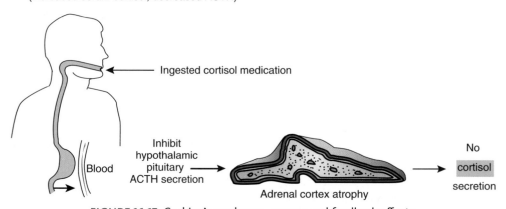

FIGURE 16-17 Cushing's syndrome—causes and feedback effects.

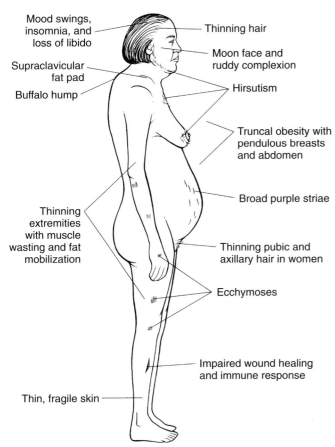

Mood swings, insomnia, and loss of libido

Thinning hair

Moon face and ruddy complexion

Supraclavicular fat pad

Buffalo hump

Hirsutism

Truncal obesity with pendulous breasts and abdomen

Broad purple striae

Thinning extremities with muscle wasting and fat mobilization

Thinning pubic and axillary hair in women

Ecchymoses

Impaired wound healing and immune response

Thin, fragile skin

FIGURE 16-18 Cushing's syndrome—typical appearance. *(From Monahan FD, Drake T, Neighbors M:* Nursing Care of Adults, *Philadelphia, 1994, Saunders.)*

TABLE 16-6	Comparison of Addison's Disease and Cushing's Syndrome
Addison's Disease (Adrenal Insufficiency)	**Cushing's Syndrome**
Deficit of corticosteroids (glucocorticoids, mineralocorticoids)	Excess glucocorticoids (cortisol)
High risk of infection	High risk of infection
Poor stress response	Poor stress response
Weight loss, fatigue	Moon face, buffalo hump, obese trunk, muscle wasting in limbs, osteoporosis
Anorexia, nausea, diarrhea	Striae, bruising of skin, high risk of infection
Hypotension, syncope	Hypertension, glucose intolerance
Hyperpigmentation	Fatigue, weakness, delayed healing

CASE STUDY A

Diabetes Mellitus Type 1

Mr. M. has had Type 1 diabetes for 15 years. He has just been admitted to the hospital with severe pyelonephritis, a kidney infection.
1. Describe the pathophysiology of Type 1 diabetes.
2. Explain why urinary tract infections are common in people with diabetes. Explain how acute renal failure could develop.

Mr. M. has had the infection for a week and has developed mild ketoacidosis because of the infection. Analysis of arterial blood gases indicates that his serum bicarbonate level is low, and his serum pH is just below normal range.
3. Explain why infection may lead to ketoacidosis.
4. Describe the characteristics of Mr. M.'s respirations that you would expect to observe while ketoacidosis is present. Include the rationale for your answer.
5. If Mr. M.'s serum pH continues to decrease below normal, how would that pH affect cell and organ function?
6. Mr. M. is voiding large volumes of urine (polyuria). Explain the reason for this.
7. Describe three signs of excessive fluid loss.
8. Mr. M.'s vision has deteriorated in the last 3 years because of retinopathy. Explain how retinopathy impairs vision.
9. Describe two problems related to diabetes that Mr. M. might encounter because of his reduced vision.

CASE STUDY B

Diabetes Mellitus Type 2

Mr. F. was diagnosed with Type 2 diabetes mellitus at age 46. At that time, he was overweight, enjoyed foods with high carbohydrate and fat content, and led a sedentary life. His family history indicated that his mother and his brother had diabetes. Weight loss, appropriate diet, and exercise were recommended to reduce blood glucose levels.
1. List the factors contributing to diabetes mellitus in this case.

At age 50, Mr. F. noticed that his vision was cloudy, particularly in one eye. Cataracts were removed from both eyes.
2. Describe a cataract and explain how diabetes promotes cataract formation.
3. Glyburide (DiaBeta) was prescribed at this time. Describe the action of this drug.

At age 56, a blister developed on the heel of one foot, which did not heal. An ulcer formed and persisted. Finally the foot was placed in a cast for 13 weeks to promote healing.
4. Explain several factors contributing to the delayed healing in Mr. F.
5. Why was it necessary in this case, to remove the cast and replace it each week?

Peripheral neuropathy with total loss of sensory function had developed in both feet. Motor function was not directly affected. Orthopedic shoes were ordered and arrangements made for a podiatrist to provide regular foot care.

6. Why is it essential that Mr. F. examine his feet carefully each day?

At this time body weight had again increased substantially and blood pressure was elevated. Fosinopril (Monopril) was prescribed, along with recommendations for weight loss and regular exercise.

7. Describe the usual manifestations of hypertension.

At age 60, routine monitoring during a workout at the health club indicated atrial fibrillation. During consultation, the cardiologist also noted his blood pressure was very high.

8. State the purpose of the following medications prescribed at this time (see Chapter 18): fosinopril (Monopril), atorvastatin (Lipitor), amlodipine (Norvasc), warfarin (Coumadin), and sotalol (Sotacor).

Since that time, continued regular exercise and dietary modification have maintained weight at recommended levels. Blood pressure is within normal range, HbA$_{1c}$ is below 7, and atrial fibrillation is controlled.

9. What does this HbA$_{1c}$ value mean?
10. Why does Mr. F. bruise easily? What precautions would be advisable at this time?
11. Briefly review the effects of diabetes over time in this case.

CASE STUDY C

Gestational Diabetes Mellitus

Following delivery of the second child, blood pressure and blood glucose remained elevated in C.S., leading to a diagnosis of Type 2 diabetes. In addition to regular exercise, metformin was prescribed and a nutritionist developed an appropriate diet.

1. Describe the pathophysiology of Type 2 diabetes.
2. Briefly describe how diet, exercise, and this drug each contribute to reduction of blood glucose.
3. Explain how stressors might affect blood glucose levels and blood pressure.

Hydrochlorothiazide (Hydro DIURIL) and irbesartan (Avapro) were prescribed to reduce blood pressure.

4. Why is persistent elevated blood pressure a serious concern in a patient (see Chapter 12)?

Several years later, C.S. experienced an episode of severe pain leading to a diagnosis of renal calculi and hypercalcemia related to an additional metabolic abnormality.

5. How does hypercalcemia cause renal calculi, and how do renal calculi cause severe pain (see Chapter 18)?

Dietary restrictions on calcium intake and increased fluid intake were recommended to reduce the risk of additional calculi.

6. How might reduced calcium intake affect C.S.?
7. Following a routine checkup and laboratory tests 2 years later, simvastatin (Zocor) was prescribed. Why is a cholesterol-lowering agent useful in the treatment of diabetes?

8. A daily low dose of enteric-coated ASA was recommended. Why is this helpful in diabetics?

Recently blood glucose levels have been elevated. Medication was changed to glyburide, but side effects in C.S. were marked. A combination of metformin and rosiglitazone has been prescribed as well as regular exercise and careful dietary control.

9. Explain why it is important to maintain low blood glucose levels.
10. Suggest several reasons why blood glucose levels may increase periodically.

CASE STUDY D

Pituitary Adenoma and Acromegaly

C.M., age 20 years, was admitted to emergency with severe headache, photophobia, drowsiness, and slight neck rigidity, suggestive of meningitis. Her medical history indicated good general health. She had been treated for carpal tunnel syndrome 3 years before, and she had noted an increase in hand and foot sizes over the past several years. In the past week, she had experienced severe headaches associated with nausea and vomiting.

Tests on CSF did not confirm meningitis. Blood tests indicated low levels of thyroxine, cortisol, and gonadotropins, but high levels of growth hormone. Radiographic tests showed a space-occupying lesion in the sella turcica. A diagnosis of pituitary adenoma with acromegaly was established. The acute episode had resulted from infarction of the pituitary gland (pituitary apoplexy).

C.M. recovered from the infarction, and was discharged from the hospital. The infarction had reduced the GH secretion to some extent. Thyroxine and cortisol levels were low normal; no replacement therapy was recommended at this time.

1. Define adenoma and describe the location of the pituitary gland.
2. Explain the rationale for the neurologic signs and symptoms leading to admission (see Chapter 14).
3. Explain the effects of acromegaly in C.M. How long was the adenoma likely present?
4. Explain the low blood levels of thyroxine, gonadotropins, and cortisol.

Two years later C.M. was experiencing temporary paresthesias in both hands in the morning. Also headaches had become more frequent and were accompanied by visual signs such as spatial distortion. Cold sensitivity and fatigue persisted. She felt her foot size had increased, but not her hand size. No other abnormalities were apparent.

5. Suggest a reason for these manifestations.

A 6-month course of bromocriptine (Parlodel—a dopamine agonist that reduces GH secretion and shrinks the tumor) was ordered, which did reduce GH levels to some extent. However, after medication was discontinued, headaches, nausea, hot flashes, and paresthesias recurred. Several months later, a course of radiotherapy to the pituitary commenced and resulted in lower GH levels and symptomatic improvement.

6. How would radiotherapy reduce the symptoms?

Tests a few months later indicated T$_4$, cortisol, and LH levels were below normal. T$_4$ replacement therapy was commenced. C.M. was given a supply of prednisone to take in the event of illness or increased stress.

7. Why is it necessary to maintain T$_4$ levels? Why is increased cortisol required during stress?

Because of continued amenorrhea (lack of menstruation) since the pituitary infarction, a course of Pergonal (gonadotropins) was given to induce ovulation when pregnancy was desired. A healthy male infant was delivered. Hydrocortisone replacement was taken throughout the pregnancy.

8. Explain how the pituitary infarction caused amenorrhea.

A few years later, Type 2 diabetes mellitus developed, controlled by diet.

9. How does acromegaly predispose to Type 2 diabetes?

No further signs of acromegaly have occurred. Thyroxine replacement continues and hydrocortisone is available in the event of illness. Complete evaluation of endocrine function, including Hydrocortisone Day Curve, continues on an annual basis to monitor replacement hormone requirements.

10. Explain why hormone levels require frequent monitoring.

CHAPTER SUMMARY

Together with the nervous system, the endocrine system is responsible for maintaining homeostasis in the body and controlling any necessary changes. Endocrine glands secrete hormones into the circulating blood for transport to the target cells. Endocrine disorders usually result from an excess or a deficit of a specific hormone, often caused by a benign adenoma.

Insulin

- *Diabetes mellitus* is caused by a deficit of insulin secretion or increased tissue resistance to insulin action, leading to abnormal carbohydrate, fat, and protein metabolism. Type 1, or insulin-dependent diabetes, requires insulin replacement and is subject to acute complications such as hypoglycemic shock. Type 2, or non-insulin dependent diabetes, a milder form, may be controlled by diet, exercise, or oral hypoglycemics, but long-term complications such as vascular and nerve degeneration are common. Early signs include polyuria, polydipsia, polyphagia, hyperglycemia, and glucosuria.

Parathyroid Hormone

- *Calcium* levels in the blood may be altered by many factors, such as renal disease, immobility, bone disease, and malabsorption syndromes, as well as by parathyroid hormone.
- *Hypoparathyroidism* leads to hypocalcemia with tetany and possible cardiac arrhythmias.
- *Hyperparathyroidism* is a cause of osteoporosis and renal calculi.

Pituitary Hormones

- Pituitary tumors may affect the level of one or more hormones, and may stimulate secretion or impair secretion.
- A pituitary disorder may alter *tropic hormone* levels, affecting the activity of glands such as the thyroid.
- A deficit of GH is one cause of *dwarfism.*
- Excess GH causes *gigantism* in children, *acromegaly* in adults.
- *Diabetes insipidus* results from a deficit of ADH, causing dehydration.

Thyroxine and Triiodothyronine (T$_3$ and T$_4$)

- *Goiter* refers to an enlargement of the thyroid gland that can develop with both hypothyroid and hyperthyroid conditions.
- *Graves' disease* is an example of *hyperthyroidism*, an autoimmune disorder manifested by signs of hypermetabolism, goiter, and exophthalmos.
- Severe *hypothyroidism* is present in *Hashimoto's thyroiditis*, an inflammatory autoimmune disorder, and *cretinism*, an untreated congenital condition impairing mental and physical development, or in *myxedema* with hypometabolism in adults.

Adrenal Glands

- *Pheochromocytoma* is a benign tumor of the adrenal medulla, important as a treatable cause of hypertension.
- *Cushing's syndrome* is caused by excess glucocorticoids resulting from a pituitary or adrenal cortical tumor, an ectopic tumor, or ingestion of glucocorticoids. The major effects include catabolic action on bone, muscle, and skin, and depressed inflammatory and immune responses.
- *Addison's disease* results from a deficit of glucocorticoids, mineralocorticoids, and androgens, affecting blood glucose levels, fluid and electrolyte balance, and the stress response.

STUDY QUESTIONS

1. Why may a spontaneous fracture occur in persons with hyperparathyroidism?
2. Compare the effects of hypocalcemia on skeletal muscle and cardiac muscle.
3. Explain why a teenager with diabetes mellitus would be more likely than an older adult to have acute complications.
4. Compare the signs of diabetic ketoacidosis and hyperosmolar hyperglycemic nonketotic coma.
5. How would the characteristics of the urine differ in untreated diabetes mellitus and diabetes insipidus?
6. Compare three manifestations that differ in hyperthyroidism and hypothyroidism.
7. Explain why glucocorticoids are considered catabolic hormones and list two specific catabolic effects.
8. Explain why untreated Addison's disease could be life threatening.
9. Describe the effects of hyperaldosteronism.
10. State the hormone imbalance involved in each of the following and list two significant effects of each condition:
    a. Gigantism
    b. Cretinism
    c. Pheochromocytoma
    d. Myxedema
    e. Acromegaly
    f. Diabetes insipidus

ADDITIONAL RESOURCES

Guyton AC, Hall JE: *Textbook of Medical Physiology*, ed 10, Philadelphia, 2001, Saunders.
Journal of Diabetes and Its Complications

Web Sites

http://www.diabetes.org *American Diabetes Association*
http://www.gghjournal.com *Growth, Genetics & Hormones (a journal)*

http://www.idf.org *International Diabetes Federation*
http://www.joslin.org *Joslin Diabetes Center*
http://www.endocrine.niddk.nih.gov/ *National Endocrine and Metabolic Diseases Information Service*

Digestive System Disorders

LEARNING OBJECTIVES

After studying this chapter, the student is expected to:

1. Describe the various causes of vomiting and the vomiting process.
2. Differentiate diarrhea from constipation.
3. Differentiate cleft lip from cleft palate.
4. Describe the common oral infections and periodontal disease.
5. Explain the common causes of dysphagia.
6. Differentiate the types of hiatal hernias and explain their effects.
7. List the causes of acute gastritis and describe the common signs.
8. Compare the effects of acute gastritis, chronic gastritis, and gastroenteritis.
9. Describe the etiology, the signs, and possible complications of peptic ulcers.

10. Describe the pathophysiology, etiology, and early signs of gastric cancer.
11. Explain how dumping syndrome develops and list the signs associated with the syndrome.
12. Explain how pyloric stenosis interferes with normal function, and list the common manifestations.
13. Describe how gallstones develop and the signs of obstruction.
14. Differentiate the types of jaundice.
15. Compare the types of infectious hepatitis.
16. Describe the common manifestations of hepatitis.
17. Explain why the cause of toxic hepatitis should be identified quickly.
18. Differentiate the types of cirrhosis.
19. Describe the pathophysiology and manifestations of cirrhosis.

LEARNING OBJECTIVES—*continued*

20. Describe the pathophysiology, signs, and possible complications of acute pancreatitis.
21. Explain how gluten toxicity may affect individuals with celiac disease.
22. Describe the signs of malabsorption.
23. Compare Crohn's disease with ulcerative colitis.
24. Describe the symptoms and the various causes of irritable bowel syndrome.
25. Describe the stages in the development of acute appendicitis and the signs associated with each stage.
26. Explain how diverticulosis and diverticulitis develop.
27. Describe the causes and possible characteristics of colorectal cancer.
28. Relate the location of colorectal cancer to the possible signs.
29. Describe the common causes of intestinal obstruction.
30. Differentiate the causes and significant signs of mechanical obstruction from those of paralytic ileus.
31. Explain the progressive effects of intestinal obstruction and the related signs.
32. Differentiate chemical peritonitis from bacterial peritonitis, including causes for each.
33. Describe the pathophysiology of peritonitis and possible complications.

KEY TERMS

abscesses	fecalith	ileostomy	rugae
adhesions	gastrectomy	impaction	sinusoids
autodigestion	gluconeogenesis	mastication	splenomegaly
bolus	glycogen	melena	steatorrhea
calculi	hematemesis	mesentery	stricture
cholestasis	hepatocytes	multiparity	tenesmus
chyme	hepatotoxins	occult	ulcerogenic
colostomy	hyperbilirubinemia	pruritus	
exocrine	icterus	retroperitoneal	

Review of the Digestive System

The general purpose of the digestive system is to efficiently process ingested food and fluids and the various secretions from glands. First they are broken down into their separate constituents; then the desired nutrients, water, and electrolytes are absorbed into the blood for use by the cells, and waste elements are eliminated from the body. Within this system, the liver can reassemble the component nutrients into new materials as they are needed by the body. For example, the proteins in milk are digested by enzymes in the digestive tract, producing the component amino acids, which are then absorbed into the blood. The individual amino acids are used by the liver cells to produce new proteins, such as albumin or prothrombin, or they may circulate unchanged in the blood to be taken up by individual cells as necessary.

Structures and Their Functions

The digestive system, sometimes called the gastrointestinal tract, alimentary tract, or gut, consists of a long hollow tube which extends through the trunk of the body, and its accessory structures: the salivary glands, liver, gallbladder, and pancreas (Fig. 17-1). The digestive tract is divided into two sections, the *upper* tract, consisting of the mouth, esophagus, and stomach, and the *lower* tract, consisting of the intestines.

Although variations occur along the tube, the wall of the gut basically has five continuous layers:

1. The inner layer is the mucosa, which includes the important mucus-producing cells. *Mucus* protects the tissues and facilitates the passage of the contents along the tube. The *epithelial* cells of the mucosa have a rapid turnover rate because of the "wear-and-tear" associated with the food and secretions passing along the tract.
2. The submucosal layer is composed of connective tissue, including blood vessels, nerves, lymphatics, and secretory glands.
3. *Circular* smooth muscle fibers.
4. *Longitudinal* smooth muscle fibers.

These two smooth muscle layers are responsible for transport or motility in the tract.

5. The outer layer of the wall comprises the visceral peritoneum, or *serosa*.

The *peritoneum* is a large serous membrane in the abdominal cavity (see Ready Reference 1). The *parietal* peritoneum covers the abdominal wall and the superior surface of the urinary bladder and uterus, and then continues, reflecting back to form the *visceral* peritoneum, which encases the organs, such as the stomach and intestine. This arrangement creates a double-walled membrane in the abdominal cavity, which is similar to the pleural and pericardial membranes. Pain receptors connected to spinal nerves are located in the parietal peritoneum.

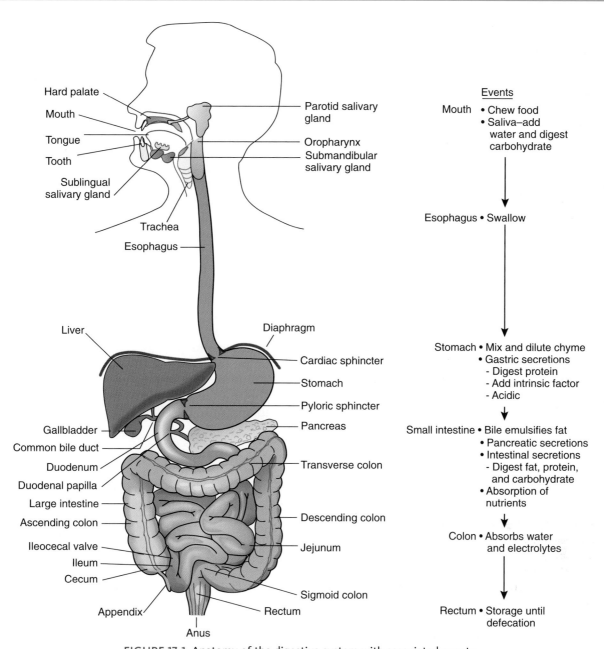

FIGURE 17-1 Anatomy of the digestive system with associated events.

The *peritoneal cavity* refers to the *potential* space between the parietal and visceral peritoneum. A small amount of serous fluid is present in the cavity to facilitate the necessary movement of structures such as the stomach. Numerous lymphatic channels drain excessive fluid from the cavity.

Because serous membranes are normally thin, somewhat permeable, and highly vascular, the peritoneal membranes are useful as an exchange site for blood during peritoneal dialysis in patients with kidney failure (see Chapter 18). However, such an extensive membrane may also facilitate the spread of infection or malignant tumor cells throughout the abdominal cavity or into the general circulation.

The mesentery is a double layer of peritoneum that supports the intestines and conveys blood vessels and nerves to supply the wall of the intestine. The mesentery attaches the jejunum and ileum to the posterior (dorsal) abdominal wall. This arrangement provides a balance between the need for support of the intestines and the need for considerable flexibility to accommodate peristalsis and varying amounts of content.

The greater *omentum* is a layer of fatty peritoneum that hangs from the stomach like an apron over the anterior surface of the transverse colon and the small intestine. The lesser omentum is part of the peritoneum that suspends the stomach and duodenum from the liver. When inflammation develops in the intestinal wall, the greater omentum, with its many lymph nodes, tends to adhere to the site, walling off the inflammation and temporarily localizing the source of the problem. Inflammation of the omentum and peritoneum may lead to scar tissue and the formation of adhesions between structures in the abdominal cavity, such as loops of intestine, restricting motility and perhaps leading to obstruction.

The kidneys and pancreas are located posterior to the stomach against the abdominal wall and *behind* the parietal peritoneum. They are covered with peritoneum only on the anterior surface and are therefore referred to as retroperitoneal organs.

Upper Gastrointestinal Tract
Oral Cavity
Food and fluid are taken into the body through the mouth, where the initial phase of mechanical breakdown and digestion takes place, and are then stored in the stomach, where processing continues. The mouth is separated from the nasal cavity by the hard and soft palates. A large variety of microorganisms make up the resident flora of the mouth. In the mouth, or oral cavity (Fig. 17-2), mastication takes place as the teeth break down solid food and mix it with saliva. Salivary secretions from the parotid, sublingual, and submandibular glands enter the mouth through the salivary ducts, moisturizing and lubricating (with mucins) the food particles and facilitating the passage of solid material down the esophagus to the stomach. Saliva also contains the enzyme amylase, which begins the digestion of carbohydrate in the mouth (Table 17-1). Perhaps you have noted how chewing crackers can bring a sweet taste in the mouth as the starch is broken down. The tongue and cheeks facilitate the movement and mixing of the food in the mouth. Chewing is usually considered a *voluntary* action, but reflex chewing can occur if voluntary control is lost.

Esophagus
When food is ready to be swallowed, the tongue pushes the bolus or ball of food back to the pharyngeal wall, where receptors of the trigeminal and glossopharyngeal nerves relay the information to the swallowing center in the medulla. Because the reflex is activated at this point, *swallowing* (or *deglutition*) becomes an *involuntary* activity. The swallowing center coordinates the actions required to move food or fluid into the stomach, without *aspiration* into the lungs, by means of cranial nerves V, IX, X, and XII in the following steps:
- The soft palate is pulled upward.
- The vocal cords are approximated.
- The epiglottis covers the larynx.
- Respiration ceases.
- The bolus is seized by the constricted pharynx.
- As the bolus of food moves into the esophagus, distending the wall, peristalsis is initiated, pushing the food down the esophagus.
- The distal part of the esophagus passes through the hiatus (opening) in the diaphragm to join the stomach in the abdominal cavity.
- The lower esophageal (gastroesophageal, or cardiac) sphincter relaxes in advance of the bolus, allowing it to drop into the stomach.

TABLE 17-1	Major Digestive Enzymes and Their Actions	
Enzyme	Source	Action
Salivary amylase	Parotid gland	Splits starch and glycogen into disaccharides
Pepsin	Gastric chief cells	Initiates splitting of proteins
Pancreatic amylase	Pancreas	Splits starch and glycogen into disaccharides
Pancreatic lipase	Pancreas	Splits triglycerides into fatty acids and monoglycerides
Trypsin, chymotrypsin, carboxypeptidase	Pancreas	Splits proteins into peptides
Pancreatic nucleases	Pancreas	Splits nucleic acids into nucleotides
Intestinal peptidase	Intestinal mucosa	Converts peptides into amino acids
Intestinal lipase	Intestinal mucosa	Converts fats into fatty acids and glycerol
Intestinal sucrase, maltase, lactase	Intestinal mucosa	Converts disaccharides into monosaccharides

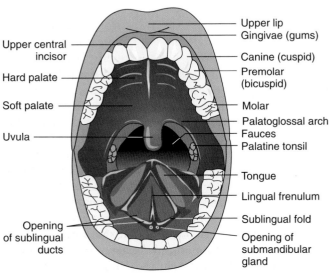

Upper lip
Gingivae (gums)
Upper central incisor
Hard palate
Soft palate
Uvula
Canine (cuspid)
Premolar (bicuspid)
Molar
Palatoglossal arch
Fauces
Palatine tonsil
Tongue
Lingual frenulum
Sublingual fold
Opening of sublingual ducts
Opening of submandibular gland

FIGURE 17-2 The oral cavity.

The pressure in this sphincter normally prevents *reflux* of gastric contents back up the esophagus. The esophagus is composed of skeletal muscle at the superior end that is gradually replaced by smooth muscle fibers. The entire tube is lined with mucous membrane and is closed, except when swallowing is in progress.

Stomach

The stomach is an expansible muscular sac that acts as a reservoir for food and fluid. The stomach can hold 1.0 to 1.5 liters of food and fluid. When empty, the stomach wall falls into folds, or rugae. The outer surface is covered by visceral peritoneum. The wall of the stomach consists of *three* smooth muscle layers—longitudinal and circular layers and an additional oblique muscle layer—plus the mucosa and submucosa. The epithelial cells of the mucosa are tightly packed together to prevent penetration of acid or pepsin into the wall. Numerous glands are located in the mucosa, and there is a layer of thick protective mucus covering the inner surface.

Constant mixing and churning of food occurs as secretions are added from the gastric glands. These secretions dilute the gastric contents, or chyme, and initiate the digestion of protein. The gastric glands located in the fundus of the stomach contain parietal cells that secrete *hydrochloric acid* and chief cells that secrete *pepsinogen*, which is converted to the active form, pepsin, by the action of hydrochloric acid. *Intrinsic factor*, required for the absorption of vitamin B_{12} in the ileum, is also produced by the parietal cells (see Chapter 10 for discussion of pernicious anemia). The gastric secretions act as a defensive mechanism because of the highly acidic pH (around 2), which destroys many microorganisms that enter the stomach from the resident flora in the mouth or from food or utensils. Protective mucus is secreted by glands in the cardiac and pyloric areas. Also, enteroendocrine cells in the glands secrete a variety of chemicals, the most important of which is the hormone *gastrin*, which is released when food enters the stomach and then stimulates the parietal and chief cells.

Depending to some extent on the type of food ingested, gastric emptying proceeds slowly, with small amounts of chyme (1 to 3 mL) passing intermittently through the pyloric sphincter into the duodenum. Secretions from the liver and the exocrine pancreas are added to the chyme in the duodenum through the ampulla of Vater and duodenal papilla (see Fig. 17-18).

Liver

The liver is located in the upper right quadrant (URQ) of the abdomen under the diaphragm and serves as the "metabolic factory" of the body. It is a large organ covered by a fibrous capsule, distention of which causes a dull, aching pain. The liver cells can regenerate, but if the organizational structure of the lobule, with its unique arrangement of blood vessels and bile ducts, is altered by necrosis and scar tissue, the regenerated areas may not be functional.

The hepatocytes, or liver cells, are arranged in lobules, and each lobule has plates of cells radiating from central veins, which eventually drain blood back into the general circulation through the hepatic veins and inferior vena cava (see Fig. 17-20). Channels or sinusoids filled with blood from two sources pass between the plates of hepatocytes. Entering the sinusoid is blood from branches of the hepatic artery, carrying oxygen to the liver cells; venous blood from the portal vein, which transports nutrients absorbed from the stomach and intestines (hepatic portal circulation); as well as from the pancreas and spleen. The arterial and venous blood mix and flow slowly through the sinusoids, permitting the hepatocytes to do their jobs. The sinusoids are lined with endothelial cells and Kupffer cells, which remove and phagocytose any foreign material and bacteria from the digestive tract before the blood enters the general circulation.

As blood flows through the sinusoids, many substances are exchanged to facilitate liver functions. Absorbed nutrients are taken up by the hepatocytes to be stored (e.g., the minerals iron and copper, or vitamins A, B_6, B_{12}, D, and K, and folic acid). Many blood components such as iron or amino acids are monitored, and those that have been depleted as the blood circulates through the body are replaced. Blood glucose levels are maintained; glucose is essential for brain function.

In conjunction with the hormone insulin, the liver responds to high levels of blood glucose by glycogenesis, converting glucose to glycogen, which is stored in the liver. Alternatively, the hepatocytes break down liver glycogen to glucose (glycogenolysis) when blood glucose levels drop and glucagon secretion increases. Gluconeogenesis, the conversion of protein and fat into glucose, may take place when blood glucose levels drop, under the influence of hormones such as cortisol or epinephrine.

Conversion of one amino acid into another takes place as needed to maintain the amino acid pool in the blood and meet the body's needs. Synthesis and control of blood levels of other materials, such as plasma proteins, clotting factors, or lipoproteins, is accomplished. Synthesis of cholesterol occurs in the liver for use in the production of steroid hormones, such as cortisol or the sex hormones, and bile salts.

Hormones, such as aldosterone and estrogen, are inactivated and prepared for excretion. Ammonia, a nitrogen waste resulting from protein metabolism in the intestine or liver, is removed from the blood and converted to urea, enabling it to be excreted by the kidneys. Drugs and alcohol are detoxified before excretion. The detoxification process makes such substances less harmful and increases the solubility of many substances, facilitating their excretion.

Damaged or old erythrocytes are removed from the blood to facilitate the recycling of iron and protein from hemoglobin (see Figs. 10-7 and 17-21). The liver serves as a blood reservoir because it is capable of releasing a large quantity of blood into the general circulation when blood volume is depleted.

The hepatocytes of the liver constantly produce *bile*, a mixture of water, bile salts, bile pigment (conjugated bilirubin), cholesterol, and electrolytes, including bicarbonate ions. Bile is vital for digestion and serves as a vehicle for the removal of bilirubin and excess cholesterol from the body. The bile salts, formed from cholesterol, are essential for the emulsification of fats and fat-soluble vitamins (vitamins A, D, E, and K) before they can be absorbed from the intestine. The majority of the bile salts are reabsorbed from the distal ileum and recycled to the liver through the enterohepatic circulation. Bicarbonate ions in bile assist in neutralizing gastric acid, increasing the pH of the small intestine so that intestinal and pancreatic enzymes can function.

Bile is an exocrine secretion, flowing through small canaliculi in the liver and draining into larger ducts until it reaches the right or left hepatic duct and then the common bile duct. A sphincter in this duct usually directs the flow of bile into the gallbladder for storage but may allow it to flow onward into the duodenum. After surgical removal of the gallbladder, the storage facility is lost, but bile is *constantly* secreted by the liver and small amounts continuously enter the duodenum.

Pancreas

The pancreas lies posterior to the stomach, with its larger end or "head" adjacent to the duodenum. The cells of the exocrine pancreas are arranged in lobules throughout the organ; they secrete digestive enzymes, electrolytes, and water into tiny ducts, which eventually drain into the main pancreatic duct that traverses the length of the pancreas. The pancreatic duct, carrying secretions from the exocrine pancreas, joins the common bile duct and then enters the duodenum.

The major proteolytic enzymes in pancreatic secretions are trypsin and chymotrypsin, carboxypeptidase, and ribonuclease (see Table 17-1). Also, pancreatic amylase aids in the digestion of carbohydrates and lipase helps to digest fats. The enzymes are secreted in inactive form and are activated after they enter the duodenum. A trypsin inhibitor is produced by the pancreatic cells to reduce the risk of enzyme activation within the pancreas. Pancreatic secretions also contain bicarbonate ion, which assists in the neutralization of hydrochloric acid in the duodenum.

Lower Gastrointestinal Tract

Small Intestine

The small intestine has three sections, the duodenum, the jejunum, and the ileum, moving in a proximal to distal direction. The contents move slowly along the tube, influenced by both mixing and propulsive movements of the wall. Digestion continues in the duodenum while many enzymes are added to the chyme and an alkaline pH is attained. The ileum is the major site of absorption of nutrients.

The significant feature of the small intestine is the presence of plicae circulares, transverse folds of the mucosa covered with *villi* and *microvilli* (see Fig. 17-32A). These numerous tiny projections greatly increase the absorptive surface area of the small intestine. Each villus is supplied with a capillary network, nerves, and a lacteal, which is a terminal lymphatic vessel that is essential for the absorption of lipids. At the base of the villi are the intestinal crypts, deep pockets from which new epithelial cells (simple columnar absorptive cells) arise. Cells in the crypts produce fluid with a pH of around 7; as well as enzymes such as enterokinase, which activate pancreatic proenzymes; and hormones, such as cholecystokinin. Other enzymes produced by the cells of the intestinal mucosa include peptidases, nucleosidases, lipase, sucrase, maltase, and lactase. Many goblet cells in the mucosa secrete large quantities of mucus into the intestine to protect the intestinal wall and buffer the acid chyme.

Large Intestine

The ileocecal valve marks the entry point from the ileum into the large intestine or colon. Hanging down at this point is a pouch, the cecum, from which the blind-ending appendix (vermiform appendix) extends. Moving superiorly from the cecum is the ascending colon, which becomes the transverse colon and then passes down the left side as the descending colon. This structure terminates as the sigmoid colon, rectum, and anal canal. The anus is the opening to the exterior.

Absorption of large amounts of water and electrolytes takes place in the colon. This "recycling" process is of critical importance in maintaining the fluid and acid-base balances in the body, because large volumes of fluids and ions, such as bicarbonate and sodium, are recovered from the added secretions and ingested fluids. General digestion and absorption of nutrients ceases in the colon. Resident bacteria assist in further breakdown of certain food materials (one cause of intestinal gas) and convert bilirubin to urobilinogen, which gives the feces the typical brown color. In the ileum, large masses of lymphoid tissue, called Peyer's patches, limit the spread of these bacteria into the small intestine. Some of these bacteria are beneficial to the human host, synthesizing vitamin K, for example, which is required for the production of clotting factors, such as prothrombin and fibrinogen, in the liver.

Colonic movements are slow to allow absorption of fluid and formation of the solid feces. The transverse and descending colon are marked by *mass movements*, strong peristaltic contractions that occur several times daily. Large pouches, or haustra, in the colon wall allow for expansion as more solid material collects.

Feces consist primarily of fiber and other indigestible material, sloughed mucosal cells, and bacteria. Increased bulk or fiber in the intestine increases intestinal motility and the rate of passage, leading to a larger fecal mass and thus, more frequent defecation, or bowel movements.

The rectum stores the solid feces until sufficient distention of the rectal wall stimulates the *defecation reflex* as follows:

1. Sensory nerve impulses from the stretch receptors in the rectal wall are transmitted to the sacral spinal cord.
2. The sacral parasympathetic nerves transmit motor impulses, which stimulate peristalsis and relax the internal anal sphincter.
3. Pelvic muscles contract and voluntary relaxation of the external anal sphincter allows defecation to occur.
4. Elimination of feces can be assisted by increasing intra-abdominal pressure through voluntary contraction of the abdominal muscles and the diaphragm.
5. If, under voluntary control, the external anal sphincter remains closed, the defecation reflex subsides temporarily. As the fecal mass increases, the reflex is stimulated again.

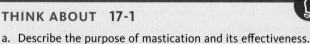

THINK ABOUT 17-1

a. Describe the purpose of mastication and its effectiveness.
b. Where are carbohydrates digested? Name the enzymes responsible.
c. Explain why the liver is referred to as the "metabolic factory" of the body.
d. State the likely times of glycogenolysis or glycogenesis relative to food intake or lack of intake.
e. Explain why the contents of the small intestine are relatively liquid and the contents of the descending colon are solid.
f. Describe one unique structural feature and the purpose of each of the following: mouth, stomach, small intestine, pancreas, and rectum.
g. Explain the functions of mucus in the digestive tract.

Neural and Hormonal Controls

Stimulation of the *parasympathetic nervous system* (PNS), primarily through the vagus nerve (cranial nerve X), results in *increased motility*, or peristalsis, and *increased secretions* in the digestive system (Table 17-2; see also Chapter 14). During the initial cephalic phase before eating, pleasant smells, thoughts, or the sight of food can effect PNS stimulation. Conversely, emotions such as fear or anger stimulate the sympathetic nervous system (SNS), which inhibits gastrointestinal activity. Sympathetic nervous system activity also causes vasoconstriction, leading to reduced secretions and regeneration of epithelial cells.

The PNS, through the facial (cranial nerve VII) and glossopharyngeal (cranial nerve IX) nerves, maintains a continuous flow of saliva in the mouth, which is essential to keep the tissues moist, effect a continuous cleansing action, and facilitate speech. A dry mouth for any reason leads to a sensation of thirst, a protection against dehydration. The sight, thought, or presence of food in the mouth stimulates increased salivary secretions, and these secretions usually continue for a time after swallowing, which is helpful in cleansing the mouth and teeth.

When food reaches the stomach, distention or stretching of the stomach and the increased pH caused by food intake activate the PNS, increasing peristalsis and gastric secretions. Peripheral nervous system stimulation also increases bile and pancreatic secretions. As digestion in the stomach progresses, peristaltic movements force small amounts of chyme, 2 to 3 mL at a time, into the duodenum. Depending on the amount and type of food involved, the stomach empties within 2 to 6 hours after a meal. Fluids pass through rapidly, whereas fats progress slowly. The presence of food in the intestine stimulates intestinal activity but inhibits gastric activity, through the *enterogastric reflex*, to prevent overloading of the duodenum and to allow sufficient time for intestinal digestion and absorption. Food passes through the small intestine at a fairly constant rate. After eating, a reflex increase in peristalsis around the ileocecal valve occurs, which moves the ileal contents into the cecum and colon. These anticipatory actions make the digestive tract into an efficient production line. Peristaltic movements in the colon are usually slow. The gastrocolic reflex stimulates a mass movement of the contents from the colon into the rectum when food enters the stomach.

Hormones play a major role in the process of digestion and absorption (see Table 17-2). *Gastrin* is secreted by mucosal cells in the pyloric antrum of the stomach in response to distention of the stomach or the presence of substances such as partially digested protein, alcohol, or caffeine in the stomach. Gastrin enters the blood and circulates, then returns to stimulate the gastric cells to increase secretions, increase gastric motility, and relax the pyloric and ileocecal sphincters, thus promoting stomach emptying.

In the presence of the chemical histamine that is released from local mast cells, stimulation of the parietal cells by the PNS or gastrin leads to increased secretion of hydrochloric acid. The histamine receptors on parietal cells are *histamine2 (H2) receptors*, not the histamine$_1$ (H$_1$) receptors on cells involved in allergic responses.

When chyme enters the duodenum, mucosal cells release hormones. Secretin and cholecystokinin (CCK) are two important ones. *Secretin* decreases gastric secretions and increases the bicarbonate ion content of pancreatic secretions and bile when the chyme is

TABLE 17-2	Major Controls in the Digestive Tract and Their Effects		
Hormone	Source	Stimulus	Effects
Gastrin	Gastric cells	Food in the stomach Protein, caffeine, or high pH of chyme	Increases gastric secretions and motility and promotes gastric emptying
Cholecystokinin	Intestinal mucosal cells	Protein and fat in the duodenum	Inhibits gastric secretions and motility; stimulates pancreatic enzyme secretion; stimulates gallbladder contractions and release of bile
Secretin	Intestinal mucosal cells	Acidic chyme in the duodenum	Stimulates bile and pancreatic secretions with high bicarbonate content
Neural Controls	**Source**	**Stimulus**	**Effects**
Parasympathetic nervous system	Vagus nerve	Taste food	Increases secretions and peristalsis
Sympathetic nervous system	SNS	Stress	Decreases secretions and peristalsis Stimulates vasoconstriction in the mucosa

highly acidic. *Cholecystokinin* inhibits gastric emptying, stimulates pancreatic secretions with increased digestive enzymes, and stimulates contraction of the gallbladder to increase bile flow into the duodenum. Variations in the digestive secretions and the rate of flow of chyme through the tract depend on the amount and type of food entering the digestive tract. For example, gastric emptying is delayed when the duodenum is full or when a meal high in fat content is ingested.

APPLY YOUR KNOWLEDGE   17-1

How might a severe neck injury have adverse effects on the digestive system?

Digestion and Absorption

Nutrients are broken down chemically into simple molecules that are absorbed along with electrolytes and water into the blood and transported to the liver through the hepatic portal system.

Complex *carbohydrates*, such as starches, are digested first in the mouth and then in the intestine. They are broken down by enzymes into simple sugars (monosaccharides) that are absorbed in the intestine, primarily in the jejunum and ileum. Glucose and galactose are absorbed by a co-transport mechanism with sodium that is already bound to a transport protein. Fructose is absorbed by facilitated diffusion. The process of active transport for sodium requires cellular energy (stored by adenosine triphosphate [ATP]), and therefore healthy cells with a good blood supply. On occasion, when a highly concentrated solution of glucose enters an empty stomach, glucose may diffuse quickly from the stomach into the blood. This rapid action can be effective in reversing hypoglycemia in a person with diabetes mellitus.

Proteins are first split into *peptides*, or short chains of amino acids, in the stomach and intestine and then further broken down by peptidases into *amino acids*, many of which are absorbed by a sodium co-transport system in the small intestine.

Lipids, or *fats*, primarily triglycerides, must first be emulsified (dispersed into tiny droplets) by bile (the bile salt component) in the small intestine; enzymes then act on the fats, forming monoglycerides and free fatty acids. These lipid-soluble molecules can diffuse across the cell membrane. Many recombine to form triglycerides again. Then, bound to protein, the lipids form *chylomicrons*, most of which diffuse into the lacteals or lymph capillaries in the microvilli. The lacteals join the lymphatic circulation, which empties into the general circulation. Eventually the lipids reach the liver or adipose cells. Short-chain fatty acids may diffuse directly into the blood. *Fat-soluble vitamins* (e.g., vitamins A, D, E, and K) or other lipid-soluble materials do not require digestion but are absorbed with the fats. If for any reason lipids are not absorbed, large molecules, such as fat-soluble vitamins, cannot be absorbed. For example, this problem may occur when individuals consume mineral oil as a laxative on a regular basis. Mineral oil remains in the intestine, and the fat-soluble vitamins are excreted with the oil.

Very small lipid-soluble molecules, such as alcohol, may be absorbed from the empty stomach into the blood by simple diffusion through the cell membranes. This promotes a high blood alcohol level within a short time after ingestion. The presence of food in the stomach delays such absorption.

Water-soluble vitamins (e.g., vitamins B and C) and *minerals* (e.g., iron, copper, and zinc) diffuse into the blood. Vitamin B_{12} must be bound to intrinsic factor before absorption. *Electrolytes* (Na^+, K^+, Cl^-, HCO_3^-, and so on) may be absorbed by active transport or diffusion into the blood. *Water* is absorbed by osmosis. About

7000 mL of water is secreted into the digestive tract each day, and approximately 2300 mL is ingested in food and fluids. Of this amount, only 50 to 200 mL leaves the body in the feces. It is obvious that severe vomiting or diarrhea can quickly interrupt the recycling mechanism and affect fluid and electrolyte balance in the body.

Drugs are primarily absorbed in the intestine, although some small acidic molecules, such as aspirin, may be absorbed in the stomach. Other small molecules may be absorbed through the oral mucosa. Some drugs are broken down by digestive enzymes. The presence of certain foods or drugs, such as antacids, can interfere with absorption of other drugs. Large amounts of food in the stomach and intestine can also delay absorption of drugs.

THINK ABOUT 17-2

a. Describe how the PNS affects the digestive tract, and name the major nerve responsible.
b. Give two reasons why it is important to control the rate of flow of chyme through the digestive tract.
c. State the source and purpose of gastrin.
d. State the final form in which carbohydrate and protein are absorbed into the blood.
e. Describe three general ways in which absorption of nutrients could be impaired.

Common Manifestations of Digestive System Disorders

Anorexia, Nausea, Vomiting, and Bulimia

The manifestations of anorexia, nausea and vomiting, may be signs of digestive system disorders or other conditions elsewhere in the body. For example, systemic infection, uremia (kidney failure), emotional responses such as fear, motion sickness, pressure in the brain, over-indulgence in food, drugs, or pain may initiate these signs. However, nausea and vomiting are common indicators of gastrointestinal disorders, and the characteristics of the vomitus and the vomiting pattern can be helpful in diagnosis. Vomiting is also considered a body defense because it removes noxious substances from the body. In addition, anorexia and vomiting can contribute to serious complications, such as dehydration, acidosis, and malnutrition.

Anorexia (loss of appetite) often precedes nausea and vomiting. Nausea is a generally unpleasant subjective feeling, which may be stimulated by distention, irritation, or inflammation in the digestive tract. Often, increased salivation, pallor, sweating, and tachycardia may occur with nausea and vomiting.

Vomiting, or emesis, is the forceful expulsion of chyme from the stomach and sometimes from the intestine. The vomiting center in the medulla coordinates the activities involved in vomiting (Fig. 17-3). The vomiting center is activated by many conditions, among which are:

- Distention or irritation in the digestive tract
- Stimuli from various parts of the brain in response to unpleasant sights or smells, or ischemia
- Pain or stress
- The vestibular apparatus of the inner ear (motion sickness)
- Increased intracranial pressure (see Chapter 14), causing sudden *projectile* vomiting without previous nausea or food intake
- Stimulation of the chemoreceptor trigger zone in the medulla by drugs, toxins, and chemicals

Drugs may also cause vomiting by direct irritation of the digestive mucosa. Toxins may result from infecting microorganisms anywhere in the body. Toxic chemicals may be endogenous, as in kidney failure, or exogenous (i.e., from external sources).

The *vomiting reflex* includes the following involuntary activities:

1. Taking a deep breath
2. Closing the glottis and raising the soft palate
3. Ceasing respiration, which minimizes the risk of aspiration of vomitus into the lungs, where it may cause significant inflammation and obstruction of the airways
4. Relaxing the gastroesophageal sphincter
5. Contracting the abdominal muscles, which squeezes the stomach against the diaphragm and forces the gastric contents upward and out of the mouth
6. Promoting expulsion of the contents of the stomach by reverse peristaltic waves in the proximal duodenum and antrum

Retching may precede vomiting and involves the same reflex, but the chyme ascends in the esophagus and then falls back into the stomach. This process may take place several times before complete vomiting occurs.

Recurrent vomiting can be exhausting and painful because the strong muscle contractions continue with each episode and the source of renewed energy—food— is not available. There is an increased risk of *aspiration* when the person is supine or unconscious or when the vomiting reflex is depressed by drugs, because the barriers to the respiratory tract may not be completely closed off or the vomitus may not be completely expelled. The cough reflex may also be suppressed. This is a common problem with postoperative vomiting or vomiting after heavy alcohol intake.

The characteristics of vomitus can be significant:

- The presence of blood leads to vomitus resembling "coffee grounds," or hematemesis, a brown, granular material resulting from the partial digestion in the stomach of protein in the blood. If hemorrhage is extensive, then red blood may be obvious in the vomitus. Blood, as a "foreign material," is irritating to the gastric mucosa.

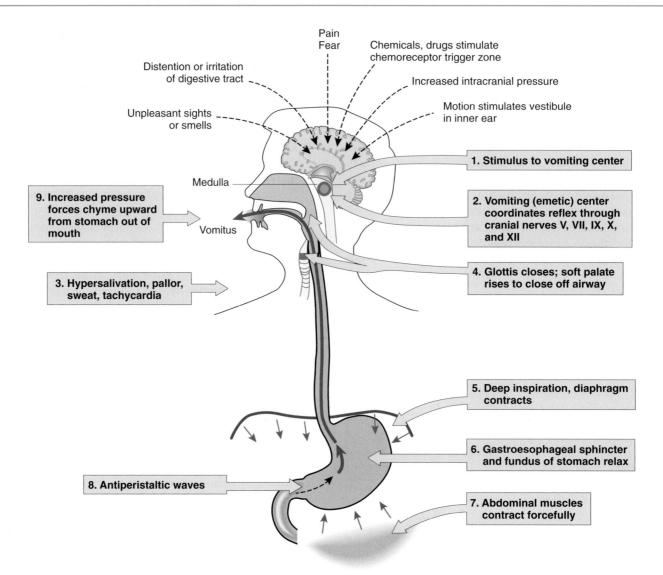

Pain
Fear

Chemicals, drugs stimulate
chemoreceptor trigger zone

Distention or irritation
of digestive tract

Increased intracranial pressure

Unpleasant sights
or smells

Motion stimulates vestibule
in inner ear

1. Stimulus to vomiting center

Medulla

9. Increased pressure forces chyme upward from stomach out of mouth

2. Vomiting (emetic) center coordinates reflex through cranial nerves V, VII, IX, X, and XII

Vomitus

4. Glottis closes; soft palate rises to close off airway

3. Hypersalivation, pallor, sweat, tachycardia

5. Deep inspiration, diaphragm contracts

6. Gastroesophageal sphincter and fundus of stomach relax

8. Antiperistaltic waves

7. Abdominal muscles contract forcefully

FIGURE 17-3 The vomiting or emetic reflex.

- Yellow- or greenish-stained vomitus usually contains bile from the duodenum.
- A deeper brown color may indicate content from the lower intestine, typical of recurrent vomiting in persons with intestinal obstruction.
- Recurrent vomiting of undigested food from previous meals indicates a problem with gastric emptying, such as pyloric obstruction

Bulimia is an eating disorder in which an individual binges and overeats followed by inducing vomiting, taking laxatives, or starving themselves to avoid weight gain. Although clinically considered a behavioral disorder, the results have a significant adverse effect on the digestion process and some of its structures. Damage to structures of the oral cavity such as the oral mucosa and the teeth are often evident as regular vomiting exposes the structures to stomach acid. Many who suffer from bulimia also experience anorexia. The exact cause is not known but studies have revealed multiple factors that could be involved. In addition to visible damage to structures of the oral cavity, other complications can include: tears of the esophagus, constipation, diarrhea, and electrolyte/nutritional imbalances and deficiencies. Treatment methods include counseling and support groups as well as psychotherapy, nutritional therapy, and antidepressive drugs.

Diarrhea

Diarrhea is an excessive frequency of stools, usually of loose or watery consistency, and may be acute or chronic. The presence of blood, mucus, or pus in the stool may be helpful in diagnosing or monitoring a disease. Diarrhea is frequently accompanied by nausea and vomiting when infection or inflammation of the digestive tract develops, but in other cases it occurs alone. Often, diarrhea is accompanied by cramping pain. Severe or prolonged diarrhea may lead to dehydration, electrolyte imbalance, acidosis, and malnutrition.

Diarrheal diseases, often referred to collectively as enterocolitis, can be classified in different ways. Some common types are the following:

- Large-volume diarrhea (secretory or osmotic) leads to a watery stool, resulting from increased secretions into the intestine. This type of diarrhea is often related to infections or a short transit time, which limits reabsorption, or to increased osmotic pressure of the intestinal contents, causing them to retain water. A common cause of osmotic diarrhea is lactose intolerance, in which lactose remains undigested and unabsorbed inside the intestine, thereby increasing the osmotic pressure of the contents.
- Small-volume diarrhea often occurs in people with inflammatory bowel disease, and the stool may contain blood, mucus, or pus. The diarrhea may be accompanied by abdominal cramps and urgency. The differentiation between the two types of diarrhea is not always marked.
- Steatorrhea is "fatty diarrhea," marked by frequent bulky, greasy, loose stools, often with a foul odor. These stools are characteristic of malabsorption syndromes, such as celiac disease or cystic fibrosis, in which the food intake is not digested or absorbed. Fat is usually the first dietary component affected, and the presence of fat interferes with the digestion of other nutrients. The abdomen is often distended because of the bulk remaining in the intestines. Malnutrition is apparent in other tissues, unless disguised by edema caused by hypoproteinemia.
- *Blood* may occur in a normal stool or with diarrhea or constipation or with inflammatory conditions:
  - *Frank* blood refers to red blood, often on the surface of the stool. This blood usually results from lesions in the rectum or anal canal; it has not been "digested."
  - Occult blood refers to small, hidden amounts of blood that are not visible to the eye but are detectable on tests of a stool specimen (e.g., the guaiac test). This may be caused by small bleeding ulcers in the stomach or small intestine.
  - Melena is a dark-colored (tarry) stool that results from significant bleeding that has occurred higher in the digestive tract; the hemoglobin has been acted on by intestinal bacteria, causing the dark color.

Gas develops normally in the digestive tract from swallowed air and digestive and bacterial action on food. Certain foods or alterations in motility also promote gas production. Excessive gas may manifest as belching (expulsion through the mouth), abdominal distention and discomfort, or flatus (expulsion through the anus).

Constipation

Bowel patterns differ among individuals, depending on factors such as diet and activity, and therefore abnormalities are relative to the individual's normal pattern. Constipation is the condition in which there are less frequent bowel movements than normal and small hard stools result. It may be an acute or chronic problem. In some individuals, periods of constipation may alternate with periods of diarrhea. In these cases, emptying of the bowel with diarrhea may lead to decreased peristalsis, which results in increased time available for reabsorption of fluid, leading to dry, hard feces. This dry mass then irritates the intestinal mucosa, leading to inflammation and increased secretions. Once the hard feces have been expelled, a period of diarrhea may follow.

Causes of constipation include:
- Increased age and weakness of the smooth muscle in the intestines
- Inadequate dietary fiber, leading to less bulk in the intestine and decreased peristalsis
- Inadequate fluid intake
- Failure to respond to the defecation reflex because of pain or inconvenient timing
- Muscle weakness and inactivity, which impede defecation
- Neurologic disorders, such as multiple sclerosis or spinal cord trauma, which predispose the individual to constipation
- Drugs, such as opiates (e.g., codeine) and other central nervous system depressants or anticholinergics (drugs that block the PNS), which slow peristalsis
- Some antacids, iron medications, and bulk laxatives (with insufficient fluid intake), which can predispose patients to constipation
- Obstruction caused by tumors or strictures, which may delay passage and cause excessive reabsorption of fluid

Chronic constipation may lead to the development of hemorrhoids or diverticulitis. Severe constipation can lead to fecal impaction (retention of feces in the rectum and colon) and intestinal obstruction, usually indicated by pain and abdominal distention. In some cases, watery diarrhea masks a fecal impaction because fluid pushes past a well-lodged fecal plug.

Fluid and Electrolyte Imbalances

Dehydration and *hypovolemia* are common complications of digestive tract disorders. When vomiting and diarrhea occur, perhaps combined with insufficient fluid intake, fluid shifts from the blood into the digestive tract. If the loss persists, eventually intracellular fluid is decreased (see Chapter 2). Hypovolemia with impaired circulation and cellular dehydration may cause decreased function in all tissues and organs.

Infants and elderly persons are particularly vulnerable to losses incurred with vomiting and diarrhea because of the unique proportions and distribution of fluid in the body in these individuals and the decreased ability of their kidneys to compensate quickly for losses.

Electrolytes such as sodium are lost in both vomiting and diarrhea because both mucus and enzyme secretions contain large amounts of electrolytes. Gastric secretions are high in chloride ion. Diarrhea leads to significant losses of potassium ion. (The effects of these imbalances may be reviewed in Chapter 2.)

Acid-base imbalances are common with vomiting and diarrhea. Initially, vomiting leads to loss of hydrochloric acid, resulting in *metabolic alkalosis* from loss of hydrogen ion and hypochloremia with increased serum bicarbonate levels (see Chapter 2).

If vomiting is severe, there is a change to *metabolic acidosis*. Duodenal secretions containing large quantities of bicarbonate ion are lost, ketoacidosis develops owing to a glucose deficit, and lactic acid accumulates as a result of hypovolemia and impaired tissue perfusion as well as increased muscle activity, which all lead to acidosis. Metabolic acidosis may also accompany diarrhea in the presence of heavy losses of bicarbonate ion in the stool and lack of absorption of fluid and glucose. The accompanying dehydration may limit the ability of the kidneys to respond to acidosis, leading to decompensation.

THINK ABOUT   17-3

a. Explain three specific causes of vomiting; include a variety of factors.
b. Describe the specific actions of the vomiting reflex that prevent aspiration.
c. Explain the similarities and differences between anorexia and bulimia.
d. Explain the changes in arterial blood gases to be expected in the early stage of vomiting and with diarrhea.

Pain

Pain in the digestive system is often difficult to describe in specific terms. A variety of descriptors may be applied.

Visceral pain fibers are connected to the autonomic nervous system; therefore autonomic responses, such as pallor and sweating or nausea and vomiting, frequently accompany this type of pain. Following are types of visceral pain that arise from the organs in the digestive system and are often difficult to localize:

- A burning sensation frequently accompanies inflammation and ulceration in the upper digestive tract; it is related to oral ulcerations when located in the mouth and to heartburn when substernal in location.
- A dull, aching pain (in the right upper quadrant of the abdomen) is typical of stretching of the liver capsule caused by swelling.
- Cramping or diffuse pain is characteristic of inflammation, distention, or stretching of the intestines.
- Colicky, often severe pain results from recurrent smooth muscle spasm or contraction and occurs in

response to severe inflammation or obstruction; for example, it may occur when the system attempts to propel an obstructing gallstone through the bile duct.

Somatic pain is characterized by a steady, intense, often well-localized abdominal pain, which indicates involvement or inflammation of the parietal peritoneum, which contains numerous pain receptors. This forms the basis for the "rebound tenderness" that is identified over an area of inflammation, such as that which develops with acute appendicitis. To elicit the response, pressure is applied slowly to the abdomen by the fingers, and then suddenly released, resulting in a sharp pain at the site.

Somatic pain receptors are directly linked to spinal nerves and may cause a reflex spasm of the overlying abdominal muscles, which leads to a rigid abdomen or "guarding." The patient tends to hold the body immobile with the hip joint flexed and the thigh drawn up.

Referred pain is a common phenomenon and may delay diagnosis because the source of the pain is perceived as a site distant from its origin. Referred pain results when visceral and somatic nerves converge at one spinal cord level, and the source of the visceral pain is then perceived as the same as that of the somatic nerve. Common sites of referred pain may be seen in Figure 4-3.

Malnutrition

Nutritional deficits may be limited or general and have many causes related to gastrointestinal function. There may be a specific problem, such as a vitamin B_{12} deficiency linked to a lack of intrinsic factor from the gastric mucosa. Iron deficiency may be caused by malabsorption, liver damage, or a bleeding ulcer.

General malnutrition may result from chronic anorexia, vomiting, or diarrhea related to gastrointestinal malfunction or other systemic causes. For example, chronic inflammatory bowel disorders may cause anorexia, diarrhea, and malabsorption, or vomiting and diarrhea may be related to external factors such as cancer treatments (radiation and chemotherapy). "Wasting syndrome," or chronic diarrhea accompanying acquired immunodeficiency syndrome (AIDS), leads to malnutrition and dehydration. Interference with bile and pancreatic secretions by mucus plugs in persons with cystic fibrosis is another example of a systemic disease that may lead to malabsorption and malnutrition.

Special diets or "fad" diets for weight loss may result in a lack of certain required elements if a proper balance of nutrients has not been assured. For example, eight essential amino acids are required simultaneously in the diet and are present in animal products. A vegetarian diet must be carefully developed to include foods that provide these amino acids. Some weight-loss diets do not contain all necessary elements. It is recommended that a nutritionist be consulted before embarking on any new diet.

In a child, growth and development may be delayed or impaired by malabsorption or malnutrition. At any stage, the outcomes probably include chronic fatigue, reduced resistance to infection, and impaired healing.

Obesity occurs when the energy value of food consumed is greater than that required by the body. The standard assessment for obesity is determination of body mass index (BMI). In an adult a BMI greater than 30 is indicative of obesity; BMI charts are inside the back cover of the text. See Chapter 23 for a discussion of adolescent obesity. Obesity may be related to ingestion of foods high in fats and simple sugars and low in fiber. Such a diet is often seen in individuals experiencing poverty, as fresh fruits and vegetables are too expensive to be included in the diet. It is currently estimated that one in four Americans is obese. Major complications of obesity include hypertension, atherosclerosis, Type 2 diabetes, obstructive sleep apnea, arthritis, and congestive heart failure. The current epidemic of obesity among adolescents and adults is expected to increase the need for health care services significantly.

Basic Diagnostic Tests

Radiographs are useful diagnostic tools in digestive system disorders. X-ray films, often using a contrast medium such as barium (in oral solution or enema), are useful in outlining many gastrointestinal system structures and abnormalities, and ultrasound may demonstrate unusual masses.

Computed tomography (CT) scans and magnetic resonance imaging (MRI) can be used to check liver and pancreatic abnormalities. Radioactive elements may be used in tracer studies when the uptake of a particular molecule is being analyzed. Techniques such as fiberoptic endoscopy allow improved visualization or biopsy of various segments of the digestive tract, such as the esophagus. Sigmoidoscopy and colonoscopy have become routine preventive and monitoring tools for cancer.

Laboratory analysis of stool specimens or gastric washings can provide evidence of infection, bleeding, tumors, or malabsorption problems. Specimens may need to be repeated over a prescribed time period, particularly if a parasitic infection is suspected.

Blood tests can be used to check liver function by evaluating serum protein levels, clotting times, serum liver enzymes, and bilirubin levels. Pancreatic problems may be detected by serum enzyme levels or stool analysis for enzymes and fat content. Blood tests can also be used to monitor tumor markers, for example, carcinoembryonic antigen (CEA) in patients with colon cancer, although these tests cannot stand alone as diagnostic tools or monitoring devices. It is usual for the patient

to experience a variety of tests before a diagnosis can be made.

Common Therapies and Prevention

Many digestive tract disorders require a team approach to assist with the many facets of the disease:

1. *Dietary modifications* are helpful in the treatment of many gastrointestinal disorders. For example, a gluten-free diet is recommended for people with celiac disease, thus removing the source of the problem. Reduced intake of alcohol and coffee (containing caffeine) may promote the healing of ulcers, and increased fiber and fluid intake may reduce constipation. Limited fat content with increased caloric intake and vitamin supplements are recommended for patients with many malabsorption syndromes. A diet that is restricted in calories is important in dealing with obesity and is usually paired with an exercise program. Other factors in the diet, such as the type of fat, the inclusion of antioxidants, and the vitamin and mineral content, are of concern to many with respect to prevention of disease.
2. *Stress reduction* techniques are useful in many patients with peptic ulcer or chronic inflammatory bowel disorders, in which exacerbations have been shown to be stress-related. These techniques are also important in the treatment of adolescents or teenagers with digestive tract disorders because their social activities and body image may be affected by the disease. Severe or prolonged stress, whether resulting from a physical stressor such as infection or trauma or an emotional stressor such as fear or anger, does affect the digestive tract. These effects result from stimulation of the SNS, leading to vasoconstriction and ischemia of the mucosa, with subsequent inflammation and ulceration. Also, SNS stimulation decreases peristalsis, resulting in prolonged contact of secretions and irritants with the mucosa. The stress response also promotes glucocorticoid secretion, which has catabolic effects if it is continued over a long term. High cortisol levels lead to reduced regeneration of the mucosa and delayed healing of lesions. A stressful environment predisposes the individual to poor nutritional habits, such as increased caffeine intake and indulgence in snack foods.
3. *Drugs* are used to treat many gastrointestinal disorders, and a great variety of medications are available to treat the diverse types of gastrointestinal problems. Examples of common medications are summarized in Table 17-3.

Many individuals treat themselves for minor digestive discomfort. It is always important to check specifically on self-prescribed medications when taking a patient history because many individuals do not think that over-the-counter drugs are of any importance. Such medications may mask signs of disease or may

TABLE 17-3   Examples of Drugs Used in Digestive System Disorders

Classification	Example	Action
Antiemetic	Dimenhydrinate (Dramamine) Prochlorperazine (Stemetil)	Reduces vomiting resulting from drugs, motion sickness, and radiation treatment
Antidiarrheal	Loperamide (Imodium) Codeine, paregoric	Reduces intestinal motility
Anti-inflammatory	Prednisone (Deltasone—a glucocorticoid) Sulfasalazine (Azulfidine)	Reduces inflammation Prednisone blocks immune response Sulfasalazine has antibacterial action
Acid-reduction	Ranitidine (Zantac): blocks H_2 receptors Lansoprazole (Prevacid): proton (H^+) pump inhibitor	Reduces secretion of hydrochloric acid in the stomach
Antimicrobial	Clarithromycin (Biaxin) Metronidazole (Flagyl) Tetracycline Cefoperazone Amoxicillin	Combination therapy for *Helicobacter pylori* infection Drugs as indicated by culture and sensitivity
Coating Agent	Sucralfate (Carafate)	Covers ulcer to allow healing
Antacid	Aluminum-magnesium combinations (Maalox)	Reduces hyperacidity
Laxative	Psyllium (Metamucil) (bulk) or docusate sodium (Colace) (stool softener)	With water, increases fecal bulk and intestinal motility
Anticholinergics	pirenzepine, propantheline bromide	reduces PNS activities—reduced secretions and mobility
Histamine-2 blockers	Tagamet, Zantac	Inhibits acid production in stomach
Proton Pump Inhibitors	Prevacid, Prilosec	reduce gastric secretions

be the cause of a problem. If possible, it is better to identify and treat the cause of a problem rather than the symptoms.

- Antacids are a common medication used for many purposes. The primary component of antacids is usually calcium carbonate, aluminum hydroxide, magnesium hydroxide, or a combination of these. Examples are Maalox or Gelusil.
- Antiemetics, taken to relieve vomiting, include drugs such as dimenhydrinate (Dramamine, Gravol) or phenothiazines such as prochlorperazine (Compazine). Cannabinoids such as nabilone (Cesamet) may be a successful antiemetic for chemotherapy-induced vomiting.
- Laxatives or enemas, of which there are many types, are used to treat acute constipation. Fluid intake should be *increased* while taking these medications. Bulk supplements (e.g., psyllium hydrophilic mucilloid [Metamucil]) or stool softeners (e.g., docusate sodium [Colace]) are helpful, particularly for recurrent constipation and are less likely to cause adverse effects than other laxatives. Chronic constipation is best treated by the addition of fiber and fluid to the diet, rather than persistent use of laxatives, which may aggravate the problem.
- Antidiarrheals, such as loperamide (Imodium), or narcotics, such as codeine or paregoric, may reduce peristalsis and relieve cramps when diarrhea is not relieved by dietary changes.

- Infections causing diarrhea are frequently self-limiting, but specific antimicrobial drugs may be required in some cases.
- Sulfasalazine (Salazopyrin or Azulfidine), an anti-inflammatory and antibacterial agent, may be used to treat acute episodes of inflammatory bowel disease.
- Antibacterials, such as clarithromycin (Biaxin) or azithromycin (Zithromax), are effective against *Helicobacter pylori* infection and are usually combined with a proton pump inhibitor such as omeprazole (Prilosec). Metronidazole is primarily used when treating protozoal infections.
- Sucralfate (Carafate or Sucrate) is a coating agent, used to enhance the gastric mucosal barrier against irritants, allowing ulcers to heal.
- Anticholinergic drugs reduce PNS activity and may be used to reduce secretions and motility. Examples include pirenzepine, which inhibits gastric acid, and propantheline bromide, which decreases gastrointestinal motility and spasm as well as reducing gastric acid.
- Histamine$_2$ blockers (H_2 receptor antagonist drugs), such as cimetidine (Tagamet) or ranitidine (Zantac) may be useful in some cases of ulcers.
- Proton (acid) pump inhibitors, such as lansoprazole (Prevacid) or omeprazole (Prilosec or Losec), are a newer group of drugs that reduce gastric secretions by interfering with the exchange of H^+ and K^+ in the

stomach. They are used in combination with antibacterials to treat *H. pylori* infection.

> **THINK ABOUT 17-4**
>
>
>
> a. Describe and state the mechanism of referred pain and colicky pain.
> b. Describe the vomiting reflex, noting possible causes of aspiration during vomiting.
> c. Explain why altered blood clotting times and serum protein levels may indicate the presence of liver disease.
> d. Explain how the use of over-the-counter medications may exaggerate or mask symptoms and sometimes exacerbate the disorder.
> e. Explain how regular use of bulk laxatives can promote peristalsis and relieve constipation.

> **APPLY YOUR KNOWLEDGE 17-2**
>
> Explain why using an antiprotozoal drug like metronidazole may be more stressful on the body than most antibacterial drugs?

Upper Gastrointestinal Tract Disorders

Disorders of the Oral Cavity

Congenital Defects

Cleft lip and cleft palate are common developmental abnormalities of the mouth and face and arise in the second or third month of gestation (Fig. 17-4). Cleft lip and cleft palate appear to be multifactorial in origin and are related to a number of inherited and environmental

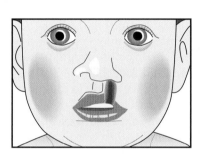

A Unilateral cleft lip (complete)

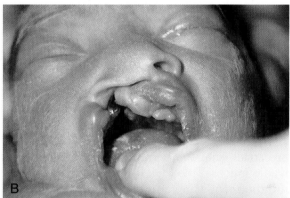

B

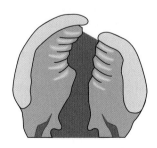

C Unilateral cleft palate and lip (complete)

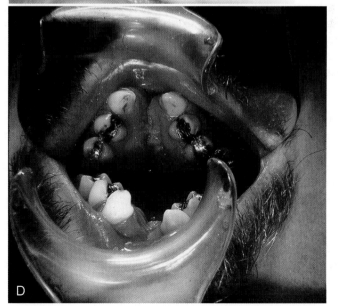

D

FIGURE 17-4 **Cleft Lip and Palate A,** Unilateral cleft lip. **B,** Unilateral cleft lip. **C,** Unilateral cleft palate and lip. **D,** Following surgical repair of cleft palate and lip. Note suture line on palate and missing anterior teeth that interfere with speech and eating. (*B from Behrman RE, Kliegman RM, Arvin AM: Slide Set for Nelson Textbook of Pediatrics, 15th ed. Philadelphia, Saunders, 1996. D, Courtesy Evie Jesin, George Brown College of Applied Arts and Technology, Toronto, Ontario, Canada.*)

factors. One or both defects may be present in various degrees of severity. Cleft lip, which may be unilateral or bilateral (on either side of the midline), results from failure of the maxillary processes to fuse with the nasal elevations or failure of the upper lip to fuse at some time between 4 and 8 weeks of fetal development.

Cleft palate involves failure of the hard and soft palates to fuse between 7 and 12 weeks of gestation, creating an opening between the oral cavity and the nasal cavity. The infant has feeding problems because there is insufficient force developed in the mouth to suck, and a high risk of aspirating fluid into the respiratory passages. Speech development is also impaired. Temporary measures include the use of special nipples or dental appliances that close off the nasal cavity. Surgical repair of the defect is necessary and additional plastic surgery to correct growth defects or improve appearance is usually indicated (see Fig. 17-4D). Therapy with a speech-language pathologist and orthodontist promotes normal development. A multidisciplinary team is frequently required over a prolonged period when major clefts are present.

Inflammatory Lesions

Aphthous ulcers (aphthous stomatitis or canker sores) are a common problem. A member of the resident flora of the oral cavity, *Streptococcus sanguis*, may be involved. These ulcers often accompany fevers, stress, or ingestion of certain foods.

Aphthous ulcers are small, shallow, painful lesions occurring on the movable mucosa, the buccal mucosa, the floor of the mouth, the soft palate, and the lateral borders of the tongue. Initially a red macule appears, accompanied by a tingling sensation. Central ulceration develops, with a punched-out whitish appearance surrounded by a red border. The ulcers heal spontaneously in a week or so.

Infections

The oral cavity has a large and varied resident flora (microflora), including many types of bacteria in addition to fungi, viruses, and protozoa. These microorganisms thrive in the crevices of the mouth, where it is moist and warm and food particles provide plentiful nutrients. They generally are harmless; however, they may cause opportunistic infections, such as candidiasis, or cause secondary infection when there are open lesions in the oral cavity. The oral cavity and pharynx may also harbor pathogens in certain individuals (carriers).

Some of the resident bacteria, particularly strains of *Viridans Streptococcus* (a-hemolytic streptococci), are of concern when they enter the blood when the body's defenses may be compromised, for example, when the mucosal barrier is broken during dental procedures, and the circulation and replication of the organisms can subsequently cause a transient bacteremia. For some individuals with damaged heart valves or a prosthesis, this can be dangerous, because infection (bacterial endocarditis, see Chapter 12) can result. Therefore prophylactic medication with amoxicillin or an alternative is sometimes recommended when there is a risk of bacteremia. (Current recommendations are available from the American Dental Association and the American Heart Association.)

Candidiasis

Candida albicans, often part of the normal resident flora of the mouth, is an opportunist under certain conditions. *Oral candidiasis* (thrush) is a common fungal infection that occurs in individuals who have received broad-spectrum antibiotics, cancer chemotherapy, or glucocorticoids and in those who have diabetes or are immunosuppressed. It is often an initial indication of infection in AIDS patients and may extend into the esophagus in such cases. The infection may also be seen in young infants as they develop resident flora, or it may be transmitted by the mother. Chronic infection on the palate is seen in persons with dentures that are poorly fitted or worn at night (Fig. 17-5A).

Candidal infection may appear as a red, swollen area as in Figure 17-5A or as irregular patches of a white curd-like material (see Fig. 17-5B) on the mucosa or tongue that can be wiped off (a diagnostic clue) to reveal erythema at the base.

Nystatin (Mycostatin), a topical antifungal agent, is the usual treatment.

Herpes Simplex Type 1 Infection

Herpetic stomatitis may be associated with *herpes labialis* (cold sores or fever blisters). Herpes infection is usually caused by herpes simplex virus type 1 (HSV-1) and is transmitted by kissing or close contact, often in childhood. The initial infection is frequently asymptomatic, but the virus remains dormant in the body in a sensory ganglion, often the trigeminal nerve ganglion.

When activated by stress, trauma, or another infection (such as a common cold), the virus migrates along the nerve to the skin or mucosa around the mouth, causing a burning or stinging sensation at the site, which is followed by development of vesicles (blisters) as the virus reproduces and causes necrosis of the host cells (see Fig. 8-9). These vesicles rupture, leaving a shallow, painful ulcer, which releases a clear fluid containing many organisms and then crusts over. The lesions heal spontaneously in 7 to 10 days, when the virus again migrates along the trigeminal nerve to the sensory ganglion, where it enters a latent stage. Recurrences are common. In immunosuppressed patients, multiple lesions may develop in the oral cavity and pharynx (herpetic gingivostomatitis).

HSV-1 is often present in the saliva for some time after the vesicle has healed. Although no cure is available at present, the acute stage may be alleviated

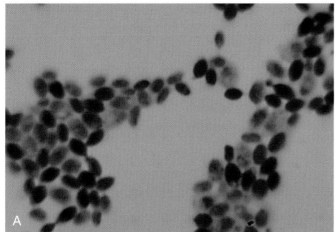

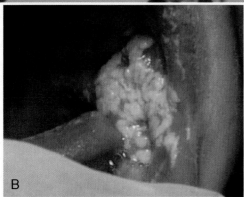

FIGURE 17-5 Thrush. **A**, Micrograph of the fungus *Candida albicans* in the yeast form (this fungus can also form filamentous mycelia) that is responsible for an oral infection called *thrush*. *C. albicans* can also cause vaginal infections in women. *(From VanMeter K, Hubert R: Microbiology for the Healthcare Professional, St. Louis, 2010, Elsevier.)* **B**, Oral candidiasis illustrating the white plaques. *(From Zitelli BJ, Davis HW: Atlas of pediatric physical Diagnosis, ed 4. St. Louis, 2002, Mosby.)*

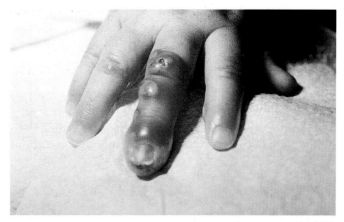

FIGURE 17-6 Herpetic whitlow. *(Courtesy of Mark Drapkin, Newton Wellesly Hospital, Newton, Massachusetts. From Stone DR, Gorbach SL: Atlas of Infectious Diseases, Philadelphia, 2000, Saunders.)*

somewhat by prompt use of antiviral medications (e.g., topical acyclovir [Zovirax]), thus decreasing the shedding of the virus, the risk of transmission, and the discomfort.

Herpes simplex virus may spread to the eyes, causing conjunctivitis and keratitis (see Chapter 15), either by contaminated fingers or through droplets sprayed from the mouth, for example, during dental treatment. Dental personnel are also vulnerable to *herpetic whitlow*, an acute and painful infection of the finger (Fig. 17-6).

Syphilis
Syphilis may cause oral lesions that contain microorganisms and are highly contagious during the first and second stages (see Chapter 19). The primary stage is characterized by a chancre, a painless ulcer usually found on the tongue, lips, or palate. The lesion heals spontaneously (without treatment) in a week or two. The second stage may be manifested by red macules or papules on the palate, similar to the typical skin rash occurring at this stage, or by mucous patches—multiple,

irregular, loose, white necrotic material on the mucosa, which is highly infectious. Again, this lesion heals spontaneously. Because these lesions may be missed, immediate treatment of the infection and control of transmission may be hampered.

Both stages of syphilis are treated with long-acting penicillin, usually by injection, because the organism, *Treponema pallidum*, also exists in the general circulation of the individual.

Dental Problems
Caries
Dental caries (tooth decay or cavities) is an infection involving *Streptococcus mutans* (as the initiator), followed by increased numbers of *Lactobacillus* and other acid-producing resident flora in the oral cavity. These bacteria act on sugars in ingested food to create large quantities of lactic acid that dissolve the minerals (calcium and phosphate) in tooth enamel, leading to erosion of the tooth surface and cavity formation. If untreated, bacterial action and decay may continue to penetrate the tooth surface until the internal structures of the tooth are infected (pulpitis) or periapical abscesses form at the root of the tooth.

Caries is promoted by frequent intake of sugar and acids such as carbonic acid in soft drinks and by the presence of multiple pits or fissures in the tooth surface. Xerostomia (dry mouth), plaque formation, and periodontal disease also increase the incidence. Fluoride, as an anticaries treatment, decreases the solubility of the minerals in enamel (fluorapatite replaces hydroxyapatite) and enhances the remineralization process. Excessive fluoride ingestion during tooth maturation can, however, cause hypocalcification of tooth enamel.

Periodontal Disease
The periodontium consists of the gingivae (gums) and the anchoring structure for the teeth, which includes

the alveolar bone around the teeth, the cementum (or outer covering of the root of the tooth), and the periodontal ligament joining the cementum to the bone. Periodontitis is the infection and damage to the periodontal ligament and bone by microorganisms, and subsequent loosening and possible loss of the teeth. There are currently eight categories of periodontal disease, ranging from mild gingival disease to severe periodontitis. Periodontal disease is often caused by poor oral hygiene, but can also be aggravated by systemic diseases and medications.

Gingivitis

Normally the gingivae, or gums surrounding the teeth, are firm, light pink with a stippled appearance, and well-shaped, and anchor the teeth firmly (Fig. 17-7A). Changes in the gingivae may reflect local or systemic problems. Gingivitis, or inflammation of the gingiva,

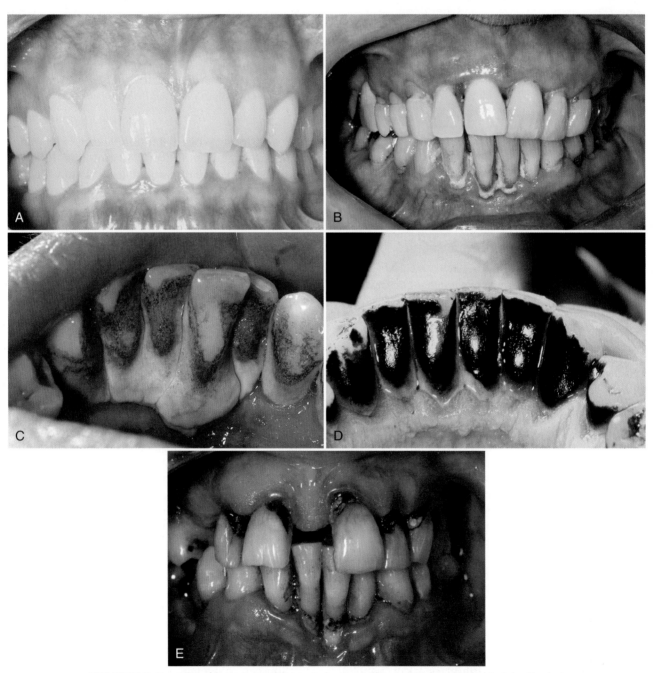

FIGURE 17-7 **Dental Problems A,** Healthy periodontium. The gingiva (gum) is light pink, stippled, and firm around the teeth. **B,** Toothbrush trauma. Improper brushing has led to loss of tooth substance and grooving of the root. **C,** Calculus or calcified plaque on tooth surface. **D,** Smoking leads to extensive calculus, staining on the teeth, and increased risk of periodontal disease. **E,** Severe periodontal disease with bone loss and caries in the root of the tooth. *(**A-E,** Courtesy Evie Jesin, George Brown College of Applied Arts and Technology, Toronto, Ontario, Canada.)*

causes the gingival tissue to become red, soft, and swollen and to bleed easily. This may result from accumulated plaque, which is a mass of bacteria and debris adhering to the tooth, particularly near the gingivae. The involved microbes secrete substances that enable them to adhere to the tooth surface and to plaque. Calculus, or tartar, refers to calcified plaque, which is more irritating to tissue because of its hard, rough surface (see Fig. 17-7C). Poor oral hygiene also predisposes to gingivitis. However, toothbrush trauma (see Fig. 17-7B), resulting from improper or excessive brushing or use of abrasives, can create extensive grooving on the tooth surface, increase plaque retention and damage to the gingivae, and increase tooth sensitivity.

Systemic factors can alter the gingivae. Development of a dark line on the gingival margin is an indicator of lead poisoning (see Chapter 28). Overgrowth (sometimes called pregnancy tumor) may occur from hormonal changes associated with pregnancy or the use of oral contraceptives. Gingival hyperplasia occurs with long-term use of drugs, such as phenytoin (Dilantin) or cyclosporine (see Fig. 14-27).

Necrotizing periodontal disease, also called trench mouth (formerly acute necrotizing ulcerative gingivitis, ANUG) is a common infection caused by anaerobic opportunistic bacteria in individuals in whom tissue resistance is decreased by stress, smoking, disease, or nutritional deficits. The gingivae around the mandibular anterior teeth (lower jaw) are affected, showing white pseudomembranous necrotic areas surrounded by red and swollen areas. The gingivae are painful and bleed easily. Débridement and antibiotics may be needed.

Periodontitis

More serious forms of periodontal disease develop when there is an increase in activity of gram-negative anaerobic bacteria as they enter the plaque. Major destructive microbes in periodontal disease include *Porphyromonas gingivalis* (formerly *Bacteroides oralis*) *Actinobacillus actinomycetemcomitans* and *Bacteroides forsythus*. These microbes secrete toxins and enzymes destructive to the tissues and white blood cells (WBCs). Such infection is not contagious.

In addition to poor oral hygiene, periodontitis is aggravated by smoking, which promotes calculus formation (see Fig. 17-7D); cancer and chemotherapy; diabetes mellitus with decreased tissue resistance and poor healing (see Fig. 16-8A); and HIV infection (AIDS), in which periodontitis is rapidly progressive and often resistant to treatment (see Fig. 17-17D).

When periodontal disease develops, plaque and calculus have progressed on the tooth beneath the gingival margin, causing inflammation in the tissues around the root of the tooth. The subgingival areas are colonized by these gram-negative anaerobic bacteria, which ultimately destroy the periodontal attachment of the tooth and the surrounding alveolar bone. An enlarging

periodontal pocket forms around the tooth, promoting more anaerobic bacterial activity and active infection. The mucosa is red and swollen and bleeds easily, and the teeth feel loose (see Fig. 17-7E). Major treatment, including drugs and surgical procedures, is required to eradicate the infection and prevent loss of teeth.

Hyperkeratosis

An example of hyperkeratosis is *leukoplakia*, a whitish plaque or epidermal thickening of the mucosa that occurs on the buccal mucosa, palate, lower lip or tongue (Fig. 17-8). The cause cannot always be identified but may be related to smoking or chronic irritation. These lesions require monitoring because, in some cases, epithelial dysplasia beneath the plaque develops into squamous cell carcinoma.

Cancer of the Oral Cavity

The common cancer of the oral cavity is *squamous cell carcinoma*. These cancers are more common in persons older than age 40, particularly smokers, those with

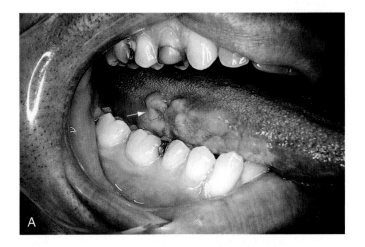

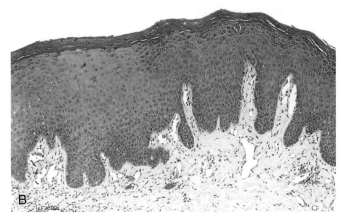

FIGURE 17-8 Leukoplakia. **A,** Leukoplakia of the tongue in a smoker. **B,** Leukoplakia with marked epithelial thickening and hyperkeratoosis. *(From Kumar V, et al: Robbins basic pathology, ed 8, Philadelphia, 2007, Saunders-Elsevier.)*

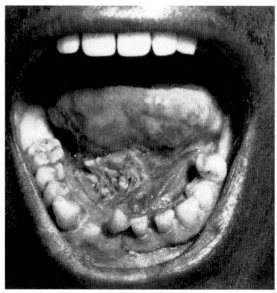

FIGURE 17-9 Squamous cell carcinoma on the floor of the mouth under the tongue. *(From Odom RB, James WD, Berger TG:* Andrews' Diseases of the Skin, *ed 9, Philadelphia, 2000, Saunders.)*

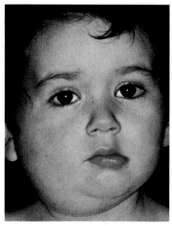

FIGURE 17-10 This young boy with mumps has unilateral parotid swelling on the right side. *(From Patton KT, Thibodeau GA:* Anatomy & Physiology, *ed 8, St. Louis, 2013, Mosby.)*

pre-existing leukoplakia, or those with a history of alcohol abuse.

Malignant tumors inside the oral cavity have a poor prognosis because they tend to be hidden and painless. Routine dental care is important in identifying these lesions in an early stage. Common sites are the floor of the mouth and the lateral borders of the tongue (Fig. 17-9). There may be multiple lesions. The carcinoma appears initially as a whitish thickening and then develops into either a nodular mass or an ulcerative lesion, which persists. Intraoral cancer spreads first to the regional lymph nodes and nodes in the neck.

Kaposi's sarcoma may occur in patients with AIDS. The typical lesion is a brownish or purple macular lesion, usually on the palate, which eventually becomes a nodular mass.

Lip cancer (usually on the lower lip) is obvious and accessible and has a good prognosis. It usually spreads locally. This cancer is common in smokers, particularly pipe smokers.

Salivary Gland Disorders

Sialadenitis refers to inflammation of the salivary glands, infectious or noninfectious. The parotid gland is most frequently affected, both by infectious agents and tumors. Bacterial infection may spread from the mouth. Mumps, infectious parotitis, is a viral infection leading to marked, usually bilateral, swelling of the gland (Fig. 17-10). Although a vaccine has been available for more than a decade, mumps outbreaks have occurred in college-aged adults; in such outbreaks revaccination is recommended to limit the spread of the disease.

Noninfectious parotitis may develop in debilitated or elderly patients who lack adequate fluid intake and mouth care. Tumors such as benign adenomas tend to

affect the parotid glands of older individuals. The most frequent malignant tumor of the salivary gland is mucoepidermoid carcinoma, occurring primarily in the parotid glands.

THINK ABOUT 17-5

Prepare a chart comparing the cause and characteristics of one inflammatory disorder, one infectious disorder, and one tumor of the oral cavity.

Dysphagia

Dysphagia, or difficulty in swallowing (Fig. 17-11), has many causes. It may result from a neurologic deficit, a muscular disorder, or a mechanical obstruction. Dysphagia may present as pain with swallowing, an inability to swallow larger pieces of solid material, or difficulty in swallowing liquids, depending on the cause of the problem.

Neurologic causative factors include infection, stroke, brain damage, and *achalasia*, which results from failure of the lower esophageal sphincter to relax owing to loss of innervation. This leads to accumulation of food and dilation of the lower esophagus as entry of food into the stomach is delayed. Often chronic inflammation develops in the esophagus, and reflux of this food may lead to aspiration when the person assumes a supine position. There is an increased risk of esophageal carcinoma in an individual who has had long-term achalasia.

Muscle impairment may result from muscular dystrophy.

Mechanical obstructions include the following:
- *Congenital atresia* is a developmental defect in which the upper and lower esophageal segments are separated; the upper section ends in a blind pouch. Reflux of feedings occurs in the infant with congenital

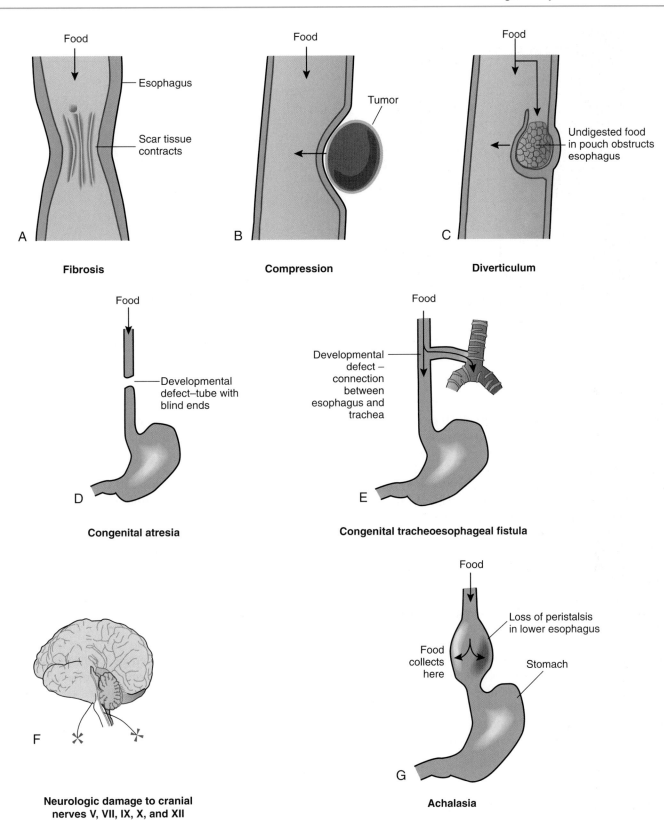

FIGURE 17-11 Causes of dysphagia.

atresia, leading to aspiration. In many cases there is a connecting fistula from one of the segments to the trachea. Surgical correction is required as soon as possible to prevent aspiration and provide fluid and nutrients to the infant.

- Stenosis, or narrowing of the esophagus, may be a developmental or acquired defect; the acquired form is usually secondary to fibrosis accompanying chronic inflammation, ulceration (esophagitis), or radiation therapy. Stenosis or stricture may also

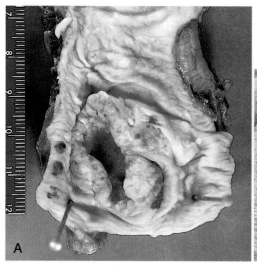
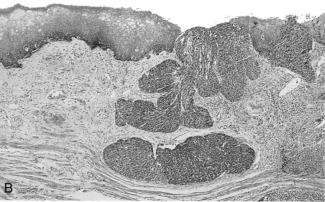

FIGURE 17-12 Esophageal squamous cell carcinoma. **A,** Large ulcerated squamous cell carcinoma of the esophagus. **B,** Low power view of cancer invasion of the submucosa. *(From Kumar V, et al: Robbins basic pathology, ed 8, Philadelphia, 2007, Saunders-Elsevier.)*

result from scar tissue that formed after accidental ingestion of corrosive chemicals, such as lye or other cleaning materials. Accidental ingestion of such damaging substances should not be treated by inducing vomiting to remove the chemical because this would cause additional tissue damage. Stenosis may require treatment with repeated mechanical dilation by bougies or surgery if food intake is severely limited by the obstruction.

- Esophageal *diverticula* are outpouchings of the esophageal wall that result either from congenital defects or inflammation. The accumulated food in the pouch obstructs the flow of food down the esophagus; causes irritation, inflammation, and scar tissue in the wall; and often is regurgitated upward at a later time, with the possibility of aspiration into the respiratory tract. Signs of diverticula include dysphagia, foul breath, chronic cough, and hoarseness. Occasionally, ulcers may form in the esophageal wall and bleed.
- *Tumors* may be internal or external. External tumors are located outside the esophagus, perhaps in a mediastinal lymph node, and compress the esophagus.

Esophageal Cancer

Esophageal cancer is primarily *squamous cell carcinoma* and is most commonly found in the distal esophagus. Tumors in the esophagus either form circumferential strictures or grow out into the lumen of the esophagus; both types cause significant dysphagia in later stages (Fig. 17-12).

Esophageal cancer is associated with chronic irritation; for example, from chronic esophagitis, achalasia, hiatal hernia, alcohol abuse, and smoking. Unfortunately,

the initial signs of dysphagia occur relatively late in the course of the disease, and the prognosis currently is poor.

Hiatal Hernia

In patients with hiatal hernia, part of the stomach protrudes through the opening (hiatus) in the diaphragm into the thoracic cavity. Normally the digestive tract is loosely attached to the diaphragm. There are two types of hiatal hernia (Fig. 17-13). With a *sliding* hernia, the more common type, a portion of the stomach and the gastroesophageal junction move above the diaphragm, particularly when the person is in the supine position. In the standing position, the herniated portion slides back down into the abdominal cavity. In a *rolling* or *paraesophageal* hernia, part of the fundus of the stomach moves up through an enlarged or weak hiatus in the diaphragm. In this type of hernia, the blood vessels in the wall of the stomach may be compressed, leading to ulceration.

Food often lodges in the pouch created by the herniated portion, resulting in inflammation of the mucosa, reflux of food up the esophagus, and dysphagia, as the mass of food enlarges and obstructs the passageway. Chronic esophagitis eventually may cause fibrosis and stricture. Often an incompetent gastroesophageal sphincter is seen in individuals with hiatal hernia, which increases the risk of reflux.

Factors contributing to hiatal hernia include shortening of the esophagus, weakness of the diaphragm, or increased abdominal pressure (e.g., from pregnancy).

The signs of hiatal hernia include *heartburn* or *pyrosis*, a brief substernal burning sensation, often accompanied by a sour taste in the mouth, which occurs after meals

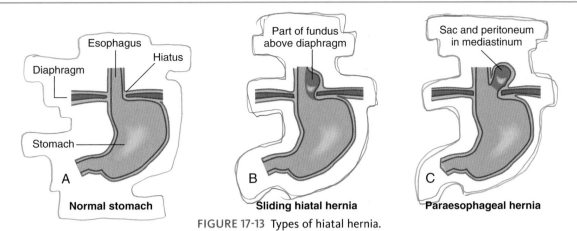

FIGURE 17-13 Types of hiatal hernia.

and results from reflux of the gastric contents up the esophagus. Frequent belching (gas) often accompanies this regurgitation. The discomfort is increased by lying down after eating, bending over, or coughing. Dysphagia is common, either because of inflammation of the esophagus or because the mass of food collected in the pouch compresses the esophagus. Persistent, mild, substernal chest pain after meals is a frequent complaint because of inflammation or distention of the pouch. The symptoms can often be reduced by eating frequent, small meals and avoiding a recumbent position after meals.

Gastroesophageal Reflux Disease

Gastroesophageal reflux disease (GERD) involves the periodic flow of gastric contents into the esophagus. It is often seen in conjunction with hiatal hernia as well as other conditions. The severity of GERD depends on the competence of the lower esophageal sphincter (LES) or the relative pressures on either side of the LES. For example, either a decrease in LES pressure or an increase in intra-abdominal pressure allows more of the gastric contents to reflux back into the esophagus. Delayed gastric emptying may also be a factor.

Episodes of reflux causing heartburn frequently occur 30 to 60 minutes after eating or at night. Frequent reflux of gastric acid leads to inflammation and ulceration of the mucosa, and eventual fibrosis and stricture in the esophagus. Eliminating factors that reduce LES pressure, such as caffeine, fatty foods, alcohol intake, cigarette smoking, and certain drugs, may relieve the discomfort. Avoidance of spicy foods and use of medication may reduce reflux and inflammation.

Gastritis

Gastritis is an inflammation of the stomach that may occur in many forms. Gastritis may be acute or chronic; these terms represent two different diseases. Acute gastritis may be a mild, transient irritation with only vague signs, or it may be a more severe ulcerative or hemorrhagic episode.

Acute Gastritis

In acute gastritis, the gastric mucosa is inflamed and appears red and edematous. It may be ulcerated and bleeding if the mucosal barrier (the tightly packed epithelial cells and layer of thick mucus) is severely damaged or the circulation is poor, which reduces tissue resistance.

Acute gastritis may result from:
- Infection by many types of microorganisms (e.g., bacteria and viruses)
- Allergies to foods such as shellfish or drugs
- Ingestion of spicy or irritating foods, such as hot peppers, particularly if the person is unaccustomed to a spicy diet
- Excessive alcohol intake
- Ingestion of aspirin or other ulcerogenic drugs (especially on an empty stomach)
- Ingestion of corrosive or toxic substances
- Radiation or chemotherapy

■ *Signs and Symptoms*

The basic signs of gastrointestinal irritation are present. Anorexia, nausea, or vomiting develops, the severity of which varies with the particular situation. Hematemesis indicates ulceration and bleeding in the stomach. Epigastric pain, cramps, or general discomfort may be present. Depending on the cause, other signs may be present; for example, fever and headache usually accompany infection. In some cases, particularly with infections, diarrhea may develop (see next section, Gastroenteritis).

Acute gastritis is usually self-limiting, with complete regeneration of the gastric mucosa in a day or two. In persons with severe or prolonged vomiting, there is a danger of dehydration, electrolyte loss, and metabolic acidosis, all of which require supportive treatment. Certain infections may require treatment with antimicrobial drugs.

Gastroenteritis

Gastroenteritis is the involvement of the stomach and the intestines in an inflammatory process. It is usually caused by infection but may also result from allergic

TABLE 17-4 Common Infections Transmitted by Food and Water

Pathogen	Source	Incubation	Pathophysiology	Manifestations
Staphylococcus aureus	Food handlers Inadequate cooking or refrigeration of custards, salad dressing, cold meats	1-7 hr (2-4, average)	Enterotoxin (exotoxin), heat-stable	Sudden severe nausea, vomiting, and cramps; sometimes diarrhea Subnormal body temperature and low blood pressure
Escherichia coli (traveler's diarrhea)	Fecal contamination of food and water	10-12 hr	Various strains may release enterotoxins (increase secretions) or invade the mucosa	Profuse watery diarrhea, sometimes with blood or mucus Vomiting and abdominal cramps often present
Salmonella species	Fecal contamination of food or undercooked or raw eggs, poultry, shellfish Contaminated work surfaces	6-72 hr	Organisms multiply in intestine, causing inflammation and ulceration	Sudden diarrhea, abdominal pain, and fever Sometimes vomiting
Rotavirus	Oral-fecal (infants)	24-72 hr	Inflammation and loss of villi	Vomiting, severe watery diarrhea, fever
Norwalk virus	Oral-fecal (adults/older children) shellfish, fomites	24-48 hr	Damage villi	Vomiting, diarrhea, and cramps, headache, fever
Entamoeba histolytica (amebic dysentery)	Fecal contamination of water and vegetables	2-4 wk	Protozoan parasite with cyst stage and active trophozoite stage; may invade mucosa, causing abscesses	Diarrhea with blood and mucus, may alternate with constipation Fever and chills
Listeria sp.	Found in soil and water	30-70 days	Granulomas	Flu-like with diarrhea.
Clostridium botulinum	Spores in poorly canned food or prepared meat	12-36 hr	Neurotoxin (exotoxin) causes nerve paralysis	Visual problems, dysphagia, then flaccid paralysis and respiratory failure Possibly early vomiting or diarrhea
Campylobacter sp.	Handling raw poultry, undercooked poultry, raw milk, contaminated water	2-5 days	infection causes tissue damage to the ileum, jejunum and colon	diarrhea, nausea

reactions to foods or drugs. Inflammation of the gastric mucosa stimulates vomiting, whereas diarrhea results when the inflammation of the intestines causes increased motility, impaired absorption, and in some cases, increased secretions. Nausea and abdominal cramps are usually present. Fever and malaise are common.

Many microorganisms may be transmitted by fecally contaminated food and water. Common causes of food-borne infections are summarized in Table 17-4. Most infections are mild and self-limiting, but occasionally serious illness results when the host is immunosuppressed or the agent is more virulent.

Often a food- or water-borne illness will involve a large number of cases; in some outbreaks entire communities may be infected. It is imperative that in times of disaster clear instructions be given about the safety of food and water. Safe sanitation must be put in place as quickly as possible to prevent further illness requiring the use of scarce health resources.

Some infections are seasonal or occur as epidemics. For example, rotaviruses cause serious infection, with vomiting and watery diarrhea, sometimes with ulceration and bleeding, in young children in temperate climates during the winter months. Epidemics of viral gastroenteritis are common in daycare centers and institutions. Careful handwashing and food handling can reduce outbreaks.

The infection is usually self-limiting, although supportive treatment may be needed for fluid and electrolyte losses, particularly in young children and the elderly. A stool culture is helpful in identifying the causative organism in persistent cases.

Infection by *Clostridium difficile* in patients on broad-spectrum antibiotics causes severe enteritis. This gram-positive bacillus exists as a spore until it reaches the colon. The vegetative form damages the intestinal mucosa, causing diarrhea that is sometimes mild, and other times severe. Outbreaks have occurred in many hospitals, resulting in some fatalities.

Escherichia coli *Infection*

Escherichia coli (*E. coli*) is usually a harmless microbe that is normally resident in the intestine. Some infective types can adhere to the mucosa and secrete an enterotoxin, causing gastroenteritis, particularly among children in nursery schools or travelers in the form of common "traveler's diarrhea." Some strains are invasive and cause five forms of intestinal disease.

- Enterotoxigenic *E. coli* (ETEC) causes diarrhea in infants and travelers in countries in which proper sanitation is lacking. Organism colonizes the small intestine and produces enterotoxins that may cause minor discomfort to severe cholera-like symptoms.
- Enteroinvasive *E. coli* (EIEC) penetrates and reproduces in and destroys the epithelial cells of the colon. The organism does not produce enterotoxins but causes severe diarrhea and fever.
- Enteropathogenic *E. coli* (EPEC) is very similar to EIEC; however, it is reported to produce and enterotoxin similar to *Shigella*.
- Enteroaggregative *E. coli* (EAggEC) produces persistent diarrhea in young children. In addition to producing an enteroaggregative heat stabile toxin, it also produces a hemolysin produced by strains that commonly cause urinary tract infections.
- Enterohemorrhagic *E. coli* (EHEC) is caused by a specific strain O157:H7. These highly virulent strains are present in cows, and infection has arisen from food and water contaminated with these strains, such as water runoff from contaminated pastures into wells, partially cooked ground beef or unpasteurized milk, or from contamination by other oral-fecal routes (e.g., diapers or direct contact). These strains of *E. coli* release verocytotoxins (*Shigella*-like toxins) in the intestine, which cause damage to the mucosa and to the blood vessel walls, and subsequently may affect blood vessels in the kidneys and elsewhere.

The onset is acute, with severe watery diarrhea and cramps, progressing to bloody diarrhea and lasting up to a week. In some individuals, the toxin is absorbed and circulates to cause hemolysis of blood cells, leading to anemia and thrombocytopenia, and also acute renal failure, requiring dialysis (see Chapter 18). A few individuals have experienced neurologic effects, such as seizures. Deaths have occurred, particularly in young children and elderly persons. The diagnosis depends on identification of these particular strains from stool samples (usually only the microbial class is identified in the routine laboratory test).

Chronic Gastritis

Chronic gastritis is characterized by atrophy of the mucosa of the stomach, with loss of the secretory glands. The loss of the parietal cells leads to achlorhydria and lack of secretion of intrinsic factor, which is required for the absorption of vitamin B_{12}. Infection with *Helicobacter pylori* is often present.

Chronic gastritis is often seen in individuals with chronic peptic ulcers, those who abuse alcohol, and the elderly. Autoimmune disorders, for example, pernicious anemia, are associated with a type of chronic gastric atrophy. Many cases are idiopathic.

The signs of chronic gastritis, which are often vague, include mild epigastric discomfort, anorexia, or intolerance for certain foods, usually spicy or fatty foods.

Persons with chronic gastritis have an increased risk of peptic ulcers and gastric carcinoma. Treatment involves appropriate antibiotics and proton pump inhibitors.

> **THINK ABOUT 17-6**
>
> a. Explain how each of the following entities causes dysphagia: achalasia, cancer of the esophagus, atresia.
> b. Explain how chronic reflux of gastric contents into the esophagus may cause hiatal hernia.
> c. Define pyrosis.
> d. Explain how prolonged vomiting leads to acidosis and dehydration.
> e. What is indicated by occult blood in the stool of a person with gastroenteritis?

Peptic Ulcer

Gastric and Duodenal Ulcers

It is estimated that 25 million Americans will have peptic ulcer during their lifetime and the incidence rate in the United States is somewhere between 500,000 and 850,000 cases per year. About one million hospitalizations occur annually with 6500 deaths per year due to peptic ulcer disease. Although incidence rates are dropping in some areas, the prevalence rate is 14.5 million people in the United States. This disease has caused significant disability and illness in the past and continues to require hospitalization and surgery in patients who do respond to drug treatment.

■ *Pathophysiology*

Peptic ulcers occur most commonly in the proximal duodenum (duodenal ulcers), but are also found in the antrum of the stomach (gastric ulcers) or lower esophagus (Figs. 17-14 and 17-15). Peptic ulcers usually appear as single, small, round cavities with smooth margins that penetrate the submucosa. Once acid or pepsin penetrates the mucosal barrier, the tissues are exposed to continued damage because acid diffuses into the gastric wall. Ulcers may erode more deeply into the muscularis and eventually may perforate the wall. An area of inflammation surrounds the crater. When the erosion invades a blood vessel wall, bleeding takes place. Bleeding may involve persistent loss of small amounts of blood or massive hemorrhage, depending on the size of the blood vessel involved. Chronic blood loss may be detected by the presence of iron deficiency anemia or occult blood in the stool; one of these may be the first indicator of peptic ulcer.

The mucosal barrier is composed essentially of the tightly packed epithelial cells with tight junctions that can regenerate quickly and are covered by a thick layer of bicarbonate-rich mucus. The development of peptic ulcers begins with a breakdown of the mucosal barrier, which results from an imbalance between the mucosal

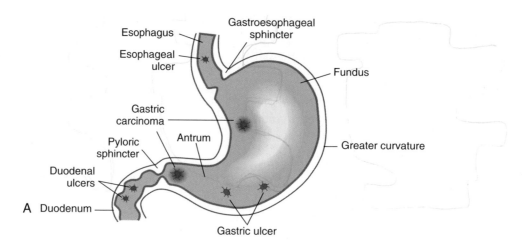

Common locations

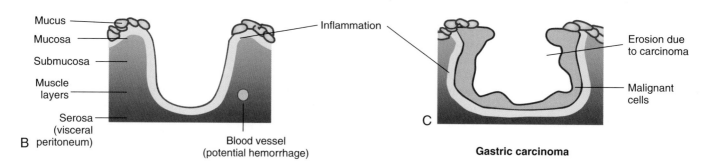

Peptic ulcer   **Gastric carcinoma**

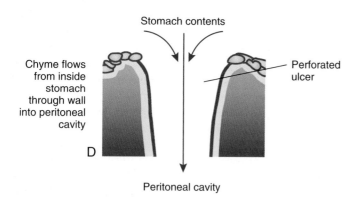

Perforated ulcer

FIGURE 17-14 **Peptic Ulcer** A, Typical locations of peptic ulcer and gastric carcinoma. **B-C,** Comparison of peptic ulcer and carcinoma. **D,** Perforated ulcer.

defense system and forces that are potentially damaging to it. Given the material that is ingested by the stomach and the fact that the powerful and highly acidic gastric secretions can digest protein in food, it is remarkable that the gastric defenses can maintain the integrity of the tissues as well as they do.

Many factors may contribute to the decreased resistance of the mucosa or excessive hydrochloric acid or pepsin secretion. Impaired mucosal defenses seem to be a more common condition in gastric ulcer development,

whereas increased acid secretion is a predominant factor in duodenal ulcers.

Currently considered to be of major significance is infection with the bacterium *Helicobacter pylori*, found in most persons with peptic ulcer disease, although its precise role is not totally understood. Not all persons with *H. pylori* infection develop ulcers, but eradication of the infection promotes rapid healing of the ulcer. *Helicobacter pylori* is known to secrete cytotoxins and the enzymes protease, phospholipase, and urease

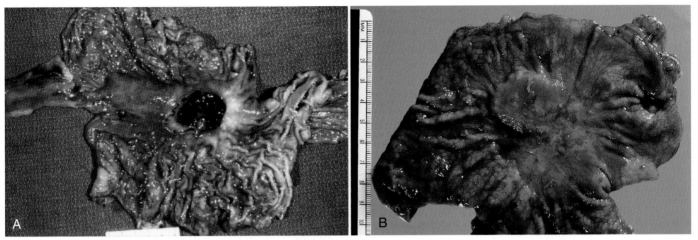

FIGURE 17-15 **A,** Bleeding peptic ulcer. *(Courtesy of RW Shaw, North York General Hospital, Toronto, Ontario, Canada.)* **B,** Early gastric cancer (superficial adenocarcinoma of the stomach). Note the flat surface of the tumor and absence of rugae. *(From Cooke RA, Stewart B.* Colour Atlas of Anatomical Pathology, *ed 3, Sydney, 2004, Churchill Livingstone).*

(which releases ammonia), all of which cause damage to mucosal defenses.

In addition, the mucosal barrier may be damaged by the following:

• An inadequate blood supply (e.g., vasoconstriction caused by stress, smoking, or shock; circulatory impairment in elderly persons; scar tissue; or severe anemia), which interferes with the rapid regeneration of the epithelium and the production of sufficient mucus, as well as reducing the secretion of alkaline bicarbonate ions in the protective mucus and reducing secretion of protective prostaglandins
• Excessive glucocorticoid secretion or medication (e.g., prednisone with its catabolic effects)
• Ulcerogenic substances that break down the mucus layer, such as aspirin, nonsteroidal anti-inflammatory drugs (NSAIDs), or alcohol
• Atrophy of the gastric mucosa (chronic gastritis)

Increased acid-pepsin secretions are associated with:

• Increased gastrin secretion
• Increased vagal stimulation or increased sensitivity to stimuli
• Increased number of acid-pepsin secretory cells in the stomach (a genetic anomaly)
• Increased stimulation of acid-pepsin secretion by alcohol, caffeine, or certain foods
• Interference with the normal feedback mechanism that reduces acid-pepsin secretion when the stomach is empty
• Rapid gastric emptying

Severe or prolonged stress appears to affect both sides of the balance, reducing mucosal blood flow and motility, leading to stasis of chyme, and increasing glucocorticoid effects. Also, stress may promote behaviors that are often implicated in ulcer development, such as increased caffeine and alcohol intake, cigarette smoking,

and altered eating patterns, which often include both irregular hours for meals and ingestion of irritating foods.

Healing of peptic ulcers is difficult because the lesion cannot be isolated from the irritants in the environment. During the healing process, granulation tissue forms deep in the cavity, and new epithelial tissue regenerates from the edges. This granulation tissue often breaks down because it is subject to damage by the chyme. Because a longer time is often required for healing, more fibrous scar tissue develops at the site. The ulcers tend to recur because predisposing factors remain or the scar tissue itself interferes with the blood supply to the area.

Several complications may accompany peptic ulcer. The ulcer may erode a blood vessel, causing *hemorrhage*, a common complication (Fig. 17-14*B*). Rupture of a small blood vessel causes continued loss of small amounts of blood, usually apparent as occult blood in the stool, whereas erosion of a large blood vessel leads to massive hemorrhage, indicated by hematemesis and shock. Hemorrhage may be the first sign of a peptic ulcer.

A second potential complication, *perforation*, occurs when the ulcer erodes completely through the wall, allowing chyme to enter the peritoneal cavity (see Fig. 17-14*D*). This process results in chemical *peritonitis*, inflammation of the peritoneal membranes and other structures in the abdominal cavity. Eventually this inflammation causes increased permeability of the intestinal wall, passage of bacteria and their toxins into the peritoneal cavity, and bacterial peritonitis. Hemorrhage is not necessarily present when perforation occurs.

Third, *obstruction* of the digestive tract may result later from stricture caused by scar tissue around the pylorus or duodenum, particularly in people with protracted or recurrent ulceration.

■ Etiology

Infection with *H. pylori* is considered an underlying cause of the majority of cases of peptic ulcers. Peptic ulcers are more common in men than women, and people in developed countries have a higher incidence, perhaps because of lifestyle factors. A genetic factor seems to be involved in the frequent familial incidence of duodenal ulcers; also, these ulcers are more common in persons with blood group O. Gastric ulcers are more common in older individuals, those with scar tissue present, and those who regularly take ulcerogenic anti-inflammatory medications (aspirin or NSAIDs). Multiple factors, such as those listed, are usually involved in the cause.

■ Signs and Symptoms

Epigastric burning or aching pain is common with ulcers, usually 2 to 3 hours after meals and at night. This cyclic pain is often relieved by ingestion of food or antacids. Intake of spicy foods may initiate pain at mealtime. Heartburn, nausea, vomiting, and weight loss may occur. Vomiting is most likely to occur after intake of alcohol or particularly irritating food. In some patients, weight gain occurs because the person discovers that more frequent food intake relieves the discomfort between meals.

Iron-deficiency anemia or the presence of occult blood in the stool may be a diagnostic indicator.

■ Diagnostic Tests

Fiberoptic endoscopy or barium x-ray may be used for diagnosis. Biopsy may be done endoscopically.

■ Treatment

Drug therapy usually consists of a combination of drugs, including two or three antimicrobial drugs and medication to reduce acid secretion, for example, Helidac. Antimicrobial therapy may include clarithromycin, tetracycline, metronidazole, and bismuth subsalicylate to eradicate *H. pylori*. An H_2 receptor-antagonist, such as cimetidine (Tagamet), or the proton (H^+) pump inhibitor omeprazole (Prilosec), reduces gastric secretions (see Table 17-3). In some individuals, a coating agent, such as sucralfate, may be helpful, or antacids may provide symptomatic relief. Cures rates of 90% have been reported with appropriate drug treatment.

Reducing exacerbating factors such as excessive coffee intake is also useful. Vagotomy may be performed to reduce acid secretions in refractory cases. Surgery (partial gastrectomy or pyloroplasty) may be required in patients with perforated or bleeding ulcers.

Stress Ulcers

Stress ulcers result from severe trauma, such as burns or head injury, or occur with serious systemic problems, such as hemorrhage or sepsis. Ulcers in the presence of burns are often called Curling's ulcers, those seen with

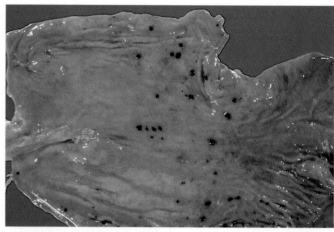

FIGURE 17-16 Multiple stress ulcers of the stomach, highlighted by dark digested blood on their surfaces. *(From Kumar V, Abbas AK, Fausto M: Robbins and Cotran Pathologic Basis of Disease, ed 7, Philadelphia, 2005, Saunders.)*

head injury are termed Cushing's ulcers, and others may be referred to as ischemic ulcers.

Multiple ulcers, usually gastric ulcers, form within hours of the precipitating event, as the blood flow to the mucosa is greatly reduced, leading to reduced secretion of mucus and epithelial regeneration (Fig. 17-16). The mucosal barrier is lost, and acid diffuses into the mucosa. In people with Cushing's ulcers, increased vagal stimulation of acid secretion often occurs. The first indicator of stress ulcers is usually hemorrhage because of the rapid onset and masking by the primary problem. Prophylactic medications are usually administered as soon as possible to minimize the risk of stress ulcer development in cases of trauma.

Gastric Cancer

■ Pathophysiology

Gastric cancer arises primarily in the mucous glands; most tumors occur in the antrum or pyloric area and some affect the lesser curvature of the stomach or cardia (see Figs. 17-14 and 17-15). Recently there has been an increase in tumors in the upper stomach near the entrance to the esophagus. Adenocarcinoma occurs most frequently. The lesion is most often an ulcerative type with an irregular crater and a raised margin. Other forms of gastric cancer may infiltrate the gastric wall, causing thickening, or may appear as a protruding mass or polyp. Early gastric carcinoma is a lesion confined to the mucosa and submucosa, whereas advanced gastric carcinoma involves the muscularis layer. Eventually the tumor extends into the serosa and spreads to the lymph nodes (regional and supraclavicular) and to the liver and ovaries. Gastric cancer is asymptomatic in the early stages and usually is not diagnosed until it is well advanced, at which point the prognosis is poor.

◼ Etiology

Geographic differences are marked in the development of gastric carcinoma, for which there is a high incidence in Japan, Iceland, Chile, and Hungary, but a significant decline (21,000) is evident in the United States, perhaps due to dietary changes. Japan has instituted a screening program for gastric carcinoma in an effort to improve the statistics in that country.

Helicobacter pylori infection is associated with a higher risk of gastric carcinoma. Diet also appears to be a key factor, and a move to a different geographic location may result in a change in risk level. Food preservatives, such as nitrates or nitrites, and smoked foods increase the risk. Genetic influences play a role; the risk is increased in family members and individuals with blood group A. The presence of chronic atrophic gastritis or polyps in an individual also increases the likelihood of cancer.

◼ Signs and Symptoms

Manifestations are usually vague and mild until the cancer is advanced. The initial signs include anorexia, feelings of indigestion or epigastric discomfort, weight loss, fatigue, or a feeling of fullness after eating. Incidental tests may reveal occult blood in the stool or iron-deficiency anemia and precipitate a search for the cause and earlier diagnosis.

◼ Treatment

Diagnosis is frequently late because of the vague symptoms and tendency for individuals to self-treat. The prognosis is varies with the stage of the cancer; those with stage I disease have a 78% survival rate and those in stage III have an 8% survival rate. Survival rates for those with metastatic disease are less than 7%. Surgery (gastric resection) combined with chemotherapy and radiation is the usual treatment and may relieve symptoms when used as a palliative measure. Vitamin B_{12} injections are usually required after gastrectomy.

Dumping Syndrome

Dumping syndrome, in which control of gastric emptying is lost, may occur after gastric resection (e.g., partial gastrectomy) because the pyloric sphincter is removed. Large quantities of ingested food are rapidly "dumped" into the intestine.

The storage stage in the stomach, which includes appropriate dilution of chyme by gastric secretions, is missed. The hyperosmolar chyme draws more fluid from the vascular compartment into the intestine (Fig. 17-17), adding to the intestinal distention and increasing intestinal motility. These changes lead to signs that occur *during or shortly after meals*, including abdominal cramps, nausea, and diarrhea. The concurrent hypovolemia causes dizziness or weakness, rapid pulse, and sweating.

In addition, individuals with dumping syndrome may experience *hypoglycemia 2 to 3 hours after meals*. The rapid gastric emptying and absorption leads to high blood glucose levels and increased insulin secretion, which results in a rapid drop in blood glucose level with no reserve nutrients advancing slowly from the stomach. Rebound hypoglycemia then develops several hours after eating, with tremors, sweating, and weakness.

These problems can usually be resolved by dietary changes, including consumption of frequent small meals that are high in protein and low in simple carbohydrates. Also, fluids should be taken between meals rather than with meals. These measures reduce the hypertonicity of the chyme and the fluctuations in blood glucose. In some cases, medication may be used to decrease intestinal motility.

Pyloric Stenosis

Narrowing and obstruction of the pyloric sphincter may be a developmental defect in infants, or it may be acquired later in life, usually because of the presence of fibrous scar tissue. In the congenital form, the pyloric muscle is hypertrophied and can be palpated as a hard mass in the abdomen.

Signs of stenosis usually appear within several weeks after birth, first as episodes of regurgitation of some food and then as projectile vomiting occurring immediately after feeding. Vomitus may be ejected some distance from the infant and does not contain bile. Stools become small and infrequent. The infant fails to gain weight, is dehydrated, and is irritable because of persistent hunger. Surgery is required to remove the obstruction.

In persons with acquired pyloric obstruction, interference with gastric emptying leads to a persistent feeling of fullness and then to an increased incidence of vomiting with or after meals. The vomitus typically contains food from previous meals.

THINK ABOUT 17-7

a. Explain why infection was not thought to be the cause of peptic ulcer in the past.

b. Explain three factors that predispose to peptic ulcer formation.

c. Explain why the prognosis for gastric cancer is poor.

d. Explain why dizziness, weakness, and tachycardia may occur: (1) immediately after a meal in a postgastrectomy patient; (2) 2 to 3 hours after eating.

Disorders of the Liver and Pancreas

Gallbladder Disorders

The gallbladder and biliary tract are frequently affected by one or more interrelated problems involving the

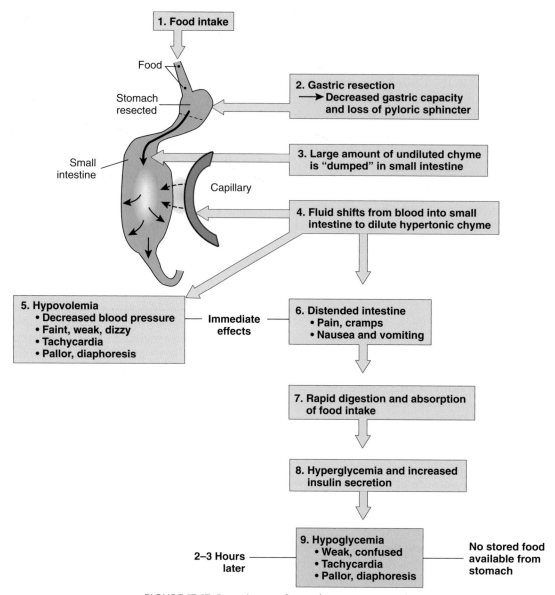

FIGURE 17-17 Dumping syndrome (postgastrectomy).

formation of gallstones (Fig. 17-18). At least 10% of the population has gallstones and 500,000 surgical procedures are done per year in the United States to treat gallbladder disease.

- *Cholelithiasis* refers to formation of gallstones, which are masses of solid material or calculi that form in the bile.
- *Cholecystitis* refers to inflammation of the gallbladder and cystic duct.
- *Cholangitis* is inflammation usually related to infection of the bile ducts.
- *Choledocholithiasis* pertains to obstruction by gallstones of the biliary tract.

■ *Pathophysiology*

Gallstones vary in size and shape and may form initially in the bile ducts, gallbladder, or cystic duct. They may consist primarily of cholesterol or bile pigment

(bilirubin) or may be of mixed content, including calcium salts (Fig. 17-19). The content of the stone depends on the primary factor predisposing to calculus formation. Cholesterol stones appear white or crystalline, whereas bilirubin stones are black.

Small stones may be "silent" and excreted in the bile, whereas larger stones are likely to obstruct the flow of bile in the cystic or common bile ducts, causing pain. Note the comparative size of the stones and the bile ducts (see Fig. 17-16).

Gallstones tend to form when the bile contains a high concentration of a component such as cholesterol or there is a deficit of bile salts. Inflammation or infection in the biliary structures may provide a focus for stone formation or may alter the solubility of the constituents, fostering the development of a calculus. Whether inflammation or infection is primary or secondary to stone formation is not always clear. Once a focus or nucleus

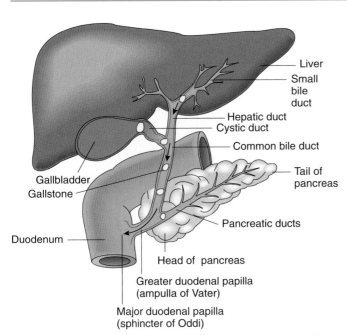

FIGURE 17-18 The biliary ducts and pancreas with possible locations of gallstones.

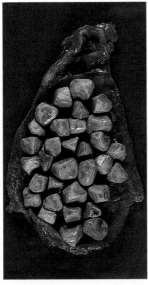

FIGURE 17-19 Resected gallbladder containing mixed gallstones. *(From Kissane JM, ed: Anderson's pathology, ed 9, St Louis, 1990, Mosby.)*

forms, the stone tends to grow, as additional solutes are deposited on it, particularly if bile flow is sluggish.

The presence of gallstones may cause irritation and inflammation in the gallbladder wall (cholecystitis), and this susceptible tissue may then be infected. Infecting organisms are usually *Escherichia coli* or enterococci, which gain access to the gallbladder through the sphincter of Oddi or from the portal veins or adjacent lymph nodes.

When a stone obstructs bile flow in the cystic or common bile duct, biliary colic develops, consisting of severe spasms of pain resulting from strong muscle contractions attempting to move the stone along. Obstruction of the biliary system at the sphincter of Oddi may

also cause pancreatitis because the pancreatic secretions are backed up or bile refluxes into the pancreatic ducts.

■ *Etiology*

Cholesterol gallstones occur twice as often in women as men. They tend to develop in individuals with high cholesterol levels in the bile. Factors that indicate a high risk for gallstones include obesity, high cholesterol intake, multiparity (several children), and the use of oral contraceptives or estrogen supplements. Bile pigment stones are more common in individuals with hemolytic anemia, alcoholic cirrhosis, or biliary tract infection.

■ *Signs and Symptoms*

Gallstones are frequently asymptomatic. However, larger calculi may obstruct a duct at any time, causing sudden severe waves of pain (biliary colic) in the upper right quadrant of the abdomen or epigastric area, often radiating to the back and right shoulder. Nausea and vomiting are usually present. The pain increases for some time and then may decrease if the stone moves on. If the pain continues, and jaundice develops as the bile backs up into the liver and blood, surgical intervention may be necessary. There is also a risk of a ruptured gallbladder if obstruction persists. Acute cholecystitis is usually associated with some degree of obstruction and inflammation. Severe pain is often precipitated by eating a fatty meal; fever, leukocytosis, and vomiting accompany the pain.

Chronic cholecystitis is manifested by milder signs, although the course may be punctuated by acute episodes. Signs often include intolerance to fatty foods, excessive belching, bloating, and mild epigastric discomfort.

■ *Treatment*

The gallbladder and gallstones may be removed using laparoscopic surgery. In many cases, the stones are fragmented by such methods as extracorporeal shock wave lithotripsy (using high-energy sound waves), sometimes assisted by administration of bile acids or drugs to break down the stone.

THINK ABOUT 17-8

a. Differentiate cholelithiasis from choledocholithiasis.
b. Explain three factors predisposing to cholesterol gallstones.
c. Describe how a cholesterol stone forms.
d. Describe the pain typical of an acute episode of gallstone obstruction and give the rationale for it.

Jaundice

Jaundice (icterus) refers to the yellowish color of the skin and other tissues that results from high levels of bilirubin in the blood. The color is usually apparent first

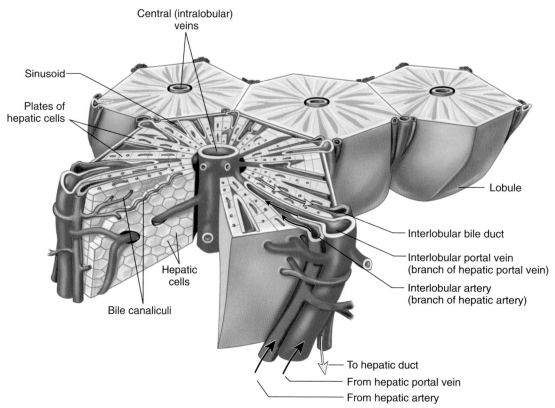

FIGURE 17-20 Structure of liver lobule. *(From Patton KT, Thibodeau GA: Anatomy & Physiology, ed 8, St. Louis, 2013, Mosby.)*

in the sclera, or white area of the eye. Bilirubin is a product of the hemolysis of red blood cells (RBCs) and the breakdown of hemoglobin (see Fig. 17-4).

Jaundice or hyperbilirubinemia is not itself a disease but rather is a sign of many different types of primary disorders. These disorders are classified in three groups (Fig. 17-21):

1. *Prehepatic* jaundice results from excessive destruction of red blood cells and is characteristic of hemolytic anemias or transfusion reactions. Liver function is normal but is unable to handle the additional bilirubin. *Physiologic jaundice of the newborn* is common 2 to 3 days after birth. Increased hemolysis of red blood cells combined with the immature infant liver leads to a transient mild hyperbilirubinemia.

2. *Intrahepatic* jaundice occurs in individuals with liver disease, such as hepatitis or cirrhosis. It is related to impaired uptake of bilirubin from the blood and decreased conjugation of bilirubin by the hepatocytes.

3. *Posthepatic* jaundice is caused by obstruction of bile flow into the gallbladder or duodenum and subsequent backup of bile into the blood. Congenital atresia of the bile ducts, obstruction caused by cholelithiasis, inflammation of the liver, or tumors all result in posthepatic jaundice.

The type of jaundice present in an individual may be indicated by increases in the serum bilirubin level and changes in the stools (see Fig. 17-21). For example, serum levels of unconjugated bilirubin (indirect-reacting) are elevated in prehepatic jaundice, whereas posthepatic jaundice results from increased amounts of conjugated bilirubin (direct) in the blood. In patients with liver disease, both intrahepatic and posthepatic jaundice may be present because inflammation or infection both impairs hepatocyte function and obstructs the bile canaliculi, leading to elevations in the blood of both unconjugated and conjugated bilirubin. In persons with posthepatic jaundice, the obstruction prevents bile from entering the intestine, interfering with digestion and resulting in a light-colored stool. Also, the bile salts that enter the blood and tissues as bile backs up cause irritation and pruritus (itching) of the skin. Treatment depends on removing the cause. Phototherapy is effective in mild forms, whereby exposure to ultraviolet light promotes the conjugation of bilirubin.

Hepatitis

Hepatitis refers to inflammation of the liver. It may be idiopathic (fatty liver) or result from a local infection (viral hepatitis), from an infection elsewhere in the body (e.g., infectious mononucleosis or amebiasis), or from chemical or drug toxicity. Mild inflammation impairs hepatocyte function, whereas more severe inflammation and necrosis may lead to obstruction of blood and bile

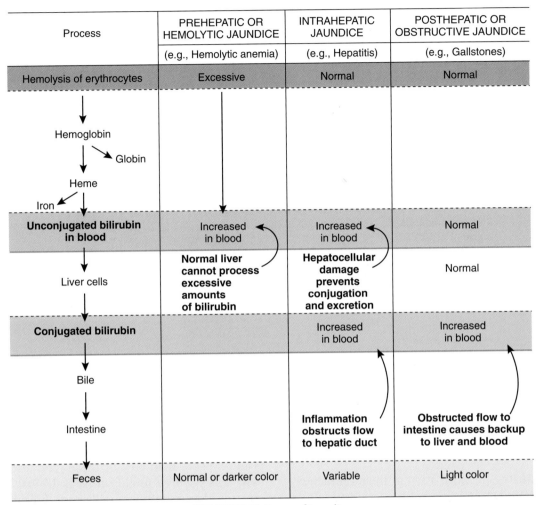

Process	PREHEPATIC OR HEMOLYTIC JAUNDICE	INTRAHEPATIC JAUNDICE	POSTHEPATIC OR OBSTRUCTIVE JAUNDICE
	(e.g., Hemolytic anemia)	(e.g., Hepatitis)	(e.g., Gallstones)
Hemolysis of erythrocytes	Excessive	Normal	Normal
Unconjugated bilirubin in blood	Increased in blood	Increased in blood	Normal
Liver cells	**Normal liver cannot process excessive amounts of bilirubin**	**Hepatocellular damage prevents conjugation and excretion**	Normal
Conjugated bilirubin		Increased in blood	Increased in blood
Intestine		**Inflammation obstructs flow to hepatic duct**	**Obstructed flow to intestine causes backup to liver and blood**
Feces	Normal or darker color	Variable	Light color

FIGURE 17-21 Types of jaundice.

flow in the liver and impaired liver cell function. Given the many functions of the liver, damage to the liver cells has extensive effects in the body. Fortunately, the liver has a good functional reserve and excellent regenerative powers.

Viral Hepatitis

■ Pathophysiology

Although a number of viruses may affect the liver cells, hepatitis is considered to result from infection by a group of viruses that specifically target the hepatocytes. These include hepatitis A virus (HAV), hepatitis B virus (HBV), hepatitis C virus (HCV), hepatitis D virus (HDV), and hepatitis E virus (HEV). There are other viruses causing hepatitis that have not yet been fully identified, meanwhile they have been temporarily designated F and G or non A-E hepatitis virus.

The liver cells are damaged in two ways—by direct action of the virus (e.g., hepatitis C) or cell-mediated immune responses to the virus (e.g., hepatitis B). Cell injury results in inflammation and necrosis in the liver. Both the hepatocytes and the liver appear swollen, and diffuse necrosis may be present. With severe inflammation, biliary stasis may develop, leading to backup of bile into the blood.

The degree of inflammation and damage varies. Many cases are mild and are not identified. Some cases show a few manifestations but not jaundice; in other cases fulminant hepatitis develops with massive necrosis and liver failure. Depending on the severity of the inflammation, the hepatic cells may regenerate, or fibrous scar tissue may form in the liver. Scar tissue often obstructs the channels used for blood and bile flow, interfering with the unique organization of the liver lobule, and leading to further damage from ischemia.

Chronic inflammation occurs with hepatitis B, C, and D and is defined as persistent inflammation and necrosis of the liver for more than 6 months. This type of disease eventually causes permanent liver damage (fibrosis) and cirrhosis. There is also an increased incidence of hepatocellular cancer associated with chronic hepatitis.

Hepatitis B, C, and D may exist in a carrier state, in which asymptomatic individuals carry the virus in their hepatocytes but can transmit the infection via their blood or body fluids to others. Carriers may

TABLE 17-5	Types of Hepatitis				
Disease	Agent	Transmission	Incubation Period	Serum Markers	Carrier/Chronic
Hepatitis A (infectious)	HAV (RNA virus)	Oral-fecal	2-6 wk	anti-HAV IgM anti-HAV IgG	None
Hepatitis B (serum)	HBV (DNA double-strand virus)	Blood and body fluids	1-6 mo (average, 60-90 days)	HBsAg anti-HBs HBcAb IgM HBcAb IgG HBeAg, HBeAb	Carrier and chronic
Hepatitis C	HCV (RNA virus)	Blood and body fluids	2 wk-6 mo (average, 6-9 wk)	anti-HCV	Carrier and chronic
Hepatitis D, chronic (delta)	HDV (defective RNA virus requires presence of HBV)	Blood and body fluids	2-10 wk	anti-HDV IgM anti-HDV IgG	Chronic
Hepatitis E	HEV (RNA virus)	Oral-fecal contamination	2-9 wk	HE Ag	None
Toxic hepatitis	Hepatotoxins; chemicals or drugs	Direct exposure	Days to months	N/A	Acute or chronic
Chronic noninfectious hepatitis	Autoimmune, metabolic, idiopathic	N/A	N/A	Various autoantibodies	Chronic

N/A, not applicable

be individuals who have never had active disease or have a chronic low-grade infection.

■ Etiology

The viruses causing hepatitis vary in their characteristics, mode of transmission, incubation time, and effects. These are summarized in Table 17-5.

■ **Hepatitis A.** Also called *infectious hepatitis*, hepatitis A is caused by a small RNA virus called the hepatitis A virus, or HAV. It is transmitted primarily by the oral-fecal route, often from contaminated water or shellfish. Outbreaks may occur in daycare centers. Sexual transmission has occurred in the homosexual population. Hepatitis A has a relatively short incubation period of 2 to 6 weeks. Hepatitis A causes an acute but self-limiting infection and does not have a carrier or chronic state.

Fecal shedding of the virus (the contagious period) begins several weeks before the onset of signs (Fig. 17-22*A*). At this time, the first antibodies, IgM-HAV, appear, followed shortly by the second group of antibodies, IgG-HAV, which remain in the serum for years, providing immunity against further infection. A vaccine is available for those who are traveling to an endemic area or anyone with any liver disease; this vaccine is administered to both children and adults. Gamma globulin provides temporary protection and may be administered to those just exposed to HAV.

■ **Hepatitis B.** In 2006 the Centers for Disease Control received reports of 4758 new cases in the United States, but estimate the occurrence rate is 10 times that number,

with many cases being asymptomatic. Further, there are more than 1 million carriers in the country, and 4000 to 5000 deaths annually from associated cirrhosis and cancer. More than 50% of those who test HIV-positive are also positive for hepatitis B. Global estimates are over 2 billion, with 350 million of those being carriers. Unfortunately, 50% of cases are asymptomatic, facilitating transmission to others.

Formerly called *serum hepatitis*, this form of hepatitis is caused by the hepatitis B virus (HBV), a partially double-stranded DNA virus. The whole virion is often called a Dane particle. This virus is more complex and consists of three antigens—two core antigens (HBcAg and HBeAg) and one surface antigen (HBsAg). Each antigen stimulates antibody production in the body (see Fig. 17-22). These serum antigens and antibodies are useful in diagnosing and monitoring the course of hepatitis, including the development of chronic hepatitis. For example, large amounts of HBsAg are produced by infected liver cells early in the course of the infection. When this antigen persists in the serum, it poses a high risk of continued active infection and damage to the liver (chronic disease). A carrier state is also common for HBV, in which the individual is asymptomatic but is contagious for the disease.

Hepatitis B has a relatively long incubation period, averaging about 2 months. Long incubation periods make it more difficult to track sources and contacts for infections. A "window," or prolonged lag time, occurs before the serum markers or symptoms become present, during which time the virus cannot be detected but can be transmitted to others.

A. Hepatitis A

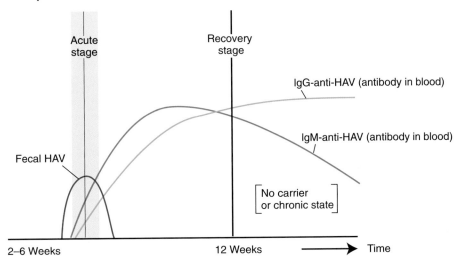

B. Hepatitis B — Acute

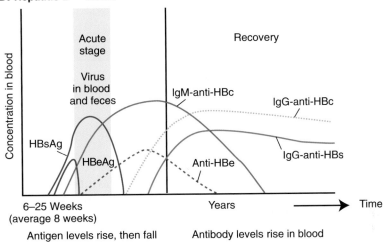

C. Hepatitis B — Chronic Infection

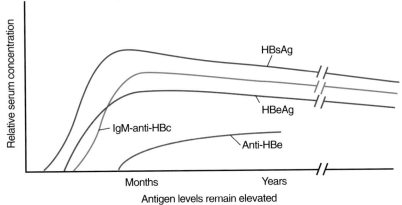

FIGURE 17-22 Serologic changes seen with hepatitis.

Hepatitis B virus infection is transmitted primarily by infected blood but is found in many body secretions. Blood transfusions are currently processed to reduce the risk of transmission. Intravenous drug abusers have a high incidence of HBV infection. Hemodialysis increases the risk, as does exposure to blood or body fluids in health care workers if barrier precautions are not taken. Sexual transmission has been noted, and HBV can be passed to the fetus during pregnancy. Activities such as tattooing and body piercing may transmit the virus. An HBV vaccine is available for long-term protection for those in high-risk groups, including health professionals, and is now routinely administered to children. Hepatitis B virus immune globulin is available as a temporary measure.

■ *Hepatitis C.* Formerly called non-A-non-B (or NANB) hepatitis, hepatitis C is the most common type of hepatitis transmitted by blood transfusions. The virus is a single-stranded RNA virus. Approximately half the cases enter a chronic disease state. The World Health Organization estimates that there are 130 to 170 million people infected globally, and the CDC estimates the prevalence rate in the United States to be 3.2 million cases. Hepatitis C virus infection increases the risk of hepatocellular carcinoma. This form of hepatitis may exist in a carrier state.

■ *Hepatitis D.* The agent for hepatitis D is also called delta virus. This incomplete RNA virus requires the presence of hepatitis B virus (HBsAg) to replicate and produce active infection. Hepatitis D virus infection usually increases the severity of HBV infection. Hepatitis D virus is also transmitted by blood; there is a high incidence of infection in intravenous drug abusers.

■ *Hepatitis E.* Hepatitis E is caused by HEV, a single-stranded RNA virus, and is spread by the oral-fecal route. It is similar to HAV and lacks a chronic or carrier state. It is more common in countries in Asia and Africa, where it causes a fulminant hepatitis that produces a high mortality rate in pregnant women.

■ *Signs and Symptoms*

The manifestations of acute hepatitis vary from mild or asymptomatic to severe disease that is often rapidly fatal. The course of hepatitis has three stages: first, the preicteric or prodromal stage; next, the icteric or jaundice stage; and last, the posticteric or recovery stage (Fig. 17-23).

1. Onset of the *preicteric* stage may be insidious, with fatigue and malaise, anorexia and nausea, and general muscle aching. Sometimes fever, headache, a distaste for cigarettes, and mild upper right quadrant discomfort are present. Serum levels of liver enzymes (e.g., aspartate aminotransferase [AST] or alanine aminotransferase [ALT]) are elevated.

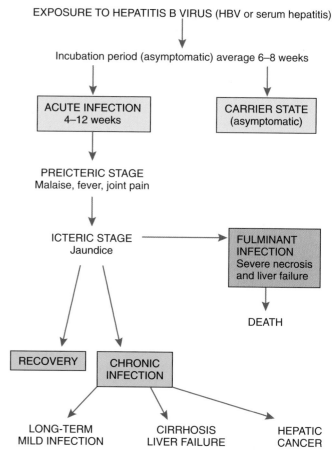

FIGURE 17-23 The course of hepatitis B infection.

2. The *icteric* stage marks the onset of jaundice as serum bilirubin levels rise. As biliary obstruction increases, the stools become light in color, the urine becomes darker, and skin becomes pruritic. The liver is tender and enlarged (hepatomegaly), causing a mild aching pain. In severe cases, blood clotting times may be prolonged, because the synthesis of blood clotting factors is impaired. This stage tends to last longer in patients with hepatitis B.

3. The *posticteric* or recovery stage is marked by a reduction in signs, although this period may extend over some weeks. On average, the acute stage of hepatitis A lasts 8 to 10 weeks, whereas hepatitis B is prolonged over 16 weeks.

■ *Treatment*

There is no method of destroying hepatitis viruses in the body at this time. Gamma globulin, if available, may be helpful when given early in the course. Supportive measures such as rest and a diet high in protein, carbohydrate, and vitamins are most useful.

Chronic hepatitis B and C may be treated with interferon α and lamivudine (Epivir or 3TC) to decrease viral replication, although this treatment is effective in only 30% to 40% of individuals. A combination of slow-acting interferon and the antiviral drug, Ribavirin, have reduced the rate of viral replication in 80% of HCV patients. Otherwise, gradual destruction of the liver occurs, leading to cirrhosis or hepatocellular cancer.

Toxic or Nonviral Hepatitis

A variety of hepatotoxins, such as chemicals or drugs, may cause inflammation and necrosis in the liver. These reactions may be direct effects of the toxins or an immune response (hypersensitivity) to certain materials. Toxic effects may result from sudden exposure to large amounts of a substance or from long-term exposure, perhaps in the workplace. Hepatotoxic drugs include acetaminophen, halothane, phenothiazines, and tetracycline. Toxic chemicals include solvents such as carbon tetrachloride, toluene, or ethanol. Reye's syndrome, which occurs when aspirin is used in the presence of viral infections, also causes toxic effects on the liver. Hepatocellular damage can result from either of two processes, inflammation with necrosis, or cholestasis (obstructed flow of bile). The signs of toxicity are similar to those of infectious hepatitis. The toxic chemical must be removed from the body as quickly as possible to reduce the risk of permanent liver damage.

THINK ABOUT 17-9

a. Explain how prehepatic jaundice might develop and the expected change in serum bilirubin.

b. Describe the difference between hepatitis A-E with regard to type/structure of the virus and transmission.

c. Describe how serum markers may indicate the presence of chronic viral hepatitis.

d. Explain why the individual who is a carrier for HBV is considered a threat to public health.

Cirrhosis

Cirrhosis is a disorder in which there is progressive destruction of liver tissue leading eventually to liver failure when 80% to 90% of the liver has been destroyed. It is the end result of a number of chronic liver diseases. About 28,000 persons die each year in the United States, and 50% of these deaths are alcohol related.

Cirrhosis may be classified by the structural changes that take place (e.g., micronodular or macronodular) or the cause of the disorder. In some cases, cirrhosis may be linked to specific underlying disorders, particularly congenital problems or inherited metabolic disorders. The four general categories of cirrhosis based on cause are:

1. Alcoholic liver disease (the largest group, also called portal or Laënnec's cirrhosis)
2. Biliary cirrhosis, associated with immune disorders and those causing obstruction of bile flow, for example, stones or cystic fibrosis, in which mucous plugs form in the bile ducts

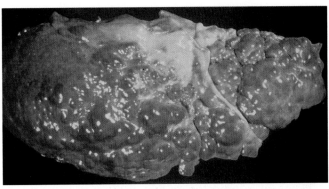

FIGURE 17-24 Cirrhosis resulting from chronic viral hepatitis. Note the broad scar and nodular surface. *(From Kumar V, Abbas AK, Fausto M: Robbins and Cotran Pathologic Basis of Disease, ed 7, Philadelphia, 2005, Saunders.)*

3. Postnecrotic cirrhosis, linked with chronic hepatitis or long-term exposure to toxic materials
4. Metabolic, usually caused by storage disorders such as hemochromatosis

■ *Pathophysiology*

Cirrhosis is a disorder in which the liver demonstrates extensive diffuse fibrosis and loss of lobular organization (see Fig. 17-20). Nodules of regenerated hepatocytes may be present but are not necessarily functional because the vascular network and biliary ducts are distorted (Fig. 17-24). Even if the primary cause is removed, further damage is likely because fibrosis interferes with the blood supply to liver tissues or the bile may back up, leading to ongoing inflammation and damage. Initially the liver is enlarged, but it becomes small and shrunken as fibrosis proceeds. In many cases degenerative changes are asymptomatic until the disease is well advanced.

Liver biopsy and serologic tests may determine the cause and extent of the damage. The progressive changes that occur in biliary and postnecrotic cirrhosis are directly linked to inflammation, necrosis, and fibrosis associated with the primary condition.

In patients with *alcoholic liver disease*, or portal cirrhosis, there are several stages in the development of hepatocellular damage related to the effects of alcohol. Alcohol and its metabolites, such as acetaldehyde, are toxic to the liver cells and alter many metabolic processes in the liver. Secondary malnutrition may aggravate the damaging effects on liver cells.

1. The initial change in alcoholic liver disease is the accumulation of fat in liver cells, causing *fatty liver*. Other than enlargement of the liver or hepatomegaly, this stage is asymptomatic and is reversible if alcohol intake is reduced.
2. In the second stage, *alcoholic hepatitis*, inflammation and cell necrosis occur. Fibrous tissue forms, an irreversible change. Acute inflammation may develop when alcohol intake increases or binge drinking

becomes more excessive. This second stage may also be asymptomatic, or it may manifest with mild symptoms, such as anorexia, nausea, and liver tenderness. In some patients, after an episode of excessive alcohol intake, there may be sufficient damage to precipitate liver failure, encephalopathy, and death.

3. The third stage, or *end-stage cirrhosis*, is reached when fibrotic tissue replaces normal tissue, significantly altering the basic liver structure to the extent that little normal function remains. Signs of portal hypertension or impaired digestion and absorption are the usual early indicators of this stage.

The pathophysiologic effects of cirrhosis evolve from two factors: the loss of liver cell functions and interference with blood and bile flow in the liver.

Major functional losses in persons with cirrhosis include:

- Decreased removal and conjugation of bilirubin
- Decreased production of bile
- Impaired digestion and absorption of nutrients, particularly fats and fat-soluble vitamins
- Decreased production of blood clotting factors (prothrombin, fibrinogen) and plasma proteins (albumin)
- Impaired glucose/glycogen metabolism
- Inadequate storage of iron and vitamin B_{12}
- Decreased inactivation of hormones, such as aldosterone and estrogen
- Decreased removal of toxic substances, such as ammonia and drugs

These changes are linked with clinical signs in Table 17-6.

Altered blood chemistry, including abnormal levels of electrolytes or amino acids, and excessive ammonia or other toxic chemicals affect the central nervous system, leading to *hepatic encephalopathy*. Serum ammonia levels correlate well with the clinical signs of encephalopathy. Ammonia is an end product of protein metabolism in the liver or intestine, and then is converted by liver cells into urea for excretion by the kidneys. The ingestion of a meal high in protein or an episode of bleeding in the digestive tract may cause a marked elevation in serum ammonia concentration and may precipitate severe encephalopathy.

The second group of effects is related to obstruction of bile ducts and blood flow by fibrous tissue as follows:

- Reduction of the amount of bile entering the intestine, impairing digestion and absorption
- Backup of bile in the liver, leading to obstructive *jaundice* with elevated conjugated and unconjugated bilirubin levels in the blood
- Blockage of blood flow through the liver, leading to high pressure in the portal veins, or *portal hypertension* (Fig. 17-25 and Fig. 12-26)
- Congestion in the spleen (splenomegaly), increasing hemolysis
- Congestion in intestinal walls and stomach, impairing digestion and absorption

TABLE 17-6	Common Manifestations of Liver Disease
Signs or Symptoms	**Pathophysiology**
Fatigue, anorexia, indigestion, weight loss	Metabolic dysfunction in the liver, such as decreased gluconeogenesis; decreased bile for digestion and absorption; portal hypertension, leading to edema of intestinal wall and interfering with digestion and absorption
Ascites	Portal hypertension, elevated aldosterone and ADH levels, decreased serum albumin level, lymphatic obstruction in liver
General edema	Elevated aldosterone and ADH levels, decreased serum albumin level
Esophageal varices, hemorrhoids	Portal hypertension and collateral circulation
Splenomegaly	Portal hypertension
Anemia	Decreased absorption and storage of iron and vitamin B_{12}, malabsorption, splenomegaly, bleeding
Leukopenia, thrombocytopenia	Splenomegaly, possible bone marrow depression by ammonia and other toxins
Increased bleeding, purpura	Decreased absorption of vitamin K, decreased production of clotting factors by liver, thrombocytopenia
Hepatic encephalopathy, tremors, confusion, coma	Metabolic dysfunction with inability to remove ammonia from protein metabolism and other toxic substances
Gynecomastia, impotence, irregular menses	Impaired inactivation of sex hormones (e.g., estrogen) leads to imbalance
Jaundice	Impaired extraction and conjugation of bilirubin; decreased production of bile and obstruction of bile flow
Pruritus	Bile salts in the tissues resulting from biliary obstruction

ADH, antidiuretic hormone.

- Development of *esophageal varices* (see Fig. 17-25 & Fig. 17-26)
- Development of ascites, an accumulation of fluid in the peritoneal cavity that causes abdominal distention and pressure

Because the esophageal veins have several points of anastomosis, or collateral channels to join with the gastric veins, the increased pressure of blood extends into the esophageal veins, creating large distended and distorted veins (varicose veins or varices) near the mucosal surface of the esophagus. These veins are easily torn by food passing down the esophagus. Hemorrhage of these esophageal varices is a common complication of cirrhosis.

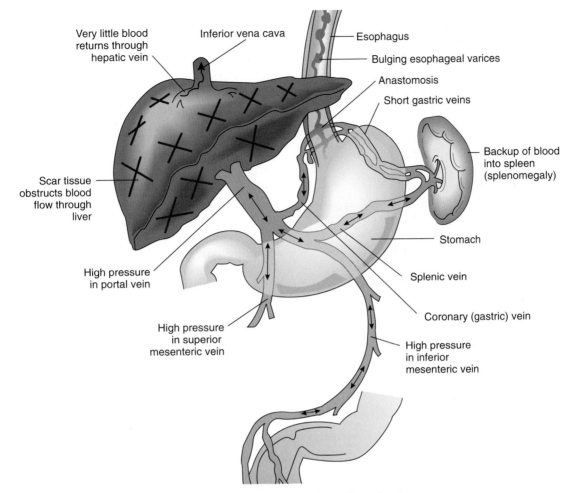

FIGURE 17-25 Development of esophageal varices.

The high pressure in the portal veins and lymphatics, in conjunction with other factors, also affects fluid shifts in the hepatic portal system, leading to *ascites* (Fig. 17-27). Portal hypertension increases the hydrostatic pressure in the veins and lymphatics; the increased serum aldosterone levels result in increased sodium ion and water in the extracellular compartment; and the decreased serum levels of albumin lower the plasma osmotic pressure. All these factors contribute to a shift of fluid out of the blood and into the peritoneal cavity.

■ *Signs and Symptoms*

Initial manifestations of cirrhosis are often mild and vague and include such signs as fatigue, anorexia, weight loss, anemia, and diarrhea. Dull aching pain may be present in the upper right quadrant of the abdomen.

As cirrhosis advances, ascites and peripheral edema develop, increased bruising is evident, esophageal varices form, and eventually jaundice and encephalopathy occur (see Table 17-6). An imbalance in sex hormone levels secondary to impaired inactivation mechanisms leads to spider nevi on the skin, testicular atrophy,

impotence, gynecomastia, and irregular menses. Complications involve ruptured esophageal varices, leading to hemorrhage, circulatory shock, and acute hepatic encephalopathy.

Acute encephalopathy manifests as asterixis, a "hand-flapping" tremor, and confusion, disorientation, convulsions, and coma. Chronic encephalopathy is characterized by personality changes, memory lapses, irritability, and disinterest in personal care.

Another complication of cirrhosis is the presence of frequent infections, often respiratory or skin infections. These infections are encouraged by excessive fluids in the tissues that interfere with the diffusion of nutrients and thus lead to delayed tissue regeneration and healing. Also, decreased protein availability in the body and anemia impair tissue maintenance. Pruritus causes scratching of the skin that may damage the skin barrier, leading to infection.

A summary of the effects of cirrhosis and liver failure is illustrated in Figure 17-28.

■ *Treatment*

Supportive or symptomatic treatment, such as avoiding fatigue and exposure to infection, is necessary.

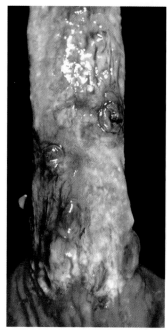

FIGURE 17-26 Esophageal varices. *(From Kumar V, et al: Robbins basic pathology, ed 9, Philadelphia, 2013, Elsevier-Saunders.)*

Dietary restrictions include restrictions on protein and sodium intake. High carbohydrate intake and vitamin supplements are necessary.

Serum electrolytes may have to be balanced, possibly requiring the use of diuretics (e.g., furosemide) to reduce body fluids. Paracentesis to remove excess fluid may be necessary, followed by albumin transfusions to prevent third spacing of fluid. Antibiotics such as neomycin are useful to reduce intestinal flora and control serum ammonia levels. Ruptured esophageal varices need emergency treatment. Portocaval shunts may be used to reduce portal hypertension.

Liver transplants provide another option (see Chapter 7). Many tests are required before transplant to determine the tissue match and general health status. Transplanting part of the liver from a suitable living donor (LDLT) has become more common because the wait time is less than that for a cadaver donor (about 18,000 persons await liver transplant, only 5000 cadaver organs will likely be available). The liver tissue is able to grow in both donor and recipient providing a complete functional organ for both. This process was first used successfully in children, in whom size of the transplant is an issue, and now is being used in adults. It is riskier in adults because more donor tissue (half the liver) is required. Currently living donor liver transplant is the standard practice in pediatric transplants and adult to

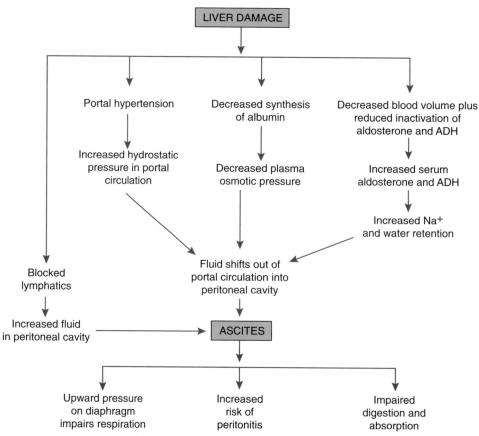

FIGURE 17-27 Development of ascites with cirrhosis.

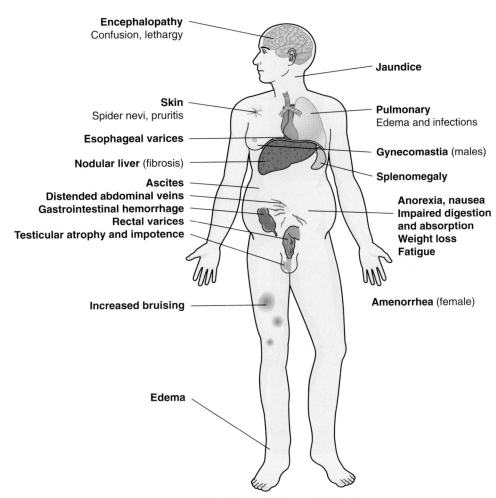

Encephalopathy
Confusion, lethargy

Jaundice

Skin
Spider nevi, pruritis

Pulmonary
Edema and infections

Esophageal varices

Gynecomastia (males)

Nodular liver (fibrosis)

Splenomegaly

Ascites
Distended abdominal veins
Gastrointestinal hemorrhage
Rectal varices
Testicular atrophy and impotence

Anorexia, nausea
Impaired digestion
and absorption
Weight loss
Fatigue

Increased bruising

Amenorrhea (female)

Edema

FIGURE 17-28 Effects of advanced cirrhosis.

adult transplants are being done in all major transplant centers in the United States.

Liver Cancer

Although secondary tumors are very common in the liver, primary malignant tumors are relatively rare, making up less than 2% of all cancers. However the number of cases and deaths are climbing for unknown reasons. The American Cancer Society has predicted 22,620 new cases and 18,160 deaths in the United States in 2009. There has not been a significant decrease in either incidence or mortality rates for liver cancer.

The most common primary tumor is hepatocellular carcinoma, developing in cirrhotic livers (Fig. 17-29). Cirrhosis may be secondary to metabolic disorders or hepatitis. Tumors may also result from prolonged exposure to carcinogenic chemicals. Secondary or metastatic cancer often arises from areas served by the hepatic portal veins or that spread along the peritoneal membranes (see Fig. 20-6 for photograph of metastatic liver cancer).

The signs of liver cancer initially are mild and general and similar to those of other liver diseases; they include anorexia and vomiting, fatigue, weight loss, and hepatomegaly. Portal hypertension and splenomegaly are

common. Paraneoplastic syndromes occur with this cancer, with tumor cells producing substances similar to erythropoietin, estrogen, or insulin (see Chapter 20). Because of the minimal early indications, the cancer is usually advanced at diagnosis. Chemotherapy is the usual treatment. If the tumor is localized, a lobectomy or radiofrequency ablation procedure may be used to remove it.

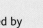

THINK ABOUT 17-10

a. Explain how the structure of the liver is altered by cirrhosis.
b. At which stage(s) is alcoholic liver disease reversible and why?
c. State the rationale for each of the following manifestations of cirrhosis: excessive bleeding, ascites, jaundice, and weight loss.
d. Explain why a transplanted liver (portion) is able to grow and function but a cirrhotic liver cannot.

Acute Pancreatitis

■ *Pathophysiology*

Pancreatitis is an inflammation of the pancreas resulting from autodigestion of the tissues. It may occur in acute

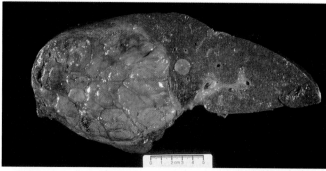

FIGURE 17-29 Hepatocellular carcinoma. A large tumor *(left)* in a noncirrhotic liver, with a small metastatic tumor nearby. *(From Kumar V, Abbas AK, Fausto M: Robbins and Cotran Pathologic Basis of Disease, ed 7, Philadelphia, 2005, Saunders.)*

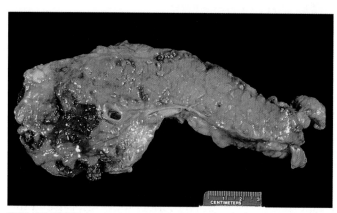

FIGURE 17-30 Acute pancreatitis. Note the dark areas of hemorrhage in the head of the pancreas and a pale area of fat necrosis around the upper left pancreas. *(From Kumar V, Abbas AK, Fausto M: Robbins and Cotran Pathologic Basis of Disease, ed 7, Philadelphia, 2005, Saunders.)*

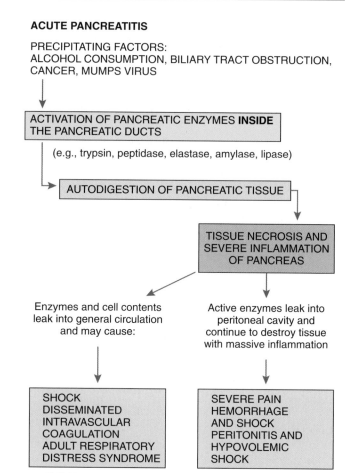

ACUTE PANCREATITIS

PRECIPITATING FACTORS:
ALCOHOL CONSUMPTION, BILIARY TRACT OBSTRUCTION, CANCER, MUMPS VIRUS

ACTIVATION OF PANCREATIC ENZYMES **INSIDE** THE PANCREATIC DUCTS

(e.g., trypsin, peptidase, elastase, amylase, lipase)

AUTODIGESTION OF PANCREATIC TISSUE

TISSUE NECROSIS AND SEVERE INFLAMMATION OF PANCREAS

Enzymes and cell contents leak into general circulation and may cause:

Active enzymes leak into peritoneal cavity and continue to destroy tissue with massive inflammation

SHOCK
DISSEMINATED INTRAVASCULAR COAGULATION
ADULT RESPIRATORY DISTRESS SYNDROME

SEVERE PAIN
HEMORRHAGE AND SHOCK
PERITONITIS AND HYPOVOLEMIC SHOCK

FIGURE 17-31 Pathophysiology of acute pancreatitis.

or chronic form. Acute pancreatitis is considered a medical emergency.

The autodigestion follows premature activation of the pancreatic proenzymes within the pancreas itself. It appears that activation of the proenzyme trypsinogen into trypsin is the trigger; in turn, trypsin converts other proenzymes and chemicals into active forms. The activated enzymes, trypsin, and the proteases amylase and lipase digest the pancreatic tissue, leading to massive inflammation, bleeding, and necrosis (Fig. 17-30).

The pancreas is composed of delicate tissue and lacks a fibrous capsule that might contain the effects of autodigestion. In some cases, pseudocysts or pancreatic abscesses may develop if the local inflammatory response is successful in localizing the injury. Otherwise, destruction by trypsin and other enzymes progresses into tissues surrounding the pancreas. Lipase causes fat necrosis, binding calcium ions (see pancreatic calcification in x-ray in Ready Reference 5). Blood vessels are eroded by elastase (a protease), leading to hemorrhage.

Damaging products, for example, cytokines and prostaglandins, released by tissue necrosis lead to widespread inflammation of the peritoneal membranes, or *chemical peritonitis*. The inflammatory response, including vasodilation and increased capillary permeability, leads to hypovolemia and circulatory collapse.

Severe pain, caused by the autodigestion of nerves and the inflammation, contributes to shock (neurogenic shock). Chemical peritonitis results in bacterial peritonitis as intestinal bacteria escape through the more permeable membranes (see Fig. 17-44).

Septicemia or general sepsis may result from the escape of bacteria and toxins from the intestines into the general circulation if the inflammatory process is not controlled quickly.

Other complications, which may cause death, are adult respiratory distress syndrome and acute renal failure.

The process is summarized in Figure 17-31.

■ *Etiology*

Although many factors may precipitate acute pancreatitis, the two major causes are gallstones and alcohol abuse. Gallstones may obstruct the flow of bile and pancreatic secretions into the duodenum or cause reflux of bile into the pancreatic duct, thus activating trypsinogen. Alcohol appears to stimulate an increased secretion of pancreatic enzymes and to contract the sphincter of Oddi, blocking flow, but there may be other mechanisms. Alcoholics may have chronic pancreatitis, and the acute episode may be an exacerbation of the chronic form, rather than a separate entity.

Signs and Symptoms

Sudden onset of acute pancreatitis may follow intake of a large meal or a large amount of alcohol.

- Severe epigastric or abdominal pain radiating to the back is the primary symptom. Pain increases when the individual assumes a supine position.
- Signs of shock—low blood pressure, pallor and sweating, and a rapid but weak pulse—develop as inflammation and hemorrhage cause hypovolemia.
- Low-grade fever is common until infection develops, when body temperature may rise significantly.
- Abdominal distention and decreased bowel sounds occur as peritonitis leads to decreased peristalsis and paralytic ileus.

Diagnostic Tests

Serum amylase levels rise within the first 12 to 24 hours and fall after 48 hours. Serum lipase levels are also elevated and remain so for approximately a week.

Hypocalcemia is common after calcium ions bind to fatty acids in areas of fat necrosis. Leukocytosis is an indicator of inflammation and infection.

Treatment

All oral intake is stopped, and bowel distention is relieved to reduce pancreatic stimulation. Shock and electrolyte imbalances are treated. Analgesics, such as meperidine, may be given for pain relief (but not morphine, which causes spasm of the sphincter of Oddi). The mortality rate is around 20%, and higher in individuals with concomitant diseases or elderly persons.

Pancreatic Cancer

Pancreatic (exocrine) cancer is increasing in incidence in North America with an estimated 42,470 cases and 35,240 deaths in the United States for 2009. The major established risk factor appears to be cigarette smoking. Pancreatitis and dietary factors have also been implicated. The common form of the neoplasm is adenocarcinoma, which arises from the epithelial cells in the ducts.

A tumor at the head of the pancreas usually causes obstruction of biliary and pancreatic flow, leading to weight loss and jaundice as early manifestations. Cancer of the body and tail of the pancreas frequently remains asymptomatic until it is well advanced and involves the nearby structures, such as the liver, stomach, lymph nodes, or posterior abdominal wall and nerves. Pain becomes very severe as the cancer progresses, eroding tissues.

Unless the tumor is diagnosed early and can be removed surgically, it is usually not diagnosed until later in the disease. Metastases occur early and effective treatments for metastatic disease are still in clinical research trials. Mortality is close to 95%. Liver failure, resulting from hepatobiliary obstruction, is often the cause of death.

> **THINK ABOUT 17-11**
>
> a. Explain why the liver is a common site of secondary cancer.
> b. Explain the concept of autodigestion and describe two specific effects of this process in the pancreas.

Lower Gastrointestinal Tract Disorders

Celiac Disease

Celiac disease, also called celiac sprue or gluten enteropathy, is a malabsorption syndrome that is considered to be primarily a childhood disorder. However, it may also occur in adults, usually at middle age. There is a related disorder, tropical sprue, which is bacterial in origin and often occurs in epidemics in tropical areas.

Celiac disease appears to be linked to genetic factors and consists of a defect in the intestinal enzyme that prevents further digestion of gliadin, a breakdown product of *gluten*. Gluten is a constituent of certain grains: wheat, barley, rye, and oats. The combination of a digestive block with an immunologic response in the person results in a toxic effect on the intestinal villi. The villi atrophy, resulting in decreased enzyme production and less surface area available for absorption of nutrients (Fig. 17-32). Thus, the end result of celiac disease is malabsorption and malnutrition.

In an infant, the first signs of the disorder usually appear as cereals are added to the diet, around 4 to 6 months of age. Malabsorption syndromes are manifested by steatorrhea, muscle wasting, and failure to gain weight. Irritability and malaise are common.

The condition can be diagnosed by a series of blood tests (celiac blood panel) checking for autoantibodies, a duodenal biopsy, and lastly, adopting a gluten-free diet to assess if health improves under the new conditions.

Fortunately celiac disease can usually be treated by maintaining a gluten-free diet, using corn and rice for grains. The intestinal mucosa returns to normal after a few weeks without gluten intake. Patients should be monitored because of an increased incidence of intestinal lymphoma.

Chronic Inflammatory Bowel Disease

Crohn's disease and ulcerative colitis are chronic inflammatory bowel diseases, the causes of which are unknown. Prevalence is estimated in the range of 500,000 cases in the United States, ranging from mild to severe. A genetic factor appears to be involved because there is a high familial incidence and inflammatory bowel

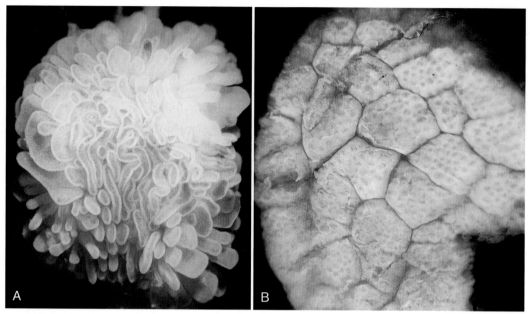

FIGURE 17-32 **A**, Normal small intestinal mucosa with villi appearing as fingers and leaves. **B**, Celiac disease-flat intestinal mucosa with total villus atrophy. *(From Cooke RA, Stewart B: Colour Atlas of Anatomical Pathology, ed 3, Sydney, 2004, Churchill Livingstone.)*

disease (IBD) is much more common among certain groups, namely whites, particularly Ashkenazi Jews (from Eastern Europe). Investigative studies on an immunologic abnormality continue because many individuals have high levels of various antibodies or HLA and a cytokine, interleukin (IL) in the blood, and T-lymphocytes that are cytotoxic to the mucosa. Two genes have been identified, which, if defective, are linked to Crohn's disease. In many patients, particularly those with ulcerative colitis, there are manifestations of immune abnormalities elsewhere in the body, including iritis, ankylosing spondylitis, arthritis, and nephrolithiasis.

There are many similarities between Crohn's disease and ulcerative colitis, and there may be an overlap in their clinical presentation in some individuals (Table 17-7). Both diseases occur in males and females. Crohn's disease often develops during adolescence, whereas ulcerative colitis more frequently appears in the second or third decade. These diseases are characterized by remissions and exacerbations as well as considerable diversity in the severity of clinical effects.

Crohn's Disease (Regional Ileitis or Regional Enteritis)

▪ Pathophysiology

Crohn's disease may affect any area of the digestive tract, but occurs most frequently in the small intestine, particularly the terminal ileum and sometimes the ascending colon. Inflammation occurs in a characteristic distribution called "skip lesions," with affected segments clearly separated by areas of normal tissue (Fig. 17-33).

TABLE 17-7	Inflammatory Bowel Disease	
Characteristic	Crohn's Disease	Ulcerative Colitis
Region affected	Terminal ileum, sometimes colon	Colon, rectum
Distribution of lesions	Transmural, all layers Skip lesions	Mucosa only Continuous, diffuse
Characteristic stool	Loose, semi-formed	Frequent, watery, with blood and mucus
Granuloma	Common	No
Fistula, fissure, abscess	Common	No
Stricture, obstruction	Common	Rare
Malabsorption, malnutrition	Yes	Not common

Initially inflammation occurs in the mucosal layer with the development of shallow ulcers. The ulcers tend to coalesce to form fissures separated by thickened elevations or nodules, giving the wall a typical "cobblestone" appearance. The progressive inflammation and fibrosis may affect all layers of the wall (transmural), leading eventually to a thick, rigid "rubber hose" wall. This change leaves a narrow lumen ("string sign"), which may become totally obstructed. Granulomas indicative of chronic inflammation may be found in the wall and the regional lymph nodes. The damaged wall impairs the ability of the small intestine to process

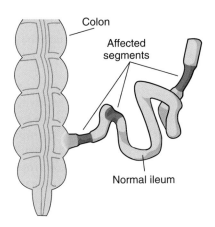

A. "Skip lesions" — distribution of affected segments alternating with normal segments of bowel

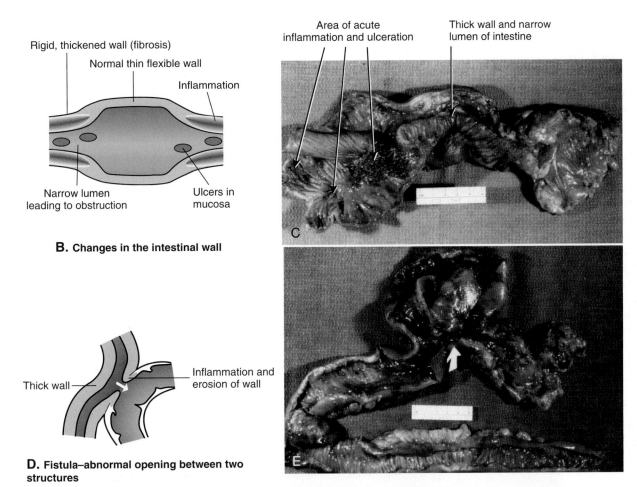

B. Changes in the intestinal wall

D. Fistula–abnormal opening between two structures

FIGURE 17-33 Regional ileitis (Crohn's disease). **A,** "Skip lesions." **B,** Narrowing and obstruction. **C,** Photograph showing narrowing ("garden-hose") and inflammation-ulceration of bowel. **D,** Diagram of fistula. **E,** Photograph showing fistula between sections of intestine. *(C and E courtesy of RW Shaw, North York General Hospital, Toronto, Ontario, Canada.)*

and absorb food. The inflammation also stimulates intestinal motility, decreasing the time available for digestion and absorption.

Interference with digestion and absorption in the small intestine may lead to hypoproteinemia, avitaminosis, malnutrition, and possibly steatorrhea.

Other complications are common. Adhesions between two loops of intestine may develop when the subserosa is inflamed. The ulcers may penetrate the intestinal wall, causing abscesses to form. Fistulas, a connecting passage between two structures, may form as the ulcer erodes through the intestinal wall. Fistulas may be found between two loops of intestine (see Fig. 17-33D), the intestine and the bladder, or the intestine and the skin. Perianal fissures and fistulas are common.

Signs and Symptoms

The course of Crohn's disease is variable. Exacerbations are marked by diarrhea with cramping abdominal pain. The stool is typically soft or semi-formed. Melena may occur if the ulcers erode blood vessels. Pain and tenderness are often centered in the right lower quadrant.

Anorexia, weight loss, anemia, and fatigue are associated with malabsorption and malnutrition. Children experience delayed growth and sexual maturation resulting from lack of adequate protein and vitamins, particularly fat-soluble vitamins A and D. Treatment with glucocorticoids also hampers growth. In addition, many psychological implications are characteristic of this type of chronic illness.

Ulcerative Colitis

Pathophysiology

The inflammation commences in the rectum and progresses in a continuous fashion proximally through the colon. The small intestine is rarely involved.

The mucosa and submucosa are inflamed, commencing at the base of the crypts of Lieberkühn (mucus-secreting goblet cells). The tissue becomes edematous and friable, and ulcerations develop (Fig. 17-34). In an attempt to heal, granulation tissue forms, but it is vascular and fragile and bleeds easily. When the ulcers coalesce, large areas of the mucosa become denuded, but there are residual "bridges" of intact mucosa over the ulcers. This tissue destruction interferes with the absorption of fluid and electrolytes in the colon.

In severe acute episodes, a serious complication, *toxic megacolon*, may develop, as inflammation impairs peristalsis, leading to obstruction and dilation of the colon, usually the transverse colon. A concern with long-term ulcerative colitis is the increased risk of colorectal carcinoma, which may be predicted by detection of metaplasia and dysplasia in the mucosa.

Signs and Symptoms

Diarrhea is present, consisting of frequent watery stools marked by the presence of blood and mucus and accompanied by cramping pain. During severe exacerbations, blood and mucus alone may be passed frequently, day or night, accompanied by tenesmus (persistent spasms of the rectum associated with a need to defecate). Rectal bleeding may be considerable and contributes to severe iron deficiency anemia. Fever and weight loss may be present.

Treatment of Irritable Bowel Disease

- Exacerbations are often precipitated by physical or emotional stressors. It is helpful to identify and remove, if possible, the specific factors that apply in each individual. It is beneficial to use a team approach to the treatment of IBD because treatment involves multiple aspects of care.
- Specific measures usually include anti-inflammatory medications, such as sulfasalazine (sulfapyridine with 5-aminosalicylic acid) or glucocorticoids. These drugs may be administered systemically, both orally and parenterally, or topically, as an enema or suppository. In some refractive cases, other immunosuppressive agents may be used.
- Antimotility agents, such as loperamide or anticholinergic drugs (see Table 17-3), are used for symptomatic relief in mild or moderate cases.
- Nutritional supplements are frequently required, particularly during acute episodes. Total parenteral nutrition (intravenous) may be required during severe exacerbations. The recommended diet is usually high in protein, vitamins, and calories but low in fat. Low-bulk diets reduce intestinal stimulation during exacerbations.

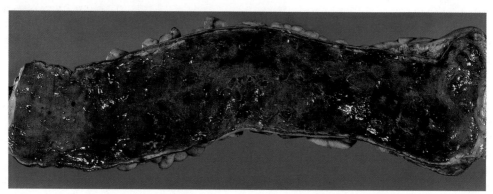

FIGURE 17-34 Acute ulcerative colitis. The mucosa is red, edematous, ulcerated, and bleeding. (*From Cooke RA, Stewart B:* Colour Atlas of Anatomical Pathology, *ed 3, Sydney, 2004, Churchill Livingstone.*)

- Antimicrobials, including metronidazole or ciprofloxacin, are required for secondary infection.
- Immunotherapeutic agents, such as azathioprine, are effective as long-term therapy.
- Surgical resection, usually ileostomy or colostomy, procedures that create an artificial opening on the surface of the abdomen, is necessary for complications, such as obstruction or fistulas, or for severe exacerbations that do not respond to medication. In some cases, surgical intervention may provide a temporary rest for the intestine and can be reversed to normal anatomy later.

THINK ABOUT 17-12

a. Explain the characteristics of steatorrhea.
b. Explain how the pathologic changes seen in celiac disease lead to malabsorption.
c. Prepare a chart comparing Crohn's disease and ulcerative colitis by location and characteristics of the lesions, manifestations, and potential complications.
d. Explain several ways in which an adolescent's growth and development could be impaired by Crohn's disease.

Irritable Bowel Syndrome

Irritable bowel syndrome (IBS) is a gastrointestinal disorder with manifestations of abdominal pain/discomfort, and changes in normal bowel habits. This disorder affects up to 20% of the worldwide population and statistics show it is more common in young and middle-aged women. The types of IBS are identified based on the primary symptoms of diarrhea, constipation, and/or pain.

▦ *Pathophysiology*

The different types of IBS are:

- Abnormal gastrointestinal motility and secretion: Those with diarrhea-type IBS experience rapid transit time of feces through the bowel, whereas those with constipation/bloating IBS have delayed transit time through the bowels. The cause may be due to hypersensitivity or the effect of serotonin on the enteric nervous system.
- Visceral hypersensitivity: causes increased sensitivity to visceral pain. Causes are similar to those of abnormal motility and secretion but may also include the involvement of activated mast cells and T-lymphocytes and effects on the autonomic and central nervous systems in processing information, resulting in increased pain.
- Postinfectious IBS: may cause low grade inflammation and abnormal immune response in the gut. Often associated with bacterial enteritis.

- Overgrowth of flora: may cause constipation and bloating due to methane gas production. This gas production is a result of the overgrowth of the normal intestinal flora found in the gut.
- Food allergy or intolerance: Certain food antigens may activate the immune response in the mucosa, causing a hypersensitivity reaction and IBS symptoms.
- Psychosocial factors: The IBS symptoms in this case may be caused by factors such as emotional stress, which in turn affects the autonomic nervous system, the neuroendocrine pathway, and pain responses.

▦ *Signs and Symptoms*

Manifestations of IBS may include: lower abdominal pain, diarrhea, constipation, alternating diarrhea and constipation, gas, bloating, and nausea. There may also be fecal urgency and incomplete evacuation of the bowels. After defecation the symptoms usually subside.

▦ *Diagnosis*

Diagnosis of IBS is based on the established signs and symptoms and the exclusion of any structural or metabolic problems that can produce similar manifestations. Test for food allergies, bacterial or parasitic infections, and problems such as lactose intolerance may also be used to confirm the disorder. A protocol referred to as Rome III criteria has been established as a guideline for diagnosing IBS.

▦ *Treatment*

There is no single cure for IBS. The treatment is individualized to address the specific symptoms. These treatments may include laxatives, fiber supplements, antidiarrheal medication, antidepressants, analgesics for pain, antispasmodic medication, and medications to balance the serotonin levels. Because of the variety of causes, research into new treatments and therapies are ongoing.

Appendicitis

A common acute problem in young adults, occurring in 10% of the population, appendicitis is an inflammation and infection in the vermiform appendix (see Fig. 17-1).

▦ *Pathophysiology*

The development of appendicitis usually follows a pattern that correlates with the clinical signs, although variations may occur because of the altered location of the appendix or underlying factors.

1. Obstruction of the appendiceal lumen by a fecalith, gallstone, or foreign material or from twisting or spasm is commonly an initiating factor.
2. Fluid builds up inside the appendix and microorganisms proliferate.

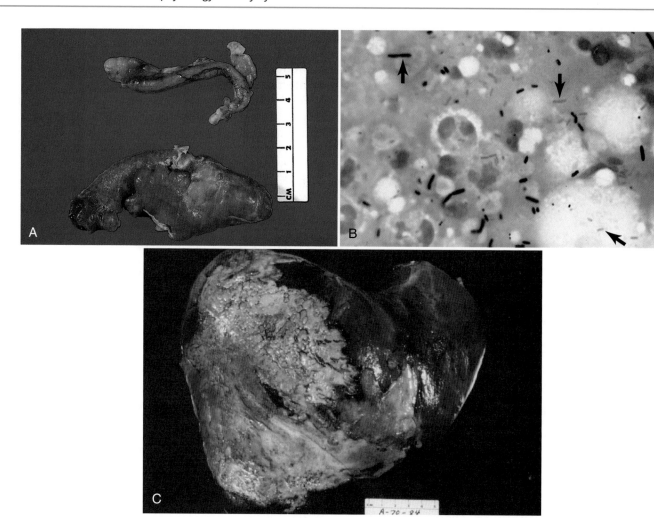

FIGURE 17-35 **A,** Acute appendicitis. Below is the inflamed appendix, red, swollen, and covered with fibrinous exudate. A normal appendix is shown above. **B,** Smear of drainage from a ruptured appendix showing infection by fecal flora and gram-positive and gram-negative bacteria. **C,** Liver affected by acute peritonitis resulting from a ruptured appendix. Note: The liver is covered by a purulent exudate. (**A** from Kumar V, Abbas AK, Fausto M: Robbins and Cotran Pathologic Basis of Disease, ed 7, Philadelphia, 2005, Saunders; **B** from Mahon CR, Manuselis G: Textbook of Diagnostic Microbiology, ed 2, Philadelphia, 2000, Saunders; **C** courtesy of RW Shaw, North York General Hospital, Toronto, Ontario, Canada.)

3. The appendiceal wall becomes inflamed and purulent exudate forms. The appendix is swollen. Blood vessels in the wall are compressed (Fig. 17-35).

4. The increasing congestion and pressure within the appendix leads to ischemia and necrosis of the wall, resulting in increased permeability.

5. Bacteria and toxins escape through the wall into the surrounding area. This breakout of bacteria leads to abscess formation or localized bacterial peritonitis.

6. An abscess may develop when the adjacent omentum temporarily walls off the inflamed area by adhering to the appendiceal surface. In some cases, the inflammation and pain subside temporarily but then recur.

7. Localized infection or peritonitis develops around the appendix and may spread along the peritoneal membranes.

8. Increasing pressure inside the appendix causes increased necrosis and gangrene in the wall (infection in necrotic tissue). The wall of the appendix appears blackish.

9. If the appendix ruptures or perforates, it releases its contents into the peritoneal cavity. This leads to generalized peritonitis, which may be life threatening (see Fig. 17-35C).

Signs and Symptoms

Sometimes appendicitis develops "silently" or manifests with significant variations. In classic cases, a sequence of signs occurs, as follows:

• General periumbilical pain related to the inflammation and stretching of the appendiceal wall occurs initially.

• Nausea and vomiting are common.

• Pain becomes more severe and localized in the lower right quadrant (LRQ) of the abdomen (Fig. 17-36).

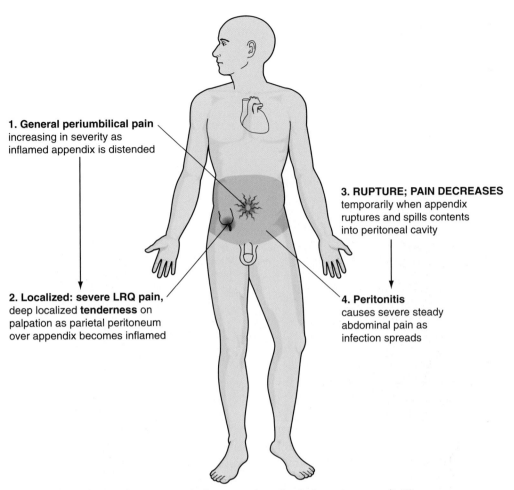

1. General periumbilical pain
increasing in severity as
inflamed appendix is distended

3. RUPTURE; PAIN DECREASES
temporarily when appendix
ruptures and spills contents
into peritoneal cavity

2. Localized: severe LRQ pain,
deep localized **tenderness** on
palpation as parietal peritoneum
over appendix becomes inflamed

4. Peritonitis
causes severe steady
abdominal pain as
infection spreads

FIGURE 17-36 Typical progression of pain in acute appendicitis.

- Lower right quadrant tenderness develops (classically at McBurney's point, midway between the umbilicus and the iliac crest). Localized pain results from involvement of the parietal peritoneum over the appendix. The location of the appendix does vary among individuals, and this can be diagnostically misleading.
- If rupture occurs, the pain usually subsides temporarily as the pressure is relieved.
- Pain recurs as a steady, severe abdominal pain as peritonitis develops.
- Low-grade fever and leukocytosis occur as inflammation develops.
- Signs indicating the onset of peritonitis include a rigid "boardlike" abdomen, tachycardia, and hypotension.

Treatment
Surgical removal of the appendix and administration of antimicrobial drugs are the standard treatment.

Diverticular Disease

Diverticular disease refers to various problems related to the development of diverticula (singular, diverticulum). Diverticula may be congenital or acquired.

- *Diverticulum* is a herniation or outpouching of the mucosa through the muscle layer of the colon wall, frequently in the sigmoid colon.
- *Diverticulosis* is asymptomatic diverticular disease. Usually multiple diverticula are present (Fig. 17-37).
- *Diverticulitis* refers to inflammation of the diverticula. It is a common problem in the Western world, affecting primarily older individuals.

Pathophysiology
Diverticula form at gaps between bands of longitudinal muscle that coincide with openings in the circular muscle bands that permit passage of blood vessels through the wall. Longitudinal muscle also occurs in three bands, rather than as a continuous sheet. Congenital weakness of the wall may also be a contributing factor.

These weaker areas of the wall bulge outward when pressure is increased, frequently inside the lumen of the intestine, for example, in the presence of strong muscle contractions. Consistently low-residue diets, irregular bowel habits, and aging lead to chronic constipation and then to muscle hypertrophy in the colon, with elevated intraluminal pressures, and finally to the gradual development of diverticula.

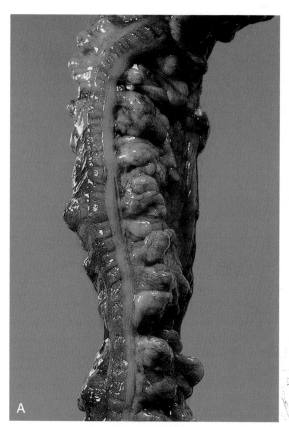

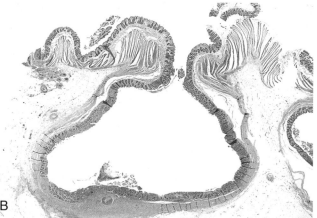

FIGURE 17-37 **A**, Diverticulosis of the sigmoid colon. *(From Cooke RA, Stewart B:* Colour Atlas of Anatomical Pathology, *ed 3, Sydney, 2004, Churchill Livingstone).* **B**, Low-power micrograph of diverticulum of the colon showing protrusion of mucosa and submucosa through the muscle wall. *(From Kumar V, et al:* Robbins basic pathology, *ed 8, Philadelphia, 2007, Saunders-Elsevier.)*

Potential complications include intestinal obstruction, perforation with peritonitis, and abscess formation.

■ Signs and Symptoms

In many cases, diverticular disease remains asymptomatic. Sometimes there is mild discomfort, diarrhea, or constipation and flatulence, which can be excused for other reasons. With diverticulitis, inflammation, related to stasis of feces in the pouches, develops in the diverticula. Lower left quadrant cramping or steady pain and tenderness with nausea and vomiting indicate inflammatory disease. A slight fever and elevated white blood cell count accompany the discomfort.

■ Treatment

During acute episodes of diverticulitis, food intake is reduced, and antimicrobial drugs are taken as required. Diverticular disease is treated by increasing the bulk in the diet, omitting foods such as seeds or popcorn, and encouraging regular bowel movements without constipation.

Colorectal Cancer

In the United States, colorectal cancer ranks high as a lethal cancer in individuals older than age 50 and is the second leading cause of cancer-related deaths. The numbers estimated for 2009 to 2012 include 143,460

persons to be diagnosed and 51,690 deaths. Overall 1 in 19 North Americans will develop colon cancer if preventive measures do not improve. Many of the deaths could be prevented by early treatment of precancerous lesions such as polyps, and early detection of malignancy. The American Cancer Society recommends fecal tests for occult blood (FOBT), every year for those more than 40 years old and a sigmoidoscopy every 3 to 5 years for those more than 50 years old. Following a survey, the CDC and American Cancer Society are promoting a routine screening for all persons greater than age 50, to include FOBT, sigmoidoscopy, and colonoscopy, to ensure more early detection and treatment. For specific information on the tests that are being used and the rationale for the use of each, see the American Cancer Society web site. Video camera capsules have been tested for identification of polyps and malignancies in the GI tract; these require the same bowel preparation as do more invasive procedures. The United States Congress has mandated screening for colorectal cancer as part of the "Welcome to Medicare" physical to be done within 6 months of qualifying for Medicare benefits. Malignant tumors are rare in the small intestine.

■ Pathophysiology

Most malignant neoplasms develop from adenomatous polyps, of which there are a diversity of types. A polyp

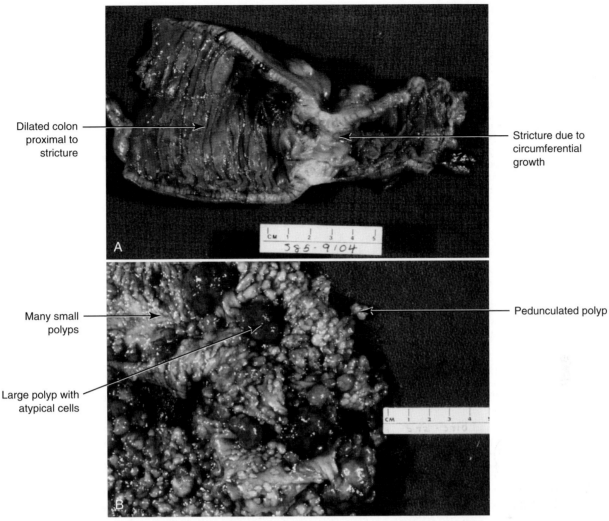

Dilated colon proximal to stricture

Stricture due to circumferential growth

Many small polyps

Large polyp with atypical cells

Pedunculated polyp

FIGURE 17-38 Colorectal cancer. **A,** Circumferential malignant growth (cancer) obstructing flow of feces and causing proximal dilation of the colon. **B,** Polyposis and malignant changes. *(Courtesy of RW Shaw, North York General Hospital, Toronto, Ontario, Canada.)*

is a mass, often on a stem, that protrudes into the lumen, and many polyps represent genetic abnormalities (Fig. 17-38). As polyps increase in size, they carry an increased risk of dysplasia and malignant changes.

These adenocarcinomas are distributed about equally in the right (or ascending) colon, the left (or descending) colon, and the distal sigmoid colon and rectum. In recent years, an increasing number of tumors have been found in the right colon using barium enema or CT scans. Lesions in this location are more difficult to diagnose at an early stage because routine rectal digital examination or proctosigmoidoscopy do not suffice. Tumors in the sigmoid colon and rectum are more easily accessible.

Carcinomas may manifest differently; for example, as circumferential or annular constrictive "napkin-ring" growths, which are common in the left colon, or as projecting polypoid masses, which are common in the right colon. Flat ulcerating lesions occur less frequently. All types of carcinomas invade the wall, the mesentery, and the lymph nodes and metastasize to the liver. Staging is

based on the degree of local invasion, lymph node involvement, and presence of distant metastases (see Chapter 20).

Most adenocarcinomas release carcinoembryonic antigen (CEA) into the blood. Detection of this antigen has limited value as a screening tool because it is also elevated in other conditions, such as ulcerative colitis. However, presence of the antigen is useful to monitor for recurrence after removal of a tumor.

■ *Etiology*

This cancer occurs primarily in persons greater than age 55. It is more common in the Western hemisphere. The presence of familial multiple polyposis or long-term ulcerative colitis in a patient increases the risk of cancer developing, often at a younger age. Genetic factors are responsible for the increased occurrence of colorectal cancer among close relatives.

Environmental factors, such as diet, also appear to play a major role in carcinogenesis. Diets high in fat,

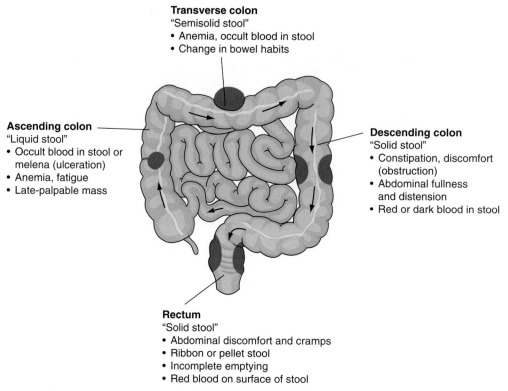

Transverse colon
"Semisolid stool"
• Anemia, occult blood in stool
• Change in bowel habits

Ascending colon
"Liquid stool"
• Occult blood in stool or
  melena (ulceration)
• Anemia, fatigue
• Late-palpable mass

Descending colon
"Solid stool"
• Constipation, discomfort
  (obstruction)
• Abdominal fullness
  and distension
• Red or dark blood in stool

Rectum
"Solid stool"
• Abdominal discomfort and cramps
• Ribbon or pellet stool
• Incomplete emptying
• Red blood on surface of stool

FIGURE 17-39 Common signs and symptoms of colorectal cancer related to location.

sugar, and red meat are thought to produce carcinogenic substances, particularly long term. Low-fiber diets increase risk because they prolong the contact time of the mucosa with carcinogens.

■ Signs and Symptoms

Although most carcinomas remain asymptomatic until they are well advanced, the initial signs of colorectal cancer depend largely on the location of the growth and the characteristics of the feces at that location in the colon (Fig. 17-39). For example, an annular lesion in the rectosigmoid area, where the fecal mass is relatively solid, causes partial obstruction with dilation of the proximal colon (see Fig. 17-38). Vague cramping pain, small flat pellets or "ribbon" stool, and a feeling of incomplete emptying are common signs of cancer in this location.

Cancer in the right colon, where the fecal material is liquid, does not cause obstruction but often manifests only as general systemic signs, such as fatigue, weight loss, or iron deficiency anemia.

An unexplained change in bowel habits, such as alternating diarrhea and constipation, may be a sign of malignancy. Bleeding may be indicated by occult blood or melena if it arises from the proximal colon. Frank (red) blood and mucus on or near the surface of the stool usually signify bleeding from a lesion in the rectum.

■ Treatment

Colorectal cancer is treated by surgical removal of the involved area, usually requiring a colostomy, an artificial opening into the abdominal wall where feces may be continually collected in a bag (Fig. 17-40). Both curative and palliative surgery may be accompanied by radiation and chemotherapy. Chemotherapy may be used in conjunction with radiation after surgery. Current recommendations are for the use of two drugs in a protocol that may include oral medication as well as intravenous drugs. The choice of drug protocol will depend on the stage of the cancer and the patient's overall health history. A new drug treatment, cetuximab, targets growth factor signals responsible for cell reproduction.

Early diagnosis is essential. Localized lesions (Dukes stage A or TNM stage I cancer) confined to the mucosa carry a 5-year survival rate of greater than 90%. Once lymph nodes are involved (Dukes stage C or TNM stage III), the 5-year survival rate drops significantly.

THINK ABOUT 17-13

a. Describe, in the order in which they develop, each stage of the pain seen with acute appendicitis, including the location and type of pain and the reason for it.
b. Define the term *diverticulitis* and explain how diverticula develop and become inflamed.
c. State two factors that predispose a patient to colorectal cancer.
d. Explain why the signs of colorectal cancer vary with the location of the tumor.

Sigmoid Colostomy—made from the sigmoid part of the colon
- Output: Fully formed stool
- Pouch: One-piece drainable,
          One-piece closed,
          Two-piece drainable,
          Two-piece closed, or
          Stomacap (if you irrigate)

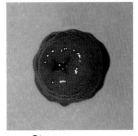

Stoma
- Not painful
- Aways red and moist
B • May bleed easily

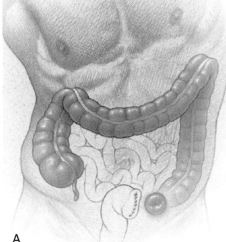

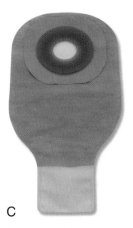

FIGURE 17-40 Colostomy. **A**, sigmoid colostomy. A surgically created opening into the colon through the abdominal wall. **B**, The stoma is the new opening on the abdomen. It is always red and moist, is not painful, but may bleed easily. **C**, A plastic pouch to collect stools is attached to the stoma. *(Courtesy of Hollister Incorporated, Patient Education Series.)*

Intestinal Obstruction

Intestinal obstruction refers to a lack of movement of the intestinal contents through the intestine. Because of its smaller lumen, obstructions are more common and occur more rapidly in the small intestine, but they can occur in the large intestine as well. Depending on the cause and location, obstruction may manifest as an acute problem or a gradually developing situation. For example, twisting of the intestine could cause sudden total obstruction, whereas a tumor leads to progressive obstruction.

Intestinal obstruction occurs in two forms. *Mechanical* obstructions are those resulting from tumor, adhesions, hernias, or other tangible obstructions (Fig. 17-41). *Functional*, or adynamic, obstructions result from neurologic impairment, such as spinal cord injury or lack of propulsion in the intestine, and are often referred to as *paralytic ileus*. Although the end result can be the same, these types manifest somewhat differently and require different treatment.

■ *Pathophysiology*
When mechanical obstruction of the flow of intestinal contents occurs, a sequence of events develops (Fig. 17-42) as follows:

1. Gases and fluids accumulate in the area proximal to the blockage, distending the intestine. Gases arise primarily from swallowed air, but also from bacterial activity in the intestine.
2. Increasingly strong contractions of the proximal intestine occur in an effort to move the contents onward.
3. The increasing pressure in the lumen leads to more secretions entering the intestine and also compresses the veins in the wall, preventing absorption, as the intestinal wall becomes edematous.
4. The intestinal distention leads to persistent vomiting with additional loss of fluid and electrolytes. With small intestinal obstructions, there is no opportunity to reabsorb fluid and electrolytes, and hypovolemia quickly results.
5. If the obstruction is not removed, the intestinal wall becomes ischemic and necrotic as the arterial blood supply to the tissue is reduced by pressure. If twisting of the intestine (e.g., volvulus) has occurred or immediate compression of arteries (e.g., intussusception or strangulated hernia) results from the primary cause of obstruction, the intestinal wall becomes rapidly necrotic and gangrenous.

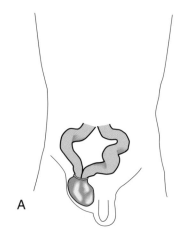

Inguinal hernia

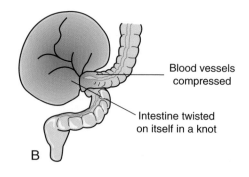

Blood vessels
compressed

Intestine twisted
on itself in a knot

Volvulus

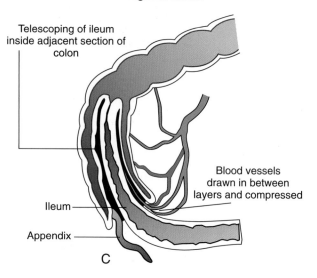

Telescoping of ileum
inside adjacent section of
colon

Blood vessels
drawn in between
layers and compressed

Ileum

Appendix

Intussusception

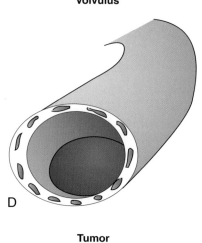

Tumor

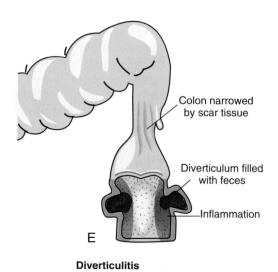

Colon narrowed
by scar tissue

Diverticulum filled
with feces

Inflammation

Diverticulitis

FIGURE 17-41 **A-E,** Causes of intestinal obstruction.

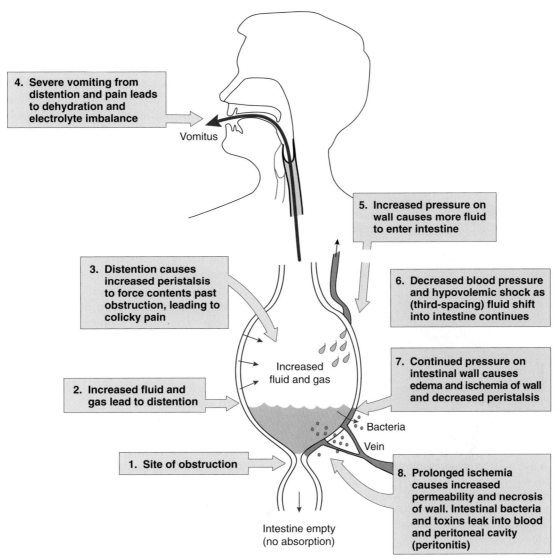

FIGURE 17-42 Effects of intestinal obstruction.

6. Ischemia and necrosis of the intestinal wall eventually lead to decreased innervation and cessation of peristalsis. A decrease in bowel sounds indicates this change.

7. The obstruction promotes rapid reproduction of intestinal bacteria, some of which produce endotoxins. As the affected intestinal wall becomes necrotic and more permeable, intestinal bacteria or toxins can leak into the peritoneal cavity (peritonitis) or the blood supply (bacteremia and septicemia).

8. In time, perforation of the necrotic segment may occur, leading to generalized peritonitis.

Functional obstruction or paralytic ileus usually results from neurologic impairment. Peristalsis ceases and distention of the intestine occurs as fluids and electrolytes accumulate in the intestine. In this type of obstruction, reflex spasms of the intestinal muscle do not occur, but the remainder of the process is similar to that of mechanical obstruction.

■ *Etiology*

Functional obstruction or paralytic ileus is common in the following situations:

- After abdominal surgery, in which the effects of the anesthetic combined with inflammation or ischemia in the operative area interfere with conduction of nerve impulses
- In the initial stage of spinal cord injuries (spinal shock)
- With inflammation related to severe ischemia
- In pancreatitis, peritonitis, or infection in the abdominal cavity
- With hypokalemia, mesenteric thrombosis, or toxemia

Mechanical obstruction may result from the following:

- Adhesions (from previous surgery, infection, or radiation) that twist or constrict the intestine, the most common cause of obstruction
- Hernias (protrusion of a section of intestine through an opening in the muscle wall) (Fig. 17-43)

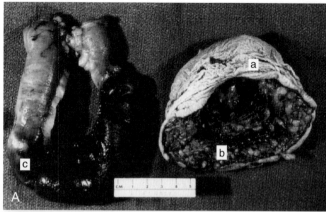

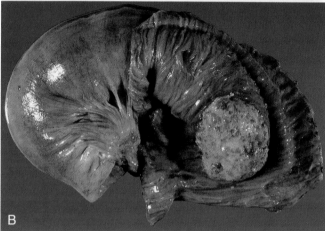

FIGURE 17-43 **A**, Hernia with infarcted intestine. The sac consists of the abdominal wall covered by skin *(a)* at a site weakened by scar tissue, forming a protrusion into which a loop of intestine is compressed *(b)*. This protrusion obstructs the blood flow to the intestinal wall *(c)* (black infarcted area) as well as the flow of feces inside the intestine. *(Courtesy of RW Shaw, North York General Hospital, Toronto, Ontario, Canada.)* **B**, Intussusception due to an adenocarcinoma (light-colored circular mass) causing acute intestinal obstruction. *(B, From Cooke RA, Stewart B: Colour Atlas of Anatomical Pathology, ed 3, Sydney, 2004, Churchill Livingstone).*

- Strictures caused by scar tissue
- Masses, such as tumors or foreign bodies
- Intussusception (the telescoping of a section of bowel inside an adjacent section)
- Intussusception may occur secondary to polyps or tumors that pull a section of bowel forward with them (see Fig. 17-41C)
- Volvulus (twisting of a section of intestine on itself), which may be linked to adhesions; in many cases, the cause of intussusception or volvulus is unknown
- Hirschsprung's disease, or congenital megacolon, a condition in which parasympathetic innervation is missing from a section of the colon, impairing motility and leading to constipation and eventually obstruction; Hirschsprung's disease often occurs in conjunction with other anomalies
- Gradual obstruction from chronic inflammatory conditions, such as Crohn's disease or diverticulitis

■ *Signs and Symptoms*
With mechanical obstruction of the small intestine, severe colicky abdominal pain develops as peristalsis increases initially. Borborygmi (audible rumbling sounds caused by movement of gas in the intestine) and intestinal rushes can be heard as the intestinal muscle forcefully contracts in an attempt to propel the contents forward. The signs of paralytic ileus differ significantly in that bowel sounds decrease or are absent, and pain is steady.

Vomiting and abdominal distention occur quickly with obstruction of the small intestine. Vomiting is recurrent and consists first of gastric contents and then bile-stained duodenal contents. No stool or gas is passed.

Restlessness and diaphoresis with tachycardia are present initially. As hypovolemia and electrolyte imbalances progress, signs of dehydration, weakness, confusion, and shock are apparent.

Obstruction of the large intestine develops slowly and signs are mild. Constipation and mild lower abdominal pain are common, followed by abdominal distention, anorexia, and eventually vomiting and more severe pain.

■ *Treatment*
The underlying cause is treated, and fluids and electrolytes are replaced. Surgery and antimicrobial therapy are required as soon as possible for any strangulation; paralytic ileus may require decompression by suction.

Peritonitis

Peritonitis is an inflammation of the peritoneal membranes that may result from *chemical* irritation or directly from *bacterial* invasion of the sterile peritoneal cavity. Chemical irritation, unless resolved quickly, ultimately leads to bacterial peritonitis. It is usually an acute condition and requires treatment of the primary cause as well as the effects. The incidence of peritonitis and septicemia has decreased with the prophylactic use of antibiotics, but peritonitis remains a threat in many situations.

■ *Pathophysiology*
Inflammation of the peritoneal membranes may commence with the presence of chemical irritants, such as bile, chyme, or foreign objects in the peritoneal cavity. This inflammation then increases the permeability of the intestinal wall, permitting enteric bacteria to enter the peritoneal cavity (Fig. 17-44). Necrosis or perforation of the intestinal wall also allows infection directly by enteric organisms.

Initially when local inflammation develops in the abdominal cavity, the peritoneum and omentum tend to produce a thick, sticky exudate, which helps the adjacent tissues to stick together and temporarily seal the area, localizing the source of the problem. In some cases the inflammation subsides and an abscess forms that

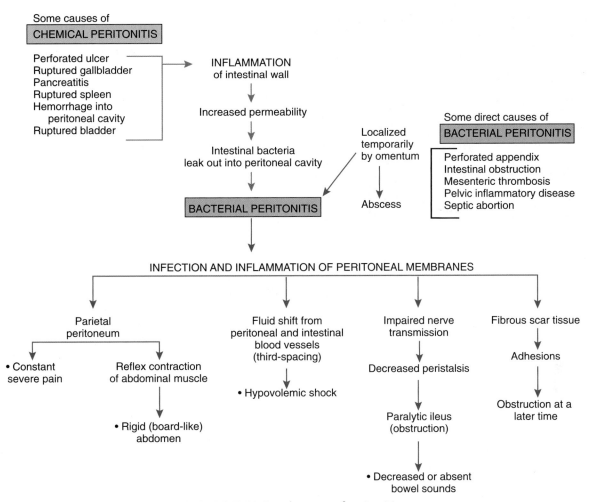

FIGURE 17-44 Development of peritonitis.

may flare up at a later time. This local inflammation may also reduce peristalsis in the area, decreasing the risk of spreading toxins or bacteria at the time. However, unless the original cause of the problem is removed, it is likely that the inflammation or infection will spread.

The peritoneum consists of a large sterile expanse of highly vascular tissue that covers the viscera and lines the abdominal cavity. This peritoneal structure provides a means of rapid dissemination of irritants or bacteria throughout the abdominal cavity. Abdominal distention is evident, and the typical rigid, boardlike abdomen develops as reflex abdominal muscle spasm occurs in response to involvement of the parietal peritoneum.

Whatever the cause, this membrane is rapidly involved in the inflammatory response, which leads to vasodilation and increased permeability. The membrane becomes edematous and red. The many blood vessels in the membranes can leak large volumes of fluid into the peritoneal cavity. Hypovolemic shock results as this process of "third-spacing" occurs (see Chapter 12). The fluid, protein, and electrolytes sequestered in the peritoneal cavity are not recycled into the circulating blood and therefore are of no value to maintenance of body fluid balance. This fluid becomes purulent as infection spreads. Nausea and vomiting, resulting from the intestinal irritation and pain, add to the fluid loss. Two complications may develop if intervention is delayed. When inflammation persists, nerve conduction is impaired, and peristalsis decreases, leading to obstruction of the intestines (paralytic ileus). The inflamed membranes permit intestinal bacteria and toxic materials to migrate into the blood and then into the general circulation, which may lead to septicemia.

■ *Etiology*
Peritonitis develops secondarily to many conditions, some of which are the following:
- Chemical peritonitis may result from the enzymes released with pancreatitis, urine leaking from a ruptured bladder, chyme spilled into the peritoneal cavity from a perforated ulcer, bile escaping from a perforated gallbladder or from blood or any other foreign material in the cavity.
- Bacterial peritonitis may be caused by direct trauma affecting the intestines (e.g., penetrating injury), a ruptured appendix, or intestinal obstruction, particularly when blood vessels are compressed and the wall becomes gangrenous.

- Any abdominal surgery may lead to peritonitis if foreign material remains in the abdomen or infection develops at the site.
- Pelvic inflammatory disease in women, in which infection ascends through the uterus and into the fallopian tubes, which provide direct access to the peritoneal cavity, may result in peritonitis (see Chapter 19).

■ Signs and Symptoms

Sudden, severe, generalized abdominal pain occurs with localized tenderness at the site of the underlying problem. The pain tends to increase with any movement, and the individual often restricts breathing. Vomiting is common. Signs of dehydration and hypovolemia, including decreased skin turgor, dry buccal mucosa, pallor, low blood pressure, agitation, and tachycardia are present. Fever and leukocytosis occur as the inflammation and infection develop. Abdominal distention is common, and a rigid abdomen signals involvement of the parietal peritoneum. Decreased bowel sounds indicate the onset of paralytic ileus and secondary obstruction.

■ Treatment

Depending on the primary cause of the peritonitis, surgery is often required to correct the cause and drain sites of infection. Massive doses of antimicrobial drugs that are specific for the major causative organism, which is usually of enteric origin, are needed, as well as replacement of fluids and electrolytes. Nasogastric suction to relieve abdominal distention is often required, as is treatment to combat paralytic ileus, when appropriate.

The prognosis depends on the underlying cause and the rapidity of treatment.

THINK ABOUT   17-14

a. Explain why the characteristics of the pain differ with mechanical and functional obstruction.
b. Explain how each of the following conditions causes an intestinal obstruction: (1) intussusception; (2) adhesion; (3) inguinal hernia.
c. Explain: (1) how an obstruction can lead to bacterial peritonitis; (2) how peritonitis can lead to obstruction.
d. Explain the cause of hypovolemic shock with peritonitis.
e. What factors lead to metabolic acidosis in bacterial peritonitis?

CASE STUDY A

Gastroenteritis

Baby K., age 14 months, has vomiting and diarrhea and is crying continuously because of what appears to be severe abdominal pain. The suspected cause is gastroenteritis caused by

Staphylococcus aureus from milk custard that had not been properly stored.
1. Briefly describe how *S. aureus* in the custard could cause vomiting and diarrhea.
2. Describe the fluid and electrolyte imbalances that can be expected in Baby K.
3. What arterial blood gas levels would you expect to find in this child with gastroenteritis?
4. Describe the signs of dehydration that can be expected in a child.
5. Explain the process and factors involved by which a young child can quickly develop vascular collapse if vomiting and diarrhea are severe.
6. Explain why water alone would not be adequate treatment for the child.

CASE STUDY B

Peptic Ulcer and Peritonitis

Ms. X., age 76, has been admitted through the emergency department with severe generalized abdominal pain and vomiting. No significant findings were immediately evident to indicate a cause. Six hours later, Ms. X.'s blood pressure began to drop, and her pulse was rapid but thready. Exploratory abdominal surgery revealed a perforated gastric ulcer and peritonitis.
1. Describe the process by which an ulcer develops.
2. Suggest several possible factors contributing to ulcer formation.
3. Explain why peptic ulcer may not be diagnosed in an early stage of development.
4. Describe the process of perforation of an ulcer and the development of bacterial peritonitis.
5. Explain why Ms. X. showed signs of shock.
Following surgery, Ms. X. had no bowel sounds, and her abdomen was distended.
6. Describe how paralytic ileus could have developed.
Ms. X. was given antibiotics, intravenous fluids, and intravenous alimentation (total parenteral nutrition).
7. Explain the reason for each of these treatments.
8. Explain why older individuals may have difficulty in compensating for fluid and electrolyte imbalances.
9. List other potential complications of immobility for which Ms. X. is at risk during a prolonged recovery.

CASE STUDY C

Hepatitis B and Cirrhosis

J.B., age 35, has had chronic hepatitis B for 9 years. The origin of his acute infection was never ascertained.
1. Describe the pathophysiology of acute hepatitis B infection.
2. If J.B. had known about his exposure, could any treatment measures have been undertaken at the time?
3. Describe two signs of the preicteric stage and three signs of the icteric stage of acute hepatitis B infection.
4. What serum markers remain high when chronic hepatitis B is present?
5. Explain the circumstances under which J.B. could transmit

the virus (including the various stages of the disease [preicteric, icteric, and so on] as well as the mode of transmission).

6. Explain how cirrhosis develops from chronic hepatitis B.
7. Explain why the early stage of cirrhosis is relatively asymptomatic.

J.B.'s cirrhosis is now well advanced. He has developed ascites, edema in the legs and feet, and esophageal varices. His appetite is poor, he is fatigued, and he has frequent respiratory and skin infections. Jaundice is noticeable.

8. What factors predispose J.B. to each of the manifestations listed in the preceding?
9. If a cure for hepatitis B were discovered at this point, how would this affect J.B.'s prognosis?

J.B. has been admitted with hematemesis and shock resulting from ruptured esophageal varices.

10. Explain why each of the following events occur: (1) excessive bleeding from trauma; (2) increased serum ammonia levels; (3) hand-flapping tremors and confusion.

CASE STUDY D

Crohn's Disease

Mr. P.T., age 19, has had Crohn's disease, affecting the ileum and part of the jejunum, for 5 years and has had numerous exacerbations. Several members of his extended family have a history of Crohn's disease.

1. Describe the pathophysiology of Crohn's disease.
2. Suggest several possible exacerbating factors for Crohn's disease.
3. Describe the common signs of an exacerbation.
4. Explain how nutritional deficits may occur with Crohn's disease.
5. P.T. has delayed growth. (He is much shorter than his classmates.) Suggest several specific contributing factors to retarded growth in a young person.
6. P.T. has developed a fistula between the ileum and the bladder. Describe the effect of a fistula.

There is considerable risk of intestinal obstruction developing in P.T. at some point in the near future.

7. Explain how this obstruction could gradually form.
8. Suggest several manifestations, with the reason for each, of an acute obstruction in the ileum.
9. Describe the potential complications of an intestinal obstruction that is not treated promptly.

CASE STUDY E

Colon Cancer

This case study incorporates several general aspects of malignant tumors (refer to Chapter 20 if necessary). Not all details can be included, but the events provide an opportunity to integrate information.

Mrs. R.C., age 82, has a history of uterine cancer 12 years ago. A hysterectomy was performed at that time, followed by radiation (an implant of radioactive material). This was deemed successful. Vaginal bleeding developed 2 years later, and a tumor located between the vagina and bladder was treated with radiation and eradicated. Since that time, she has remained relatively healthy and led an active life.

Now, Mrs. R.C. has developed some abdominal discomfort, fatigue, and loss of energy, but tests (blood tests and ultrasound) failed to reveal any specific cause or abnormality. Continued pain and indigestion, combined with knowledge of her history, prompted a repeat of the tests 3 months later, again all negative.

1. Suggest possible reasons for negative tests.

Pain continued, and occasional vomiting developed as well as inability to eat a large meal. A weight loss of 30 pounds was evident. Other illness delayed further tests for several months. A colonoscopy uncovered a malignant tumor in the upper descending colon. At this time a small opening was prepared in the intestine to allow passage of semi-liquid foods.

2. List the signs indicating intestinal obstruction. Why have these signs been slow in developing?

Two months later during surgery, a colostomy was created and healing seemed to be satisfactory. Only a small amount of the tumor had been removed. The oncologist determined that radiation was not an option given the history and chemotherapy was not effective with this malignant cell.

3. Describe possible reasons why additional treatment would not be recommended in this case.

Following surgery, food intake improved and some weight gain was achieved. However a pulmonary embolus developed several weeks after surgery and was treated with anticoagulants.

4. List the factors contributing to a pulmonary embolus in this case.

A month later, the stoma began bleeding slightly and protruding. Slight rectal bleeding also developed. The stoma became very large, painful, and unmanageable. Surgery was performed to construct another stoma. Nevertheless, loose stools were evacuated from the rectum, indicating the tumor had invaded other parts of the intestine. Following this surgery, there was increasing weakness and abdominal pain with a general decline in health until her death 6 weeks later.

5. List the evidence indicating the spread of malignant cells.
6. Briefly discuss your impressions of the events in this case history.

CHAPTER SUMMARY

The digestive system is subject to frequent transient inflammatory or infectious conditions as well as chronic disorders that cause serious malnutrition and fluid-electrolyte imbalances. The liver and pancreas perform major metabolic functions in addition to their roles in the digestion and absorption of essential nutrients.

Upper Gastrointestinal Tract

- Many *infections of the oral cavity*, including herpes simplex virus, candidiasis, and periodontal disease, cause localized pain and interfere with food intake and nutrition.

- *Acute gastritis* or *gastroenteritis* can cause serious fluid and electrolyte imbalances in infants and elderly persons. Gastroenteritis is typically caused by infections by microorganisms, many entering the tract through the consumption of contaminated water and/or food.
- *Peptic ulcer* results from erosion of the mucosal barrier and is frequently associated with infection by *H. pylori*. Serious complications include hemorrhage and perforation.
- *Dumping syndrome* may develop following gastric resection with removal of the pyloric sphincter, allowing gastric contents to enter the small intestine at a rapid rate in concentrated form.

Liver and Pancreas

- *Cholelithiasis* refers to gallstone formation, commonly due to excess cholesterol in the bile. Severe colicky pain results when gallstones obstruct a bile duct.
- *Jaundice* or *hyperbilirubinemia* is a sign of a primary problem such as hemolytic anemia or liver disease.
- *Hepatitis* includes a group of viral infections of the liver that may be differentiated by the structure of the virus, the mode of transmission and incubation period, and ability to cause chronic disease or exist in a carrier state.
- *Cirrhosis* is the end result of extensive fibrosis in the liver, thus impairing many metabolic processes, such as storage and conversion of nutrients, production of clotting factors and plasma proteins, detoxification, and bile production.

- *Acute pancreatitis* involves autodigestion of the pancreas and surrounding tissue, resulting in severe pain, hemorrhage, shock, or peritonitis.

Lower Gastrointestinal Tract

- *Crohn's disease* and *ulcerative colitis* are two forms of chronic inflammatory bowel disease of unknown cause, characterized by recurrent diarrhea.
- Irritable bowel syndrome (IBS) is a complex gastrointestinal disorder characterized by abdominal pain and changing bowel habits. There are a number of types based on the causes and symptoms. Treatment is individualized due to the variety of symptoms and underlying causes.
- Acute *appendicitis* is caused by obstruction and infection. The increasing pressure may cause rupture and generalized peritonitis.
- *Colorectal carcinoma* is a common tumor, more difficult to diagnose at an early stage if located in the ascending or transverse colon. Obstruction in the rectum or sigmoid can be detected.
- *Intestinal obstruction*, if caused mechanically by a stricture or volvulus, causes severe colicky pain, marked bowel sounds, and vomiting. With obstruction due to *paralytic ileus*, severe steady pain results and bowel sounds are absent.
- *Peritonitis* resulting from a perforated ulcer or ruptured bladder may initially be termed chemical, but infection and bacterial peritonitis follow as intestinal bacteria leak out of the intestines. Severe generalized pain and abdominal rigidity are significant signs.

STUDY QUESTIONS

1. a. List the defense mechanisms that reduce the risk of infection in the oral cavity.
    b. State the locations of resident (normal) flora in the digestive tract.
    c. State the approximate pH of gastric secretions and two purposes served by this pH level.
2. a. Explain how the liver responds to high blood glucose levels.
    b. Describe six functions of the liver (include a variety of functions).
3. a. What is the major site of absorption of water and electrolytes?
    b. Which substances are absorbed primarily by active transport and which are absorbed by osmosis?
    c. Explain why tissue damage hinders active transport.
4. Describe the location and role of the parasympathetic nervous system in defecation.
5. a. Explain the purpose of the enterogastric reflex.
    b. Describe two results of an excessively rapid flow of chyme through the digestive tract.

6. a. Name the common electrolytes lost because of diarrhea.
    b. State the major effect on the body of sodium loss and potassium loss.
    c. State and explain what arterial blood gas levels may be expected in the presence of severe vomiting.
7. Define *steatorrhea* and explain several possible causes of this manifestation.
8. Explain several ways in which severe stress can affect the digestive tract.
9. Explain how an H_2 antagonist agent affects gastric function.
10. Explain how dysphagia may result from:
    a. stricture
    b. diverticulitis
11. Explain why hiatal hernia is aggravated by:
    a. intake of a large meal
    b. lying down after a meal
12. a. Explain several mechanisms by which intestinal infection can cause diarrhea.
    b. Explain how fluid balance and acid-base balance are altered by diarrhea.

13. a. Explain why peptic ulcers often do not heal quickly but tend to persist or recur.
    b. Describe the common differences between gastric ulcer and gastric cancer.
14. a. Define cholecystitis.
    b. List factors that predispose to cholelithiasis.
    c. Trace a gallstone on its path from a bile canaliculus to the duodenum and note the different possible effects caused by obstruction at various locations.
15. a. State a common cause of posthepatic jaundice and the significant change in serum bilirubin that occurs with it.
    b. Describe the common manifestations of acute hepatitis.
16. Describe how chronic hepatitis may affect liver tissue
17. a. Describe the three common types of cirrhosis and give one cause of each.
    b. State the rationale for each of the following signs of cirrhosis: nausea, abdominal pain (upper right quadrant), esophageal varices, and hepatic encephalopathy.
18. Describe possible obstructive effects of liver cancer.
19. Explain two causes of shock resulting from acute pancreatitis.
20. a. Explain why malnutrition may develop from Crohn's disease.
    b. Explain the process by which chronic bleeding may cause anemia.

c. Explain, using an example, how a fistula develops in patients with Crohn's disease.
    d. Compare the characteristics of diarrhea typical of Crohn's disease with that of ulcerative colitis.
21. List the various symptoms and possible causes of irritable bowel syndrome.
22. Describe the pathophysiology involved in the various stages of acute appendicitis.
23. a. Explain how a long-term, low-residue diet contributes to the development of diverticula.
    b. Explain how chronic diverticulitis can cause intestinal obstruction.
24. List the common early signs of colorectal cancer, relating each to a particular site.
25. Explain why the prognosis for colorectal cancer is relatively poor.
26. Explain how intestinal obstruction results from volvulus, paralytic ileus, and tumor.
27. Explain how hypovolemia develops with intestinal obstruction.
28. a. Explain how the peritoneal membranes may provide a defense in the early stage of acute appendicitis.
    b. Explain how the structure of the peritoneal membrane may be a disadvantage after the appendix ruptures.
    c. Explain how shock develops with acute peritonitis.

ADDITIONAL RESOURCES

Beers M, Berkow R: *The Merck Manual of Diagnosis and Therapy*, ed 18, Whitehouse Station, NJ, 2006, Merck Research Laboratories.
Centers for Disease Control and Prevention: Surveillance for Acute Viral Hepatitis—United States, 2006. *MMWR* 57(No. SS-2), 2008.
Heymann DL, Ed.: *Control of Communicable Diseases Manual*, ed 17, Washington, DC, 2004, American Public Health Association.
Kumar V, Abbas AK, Fausto M: *Robbins and Cotran Pathologic Basis of Disease*, ed 8, Philadelphia, 2007, Saunders.
Patton T, Thibodeau G: *Anatomy & Physiology*, ed 7, St. Louis, 2010, Mosby.

Web Sites
http://www.ccfa.org *Crohn's and Colitis Foundation of America*
http://www.cdc.gov/ncidod/diseases/hepatitis/index.htm *Viral hepatitis (Centers for Disease Control and Prevention)*

http://www.coloncancer.org *Johns Hopkins and hereditary colorectal cancer*
http://www.csaceliac.org *Celiac Sprue Association (gluten-free diets)*
http://www.digestive.niddk.nih.gov *National Institute of Diabetes and Digestive and Kidney Diseases*
http://www.fda.gov *U.S. Food and Drug Administration*
http://www.gastro.org *American Gastroenterological Association*
http://content.nejm.org *The New England Journal of Medicine*
http://www.mayoclinic.com/
http://www.nih.gov
http://www.ibsgroup.org/

Urinary System Disorders

CHAPTER OUTLINE

LEARNING OBJECTIVES

After studying this chapter, the student is expected to:

1. Compare the etiology, pathophysiology, and manifestations of cystitis and pyelonephritis.
2. Explain the development of acute poststreptococcal glomerulonephritis, its signs and symptoms, including laboratory tests and possible complications.
3. Describe the etiology and significant manifestations of nephrotic syndrome.
4. Explain the common signs and symptoms of urinary tract obstruction.
5. List common causes of urinary calculi.
6. Explain how hydronephrosis develops and its effects on the kidney.

7. Describe the incidence and early signs of adenocarcinoma of the kidney, bladder cancer, and Wilms' tumor.
8. Explain how nephrosclerosis affects: (a) the kidney, and (b) systemic blood pressure.
9. Describe the etiology, usual age at onset, manifestations, and outcome of adult polycystic disease.
10. Compare acute and chronic renal failure with regard to common causes, pathophysiology, signs and symptoms, and possible complications.
11. Explain how peritoneal dialysis or hemodialysis substitutes for a nonfunctioning kidney, including limitations of the therapy.

KEY TERMS

anasarca	dysuria	oliguria	renal colic
anuria	frequency	osteodystrophy	retroperitoneally
azotemia	glucosuria	polyuria	ultrafiltration
calculi	hematuria	proteinuria	urgency
dialysate	nocturia	pyuria	

Review of the Urinary System

The functions of the urinary system are:
- Removal of metabolic wastes (nitrogenous and acidic)
- Removal of hormones, drugs, and other foreign material from the body
- Regulation of water, electrolytes, and acid-base balance in the body
- Secretion of erythropoietin
- Activation of vitamin D
- Regulation of blood pressure through the renin-angiotensin-aldosterone system

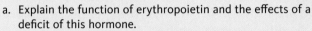

THINK ABOUT 18-1

a. Explain the function of erythropoietin and the effects of a deficit of this hormone.
b. Explain the function vitamin D and the possible effects of a deficit of this vitamin.

Structures and Anatomy

Kidneys

The two kidneys are bean-shaped structures, each the size of a fist, located behind the peritoneum (that is, retroperitoneally) on the posterior abdominal wall. The kidneys are covered by a fibrous *capsule* and are embedded in fat, with the superior portion also protected by the lower ribs (Fig. 18-1).

Inside each kidney is the *cortex*, or outer layer, in which the majority of the glomeruli are located, and the *medulla*, or inner section of tissue, which consists primarily of the tubules and collecting ducts. Inside the medulla lie the *renal pelvis* and calyces, through which urine flows into the ureter (Fig. 18-2).

Each kidney consists of over a million *nephrons*, the functional units of the kidney (Fig. 18-3). The renal corpuscle consists of Bowman's capsule (glomerular

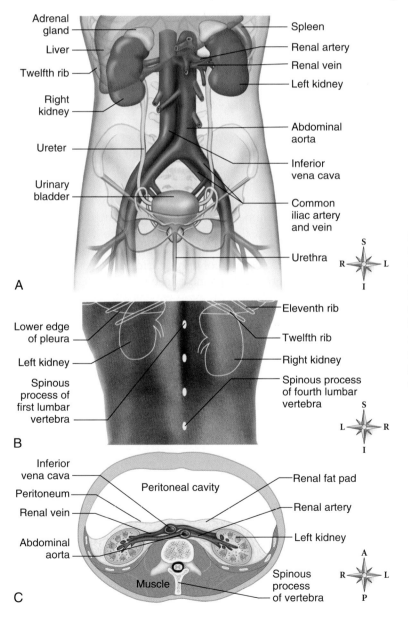

FIGURE 18-1 **Location of Urinary System Organs A,** Anterior view of the urinary organs with the peritoneum and visceral organs removed. **B,** Surface markings of the kidneys, eleventh and twelfth ribs, spinous processes of L1 to L4, and lower edge of the pleura (posterior view). **C,** Horizontal (transverse) section of the abdomen showing the retroperitoneal position of the kidneys. (**A,** From *Barbara Cousins.* **B,** *From Abrahams P, Marks S, Hutchings R:* McMinn's Color Atlas of Human Anatomy, *ed 5, Philadelphia, 2003, Mosby,* **C:** *From Patton KT, Thibodeau GA:* Anatomy & Physiology, *ed 8, St. Louis, 2013, Mosby.*)

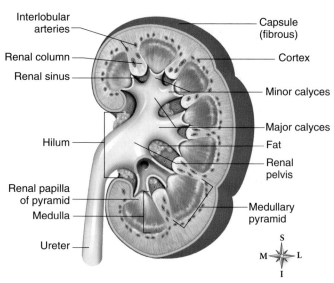

FIGURE 18-2 Internal Structure of the Kidney Coronal section of the right kidney in an artist's rendering. *(Adapted from Brundage DJ: Renal Disorders. Mosby's Clinical Nursing Series, St. Louis, 1992, Mosby.)*

TABLE 18-1	Composition of Blood, Filtrate, and Urine		
Substance	Blood	Filtrate	Urine
Water (L)	180	180	1.4
Cells	Yes	No	No
Glucose (mg/L)	1000	1000	0
Protein (mg/L)	40,000	0-trace	0-trace
Urea (mg/L)	260	260	18,000
Na^+ (mEq/L)	142	142	128
K^+ (mEq/L)	5	5	60
HCO_3^- (mEq/L)	28	28	14

capsule), which is the blind end of the proximal convoluted tubule. This capsule surrounds a network of capillaries, called the glomerulus or glomerular capillaries. These form the filtration unit for the blood.

During *filtration,* a large volume of fluid, including wastes, nutrients, electrolytes, and other dissolved substances, passes from the blood into the tubule. Cells and protein remain in the blood (Table 18-1). When the filtration pressure increases, more filtrate forms, and more urine is produced. The filtrate flows into the *tubules.* The tubule consists of three parts, the proximal convoluted tubule, the loop of Henle, and the distal convoluted tubule. Here *reabsorption* of essential nutrients, water, and electrolytes takes place and *secretion* of certain wastes and electrolytes occurs. The collecting ducts transport the urine to the renal pelvis.

Reabsorption is one process that takes place in the tubules. In the proximal convoluted tubule, most of the water is reabsorbed into the blood in the peritubular

capillaries, along with glucose and other nutrients and some electrolytes. Reabsorption of nutrients and electrolytes involves the use of *active transport* (e.g., sodium ions), which requires carrier molecules and an energy source. Sodium absorption may be linked to the *cotransport* of other molecules (e.g., glucose or amino acids with Na^+). Anions such as chloride may be reabsorbed by electrochemical gradient or by cotransport with Na^+. If a substance such as glucose is present in excessive amounts in the filtrate, there are insufficient carrier molecules in the tubules for complete reabsorption into the blood in the peritubular capillaries. Therefore the excess glucose is present in the urine. This limit on reabsorption is called the *transport* or *tubular* maximum (e.g., approximately 310 mg/min for glucose). Thus, persistent glucosuria is an indication of hyperglycemia associated with diabetes mellitus.

Water is reabsorbed by *osmosis.* As the filtrate progresses through the loop of Henle and the distal convoluted tubule, electrolytes and water are adjusted to the body's current needs.

Hormones control the reabsorption of fluid and electrolytes (see Chapters 2 and 16):
- Antidiuretic hormone (ADH) from the posterior pituitary controls the reabsorption of water by altering the permeability of the distal convoluted tubule and collecting duct.
- Aldosterone, secreted by the adrenal cortex, controls sodium reabsorption and water by exchanging sodium ions for potassium or hydrogen ions in the distal convoluted tubule.
- Atrial natriuretic hormone from the heart is the third hormone controlling fluid balance by reducing sodium and fluid reabsorption in the kidneys.

Concurrently the acid-base balance of the blood is maintained, with removal of excess acids and replacement of buffers such as bicarbonate (see Chapter 2).

Active secretion of some wastes and drugs from the blood into the filtrate also occurs in the distal tubule (Fig. 18-4).

THINK ABOUT 18-2

Which of the following substances does the body normally retain? Which does it normally excrete? (1) glucose, (2) sodium ions, (3) bicarbonate ions, (4) acids

The organization of the nephrons within a kidney is complex and must be maintained for effective renal function. The blood vessels and the collecting tubules and ducts for the filtrate must be functionally integrated to fulfill the purpose of the system. Scar tissue can interfere with blood or filtrate flow and thus can lead to secondary damage and progressive destruction of the kidney.

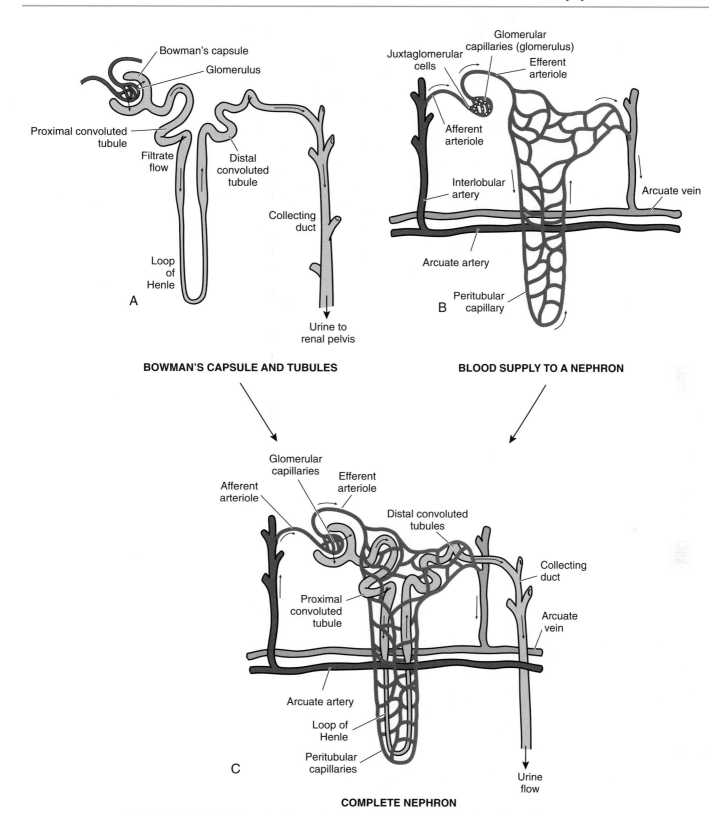

BOWMAN'S CAPSULE AND TUBULES

BLOOD SUPPLY TO A NEPHRON

COMPLETE NEPHRON

FIGURE 18-3 **The Nephron A,** Glomerulus and tubules. **B,** Blood supply to the nephron. **C,** Complete nephron.

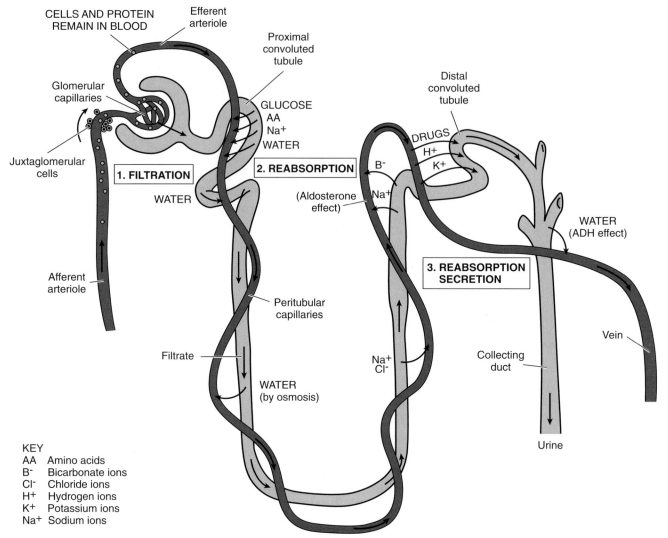

FIGURE 18-4 Schematic illustration of formation of urine.

Renal Arteries and Veins

A large amount of blood enters and leaves the kidney at the hilum through the renal artery and vein. From 20% to 25% of the cardiac output enters the renal arteries from the aorta; thus the kidneys are processing a large volume of blood at any given time. Each renal artery passes through the renal pelvis, dividing several times during its passage (see Fig. 18-2). *No anastomoses* or junctions exist between the interlobar and arcuate arteries, meaning that no alternative blood supply is available to a lobe of the kidney that is deprived of its blood supply, perhaps by an embolus (e.g., a blood clot). Any obstruction to blood flow would therefore cause that particular lobe to undergo necrosis and infarction.

The interlobar arteries divide several times, eventually forming the *afferent arterioles,* which supply the *glomerular capillaries* (see Fig. 18-3). The arrangement of blood vessels in the kidney is unique because the blood from the glomerular capillaries then flows into another arteriole, the *efferent arteriole,* and then into a second capillary network, the *peritubular capillaries* or *vasa recta.*

Therefore there are two arterioles and two sets of capillaries included in each nephron.

This blood supply also provides nourishment for the renal tissues. Note that the kidney tubules are last to receive nutrients.

To summarize the blood flow: renal artery → interlobar artery → arcuate artery → interlobular artery → afferent arteriole → glomerular capillaries → efferent arteriole → peritubular capillaries → interlobular vein → arcuate vein → interlobar vein → renal vein. The names of the blood vessels match the structures.

THINK ABOUT   18-3

a. Trace the movement of a glucose molecule in the renal artery through the kidney and into the renal vein, naming each structure and process in sequence.

b. Trace the progress of an acid waste from the distal convoluted tubule to the point of excretion.

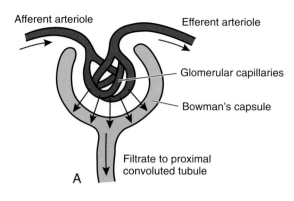

NORMAL FILTRATION

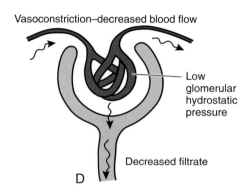

AFFERENT ARTERIOLE: DILATION

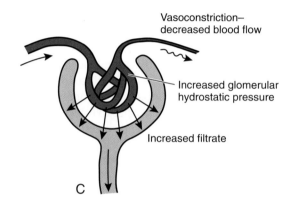

EFFERENT ARTERIOLE: CONSTRICTION

AFFERENT ARTERIOLE: CONSTRICTION

FIGURE 18-5 **Control of Glomerular Filtration Rate (GFR) A,** Normal filtration. **B,** Afferent arteriole: dilation. **C,** Efferent arteriole: constriction. **D,** Afferent arteriole: constriction.

The purpose of the dual arterioles is to control the pressure in the glomerular capillaries and consequently the glomerular filtration pressure. This pressure determines the glomerular filtration rate (GFR). By constricting or dilating the arterioles, the amount of blood in the glomerular capillaries is adjusted, and filtration is normally maintained regardless of fluctuations in the systemic blood pressure. For instance, if the afferent arteriole is dilated and the efferent arteriole is constricted, hydrostatic pressure in the glomerular capillaries will increase, and GFR will increase (Fig. 18-5).

The degree of constriction in the arterioles is controlled primarily by three factors, local *autoregulation,* the sympathetic nervous system, and the renin-angiotensin mechanism.

1. Autoregulation refers to the small, local reflex adjustments in the diameter of the arterioles that are made in response to minor changes in blood flow in the kidneys. This adjustment maintains the normal filtration rate.

2. The sympathetic nervous system (SNS) increases vasoconstriction in both arterioles when stimulated.

3. Renin is secreted by the juxtaglomerular cells in the kidney when blood flow in the afferent arteriole is

reduced for any reason (see Fig. 18-5). Through a series of enzyme reactions, renin acts on the plasma protein angiotensinogen to produce angiotensin I and as the blood passes through the lung, angiotensin converting enzyme (ACE) converts angiotensin I to angiotensin II, which is a powerful systemic vasoconstrictor.

If blood flow in the kidney is seriously impaired, as it is when blood pressure drops, both the SNS and the renin-angiotensin mechanism are activated to restore blood pressure and blood flow to vital areas.

THINK ABOUT   18-4

a. Explain the effect on hydrostatic (blood) pressure within the glomerular capillaries and on filtration if the afferent arteriole is severely constricted.

b. Explain the effect of prolonged severe vasoconstriction on the renal tissue.

c. Explain the effect of renin on filtration.

d. Explain the change in filtration if excess glucose is present in the blood entering the kidney.

Blood pressure is closely related to kidney function, and frequently it is elevated with renal disease. When the blood flow or blood pressure in the afferent arteriole decreases for *any* reason, the *renin-angiotensin-aldosterone* triad is stimulated. Angiotensin not only causes systemic vasoconstriction, it also stimulates the secretion of aldosterone. This hormone increases the reabsorption of sodium and water to increase blood volume, thus increasing blood pressure. Serum renin levels can determine whether this mechanism is a factor in hypertension (high blood pressure), in which case renin-blocking drugs (beta-adrenergic blocking drugs) can be prescribed (see Chapter 12).

When the *filtrate* has been processed in the tubules and collecting ducts, it is considered to be *urine*. Urine is transported through the collecting ducts to the renal calyces and pelvis and then into the ureters, where peristaltic movements assist its flow to the urinary bladder. The renal pelvis, calyces, ureters, and bladder are lined with transitional epithelium that is not permeable to water and can resist the irritation of constant contact with urine.

The *bladder* is composed of smooth muscle that falls in rugae, or folds, to form an expandable sac. It is located retroperitoneally in the pelvic cavity. The bladder has openings for the two ureters to bring urine in and an outlet for the urethra through which urine flows out of the body. The triangular section outlined by these three openings is called the trigone (see Fig. 18-1).

The female *urethra* is 3 to 4 cm long. It is relatively short and wide and opens onto the perineum anterior to the vagina and anus. The proximity of the urethra to these two sources promotes infection of the bladder in women.

The male urethra is about 20 cm long and passes through the penis. At the base of the male bladder is the prostate gland, which plays a role in semen production and frequently is hypertrophied in older men, obstructing urine flow (see Chapter 19 for reproductive disorders). During orgasm in the male, a sphincter closes off the flow of urine and semen is ejaculated through the urethra.

The mucosa lining the urinary tract is continuous through the urethra, bladder, and ureter to the pelvis of the kidney. Organisms can easily enter the system through the urethra, and this continuous mucosa facilitates the spread of infection through the urinary tract (an ascending infection).

Micturition (urination, voiding) occurs when a reflex is stimulated by increased pressure as the bladder distends. The reflex is transmitted by parasympathetic nerves extending to the sacral spinal cord. If the time is appropriate, under voluntary control, the external and internal sphincters of the bladder and the pelvic diaphragm relax while the bladder muscle contracts, emptying the bladder.

Incontinence and Retention

Incontinence, or the loss of voluntary control of the bladder, has many causes. Young children must learn voluntary control as the nervous system matures. *Enuresis* defines involuntary urination by a child after age 4 to 5, when bladder control can be expected. Most children have nocturnal enuresis only. The majority of cases appear to be related to factors such as a developmental delay, sleep pattern, or psychosocial aspects rather than to a physical defect. *Stress incontinence* occurs when increased intra-abdominal pressure forces urine through the sphincter. This can occur with coughing, lifting, or laughing, but occurs more frequently in women after the urogenital diaphragm has become weakened by multiple pregnancies or age. *Overflow incontinence* results from an incompetent bladder sphincter. In the elderly, a weakened detrusor muscle may prevent complete emptying of the bladder, leading to frequent emptying and incontinence. Spinal cord injuries or brain damage frequently cause a neurogenic bladder, which may be spastic or flaccid, due to interference with central nervous system (CNS) and autonomic nervous system control of the bladder emptying.

Retention is an inability to empty the bladder. It may be accompanied by overflow incontinence. Note that a spinal cord injury at the sacral level blocks the micturition reflex, resulting in retention of urine or failure to void. Retention also may occur after anesthesia, either general or spinal. Inability to control urine flow may be managed by wearing pads or briefs that contain the urine.

A *catheter* is a tube inserted in the urethra that drains urine from the bladder to a collecting bag outside the body. Catheters are common sources of infection in the urinary tract because they are irritating to the tissue and, when inserted, may be a means of introducing bacteria directly into the bladder if sterile technique is not used. Catheters prevent kidney damage due to backup of urine, collect urine, and prevent skin breakdown in the incontinent client.

THINK ABOUT 18-5

Locate the urinary bladder relative to the uterus and rectum in a woman. Briefly explain two possible implications of this location.

Diagnostic Tests

Urinalysis

The constituents and characteristics of urine may vary with dietary intake, drugs, and the care with which a specimen is handled. Urine normally is clear and straw-colored and has a mild odor. Urine pH is in the range of 4.5 to 8.0. The following lists offer general guidelines to common abnormalities noted in freshly voided specimens. An "old" specimen will not provide accurate information. See the inside front cover of this book for normal values.

Appearance
- Cloudy—may indicate the presence of large amounts of protein, blood cells, or bacteria and pus
- Dark color—may indicate hematuria (blood), excessive bilirubin content, or highly concentrated urine
- Unpleasant or unusual odor—may indicate infection or result from certain dietary components or medications

Abnormal Constituents (Present in Significant Quantities)

- Blood (hematuria)—small (*microscopic*) amounts of blood are often associated with infection, inflammation, or tumors in the urinary tract; large numbers of red blood cells (*gross* hematuria) indicate increased glomerular permeability or hemorrhage in the tract
- Protein (proteinuria, albuminuria)—indicates the leakage of albumin or mixed plasma proteins into the filtrate owing to inflammation and increased glomerular permeability
- Bacteria (bacteriuria) and pus (pyuria)—indicate infection in the urinary tract (Fig. 18-6*A*)
- Urinary *casts* (microscopic-sized molds of the tubules, consisting of one or more cells, bacteria, protein, and so on)—indicate inflammation of the kidney tubules (see Fig. 18-6*B*)
- Specific gravity indicates the ability of the tubules to concentrate the urine; a very low specific gravity (dilute urine) usually is related to renal failure (assuming normal hydration)
- Glucose and ketones (ketoacids) are found in the urine when diabetes mellitus is not well controlled (see Chapter 16)

> **THINK ABOUT 18-6**
> a. Explain the presence of the abnormal constituents of urine.
> b. Explain why hematuria and proteinuria reflect a glomerular problem rather than a tubular problem in the kidney.

Blood Tests

Like most other diseases, urinary tract disorders produce abnormalities that can be detected by various blood tests. Some of the more commonly used tests and implications are described here.

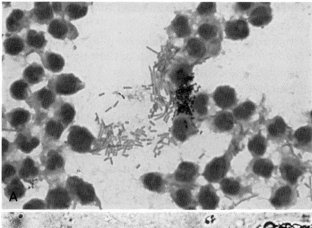
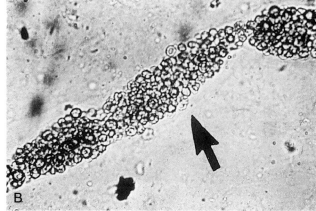
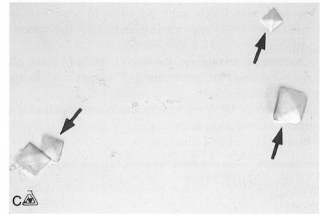

FIGURE 18-6 **A,** Urinalysis—smear shows infection with heavy purulence and presence of gram-negative and gram-positive organisms (*E. coli* and *Enterococcus faecalis*) (density of microbes 10^5/mL urine). **B,** Urinalysis—red blood cell cast. **C,** Urinalysis—calcium oxalate crystals in the urine. (**A,** *From Mahon CR, Manuselis G:* Textbook of Diagnostic Microbiology, *ed 2, Philadelphia, 2000, Saunders.* **B** *and* **C** *from Stepp CA, Woods M:* Laboratory Procedures for Medical Office Personnel, *Philadelphia, 1998, Saunders.*)

- Elevated serum urea (blood urea nitrogen [BUN]) and serum creatinine—indicate failure to excrete nitrogen wastes (resulting from protein metabolism) due to decreased GFR
- Metabolic acidosis (decreased serum pH and decreased serum bicarbonate)—indicates decreased

GFR and failure of the tubules to control acid-base balance (see Chapter 2)

- Anemia (low hemoglobin level)—indicates decreased erythropoietin secretion and/or bone marrow depression, due to accumulated wastes
- Electrolytes—depend on the related fluid balance: that is, retention of fluid if GFR is decreased may result in a dilution effect, and laboratory values are therefore not a true reflection of renal status; however, abnormal levels may still cause clinical effects and require monitoring and treatment
- Antibody level—antistreptolysin O (ASO) or antistreptokinase (ASK) titers are used for diagnosis of poststreptococcal glomerulonephritis
- Renin levels—indicate a cause of hypertension

Other Tests

- Culture and sensitivity studies on urine specimens are used to identify the causative organism and select drug treatment when infection is suspected (see Chapter 6).
- Clearance tests, such as creatinine or insulin clearance, or radioisotope studies are used to assess GFR.
- Radiologic tests, such as radionuclide imaging, angiography, ultrasound, computed tomography (CT), magnetic resonance imaging (MRI), and intravenous pyelography (IVP), may be used to visualize the structures and any abnormalities in the urinary system (see Ready Reference 5).
- Cystoscopy visualizes the lower urinary tract and may be used in performing a biopsy or remove kidney stones.
- Biopsy may be used to acquire tissue specimens to allow microscopic examination of suspicious lesions in the bladder or kidney.

> **THINK ABOUT 18-7**
>
> What is the normal pH range for the blood and urine? What serum and urine pH would indicate that acidosis had developed?

Diuretic Drugs

Diuretics, commonly referred to as "water pills," are used to remove excess sodium ions and water from the body, therefore increasing the excretion of water through the kidneys and urinary output. In turn, this reduces fluid volume in the tissues (edema) and blood. They are prescribed for many disorders other than renal disease, including hypertension, edema, congestive heart failure, liver disease, and pulmonary edema (see Chapter 12).

There are several mechanisms by which urine volume can be increased. A few examples of diuretic drugs are listed in Table 18-2. The most commonly used drug group inhibits sodium chloride reabsorption in the tubules. Examples of this group include hydrochlorothiazide (Hydro Diuril), a mild diuretic, and furosemide (Lasix), which is more potent. Hydrochlorothiazide is useful because it has an additional antihypertensive action, the mechanism for which is unknown. The major side effect of these drugs is excessive loss of electrolytes, which may cause muscle weakness or cardiac arrhythmias. Because these drugs may cause marked loss of potassium, patients may require dietary supplements such as bananas or replacement by potassium chloride tablets. Another group of diuretics, the potassium-sparing type (e.g., spironolactone [Aldactone]), may be given in combination with thiazides to minimize the risk of *hyperkalemia or hypokalemia* (high or low serum potassium levels). Many combinations of diuretics with other drugs, such as hydrochlorothiazide/propranolol or hydrochlorothiazide/quinapril, are available to treat hypertension or heart failure.

These drugs are usually administered in the morning because they often cause urinary frequency for a period of time (the need to urinate often). This may limit other morning activities and appointments. Patients taking diuretics should be observed for dizziness or *orthostatic hypotension* when moving from a supine to an upright position. Many individuals also have xerostomia, or dry mouth, with increased risk of dental caries.

TABLE 18-2 Examples of Diuretic Drugs

Name of Drug	Action	Use
hydrochlorothiazide (Hydro DIURIL)	Inhibits reabsorption of Na^+ and water in distal tubule (thiazide type)	Increase excretion of fluid in hypertension, CHF, edema
furosemide (Lasix)	Decreases reabsorption of Na^+ and water in the proximal and distal tubules and the loop of Henle (a loop diuretic)	Reduce body fluids in hypertension, CHF, edema, renal disease, liver disease
spironolactone (Aldactone)	Aldosterone antagonist, blocks reabsorption of Na^+ and K^+ in distal tubule (potassium-sparing diuretic)	Decrease Na^+ and water in body, but conserve K^+ in CHF, hypertension, liver disease
acetazolamide (Diamox)	Carbonic anhydrase inhibitor blocks reabsorption of Na^+ and secretion of H^+	Reduce fluids in CHF, glaucoma
mannitol (intravenous)	Increases osmotic pressure and water in the filtrate, reduces Na^+ absorption (osmotic diuretic)	Cerebral edema, glaucoma

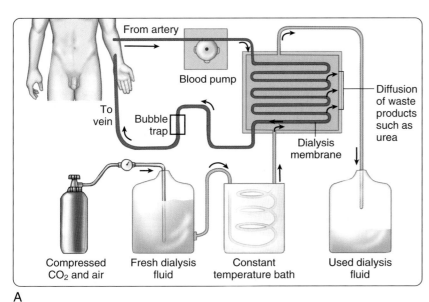

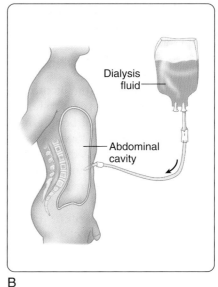

A

B

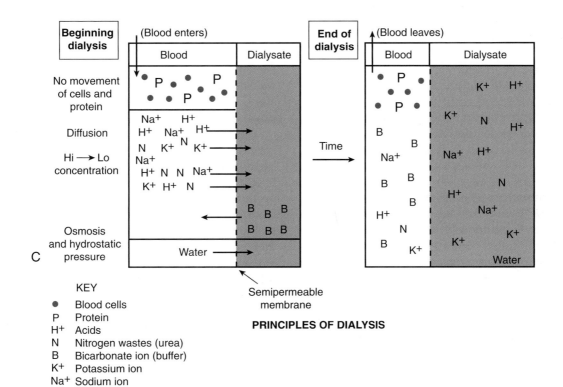

KEY

● Blood cells
P Protein
H⁺ Acids
N Nitrogen wastes (urea)
B Bicarbonate ion (buffer)
K⁺ Potassium ion
Na⁺ Sodium ion

PRINCIPLES OF DIALYSIS

FIGURE 18-7   **A,** Hemodialysis. **B,** Continuous ambulatory peritoneal dialysis (CAPD). **C,** Principles of dialysis. *(A and B From Patton KT, Thibodeau GA:* Anatomy & Physiology, *ed 8, St. Louis, 2013, Mosby)*

Dialysis

Dialysis provides an "artificial kidney," which can be used to sustain life after the kidneys fail. (There is considerable reserve in the renal system; an individual can function normally with half of one kidney.) Dialysis is used to treat someone who has acute renal failure until the primary problem has been reversed, or it can be used for patients in end-stage renal failure, perhaps until a transplant becomes available. In people with

renal transplants, it may be required if rejection occurs or between transplants (see Chapter 7 for transplants). Dialysis is a demanding procedure for both the patient and the family. Diet, particularly protein and electrolytes, and also fluid intake are severely restricted.

There are two forms of dialysis, peritoneal dialysis and hemodialysis (Fig. 18-7). *Hemodialysis* is provided in a hospital, dialysis center, or at home with special equipment and training. During the procedure, the patient's blood moves from an implanted shunt or catheter in an artery, often in the arm, through a tube to a machine where the exchange of wastes, fluid, and electrolytes takes place. A semipermeable membrane separates the patient's blood from the dialysis fluid (dialysate), and the constituents move between the two compartments. For example, wastes move from blood to the dialysate while bicarbonate ion moves into the blood from the dialysate. Blood cells and protein remain in the blood, unable to pass through the semipermeable membrane. Movement occurs by ultrafiltration, diffusion (by a concentration gradient), and osmosis. After the exchange has been completed, the blood is returned to the patient's vein. Heparin or another anticoagulant is administered to prevent clotting, requiring monitoring of blood-clotting times.

Hemodialysis is usually required three times a week, each session lasting about 3 to 4 hours. The patient may feel uncomfortable during the session because fluid and electrolyte balances change quickly, but usually he or she feels much better after the treatment. The feeling of well-being then dissipates gradually as wastes accumulate before the next treatment.

Dialysis has potential complications. The shunt may become infected, or blood clots may form. Eventually the blood vessels involved at the shunt become sclerosed or damaged, and a new site must be selected. Patients on dialysis have an increased risk of infection by the hepatitis B or C viruses or human immunodeficiency virus.

Peritoneal dialysis can be administered in a dialysis unit or at home. It may be done at night while the patient sleeps or continuously while the patient is ambulatory (this is called continuous ambulatory peritoneal dialysis). In this procedure, the peritoneal membrane, which is very large in surface area, thin, and highly vascular, serves as the semipermeable membrane. A catheter with entry and exit points is implanted in the peritoneal cavity. The dialyzing fluid is instilled through the catheter into the cavity and remains there, allowing the exchange of wastes and electrolytes to occur by diffusion and osmosis. Then the dialysate is drained from the cavity by gravity into a container. This process requires more time than hemodialysis. However, the more continuous exchange process prevents excessive and sudden changes in fluid and electrolyte levels in the body, and the components of a dialysis solution can be adapted to individual needs.

The major complication of peritoneal dialysis is infection resulting in peritonitis. Newer methods under investigation make use of charcoal absorbents and ultrafiltration techniques.

Prophylactic antibiotics are given with either form of dialysis whenever there is a risk of transient bacteremia; for example, with any invasive procedure or tissue trauma. Any additional problem occurring in the patient, such as infection, may also alter dialysis requirements.

Caution is required with many drugs because toxic levels can build up in the blood.

THINK ABOUT 18-8

Explain why a dialysis solution would initially be low in urea but high in bicarbonate content.

Disorders of the Urinary System

Urinary Tract Infections

Urinary tract infections (UTIs) are extremely common. It is estimated that 6 million Americans are affected annually. Urine generally provides an excellent medium for growth of microorganisms. Cystitis and urethritis are considered infections of the lower urinary tract, whereas pyelonephritis is an upper tract infection (Fig. 18-8). Most infections are *ascending,* arising from organisms in the perineal area and traveling along the *continuous mucosa* in the urinary tract to the bladder and then along the ureters to the kidneys. Occasionally pyelonephritis results from a blood-borne infection.

The common causative organism is *Escherichia coli,* which is one of the resident flora of the intestine (approximately 85%). The virulent forms of *E. coli* can adhere to the mucosa of the bladder by means of fimbriae or pili, and therefore are not washed out when the bladder empties. Other organisms associated with UTIs include *Klebsiella, Proteus, Enterobacter, Citrobacter, Serratia, Pseudomonas, Enterococcus,* coagulase negative *Staphylococcus, Chlamydia,* and *Mycoplasma.* In men, urethritis and prostatitis may accompany lower tract infections.

■ *Etiology*

Women are anatomically more vulnerable to infection than men because of the shortness and width of the urethra, its proximity to the anus, and the frequent irritation to the tissues. The irritation may be caused by sexual activity, baths, and the use of some feminine hygiene products. Improper hygiene practices during defecation or menstruation also increase risk.

Older men with prostatic hypertrophy and retention of urine frequently develop infection. Because the male reproductive tract shares some of the structures of the urinary tract, any infection of the prostate or testes is likely to extend to the urinary structures.

Congenital abnormalities are a common cause of infection in children, particularly where obstructions to flow or reflux are present. The elderly are at increased risk because of the tendency toward incomplete emptying, reduced fluid intake, impaired blood supply to the bladder, and immobility.

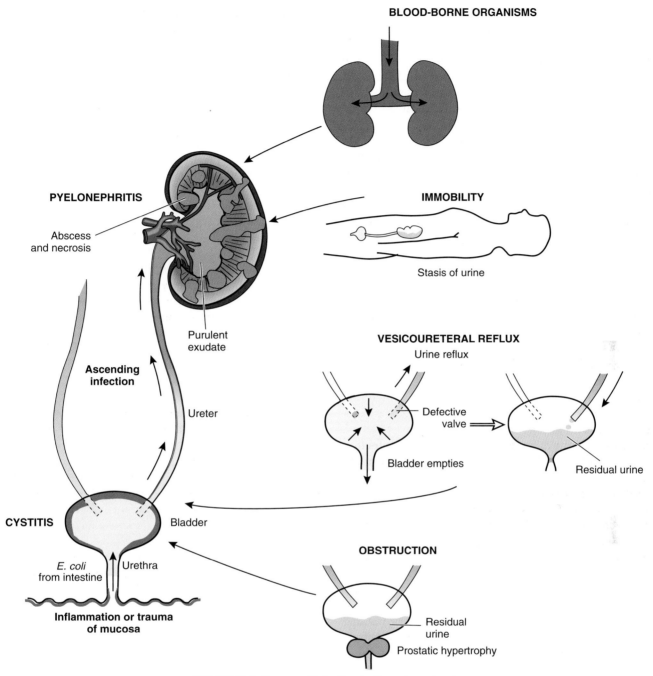

BLOOD-BORNE ORGANISMS

PYELONEPHRITIS

Abscess
and necrosis

Purulent
exudate

**Ascending
infection**

Ureter

CYSTITIS   Bladder

E. coli   Urethra
from intestine

**Inflammation or trauma
of mucosa**

IMMOBILITY

Stasis of urine

VESICOURETERAL REFLUX
Urine reflux

Defective
valve

Bladder empties

Residual urine

OBSTRUCTION

Residual
urine

Prostatic hypertrophy

FIGURE 18-8 Causes of infection in the urinary tract.

Common predisposing factors for UTIs in both men and women include incontinence with incomplete emptying of the bladder, retention of urine in the bladder, and any obstruction to urine flow, which tends to result in growth of organisms because bacteria are not promptly flushed out of the bladder by voiding. Pregnancy, scar tissue, and renal calculi (kidney stones) all contribute to infection because the urine and any contaminants do not flow freely through and out of the system. Infection may also result from decreased host resistance present with immunosuppression or diabetes mellitus (vascular impairment and glucosuria). Direct

contamination of the urethra and bladder may result from fecal incontinence. As mentioned, instruments or catheters may directly introduce bacteria into the bladder and frequently traumatize the bladder wall, breaking the barrier to infection.

THINK ABOUT   18-9

a. List several factors that would predispose a pregnant woman with diabetes to cystitis.

b. Why does male anatomy make it likely that a reproductive system infection may extend into the urinary system?

Cystitis and Urethritis

▪ *Pathophysiology*

With cystitis, the bladder wall and with urethritis, the urethra are inflamed, red, and swollen, and in some cases, ulcerated. The bladder wall is irritated and hyperreactive and bladder capacity is usually reduced.

▪ *Signs and Symptoms*

In some cases, the manifestations are very mild and may be unnoticed.

- Pain is common in the lower abdomen.
- Dysuria (painful urination), urgency (need to void immediately), frequency (short intervals between voiding), and nocturia (need for urination during sleep period) occur as the inflamed bladder wall is irritated by urine.
- Systemic signs of infection may be present (fever, malaise, nausea, and leukocytosis).
- The urine often appears cloudy and has an unusual odor.
- Urinalysis indicates bacteriuria (the presence of bacteria in the urine), pyuria, and microscopic hematuria (see Fig. 18-6A).

Pyelonephritis

▪ *Pathophysiology*

One or both kidneys may be involved. The infection extends from the ureter into the kidney, involving the renal pelvis and medullary tissue (tubules and interstitial tissue). Purulent exudate fills the kidney pelvis and calyces, and the medulla is inflamed. Abscesses and necrosis can be seen in the medulla and may extend through the cortex to the surface of the capsule. If the infection is severe, the exudate can compress the renal artery and vein and obstruct urine flow to the ureter. Bilateral obstruction is likely to result in acute renal failure (see Fig. 18-15C).

Recurrent or chronic infection can lead to fibrous scar tissue forming over a calyx, leading to loss of tubule function and hydronephrosis. If severe and bilateral, it can eventually cause chronic renal failure.

▪ *Signs and Symptoms*

- The signs of cystitis, such as dysuria, are also present, because infection is present in both kidneys and bladder.
- Pain associated with renal disease is usually a dull aching pain in the lower back or *flank* area, resulting from inflammation that stretches the renal capsule.
- Systemic signs are usually more marked in pyelonephritis.
- Urinalysis results are similar to those for cystitis except that *urinary casts*, consisting of leukocytes or renal epithelial cells, are present, reflecting the involvement of the renal *tubules*.

▪ *Treatment*

UTIs are treated promptly with antibacterial drugs such as trimethoprim-sulfamethoxazole (Bactrim, Cotrim, Septra), nitrofurantoin (Furadantin), cephalosporins (Keflex, Duricef), carbapenems (Doribax), amoxicillin and Fosfomycin which is prescribed for pregnant women. The patient is encouraged to substantially increase fluid intake. In some cases pockets of infection persist in the bladder. Therefore, it is essential to follow up on the course of antibiotics with *urinalysis* 4 to 6 weeks after the course of drugs has been completed, to ensure that the infection has been totally eradicated. Chronic cystitis tends to be asymptomatic and therefore can persist and spread to the kidneys, where it causes more damage.

The infection tends to recur unless the predisposing factors are removed. Chronic pyelonephritis often causes insidious damage, with areas of obstructive scar tissue that promote continued infection and eventually cause chronic renal failure.

Cranberry juice may be recommended as a prophylactic measure. The tannin content appears to reduce the capability of *E. coli* to adhere to the bladder mucosa.

THINK ABOUT   18-10

List the signs and symptoms of pyelonephritis that indicate that *infection* is present and mark those indicating that *kidney involvement* (local or systemic) exists.

Inflammatory Disorders

Glomerulonephritis (Acute Poststreptococcal Glomerulonephritis)

There are many forms of glomerulonephritis. A representative form of glomerular or nephritic disease is acute poststreptococcal glomerulonephritis (APSGN), which follows streptococcal infection with certain strains of group A beta-hemolytic *Streptococcus*. These infections usually originate as upper respiratory infections, middle ear infections, or "strep throat." Certain strains of *Staphylococcus* are occasionally responsible for initiating the immune disorder in the kidney.

Acute glomerulonephritis develops 10 days to 2 weeks after the antecedent infection. Primarily APSGN affects children between the ages of 3 and 7 years, especially boys.

▪ *Pathophysiology*

The antistreptococcal antibodies, formed as usual from the earlier streptococcal infection, create an antigen-antibody complex (type III hypersensitivity reaction) that lodges in the glomerular capillaries, activates the complement system to cause an inflammatory response

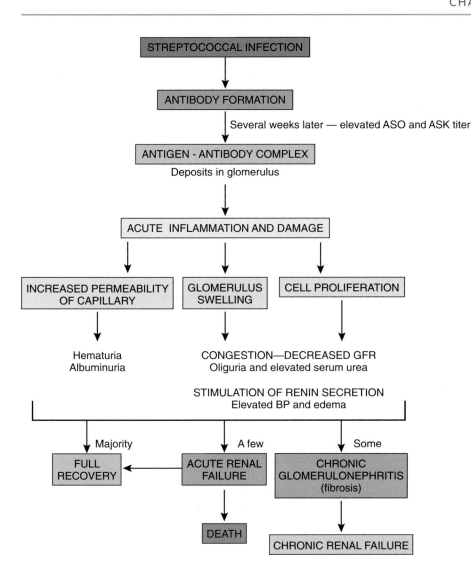

FIGURE 18-9 Development and course of poststreptococcal glomerulonephritis.

in the glomeruli of both kidneys (Fig. 18-9). (See Chapter 7 for a review of the immune response.) This leads to increased capillary permeability and cell proliferation (Fig. 18-10) and results in leakage of some protein and large numbers of erythrocytes into the filtrate. The specific mechanisms of damage are not totally clear, but immunoglobulin G and C3 (complement) are present in glomerular tissue and serum C3 is reduced.

When the inflammatory response is severe, the congestion and cell proliferation interfere with filtration in the kidney, causing decreased GFR and retention of fluid and wastes. Acute renal failure is possible if blood flow is sufficiently impaired. The decreased blood flow in the kidney is likely to trigger increased renin secretion, which leads to elevated blood pressure and edema (see Fig. 18-14). Severe prolonged inflammation causes scarring of the kidneys.

Signs and Symptoms
- The urine becomes dark and cloudy ("smoky" or "coffee-colored") because of the protein and red blood cells that have leaked into it.

- Facial and periorbital edema occur initially, followed by generalized edema as the colloid osmotic pressure of the blood drops and sodium and water are retained.
- Blood pressure is elevated owing to increased renin secretion and decreased GFR.
- Flank or back pain develops as the kidney tissue swells and stretches the capsule.
- General signs of inflammation are present, including malaise, fatigue, headache, anorexia, and nausea.
- Urine output decreases (oliguria) as GFR declines.

Diagnostic Tests
- *Blood tests* show elevated serum urea and creatinine as GFR decreases.
- Blood levels of Anti DNase B, streptococcal antibodies, ASO, and ASK are elevated.
- Complement level is decreased. It is probably a causative factor in the inflammatory damage that occurs in the kidney.
- Metabolic acidosis, with decreased serum bicarbonate and low serum pH, is present.

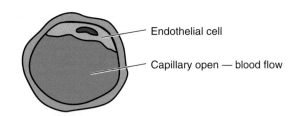

NORMAL GLOMERULUS

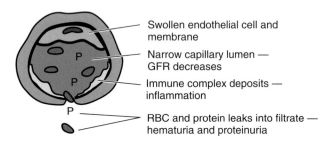

MILD GLOMERULONEPHRITIS

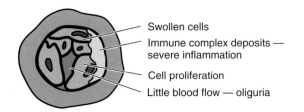

SEVERE GLOMERULONEPHRITIS

= RBC

P = PROTEIN

FIGURE 18-10 Schematic representation of changes occurring in the nephron with acute poststreptococcal glomerulonephritis.

- *Urinalysis* confirms the presence of proteinuria, gross hematuria, and erythrocyte casts (see Fig. 18-6*B*).

■ *Treatment*

Sodium restrictions may apply, and in severe cases, protein and fluid intake is decreased. Drug treatment includes glucocorticoids to reduce the inflammation, and antihypertensives to reduce high blood pressure.

In most cases, recovery takes place with minimum residual damage, although it is important to prevent future exposure to streptococcal infection and recurrent inflammation due to another hypersensitivity reaction. In children, the edema usually recedes in 5 to 10 days, and hypertension decreases in 2 to 3 weeks. Proteinuria and hematuria improve but often persist for some time. Prophylactic antibiotics may be needed. Post-recovery testing is recommended to ensure that chronic inflammation is not present.

Some cases, particularly in adults, are not easily resolved. Acute renal failure occurs in approximately 2% of cases. Chronic glomerulonephritis develops in about 10%, which gradually destroys the kidneys through end-stage renal disease or uremia.

THINK ABOUT 18-11

a. Explain the development of inflammation in the kidney with APSGN.
b. Describe the signs of APSGN related to: (1) increased glomerular permeability, and (2) decreased glomerular filtration rate.

Nephrotic Syndrome (Nephrosis)

The nephrotic syndrome is secondary to a number of renal diseases as well as to a variety of systemic disorders (e.g., systemic lupus erythematosus, exposure to toxins or drugs). However, lipoid nephrosis, also known as minimal change disease, is a primary disease in young children ages 2 to 6 years.

■ *Pathophysiology*

The pathogenesis is not well established, but the following sequence develops.

1. There is an abnormality in the glomerular capillaries and increased permeability that allows large amounts of plasma protein, primarily albumin, to escape into the filtrate.
2. This results in marked hypoalbuminemia with decreased plasma osmotic pressure and subsequent generalized edema.
3. Blood pressure may remain low or normal in many cases because of hypovolemia or it may be elevated depending on angiotensin II levels.
4. The decreased blood volume also increases aldosterone secretion, leading to more severe edema.
5. The other significant components of nephrotic syndrome are the high levels of cholesterol in the blood and lipoprotein in the urine. The cause of the hyperlipidemia and lipiduria is not totally clear, although it appears to be related to the response of the liver to heavy protein loss.

■ *Signs and Symptoms*

Urinalysis indicates marked proteinuria, lipiduria and casts (fatty, epithelial, and hyaline). Cells may be present with certain primary diseases. Urine is often frothy.

The significant sign of nephrosis is the massive edema (anasarca) associated with weight gain and pallor. This excessive fluid throughout all tissues impairs appetite (ascites), breathing (pleural effusion), and activity (swollen legs and feet). Skin breakdown and infection may develop because arterial flow and capillary exchange are impaired.

■ *Treatment*

Glucocorticoids such as prednisone are prescribed to reduce the inflammation in the kidney. Angiotensin-converting enzyme inhibitor drugs, such as ramipril, may decrease protein loss in the urine. Antihypertensive and antilipemic therapy may be required in some individuals. Nephrotic syndrome tends to recur and requires frequent monitoring and continued treatment. Recurrences may be treated with cytotoxic therapies such as cyclophosphamide. When administered long term, glucocorticoids have significant negative effects on a child's growth (see Chapter 5 for long-term effects of therapy). Sodium intake may be restricted, but protein intake is usually increased.

Urinary Tract Obstructions

In older men, the urinary tract is frequently obstructed by benign prostatic hypertrophy or prostatic cancer. These topics are discussed in Chapter 19.

Common causes of obstruction in men and women include: tumors, inflammation, scarring, stenosis, congenital defects, and renal calculi (Fig. 18-11)

Urolithiasis (Calculi, or Kidney Stones)

Kidney stones are a common problem and frequently recur if the underlying cause is not treated.

■ *Pathophysiology*

Calculi can develop anywhere in the urinary tract. Stones may be small or very large (e.g., *staghorn* calculus, a very large stone that forms in the renal pelvis and calyces in the shape of a deer's antlers).

Calculi tend to form when there are excessive amounts of relatively insoluble salts in the filtrate, or when insufficient fluid intake creates a highly concentrated filtrate. Once any solid material or debris forms, deposits continue to build up on this nidus, or focus, and eventually form a large mass. Cell debris from infection may also form a nidus. Immobility may result in calculi in the kidney because of stasis of urine resulting in chemical changes in the urine. Increasing fluid intake (at least eight glasses of water per day) can assist in removing small stones quickly from the urinary tract.

Stones usually cause manifestations only when they obstruct the flow of urine (e.g., in the ureter). Calculi

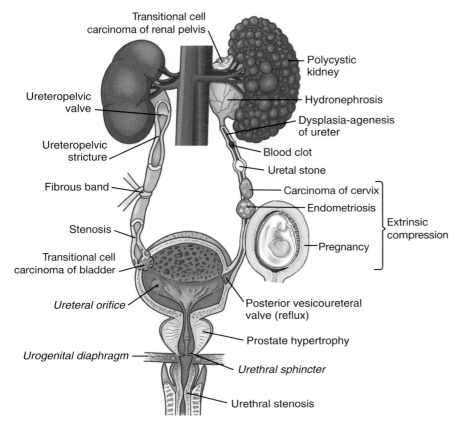

FIGURE 18-11 Major sites of urinary tract obstruction. *(From McCance KL, et al: Pathophysiolgy: The biologic basis for disease in adults and children, ed 6, St. Louis, 2010, Mosby.)*

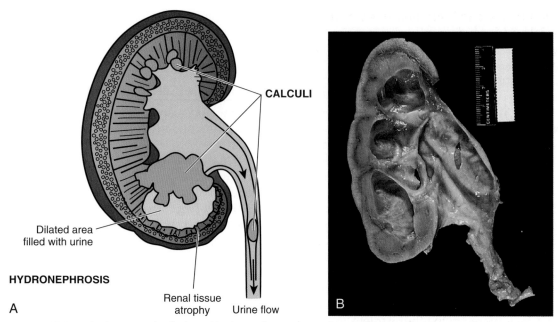

FIGURE 18-12 **A,** Renal calculi and hydronephrosis. **B,** Hydronephrosis with dilation of the renal pelvis and calyces and atrophy of renal tissue. *(From Kumar V, Abbas AK, Fausto M:* Robbins and Cotran Pathologic Basis of Disease, *ed 7, Philadelphia, 2005, Saunders.)*

may lead to infection because they cause stasis of urine in the area and also irritate the tissues. This may be an early indication of calculi formation.

When located in the kidney or ureter, calculi may cause the development of *hydronephrosis,* with dilation of calyces and atrophy of renal tissue related to the back pressure of urine behind the obstructing stone (Fig. 18-12).

■ *Etiology*

Approximately 75% of calculi are composed of calcium salts, the remainder consisting primarily of uric acid (a breakdown product of purine nucleotides) or urates, struvite (magnesium ammonium phosphate), or cystine (rare), depending on the predisposing factor. Calculi should be examined and urinalysis completed to determine the content of the stones and the predisposing factors.

Calcium stones (phosphate, oxalate, or carbonate) form when calcium levels in the urine are high owing to hypercalcemia, perhaps due to a parathyroid tumor or other metabolic disorder (see Fig. 18-6C). The solubility of calcium salts and uric acid also varies with the *pH* of the urine. Calcium stones form readily when the urine is highly alkaline. Inadequate fluid intake is a major factor in calculus formation. Calcium oxalate stones may develop in people following vegetarian diets high in oxalate that lead to increased levels of oxalate in the urine.

Uric acid stones develop with hyperuricemia (due to gout, high purine diets, or cancer chemotherapy), especially when the urine is acidic. Infection may cause

stones consisting of mixed inorganic salts, because in such cases the urine pH is alkaline and debris from the infection may act as a focus for the deposition of crystals.

THINK ABOUT 18-13

Explain how decreased fluid intake or dehydration predisposes to calculi in the urinary tract.

■ *Signs and Symptoms*

Stones in the kidney or bladder are frequently asymptomatic, unless frequent infections lead to investigation. Sometimes flank pain occurs because of distention of the renal capsule.

Obstruction of the ureter causes an attack of "renal colic," consisting of intense spasms of pain in the flank area radiating into the groin that last until the stone passes or is removed. This pain is caused by vigorous contractions of the ureter in an effort to force the stone out. The severe pain may be accompanied by nausea and vomiting, cool moist skin, and rapid pulse. Radiologic examination confirms the location of the calculi.

■ *Treatment*

Small stones can be passed eventually, the urine strained to catch stones for analysis. Newer methods of fragmentation of larger stones, such as extracorporeal shock-wave lithotripsy and laser lithotripsy, have been quite successful and have decreased the need for invasive surgery. In some cases, drugs may be used to partially dissolve the stones.

Prevention of recurrence related to specific risk factors is of primary importance. Treatment of the underlying condition, adjustment of urine pH by ingestion of additional acidic or alkaline substances, and increased fluid intake all minimize the risk of recurrence.

Hydronephrosis

This occurs as a secondary problem, a complication of calculi, but also of tumors, scar tissue in the kidney or ureter, and untreated prostatic enlargement. Developmental defects are common in the urinary tract and may cause obstruction by kinking or stenosis of a ureter. Obstructive uropathy can be diagnosed by ultrasonography in the fetus, allowing for immediate or neonatal corrective surgery, thus preventing major kidney damage.

Urine is continually forming. Any prolonged interference with urine outflow through the system results in back pressure and a dilated area filled with urine in the ureter or kidney (see Fig. 18-12*B*). In the kidney, continued buildup of urine, particularly over a prolonged period of time, causes necrosis of the tissue because of direct pressure and compression of the blood vessels. Hydronephrosis is frequently asymptomatic unless mild flank pain occurs as the renal capsule is distended, or unless infection develops. It can be diagnosed with ultrasonography, radionucleotide imaging, CT scan or IVP. If the cause is not removed, bilateral hydronephrosis could lead to chronic renal failure.

Tumors

Benign tumors are rare in the urinary tract. Malignant tumors occur primarily after age 50 years, in males by a ratio of 3:2. Smoking is a major predisposing factor.

Renal Cell Carcinoma

Renal cell carcinoma (adenocarcinoma of the kidney) is a primary tumor arising from the tubule epithelium, more often in the renal cortex (Fig. 18-13). The American Cancer Society recently estimated that there would be 65,150 new cases of renal cell carcinomas in 2013, resulting in 13,680 deaths. It tends to be asymptomatic in the early stage and often has metastasized to liver, lungs, bone, or CNS at the time of diagnosis. This cancer occurs more frequently in men and smokers.

The initial sign is usually painless hematuria, either gross or microscopic. Other manifestations include dull, aching flank pain; a palpable mass; unexplained weight loss; and anemia or erythrocytosis (depending on the tumor's effects on erythropoietin secretion).

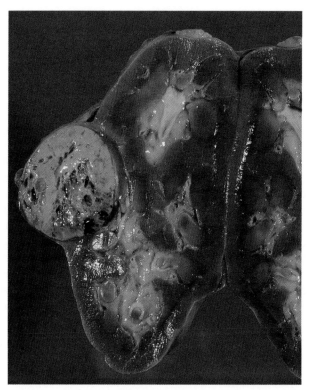

FIGURE 18-13 Renal cell carcinoma. A well-circumscribed spherical tumor is bulging through the cortical surface. Areas of hemorrhage and cysts can be seen in the tumor. *(From Cooke RA, Stewart B: Colour Atlas of Anatomical Pathology, ed 3, Sydney, 2004, Churchill Livingstone.)*

Paraneoplastic syndromes such as hypercalcemia (increased parathyroid hormone) or Cushing's syndrome (increased adrenocorticotropic hormone) are common.

This tumor tends to be silent; therefore, diagnosis is made in one third of cases after metastasis to lungs, liver, or bone has occurred. Removal of the kidney (nephrectomy) is the treatment because the tumor is usually unresponsive to radiation or chemotherapy. The 5-year survival rate varies from 96% in Stage I to 23% in Stage IV; newer treatment measures and diagnostic technology may result in higher survival rates.

Bladder Cancer

Malignant tumors of the bladder commonly arise from the transitional epithelium lining the bladder in the trigone area. This cancer often develops as multiple tumors and tends to recur. It is diagnosed by urine cytology (malignant cells in the urine) and biopsy. The tumor is invasive through the wall to adjacent structures, and it metastasizes through the blood to pelvic lymph nodes, liver, and bone. Staging categories range from an in situ tumor through the degree of bladder wall invasion to metastasis. The early sign is hematuria, gross or microscopic. Dysuria or frequency may develop and infection is common.

Bladder cancer has a high incidence in individuals working with chemicals in laboratories or industry, particularly with dyes, rubber, and aluminum. More than 50% of patients are cigarette smokers. Other predisposing factors are recurrent infection and heavy intake of analgesics.

Treatment includes surgical resection of the tumor in 90% of cases, chemotherapy, and radiation. Urinary diversion (e.g., ileal loop, the creation of an alternate internal or external urine collecting unit using part of the ileum) may be required following surgery. Photoradiation (a combination of drug and laser treatment) has been successful in some early cases. Instillation of BCG, bacillus Calmette-Guérin vaccine (a biologic response modifier intended to strengthen the immune response), into the bladder after resection has reduced recurrences of superficial tumors (see Chapter 20). Continued monitoring is necessary to detect recurrences in an early stage. Five-year survival rates vary from 85% in Stage I to 16% in Stage IV.

Vascular Disorders

Nephrosclerosis

■ *Pathophysiology*

Nephrosclerosis involves vascular changes, similar to those of arteriosclerosis, in the kidney. Some vascular changes occur normally with aging, but these excessive changes cause thickening and hardening of the walls of the arterioles and small arteries and narrowing or occlusion of the lumina of the blood vessels. Such changes reduce the blood supply to the kidney, causing ischemia and atrophy, and also stimulate the secretion of renin, ultimately increasing the blood pressure (Fig. 18-14). Continued ischemia can lead to gradual destruction of renal tissue and chronic renal failure. Often such damage is asymptomatic until a late stage.

It is often difficult to determine whether the primary lesion has developed in the kidney or it is secondary to essential hypertension (see Chapter 12), diabetes

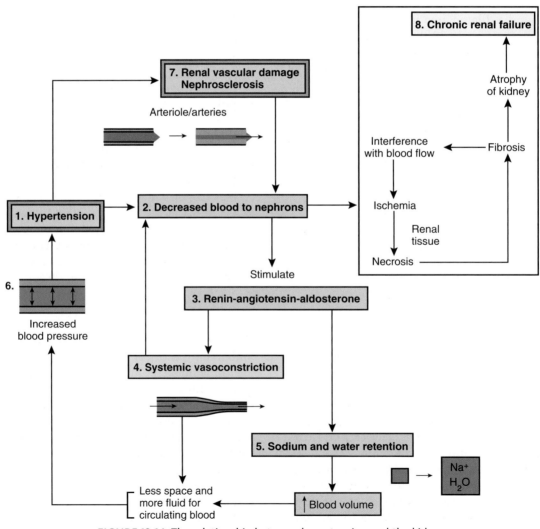

FIGURE 18-14 The relationship between hypertension and the kidney.

mellitus (see diabetic nephropathy and Fig. 16-6 in Chapter 16), or another condition. In any case, a vicious cycle can develop with the kidneys and hypertensive changes, and this must be broken to prevent renal failure or other complications of hypertension such as congestive heart failure.

▧ *Treatment*

Drugs such as antihypertensive agents, diuretics, ACE inhibitors, and beta-blockers (which block renin release) all can assist in maintaining renal blood flow and reducing blood pressure. These drugs are discussed in Chapter 12 (see Table 12-1). Sodium intake should be reduced as well.

THINK ABOUT 18-14

Explain factors that may contribute to elevated blood pressure in the client with renal disease.

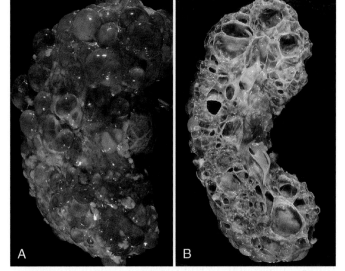

FIGURE 18-15 Polycystic Kidney (Adult Autosomal Dominant) A, External surface of enlarged kidney, showing cysts. **B,** Bisected, shows large interior cysts. *(From Kumar V, Abbas AK, Fausto M: Robbins and Cotran Pathologic Basis of Disease, ed 7, Philadelphia, 2005, Saunders.)*

Congenital Disorders

It is estimated that 10% of infants are born with an abnormality in the urinary system. Some examples follow:

- *Vesicoureteral reflux* is due to a defective valve in the bladder mentioned under urinary tract infections.
- *Agenesis* refers to a developmental failure of one kidney to develop. This is asymptomatic and usually is an incidental finding if diagnosed at all.
- *Hypoplasia,* or failure to develop to normal size, is often a unilateral defect. Sometimes it results from fibrosis in the kidney, rather than being a true developmental flaw.
- *Ectopic kidney* means that a kidney and its ureter are displaced out of normal position. A common location is lower in the abdominal or pelvic cavity. Kidney function is normal. In this position the ureter may become kinked, causing obstruction or infection.
- *Fusion* of the two kidneys during development is a common malformation, resulting in a single "horseshoe" kidney. Usually kidney function is normal.

Adult Polycystic Kidney

The most common form of this genetic disease is transmitted as an autosomal dominant gene on chromosome 16. There are no indications in the child and young adult; the first manifestations usually appear around age 40 years, when chronic renal failure becomes symptomatic and dialysis is required. This condition is responsible for about 10% of the patients with end-stage chronic renal failure. In some cases, early diagnosis is possible when high blood pressure occurs and is difficult to control or when secondary polycythemia develops due to increased erythropoietin secretion. Diagnosis can be confirmed by an abdominal CT scan or MRI.

Multiple cysts develop in both kidneys and gradually expand over the years, first enlarging the kidneys, then compressing and destroying kidney tissue until chronic renal failure occurs (Fig. 18-15). In some cases, cysts are found in other organs such as the liver or cerebral aneurysms are found.

Polycystic disease in children is transmitted as a recessive gene and is manifest at birth. However, in this case, the child is either stillborn or dies during the first months.

Wilms' Tumor (Nephroblastoma)

This is a rare tumor occurring in children. It is associated with defects in tumor-suppressor genes on chromosome 11 and may occur in conjunction with some other congenital disorders. It is usually unilateral. The tumor presents as a large encapsulated mass.

Wilms' tumor is usually diagnosed at ages 3 to 4 years, when the large abdominal mass becomes obvious (often a waistband on clothes does not fasten or a unilateral bulge appears). In some cases the child develops high blood pressure. Pulmonary metastases may be present at diagnosis.

The prognosis for the child depends on the histologic results as well as the stage of the tumor at diagnosis.

Tumors showing a favorable histology (less aggressive) have an average 5 year survival rate of 90%.

Renal Failure

Acute Renal Failure

■ *Pathophysiology*

The kidneys may fail to function for many different reasons. Either directly reduced blood flow into the kidney or inflammation and necrosis of the tubules cause obstruction and back pressure, leading to greatly reduced GFR and oliguria (reduced urine output) or anuria (no urine output).

Both kidneys must be involved. The failure is usually reversible if the primary problem is treated successfully. Dialysis may be used to replace the kidney function during this period. In some cases, the kidneys sustain a degree of permanent damage.

■ *Etiology*

Acute renal failure has numerous causes (Fig. 18-16):

- Acute bilateral kidney disease, such as glomerulonephritis, which reduces GFR
- Severe and prolonged circulatory shock or heart failure, which results in tubule necrosis. Shock associated with burns or crush injuries or sepsis frequently causes renal failure. With burns, the damaged erythrocytes break down in the circulation, releasing free hemoglobin that may accumulate in the tubules, causing obstruction. Hemoglobin also is toxic to tubule epithelium, causing inflammation and necrosis (see Chapter 5, Burns). When skeletal muscle is crushed in an accident, myoglobin is released with similar effects;
- *Nephrotoxins* such as drugs, chemicals, or toxins, which cause tubule necrosis and obstruction of blood flow. Industrial chemicals such as the solvent carbon tetrachloride may cause acute renal failure when exposure is intense. Long-term low-level exposures may cause gradual damage, eventually leading to chronic renal failure. The list of frequently used drugs possibly causing tubule damage is growing longer and now includes sulfa drugs, phenacetin, nonsteroidal anti-inflammatory drugs, acetaminophen and aspirin, and penicillin. When patients take these drugs, fluid intake should be greatly increased to reduce the risk of kidney damage.
- Occasionally mechanical obstructions such as calculi, blood clots, or tumors, which block urine flow beyond the kidneys and cause acute renal failure

■ *Signs and Symptoms*

Acute renal failure usually develops rapidly. Blood tests show elevated serum urea nitrogen (BUN) and creatinine as well as metabolic acidosis and hyperkalemia, confirming the failure of the kidneys to remove wastes.

■ *Treatment*

It is important to reverse the primary problem as quickly as possible to minimize the risk of necrosis and permanent kidney damage, with uremia (see chronic renal failure).

Dialysis may be used to normalize body fluids and maintain homeostasis during the *oliguric* stage. Recovery from acute renal failure is evidenced by increased urine output (*diuretic* stage). It may take a few months before the epithelium lining the renal tubules recovers totally, so fluid and electrolyte balance may not return to normal for some time.

> **THINK ABOUT   18-15**
>
> Focusing on the circulation through the nephron, explain why severely decreased blood flow in the afferent arteriole could cause tubule necrosis and obstruction.

Chronic Renal Failure

Chronic renal failure is the gradual irreversible destruction of the kidneys over a long period of time. It may result from chronic kidney disease, such as bilateral pyelonephritis or congenital polycystic kidney disease, or from systemic disorders such as hypertension or diabetes. As mentioned, long-term exposure to nephrotoxins is a cause. The gradual loss of nephrons is asymptomatic until it is well advanced because the kidneys normally have considerable reserve function. Once advanced, the progress of chronic renal failure may be slowed but cannot be stopped because the scar tissue and loss of functional organization tend to cause further degenerative changes.

■ *Pathophysiology*

Chronic renal failure has several stages (Fig. 18-17), progressing from decreased renal reserve, to insufficiency, to end-stage renal failure or uremia. In the early stages of *decreased reserve* (around 60% nephrons lost) there is a decrease in GFR, serum creatinine levels that are consistently higher than average but within normal range, serum urea levels that are normal, and no apparent clinical signs. The remaining nephrons appear to adapt, increasing their capacity for filtration.

The second stage (around 75% nephrons lost), or that of *renal insufficiency,* is indicated by a change in blood chemistry and manifestations. At this point, GFR is decreased to approximately 20% of normal, and there is significant retention of nitrogen wastes (urea and creatinine) in the blood. Tubule function is decreased, resulting in failure to concentrate the urine and control the secretion and exchange of acids and electrolytes. Osmotic diuresis occurs as the remaining functional

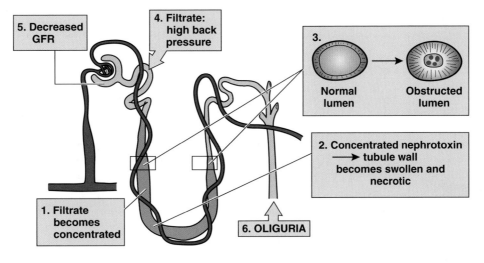

5. Decreased GFR

4. Filtrate: high back pressure

3.

Normal lumen → Obstructed lumen

2. Concentrated nephrotoxin → tubule wall becomes swollen and necrotic

1. Filtrate becomes concentrated

6. OLIGURIA

A   **NEPHROTOXINS**

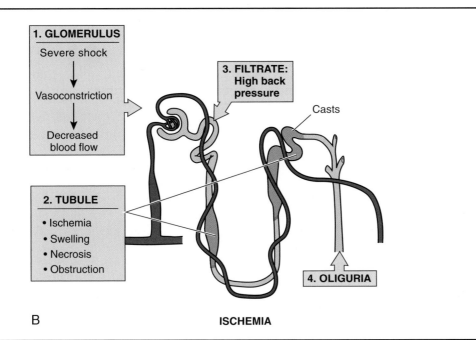

1. GLOMERULUS

Severe shock
↓
Vasoconstriction
↓
Decreased blood flow

3. FILTRATE: High back pressure

Casts

2. TUBULE

• Ischemia
• Swelling
• Necrosis
• Obstruction

4. OLIGURIA

B   **ISCHEMIA**

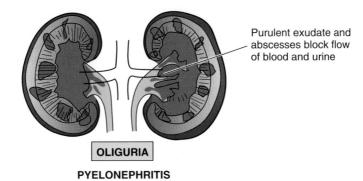

Purulent exudate and abscesses block flow of blood and urine

OLIGURIA

C   **PYELONEPHRITIS**

FIGURE 18-16 **Causes of Acute Renal Failure A,** Nephrotoxins. **B,** Ischemia. **C,** Pyelonephritis.

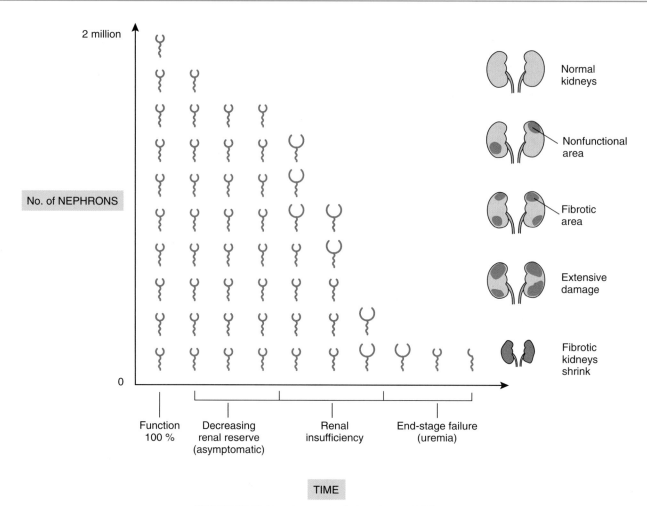

FIGURE 18-17 Development of chronic renal failure.

nephrons filter an increased solute load. This stage is marked by excretion of large volumes of dilute urine (low fixed specific gravity). Erythropoiesis is decreased, and the patient's blood pressure is elevated. The cardiovascular system must compensate for these effects (see Chapter 12).

Uremia, or *end-stage renal failure* (more than 90% nephrons lost), occurs when GFR is negligible. Fluid, electrolytes, and wastes are retained in the body, and all body systems are affected. In this stage, marked oliguria or anuria develops. Regular dialysis or a kidney transplant is required to maintain the patient's life. A comparison of acute and chronic renal failure may be found in Table 18-3.

■ *Signs and Symptoms*
The *early* signs of chronic renal failure include:
- Increased urinary output (polyuria), manifested as frequency and nocturia
- General signs such as anorexia, nausea, anemia, fatigue, unintended weight loss, and exercise intolerance

TABLE 18-3	Comparison of Acute Renal Failure and Chronic Renal Failure	
Characteristic	Acute Renal Failure	Chronic Renal Failure
Causes	Severe shock	Nephrosclerosis
	Burns	Diabetes mellitus
	Nephrotoxins, massive exposure	Nephrotoxins, long-term exposure
	Acute bilateral kidney infection or inflammation	Chronic bilateral kidney inflammation or infection
		Polycystic disease
Onset	Sudden, acute	Slow, insidious
Early signs	Oliguria, increased serum urea	Polyuria with dilute urine
		Anemia, fatigue, hypertension
Progressive signs	Recovery—increasing urine output	End-stage failure or uremia
	If prolonged failure—uremia	Oliguria, acidosis, azotemia

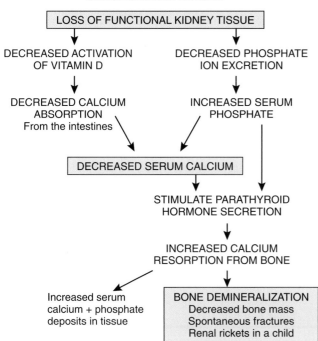

OSTEODYSTROPHY WITH CHRONIC RENAL FAILURE

LOSS OF FUNCTIONAL KIDNEY TISSUE

DECREASED ACTIVATION OF VITAMIN D

DECREASED PHOSPHATE ION EXCRETION

DECREASED CALCIUM ABSORPTION
From the intestines

INCREASED SERUM PHOSPHATE

DECREASED SERUM CALCIUM

STIMULATE PARATHYROID HORMONE SECRETION

INCREASED CALCIUM RESORPTION FROM BONE

Increased serum calcium + phosphate deposits in tissue

BONE DEMINERALIZATION
Decreased bone mass
Spontaneous fractures
Renal rickets in a child

FIGURE 18-18 The development of osteodystrophy in chronic renal failure.

- Bone marrow depression and impaired cell function caused by increased wastes and altered blood chemistry
- High blood pressure

As the kidneys fail completely (end-stage failure), *uremic* signs appear:

- Oliguria
- Dry, pruritic, and hyperpigmented skin, easy bruising
- Peripheral neuropathy—abnormal sensations in the lower limbs
- Impotence and decreased libido in men, menstrual irregularities in women
- Encephalopathy (lethargy, memory lapses, seizures, tremors)
- Congestive heart failure, arrhythmias
- Failure of the kidney to activate vitamin D for calcium absorption and metabolism, combined with urinary retention of phosphate ion, leading to hypocalcemia and hyperphosphatemia with osteodystrophy (Fig. 18-18), osteoporosis, and tetany (see Chapters 9 and 16)
- Possibly uremic frost on the skin and a urinelike breath odor in the terminal stage or if infection is present
- Systemic infections such as pneumonia (common), owing to poor tissue resistance related to anemia, fluid retention, and low protein levels

■ *Diagnostic Tests*

Anemia, acidosis, and azotemia are the key indicators of chronic renal failure.

1. Metabolic acidosis becomes decompensated (serum pH below 7.35) in the late stage as GFR declines and tubule function is lost (see Chapter 2).
2. Azotemia refers to the presence of nitrogen wastes in the blood, as indicated by elevated serum creatinine and urea levels.
3. Anemia becomes severe.
4. Serum electrolyte levels may vary depending on the amount of water retained in the body. Usually hyponatremia and hyperkalemia occur, as well as hypocalcemia and hyperphosphatemia.

■ *Treatment*

Chronic renal failure affects all body systems, as indicated earlier. It is difficult to maintain homeostasis of fluids, electrolytes, and acid-base balance. Drugs are available to stimulate erythropoiesis and reduce phosphate levels. As well, specific drugs may be required to treat hypertension, arrhythmias, heart failure, and other complications. Drug dosages need to be carefully considered and adjusted if necessary in patients with uremia because of the kidney's decreased ability to excrete drugs in a timely manner.

Clients are subject to many complications, which in turn affect the uremia. For instance, a simple infection increases the wastes in the body, compromising all body systems. Intake of fluid, electrolytes, and protein must be restricted because the kidneys are limited in their ability to excrete excess wastes and fluid. Children with kidney failure have retarded growth and renal rickets.

In the uremic stage, dialysis or a transplant is required. Organ transplants are discussed in Chapter 7.

THINK ABOUT 18-16

a. Compare acute and chronic renal failure with respect to cause, reversibility, and urinary output at onset.

b. If uremia is untreated or if complications occur, metabolic acidosis can become decompensated. What change occurs in serum pH at this point, and what is the effect on overall cell metabolism in the body?

c. Why is there an increased risk of drug toxicity in the later stages of renal failure?

CASE STUDY A

Nephrosclerosis and Chronic Renal Failure

Mr. H., age 68 years, has a long history of hypertension. He has had more headaches recently, his legs and feet are swollen, and he has noticed that more frequent voiding, both during the day and at night, is necessary. He constantly feels tired and does not feel hungry. Mr. H.'s blood pressure is 170/110, his pulse is 94, and he has gained 12 pounds in the last 2 months. Diagnostic test findings related to the blood and urine include elevated serum creatinine and urea levels, low serum bicarbonate, low hemoglobin and hematocrit, and low serum sodium. The urine contains protein and has a very low specific gravity. The diagnosis is renal insufficiency or chronic renal failure due to nephrosclerosis.

1. Describe how nephrosclerosis leads to chronic renal failure.
2. Explain the cause of the edema and the weight gain.
3. State three factors contributing to fatigue.
4. Explain why Mr. H.:
   a. is voiding frequently.
   b. has a very dilute urine.
5. Explain why Mr. H. has:
   a. high blood pressure.
   b. anemia.
   c. metabolic acidosis.
6. List the signs indicating that Mr. H. has progressed into uremia or end-stage renal failure.
7. List three reasons why development of pneumonia is a high risk in Mr. H.

has noticed that he is not producing as much urine and thinks that this is due to decreased fluid intake during work. His partner contacts his doctor and takes him to the emergency department as directed. When seen in the emergency clinic, his blood pressure is 170/96, he has an abnormal pulse, and blood tests reveal elevated BUN, K^+ and creatinine levels. Further tests lead to a diagnosis of acute renal failure due to tubular necrosis.

1. What are possible causes of acute renal failure in this case?
2. How have the kidneys been damaged; will they recover normal function?
3. What is the cause of nausea and fatigue?
4. Explain how hypertension has developed in G.R.
5. Explain the cause of oliguria.
   G.R. is hospitalized and treated with steroid medication and emergency hemodialysis. Four days later he begins to void large volumes of urine.
1. What is the significance of diuresis in this case?
2. What can G.R. expect in the future; what changes need to be made in regard to his work to prevent recurrence of acute renal failure or the development of chronic renal failure in the future?

CASE STUDY B

Acute Poststreptococcal Glomerulonephritis

D.K., age 4 years, has been diagnosed with APSGN 1 month after he was ill with tonsillitis. His face, abdomen, and legs are swollen, and he is not interested in his toys. He is short of breath when he moves about. His urine is dark and cloudy and is scant in volume.

1. Explain how D.K.'s tonsillitis is probably related to the development of APSGN.
2. Explain why his urine is dark.
3. State two other significant characteristics you would expect to find in the urine.
4. State three abnormalities likely to be found on examination of D.K.'s blood and explain the reason for each.
5. Explain why D.K. is producing very small amounts of urine.
6. Explain why acute renal failure could develop.

CASE STUDY C

Nephrotoxicity

G.R. is a successful collage artist. He works with adhesives, paints, and solvents, which often must be heated to produce textured artworks. During the summer months he works out of doors and in the colder weather works in his studio, which is equipped with an exhaust fan. On very cold days he sometimes turns off the fan. He has been working very long hours to prepare for his upcoming winter show.

Several times in the past few days he has commented to his partner that he feels weak, nauseated, and unable to work. He

CHAPTER SUMMARY

Kidney disease may affect one or more of the glomeruli, the tubules, or the blood vessels of the nephrons, thus altering filtration or reabsorption and secretion and the excretion of wastes. Scar tissue may interfere with the essential organization of the nephrons within the kidney. Renal disease often has numerous systemic effects, including elevated blood pressure.

- *Dialysis,* either peritoneal or hemodialysis, may replace kidney function temporarily or long term.

Urinary Tract Infections

- *Cystitis,* infection of the bladder, may ascend along the continuous mucosa, to cause *pyelonephritis.* The common cause is *E. coli.* Urinalysis confirms the diagnosis. Follow-up testing is necessary to ensure complete eradication of the infection.
- *Urethritis* is the infection and inflammation of the urethra

Inflammatory Disorders

- *Acute poststreptococcal glomerulonephritis,* an example of a childhood inflammatory disease, is caused by an abnormal immune reaction. Mild glomerular inflammation causes leakage of erythrocytes and protein into the filtrate; severe inflammation reduces GFR and excretion of wastes.
- *Nephrosis* or *nephrotic syndrome* is associated with many abnormal conditions. Significant manifestations are severe generalized edema, proteinuria, and lipiduria.

Obstructions

- *Urinary calculi,* formed primarily of calcium salts, may obstruct urinary flow, causing hydronephrosis, and predisposition to infection.
- *Renal cell carcinoma* and *bladder cancer* are frequently manifested initially by painless hematuria.

Renal Failure

- *Acute renal failure* is reversible and may result from bilateral renal inflammation, severe shock, or nephrotoxins. It is indicated by sudden oliguria, increased serum urea, and acidosis.
- *Chronic renal failure* develops from the gradual destruction of nephrons. The process is irreversible and ultimately results in uremia with retention of body wastes and loss of homeostasis. It is asymptomatic until the stage of renal insufficiency, indicated by production of large volumes of dilute urine, increasing serum urea, elevated blood pressure, anemia, and fatigue.

STUDY QUESTIONS

1. Trace the blood flow through the kidney, naming the blood vessels in order.
2. Trace the filtrate and the major changes in it, from Bowman's capsule to the urethra.
3. If the sympathetic nervous system causes vasoconstriction in the kidney, how does this increase blood pressure? How does it affect urine output?
4. Compare the signs/symptoms of cystitis and pyelonephritis.
5. Compare the causes and pathophysiology of acute pyelonephritis, APSGN, and nephrotic syndrome.
6. How might urinary tract infections lead to calculus formation?
7. Compare the pathophysiology of acute and chronic renal failure.
8. Describe all the factors contributing to the lethargy of someone with chronic renal failure.
9. A client with chronic renal failure on hemodialysis is having extensive dental work performed. What precautions need to be taken in this case?
10. List the substances that should pass from the blood into the dialyzing fluid.
11. Why is protein intake restricted in patients with kidney disease?
12. Explain how a respiratory infection such as pneumonia can aggravate the effects of uremia?
13. Explain how a child's growth and development may be affected by chronic nephrosis and renal failure?
14. Differentiate the causes of frequent voiding associated with cystitis and with renal insufficiency.
15. Differentiate the causes of urinary retention and anuria.

ADDITIONAL RESOURCES

Urologic Clinics, a periodical published quarterly by Saunders, Philadelphia.

Patton K, Thibodeau G: *Anatomy & Physiology,* ed 7, St. Louis, 2010, Mosby.

McCance K, Huether S, Brashers V, Rote N: *Pathophysiology: The Biologic Basis for Disease in Adults and Children,* ed 6, St. Louis, 2010, Mosby.

Web Sites

http://www.kidney.org *National Kidney Foundation*
http://www.nlm.nih.gov/medlineplus/encyclopedia.html *MEDLINE Plus*

http://www.kidney.niddk.nih.gov *National Kidney and Urologic Diseases Information Clearinghouse (NKUDIC)*
http://www.mayoclinic.com *Mayo Clinic*
http://www.cancer.org *American Cancer Society*

CHAPTER 19

Reproductive System Disorders

CHAPTER OUTLINE

LEARNING OBJECTIVES

After studying this chapter, the student is expected to:

1. Describe the causes of infertility in males and females.
2. Describe the common congenital abnormalities in males and females.
3. Compare benign prostatic hypertrophy with cancer of the prostate.
4. Describe the incidence and pathophysiology of testicular cancer.
5. Compare the common menstrual disorders.
6. Describe endometriosis and its complications.
7. Explain how pelvic inflammatory disease develops and its effects.
8. Describe the breast lesions, fibrocystic breast disease, and breast cancer.
9. Compare the common benign and malignant tumors in the cervix, uterus, and ovaries.
10. Describe the common sexually transmitted diseases.

KEY TERMS

dyspareunia	hirsutism	leukorrhea	menarche
exogenous	lactation	meatus	spermatogenesis
gynecomastia			

Disorders of the Male Reproductive System

Review of the Male Reproductive System

Structure and Function

The male gonads, the *testes*, are suspended by the spermatic cord in the *scrotum*, a sac outside the abdominal cavity (Fig. 19-1). The testes constantly produce sperm and the sex hormone testosterone.

The scrotal sac consists of a layer of skin that is continuous with the skin of the perineal area plus an inner muscle layer and fascia. The scrotal covering is loose and falls into folds or rugae. A connective tissue septum separates the two testes within the scrotum. Each testis and attached epididymis is enclosed in the *tunica vaginalis*, a double-walled membrane with a small amount of fluid between the layers (see Fig. 19-1). The *spermatic cord* contains arteries, veins, and lymphatics for the testes (see Fig. 19-3).

The testes are positioned outside the abdominal cavity to provide an optimum temperature for sperm production, 2°F to 3°F (1°C to 2°C) below normal body temperature. The scrotal muscle draws the testes closer to the body whenever the environmental temperature drops. When the temperature climbs, the muscle relaxes, letting the testes drop away from the body. The fetal testes descend from the abdominal cavity through the inguinal canal into the scrotum during the third trimester of pregnancy. Then the inguinal canal closes (see Fig. 19-2).

At puberty the testes mature and begin to produce sperm and testosterone under the influence of the gonadotropins secreted by the adenohypophysis. In addition to the testes, the male reproductive system includes an extensive duct system connected to accessory glands and structures that form and transport the semen preparatory to ejaculation from the penis during sexual intercourse (see Fig. 19-1).

Spermatogenesis, the production of spermatozoa, is a continuous process. It takes approximately 60 to 70 days to complete the process of development.

1. The testes consist of many lobules containing the *seminiferous tubules*, the "sperm factories" of the body.
2. Efferent ducts conduct the multitudes of sperm into the *epididymis*, where the sperm mature.
3. Peristaltic movements in the epididymis assist the sperm to move on into the *ductus deferens* (vas deferens) and then to the *ampulla*, where the now-motile sperm may be stored for several weeks until ejaculation occurs (see Fig. 19-1). Vasectomy, which is one method of birth control, involves cutting or obstructing the vas deferens to block the passage of sperm.

When *semen* is formed at the time of emission, fluid containing many substances is gathered from the various accessory structures entering the ejaculatory duct and urethra:

- The *seminal vesicles,* located behind the bladder, provide a secretion that includes fructose to nourish the sperm.
- The *prostate gland,* which surrounds the urethra at the base of the bladder, adds an alkaline fluid to provide an optimum pH of around 6 for fertilization. (The vaginal secretions and the initial sperm-containing fluid are acidic.)

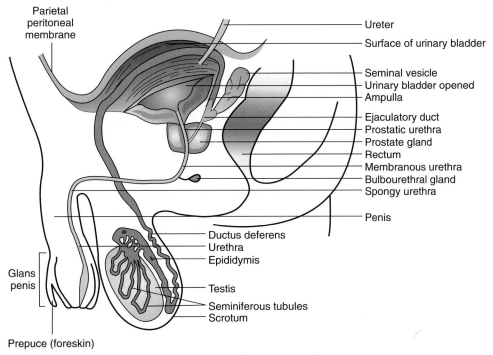

FIGURE 19-1 Anatomy of the male reproductive system.

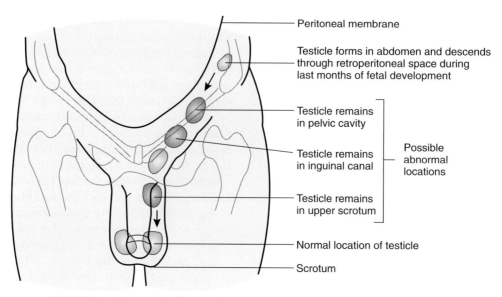

FIGURE 19-2 Cryptorchidism and possible positions of the undescended testis.

- The *bulbourethral glands* (Cowper's glands), situated near the base of the penis, secrete an alkaline mucus, which probably neutralizes any residual urine in the urethra.

The total volume of semen ejaculated at one time is 2 to 5 mL. Semen consists primarily of fluid, but contains 1 to 2 hundred million sperm.

Hormones

Gonadotropic hormones released by the adenohypophysis or anterior pituitary gland include:

- Follicle-stimulating hormone (FSH), which initiates spermatogenesis
- Luteinizing hormone (LH, or interstitial cell-stimulating hormone), which stimulates testosterone production by the interstitial cells (Leydig's cells) in the testes

Testosterone is essential for the maturation of sperm. Serum levels of testosterone provide a negative feedback system for the continuous control of gonadotropin secretions, there being no cyclic hormones in males (see Chapter 16). Other functions of testosterone include the development and maintenance of secondary sex characteristics such as male hair distribution, deeper voice, and maturing of the male external genitalia. Also, testosterone is an anabolic steroid hormone that promotes protein metabolism and skeletal muscle development, influencing the physical changes seen in the adolescent male (see Chapter 23). These steroid hormones are being abused more frequently by both males and females who are athletes or are interested in body building or altered body image. Unfortunately, serious adverse effects are associated with such use, such as liver damage, cardiovascular disease, and damage to the reproductive structures.

THINK ABOUT 19-1

a. Describe the location and function of the: (1) testis, (2) seminal vesicle, (3) epididymis.

b. Explain how testosterone levels are maintained including an explanation of negative feedback.

Congenital Abnormalities of the Penis

Epispadias and Hypospadias

Epispadias refers to a urethral opening on the dorsal (upper) surface of the penis, proximal to the glans. If the urethral defect extends proximally and affects the urinary sphincter, *incontinence* may result. Infections may result from stricture at the opening.

In some cases, this condition is associated with *exstrophy of the bladder,* which is a failure of the abdominal wall to form across the midline.

Hypospadias is a urethral opening on the ventral (under) surface of the penis. If the opening occurs in the proximal section of the penis, it is considered more severe and may be accompanied by *chordee,* ventral curvature of the penis. Other abnormalities such as cryptorchidism are often associated with hypospadias. Surgical reconstruction, which may be performed in stages, is recommended for both epispadias and hypospadias to provide normal urinary flow and normal sexual function.

Disorders of the Testes and Scrotum

Cryptorchidism

Maldescent of the testis, or cryptorchidism, occurs when one of the testes fails to descend into the normal position in the scrotum during the latter part of pregnancy (Fig. 19-2). The testis may remain in the abdominal cavity or discontinue the descent at some point in the inguinal canal or above the scrotum. In some cases, the testis assumes an abnormal position outside the scrotum; this is called an ectopic testis. In many cases, spontaneous descent occurs during the first year after birth.

The reason for maldescent is not fully understood. Possible factors include hormonal abnormalities, a short spermatic cord, or a small inguinal ring. If the testis remains undescended, the seminiferous tubules degenerate, and spermatogenesis is impaired.

Of concern is the increased risk of testicular cancer in cryptorchid testes (see Chapter 23). Therefore, surgical positioning of the testes in the scrotum before age 2 is advisable.

Hydrocele, Spermatocele, and Varicocele

Hydrocele occurs when excessive fluid collects in the potential space between the layers of the tunica vaginalis (Fig. 19-3A). This may occur around one or both testes and can be distinguished by transillumination.

Hydrocele may occur as a congenital defect in a newborn when peritoneal fluid accumulates in the scrotum. This fluid may be reabsorbed in time. The fluid may continue to escape from the peritoneal cavity if the proximal portion of the processus vaginalis, a section of peritoneal membrane, does not close off as expected following descent of the testes. Usually the scrotum fills with more fluid during the day, becoming larger and firmer, and then the fluid subsides during the night.

The other common finding in an infant in whom the processus vaginalis remains open is an inguinal hernia, which is a loop of intestine that passes through the abnormal opening (see Fig. 17-41). Such a hernia usually leads to intestinal obstruction. Surgical repair is recommended if the opening remains patent or herniation persists because there is a risk that the herniated intestinal loop may become strangulated.

Acquired hydrocele may result from scrotal injury, an infection, a tumor, or unknown causes. Acquired hydroceles are more common after middle age. Large amounts of fluid may compromise the blood supply to the testis, requiring aspiration.

A *spermatocele* is a cyst containing fluid and sperm that develops between the testis and the epididymis outside the tunica vaginalis. It may be related to an abnormality of the tubules. If the cyst is large, it may be surgically removed.

A *varicocele* is a dilated vein in the spermatic cord, usually on the left side. It frequently develops after puberty and results from a lack of valves in the veins, permitting backflow of blood and increased pressure in the veins. Varicocele may be mild, and scrotal support minimizes the heavy feeling. If it is extensive, the varicocele is painful or tender and leads to infertility because

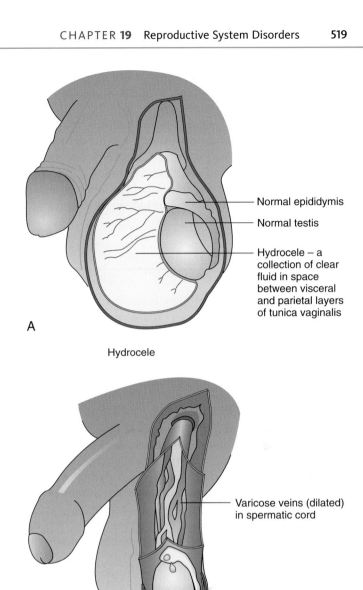

A

Hydrocele

- Normal epididymis
- Normal testis
- Hydrocele – a collection of clear fluid in space between visceral and parietal layers of tunica vaginalis

B

Varicocele

- Varicose veins (dilated) in spermatic cord

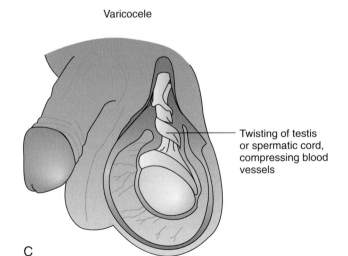

C

Torsion of testis

- Twisting of testis or spermatic cord, compressing blood vessels

FIGURE 19-3 Abnormalities of the scrotum.

of the impaired blood flow to the testes and decreased spermatogenesis. In this case, surgical treatment of the abnormal veins is necessary.

Torsion of the testis occurs when the testis rotates on the spermatic cord, compressing the arteries and veins. Ischemia develops, and the scrotum swells. Immediate treatment is required manually and surgically to restore blood flow to the testis. Testicular torsion frequently occurs during puberty, both spontaneously and following trauma.

Inflammation and Infections

Prostatitis

The National Institutes of Health recognizes four categories of prostatitis: category 1, acute bacterial; category 2, chronic bacterial; category 3, nonbacterial; and category 4, asymptomatic inflammatory prostatitis. It is considered an ascending infection or inflammation with multiple causes. The prostate is somewhat protected from ascending infection by the flushing action of urination and ejaculation and by an intact mucous membrane. Also, the prostatic secretions contain antimicrobial factors. However, the close association of the male reproductive tract with the urinary tract, including the continuous mucosa, promotes the spread of infection through the structures, and prostatitis is therefore closely associated with urinary tract infections.

The causes of the common nonbacterial form of prostatitis and prostatodynia (painful prostate) have not been established.

■ *Pathophysiology*

Acute bacterial prostatitis causes a tender, swollen gland, typically soft and boggy on palpation. The urine contains large quantities of microorganisms, pus, and leukocytes. Expressed prostatic secretions also contain many organisms, confirming the source of the infection. However, this process may be painful and may actually spread the infection or cause bacteremia in acute cases.

Nonbacterial prostatitis is indicated by large numbers of leukocytes in the urine and prostatic secretions, although the prostate gland is not markedly enlarged.

In patients with chronic prostatitis the prostate is only slightly enlarged, irregular, and firm because fibrosis is more extensive. In most cases of prostatitis the urinary tract is infected and signs of dysuria, frequency, and urgency occur. Other parts of the reproductive tract (e.g., the epididymis or testes) may be involved as well.

■ *Etiology*

Acute bacterial prostatitis is usually an *ascending* infection (it progresses up the urethra) and is caused primarily by *Escherichia coli* but sometimes by *Pseudomonas*, *Proteus*, or *Streptococcus faecalis*.

It occurs:
- In young men in association with urinary tract infections due to invasion by coliform bacteria from the intestines (see Chapter 18)
- In older men with benign prostatic hypertrophy
- In association with sexually transmitted diseases (STDs) such as gonorrhea
- With instrumentation such as catheterization
- Sometimes from hematogenous spread (through the blood)

Chronic prostatitis is usually related to repeated infection by *E. coli*.

■ *Signs and Symptoms*

Although both acute and chronic infections are manifested by dysuria, urinary frequency, and urgency, similar to cystitis, the acute infection is usually accompanied by fever and chills. Low back pain or lower abdominal discomfort may be present. Severe inflammation in the prostate may cause obstruction of the urinary flow through the urethra, resulting in a decreased urinary stream, hesitancy in initiating urination, incomplete bladder emptying, and nocturia or frequency. Systemic signs include fever, malaise, anorexia, and muscle aching. In non-bacterial prostatitis, the urinary signs are present, often intermittently, but the systemic signs are less marked.

■ *Treatment*

Antibacterial drugs such as ciprofloxacin (Cipro) are recommended for bacterial infections. Follow-up tests should confirm complete eradication. Nonbacterial prostatitis can be treated by anti-inflammatory drugs as well as by prophylactic antibacterials.

Balanitis

Balanitis is a fungal infection of the glans penis that can be transmitted during sexual activity. The fungus, *Candida albicans*, causes the infection primarily in uncircumcised males. Balanitis first appears as penile vesicles which later develop into patches that cause severe burning and itching. Diagnosis is accomplished by the identification of the presence of Candida. Treatment is done with topical antifungal medications such as Miconazole, Tolnaftate and Clotrimazole.

THINK ABOUT 19-2

a. Describe the appearance and functional changes in a baby boy with: (1) epispadias and (2) hydrocele.
b. Compare the typical signs of acute bacterial prostatitis, chronic bacterial prostatitis, and acute nonbacterial prostatitis.

Bladder

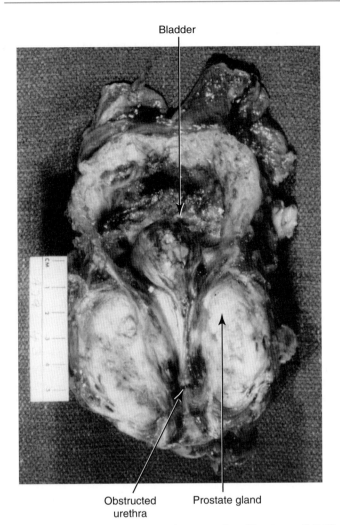

Obstructed urethra   Prostate gland

FIGURE 19-4 Benign prostatic hypertrophy. *(Courtesy of R.W. Shaw, MD, North York General Hospital, Toronto, Ontario, Canada.)*

Tumors

Benign Prostatic Hypertrophy

■ *Pathophysiology*

Benign prostatic hypertrophy (BPH) is a very common disorder in older men, with an estimated 50% of men over 65 years experiencing some form varying from mild to severe. Although called hypertrophy, the change is actually hyperplasia of the prostatic tissue with formation of nodules surrounding the urethra. These changes lead to compression of the urethra and variable degrees of urinary obstruction (Fig. 19-4). This hyperplasia appears to be related to an imbalance between estrogen and testosterone that results from the hormonal changes associated with aging. No connection between BPH and prostatic carcinoma has been identified.

Rectal examination reveals an enlarged gland. Incomplete emptying of the bladder due to the obstruction leads to frequent infections (Fig. 19-5). Continued obstruction causes a distended bladder, dilated ureters, hydronephrosis, and possible renal damage (see Chapter 18). If significant obstruction and urinary retention

BENIGN PROSTATIC HYPERTROPHY (BPH)

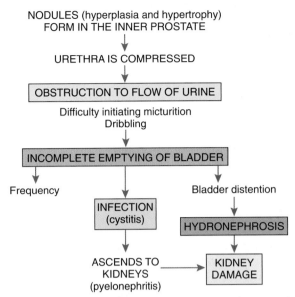

FIGURE 19-5 Complications of benign prostatic hypertrophy.

develop in the patient, surgical intervention, using one of several techniques, is required.

■ *Signs and Symptoms*

The initial signs indicate obstruction of urinary flow. Hesitancy, dribbling, and decreased force of the urinary stream are direct results of the narrowed urethra. Incomplete bladder emptying leads to frequency, nocturia, and recurrent urinary tract infection.

■ *Treatment*

Only a small percentage of cases require intervention. Drugs to reduce the androgenic effects and slow nodular growth include Avodart (dutasteride). When surgery is not desirable, alpha-adrenergic blockers such as Flomax (tamsulosin) relax smooth muscle in the prostate and bladder, resulting in increased flow of urine. A combination of Proscar (finasteride) and Cardura (doxazosin) has been shown to greatly reduce the progression of hypertrophy and possible obstruction of the urethra. Surgery may be recommended when obstruction is severe and several procedures are available. Choice depends on the man's overall health status and the degree of obstruction.

Cancer of the Prostate

Prostate cancer is common in men older than 50 years and ranks high as a cause of cancer death in men. The National Cancer Institute of the NIH estimated that in 2013 there will be 238,590 new cases of prostate cancer in the United States resulting in 29,720 deaths, which is the second leading cause of death from cancer in men. One in six men is expected to develop prostatic cancer during their lifetime.

Pathophysiology

Most tumors are adenocarcinomas arising from the tissue near the surface of the gland (rather than in the central area, as in BPH). There may be more than one focus of neoplastic cells. Tumors vary in degree of cellular differentiation; the more undifferentiated or anaplastic tumors are much more aggressive, growing and spreading at a faster rate. Many tumors are androgen dependent.

Prostate cancer is both invasive to regional tissues such as lymph nodes or urethra and, metastatic to bone (Fig. 19-6). With better screening of men older than 50 years for this cancer many individuals are being

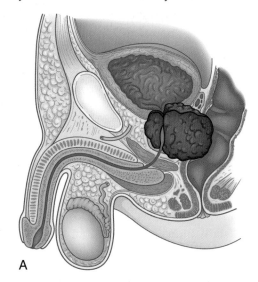

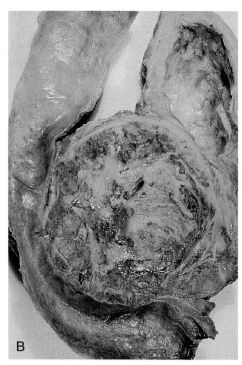

FIGURE 19-6 Carcinoma of prostate. **A,** Schematic of prostate tumor. **B,** Carcinoma of the prostate extending into the rectum and urinary bladder. *(B from Damjanov I, Linder J, editors: Pathology: a color atlas, St Louis, 2000, Mosby.)*

diagnosed in earlier stages than in the past. Five-year survival rates vary considerably: Localized cancers have a 100% survival rate, whereas regional spread reduces the rate to 89%, and distant metastases of bone or other organs have a 37% survival rate.

Etiology

Five to ten percent of prostatic cancers are caused by inherited mutations, and the mutation in the HPC1 gene has been identified as the cause of these cancers. Other causes include high androgen levels (either intrinsic or extrinsic), increased insulinlike growth factor, and recurrent prostatitis. Prostatic cancer is common in North America and northern Europe but not in countries farther east. The incidence is higher in the African-American population than in Caucasians, indicating a possible genetic factor. Testosterone receptors are found on cancer cells. Note that BPH alone does not predispose to prostatic cancer.

Signs and Symptoms

A hard nodule in the periphery of the gland, often in the posterior lobe, may be detected on digital rectal examination. The tumor tends not to cause early urethral obstruction because of its location. As the tumor develops, some obstruction occurs, producing signs of hesitancy, a decreased stream, urinary frequency, or bladder infection (cystitis).

Diagnostic Tests

Two serum markers are helpful—prostate specific antigen (PSA), which provides a useful screening tool for early detection as well as supportive data for the diagnosis, and prostatic acid phosphatase, which is elevated when metastatic cancer is present. Prostate specific antigen may be elevated with BPH or infection, so it is not diagnostic by itself and there have been false positive and false negative results. These serum markers may be useful in monitoring the effectiveness of treatment. It is recommended that all men older than age 50 be tested regularly. Men who are considered high risk for prostatic cancer due to ethnicity or family history should begin testing at age 45.

Ultrasonography using a small ultrasound probe and biopsy confirm the diagnosis. Bone scans and monoclonal antibody scans are useful for detecting early metastases.

Diagnosis is based on three criteria: an elevated PSA, abnormality on digital rectal exam, and biopsy results, which are expressed as a numeric value based on the Gleason scale, which is based on the proportion of abnormal cells present in the biopsy specimen.

Treatment

Surgery (radical prostatectomy) and radiation (including implants) are the treatments of choice. There is risk of impotence or incontinence. When the tumor is androgen sensitive, orchiectomy (removal of the testes) or antitestosterone drug therapy (e.g., flutamide [Euflex]) may be suggested to reduce hormonal effects. New chemotherapy protocols are now in clinical trials. Approximately 30% of men deemed "cured" have a recurrence of the cancer after 5 years.

Cancer of the Testes

Benign tumors of the testes are extremely rate and the majority of tumors that occur in the testes are malignant, arising from germ cells. Although testicular cancer is not common, with about 1 in 300 men being affected during their lifetime, there is concern because it occurs primarily in the 15- to 35-year-old age group, and the incidence is increasing. The cause for the increase in cases is not known. Testicular cancer is the most common solid tumor in young men. Certain types of testicular cancer may occur in other groups, such as younger children or older males. For this reason, regular monthly testicular self-examination is recommended to check for an unusual hard mass. Illustrated instructions are available from The American Cancer Society and medical clinics.

■ *Pathophysiology*

Testicular cancer may originate from one type of cell, for example, a seminoma, or may be mixed, consisting of cells from a variety of sources and with varying degrees of differentiation. A teratoma consists of a mixture of different germ cells (Fig. 19-7). A common mixed tumor is a teratoma, derived from one or more of the germ cell layers, combined with an embryonal carcinoma, which has poorly differentiated cells.

Some malignant tumors secrete human chorionic gonadotropin (hCG) or alpha-fetoprotein (AFP), which serve as a useful serum marker for both diagnosis and follow-up monitoring.

Some testicular neoplasms may spread at an early stage, for example, choriocarcinoma, whereas others, such as seminomas, remain localized for a more prolonged period. Testicular tumors follow a typical pattern when spreading, first appearing in the common iliac and para-aortic lymph nodes and then in the mediastinal and supraclavicular lymph nodes. Metastases spreading through the blood to the lungs, liver, bone, and brain occur at a later time.

Several staging systems are used, based on the extent of the primary tumor, the degree of lymph node involvement (retroperitoneal or otherwise), and the presence of distant metastases.

■ *Etiology*

This tumor has a heredity pattern with change in chromosome number 12 in some families and there is a possible relationship with infection or trauma. An established predisposing factor is *cryptorchidism,* or maldescent of the testes.

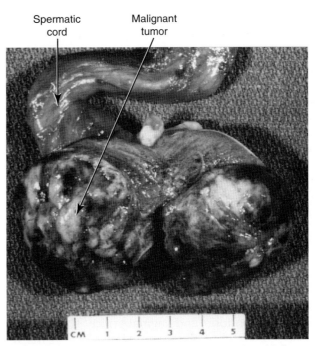

FIGURE 19-7 Cancer of the testes-spermatic cord and left testis with mixed embryonal teratoma and choriocarcinoma. *(Courtesy of R.W. Shaw, MD, North York General Hospital, Toronto, Ontario, Canada.)*

■ *Signs and Symptoms*

Testicular tumors present as hard, painless, usually unilateral masses. The testis may be enlarged or may feel heavy. Eventually there may be a dull aching pain in the lower abdomen. In some cases, hydrocele or epididymitis may develop because of inflammation, or gynecomastia (enlarged breasts) may become evident if hormones are secreted by the tumor.

■ *Diagnostic Tests*

Tests such as ultrasound, computed tomography scans, and lymphangiography, and the presence of tumor markers (e.g., AFP and hCG) are useful in diagnosis. If a solid mass is seen during diagnostic imaging, surgical removal of the entire testis is done rather than a local biopsy of the mass. This is done to reduce the possibility of spread of tumor cells.

■ *Treatment*

Treatment of testicular cancer using a combination of surgery (orchiectomy), radiation therapy, and sometimes chemotherapy has greatly improved the prognosis. Orchiectomy does not usually interfere with sexual function. However, radiation or chemotherapy may temporarily reduce fertility for a few months. Men who are scheduled for these treatments may wish to consider sperm banking before the procedure. Cancer cells are not transmitted in the semen.

Disorders of the Female Reproductive System

Review of the Female Reproductive System

Structure and Function

The female external genitalia or *vulva* include the mons pubis, labia, clitoris, and vaginal orifice. The *mons pubis* consists of the adipose tissue and hair covering the symphysis pubis. The *labia majora,* the outer fold, and the *labia minora* inside it are long, thin folds of skin extending back and down from the mons pubis, protecting the orifices. Sebaceous glands and sweat glands are located in the folds. The *clitoris* is a small projection of erectile tissue located anterior to the urethra. It is analogous to the male penis and is very sensitive to touch. In the *vagina,* the entryway to the reproductive tract, the orifice or introitus is situated between the urethral meatus (anterior) and the anus (posterior) (Fig. 19-8). The vagina is a muscular, distensible canal extending upward from the vulva to the cervix. It is lined with a mucosal membrane and falls in rugae or folds, allowing expansion during coitus (intercourse) or childbirth. The mucosa consists of stratified squamous epithelial cells, which are hormone sensitive. This mucous membrane is continuous up through the uterus and fallopian tubes, enabling the spread of infection. Following menopause and the decline in estrogen secretions, the mucosa becomes thin and fragile.

Bartholin's glands (the greater vestibular glands) are located on either side of the vaginal orifice and secrete mucus in response to sexual stimulation to facilitate penile penetration into the vagina during intercourse. Skene's glands, located by the external urethral meatus, also secrete mucus to keep the tissues moist. Both of these sets of mucus-secreting glands are easily obstructed and infected. Leukorrhea, the normal vaginal discharge, is produced by these glands; the secretions are relatively clear or whitish and contain mucus and sloughed cells. The amount fluctuates during the menstrual cycle. Before puberty and after menopause vaginal pH is around 7, but during the reproductive years it is more acidic, between 4 and 5, due to an increased population of *Lactobacillus.* The acidic pH and the thickness of the epithelium provide protection against infection.

The upper vagina surrounds the cervix, which is the lower part or neck of the uterus. The endocervical canal is the passageway between the internal os of the cervix at the uterine end and the external os at the vaginal end. The external os is a small opening filled with thick mucus that acts as a barrier to vaginal flora attempting to ascend into the uterus. The lining of the endocervical canal is continuous with that of the uterus and the vagina but differs in composition. The endocervical canal is lined with columnar epithelial cells, which change to squamous epithelium in the vagina. The point of change is known as the transformation zone or squamous-columnar junction, and this is the common site of cervical dysplasia and cancer.

The uterus is a muscular sac within which a fertilized ovum may be implanted and develop. Note the relative sizes of the uterus and other structures in Figure 19-8. The pear-shaped body of the uterus is called the corpus. It is loosely suspended by ligaments in the pelvic cavity to allow for expansion during pregnancy. Normally it is anteverted, or tipped forward, resting on the urinary bladder (see Fig. 19-8).

The uterine wall is made up of three layers: the outer perimetrium or parietal peritoneum, the thick, middle layer of smooth muscle or myometrium, and the inner endometrium. The endometrium consists of a functional layer that is responsive to hormones during the menstrual cycle and an underlying basal layer that is responsible for the regeneration of the endometrium following menses.

The two fallopian tubes (oviducts) originate near the top of the uterus, just under the fundus, the top part of the corpus. Each tube curves up and out, ending in a flared opening over the ovary. This end portion has a fringe of fimbriae, moving finger-like projections that draw the released ovum into the tube. Cilia and peristaltic movements in the fallopian tube continue to move the ovum toward the uterus. Usually the ovum is fertilized by a sperm in the distal fallopian tube, and then it continues on to the uterus, where it is implanted at a suitable site in the endometrium.

The female gonads are the ovaries, which produce the ova, one each month during the reproductive years between menarche (onset) and menopause. The two ovaries are suspended by ligaments, one on either side of the uterus. These ovaries supply the female gamete, the ovum, and the sex hormones for the female, primarily estrogen and progesterone, on a cyclic basis (Fig. 19-9).

The female breast plays a significant role in the reproductive system. It responds to cyclic hormonal changes and is responsible for lactation, the provision of breast milk to the newborn. Mammary tissue develops under the influence of increased estrogen secretion, commencing at puberty. The breast consists of 15 to 20 lobes supported by ligaments. Muscle and fatty tissue are interspersed among the lobes and their subunits, the

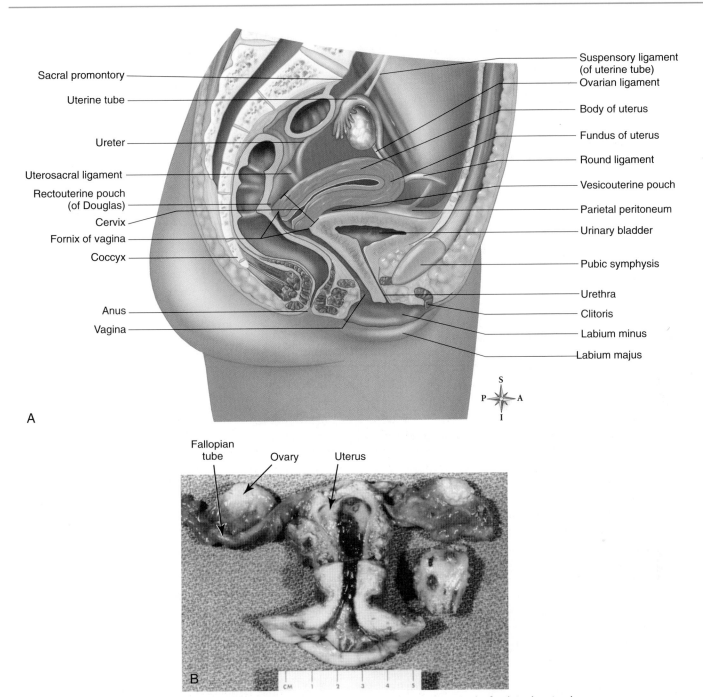

FIGURE 19-8 **Female Reproductive Organs A,** Diagram (sagittal section) of pelvis showing location of female reproductive organs. **B,** Ovaries, fallopian tubes, uterus, and vagina of a postmenopausal woman. Note the relative sizes of the structures. (**A,** *From Patton KT, Thibodeau GA: Anatomy & Physiology, ed 8, St. Louis, 2013, Mosby.* **B,** *Courtesy of R.W. Shaw, MD, North York General Hospital, Toronto, Ontario, Canada.*)

lobules and the acini. The *acini* are the basic functional units of the breast tissue, consisting of epithelial cells that secrete milk and contracting cells that move the milk into ducts. The breast tissue also has a system of collecting and ejecting ducts for milk that culminate in openings in the nipple. The breast is well supplied with blood vessels, lymphatics, and nerves. Sebaceous glands are found in the areola, the pigmented tissue surrounding the nipple (Fig. 19-10).

During the menstrual cycle, the higher estrogen and progesterone levels increase both the vascularity of the breast and the proliferation and dilation of the ducts,

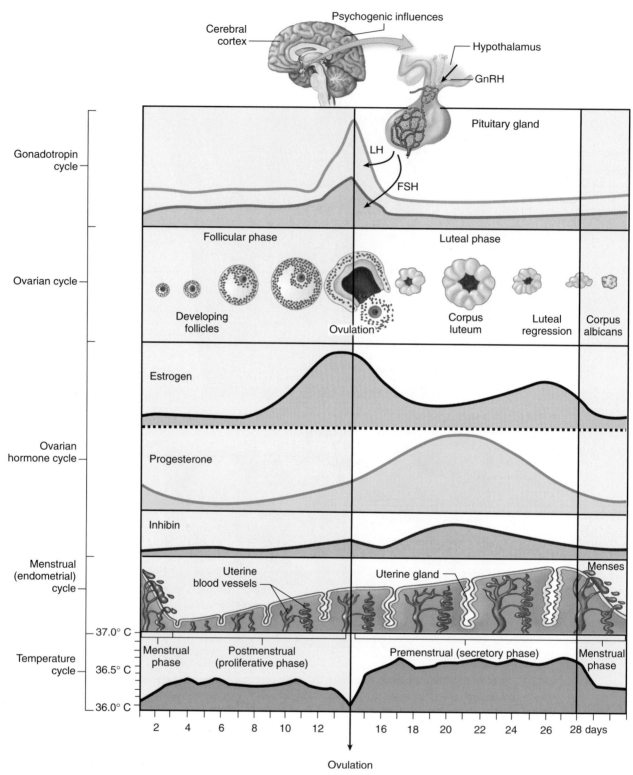

FIGURE 19-9 Female Reproductive Cycles This diagram illustrates the interrelationships among the cerebral, hypothalamic, pituitary, ovarian, and uterine functions throughout a standard 28-day menstrual cycle. The variations in basal body temperature are also illustrated. *(From Patton KT, Thibodeau GA: Anatomy & Physiology, ed 8, St. Louis, 2013, Mosby.)*

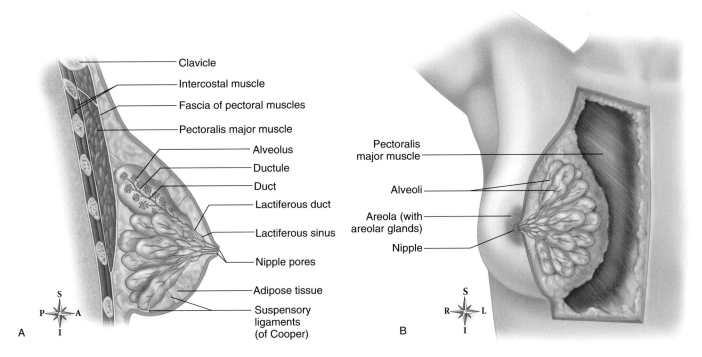

FIGURE 19-10 The Female Breast A, Sagittal section of a lactating breast. Notice how the glandular structures are anchored to the overlying skin and to the pectoral muscles by the suspensory ligaments of Cooper. Each lobule of glandular tissue is drained by a lactiferous duct that eventually opens through the nipple. **B,** Anterior view of a lactating breast. Overlying skin and connective tissue have been removed from the medial side to show the internal structure of the breast and underlying skeletal muscle. In nonlactating breasts, the glandular tissue is much less prominent, with adipose tissue making up most of each breast. *(From Patton KT, Thibodeau GA:* Anatomy & Physiology, *ed 8, St. Louis, 2013, Mosby.)*

leading to increased fullness and tenderness of the breasts premenstrually. It is recommended that breast self-examination be performed shortly after the conclusion of menses, when hormone levels are low and the breasts are small and less nodular. This examination should be performed at the same time each month to allow comparison of the normal characteristics of the breast. Postmenopausally, examination should be done at regular intervals such as the day of the month the woman's birthday falls on.

Hormones and the Menstrual Cycle

Hormonal secretions, release of ova, and associated endometrial changes occur in a cyclic pattern in women during the reproductive years (see Fig. 19-9). The average cycle is 28 days, but a range of 21 to 45 days is considered normal. Some women experience irregular cycles.

The cycle consists of:

- First, menstruation, or menses, occurs (the sloughing of the endometrial tissue that occurs when implantation of the ovum has not occurred).
- The endometrial proliferation stage follows, when increasing FSH is secreted by the anterior pituitary gland, resulting in maturation of an ovarian follicle.
- The maturing follicle secretes estrogen, causing proliferation or thickening of the functional layer of the endometrium.
- At midpoint, as LH levels greatly increase, ovulation takes place with release of the mature ovum.
- The ovarian follicle is now converted by LH into the corpus luteum, which increases production of progesterone.
- Progesterone enhances the development of endometrial blood vessels and glycogen-secreting glands in preparation for the implantation of a fertilized ovum.

If fertilization does not occur, estrogen and progesterone levels drop, and the corpus luteum and endometrium degenerate, resulting in menstruation, and beginning another cycle.

Hormonal levels fluctuate considerably in the female during the cycle, a result of complex interactions involving the hypothalamus, the anterior pituitary, and the ovary (see Chapter 16). The feedback mechanism involves estrogen and progesterone acting on the anterior pituitary gland to control the release of LH and FSH. The changes in hormone levels and basal body temperature (early morning) that occur during the cycle may be useful in determining the anticipated time of ovulation or fertile periods in women.

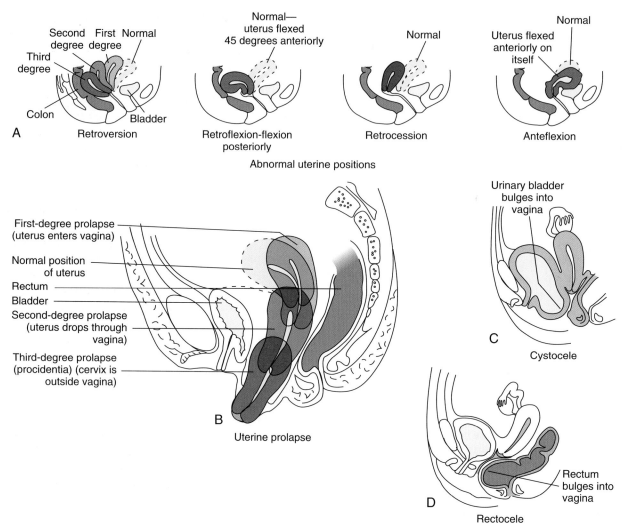

FIGURE 19-11 Structural abnormalities of the uterus.

Structural Abnormalities

The normal position of the uterus is slightly *anteverted* (tipped forward) and *anteflexed* (bent forward over the bladder), with the cervix downward and back. The position of the uterus may vary because of a minor congenital anatomic alteration, childbirth, or a pathologic condition such as scar tissue or a tumor. Examples of uterine displacement are shown in Figure 19-11*A*. A *retroverted* uterus is tipped backward. The uterus may be excessively curved or bent, either retroflexed (bent backward) or anteflexed (bent forward). In most cases, there are no deleterious effects from such changes in position. In some cases, infertility may result if the cervix is not positioned appropriately to facilitate the passage of sperm. Often malposition does not cause any symptoms. Marked retroversion may cause back pain, dysmenorrhea (painful menstruation), and dyspareunia (painful intercourse).

With aging or excessive stretching or trauma, the supporting ligaments, fascia, and muscles for the uterus, bladder, and rectum may become weakened (*pelvic relaxation*), and these organs may shift out of their normal position in the pelvis. Factors predisposing patients to this condition include difficult childbirth including prolonged labor, multiple births, birth of a large baby, and repeated pregnancies separated by short intervals. A genetic component also appears to be a factor. The effects often become apparent some years after the original injury has occurred, usually around menopause, when the decreasing hormonal levels contribute further to tissue atrophy. More than one structure may be affected in any one individual.

Uterine displacement or *prolapse* is the descent of the cervix or uterus into the vagina (see Fig. 19-11*B*).

Prolapse is classified as:
- First degree if the cervix drops into the vagina
- Second degree if the cervix lies at the opening to the vagina and the body of the uterus is in the vagina
- Third degree (procidentia) if the uterus and cervix protrude through the vaginal orifice

Although the early stage of prolapse may be asymptomatic, the more advanced stages cause discomfort and a feeling of heaviness in the vagina. Protrusion of the cervix causes irritation and infection in the cervix. Prolapse may be treated by surgery or by using a pessary to maintain the uterus in position.

A *cystocele* is a protrusion of the bladder into the anterior wall of the vagina (see Fig. 19-11*C*). The bladder cannot be emptied completely, and recurrent cystitis is common. A *rectocele* is a protrusion of the rectum into the posterior wall of the vagina (see Fig. 19-11*D*). The mass may be small or large enough to drop into the vaginal opening. Interference with defecation and a feeling of pressure in the pelvis are the common indicators. Rectocele and cystocele, if severe, require surgical repair.

Menstrual Disorders

Menstrual Abnormalities

Amenorrhea, or absence of menstruation, may be primary or secondary. In the primary condition, menarche has never occurred. This may result from a genetic disorder such as Turner syndrome (a chromosome abnormality, XO, in which the ovaries do not function). Congenital defects affecting the hypothalamus, central nervous system, or pituitary, or congenital absence of the uterus and congenital uterine hypoplasia (infantile uterus) may also interfere with the normal process. Secondary amenorrhea is the cessation of menstruation in an individual who previously experienced cycles. It frequently results from an impediment in the hypothalamic-pituitary axis. The hypothalamus may be suppressed by conditions such as tumors, stress, sudden weight loss, eating disorders, or participation in competitive sports, leading to reduced body fat. Systemic factors such as anemia or chemotherapy may also cause secondary amenorrhea.

Dysmenorrhea refers to painful menstruation and may be primary or secondary. Primary dysmenorrhea has no organic foundation and develops when ovulation commences. The majority of women experience some discomfort, but for many the pain is sufficient to interrupt normal activities. In many cases, dysmenorrhea is relieved following childbirth. The severe cramping pain is related to the excessive release of prostaglandin during endometrial shedding. This prostaglandin causes strong uterine muscle contractions and ischemia. Pain develops 24 to 48 hours before or at the onset of menses and lasts for 24 to 48 hours. In addition, nausea and vomiting, headache, and dizziness may accompany the cramps as the prostaglandins enter the systemic circulation. Some relief may be afforded by the use of a heating pad, exercise, or medications such as ibuprofen (Advil), a nonsteroidal anti-inflammatory drug, which inhibits prostaglandin synthesis. An alternative treatment is the use of oral contraceptives, which lead to anovulatory cycles that are not painful. Secondary dysmenorrhea results from pelvic disorders such as endometriosis, uterine polyps or tumors, or pelvic inflammatory disease.

Abnormal menstrual bleeding is a common concern. Examples of abnormal patterns include:
- *Menorrhagia* (increased amount and duration of flow)
- *Metrorrhagia* (bleeding between cycles)
- *Polymenorrhea* (short cycles of less than 3 weeks)
- *Oligomenorrhea* (long cycles of more than 6 weeks)

The usual cause of an altered pattern is lack of ovulation; however, this condition may also result from hormonal disorders such as thyroid abnormalities or pathologic conditions such as tumors. Any change in the woman's individual pattern is significant and should be investigated.

Premenstrual syndrome (PMS) is a condition that begins a week or so before the onset of menses and ends with the onset of menses. The cause is not completely understood, but research on hormonal factors continues. In most women PMS causes nuisance symptoms such as breast tenderness, weight gain, abdominal distention or bloating, irritability, emotional lability, sleep disturbances, depression, headache, and fatigue. Some women have increased mental concentration and activity, whereas others are lethargic. These manifestations are severe in 3% to 8% of women reporting PMS; the more severe form of the disorder is termed premenstrual dysphoric syndrome. Treatment measures are tailored to the individual and may include hormonal therapy and the use of diuretics or antidepressants as necessary.

Endometriosis

Endometriosis affects about 5 million women in the United States and is defined as the presence of endometrial tissue outside the uterus on structures such as the ovaries, ligaments, or colon (Fig. 19-12). On occasion, it may affect distant sites such as the lungs. This *ectopic* endometrium responds to cyclic hormone variations, growing during the proliferation and secretory stages of the menstrual cycle and then degenerating, shedding, and bleeding. Because there is no exit point for this blood, and blood is irritating to tissues when it does not belong there, local inflammation and pain result. The inflammation recurs with each cycle and eventually causes the development of fibrous tissue. Although it may be possible to palpate nodular tissue, the diagnosis is confirmed by laparoscopy.

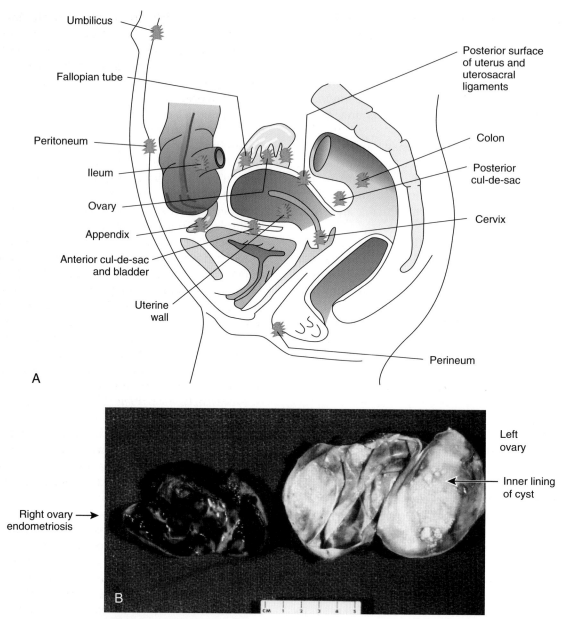

Umbilicus

Fallopian tube

Peritoneum

Ileum

Ovary

Appendix

Anterior cul-de-sac and bladder

Uterine wall

Posterior surface of uterus and uterosacral ligaments

Colon

Posterior cul-de-sac

Cervix

Perineum

A

Right ovary endometriosis

Left ovary

Inner lining of cyst

B

FIGURE 19-12 Endometriosis A, Possible ectopic sites. **B,** Endometriosis involving the right ovary (chocolate cyst) and left ovary showing the inner lining of a large cyst with excrescences. (**B,** *Courtesy of R.W. Shaw, MD, North York General Hospital, Toronto, Ontario, Canada.*)

Fibrous tissue may cause adhesions and obstruction of the involved structures, such as the urinary bladder or colon. When the uterus is pulled out of its normal position (e.g., into retroversion) by adhesions, infertility frequently results. The fallopian tube may be blocked or the ovary covered by fibrous tissue, preventing movement of the ovum into and through the tube, ultimately causing infertility. When endometrial tissue occurs on the ovary, a "chocolate cyst" develops, a fibrous sac containing old brown blood (see Fig. 19-12*B*).

The primary manifestation of endometriosis is dysmenorrhea. The pain may persist throughout menses and typically becomes more severe each month. Dyspareunia, or painful intercourse, may occur if the vagina and supporting ligaments are affected by adhesions.

The cause of endometriosis has not been established. Proposed mechanisms include migration of endometrial tissue up through the fallopian tubes into the peritoneal cavity during menstruation, development from embryonic tissue at other sites, spread of endometrium through the blood or lymph, or transplantation of tissue during surgery such as a cesarean section.

Treatment measures include hormonal suppression of the endometrial tissue, with relief of the pain associated with the monthly cycle, or surgical removal of the ectopic endometrial tissue. Pregnancy and lactation also result in amenorrhea, and atrophy of the ectopic tissue.

These measures do not cure endometriosis, but they do delay further damage and alleviate the symptoms.

THINK ABOUT 19-5

a. Describe each of the following: (1) second-degree uterine prolapse, (2) cystocele, and (3) retroversion of the uterus. Explain the secondary problems that may occur with second- or third-degree prolapse.

b. Differentiate the following terms from one another: (1) dysmenorrhea, (2) premenstrual syndrome, and (3) menorrhagia.

c. Explain the process by which endometriosis can cause infertility.

Infections and Inflammation

Many infections of the vagina (vaginitis) and cervix (cervicitis) are considered STDs and are included in the section on these diseases later in this chapter. Other inflammations of the female reproductive organs often caused by infections include salpingitis (inflammation of the oviduct or fallopian tube), urethritis (inflammation of the urethra), oophoritis (inflammation of the ovaries), and mastitis (inflammation of the mammary gland). In addition to infections caused by organisms passed on through sexual contact, other infections may arise through non–sexually transmitted organisms such as *Staphylococcus aureus*, which is the bacteria primarily responsible for toxic shock syndrome and mastitis.

Candidiasis

Candidiasis is one form of vaginitis that is not sexually transmitted. It is a yeast infection caused by *Candida albicans* (*Monilia*) and usually occurs as an opportunistic superficial infection of mucous membranes or skin (see Fig. 6-7). Infection may follow antibiotic therapy for an unrelated bacterial infection elsewhere in the body (which creates a more alkaline pH and upsets the balance of resident flora) or may develop because of decreased resistance (e.g., in immune-deficiency states), or increased glycogen or glucose levels in the secretions (e.g., with pregnancy, use of oral contraceptives, or diabetes).

Candidiasis causes red and swollen pruritic mucous membranes and a thick, white, curdlike discharge. White patches may adhere to the vaginal wall. Dysuria (painful urination) and dyspareunia (painful intercourse) may be present. An antifungal agent such as nystatin is effective treatment. To prevent recurrence, the predisposing factors need to be addressed.

Pelvic Inflammatory Disease

Pelvic inflammatory disease (PID) is an infection of the reproductive tract, particularly the fallopian tubes and ovaries. The condition includes cervicitis endometritis (uterus), salpingitis, and oophoritis. The infection may be acute or chronic. PID is a common problem and is a matter of concern because of the potential acute complications such as peritonitis and pelvic abscess as well as the long-term problems of infertility and the high risk of ectopic pregnancy.

■ *Pathophysiology*

The infection usually originates as a vaginitis or cervicitis and is polymicrobial, often involving several causative bacteria. The microbes ascend through the uterus into the fallopian tubes (Fig. 19-13). The early stage of inflammation promotes additional invasion of bacteria into the mucosa. The tubal walls become edematous, and the lumen is filled with purulent exudate, effectively obstructing the tube and restricting drainage into the uterus. The exudate drips out of the fimbriae onto the ovary and surrounding tissue. The peritoneal membranes attempt to localize the infection initially, but peritonitis may develop (see Chapter 17). Abscesses may form as the inflammatory response struggles to contain or wall off the infection. Pelvic abscesses may be life threatening if not quickly drained surgically. Infection may spread, resulting in septicemia. The most common cause of death in women with PID is septic shock.

Adhesions and strictures are common sequelae; they affect the tubes and ovaries, leading to infertility or ectopic pregnancy (implantation of the fertilized ovum in the fallopian tube). Adhesions or scar tissue may also affect the surrounding structures such as the colon.

■ *Etiology*

The majority of infections arise from sexually transmitted diseases such as gonorrhea (*Neisseria gonorrhoeae*) and chlamydiosis (*Chlamydia trachomatis*). Multiple organisms are present in many cases. Other potential agents include *Bacteroides*, *Gardnerella vaginalis*, Group B streptococci, *E. coli*, *Pseudomonas*, *Haemophilus influenza*, and *Enterococcus*.

A prior episode of vaginitis or cervicitis, often with few signs, frequently precedes the development of PID. Infection is likely to become acute during or immediately following menses, when the endometrium is more vulnerable.

Pelvic inflammatory disease may also result from insertion of an intrauterine device (IUD, a contraceptive device) or other instrument contaminated by organisms from the lower reproductive tract or other source. Any instrument or device is likely to traumatize the tissue or perforate the wall, leading to inflammation and infection (see Fig. 19-13*B*—note the adhesions around the IUD). Infection may also be associated with abortion or childbirth. Historically PID was the feared complication of illegal abortions or deliveries under primitive conditions.

Occasionally infection in the reproductive tract may result from bloodborne organisms or from an infection

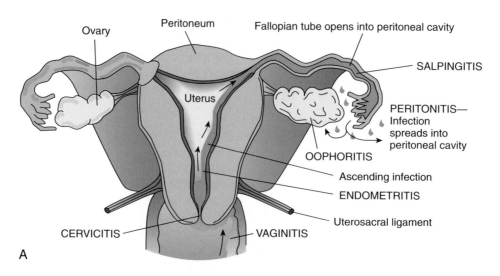

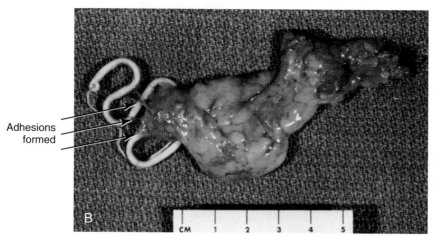

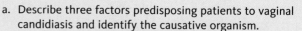

FIGURE 19-13 **Pelvic Inflammatory Disease A,** Spread of infection. **B,** Uterus perforated by intra-uterine device (IUD) leads to localized inflammation in peritoneal cavity and omentum forming adhesions around IUD. (**B,** *Courtesy of R.W. Shaw, MD, North York General Hospital, Toronto, Ontario, Canada.*)

in the peritoneal cavity related to conditions such as appendicitis.

▪ Signs and Symptoms

Lower abdominal pain is usually the first indication of PID. Pain may be sudden and severe or gradually increasing in intensity. Characteristically it is a steady pain that increases with walking. Tenderness is common during pelvic examination. Purulent discharge is evident at the cervical os. Dysuria may be noted. Fever and leukocytosis depend on which causative organisms are involved. Peritonitis is indicated by increasing abdominal distention and rigidity.

▪ Treatment

Aggressive treatment with appropriate antimicrobials such as cefoxitin and doxycycline is required. Recurrent infections are common; therefore it is recommended that sexual partners be treated with antibiotics and that follow-up examinations are scheduled to ensure complete eradication of the infection.

THINK ABOUT 19-6

a. Describe three factors predisposing patients to vaginal candidiasis and identify the causative organism.
b. Explain how infection in the vagina can cause PID.
c. List the signs of PID and the reasons for them.
d. Explain why PID is considered a serious condition.

Benign Tumors

Leiomyoma (Fibroids)

A leiomyoma is a benign tumor of the myometrium, the cause of which is unknown. These uterine tumors are common in women during the reproductive years occurring in more than 30% of women, particularly Asian and African-American women. Following menopause the tumors tend to shrink. As benign tumors, they are not considered precancerous.

Fibroids are classified by location, developing in the uterine wall (intramural), beneath the endometrium (submucosal), or under the serosa (subserosal). The two

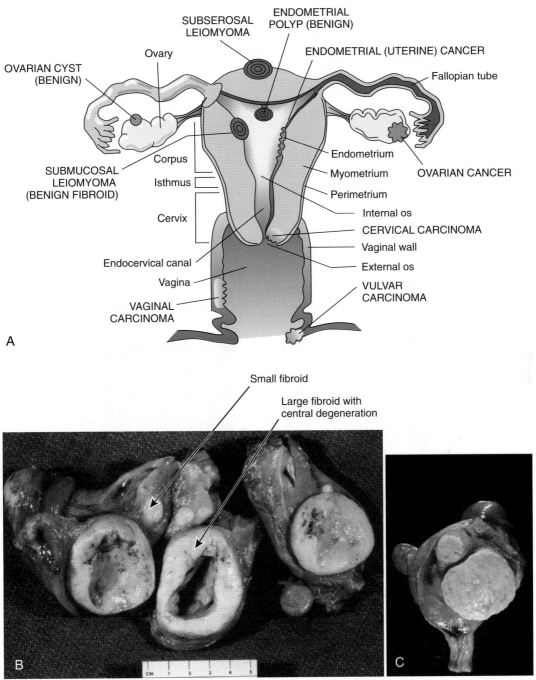

FIGURE 19-14 **A** and **B**, Types of benign uterine fibroids. (**B**, *Courtesy of R.W. Shaw, MD, North York General Hospital, Toronto, Ontario, Canada.*) **C**, Leiomyomas of the myometrium. The uterus is opened to reveal the tumors (*firm, white mass*) bulging into the cavity. (*From Kumar V, Abbas AK, Fausto M: Robbins and Cotran Pathologic Basis of Disease, ed 7, Philadelphia, 2005, Saunders.*)

latter forms may develop as polyps, the submucosal type projecting inward into the uterine cavity and the subserosal type growing outward into the pelvic cavity (Fig. 19-14).

Fibroids usually occur as multiple well-defined but unencapsulated masses, which vary widely in size. Large leiomyomas degenerate in the central region, undergoing necrosis and forming cysts. These benign tumors are hormone dependent, growing rapidly during pregnancy and decreasing in size with increasing fibrosis after menopause.

Fibroids are often asymptomatic until they grow large enough to be palpated. Abnormal bleeding such as menorrhagia may be an indicator of fibroid development. Large tumors may cause pressure on adjacent structures, leading to urinary frequency or constipation

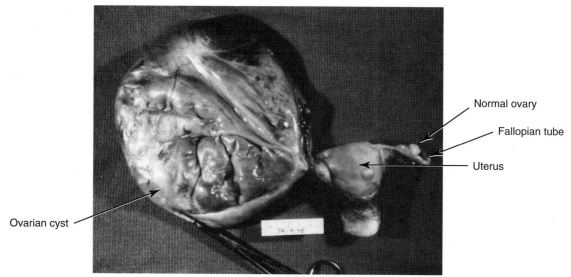

FIGURE 19-15 **A Large Ovarian Cyst** Note the relative size of the normal ovary and uterus. *(Courtesy of R.W. Shaw, MD, North York General Hospital, Toronto, Ontario, Canada.)*

and a heavy sensation in the lower abdomen. Large fibroids may interfere with implantation of the fertilized ovum or the course of pregnancy.

Treatment of large tumors involves hormonal therapy or surgery.

Ovarian Cysts

A variety of types of cysts occur frequently on the ovaries. Follicular and corpus luteal cysts are common and develop unilaterally in both ruptured and unruptured follicles. These functional ovarian cysts last approximately 8 to 12 weeks and disappear without complications. They are usually multiple, small, fluid-filled sacs located under the serosa covering the ovary. On occasion, a cyst may become large enough to cause discomfort, urinary retention, or menstrual irregularities (Fig. 19-15—compare the size of the cyst to the normal ovary). Bleeding resulting from rupture can cause more serious inflammation in the peritoneal cavity and requires surgical intervention. With a large cyst there is also risk of torsion of the ovary. Ultrasound examination or laparoscopy can be used to identify a cyst.

Polycystic Ovarian Syndrome

In *polycystic ovarian syndrome,* or Stein-Leventhal syndrome, large ovaries containing cysts and covered with a thick capsule develop (Fig. 19-16). Associated hormonal abnormalities include elevated androgen, estrogen, and LH levels and decreased FSH levels. The usual fluctuations or peaks in FSH and LH are missing. Ovulation does not occur. The basic problem is a dysfunction in the hypothalamic-pituitary control system. The cause is unknown, although in some women an inherited factor has been demonstrated. Young women manifest hirsutism, amenorrhea, and infertility. Medications such as clomiphene, an antiestrogen agent, may

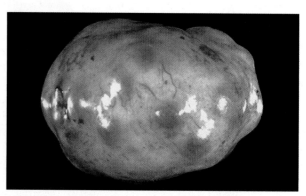

FIGURE 19-16 **Polycystic Ovary Syndrome (PCOS)** The ovary is studded with fluid-filled cysts developed from follicles that have failed to rupture. *(From Kumar V, Abbas A, Fausto N: Robbins and Cotran Pathologic Basis Of Disease, ed. 7, Philadelphia, 2005, Saunders.)*

stimulate ovulation, or surgical wedge resections of the ovaries may help to control the hormone levels. Oral contraceptives are used to reduce androgen secretions and masculinization effects. In women who have insulin resistance, treatment with an antihyperglycemic drug such as Metformin may result in ovulation.

Fibrocystic Breast Disease

Also called benign breast disease or fibrocystic change, this includes a broad range of breast lesions. There is some confusion between the normal physiologic changes in the breast that occur during the menstrual cycle and abnormal or pathologic changes. Fibrocystic disease refers to the presence of nodules or masses in the breast tissue that *change* during the menstrual cycle in response to fluctuating hormone levels, particularly estrogen. The connective tissue of the breast is gradually replaced by dense fibrous tissue. Increasing fluid in the breast during the secretory phase of the menstrual cycle accumulates in cysts bound by fibrous tissue, unable to escape. As well, the epithelial cells in the ducts proliferate in response to hormones. The cysts enlarge over time, often causing more degeneration of normal tissue.

Three categories of lesions have been designated, based on the risk of development of breast cancer. One category is nonproliferative lesions, which include microcysts and fibroadenomas. These are not considered precancerous. Fibroadenomas are specific benign tumors that appear as singular, movable masses. These tumors are usually excised.

The second category includes proliferative lesions (with epithelial hyperplasia in the ducts) in which there are no atypical cells. The risk of developing breast cancer in this group increases if there is also a family history of breast cancer.

The third category, a small one, requires monitoring, particularly if a family history of breast cancer is present. These lesions show proliferative changes with atypical cells. Breast biopsy can detect atypical cells and can differentiate benign from malignant cells.

The cysts or nodules feel firm and movable and vary in size during the cycle. The effects are more marked before menstruation, the breasts becoming heavy, painful, and tender.

Treatment is largely symptomatic but may include dietary changes such as reduction of caffeine and fat intake and drugs such as the androgen danazol. Fluid may be aspirated from cysts. Cysts may be removed if they manifest premalignant changes. Often there is some improvement after menopause.

Malignant Tumors

Neoplasms of the breast, cervix, and uterus are covered in this section. Ovarian cancer is discussed in Chapter 20 as well as in this chapter.

Carcinoma of the Breast

Carcinoma of the breast is a common malignancy in women and a major cause of death. Rarely breast cancer occurs in males. The incidence of breast carcinoma continues to increase after age 20, and more women are developing the malignancy at a younger age. The National Cancer Institute of the NIH estimates that in 2013 there will be 232,340 new female and 2240 new male cases in the United States resulting in 39,620 female and 410 male deaths. The overall incidence and mortality rate for this cancer has been increasing for a period of years, but it is now seems to be decreasing. There are currently 2.9 million survivors of breast cancer living in the United States.

■ *Pathophysiology*

Malignant tumors develop in the upper outer quadrant of the breast in approximately half the cases; the central portion of the breast is the next most common location (see Fig. 20-2). Most tumors are unilateral, although bilateral primary tumors may develop in some cases.

There are different types of breast carcinomas, but the majority arises from cells of the ductal epithelium. This cancer infiltrates the surrounding tissue and frequently adheres to the skin, causing dimpling. The tumor becomes *fixed* when it adheres to the muscle or fascia of the chest wall.

The malignant cells spread at an early stage, first to the nearby lymph nodes. Tumors in the upper outer quadrant and central breast area spread to the axillary lymph nodes. In most cases, several nodes are affected at the time of diagnosis. Widespread dissemination follows quickly, including metastases to the lungs, brain, bone, and liver (see Fig. 20-5 for illustration of breast cancer metastases).

Tumor cells are graded on the basis of the degree of *differentiation* or *anaplasia* (see Chapter 20). The tumor is then staged based on the size of the primary tumor, the involvement of lymph nodes, and the presence of metastases.

The presence of estrogen or progesterone *receptors* on the tumor cells is a major factor in determining how to treat the individual cancer. Such a tumor is hormone dependent because its growth is enhanced by the particular hormone.

■ *Etiology*

The majority of cases occur in women greater than age 50. A strong genetic predisposition has been supported by the identification of specific genes related to breast cancer, BRCA-1 and BRCA-2. Familial occurrence that is proportional to the numbers of affected relatives and the closeness of the relationships has been well documented.

The other major factor in the etiology of breast cancer is hormones—specifically, exposure to high estrogen levels. Circumstances such as a long period of regular menstrual cycles (for example, from an early menarche to late menopause), nulliparity (no children), and delay of the first pregnancy, all of which are associated with longer exposure to estrogen appear to promote cancer development. The role of exogenous estrogen in oral contraceptives or postmenopausal supplements remains controversial. Current formulations for oral contraceptives containing reduced levels of estrogens have considerably reduced the risks.

Other factors predisposing to breast carcinoma include fibrocystic disease with *atypical* hyperplasia, prior carcinoma in the uterus or in the other breast, and exposure of the chest to radiation (particularly in young women).

Lack of exercise, smoking, and a high-fat diet have been identified as risk factors in some studies. Prior abortion does not increase the risk of developing breast cancer. Considerable research continues to identify nongenetic risk factors which may be modified during the woman's life.

■ Signs and Symptoms

The usual initial sign is a single, small, hard, painless nodule. The mass is freely movable in the early stage but later becomes fixed. Other signs as the tumor becomes more advanced include dimpling of the skin, retraction of or discharge from the nipple, and a change in breast contour. Biopsy confirms the diagnosis of malignancy.

■ Treatment

Surgery, combined with radiation and chemotherapy, provides effective treatment for many cases. Surgical removal of the tumor, involving minimal tissue loss as in a lumpectomy, is the preferred method in stage 1 and stage 2, although a more radical approach involving a mastectomy may be necessary in more advanced cases. Either surgical approach may be combined with radiation after surgery. Women may opt for mastectomy and breast reconstruction if there is a strong genetic risk of recurrence of the cancer.

In addition, some lymph nodes are removed according to the existing lymphatic pathway from the tumor. The number of lymph nodes removed depends on the spread of tumor cells. (The nodes are checked during surgery.) Subsequent surgical reconstruction may be desired by some patients. Removal or radiation of lymph nodes impairs lymphatic drainage from the arm, resulting in swelling and stiffness. Physiotherapy and exercise are important in maintaining mobility and reducing swelling.

Chemotherapy and radiation (adjuvant therapy) are useful for eradicating any undetected *micrometastases* remaining in such a high-risk cancer, even with a very small localized mass, and are used as palliative measures as well. Current trials involve implants of radioactive seeds in surrounding tissue following surgery to provide localized radiation without the need for daily treatment.

If the tumor proves to be responsive to estrogen, postoperative therapy includes removal of the hormonal stimulation. In a premenopausal woman, the ovaries are removed. A sequence of hormone-blocking agents such as Tamoxifen or similar agents targeting the estrogen receptors in the tumor reduces the risk of cancer recurrence in postmenopausal women. There is some concern that selective estrogen receptor modulators inhibit estrogen receptors in breast cells, but may activate uterine cells leading to endometrial proliferation. Other targeted drug therapies include drugs to block the growth factors that stimulate mitosis in the tumor. Such drugs include trastuzumab (Herceptin) and lapatinib (Tykerb). Women with stage 3 or 4 breast cancer may receive bevacizumab (Avastin) to reduce the growth of blood vessels in secondary tumors.

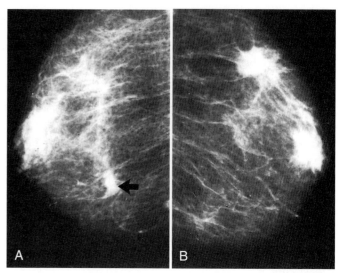

FIGURE 19-17 Mammogram showing bilateral invasive ductal carcinoma. **A**, Left breast. The larger mass was palpable. The smaller right mass was not palpable (arrow). **B**, Right breast. Multiple masses are shown. *(From Powell DE, Stilling CB: Diagnosis and detection of breast diseases, St Louis, 1993, Mosby.)*

The prognosis is relatively good for tumors without nodal involvement, but as the number of lymph nodes affected by the cancer increases, the prognosis becomes more negative. Breast cancer may recur many years later, but generally the longer the time elapsed without recurrence, the lower the risk of recurrence. Current statistics with respect to prognosis can be found on the American Cancer Society web site.

Breast self-examination is recommended for all women older than 20 years as a measure to reduce mortality and identify cancers in an early stage. Indeed, many tumors are discovered by women during breast self-examination. Recent studies have questioned this practice, citing the risk of surgical biopsy when the lump is a benign cyst. It is important to note that the comparator group in this study was women who had a yearly breast exam by a skilled practitioner familiar with breast changes. Many women do not access such professionals on a regular basis. Mammography is used as a routine screening tool because it can detect lesions before they become palpable or masses deep in the breast tissue (Fig. 19-17). Ultrasound and MRI are also used to identify and characterize masses. Diagnostic testing of exudates from the breast or fine needle ductal biopsy through the nipple is also used in some settings. Each diagnostic measure has its strengths and weaknesses. It is important for the woman to discuss screening and diagnostic measures with her physician. Routine screening is shown to reduce mortality from breast cancer.

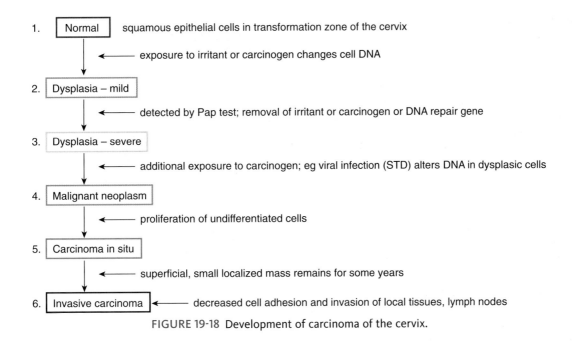

1. Normal — squamous epithelial cells in transformation zone of the cervix

   ← exposure to irritant or carcinogen changes cell DNA

2. Dysplasia – mild

   ← detected by Pap test; removal of irritant or carcinogen or DNA repair gene

3. Dysplasia – severe

   ← additional exposure to carcinogen; eg viral infection (STD) alters DNA in dysplasic cells

4. Malignant neoplasm

   ← proliferation of undifferentiated cells

5. Carcinoma in situ

   ← superficial, small localized mass remains for some years

6. Invasive carcinoma ← decreased cell adhesion and invasion of local tissues, lymph nodes

FIGURE 19-18 Development of carcinoma of the cervix.

THINK ABOUT 19-7

a. Compare the signs of fibrocystic disease and breast cancer.
b. Explain why chemotherapy and radiation may be recommended following surgery for breast cancer even when no lymph nodes appear to be involved.
c. Explain the recommended treatment for estrogen-dependent breast cancer in premenopausal and postmenopausal women.
d. Explain what is meant by "targeted therapy" for breast cancer.
e. Discuss the importance of breast cancer screening and early diagnosis.

Carcinoma of the Cervix

The number of cases of invasive cancer and the number of deaths from cervical cancer has declined by 74% with the increased use of the Papanicolaou (Pap) smear for screening and early diagnosis while the cancer is still in situ. The National Cancer Institute of the NIH estimates 12,340 new cases of cervical cancer resulting in 4030 deaths in the United States in 2013. The average age at onset for carcinoma in situ is 35, whereas invasive carcinoma manifests at approximately age 45. Nearly one in five cancers is diagnosed after age 65; thus women need to be screened after menopause. More cases are occurring in women in their twenties and thirties. Hispanic-American women have twice the risk of developing cervical cancers than women in other ethnic groups. Five-year survival rates for noninvasive cancer are close to 100%; with invasion the rate drops to 92%, and overall survival rate including later stages is 72%.

■ *Pathophysiology*

The early changes in the cervical epithelial tissue consist of *dysplasia*, which is initially mild but becomes progressively more severe (Fig. 19-18). This dysplasia usually occurs at the junction of the columnar cells with the squamous epithelial cells of the external os of the cervix (the transformation zone). The majority of cervical carcinomas arise from squamous cells.

Cervical intraepithelial neoplasia is graded from I to III based on the amount of dysplasia and the degree of cell differentiation. Grade III consists of carcinoma in situ in which many disorganized, undifferentiated, abnormal cells are present (severe dysplasia). Because the time span from mild dysplasia to carcinoma in situ may be 10 years, there are many opportunities for detection in this early stage. The Pap smear allows an examination of scrapings of the cervical cells and those that slough from the site and are present in the local secretions. These cells indicate the presence of dysplasia long before any signs of cancer appear.

Carcinoma in situ is a noninvasive stage, to be followed by the *invasive* stage. Figure 19-19 illustrates the stages. Figure 19-19A demonstrates a Pap test, B shows an early stage of invasion, and C the advanced stage, a protruding mass.

Invasive carcinoma has varying characteristics, sometimes appearing as a protruding nodular mass or perhaps as ulceration, and sometimes infiltrating the wall. Eventually all characteristics are present in the lesion. As the carcinoma spreads in all directions into the adjacent tissues, including the uterus and vagina, it may also invade the uterine wall and extend into the ligaments, bladder, or rectum. Metastases to lymph

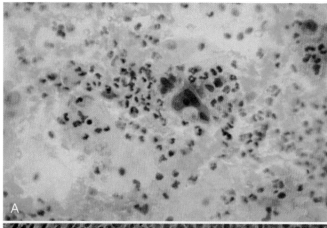

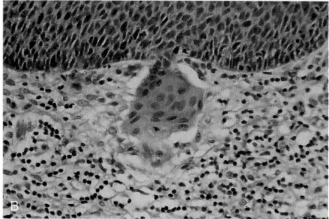

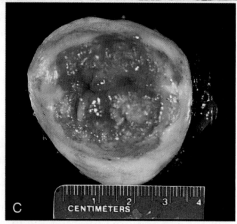

FIGURE 19-19 **Cancer of the Cervix A,** Positive Pap smear indicative of cervical cancer. *(From Christiansen JL, Grzybowski JM: Biology of Aging, St. Louis, 1993, Mosby.)* **B,** Early invasion (microscopic) occurring in a cervical neoplasm (stage I). **C,** Carcinoma well advanced, the neoplastic mass projecting above the mucosa. **(B and C** *From Kumar V, Abbas AK, Fausto M: Robbins and Cotran Pathologic Basis of Disease, ed 7, Philadelphia, 2005, Saunders.)*

nodes or distant sites occur rarely and at a very late stage. Staging of the carcinoma begins with stage 0, representing carcinoma in situ; stage I represents cancer restricted to the cervix; and stages II to IV indicate further spread to the surrounding tissues.

Etiology

Cervical cancer is strongly linked to oncogenic sexually transmitted diseases such as herpes simplex virus type 2 (HSV-2) and human papillomavirus (HPV) strains 16, 18, 31, 34, or 45. The Centers for Disease Control and Prevention (CDC) defines cervical carcinoma as a sexually transmitted infection. The virus may exert direct effects on the host cell or may cause an antibody reaction; increased viral antibodies have been associated with the increasing dysplasia. A vaccine (Gardasil) against HPV-6, HPV-11, HPV-16, and HPV-18 has been developed and shown to reduce the risk of cervical carcinoma. Gardasil immunization is recommended by the CDC for all girls before adolescence. In 2009 data from the Vaccine Adverse Event Reporting System prompted the FDA to look into reports of dangerous adverse effects being reported by users of the vaccine. Initial research confirmed the safety of the vaccine; however, the FDA is continuing to monitor safety data regarding the vaccine.

High-risk factors for cervical carcinoma include multiple sexual partners, promiscuous partners, participation in sexual intercourse during the early teen years, and a patient history of sexually transmitted disease. Other environmental factors, such as smoking, are considered as predisposing women to cervical cancer.

Signs and Symptoms

Cervical cancer is asymptomatic in the early stage but can be detected by the Pap test. The invasive stage is indicated by slight bleeding or spotting or a slight watery discharge. Anemia or weight loss may accompany the local signs.

Treatment

Biopsy is used to confirm the diagnosis. Surgery combined with radiation (either an implant of radioactive material or external radiation—see Chapter 20) is the recommended treatment. The 5-year survival rate is 100% when the carcinoma is still in situ. The prognosis for a patient with invasive carcinoma depends on the extent of spread of the cancer cells.

THINK ABOUT 19-8

a. Explain the following terms and give an example of each: (1) dysplasia, (2) carcinoma in situ, (3) carcinogenic, and (4) invasive.
b. Explain how viruses can be carcinogenic.
c. Explain why vaginal bleeding or abnormal discharge indicates a more advanced stage of cervical cancer.

Carcinoma of the Uterus (Endometrial Carcinoma)

Carcinoma of the uterus remains a common cancer in women older than 40 years, the majority of cases occurring in the 55- to 65-year age range. It is estimated that

44,192 new cases occurred in the United States in 2009 resulting in 7713 deaths. A simple screening test is not available for this cancer; the Pap test does not screen for this cancer. However, the early indicator is vaginal bleeding, which in a postmenopausal woman is a significant sign demanding investigation.

■ Pathophysiology

Some endometrial cancers are derived from connective tissue or muscle and are termed leiomyosarcomas. These tumors have a poor prognosis and frequently have metastasized to the lungs by the time diagnosis is made. For more information on sarcomas, see Chapter 9.

The majority of endometrial carcinomas are adenocarcinomas arising from the glandular epithelium. The malignant changes develop from endometrial hyperplasia, with the cells gradually becoming more atypical. Excessive estrogen stimulation appears to be the major factor in the development of hyperplasia. This cancer is a relatively slow-growing tumor and may infiltrate the uterine wall, leading to a thickened area, or it may mushroom out into the endometrial cavity (Fig. 19-20). Eventually the tumor mass fills the interior of the uterus and extends through the wall into the surrounding structures.

Endometrial cancers are graded from 1, indicating well-differentiated cells, to grade 3, indicating poorly differentiated cells.

Staging of the cancer is based on the degree of localization. In stage I, tumors are confined to the body of the uterus. In stage II, cancer is limited to the uterus and the cervix. In stage III, the cancer has spread outside the uterus but remains within the true pelvis; and in stage IV, the tumor has spread to the lymph nodes and distant organs. Five-year survival rate for stage I is 99%, stage II is 80%, stage III is 60%, and stage IV is 32%.

■ Etiology

Individuals with a history of increased estrogen levels have a higher incidence of uterine cancer. Exogenous estrogen taken by postmenopausal women is associated with an increased risk of endometrial cancer, and currently the guidelines for use and the dosage of estrogen have been reduced to minimize this danger. Other causes of hyperestrinism include infertility or the earlier ingestion of sequential oral contraceptives. The current practice of combining estrogen with progestin reduces the risk of hyperplasia in the uterus, but is still associated with increased risk of breast cancer. There is also an increased incidence of cancer in obese women and in those with diabetes or hypertension.

■ Signs and Symptoms

Painless vaginal bleeding or spotting is the key sign of endometrial cancer because the cancer erodes the surface tissues. The Pap smear is not a dependable assessment tool for detecting abnormal endometrial cells. Direct aspiration of uterine cells provides a more accurate cell sample with biopsy required to confirm the diagnosis. Late signs of malignancy include a palpable mass, discomfort or pressure in the lower abdomen, and bleeding following intercourse.

■ Treatment

Surgery and radiation constitute the usual treatment measures with chemotherapy in the later stages. When chemotherapy is used, a combination of two drugs is used.

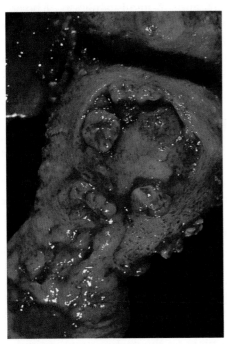

FIGURE 19-20 Endometrial adenocarcinoma presenting as a diffuse tumor involving the entire endometrial surface and projecting into the uterine cavity. *(From Kumar V, Abbas AK, Fausto M: Robbins and Cotran Pathologic Basis of Disease, ed 7, Philadelphia, 2005, Saunders.)*

> **THINK ABOUT 19-9**
>
> a. Differentiate a uterine fibroid from uterine cancer.
> b. Explain why the cure rate for cervical cancer is much better than that for ovarian cancer (refer to Chapter 20).
> c. List the tumors whose development is influenced by hormones and explain how these may be treated.

Ovarian Cancer

Ovarian cancer is of concern because only about 25% of ovarian cancer is diagnosed in the early stage, at which time the prognosis is favorable. This cancer has long been considered a silent tumor. The National cancer Institute of the NIH has estimated 22,240 new cases in the United States in 2013, resulting in an estimated 14,030 deaths. Two thirds of the women diagnosed with ovarian cancer are greater than age 55. Genetic factors have a role in its development.

There are different types of ovarian cancer tumors, which vary in virulence. These types include: serous, mucinous and endometrioid tumors. The serous tumors account for the majority of malignant cases of ovarian cancer. Early indications of ovarian cancer include feeling of bloating and fullness, indigestion, frequent urination, backache, and pain with intercourse.

The lack of a reliable screening test and the hidden nature of the cancer hinder early diagnosis. A large mass may be detected by pelvic exam. Transvaginal ultrasound CT (computerized tomography) scans, MRI (magnetic resonance imaging, pelvic exams, and CA125 (a protein whose high levels indicate ovarian cancer) tests are current tools for diagnosis. Treatment involves surgery and chemotherapy.

Infertility

Infertility or sterility affecting a couple's reproductive capacity may be caused solely by male conditions, solely by female conditions, or by combined male and female factors. Each of these categories occurs in approximately equal proportions. A couple is considered infertile after a year of unprotected intercourse fails to produce a pregnancy. Infertility occurs in approximately 15% of couples in North America.

Male problems include changes in sperm or semen, hormonal abnormalities, or physical obstruction of sperm passage. Semen analysis assesses specific characteristics such as the number, normality, and motility of sperm. Ability of the sperm to penetrate the cervical mucus and the presence of sperm antibodies are also considered.

Hormonal imbalances may result from either pituitary disorders or testicular problems. Ductal obstructions may result from congenital problems or scar tissue related to prior events such as infection. Many drugs are now available for the treatment of erectile dysfunction.

Decreased fertility has many possible causes:
- Infertility may be associated with hormonal imbalances resulting from altered function of the hypothalamus, anterior pituitary gland, or ovaries. Altered function may occur following the use of oral contraceptives. For example, the feedback system may not be functioning or may be suppressed by stress, extreme exercise or training, or the ovaries may be abnormal (e.g., in the Stein-Leventhal syndrome).
- Increasing age of the parents at the time of the first attempt at conception is another possible cause.
- Structural abnormalities may prevent pregnancy, for example, a small or bicornuate (divided) uterus or uterine fibroids.
- The fallopian tubes, epididymis, or vas deferens may be obstructed by scar tissue resulting from infection or endometriosis.
- Infection of the testes may "burn out" sperm-producing cells.
- Chemotherapy may reduce viability of sperm or ova.
- Workplace toxins and environmental pollutants may reduce viable sperm.
- Access of viable sperm may be reduced by a change in vaginal pH due to infection or the use of douches, excessively thick cervical mucus, or the development of antibodies in the woman to particular sperm.
- Recent evidence implicates cigarette smoking by either the male or female partner and second-hand smoke as a deterrent to pregnancy.

It is estimated that 25% of fertilized ova fail to implant and develop into a viable embryo. The reasons for this are many and may include chromosomal or genetic anomalies. Because the woman is not aware of the fertilization, little if any research is available on such implantation failures.

A broad range of tests is available to assess each group of factors in a progressively more detailed manner. It is usual to test the male partner first since the tests are not invasive.

The woman's general health status is investigated to rule out any systemic causes. The woman may record basal body temperature, times of intercourse, and menstrual cycles to determine the optimal time for fertilization. Physical abnormalities may be assessed by means of a pelvic examination and by tests such as ultrasound, computed tomography scans, or laparoscopy. Hysteroscopy is another method of detecting uterine abnormalities. Tubal insufflation (using gas and a pressure measurement) or a hysterosalpingogram (radiograph or x-ray with contrast material) can ascertain the patency of the tubes and uterus. Evaluation of hormone levels throughout the cycle requires extensive testing. Other possible factors such as cervical mucus and the presence of sperm antibodies require specific tests. Frequently a combination of factors contributes to infertility; therefore it is best to conduct a range of tests.

Sexually Transmitted Diseases

Sexually transmitted diseases (STDs), formerly called venereal diseases, encompass a broad range of infectious diseases that are spread by sexual contact. Although the incidence of gonorrhea has decreased a little, the incidence of other STDs has increased, resulting in an overall increase. The actual figures are probably much higher than those stated because many cases of STD are not reported. The increased numbers have been attributed to societal changes in many countries, including factors such as increased participation in premarital sex, particularly among young adults; an increased divorce rate; and an increased number of sexual partners on the part of some individuals. Many people do not take protective measures against STDs, especially when hormonal contraceptives are used to prevent pregnancy. In addition to the standard STDs such as gonorrhea, syphilis, and chlamydial infection,

TABLE 19-1   **Sexually Transmitted Diseases**

Infection	Cause	Signs	Complications	Treatment/Cure
Chlamydia	Chlamydia C. trachomatis	Mild dysuria and discharge or asymptomatic	Arthritis Females—PID and infertility Neonates—conjunctivitis and pneumonia	Antimicrobial therapy, e.g., azithromycin Retest for eradication
Gonorrhea	Bacterium N. gonorrhoeae	Dysuria and discharge Mild or asymptomatic in women	Arthritis Male—prostatitis and epididymitis Female—PID and infertility Neonates—conjunctivitis	Antibacterial drugs (penicillin or ceftriaxone + doxycycline) Some drug-resistant strains Retest for eradication
Syphilis	Bacterium T. pallidum	Primary Syphilis—Painless ulcer or chancre at site of entry Secondary Syphilis—Rash, fever, headache	Tertiary Syphilis— Gumma, neurosyphilis, or cardiovascular system damage Congenital syphilis in child	Penicillin G—long-acting Retest for eradication
Genital Herpes	Virus Herpes simplex 2 (HSV-2)	Vesicles and ulcers	Recurs Meningitis Fetus/neonate damage	No cure Antiviral drug, e.g., oral acyclovir, reduces activity and shedding
Genital Warts	Virus Human papillomavirus (HPV)	Soft gray mass or polyp	None	Can be removed, but rarely cured
Trichomoniasis	Protozoa T. vaginalis	Asymptomatic, or women may have discharge and dysuria	None	Antimicrobial drugs, e.g., metronidazole

there is evidence that infections such as hepatitis B may be spread by sexual contact. HIV is spread by both heterosexual and homosexual exchange of body fluids.

Among the many concerns about STDs:

1. Immunity against recurrent infection is not achieved during the first infection with many STDs; therefore recurrent infections are common.
2. Because more than one STD may be present in any one individual at a given time, careful testing and diagnosis to uncover the presence of second infections are necessary.
3. Frequently STDs are asymptomatic, particularly in women, thus promoting the spread of infection by persons who are unaware that they are carrying the microbes.
4. No cure is available for viral STDs such as herpes or human immunodeficiency virus (HIV; see discussion of HIV-AIDS in Chapter 7), although drugs are available that may help to limit the acute stage of infection.
5. Drug-resistant microorganisms are becoming increasingly common, thus raising the inherent risks associated with STDs.
6. Infections may be transmitted by an infected mother to a fetus or newborn, frequently resulting in congenital defects or death or disability for the child.
7. Partners of an infected person are difficult to trace, notify, and treat.
8. Condoms are often not used or used improperly in high-risk situations. The abuse of alcohol and the use of date rape drugs has increased the incidence of unprotected sex.

In this section, several of the more common STDs are discussed. A summary may be found in Table 19-1.

Bacterial Infections

Chlamydial Infection

Chlamydial infection is considered one of the most common STDs and the leading cause of PID. The pathogen is the bacterium *Chlamydia trachomatis*, a gram-negative obligate intracellular parasite, which requires a host cell to reproduce (see Fig. 6-6). As in gonorrhea, chlamydiae invade the epithelial tissue of the urogenital tract, causing inflammation.

In most males chlamydial infection becomes evident in several weeks after exposure as urethritis (nongonococcal urethritis) and epididymitis. Manifestations of urethritis include dysuria, itching, and a whitish discharge from the penis. Epididymitis manifests as a painful, swollen scrotum, usually unilateral, accompanied by fever. The inguinal lymph nodes are swollen. Proctitis (rectal inflammation with bleeding and discharge) may occur in anyone practicing anal intercourse.

Females are often asymptomatic until PID develops. A few experience urethritis, bartholinitis, cervicitis, or salpingitis. Signs of urethritis include dysuria and urinary frequency. Infection in Bartholin's glands causes a purulent discharge and cyst formation. Cervicitis may be asymptomatic, or a purulent discharge with inflamed tissues may be evident at the cervical os. Spread to the fallopian tubes leads to the development of PID.

Newborns may be infected during passage through the cervix and vagina, resulting in infection in the eyes (conjunctivitis) or in the lungs because of aspiration of infected secretions (pneumonia). The usual treatment for chlamydial infection is tetracycline or azithromycin for the infected person and any sexual partners. Chlamydia and gonorrhea are often seen together in the same client and thus newer protocols call for treatment of both infections simultaneously with a combination of doxycycline and azithromycin.

Gonorrhea

Gonorrhea is caused by *N. gonorrhoeae*, a gram-negative aerobic diplococcus (gonococcus). Many strains of *N. gonorrhoeae* have become resistant to penicillin and tetracycline. The bacteria use pili to attach to the epithelial cells and then damage the mucosa, causing an inflammatory reaction and formation of a purulent exudate.

The most common site of inflammation in males is the urethra, which results in dysuria and a purulent urethral discharge. Epididymitis may follow (Fig. 19-21). Some men are asymptomatic. In females, the infection usually involves the endocervical canal and frequently is asymptomatic. It may also affect Skene's and Bartholin's glands, causing more visible manifestations. Pelvic inflammatory disease, a serious complication, frequently follows as the infection ascends along the mucosa. Females may experience infection in the anus and rectum when infected exudate spreads from the vagina.

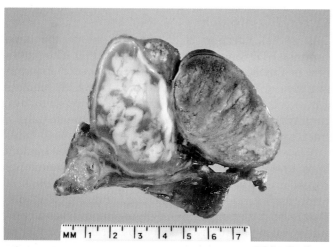

FIGURE 19-21 Acute epididymitis caused by gonococcal infection. *Left,* the epididymis is necrotic and replaced by an abscess. Normal testis is seen on the right. *(From Kumar V, Abbas AK, Fausto M: Robbins and Cotran Pathologic Basis of Disease, ed 7, Philadelphia, 2005, Saunders.)*

Women are prone to develop bacteremia and gonococcal arthritis, with multiple joint inflammations.

Orogenital contact leads to pharyngeal infection manifested as pharyngitis, tonsillitis, or lymphadenopathy. Gonococcal conjunctivitis may be seen in Figure 15-3. The newborn may become infected during the birth process, resulting in the eye infection called ophthalmia neonatorum.

Considering the resistant strains of the organism, the suggested drugs are ceftriaxone and doxycycline. Culture and sensitivity tests may be required to determine effective drugs.

Syphilis

The prevalence of syphilis had been decreasing in the period between 1990 and 2000. The rate increased from 2001 to 2009 but again showed a decrease in 2010. Reasons for the increase vary but it has also been noted that there has been an increase in antibiotic resistant strains of the pathogen. The causative organism of syphilis is *Treponema pallidum,* an anaerobic spirochete (so called because of its corkscrew shape). Dark-field or electron microscopy is required for identification (Fig. 19-22*A*). Serum antibodies also provide a diagnostic test.

Syphilis is a systemic infection that consists of four stages, and the organism can be isolated from lesions in the first two stages.

1. The *primary* stage is identifiable by the presence of a *chancre,* a painless, firm, ulcerated nodule that develops at the point of contact on the skin or mucosa about 3 weeks after exposure (see Fig. 19-22*B*). The organisms reproduce in the chancre and initiate an immune response. This lesion heals spontaneously (without treatment) in several weeks. Such lesions are frequently missed because they may not be visible (e.g., they may be in the cervix in the female) and are asymptomatic. Regional lymphadenopathy may also be present in this stage.

2. By the time the chancre heals, the organisms have entered the general circulation, and if untreated, the *second stage* of the infection begins with a widespread symmetric rash, usually maculopapular and reddish, on the skin and mucous membranes, particularly the palate. This typical rash may be found on the palms of the hands and the soles of the feet. Mucous patches (loose, white, necrotic material) may appear on the tongue. General signs of infection—malaise, low-grade fever, sore throat, stomatitis, and anorexia—are common. Again, these lesions are self-limiting and disappear spontaneously in a few weeks.

3. The patient then enters the *latent stage,* which may persist for years. Sometimes the skin lesions recur, but usually the person is asymptomatic, although serologic evidence of disease remains.

4. Some untreated patients never develop *tertiary syphilis,* and treatment has reduced the incidence of this stage. The typical lesion of this stage is the *gumma,*

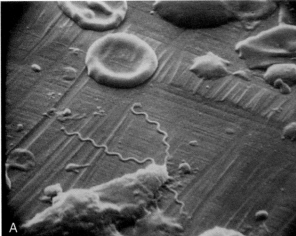

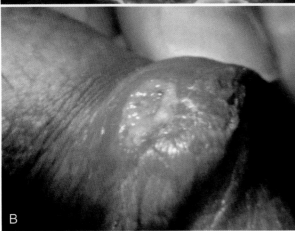

FIGURE 19-22 **Syphilis A,** Scanning electron micrograph shows *Treponema pallidum* (thin spirals) adjacent to an erythrocyte. **B,** Penile syphilitic chancre, painless papule with central ulceration at the inoculation site on the penis. *(From Mahon CR, Manuselis G: Textbook of Diagnostic Microbiology, ed 2, Philadelphia, 2000, Saunders.)*

an area of necrosis and fibrosis. Bone gummas lead to destruction (e.g., in the hard palate) and pathologic fractures, whereas gummas in the liver manifest as nodules similar to those of cirrhosis. The cardiovascular system is most frequently affected by gummas, showing damage to the arterial wall and development of aortic aneurysms. Neurosyphilis damages the central nervous system, resulting in dementia, blindness, and motor disabilities (tabes dorsalis). A concern with syphilis is the development of *congenital syphilis* if the fetus is infected after the fourth month of gestation. The child may die in utero or survive with active infection or multiple abnormalities, particularly in the bones (e.g., saddlenose). Malformations of the teeth (e.g., Hutchinson's incisors and mulberry molars) are typical. Inflammation and fibrosis damage the liver and lungs.

Transmission occurs by contact with exudate from the skin and mucosal lesions or by body fluids, including semen, blood, and vaginal secretions, during sexual contact. It is likely that syphilis can be transmitted during the first few years of the latent stage as well as during the first two stages.

Treatment consists of long-acting penicillin or azithromycin for resistant microbes.

THINK ABOUT 19-10

a. Describe the causative organisms for: (1) chlamydial infection, (2) gonorrhea, and (3) syphilis.
b. Explain how salpingitis may develop in women with chlamydial infection.
c. Compare syphilis and gonorrhea in terms of the early signs, distribution of organisms, and potential long-term effects if untreated.
d. Give two reasons why STDs are difficult to control (i.e., why it is difficult to reduce the incidence).

Viral Infections

Viral STDs constitute a serious problem because antiviral agents reduce the severity of the acute stage of infection by inhibiting viral reproduction and shedding of viruses, but they usually do not eradicate the infection.

HIV-AIDS may be considered an STD in some cases and has been described under Immune Deficiency in Chapter 7.

Genital Herpes

Herpes genitalis is usually caused by HSV-2, although some cases result from HSV-1. Herpes simplex virus type 1 is the agent that also causes herpes labialis, or cold sores (discussed in Chapter 8), and may cause genital lesions if oral sex is practiced or if it is autoinoculated by the hands. The lesions are similar. Usually a tingling and burning sensation at the site precedes the appearance of the actual lesion. The lesion characteristic of herpes is a vesicle (blister) surrounded by an erythematous area (Fig. 19-23). The vesicle ruptures after several days, leaving a painful ulcerated area and watery exudate. Eventually a crust forms over the ulcer, and it heals spontaneously in 3 to 4 weeks. Sometimes the initial episode is very mild and not noticed. In women, the lesion is usually found on the cervix, vulva, or urethra. Men have lesions on the penis, scrotum, or urethra. Vesicles may also appear on the buttocks or thighs.

Systemic signs may be present during the acute stage, including fever, headache, and lymphadenopathy.

Following this acute stage, the herpes virus usually migrates along the dermatome to the dorsal sacral root ganglion and there enters a latent stage. Body secretions may contain viruses for a time after the visible lesion heals.

When reactivated, the virus migrates back to the mucosa or skin and enters the host cells for replication, forming a new vesicle. Reactivation may be triggered by

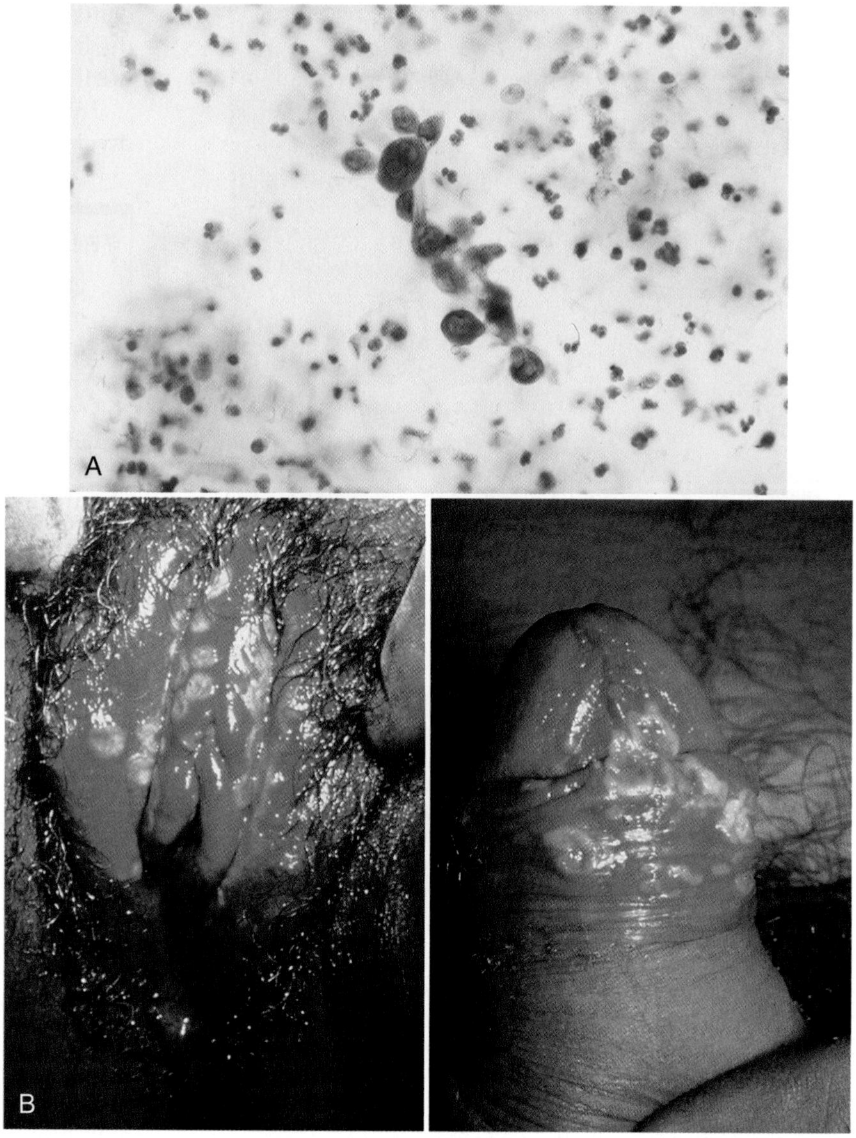

FIGURE 19-23 **Genital herpes. A,** Herpes simplex virus in a cervical specimen. Infected cervical cells stain brown. *(From de la Maza LM, Pezzlo MT, Baron EJ:* Color Atlas of Diagnostic Microbiology. *St. Louis, 1997, Mosby.)* **B,** Genital herpes in the female and male. Note the blisters and ulceration. *(From Behrman RE, Kliegman RM, Arvin AM:* Slide Set, Nelson Textbook of Psediatrics, *ed 15, Philadelphia, 1996, Saunders.)*

many factors, such as respiratory infections or stress. Recurrent herpes is more common with HSV-2 than with HSV-1. Prodromal signs, such as tingling or burning, signal recurrence before the lesion appears.

The fluid in the vesicles contains many viruses and may spread the infection to the eyes or skin elsewhere if caution and careful handwashing are not practiced. Active lesions in the vagina or cervix may transmit herpes virus to an infant during a vaginal delivery, frequently causing death or severe central nervous system damage. Delivery by cesarean section is advocated.

Cervical cancer frequently develops in women with genital herpes. Frequent Pap tests are suggested to monitor any tissue changes.

An antiviral agent such as acyclovir (Zovirax) may be applied topically or taken orally to lessen the active stage of infection and reduce the shedding of viruses to some extent; drug-resistant strains of HSV have been identified. This treatment may lessen the symptoms but does not cure the infection.

Condylomata Acuminata (Genital Warts)

Certain types of HPV cause genital warts, an STD that is increasing in frequency. Human papillomavirus is a circular, double-stranded DNA virus. There are many types of HPV, of which several affect the genital tract. Several of these types also are considered to be a cause of cervical cancer. The incubation period for this infection may be as long as 6 months, and the disease may be asymptomatic, depending on the location of the lesions. Pregnancy promotes the growth and spread of genital warts.

The condylomata, or warts, vary in appearance from soft, fleshy projections or cauliflower-like masses to flat lesions, to small pointed masses. Flat condylomata require preliminary treatment with acetic acid before they can be visualized. Biopsy is useful in differentiating condylomata from other causes of dysplasia or hyperkeratoses. In women the lesions may be present in the cervix or vagina, and in men they frequently are found on the penis.

Genital warts may be removed by a number of different methods including surgery, laser, cryotherapy, and topical caustics, but they tend to recur.

Protozoan Infection

Trichomoniasis

Trichomoniasis is caused by *Trichomonas vaginalis,* an anaerobic flagellated protozoan, an extracellular parasite (see Fig. 6-8). The infection is usually asymptomatic in men, the organisms residing primarily in the urethra. In women the infection may be subclinical and then flare up when the microbial balance of the vagina shifts.

Trichomoniasis is a localized infection, the organism attaching to the squamous epithelium of the vaginal and urethral mucosa and to Bartholin's glands. Active infection causes a copious yellowish, foul-smelling discharge as well as inflammation and itching of the mucosa. Systemic treatment of both partners is necessary with drugs such as metronidazole (Flagyl) or tinidazole.

THINK ABOUT 19-11

a. Describe the causative organism and its classification for: (1) trichomoniasis, and (2) genital herpes.
b. Compare the early manifestations of chlamydial infection, syphilis, and genital herpes.
c. Explain why genital herpes tends to recur.

CASE STUDY A

Benign Prostatic Hypertrophy

Mr. Humpert, age 71, presented to his physician with dysuria, urinary frequency, and urgency. Following urinalysis, cystitis was diagnosed. Benign prostatic hypertrophy was noted.

1. What is the purpose of the prostate gland?
2. Describe the changes that occur in the prostate with BPH and the reason for these changes.
3. Explain how BPH predisposes a patient to cystitis.
   The infection was treated with antibacterial drugs, and Mr. H. was asked to return for follow-up.
4. List the manifestations of BPH, along with the reasons for them, that Mr. H. is likely to experience as the disease continues to develop.
   As the disease progresses, Mr. H. is reluctant to consider surgical treatment.
5. Is there a high risk of developing a prostatic malignancy if treatment is delayed?

CASE STUDY B

Breast Cancer

Mrs. Ann Thompson, age 52, felt a small, hard, painless lump in the upper outer quadrant of her left breast during regular breast self-examination. Her mother and a cousin had had breast cancer. Mrs. A.T. has no children and still has menstrual cycles. After seeing her physician and having a mammogram, a biopsy was scheduled, which confirmed that the nodule was malignant.

1. List the factors in the patient's history that increase the risk of developing breast cancer.
2. Describe other possible signs of breast cancer.
3. Explain why this lump is not typical of a benign condition.
   A lumpectomy was performed on Mrs. A.T. and a number of axillary lymph nodes were removed.
4. Explain why the axillary lymph nodes were removed.
5. The tumor cells tested positive for estrogen receptors. Explain the significance of this information and the implications for Mrs. A.T.
6. Mrs. A.T.'s lung and bone scans were negative. Explain the purpose of these scans.
   Only two of the axillary lymph nodes were positive for tumor cells. The prognosis appeared good, but the oncologist recommended a course of radiation and chemotherapy (refer to Chapter 20).
7. Explain why additional treatment is recommended in this case.
8. Explain why Mrs. A.T. will have an increased risk of infection after she starts the radiation and chemotherapy treatments.
9. Explain why Mrs. A.T. will have to undergo frequent mammograms and check-ups for the next few years.

CASE STUDY C

Gonorrhea and PID

P.J., age 23 years, tested positive for gonorrhea 6 months ago. She had no signs of infection, but her partner had been diagnosed and was being treated for gonorrhea. In this case, the penicillinase-producing organisms proved to be resistant to penicillin, and treatment continued with ceftriaxone.

1. Describe the usual signs of gonorrhea in a male.
2. Explain the meaning of the term *drug-resistant* as it relates to microbes and how it might be determined (see Chapter 6).
   Six months later, P.J. was admitted to the emergency department with severe abdominal pain and vomiting. A purulent cervical discharge was obvious, and initial examination of the exudate indicated infection by *N. gonorrhoeae* as well as other microorganisms. A tentative diagnosis of PID was given.
3. Describe how gonorrhea leads to PID.
4. Explain why peritonitis is a potential complication of PID.
5. Give several reasons why infertility may be a sequela to PID.

CHAPTER SUMMARY

The reproductive systems of the male and female consist of the gonads, or testes and ovaries, respectively, combined with a complex system of ducts and auxiliary structures. In the male, the reproductive system shares some parts with the urinary system. Reproductive function is dependent on close links with the endocrine, cardiovascular, and nervous systems. Unfortunately, the reproductive systems are a major site of malignant tumors and infections.

Disorders of the Male Reproductive System

- *Torsion of the testis* must be treated quickly to prevent ischemic damage.
- *Prostatitis* may be associated with urinary tract infections and STDs.
- *Benign prostatic hypertrophy* occurs in older men, causing urinary obstruction, but is not associated with malignancy.
- *Cancer of the prostate* may be androgen dependent and usually metastasizes at an early stage to bone.
- Testicular self-examination for early detection of *testicular cancer* is recommended for young men.

Disorders of the Female Reproductive System

- *Endometriosis* is a cause of dysmenorrhea and infertility.

- *Candidiasis* is a frequent opportunistic vaginal infection in women.
- *Pelvic inflammatory disease* is a serious bacterial infection caused by microbes such as chlamydia ascending into the fallopian tubes and entering the peritoneal cavity to cause peritonitis and later, strictures, adhesions, and infertility.
- Some forms of *fibrocystic breast disease* require monitoring for malignant cell changes.
- Routine screening to ensure early detection is recommended for *breast cancer*, particularly in women with family history. The tumor usually manifests initially as a single, hard, painless nodule.
- Incidence of *cervical cancer* is increasing because of viral STDs, although early detection with Pap tests has improved the prognosis.

Infertility and Sterility

- Causes may be based in the male or the female or in a combination of factors, related to production of ova or sperm, structural defects, or hormone imbalances.

Sexually Transmitted Diseases

- These infections include chlamydia, gonorrhea, syphilis, herpes, genital warts, and trichomoniasis. They have increased in numbers, with more drug-resistant microbes and viral infections making control difficult.

STUDY QUESTIONS

1. Describe the structure and function of the:
   a. Scrotum
   b. Spermatic cord
   c. Prostate gland
2. List the functions of testosterone.
3. Describe the altered function resulting from:
   a. Hypospadias
   b. Cryptorchidism
4. Explain why BPH occurs in older males.
5. List the signs of BPH.
6. Compare the typical sites of metastasis for prostatic and testicular cancer.
7. State and explain one significant effect of cystocele.
8. Explain the cause of pain resulting from:
   a. Endometriosis
   b. Primary dysmenorrhea
9. Explain the potential problem resulting from the break in continuity between the fallopian tubes and the ovaries.
10. Describe the structure and purpose of each layer in the uterine wall.
11. Describe the defenses against infection in the female reproductive tract.
12. Describe the effects of increased estrogen secretion during the menstrual cycle.
13. Describe the causative organism and the manifestations of vaginal candidiasis.
14. Explain how an abscess may develop with PID.
15. Explain why most forms of fibrocystic breast disease are not considered precancerous, but some lesions require monitoring.
16. List the disorders characterized by pain related to the menstrual cycle.
17. Define the terms *invasive* and *metastatic* and give an example of each from the reproductive disorders.
18. Compare the early signs and the reasons for them of:
    a. Cervical cancer
    b. Uterine cancer
    c. Ovarian cancer (refer to Chapter 5)
19. List three hormone-dependent reproductive disorders and describe the role of the hormone in each case.
20. Name and describe the characteristics of the organism causing chlamydial infection.

21. Explain, using specific examples, two reasons why STDs may go undetected.
22. Describe the manifestations of the secondary stage of syphilis.
23. Explain how antiviral agents may reduce the transmission of herpes simplex virus.

24. List the STD and the organism that causes a:
    a. Chancre
    b. Vesicle
    c. Gumma
    d. Purulent exudate
    e. Pharyngitis
    f. Wart

ADDITIONAL RESOURCES

Copstead-Kirkorn LE: *Pathophysiology*, ed 4, Philadelphia, 2009, Saunders.

Heynman DL, editor: *Control of Communicable Diseases Manual*, ed 18, Washington, DC, 2004, American Public Health Association.

National Cancer Institute—Cancer Information Service: 1-800-4-CANCER (1-800-422-6237)

Patton K, Thibodeau G: *Anatomy and Physiology*, ed 7, St. Louis, 2010, Mosby.

Kumar V, Abbas A, Fausto N, Mitchell R: *Robbins Basic Pathology*, ed 8, Philadelphia, 2007, Saunders.

Web Sites

http://www.cdc.gov/cancer/prostate *Centers for Disease Control and Prevention-Information on Prostate cancer*

http://www.nlm.nih.gov/medlineplus/tutorials/whatisprostatecancer/htm/index.htm

http://www.cancer.gov/cancertopics/ *National Cancer Institute—Cancer Topics*

http://familydoctor.org/165.xml *American Academy of Family Physicians-Information on STIs*

http://www.cdc.gov/std *Centers for Disease Control and Prevention-Sexually Transmitted Diseases*

http://www.webmd.com/ *WebMD*

http://www.emedicinehealth.com/ *eMedicine health*

SECTION IV
Biological Factors Contributing to Pathophysiology

Neoplasms and Cancer

CHAPTER OUTLINE

LEARNING OBJECTIVES

After studying this chapter, the student is expected to:

1. Distinguish between benign and malignant tumors, their characteristics, and terminology.
2. List the warning signs of cancer.
3. Explain the local and systemic effects of cancer.
4. Describe common diagnostic tests.
5. Discuss the spread of malignant tumors by invasion, metastasis, and seeding and relate them to the staging of cancer.
6. Describe the stages involved in carcinogenesis, specific risk factors, and possible preventive measures.
7. Explain the host defenses against cancer.
8. Discuss possible treatment measures, including radiation and chemotherapy, as well as nutrition.
9. Describe and differentiate among three examples of malignant tumors: skin cancer, ovarian cancer, and brain cancer.

KEY TERMS

anemia	cytologic	mutation	radiofrequency ablation
angiogenesis	differentiation	nadir	radioisotopes
antineoplastic	infiltrate	oncology	remission
apoptosis	leukopenia	palliative	recurrence
atypical	metastasis	pneumonia	seeding
biopsies	micrometastases	prognosis	thrombocytopenia
chromosomes	mitosis	prophylactic	total parenteral nutrition

Review of Normal Cells

The cell is the functional and structural unit in the human body. Cells vary in their degree of development, depending on the differentiation or specialization required for a particular cell's function; for example, neurons or cardiac muscle cells are highly developed, whereas fibroblasts are less so. Normally cells are organized in an orderly arrangement in a tissue and differentiated to fulfill that tissue's purpose. When cells become disorganized or undifferentiated or their growth becomes uncontrolled, their specialized functions are lost.

Every cell has an outer *plasma membrane,* enclosing the fluid cytoplasm or intracellular fluid. The membrane is semipermeable, controlling passage of materials into and out of the cell. It also maintains the cell's shape. The *nucleus* of the cell consists of DNA, the genetic material that controls the particular cell's function and structure, enclosed in the nuclear membrane. The *cytoplasm* contains various nutrients, proteins, glucose, and electrolytes required for cell metabolism. Additional substances are present, depending on the cell's function; for example, glycogen in liver cells or lipids in fat cells. Other structures are located in the cytoplasm, such as ribosomes, granules that produce proteins; mitochondria providing energy in the form of ATP for cell activities; lysosomes containing digestive enzymes, to break down unwanted materials; and the Golgi complex to process and release proteins. Organelles inside the cell have many metabolic functions, such as the synthesis of protein or transport of cell products and wastes outside the cell membrane.

The plasma membrane includes special protein molecules or receptors for substances such as hormones, chemical transmitters, or drugs, which affect the cell's function. Cells may communicate with each other by chemicals or by forming protein channels between cells. Research is focused on this communication, seeking to learn the "what and how" of the transfer between cells and whether this knowledge could lead to the prevention of some diseases or new treatments. Cell membranes also have specialized mechanisms to adhere to each other and maintain an organized arrangement in a tissue or organ.

Regulator genes control mitosis for different types of cells. Growth factors such as cytokines signal proliferation, whereas inhibitors inside cells prevent excessive growth. During its lifespan, each cell follows the basic cell cycle of growth and reproduction or mitosis. (See Fig. 20-10 for a schematic drawing of the cell cycle.) The timing of each event varies with the specific cell type. Epithelial cells that reproduce rapidly may complete the cycle in a few hours. Other cells spend months completing one cycle. Genetic control over growth and reproduction is exerted through *DNA,* and the daughter cells are identical to the parent cell. If DNA is altered in the parent cell, this mutation is passed on to the daughter cells.

Different cells experience different life spans; for example, erythrocytes live for approximately 120 days, but some leukocytes survive only a few days. Highly specialized cells such as neurons cannot undergo mitosis, but they have a long life span of many years. Epithelial cells usually replicate very rapidly because of the demand for replacement caused by constant "wear and tear" on surface tissues. There are usually several layers of tightly packed cells, the upper layers being sloughed off or shed and replaced by regenerating cells from the lower layers. Some types of cells can increase their reproductive rate on demand; for example, bone injury increases osteoblast activity. Cell reproduction always requires an adequate blood supply to the area and sufficient quantities of essential nutrients such as amino acids, glucose, and oxygen. Normally, cell growth and reproduction are also subject to stimuli such as hormones and inhibition by contact with nearby cells.

APPLY YOUR KNOWLEDGE   20-1

Discuss several ways by which the normal process of cell replication can be altered, and state outcomes.

Cellular aging occurs naturally over time and results in an altered structure of the cell, decreased function, and, in time, cell death. The processes of cellular aging and changes in cell control systems are not fully understood. Certain cells undergo apoptosis, programmed cell death (see Chapter 1). Current theories on the aging process focus on a programmed number of reproductive cycles available for a specific cell type and the effects of wear and tear causing cell damage (see Chapter 24).

Changes in DNA can alter cell structure and function or cause cell death. DNA can mutate spontaneously during mitosis or as a result of exposure to chemicals, viruses, radiation, and other environmental hazards. Rapid rates of mitosis associated with tissue trauma or other stimuli may increase the risk of errors occurring in the chromosomes, cell enzymes, or cell components. Mutant cells may change function as well as lose control of mitosis. Seriously defective cells usually die or are destroyed by the immune system.

THINK ABOUT   20-1

a. Which types of cells have rapid rates of mitosis?
b. Which cells never undergo mitosis? What is the result of tissue damage in tissues such as these?

Benign and Malignant Tumors

A neoplasm or tumor is a cellular growth that is no longer responding to normal body controls. The cells

TABLE 20-1 Tumor Nomenclature

Root	Suffix	Example
Fatty tissue: lip-	Benign: -oma	Lipoma: benign tumor of fatty tissue
Gland tissue: adeno-	Malignant epithelial tissue: -carcinoma	Adenocarcinoma: malignant tumor of epithelial lining of a gland
Fibrous tissue: fibro-	Malignant connective tissue: -sarcoma	Fibrosarcoma: malignant tumor of fibrous tissue

TABLE 20-2 Characteristics of Benign and Malignant Tumors

	Benign Tumors	Malignant Tumors
Cells	Similar to normal cells	Varied in size and shape with large nuclei
	Differentiated	Many undifferentiated
	Mitosis fairly normal	Mitosis increased and atypical
Growth	Relatively slow Expanding mass	Rapid growth Cells not adhesive, infiltrate tissue
	Frequently encapsulated	No capsule
Spread	Remains localized	Invades nearby tissues or metastasizes to distant sites through blood and lymph vessels
Systemic effects	Rare	Often present
Life-threatening	Only in certain locations (e.g., brain)	Yes, by tissue destruction and spread of tumors

continue to reproduce when there is no need for them. This excessive growth deprives other cells of nutrients. Many neoplasms are unable to function as normal tissue cells because they consist of atypical (abnormal) or immature cells. The characteristics of each tumor depend on the specific type of cell from which the tumor arises, resulting in a unique appearance and growth pattern. The expanding mass creates pressure on surrounding structures.

Nomenclature

Tumors are named according to a system (Table 20-1). The root word, such as *chondro,* is the cell of origin, in this case cartilage. Depending on the type of tissue in which a tumor is located, the suffix indicates malignant tumors (*carcinoma* for epithelial tissue, *sarcoma* for connective tissue). The suffix *oma* alone indicates a benign tumor, e.g., lipoma. However, a number of neoplastic disorders have acquired unique names that are recognized in medical practice. Examples include Hodgkin disease, Wilms tumor, and leukemia. Oncology is the study of malignant tumors, otherwise known as cancer.

THINK ABOUT 20-2

a. What does the term *chondroma* mean? Neuroma? Adenocarcinoma?

b. What term is applied to a malignant bone tumor? (Hint: Bone is osteo.)

Characteristics of Benign and Malignant Tumors

Characteristics of specific tumors vary considerably depending on the cell of origin. The general characteristics of each type are summarized in Table 20-2. *Benign* tumors usually consist of differentiated cells that reproduce at a higher than normal rate. The benign tumor is often encapsulated and expands but does not spread (Fig. 20-1). It is usually freely moveable on palpation. Tissue damage results from compression of adjacent structures such as blood vessels. A benign tumor is not

considered life threatening unless it is in an area such as the brain where the pressure effects can become critical.

By comparison, *malignant* tumors are usually made up of undifferentiated, nonfunctional cells that do not appear organized. The cells tend to reproduce more rapidly than normal and often show abnormal mitotic figures. These cells have lost cellular connections with each other, and reproduction is not inhibited in the presence of other similar cells. Tumor cells infiltrate or spread into surrounding tissue and may easily metastasize or break away to spread to other organs and tissues (Fig. 20-2).

Malignant Tumors: Cancer

Pathophysiology

A tumor manifests as an enlarging space-occupying mass composed of more primitive or *dysplastic* cells. Normal organization, growth inhibition, contact controls, and cell-cell communication are absent. Cell membranes, including surface antigens, are altered. The expanding mass compresses nearby blood vessels, leading to necrosis and an area of inflammation around the tumor, and increases pressure on surrounding structures. Malignant cells do not adhere to each other but often break loose from the mass, infiltrating into adjacent tissue. Tumor cells often secrete enzymes such as

Benign Tumor

Malignant Tumor

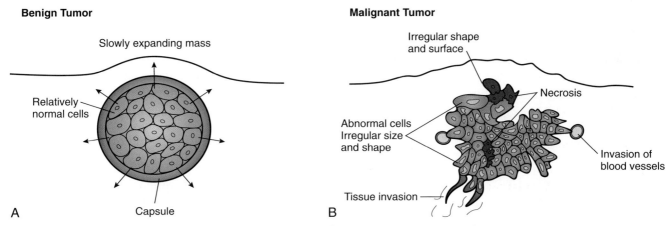

FIGURE 20-1 Characteristics of benign and malignant neoplasms.

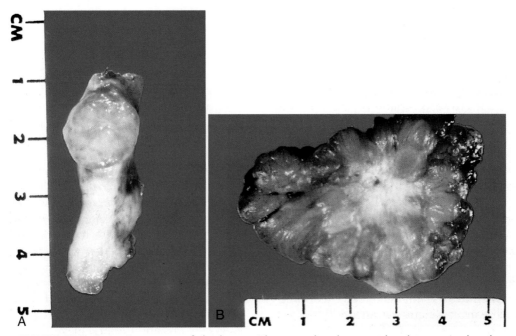

FIGURE 20-2 **A**, Benign tumor of the breast. The tan-colored encapsulated tumor is sharply demarcated from the whiter breast tissue. **B**, Malignant tumor of the breast. Cut section of an invasive ductal carcinoma that is infiltrating the surrounding breast tissue. *(From Kumar V, Abbas AK, Fausto M:* Robbins and Cotran Pathologic Basis of Disease, *ed 7, Philadelphia, 2005, Saunders.)*

collagenase, which break down protein or cells, adding to the destruction and facilitating the tumor's spread into adjacent tissue. Inflammation and the loss of normal cells lead to a progressive reduction in organ function.

As a tumor mass enlarges, the inner cells are frequently deprived of blood and nutrients and die. This necrosis can lead to more inflammation and infection at the site. Some cancer cells secrete growth factors, which stimulate angiogenesis, the development of new capillaries in the tumor, thus promoting tumor development. Antiangiogenesis factors have also been located and several new drugs are based on this blocking action. These drugs are of limited effect in clients receiving chemotherapy because the reduction in blood vessel

development impairs the delivery of chemotherapy agents to the tumor. Tumor cells may increase the uptake of nutrients or "trap" nutrients, depriving normal cells and preventing any tissue regeneration.

Some neoplasms develop very rapidly, whereas others remain in situ for a long time. In situ refers to neoplastic cells in a preinvasive stage of cancer that may persist for months or years. This condition offers an excellent opportunity for early diagnosis of cervical cancer and certain oral cancers.

Grading of tumors is based on the degree of differentiation of the malignant cells—a grade I tumor has well-differentiated cells similar to the original cells, whereas a grade IV tumor is undifferentiated with cells varying in size and shape (anaplasia); this type of tumor is considered highly malignant and likely to progress quickly.

THINK ABOUT   20-3

a. Why is infection likely to occur at the tumor site?
b. Explain the characteristics of undifferentiated cells.
c. How are cells in a biopsy specimen from a tumor identified as malignant?

Effects of Malignant Tumors

All health care workers should be aware of the early indicators of possible malignancies. The classic warning signs of cancer are listed in the box below.

WARNING SIGNS OF CANCER

1. Unusual bleeding or discharge anywhere in the body.
2. Change in bowel or bladder habits (e.g., prolonged diarrhea or discomfort).
3. A change in a wart or mole (i.e., color, size, or shape).
4. A sore that does not heal (on the skin or in the mouth, anywhere).
5. Unexplained weight loss.
6. Anemia or low hemoglobin, and persistent fatigue.
7. Persistent cough or hoarseness without reason.
8. A solid lump, often painless, in the breast or testes or anywhere on the body.

Even if cancer is not present, any of these signs could be the indicator of some other disease process, so it should be checked by a physician. A critical observation can save a life. Sometimes a client may need encouragement to have such warning signs investigated.

Local Effects of Tumors

- *Pain* is not usually an early symptom of cancer; rather, it occurs when the tumor is well advanced. Pain is a warning of a problem; therefore it is helpful if it occurs early, but this is rare. The severity of the pain depends on the type of tumor and its location. Pain may be caused by direct pressure of the mass on sensory nerves, particularly where space is restricted (e.g., bone cancer). Dull, aching pain results from the stretching of a visceral capsule such as occurs in the kidney or liver. Inflammation also contributes to pain because of increased pressure on the nerves and the irritation of nerve endings by chemical mediators (see Chapter 5). Secondary causes of pain include infection, ischemia, and bleeding. Blood can be "irritating" to tissues and, if it collects in an area, can cause pressure on nerves (see Chapter 4).
- *Obstruction* can result when a tumor compresses a duct or passageway from an external position or grows inside a passageway or around a structure (Fig. 20-3). Obstruction may occur in ducts or tubes in the body such as those in the digestive tract. Blood supply or lymphatic flow may be restricted, leading to ulceration and edema. Air flow in the bronchi or nerve conduction may be blocked. Obstructions can cause serious complications for the patient, even in the early stage. In the late stage prevention of obstruction may form the rationale for continuing palliative treatment.
- Tissue necrosis and ulceration may lead to infection around the tumor, particularly in areas where normal flora can become opportunistic. For example, infection is likely to be associated with cancer in the oral cavity. Host resistance to microbial invasion is often reduced with cancer.

Systemic Effects of Malignant Tumors

Systemic or general effects of cancer include the following:

- *Weight loss* and *cachexia* (severe tissue wasting) occur with many malignancies. Contributing factors include anorexia, fatigue, pain, stress, and the increased demands placed on the body by reproducing tumor

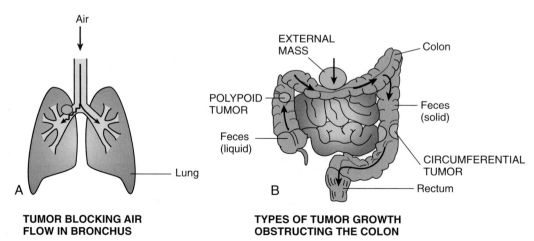

TUMOR BLOCKING AIR FLOW IN BRONCHUS

TYPES OF TUMOR GROWTH OBSTRUCTING THE COLON

FIGURE 20-3 **A** and **B**, Obstruction by tumors.

cells (nutrient trapping), altered carbohydrate and protein metabolism, and cachectic factors produced by macrophages in response to the tumor. This in turn leads to added fatigue and weakness and tissue breakdown.

- Anemia or decreased hemoglobin is a common problem resulting from anorexia and decreased food intake, chronic bleeding with iron loss, and bone marrow depression. Anemia decreases the oxygen available to cells, leading to fatigue and poor tissue regeneration.
- *Severe fatigue* caused by inflammatory changes, cachexia, anemia, stress, and treatment schedules. Psychological factors involved in facing a life-threatening illness can also lead to fatigue and depression.
- *Infections* such as pneumonia occur frequently as host resistance declines. Tissue breakdown develops and the immune system is less effective. The host's immobility contributes to infection in the lungs because of stasis of secretions in the lungs and a weaker cough effort.
- *Bleeding* may occur because the tumor cells may erode the blood vessels or cause tissue ulceration. Bone marrow depression and hypoproteinemia may contribute to poor clotting. Chronic bleeding is common in the digestive tract, where the mucosa fails to regenerate quickly. Chronic blood loss leads to iron deficiency anemia (see Chapter 10).
- *Paraneoplastic syndromes* are additional problems associated with certain tumors, such as bronchogenic carcinoma in the lungs. Tumor cells release substances that affect neurologic function or blood clotting or have hormonal effects. For example, the cells of a bronchogenic carcinoma may produce adrenocorticotropic hormone, leading to the manifestations of Cushing's syndrome in the patient. This syndrome may confuse the diagnosis of cancer, complicate the monitoring and treatment of the patient, and cause change in body image.

THINK ABOUT 20-4

a. Differentiate local from systemic signs of malignant neoplasms and include an example of each.
b. Explain the systemic effects of malignant tumors with regard to: (1) pain, (2) bleeding, (3) weight loss, and (4) fatigue.

Diagnostic Tests

Tests are important in the early detection of cancer and in long-term monitoring of the patient subsequent to the diagnosis. Routine screening tests and self-examination programs need to be promoted, especially in high-risk clients. Frequent monitoring during and after treatment as well as ongoing follow-up are important in assessing the effectiveness of treatment and providing warning of recurrence.

A diagnostic test is not usually 100% reliable by itself because there may be false-negative or false-positive results. The only definitive test for malignancy requires examination of the tumor cells themselves. Other results should be assessed in conjunction with associated data. The following are selected types of tests used for the diagnosis of cancer:

1. *Blood tests* are important both as an indicator of a problem and in monitoring the effects of chemotherapy and radiation. Hemoglobin and erythrocyte counts may be low, a general sign of cancer. In some types of cancer, such as leukemia, the cell characteristics are diagnostic when confirmed by a bone marrow examination. Therapy frequently results in thrombocytopenia, erythrocytopenia, and leukopenia, and these may limit treatment if cell counts fall too low.
2. *Tumor markers* are substances, enzymes, antigens, or hormones, produced by some neoplastic cells. These tumor cell markers can be used to screen high-risk individuals, confirm a diagnosis, or monitor the clinical course of a malignancy. Examples include carcinoembryonic antigen for colon cancer, human chorionic gonadotropin for testicular cancer, alpha-fetoprotein for hepatocellular cancer, CA125 for ovarian cancer, and prostate specific antigen for prostate cancer. Many of these substances are present with other diseases; therefore their presence does not necessarily indicate a positive diagnosis. Chromosome markers, such as Philadelphia chromosome for chronic myelocytic leukemia, are also useful. Specific genes have been linked to certain cancers, such as BRAC-1, which is associated with higher probability of breast or ovarian cancer. Genetic testing does not indicate whether a cancer is present or whether one will develop in the future; it simply indicates increased risk.
3. *X-ray, ultrasound, magnetic resonance imaging* and *computed tomography (CT)* scans are methods of examining changes in tissues or organs (see Ready Reference 5 for information on these tests). In some cases radioisotopes may be used during these procedures to trace metabolic pathways and assess function.
4. *Cytologic* tests are used to screen high-risk individuals, confirm a diagnosis, or follow a clinical course and monitor change. *Histologic* and *cytologic examinations* are used to evaluate biopsies of suspicious masses and check sloughed cells in specific tissues (exfoliative cytology). This is the only dependable confirmation of malignancy. An accurate evaluation depends on good technique and preservation of the specimen. For example, a regular Pap test examining cervical cells is a screening tool for cell changes indicating the development of cervical cancer. Increased use of this test has led to early detection and a greatly

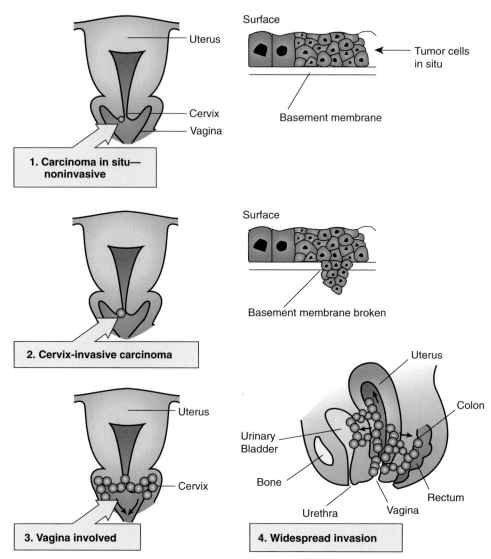

FIGURE 20-4 Invasive carcinoma of the cervix.

improved prognosis for cervical cancer patients. Breast biopsy may be done by an interventional radiologist using ultrasound to visualize the mass and a wide bore needed to extract a tissue sample for histologic examination. This is done in the ultrasound laboratory often immediately after a mass is detected by mammography. It is relatively painless and the woman returns to normal activity shortly after the test.

Spread of Malignant Tumors

Tumors spread by one or more methods depending on the characteristics of the specific tumor cells. They produce *secondary* tumors that consist of cells identical to the *primary* (parent) tumor. Many cancers have spread prior to diagnosis, and this factor must be considered before treatment begins. There are three basic mechanisms for the spread of cancer:

- *Invasion* refers to local spread, in which the tumor cells grow into adjacent tissue and destroy normal cells (Fig. 20-4). Tumor cells are loosely attached to other cells and also secrete lytic enzymes that break down tissue. The origin of the word *cancer* is the Latin word meaning "crablike," a good image of an invasive tumor.

- Metastasis means spread to distant sites by blood or lymphatic channels. In this case the tumor cells erode into a vein or lymphatic vessel, travel through the body, and eventually lodge in a hospitable environment to reproduce and create one or more secondary tumors (Fig. 20-5). Only a few tumor cells survive this transfer, but it only takes a few to start a new tumor. Frequently the first metastasis appears in the regional lymph nodes, which localize the tumor cells for a time. These lymph nodes are checked at the time of surgery, and often several are removed. Usually the lymph nodes are removed or treated to eradicate any micrometastases that may be missed, particularly in cancers that are known to spread at an early stage (e.g., breast cancer). Many cancers spread by normal

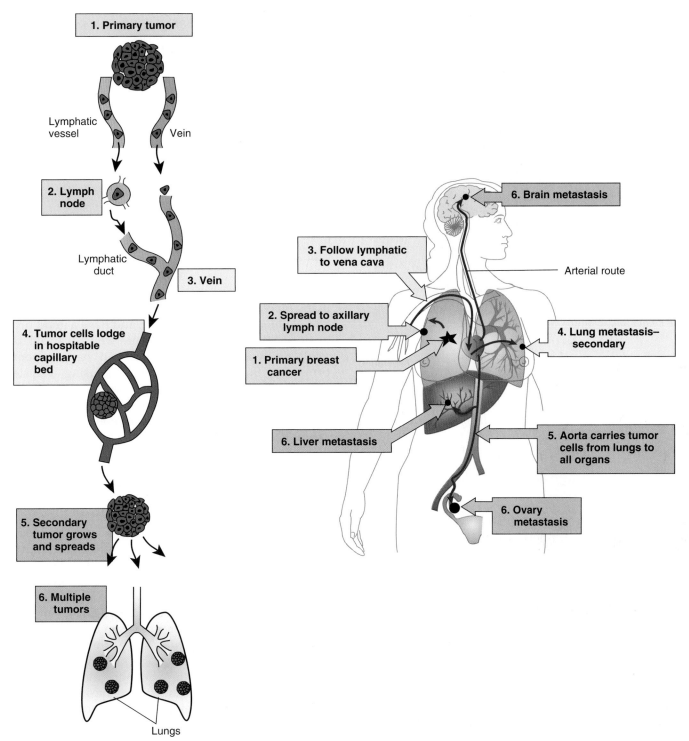

FIGURE 20-5 Metastatic breast cancer.

venous and lymphatic flow, and therefore the lungs and liver are common secondary sites for many tumors (Fig. 20-6). Note the large number of secondary tumors in the liver shown in this figure. However, some cancers are more selective and spread to unusual sites.

• Seeding refers to the spread of cancer cells in body fluids or along membranes, usually in body cavities.

Again, the tumor cells break away and travel easily with the movement of fluid and tissue. An example is ovarian cancer, in which the large peritoneal membrane encourages dispersion of the tumor cells throughout the peritoneal cavity (Fig. 20-7). Malignant cells may also be dislodged from the tumor if excessive handling occurs during diagnostic procedures or surgery, leading to further spread.

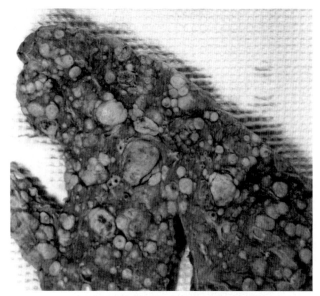

FIGURE 20-6 Liver with multiple metastatic tumors. *(Courtesy of Paul Emmerson, Toronto, Ontario, Canada.)*

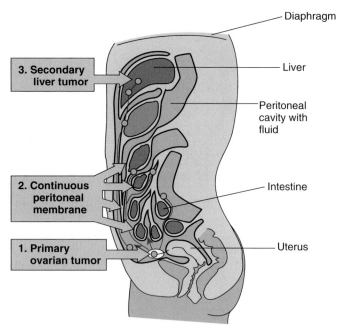

FIGURE 20-7 Ovarian cancer spread by seeding throughout the peritoneal cavity.

Staging of Cancer

Staging of cancer is a classification process applied to a specific malignant tumor at the time of diagnosis. It may be repeated at critical points. The staging system describes the extent of the disease at the time and therefore provides a basis for *treatment* and prognosis. Staging systems are based on the:

- Size of the primary tumor (T)
- Extent of involvement of regional lymph nodes (N)
- Spread (invasion or metastasis) of the tumor (M)

A simplified version of staging is presented in Box 20-1. Subgroups for each stage have also been established for

---

BOX 20-1	Example of Staging-Breast Cancer
T	Size of tumor
N	Involvement of lymph nodes
M	Presence of metastasis

Breast Cancer

Stage I: T_1—tumor 2 cm or less in diameter; N_0—no lymph nodes involved; M_0—no metastasis

Stage II: T_0 to T_2—tumor less than 5 cm in diameter; N_1—nodes involved; M_0—no metastasis

Stage III: T_3—tumor larger than 5 cm in diameter; N_1 or N_2—nodes involved; tumor may be fixed; M_0—no metastasis

Stage IV: T_4—tumor any size but fixed to chest wall or skin; N_3—clavicular nodes involved (spread); M_1—metastasis present

---

many types of cancer. Generally stage I tumors are small and well localized, easy to treat, and have a good prognosis, whereas stage IV tumors are well advanced, difficult to treat at multiple sites, and have a poorer prognosis. Some tumors are staged using a system similar to that shown, but the terminology is different. Information on staging of a particular type of tumor is easily available on web sites maintained by the American Cancer Society or the Canadian Cancer Society.

Etiology

Carcinogenesis

Research is proceeding into the various genes responsible for cell growth and replication and the mechanisms that activate or inhibit the activities of these genes. Discoveries to date include genes that repair DNA, genes that program cell death (apoptosis), genes that cause cancer (oncogenes), and tumor-suppressor genes. Changes in cell DNA are at the root of malignant transformation (see Fig. 21-2 for a diagram of DNA).

Carcinogenesis is the process by which normal cells are transformed into cancer cells. Malignant tumors develop from a sequence of changes over a relatively long period of time. A combination of factors or repeated exposure to a single risk factor leads to changes that activate or change gene expression, leading to transformation of the normal cell into a malignant cell. Some specific cancers have well-established risk factors (e.g., bronchogenic carcinoma or lung cancer and cigarette smoking). The multiplicity of developmental steps in carcinogenesis is supported by the fact that not all cigarette smokers develop cancer. It is difficult to establish precise predisposing or causative (etiologic) factors for each cancer, because it takes many years to gather sufficient documentation, and frequently multiple factors are involved. The role of oncogenic viruses has been confirmed with evidence that particular strains of human papillomavirus are agents of carcinogenesis in

TABLE 20-3 Risk Factors	
Risk Factors (Carcinogen)	Example
Genetic Factors: Oncogenes that regulate all growth	Breast cancer: high family incidence; retinoblastoma: inherited Leukemia: chromosomal abnormalities
Viruses: Oncogenic viruses alter host cell DNA	Hepatic cancer: hepatitis virus Cervical cancer: papilloma virus (HPV) or herpes simplex II; Kaposi's sarcoma: HIV
Radiation: Ultraviolet rays (sun), x-rays, gamma rays, and radioactive chemicals cause cumulative chromosomal damage in cells	Skin cancer: sun exposure Leukemia: radiation exposure
Chemicals: Exposure to both natural and synthetic products in excess may be hazardous; the effects of carcinogenic agents depend on the amount and duration of exposure	Lung cancer: asbestos, nickel Leukemia: solvents (e.g., benzene) Bladder cancer: aniline dyes and rubber
Biologic Factors: Chronic irritation and inflammation with increased mitosis	Colon cancer: ulcerative colitis; oral cancer: leukoplakia
Age: increasing	Many cancers are more common in older persons
Diet: natural substances, additives, or processing methods	Colon cancer: high-fat diet; gastric cancer: smoked foods
Diet: natural substances, additives, or processing methods	Colon cancer: high-fat diet; gastric cancer: smoked foods
Hormones	Endometrial cancer: estrogen

cervical cancer. Exposure to radiation continues to lead to leukemia, and ultraviolet radiation (sun) leads to skin cancer. Also, the incidence of some cancers has changed without adequate explanation. Diagnostic techniques continue to improve and as more data become available statistical and etiologic relationships change.

The stages in carcinogenesis have been organized into:

1. *Initiating* factors or procarcinogens cause the first irreversible changes in the cell DNA. Genetic changes or exposure to an environmental risk may cause this first mutation (Fig. 20-8). This initial change does not create an active neoplasm.
2. Exposure to *promoters* later causes further changes in DNA, resulting in less differentiation and an increased rate of mitosis. Dysplasia or anaplasia may be evident at this time. This process may lead to development of the tumor. Promoters include hormones and environmental chemicals. The prolonged time interval and multiple factors involved complicate efforts by researchers to establish risk factors for many cancers.
3. Continued exposure and changes in DNA result in a malignant tumor that is capable of growth and invasion of local tissue.
4. Changes in the regulation of growth result in cells that are capable of detaching from the tumor and spreading to distant sites (metastasis).

The process of carcinogenesis varies greatly with respect to time. Some tumors develop relatively rapidly, whereas others require decades to develop to the point at which they can be diagnosed. Knowing the speed with which tumor cells reproduce and spread is significant in making treatment decisions. Tumors that metastasize readily and exhibit cells that reproduce quickly are described as "aggressive."

Risk Factors and Prevention

Risk factors are summarized in Table 20-3. Risk factors associated with geographic areas or ethnic groups may relate to environmental influences or diet as well as genetic variables.

Some risk factors such as foods can be avoided. Other factors, such as genetic predisposition, cannot be avoided but can be addressed by encouraging frequent screening and therefore early diagnosis.

The list "Seven Steps to Health" (Box 1-1) includes some specific measures to reduce the common risk factors for cancer such as limiting sun exposure, ensuring regular medical and dental examinations and screening, or altering diet. For example, increasing fiber content in the diet and reducing fats decreases the risk of breast cancer. Deeply pigmented fresh fruits and vegetables provide antioxidants such as vitamins A and E, chemicals that protect cells against damaging substances called free radicals. Free radicals form in cells from exposure to radiation or certain products from metabolic processes. Foods containing antioxidants are now promoted to offset this problem.

THINK ABOUT 20-5

a. Suggest possible reasons for the increased incidence of many cancers in the elderly.
b. Why may it take several years for developments in tumor marker research to result in diagnostic technologies and treatments?

Host Defenses

Cancer suppressor genes present in the body can inhibit neoplastic growth. The immune system appears to offer

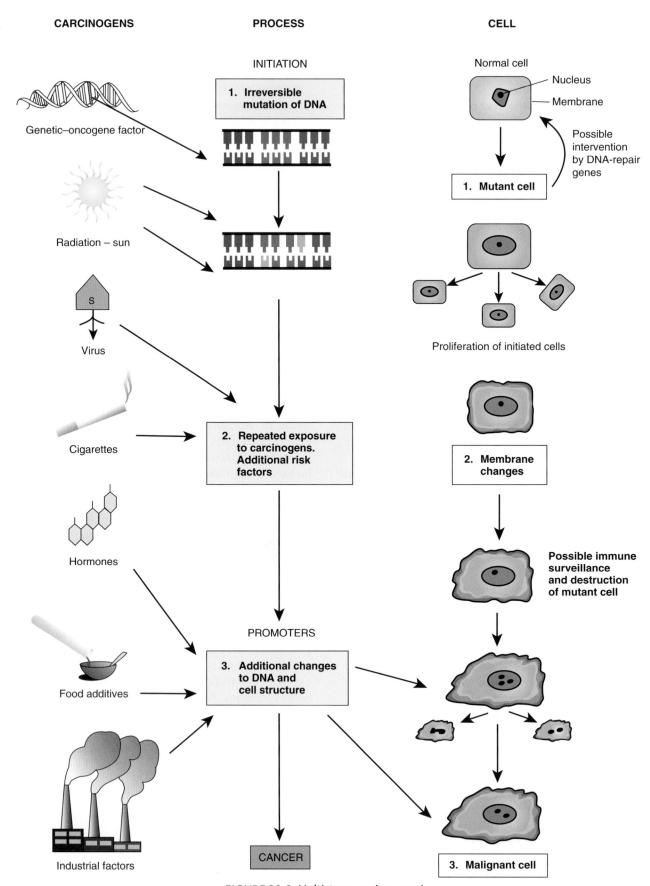

FIGURE 20-8 Multistage carcinogenesis.

protection by reacting to changes in the membranes of some tumor cells, which are seen as "foreign." The immune response includes both cell-mediated and humoral immunity (see Chapter 7). Cytotoxic T lymphocytes, natural killer cells, and macrophages are involved in immune surveillance and the destruction of "foreign" or abnormal cells. Temporary or long-term immunodeficiency has been shown to increase the risk of cancer. For example, human immunodeficiency virus (HIV) infection or acquired immunodeficiency syndrome (AIDS) decreases the number of T lymphocytes. Cancers such as Kaposi's sarcoma and lymphomas occur frequently in AIDS patients (see Chapter 7).

Treatment

Basic treatment measures are surgery, chemotherapy, immunotherapy, or radiation, or a combination thereof, depending on the specific cancer. Not all cancer cells are sensitive to radiation or chemotherapy. Hematopoietic cancers such as leukemia are treated by chemotherapy because the cancer cells are dispersed in the blood. Solid tumors are frequently removed by surgery, which is then followed by chemotherapy or radiation (or both) if the tumor cells are sensitive to these therapies. Immunotherapy stimulates the patient's immune system to target the cancer and attack it.

Treatment may be:

- *Curative* if the tumor is small and localized, or
- Palliative if the cancer is advanced. Palliative treatment is intended to reduce the manifestations and complications related to the cancer and to prolong life. For example decreasing the size of a tumor may lessen the pressure on a nerve, relieving pain, or reduce pressure on the esophagus or bronchus.

Adjuvant therapy is additional prophylactic (preventative) treatment used in cancers that are known to metastasize early in their development, producing secondary tumors that are too small to be detected (micrometastases). For example, following apparent complete removal of a localized breast tumor with no evidence of spread, chemotherapy and radiation may be administered as a precaution in case a few cancer cells have broken away to a lymph node or adjacent tissue.

Chemotherapy and *radiation therapy* are administered in repeated doses at intervals that maximize tumor cell death but minimize the effects on normal tissues. Not all cancer cells are destroyed in one treatment. In solid tumors only the surface layers are affected during each treatment. Between treatments, the tumor may grow slightly (Fig. 20-9). Therefore, treatment continues for a long time, whether curative or palliative.

It is important that any infections, dental problems, or other potential complications be treated before commencing therapy. For example, any loose or extensively damaged teeth might be removed, caries and periodontal disease treated, and a good oral hygiene program

instituted. During therapy it is risky to implement major procedures because of the tendency toward hemorrhage and the possibility of severe infection as a result of immunosuppression and poor healing capabilities of the patient.

Other therapeutic measures may involve nutritional counseling, physiotherapy, occupational therapy, or assistance with other specific problems such as speech therapy. Associated with physical treatment measures is the need to support the client psychologically. The thought of cancer brings great fear and anxiety to clients, fear of death, fear of the treatment and disfigurement, and anxiety related to long-term disability. Many factors are involved. Some clients have a substantial support system, whereas others do not. Treatment can last for months or years, and monitoring continues for a lifetime.

THINK ABOUT 20-6

Suggest some benefits to the patient who chooses to have palliative treatment rather than curative radiation therapy.

Surgery

Surgery involves the removal of the tumor and surrounding tissue, including the nearby lymph nodes if required. The tumor cells and the boundaries are checked to confirm the diagnosis and to ensure their complete removal. The surgical approach may involve the use of a laparoscope and several small incisions. This approach minimizes tissue damage and improves recovery time for the patient.

In some cases removal of adequate surrounding tissue may result in considerable impact on function, for example, in the brain or with skeletal muscle damage. Sometimes complete removal of the tumor may be impossible, but reducing the size of the mass may prevent complications and alleviate some symptoms.

An alternative to surgery for small single tumors in the lungs or liver is radiofrequency ablation. This process is less invasive, easier for the patient to tolerate, and does not require the loss of an entire lobe of the organ as may happen with surgery. An interventional radiologist uses CT scans and ultrasound to guide and needle and electrodes into the tumor. Heat is supplied in the form of radio waves to destroy the malignant cells and tissue immediately surrounding the tumor.

Radiation Therapy

Radiation may be used alone (e.g., for some lymphomas) or combined with other therapies to treat radiosensitive tumors. Radiotherapy causes mutations or alterations in the targeted DNA, thus preventing mitosis or causing immediate cell death. Radiation also damages blood vessels, cutting off blood supply to the tumor cells

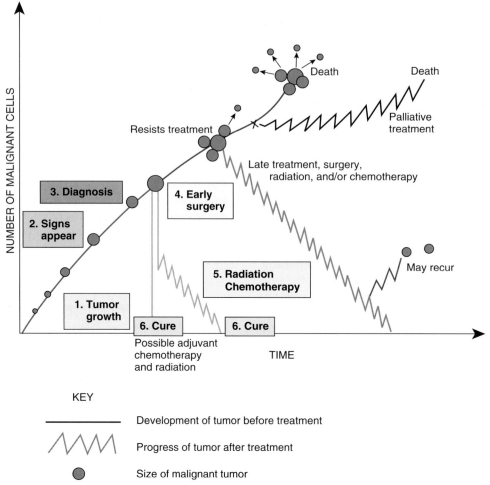

FIGURE 20-9 The effects of treatment on a solid tumor.

and starving them. Radiation is most effective on cells undergoing DNA synthesis or mitosis; therefore it destroys the more rapidly dividing cells in the body, both tumor cells and normal cells (radiosensitive cells). Some types of cancer are radioresistant or unresponsive to radiation. Radiation may be used before surgery to shrink a tumor or destroy loose surface cells, or may be begun after healing of the surgical site (approximately 6 weeks).

Ionizing radiation consists of either electromagnetic waves such as x-rays or gamma rays (from radioactive substances such as radium or cobalt) or high-energy, penetrating particles (electrons, protons). There are several methods of administration:

- External sources, such as a cobalt machine, deliver radiation for a short period of time to a specific site in the body. This method frequently requires the client to have daily treatments for a 6-week period on an outpatient basis. No radiation remains in the body following treatment.
- Internal insertion of radioactive materials at the tumor site may be used to treat specific cancers such as cervical or oral tumors. This is accomplished by sealing the radioisotope (e.g., radium) in a "seed" or

needle and implanting the device at the site (brachytherapy).

Brachytherapy is now being used to treat breast cancer in the early stages when radioactive material is implanted in surrounding tissue following removal of the tumor. If this method proves successful over time, it would replace the daily administration required now for this high-risk cancer.

- Another method is to instill a radioisotope (e.g., ^{198}Au or radioactive gold salt) in a solution in a body cavity, such as the pleural cavity, to control excessive inflammatory exudate or blood from the tumor. These clients must be monitored to ensure that there is no leakage or loss of radioactive materials. For certain cancers, radioisotopes may be given orally (e.g., ^{131}I [radioactive iodine] for thyroid cancer because iodine goes directly to the thyroid gland).

Precautions are required when clients have internal sources of radiation to minimize radiation exposure of other persons. Minimal risk is incurred when the half-life (period when significant radiation is emitted) of a specific radioisotope is short, the cumulative time of exposure is as short as possible, the distance between the source and the individual is great, and shielding materials (e.g., lead aprons), which block penetration by radiation, are used to protect body regions not affected by the cancer.

Adverse effects of radiation depend on the dose and extent of penetration of radiation into the body. Normal cells that rapidly reproduce, such as those in the skin and mucosa (epithelial cells), bone marrow, and gonads are also damaged by radiation.

1. *Bone marrow depression* is the most serious negative effect, so blood cell counts are constantly monitored. Decreased leukocytes greatly increase the risk of infection, decreased platelets may cause excessive bleeding, and decreased erythrocytes contribute to fatigue and tissue breakdown. If blood cell counts are reduced to a critical level, treatment may need to be postponed or blood transfusions may be necessary. Pneumonia and septicemia are common life-threatening complications because body defenses are reduced.
2. Epithelial cell damage includes damage to blood vessels (*vasculitis*) and skin. Skin becomes inflamed (as in a sunburn), and hair loss (alopecia) occurs. The mucosa of the digestive tract is damaged, resulting in some nausea, vomiting, and diarrhea, and the attendant risk of malnutrition and dehydration. Also, inflammation and ulceration in the digestive tract may lead to bleeding, as indicated by melena or hematemesis (blood in the stool or vomitus). With head or neck radiation, the oral mucosa may become ulcerated, and xerostomia (dry mouth) may develop, thereby making it more difficult for the client to eat many foods and increasing the risk of damage to teeth. Swelling may impair swallowing and ventilation.
3. Abdominal radiation is likely to damage the ovaries or testes, leading to sterility or the risk of teratogenesis. Sperm banking or egg retrieval and storage should be discussed with the client before starting treatment.
4. In addition, radiation often produces a nonspecific fatigue and lethargy accompanied by mental depression.

Long-term effects of radiation are related to inflammation, necrosis, and scar tissue along the pathway of the radiation and at the tumor site. At some later time, scar tissue may cause adhesions or obstruction and other secondary problems (see Chapter 5).

THINK ABOUT 20-7

a. Explain why the client with cancer may lack adequate nutrition to maintain normal tissue needs.
b. Explain the adverse effects radiation therapy can have on a patients' immune system, digestion, reproductive functions and possible congenital issues.

Chemotherapy

Some types of cancer cells respond well to certain antineoplastic drugs, whereas other types of cells are resistant to this therapy. Chemotherapy may be used alone (as in leukemias), or may be combined with surgery or radiation. Drugs are most effective against the most rapidly reproducing cells and on small tumor masses. Usually therapy commences approximately 6 weeks following surgery, allowing time for some recovery.

In most treatment protocols, a combination of two to four drugs, each from a different classification, is given to a patient at periodic intervals. The classifications include antimitotics, antimetabolites, alkylating agents, and antibiotics. The drugs interfere with protein synthesis and DNA replication at different points in the tumor cell cycle, thus destroying the cells. A cell cycle is essentially a mini life cycle of growth and reproduction. The choice of drugs and the timing sequence depend on the cell cycle of the particular tumor cell. So each type of cancer is matched to a specific drug treatment. When each drug acts at a different point in the cell cycle, the maximum number of malignant cells can be destroyed.

Figure 20-10 illustrates the combination of:
- *A*driamycin (doxorubicin), an antitumor antibiotic that binds DNA and inhibits synthesis of nucleic acids, acting primarily on cells in the S phase (DNA synthesis) but with some activity in other stages (e.g., altering the cell membrane)
- *B*leomycin, also an antitumor antibiotic that inhibits DNA synthesis
- *V*inblastine, a cell-cycle–specific antimitotic drug that acts on cells in the M stage (mitosis)
- *D*acarbazine, an alkylating agent nonspecific drug acting at several points in the cycle

This combination is the "ABVD" regimen for treating Hodgkin's lymphoma, still the most effective drug treatment for this cancer, although many other combinations have been tried. This combination of drugs is administered intravenously on day 1 and day 15, and then repeated every 4 weeks. Every 4 weeks, Hydrocortisone may be added to the combination of drugs.

There are a large number of specific protocols, and new ones are being researched constantly in an effort to improve effectiveness and minimize adverse effects. Research on adjuvant carrier molecules, which increase cellular uptake of chemotherapy drugs, is providing information on more effective delivery of such drugs. High doses of the drugs are administered to maximize damage to the tumor; then a rest period is provided to allow recovery of normal tissues. A cycle may be repeated at specific weekly or monthly intervals. Many drugs are administered intravenously on an outpatient basis. Lower dosages or milder drugs may be used as palliative therapy.

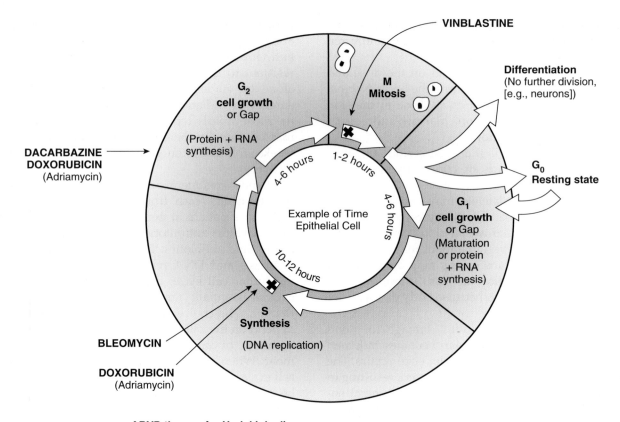

FIGURE 20-10 The cell cycle and chemotherapy.

Adverse effects (side effects) may be quite marked with drug therapy. As with radiation, the normal cells are also damaged, most commonly the skin and mucosa, bone marrow, and gonads. The need to minimize adverse effects is another factor in choosing the combination. For example, not all the drugs in a combination can seriously depress the bone marrow, but rather, one of the drugs in the combination may cause nausea or hair loss.

• Bone marrow depression is the limiting factor with chemotherapy, and dangerously low blood counts may require transfusions or cessation of therapy until the bone marrow recovers. Blood tests are taken before each treatment to check cell count. The nadir, or point of lowest cell count (neutropenia or leukopenia), may occur at different points in the cycle depending on the particular drug. If the count is too low, treatment may need to be postponed, and antibiotics or hospitalization may be required. Hemorrhage is a major risk with thrombocytopenia. Infections are common with neutropenia, septicemia with tumors in the gastrointestinal tract, and pneumonia with lung cancers. Skin infections are common,

particularly if immobility or malnutrition has led to skin breakdown. Of course, in cases in which the blood cells are already reduced in number or function, as with the leukemias, the effects of chemotherapy can be critical.

• Vomiting may occur during or shortly after treatment owing to direct chemical stimulation by the drug of the emetic or vomiting center in the brain. Vomiting may continue after treatment in response to the mucosal inflammation and damage in the digestive tract. In some cases, nausea and vomiting develop before chemotherapy administration related to anxiety or past experience.

Antiemetic drugs such as ondansetron (Zofran) may be helpful in decreasing vomiting. Alternatives include dexamethasone (Decadron) and prochlorperazine (Stemetil).

• Epithelial cells are easily damaged because of the ongoing mitosis. Hair loss (*alopecia*) and breakdown of skin and mucosa occur frequently. Stomatitis in the mouth and diarrhea are common problems and contribute to malnutrition. Candidal infections are common in the mouth.

- In addition, some antineoplastic drugs have unique damaging effects in specific areas; for example, fibrosis in the lungs or damage to myocardial cells.

THINK ABOUT 20-8

Explain several ways by which the treatment of cancer by chemotherapy may temporarily create additional health problems for the patient.

Other Drugs

Hormones are frequently prescribed during cancer treatment in addition to the basic treatment. A glucocorticoid such as prednisone is used to decrease mitosis and increase erythrocyte counts (see Chapter 5). For the patient, these drugs improve appetite and a sense of well-being. They also decrease inflammation and swelling around the tumor.

Sex hormones are beneficial when tumor growth is dependent on such hormones; for example, estrogens may slow the growth of prostate cancer. Hormone-blocking agents are often effective in reducing tumors and preventing recurrences. Tamoxifen is an example of an estrogen-blocking agent used in clients with estrogen-dependent breast cancer; it has been particularly useful in postmenopausal women. Other related agents are being assessed for long-term effects. A newer drug, exemestane (Aromasin), has been useful with fewer side effects in advanced cases of postmenopausal, hormone-dependent breast cancer in which tamoxifen is not effective. This drug blocks the conversion, by the enzyme aromatase, of androgens to estrogens.

Biologic response modifiers are agents that augment the natural immune response in the body to improve surveillance and removal of abnormal cells. Included in this group are a natural product of human cells, interferon, and bacillus Calmette-Guérin (BCG) vaccine (for tuberculosis). Interferon has not been as effective as expected, primarily due to undesirable and often dangerous side effects such as negative effects on areas of the immune system, but investigation into this area continues. The BCG vaccine may be injected near the tumor or instilled in a cavity such as the bladder when cancer is present. It stimulates the movement of macrophages and T lymphocytes to the site, where they may destroy the tumor cell. Other than BCG for treatment of bladder cancer, these are not a first-line treatment at this time.

Identifying and acting on molecular targets, perhaps in the immune response, is seen as a way of developing new drugs with fewer side effects. Trastuzumab (Herceptin) is used to treat advanced breast cancer. It is an antibody that binds cell receptor sites, blocking growth signals and stimulating immune defenses. Another new group achieving a favorable response consists of drugs

with antibody action, labeled with radioisotopes. An example is tositumomab (Bexxar) used for non-Hodgkin's lymphoma. It exerts antibody action against antigen on the tumor cells, destroying the cells. In this case, radioactive iodine has a half-life of 8 days. There have been reports of allergic reactions.

Another focus for investigation is the *angiogenesis inhibitor drug* group (e.g., angiostatin or endostatin). Angiogenesis means new blood vessels, and as a tumor grows and spreads, so must new blood vessels. Anti-angiogenesis drugs block the stimulus for endothelial cell (blood vessel walls) growth by various mechanisms and therefore reduce local blood flow and starve the tumor cells. It was hoped that these drugs would have fewer adverse effects and could be combined with traditional chemotherapy for more effective treatment. To date the results have not met expectations, possibly because blocking the growth of blood vessels also reduces the delivery of chemotherapy to the cells in the tumor. Bevacizumab (Avastin) has prolonged the life of individuals with colorectal cancer. It has antibody activity against vascular endothelial growth factor, secreted by many tumor cells and required to form blood vessels.

Analgesics for pain control are an important part of therapy, particularly when cancer is advanced (see Chapter 4). Determining the cause of the pain is important because this determines the therapeutic approach. In some cases, a specific factor such as infection or muscle spasm can be treated, leading to pain reduction. Radiation treatment can relieve nerve compression.

For analgesics, a stepwise approach is frequently adopted. This involves using mild drugs in low doses initially, then increasing the dose, then changing to a stronger analgesic, and ultimately using morphine. Multiple-drug "cocktails" are often effective as the pain intensity increases. Very high doses of narcotics may be administered as tolerance builds. Self-administration or implanted units providing continuous infusion are helpful in long-term pain control. Dependency is currently less of a concern, but narcotic analgesics do have a number of significant side effects. These include nausea, constipation, drowsiness, and respiratory depression. Other methods for pain relief may be beneficial, as well as measures that reduce fatigue and anxiety, which can aggravate pain.

Alternative therapies are sought by many clients in whom the traditional treatments have not been successful. Research continues to study many of these, although trials have not shown significant benefit of such approaches.

Nutrition

Patients with advanced cancer are often malnourished. Contributing factors include change in taste sensations, anorexia and vomiting, sore mouth or loss of teeth, pain and fatigue, malabsorption due to inflammation in the digestive tract, altered metabolism, and nutrient trapping by the tumor. These factors may result from the tumor itself or from the effects of chemotherapy and radiation.

The use of measures such as ice and mouth rinses is suggested to reduce the discomfort of ulcers and inflammation in the mouth. Frequent small amounts of nonirritating and favorite foods are better tolerated. These small meals can be planned to be attractive to the patient and optimize protein and vitamin intake. Pain control and antiemetic drugs may increase appetite. If necessary, total parenteral nutrition may be used. It involves the administration of a nutrient mixture directly into a peripheral vein.

Complementary Therapies

Many alternative approaches are used to treat or "cure" cancer. These nonmedical therapies are referred to as complementary. They range from the use of a raw food macrobiotic diet, to the use of insulin and glucose to accompany chemotherapy. Although some complementary therapies have shown benefit when combined with medical therapy, there is no research-based evidence to show that any complementary therapy on its own will prolong life or reduce metastasis. Clients choosing to use complementary therapies should advise their oncology team that they are doing so. Cancer treatment is a complex science and the public is demanding better therapeutic outcomes, thus complementary therapy may offer hope for a better outcome. It is important that the health care worker is aware of complementary therapies and can direct patients to the appropriate information about any such treatment. Additional information on alternative or complementary therapy in general is in Chapter 3 of this text.

Prognosis

A "cure" for cancer is generally defined as a 5-year survival without recurrence after diagnosis and treatment. In some cases, several periods of remission (no clinical signs) may occur before the disease becomes terminal.

In some cases, early diagnosis and treatment limit the extent of the illness in an individual. In other cases, cancer treatment involves a prolonged period of illness with intermittent acute episodes. Information and support for the patient and family are offered by the American Cancer Society as well as cancer clinics and the many other community support groups.

The death rates for specific cancers vary. For some types of cancer, such as lung cancer, there has been no significant improvement in the outcome even with aggressive treatment. For other cancers, such as certain childhood leukemias and Hodgkin's lymphoma, effective treatment has been developed, and survival rates are much improved. Current statistics for specific cancers are available from the American Cancer Society or Canadian Cancer Society. Prognosis in a specific

individual is influenced by many factors and so is subject to change.

> **THINK ABOUT   20-9**
>
> a. From your knowledge of normal physiology, explain how good nutrition could reduce the complications or additional problems associated with cancer and its treatment.
> b. Suggest some factors other than clinical test results that could affect the prognosis or outcome for an individual with cancer.

Examples of Malignant Tumors

These examples are used to illustrate some general aspects of cancer. Additional details are provided in the appropriate chapter dealing with the affected system. For specific information on other types of cancer, refer to the body system chapter in which the affected organ/structure is discussed.

Skin Cancer

Skin cancer is visible, easily diagnosed and treated (by surgery), and develops slowly; therefore most types with the exception of malignant melanoma have an excellent prognosis. Skin cancers have the highest rate of recurrence and usually arise on the head and neck or back, areas exposed to the sun and irritation. They occur more frequently in individuals with fair skin who are over 40 years of age and live in southern climates. The number of cases is increasing, resulting in a public education campaign to reduce sun exposure and sun tanning practices.

Basal cell carcinoma is the most common form of skin cancer (see Chapter 8 for other skin cancers). The tumor appears as a pearly papule and develops a central ulceration, a "rodent ulcer" (Fig. 20-11). Significant

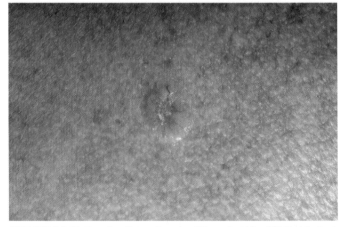

FIGURE 20-11 Basal cell carcinoma. *(From Lookingbill D, Marks J: Principles of Dermatology, ed 3, Philadelphia, 2000, Saunders.)*

characteristics of the lesion include *lack of pain or pruritus* (itching) and *persistence*—the lesion remains and grows slowly. The tumor is slowly invasive into the subcutaneous tissues.

> **THINK ABOUT 20-10**
> Explain several reasons for the good prognosis in skin cancer.

Ovarian Cancer

Ovarian cancer has a very poor prognosis, ranking high in mortality rates. The tumor is hidden in the peritoneal cavity; it is a "silent" tumor (see Fig. 20-7). Although there are many histologic types of ovarian cancer, this section deals only with the basic concepts (see Chapter 19). Hormonal and genetic factors appear to play a role in development of this cancer.

Presenting (or first) signs are vague and appear only after the tumor is well advanced and is large enough to cause pressure on the adjacent structures, such as the bladder or intestine, or when an inflammatory exudate forms in the abdominal cavity. These late signs often contribute to a late diagnosis and a delay in treatment. There are tumor markers to assist in early diagnosis and screening, but false-negatives do occur. The marker CA125 is elevated in other conditions as well as ovarian cancer, but is useful in monitoring the effectiveness of treatment. The first indications are usually altered bowel or bladder function or increased abdominal girth. The tumor spreads easily by means of the lymphatic vessels and by seeding as cancer cells pass along the peritoneal membranes or are sloughed into peritoneal fluid, traveling to the liver and other organs. The cancer also invades the uterus and pelvis. Treatment includes surgery, radiation, and chemotherapy. See Chapter 19 for further discussion.

Brain Cancer

Brain tumors may be benign or malignant. Both are space-occupying masses that create pressure inside the skull, and both are serious for this reason. Brain tumors, even when small, can cause death if they are located in the brainstem or cerebellum, where they can interfere with vital functions such as respiration. Removal of the mass may be fairly easy if it is located on the brain surface but difficult and dangerous if it is located elsewhere (Fig. 20-12). Brain tumors vary histologically, originating from neurons, neuroglial cells, blood vessels, or connective tissue. They can occur in children as well as adults (Fig. 20-13). Early indications of brain tumors are seizures or signs of pressure such as headache, drowsiness, vomiting, visual problems, or impaired motor function (see Chapter 14 for information on increased intracranial pressure). Malignant brain tumors do not metastasize outside the central nervous system because the primary tumor is usually fatal before

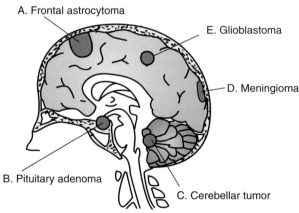
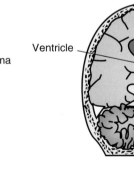

A + D. Tumors on surface of brain

B. Pituitary tumor causes neurologic dysfunction and hormonal abnormalities

C. Cerebellar tumors, even when small, can interfere with vital brain stem function

E. Tumors in the interior of the brain shift ventricles and interfere with flow of cerebrospinal fluid

F. Multiple metastases

FIGURE 20-12 Effects of brain tumors in various locations.

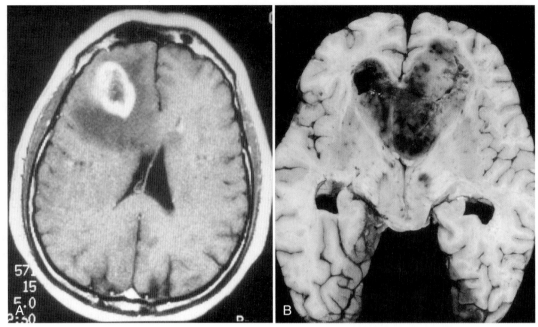

FIGURE 20-13 **A** and **B**, Brain tumor. **A**, Computed tomographic (CT) scan of a large tumor in the cerebral hemisphere, enhanced with contrast material and showing pronounced peritumoral edema. **B**, A tumor (Glioblastoma multiforme) appearing as a necrotic, hemorrhagic, infiltrating mass in the brain. *(From Kumar V, Abbas AK, Fausto M: Robbins and Cotran Pathologic Basis of Disease, ed 7, Philadelphia, 2005, WB Saunders.)*

metastasis begins. However, tumors from the breast lung or bone can metastasize into the brain, forming secondary tumors. Treatment of brain tumors may be surgery, radiation, or chemotherapy and may cause the loss of some additional brain tissue. Aftereffects of treatment may include loss of specific function and disability.

Cancer Incidences

In 2009 the CDC released information from The United States Cancer Statistics: 2009 Incidence and Mortality Report that contained official statistics for cancer incidence and mortality in 98% of the US population. This information is presented here by sex, by the three most common cancers and then the leading causes of cancer death.

Cancer among men:
- Three most common
  - Prostate Cancer—First among men of all races
  - Lung Cancer—Second among white, black, native American, and Asian men; third among Hispanic men
  - Colorectal cancer—Second among Hispanic; third among white, black, native American, and Asian men

- Leading causes of cancer deaths
  - Lung cancer—First among men of all races
  - Prostate cancer—Second among white, black, Hispanic, and native America men; fourth among Asian men
  - Liver cancer—Second among Asian men
  - Colorectal cancer—Third among men of all races

Cancer among women:
- Three most common
  - Breast cancer—First among women of all races
  - Lung cancer—Second among white, black and native American women; third among Asian and Hispanic women
  - Colorectal cancer—Second among Asian and Hispanic women; third among white, black and native American women
- Leading causes of cancer deaths
  - Lung cancer—First among white, black, Asian, and native American women; second among Hispanics
  - Breast cancer—First among Hispanic women and second among white, black, Asian, and native American women
  - Colorectal cancer—Third among women of all races

CASE STUDY A

Lung Cancer

Ms. T., a 65 year-old woman in good health, presents to her family doctor with a chronic cough. She is currently a non-smoker. A chest x-ray shows a small growth in the right lung. A blood test for lung tumor markers is negative and a bronchoscopy is scheduled to biopsy the tumor. The pathology report indicates the lung tumor is a secondary tumor from the small intestine. Ms. T. is referred to an oncologist for treatment.

1. What factors in her history indicate a risk of cancer for Ms. T.?
2. What is the significance of a negative test for tumor markers in this case?
3. How did the small intestine tumor cells reach the lungs?
4. What is the probable prognosis for Ms. T.?

CASE STUDY B

Breast Cancer

W.R., a 32-year-old woman, felt a small, hard, painless lump in her left breast during regular self-examination. The lump did not disappear during the next few days, so she went to her physician for an examination. Tests followed, and a biopsy confirmed the presence of a malignant tumor. The tumor (1.5 cm) was removed, as well as five lymph nodes, two of which contained malignant cells. No other metastases appeared to be present. Courses of radiation and chemotherapy were recommended following a 6-week recovery period, and the prognosis appeared good.

1. Which activities led to the good prognosis?
2. Why were the lymph nodes checked?
3. Why are radiation and chemotherapy recommended in this case? Describe three possible side effects of treatment.

CHAPTER SUMMARY

In the body, each cell type is distinguished by its individualized life cycle and pattern of differentiation. Neoplasm means "new growth," whereby the cells do not follow the normal growth controls. The changes are determined by biopsy and histologic examination.

- Benign neoplasms are space-occupying masses of abnormal cells, but they do not spread to distant sites and are not considered life threatening unless located in an area such as the brain.
- Malignant neoplasms (cancer) usually consist of more primitive cells that are reproducing more rapidly, and they spread by invasion or metastases. Systemic effects are present.
- Local effects relate to the pressure of the mass (e.g., ischemia and necrosis, obstruction, or pain).
- Systemic effects of malignant tumors include weight loss, anemia, fatigue, and paraneoplastic syndrome.
- Grading of a cancer is determined by the degree of differentiation and indicators of mitoses seen in the tumor cells.
- Staging of a tumor at the time of diagnosis is based on the size of the primary tumor, the involvement of nearby lymph nodes, and the presence of distant metastases. Staging is used as a guide to treatment and prognosis.
- Treatment may involve any or all of surgery, radiation, and chemotherapy. A cancer is considered cured after 5 years without recurrence.
- The carcinogenic process is based on exposure, first to initiating factors and later to promoters, each of which contributes to changes in cell DNA, creating a malignant neoplasm.
- Carcinogens or risk factors include genetic predisposition and environmental, biologic, and dietary factors.
- Radiation therapy may be provided by external sources such as a cobalt machine or by internal implants of material such as radioactive radium.
- Chemotherapy frequently consists of a specific combination of drugs administered (often intravenously) at intervals over a period of time. Hormones such as prednisone may be added to the regimen. The growth of some tumor cells is hormone dependent, in which case hormones may be provided or removed, as necessary. Several new approaches to drug therapy are under development.
- Adverse effects of chemotherapy and radiation include bone marrow depression causing leukopenia, anemia, and thrombocytopenia; epithelial damage causing mucosal ulceration and hair loss; and nausea and vomiting.
- Basal cell carcinoma is an example of skin cancer related to sun exposure. The prognosis is excellent because the cancer is slow growing, obvious at an early stage, and easily treated.
- Ovarian cancer has a poor prognosis because of the tumor's hidden location and lack of signs until it is large in size or metastasis has occurred, as well as its rapid growth and early spread.
- Brain tumors, both benign and malignant, result in pressure inside the skull and may be difficult to remove without causing additional brain damage.

STUDY QUESTIONS

1. Compare benign and malignant neoplasms, describing three differences.

2. How does the zone of inflammation around the tumor contribute to pain?

3. Explain why metastasis can lead to multiple secondary tumors in different sites.
4. Why may chemotherapy be recommended for a client when a cure is not likely?
5. Explain why severe thrombocytopenia can be life threatening.
6. Explain two reasons why infection may occur with cancer.
7. Describe two potential problems resulting from bleeding.
8. Describe the local effects of radiation.
9. Explain why benign brain tumors are serious.
10. Compare basal cell skin cancer and ovarian cancer by:
    a. presenting signs
    b. spread
    c. prognosis

ADDITIONAL RESOURCES

Andreoli TE, Loscalzo J, Carpenter CCJ, Griggs RC: *Andreoli and Cecil's Essentials of Medicine*, Philadelphia, 2007, Saunders.

Cancer Information Service: 1-800-422-6237.

Fischer DS, Knobf MT, Durivage HJ, Beaulieu NJ: *The Cancer Chemotherapy Handbook*, ed 6, St. Louis, 2003, Mosby.

Kumar V, Abbas AK, Fausto M: *Robbins and Cotran Pathologic Basis of Disease*, ed 8, Philadelphia, 2007, Saunders.

Mosby's Drug Consult 2006. St. Louis, 2006, Mosby.

Web Sites

http://www.americanscientist.org *American Scientist*

http://www.cancer.gov/cancerinformation *National Cancer Institute*

http://www.cancer.org *American Cancer Society*

http://jama.ama-assn.org *The Journal of the American Medical Association*

http://www.nci.nih.gov/ *National Cancer Institute*

http://www.nature.com *Nature, journal*

http://www.mayoclinic.com *Mayo Clinic*

http://ovariancancer.jhmi.edu *Johns Hopkins University*

http://www.sciam.com *Scientific American, journal*

CHAPTER 21

Congenital and Genetic Disorders

CHAPTER OUTLINE

LEARNING OBJECTIVES

After studying this chapter, the student is expected to:

1. Define congenital, genetic, chromosomal, developmental, and multifactorial disorders.
2. Describe the inheritance pattern of autosomal recessive, autosomal dominant, and X-linked recessive disorders.
3. Explain the common causes of developmental disorders and their relationship to fetal development.
4. Discuss the importance of proteomics in the development of treatments for genetic disorders.
5. Describe the benefits and risks of genetic screening programs and prenatal testing.
6. Discuss the purposes of genetic engineering and current concerns.
7. Describe the cause and effect of Down syndrome.

KEY TERMS

allele	gene penetration	karyotype	organogenesis
amniocentesis	genotype	meiosis	phenotype
anomaly	heterozygous	mitosis	polygenic
autosomes	homozygous	mutation	teratogenic
expression	incomplete dominant	neonates	trisomy

Review of Genetic Control

Genetic information for each cell is stored on chromosomes, of which there are 23 pairs in each human cell. Twenty-two pairs are autosomes, and they are numbered when arranged by size and shape in a diagnostic graphic termed a karyotype (Fig. 21-1). The 23rd pair consists of the pair of sex chromosomes; males have XY, and females have XX chromosomes. A male child receives the X chromosome from his mother and a Y chromosome from his father. A female child receives an X chromosome from each parent. During meiosis in humans, each sperm and each ovum receive only 23 chromosomes, that is, one chromosome from each pair.

When the ovum is fertilized by the sperm, the resulting zygote has 46 chromosomes, or 23 pairs containing an assortment of genetic information inherited from the parents. Because so many combinations of genes are possible, it is most unlikely that any two persons other than identical twins will have the same genes and sequence of DNA (deoxyribonucleic acid). Therefore, DNA is considered a unique identifying characteristic for an individual (Fig. 21-2).

Chromosomes are made up of many genes, which are matched for a function (allele) at a specific location on the paired chromosomes. A gene is a DNA "file" that contains information about protein synthesis in the cell. All cells in an individual's body contain the same

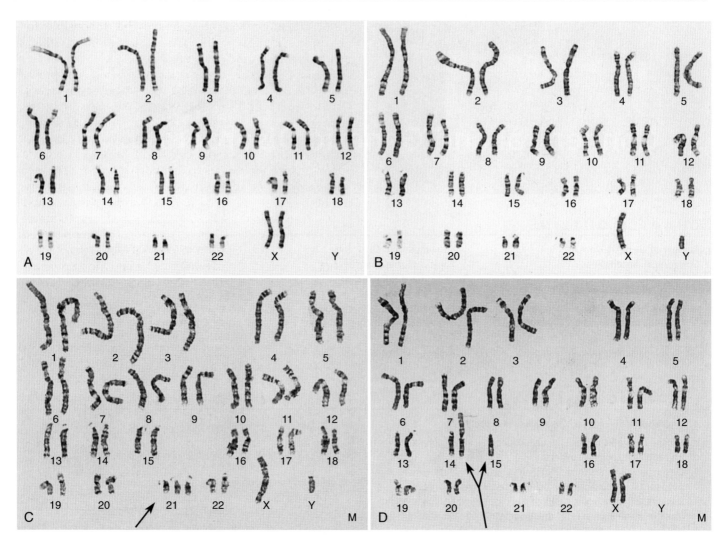

FIGURE 21-1 **Examples of Karyotypes** A, Normal female (46, XX). **B,** Normal male (46, XY). **C,** Male with Down syndrome or trisomy 21 (47, XY, + 21). **D,** Female with translocation involving chromosomes 14 and 15 (45, XX, t (14q15q)). *(Courtesy of Cytogenetics Laboratory, North York General Hospital, Toronto, Ontario, Canada.)*

chromosomes and genes for the same traits (genotype), although not all genes are active in each cell. This limited activity is referred to as *gene expression*. Usually only a small group of genes is controlling protein synthesis in a particular cell at any particular time; gene expression is related to the cell's specific function.

Genes are composed of DNA strands, which determine the function of all cells in the body. RNA (ribonucleic acid) provides the communication link with DNA during the actual synthesis of proteins and helps to maintain control of cell activity. During embryonic and fetal development, when cells are undergoing mitosis (somatic cell division), the chromosomes replicate, and each daughter cell receives a copy of DNA identical to that in the parent cell. Therefore the same genetic information is carried forward. Changes can occur because of an error in the process of meiosis or mitosis, but these are relatively rare. Such a mutation or alteration in genetic material may be spontaneous or

may result from exposure to harmful substances such as radiation, chemicals, or drugs.

Research has been directed toward "mapping" all the genes on particular chromosomes and identifying the role of each gene (Fig. 21-3). The *International Human Genome Project* (HGP) is a worldwide project conducted by geneticists that aims to identify and map all the genes on every chromosome. The first stage was completed in 2003, listing millions of base pairs in the human DNA strand. Not all genes have been sequenced in the genome to date. Although it was originally estimated that there are a total of 50,000 to 100,000 protein-coding genes in the human chromosome, current knowledge has reduced this figure to approximately 20,000 to 25,000. In addition, some DNA sequences act as regulators or "on/off switches" for gene activity, whereas other sequences have unknown functions and have been termed *junk DNA*. Repeats of base pairs in this so-called junk DNA have been identified as abnormalities leading

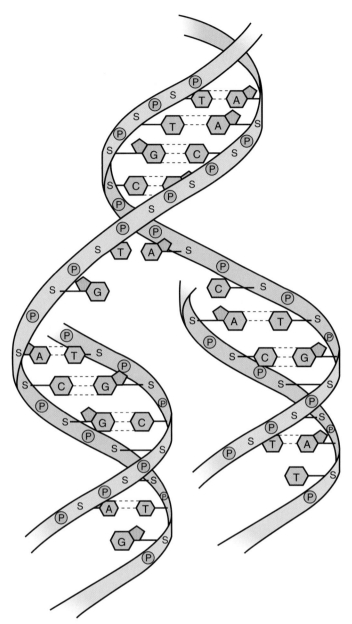

FIGURE 21-2 DNA replication. *(From Applegate E: The Anatomy and Physiology Learning System, ed 2, Philadelphia, 2000, Saunders.)*

to disease. As more information becomes available, it becomes easier to decode the DNA sequences and clarify problem areas. Now the refining, verifying, and analysis of data, and identification and functional determination of individual genes continue.

When a specific gene for a pathologic condition is identified, a DNA analysis follows, leading, to the development of a simple blood test to screen individuals for the presence of that specific gene. The genetic link to a disease may lead to improved treatment, a cure, or prevention. Many genetic conditions have been determined so far, as well as a large number of genes related to cancer and cardiovascular disease. Every year, a few more disease-causing genes are located. For some

disorders, more than one gene may be responsible; for example, each of four different genes causes four different types of Fanconi's anemia.

Genes control all physical characteristics, such as eye color or color blindness, and all metabolic processes. The effects, such as shade of eye color, vary with the gene penetration or frequency of expression of the gene among individuals carrying the gene. Inheritance of many genes for both normal characteristics and disease characteristics follows specific patterns of inheritance termed *Mendelian laws* or patterns. Mendelian inheritance includes recessive and dominant patterns and results can be predicted using algebra or Punnett squares (Fig. 21-4). Traditionally recessive genes are represented by lowercase letters and dominant genes by capital letters. Many traits such as eye color and blood type are polygenic, meaning that more than one allele determines the genotype and thus the phenotype of the individual.

THINK ABOUT 21-1

a. What are the purposes of meiosis?
b. Which pair number represents the sex chromosomes?
c. Which parent passes on the Y chromosome to the child?
d. Describe the structure, location, and function of a gene.
e. Why is DNA considered a dependable means of identification for an individual? How might this be used?
f. List three ways that genetic control (DNA) could be altered.

Congenital Anomalies

Congenital anomalies refer to disorders present at birth. Such defects include genetic or inherited disorders as well as developmental disorders.

• Genetic disorders may result from a single-gene trait or from a chromosomal defect, or they may be *multifactorial*. A few examples are listed in Box 21-1.
• Single-gene disorders are caused by a change in one gene within the reproductive cells (ova or sperm); this mutant gene is then transmitted to subsequent generations following the specific inheritance pattern for that gene. Mutations in the body cells other than the reproductive cells may cause dysfunction but are not transmitted to offspring. In some cases, the expression, or effect (phenotype), of an altered gene produces clinical signs that vary in severity depending on the penetration or activity of the gene. Clinical signs of genetic disorders are not always present at birth but may occur months or years later, for example, Huntington disease, which is seen in adults. However, children with genetic disorders do constitute a significant percentage of those who require hospital and community care. Additional information on children with genetic disorders can be found in any pediatrics textbook.

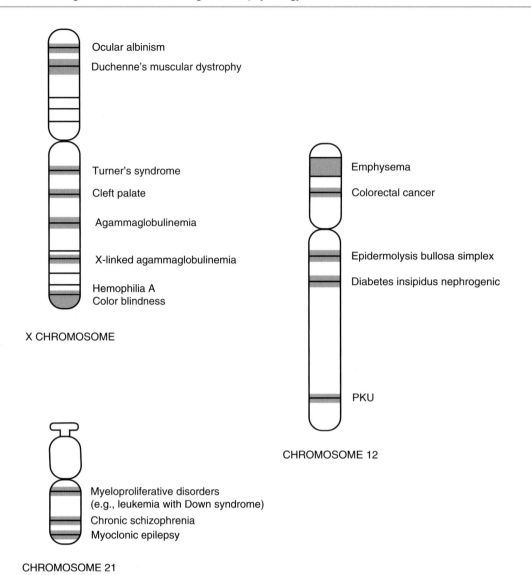

FIGURE 21-3 Examples of approximate gene locations on selected chromosomes.

BOX 21-1 Examples of Genetic Disorders and Their Inheritance

Single-Gene Disorders
Autosomal Dominant Disorders
Adult polycystic kidney disease
Huntington's chorea
Familial hypercholesterolemia
Marfan syndrome

Autosomal Recessive Disorders
Cystic fibrosis
Phenylketonuria
Sickle cell anemia
Tay-Sachs disease

X-Linked Dominant Disorders
Fragile X syndrome

X-Linked Recessive Disorders
Color blindness
Duchenne muscular dystrophy
Hemophilia A

Multifactorial Disorders
Anencephaly
Cleft lip and palate
Clubfoot
Congenital heart disease
Myelomeningocele
Schizophrenia

Chromosomal Disorders
Down syndrome
Monosomy X (Turner syndrome)
Polysomy X (Klinefelter syndrome)
Trisomy 18 (Edwards syndrome)

AUTOSOMAL RECESSIVE DISORDERS – Example: Cystic fibrosis

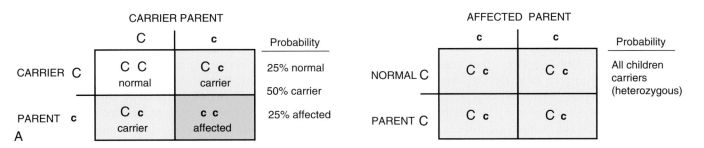

AUTOSOMAL DOMINANT DISORDERS – Example: Huntington's chorea

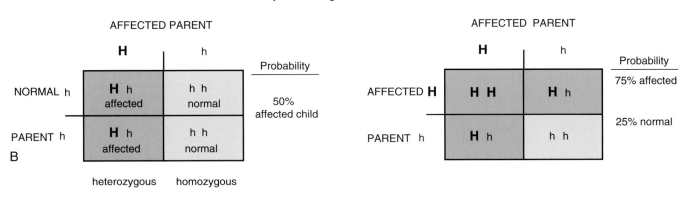

X-LINKED RECESSIVE DISORDERS – Example: Duchenne's muscular dystrophy

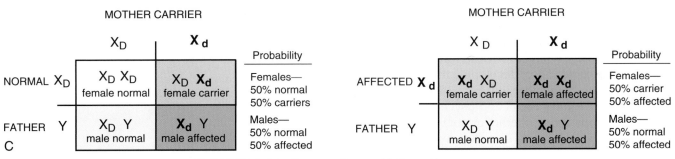

FIGURE 21-4 Inheritance patterns with Punnett squares.

- Chromosomal *anomalies* usually result from an error during meiosis, when the DNA fragments are displaced or lost, thus altering genetic information (e.g., Down syndrome). This may be spontaneous or result from exposure to a damaging substance. During meiosis, genes are often redistributed during the process of "crossover" in which chromosomes may swap portions. There may be an error in chromosomal duplication or reassembly, resulting in abnormal placement of part of the chromosome (a translocation), altered structure (deletion), or an abnormal number of chromosomes. This change is reflected in the expression of genes in the child. These birth defects are more common when the mother is greater than age 35. New research has also identified a higher risk in children of older fathers. Such errors are a common cause of spontaneous abortions during the first trimester of pregnancy. Chromosomal anomalies are found in approximately 7 in 1000 births.

- Other congenital or developmental disorders result from premature birth, a difficult labor and delivery, or exposure to a damaging agent during fetal development. The defect may be limited to one organ, or it may affect the functions of many organs. Such congenital disorders often do not have a genetic component, but because they present at birth, they are termed *congenital* or *developmental*.

Developmental defects may be spontaneous errors or may result from exposure to environmental factors in utero. The DNA of the embryonic cells may be altered easily because rapid mitosis and differentiation take place during the first months of embryonic development. During this period replication of DNA occurs frequently and the possibility of damage is significant. Maternal nutrition may also affect development. For example, low folic acid levels in the mother are a factor in the occurrence of spina bifida in the embryo.

- Teratogenic agents—agents that cause damage during embryonic or fetal development—are often difficult to define. Many reports must be collated before a cause is identified. Often the reports do not point to a single factor, and scientific experiments on humans to verify the data are not ethically feasible. For example, the effects of the drug thalidomide were not realized for a long time, and during this time many children were born with missing limbs. Since then, women have been advised to refrain from using any drugs or chemicals during the childbearing years unless recommended by a physician. Teratogenic agents may be present in the workplace; women of childbearing years should be especially careful in following all health and safety recommendations in the workplace.

- Multifactorial disorders, affecting approximately 10% of the population, are more complex. They may be polygenic (caused by multiple genes), or they may be the result of an inherited tendency toward a disorder that is expressed following exposure to certain environmental factors. A combination of factors is required for the problem to be present, whether at birth or later in life. Frequently the predisposing factors of a disorder such as atherosclerosis (heart and vascular disease), certain cancers (e.g., breast cancer), or schizophrenia (a psychiatric disorder) include a *familial tendency*, which means that family members have an increased risk of developing the disorder, but not every family member will have the disease.

Genetic disorders have social and psychological implications. Decisions about whether or not to bear children when there is a risk of such disorders frequently create ethical dilemmas for families. Social implications of the birth of a child with a genetic disease who requires specialized care and treatment is also of concern. Parents often have difficulty in adjusting to the birth of a child with an unanticipated disorder and may need continued assistance with the care of the child and any associated feelings of guilt. Social resources for the care and education of children who are disabled by a genetic disorder may not be readily available in the community or may be prohibitively expensive.

THINK ABOUT 21-2

a. What are translocation and deletion events that may occur during chromosomal duplication or assembly?
b. Differentiate congenital from genetic defects.
c. Differentiate a multifactorial disorder from a chromosomal disorder.

Genetic Disorders

Single-Gene Disorders

More than 6000 abnormalities are known, with a single-gene disorder occurring in 1:200 live births. Many disorders present few if any signs and may not be diagnosed; serious defects usually cause spontaneous miscarriage. Single-gene disorders are commonly classified by inheritance pattern, the major groups being recessive, dominant, and X-linked recessive. Examples are given in Box 21-1.

A single gene may control a limited function, such as color-blindness, or it may have widespread effects, as in cystic fibrosis or Marfan syndrome (Fig. 21-5). It is also important to realize that certain functions such as hearing may be affected by a number of different genes; for example, deafness in children is linked to approximately 16 genes.

When considering the probability that a certain child will be affected, it should be remembered that the risk is calculated individually for *each* pregnancy. For example, if the first child has Duchenne muscular dystrophy, all subsequent children will not necessarily be

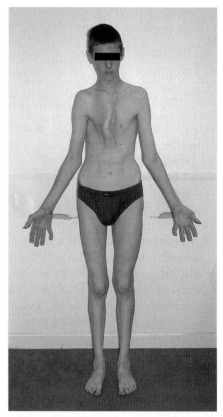

FIGURE 21-5 Clinical manifestations of Marfan syndrome. Skeletal deformities such as pectus excavatum and abnormal curvature of the thoracic spine are common findings. *(From Turnpenny P: Emory's elements of medical genetics, ed 14, Philadelphia, 2012, Churchill Livingstone.)*

normal because the abnormality has already been expressed. The situation is similar to the probability, approximately 50% with each pregnancy, of having a boy or a girl, even if the parents have already produced four boys!

Autosomal Recessive Disorders

Autosomal recessive disorders include a variety of conditions, such as cystic fibrosis, which affects the exocrine glands, primarily the lungs and pancreas; sickle cell disease, which involves defective hemoglobin; and phenylketonuria (PKU), in which a metabolic enzyme is missing. In recessive disorders, both parents must pass on the defective gene (see Fig. 21-4A) to produce an affected (homozygous) child. Male and female children are affected equally. If the child is heterozygous (that is, if one normal gene and one disease gene are present in the pair), then that child is a carrier and shows no clinical signs of disease. In this case, the genotypes of the parents determine the risk of transmitting the defect to the child.

In each pregnancy, in which each parent is heterozygous for the recessive disease trait, the probability of inheritance is:

- 25% that the child will be born with the unaffected genotype
- 50% that the child will be born with the carrier genotype
- 25% that the child will be born with the affected or disease genotype

If only one parent carries the recessive gene for the disease, there is a 50% probability of the child being a carrier and a 50% probability of having the unaffected genotype.

Interestingly, some of these disease-causing genes appear to provide additional resistance to other diseases. For example, carriers of the sickle cell gene have demonstrated increased resistance to malaria.

Many of these recessive gene disorders involve an *enzyme defect* that causes toxic metabolites to accumulate inside cells or in the blood and tissues, interfering with cell function and possibly causing death. These disorders may also be called *storage disease* or *inborn errors of metabolism*. For example, PKU is defined as a deficiency of the enzyme phenylalanine hydroxylase, an enzyme required to convert phenylalanine into tyrosine, resulting in toxic levels of phenylalanine, which results in brain damage if phenylalanine is present in the diet.

Some genes do not wholly fit either the recessive or the dominant pattern. For example, the gene for sickle cell disease is transmitted as a recessive, but may also be referred to as incomplete dominant because heterozygotes may display some clinical signs (sickle cell trait), whereas homozygotes show the full range of expression (sickle cell anemia). Further discussion of sickle cell disease may be found in Chapter 10.

THINK ABOUT 21-3

a. State the probability as a percentage value of a child of two carrier parents being affected by Tay-Sachs disease.
b. State the probability as a percentage value that a child will be the carrier of a recessive gene when the mother is a carrier and the father is normal.

Autosomal Dominant Disorders

In autosomal dominant disorders, the presence of the defect in only one of the alleles produces clinical expression of the disease. An affected parent has a 50% probability of passing the disorder on to each child regardless of the gender of the child (see Fig. 21-4B). There are no carriers, and unaffected persons do not transmit the disorder.

Some of these conditions do not become evident clinically until mid-life, and because diagnostic tests are not always available, the defective gene may already have been passed on to the next generation before the disease is diagnosed. A screening program is available to detect the presence of the gene for Huntington's disease, a condition in which brain degeneration does not develop until mid-life (see Chapter 14).

X-Linked Dominant Disorders

Fragile X syndrome is the most common cause of mental retardation, cognitive deficit, and learning disorders in North America. One in 4000 boys are affected and one in 8000 girls have been identified with the disorder. Social and behavioral problems are often present and may account for the higher identification in males. One-third of affected males exhibit autistic behaviors and one-sixth experience seizures. The mutation responsible for Fragile X syndrome is inherited as a dominant allele carried on the X chromosome, thus males and females can be affected. The mutation causes the affected X chromosome to appear constricted or broken.

X-Linked Recessive Disorders

Alleles for sex-linked recessive disorders are usually carried by the X chromosome. (The Y chromosome does not carry the same genes as does the X.) The genes for X-linked disorders are recessive but are manifested in heterozygous males who lack the matching normal gene on the Y chromosome. Females are carriers (without clinical signs) when they are heterozygous. Examples of X-linked recessive disorders include hemophilia A and Duchenne's muscular dystrophy.

Carrier females have a 50% chance of producing an affected male child and an equal chance of producing a carrier female child in each pregnancy. An affected male will transmit the defect to all his daughters, who become carriers, whereas his sons will neither be affected, nor be carriers. (The male passes only the normal Y chromosome to his sons.)

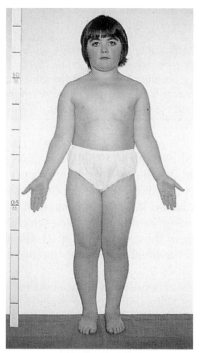

FIGURE 21-6 Typical clinical manifestations of Turner syndrome. *(From Patton KT, Thibodeau GA:* Anatomy & Physiology, *ed 8, St. Louis, 2013, Mosby.)*

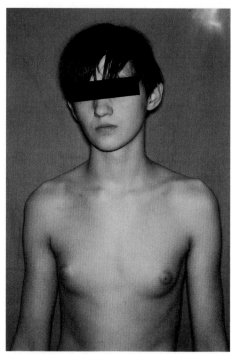

FIGURE 21-7 Typical clinical manifestations of Klinefelter syndrome. *(From Moore KL, Persuad TVN:* The Developing Human: Clinically Oriented Embryology, *ed 8, Philadelphia, 2007, Saunders, pp 466.)*

THINK ABOUT 21-4

a. Marfan syndrome is transmitted by a dominant gene. State the probability that a child with an affected parent will have the disorder.

b. State the probability of a male child being affected and of a female child being affected if the mother carries a gene for a sex-linked recessive disorder. What if it is the father who carries the gene?

c. Hemophilia A is transmitted by an X-linked recessive gene. With an affected father, what is the probability that a child will have the disease? With an affected father and a carrier mother, what is the probability?

---

polysomy X, an extra X chromosome is present (XXY), resulting in a total of 47 chromosomes in each cell. Not all males show signs and are diagnosed, but typically, testes are small and sperm are not produced. Other common chromosomal abnormalities occur when parts of chromosomes are rearranged or lost during replication.

THINK ABOUT 21-5

Differentiate a chromosomal disorder from a single-gene disorder.

Chromosomal Disorders

Down syndrome is an example of a 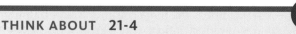 trisomy, in which there are three chromosomes rather than two in the 21 position; it is called trisomy 21 (see Fig. 21-1C). Therefore an individual with Down syndrome has 47 chromosomes. A less common form of Down syndrome exists in which part of a chromosome 21 is attached to another chromosome (translocation). Trisomy 21 change has marked effects throughout the body. Additional information is provided at the end of the chapter.

Monosomy X, or Turner syndrome (Fig. 21-6), occurs when only one sex chromosome, the X chromosome, is present. This person has only 45 chromosomes, resulting in a variety of physical abnormalities and lack of ovaries. In Klinefelter's syndrome (Fig. 21-7) or

Multifactorial Disorders

Multifactorial disorders are involving a number of genes or genetic influences combined with environmental factors. Common examples include cleft palate, congenital hip dislocation, congenital heart disease, type 2 diabetes mellitus, anencephaly, and hydrocephalus. These disorders tend to be limited to a single localized area. The same defect is likely to recur in siblings, but there is no increased risk of occurrence of other defects.

If the presence of the mutated gene can be documented, avoidance of certain environmental factors or close monitoring of the individual may minimize the risk of development of the disease. For example, genetic

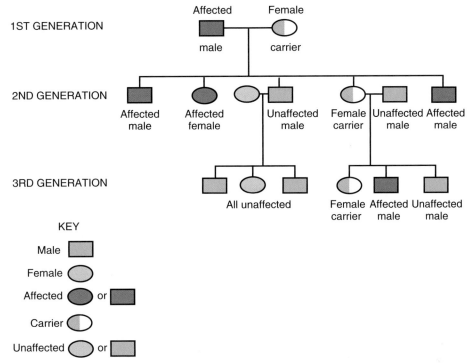

FIGURE 21-8 Family pedigree for an X-linked recessive trait.

mutations have been noted in some forms of breast cancer. Frequent periodic breast examinations are recommended in women in families in which such genes have been identified. Familial incidence can be determined by using a family pedigree and tracing the incidence of the disorder through several generations (Fig. 21-8). In colon cancer, which has shown a familial pattern, dietary changes to reduce the risk of development of tumors and early colonoscopy may reduce mortality from the cancer. Carrying a gene for a multifactorial disorder such as a cancer increases the risk of developing the disease; but because penetrance of genes differs, one cannot predict with certainty that the individual will develop cancer.

Developmental Disorders

Exposure to negative environmental influences during pregnancy and even before pregnancy such as radiation may cause changes in the sperm or ova. Evidence has been gathered about the damaging effects on the fetus of alcohol (fetal alcohol syndrome), cigarette smoking (low birthweight and increased risk of stillbirth), radiation, pharmaceuticals, cocaine abuse, and maternal infections. Chemicals such as mercury in food and water, as well as many drugs, can cross the placental barrier and damage the rapidly dividing cells of the embryo and fetus. TORCH is an acronym applied to routine prenatal screening tests for high-risk maternal infections: *T*oxoplasmosis, *O*ther (hepatitis B, mumps, rubeola, varicella, gonorrhea, syphilis), *R*ubella, *C*ytomegalovirus, and *H*erpes. Newer programs provide

integrated assessment of the TORCH diseases as well as other significant teratogenic or harmful factors.

Because many chemicals and drugs are thought to be possibly teratogenic, and because it is difficult to establish proof of such harm, it is recommended that women avoid unnecessary exposure to drugs, chemicals, or radiation during the childbearing years. In most cases, the damage to the embryo occurs in the early period before a pregnancy is suspected. A deficit or excess of particular nutrients can also lead to developmental abnormalities. The cause of specific malformations is rarely known.

Exposure to harmful influences in the first 2 weeks of embryonic life usually results in the death of the embryo. The most critical time is the *first 2 months* of development, when the cells are dividing rapidly and differentiating, organogenesis is taking place, and the basic body structures are forming (Fig. 21-9). Changes in the basic cells at this time have far-reaching effects. The effects of exposure depend on the stage of development at the precise time of the exposure. In addition to an anomaly, or a developmental abnormality, exposure to damaging substances such as cocaine may cause premature birth, a high risk of further illness in the infant (low birthweight or increased respiratory problems), and increased risk of sudden infant death syndrome.

Cerebral palsy is an example of the kind of brain damage that can occur before, during, or immediately after birth (see Chapter 14). The cause may be insufficient oxygen, the toxic effects of excessive bilirubin in the blood (jaundice), or trauma. The effects may be localized or may involve several areas of the brain.

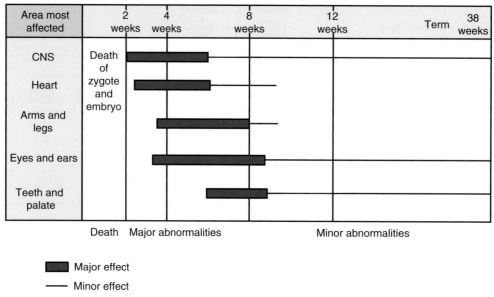

Area most affected	2 weeks	4 weeks	8 weeks	12 weeks	Term	38 weeks
CNS	Death of zygote and embryo					
Heart						
Arms and legs						
Eyes and ears						
Teeth and palate						

Death   Major abnormalities   Minor abnormalities

▬▬▬ Major effect

—— Minor effect

FIGURE 21-9 Effects of teratogens during pregnancy.

THINK ABOUT   21-6

a. At which stage of pregnancy does the highest risk of central nervous system damage occur?
b. State five substances that are thought to be teratogenic.

Diagnostic Tools

Diagnostic tests that can detect some disease-causing genes or chromosomal abnormalities in carriers, during the prenatal period, immediately after birth, or later in life when a disorder is suspected are available. Tests are not available for many disorders because either the cause or a testing procedure may not yet have been identified. Some disorders have such a low incidence rate that research and development of technology to test for the trait has not been feasible. The cost of genetic testing may be very high and thus testing is not universal. Testing is recommended for those who have a family history of a specific disease, those who have previously given birth to a child with an abnormality, and women more than 35 years of age.

Screening programs for carriers are available for many disorders, particularly when the disorder has an ethnic basis and therefore a clearly defined population to test. For example, Tay-Sachs disease is common among Ashkenazi Jews, and specific screening programs for this group have been successful in determining the carrier population, reducing the incidence, and offering reassurance and guidance to many individuals. A simple blood test can also detect carriers of sickle cell disease. Screening programs are helpful when genetic counseling is available to assist individuals or families make decisions in light of the results.

Prenatal diagnosis may offer reassurance to high-risk families; early diagnosis also provides time to plan for the special needs of an affected child or time to make an informed decision about an abortion. Birth defects that may be minor or severe occur in 1:28 live births. Prenatal diagnosis does not ensure the birth of a "perfect child" because testing does not eliminate all possibilities of defects; rather, the tests detect certain defects. Examples of prenatal testing include ultrasonography, which can visualize structural anomalies and maternal blood tests such as the triple screen, performed at 16 to 18 weeks. This test measures levels of alpha-fetoprotein (AFP), the beta subunit of human chorionic gonadotropin (hCG), and unconjugated estriol (uE3). In some areas a quadruple screen is used, which also checks levels of inhibin-A. Abnormal levels indicate a high risk of conditions such as spina bifida or Down syndrome. Follow-up amniocentesis or chorionic villus sampling may confirm the abnormality.

Methods of prenatal diagnosis include amniocentesis, or extraction of amniotic fluid from the uterus, and extraction of a sample of the chorionic villus of the fetus so as to examine a sample of fetal tissue. Chromosomal abnormalities can then be detected by growing fetal cells, harvesting them, and then examining the chromosomes or karyotype (see Fig. 21-1). DNA tests, enzyme deficits, and the presence of abnormal constituents such as AFP can also be included in this examination. These are invasive procedures and carry a slight risk to the fetus and mother. One other drawback of prenatal diagnosis is that some tests may not show conclusive results for 4 to 6 weeks and are often not done until approximately 16 to 18 weeks into the pregnancy, leaving a long period of uncertainty. Improved equipment and techniques in ultrasonography and blood tests are leading to more rapid and more definitive diagnoses, thus reducing the need for amniocentesis.

Neonates can be tested approximately 48 hours after birth, using blood from a heel prick. Most babies do not show signs of metabolic disorders at birth because the maternal kidney and liver have been active up to that time, but permanent damage to tissues can occur quickly thereafter. Mandatory screening after birth is required in many areas for congenital metabolic disorders such as PKU and hypothyroidism, in which prompt treatment can prevent mental retardation in affected children. The number of tests required varies in different areas, but may also include metabolic disorders such as sickle cell anemia, maple syrup urine disease (MSUD), galactosemia, congenital adrenal hyperplasia, biotinidase deficiency, and homocystinuria. The infection congenital toxoplasmosis is frequently included. Many hospitals offer additional optional tests for metabolic disorders. Tests for cystic fibrosis include a check for a pancreatic immunoreactive trypsinogen (IRT), which, if positive, is followed by a DNA test and additional tests. In addition, an infant may be screened for hearing loss before leaving the hospital.

Genetic Technology

Genetic Engineering and Gene Therapy

Genetic engineering refers to the laboratory practices of manipulating genes in living organisms, including microorganisms, plants and animals, and humans. Genes may be altered by changing the sequence of DNA by rearrangement, deletion, or substitution. The ultimate *goal* of gene manipulation is to remove a defective gene and supply a normal one so as to eliminate genetic defects. Recombinant DNA technology formed an early stepping stone toward this goal. A chain of DNA was split and either some of the components changed position or a new piece was added, and then the chain was joined together again. This altered DNA then produces identical specific molecules such as insulin or erythropoietin.

Gene therapy can be effective, particularly in humans, where a single gene appears to be responsible for a disease, such as cystic fibrosis, polycystic kidney, or Huntington disease. Gene therapy involves the introduction of normal genes into living target cells, sometimes by means of a harmless virus or bacterium, thus changing the cell activity or replacing missing genes. For example, insertion of a gene to supply an enzyme missing in children with severe combined immunodeficiency disease (SCID) is underway. Some gene therapies have been withdrawn from clinical trials because of unexpected death; the process of developing safe and effective gene therapy has generally been slower and more difficult than expected. It is anticipated that new treatments with a genetic basis may be sought for problems in the areas of mental illness, cancer, substance abuse, and criminal behavior. In some of these cases there is not yet a clear indication of a precise genetic component or cause to target with therapy.

Genetic Diagnosis and DNA Testing

DNA testing for genetic disorders has been used to identify genetic disorders in embryos and newborns. There have been a number of cases in which gene testing was conducted on embryos (from in vitro fertilization) to ensure birth of a child whose tissue was compatible with that of an older sibling, ill with leukemia. The child then could provide stem cells to the older sibling, saving the child's life. Preimplantation genetic diagnosis through testing of embryos has also been used to guard against the birth of a child with a serious defect.

Another benefit of gene testing is seen in the identification of individuals who possess genes that place them at high risk of colon cancer (e.g., familial polyposis). These persons can subsequently receive frequent examinations. Women who have had breast cancer, but do not possess the genes predisposing to recurrence, may not require as extensive chemotherapy and radiation after surgery for the primary cancer.

Concern has been expressed about the possible abuse of gene testing and therapy procedures and the risk of unanticipated changes in the expression of genes. In humans, instead of a cure, could altered genes cause other disorders to appear? How dependable is the information? Other concerns relate to access to personal genetic information by insurance companies, who could turn down coverage of persons on a genetic basis, police and the courts, or employers. Legislation has been drafted to protect the genetic rights of the individual, but not all jurisdictions have enacted such protections. DNA testing can be used to identify individuals because DNA is considered a unique characteristic like a "fingerprint," thereby facilitating the use of genetic markers in blood and other body fluids by forensic scientists. Another forensics application is the analysis of DNA from a crime scene to identify if the individual is male or female or carries any specific characteristics. Many questions concerning the use, possible complications, and potential for abuse of genetic testing procedures still remain to be answered.

Proteomic Research and Designer Drugs

Research has recently turned from identification of base pairs in the DNA of specific genes to the proteins that are elaborated when the gene is activated. This study is termed *proteomics* and strives to characterize all of the proteins that are significant in the metabolic pathway for expression of a particular allele. Proteomic research is being funded to determine the shape and chemical activity of these crucial proteins so as to develop drugs specific to the metabolic pathway. These research products have been referred to as "designer drugs" in the popular press. Imatinib mesylate (Gleevec) a drug specific to growth proteins in ovarian cancer and Trastuzumab (Herceptin), specific to some growth proteins in breast cancers, are examples of such drug research. Some currently used drugs interact differently in genetically different individuals; proteomic research will help to develop drugs tailored to the individual's genotype and reduce untoward side effects of commonly used medications. This research is, however, much more complex than the HGP and progress is not expected to be instantaneous; sequencing DNA base pairs in the Human Genome Program was the first of many steps in understanding and treating common diseases that have a genetic component.

THINK ABOUT   21-7

a. Explain why it would be helpful to know if one is carrying a gene associated with a disease.
b. Briefly describe two methods of prenatal diagnosis and the purpose of each.

Down Syndrome

Down syndrome, or trisomy 21, is a common chromosomal disorder, resulting in numerous defects in physical and mental development. Formerly called Down's syndrome or mongolism, it is now identified as Down syndrome in North America. The risk of bearing a child with Down syndrome increases with maternal age. For example, a woman at age 30 has a risk of approximately 1 in 1000 of bearing a child with Down syndrome, whereas at age 35 the risk increases to approximately 1 in 500 and at age 40 to 1 in 100. Whether this risk is caused by damage to the oocytes resulting from degeneration with aging or environmental agents or other factors is unknown. Recently it has been suggested that some cases may be of paternal origin. A positive triple screen test on maternal blood followed by amniocentesis can detect the disorder.

Characteristics of individuals with Down syndrome include the following (Fig. 21-10):

- The head is small and has a flat facial profile.
- The eyes are slanted, and the irises contain Brushfield spots.
- The mouth tends to hang open, revealing a large, protruding tongue and a high-arched palate.
- The hands are small and have a single palmar (simian) crease.
- The muscles tend to be hypotonic, the joints are loose, cervical abnormalities and instability are often evident, and stature is short.
- Developmental stages are delayed.

- All children are cognitively impaired, but the severity of impairment varies with the individual, and early stimulation programs are helpful.
- Sexual development is often delayed or incomplete.
- Many children have an assortment of other problems, including visual problems (cataracts, strabismus), hearing problems, obstructions in the digestive tract, celiac disease, congenital heart defects, decreased resistance to infection (immune deficit), and a high risk of developing leukemia. As the life of these children has been extended as a result of improved medical care, a marked increase in the development of Alzheimer's disease after 40 years of age has been observed.

THINK ABOUT   21-8

a. Explain the meaning of trisomy 21.
b. How is prenatal diagnosis of Down syndrome achieved?
c. Can diagnostic tests provide full information on the extent of effects of Down syndrome in an individual child at the time of birth?

CASE STUDY A

Retinoblastoma

A.L. is a healthy toddler with a normal perinatal history. Her parents notice a white spot in the pupil of one eye and request a referral to a pediatric ophthalmologist. Examination of the eye suggests that A.L. has developed a retinoblastoma, a cancer in her eye. This cancer occurs in approximately 1 in every 1500 live births and approximately 250 children are diagnosed each year in the United States. The family is referred for genetic testing and counseling. Retinoblastoma can occur because of a change in chromosome 13 or a mutation in the RB1 gene, which in its normal state prevents abnormal mitosis. A.L.'s tumor results from mutation of the RB1 gene, but neither parent shows this mutation.

1. What is the difference in the cause and inheritance of chromosomal changes compared with the inheritance of a mutation in a specific gene?
2. How did the mutation likely occur in the genes in A.L.'s tumor cells?
3. Testing of A.L.'s blood shows no evidence of the RB1 mutation; how likely is it that A.L. could transmit the mutated gene to her children?
4. How has the mutation caused growth of the tumor in A.L.'s eye?
5. What is the prognosis if the tumor is limited to the intraocular tissues?

CHAPTER SUMMARY

Congenital disorders are conditions that are present in an individual at birth but are not necessarily manifested until later in life. Included are inherited genetic

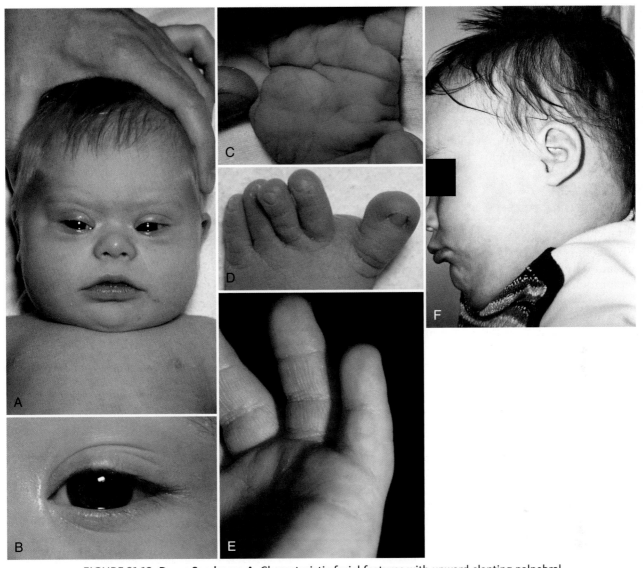

FIGURE 21-10 **Down Syndrome A**, Characteristic facial features with upward-slanting palpebral fissures, epicanthal folds, and flat nasal bridge. **B**, Brushfield spots. **C**, Bridged palmar crease, seen in some infants with Down syndrome. There are two transverse palmar creases connected by a diagonal line. **D**, Wide space between first and second toes. **E**, Short fifth finger. **F**, Small ears and flat occiput. *(From Zitelli BJ, Davis HW: Atlas of Pediatric Physical Diagnosis, ed 4, St. Louis, 2002, Mosby.)*

disorders and developmental defects resulting from damage to the child in utero or at birth. Genetic disorders are a consequence of changes in the genes that make up the 23 pairs of chromosomes in each human cell. Each gene is a DNA file that controls one or more aspects of cellular activity.

- The Human Genome Project is a multinational research effort whose goal is to identify the location, DNA sequence, and purpose of every gene so as to reduce the incidence of inherited disorders by the manipulation and replacement of defective genes.
  - Proteomics is the science of identifying the proteins associated with the expression of a particular gene so as to design drugs to replace absent proteins or inhibit damaging proteins.

- The common patterns of inheritance of single gene disorders are classified as recessive (e.g., cystic fibrosis) or X-linked recessive (e.g., hemophilia A), dominant (e.g., Huntington disease) or X-linked dominant (Fragile X syndrome).
- The probability of inheritance can be predicted using Punnett squares. The same probability exists with each pregnancy.
- Chromosomal disorders, such as Down syndrome or trisomy 21, involve an abnormal distribution of the chromosomes or dislocation of a part or loss of a chromosome. A karyotype demonstrates the arrangement of the chromosomes from an individual's cell.
- Developmental disorders are caused by damage to one or more body structures during embryonic or

fetal development, during labor and delivery, or shortly after birth. The embryonic stage, the time of organogenesis, is the most vulnerable period. Possible factors include hypoxia, viruses, radiation, and exposure to drugs or other teratogens.
- Multifactorial disorders result from a combination of genetic predisposition and exposure to certain environmental factors.
- Screening programs are available for carriers of specific genetic disorders. Ultrasonography and amniocentesis may detect certain developmental defects in the fetus. A family pedigree will assist in determining the risk of such an occurrence, justifying the testing procedure and genetic counseling.
- Down syndrome is presented as an example of a disorder affecting many body components. Abnormalities can be found in most systems and include physical appearance, skeletal structure, and intellectual development.

STUDY QUESTIONS

1. Define homozygous and heterozygous.
2. What is the purpose of a pedigree?
3. Explain why teratogens are difficult to identify.
4. Explain why a woman carrying the gene for hemophilia can produce two hemophiliac sons when she is mated to a normal male.
5. Under what conditions does a female acquire an X-linked recessive disorder?
6. Why are X-linked recessive disorders never passed from a father to a son?
7. The pedigree for Queen Victoria of England, a carrier of hemophilia A, shows the transmission to some of her descendants, including members of many royal families in Europe, such as Russia and Spain, but not Germany. Hemophilia A does not affect anyone in the present British royal family. Can you explain why hemophilia A has disappeared from one family and appeared in others?
8. What is the probability that a parent carrying a dominant trait will pass that trait on to each child?
9. How can prenatal diagnosis demonstrate the sex of an unborn child?
10. Describe briefly amniocentesis and its purpose.
11. Which of the following can be identified by an abnormal karyotype?
    a. Sickle cell disease
    b. Cystic fibrosis
    c. Monosomy X
    d. Tay-Sachs disease
    e. Huntington's chorea

ADDITIONAL RESOURCES

Applegate EJ: *The Anatomy and Physiology Learning System Textbook*, ed 2, Philadelphia, 2006, Saunders.

Copstead LE, Banasik JL: *Pathophysiology*, ed 4, St. Louis, 2010, Saunders.

Kumar V, Abbas AK, Fausto M: *Robbins and Cotran Pathologic Basis of Disease*, ed 7, Philadelphia, 2007, Saunders.

Scientific American, July 2000: A series of articles on gene technology.

Web Sites

http://www.ornl.gov/sci/techresources/Human_Genome/home.shtml *The human genome project at Genome Project Information*

http://www.familysearch.org *Family history information*

http://www.sciam.com *Scientific American journal*

http://www.ncbi.nlm.nih.gov/entrez/query.fcgi?db=OMIM *Database of genetic diseases*

http://www.modimes.org/professionals *March of Dimes*

http://learn.genetics.utah.edu/ *The University of Utah Genetic Science Learning Center*

http://www.mayoclinic.com/ *Mayo Clinic*

http://www.cdc.gov/ *Centers for Disease Control and Prevention*

Complications of Pregnancy

CHAPTER OUTLINE

LEARNING OBJECTIVES

After studying this chapter, the student is expected to:

1. Understand the stages of fetal development and the basic effects on the mother.
2. Describe the impact of maternal hormonal changes on the systems.
3. Discuss the potential problems of hypertension, thrombus formation, placental separation, and Rh incompatibility during pregnancy.

KEY TERMS

abortion
amniocentesis
amnion
amniotic fluid
auscultation
bilirubin
caries
cervical os
chorionic villi
chorionic villus sampling

differentiation
embolus
embryo
fetus
gestation
gestational age
gingivitis
gravidity
hemolysis
human chorionic gonadotropin

hypertension
hypotension
immunoglobulin
inner cell mass
jaundice
lactation
lordosis
organogenesis
ovum
parity

peritonitis
placenta
sperm
supine
teratogen
thrombus
trimesters
trophoblast
viable
zygote

Embryonic and Fetal Development

Many natural changes occur in the mother's body during embryonic and fetal development. In some cases, the mother's condition affects the child's development and growth. In other cases, the physiologic changes in the mother can initiate disease or aggravate preexisting conditions. Additional information is available in any obstetrics textbook. Infertility is discussed in Chapter 19 of this text.

Conception or fertilization of the ovum by a sperm takes place in the *oviduct* or *fallopian tube*. During the next few hours, the genetic information contained in the ovum (oocyte) is merged with that contained in the sperm to form the zygote (fertilized ovum), and many mitotic divisions occur as the zygote moves along the fallopian tube toward the uterus. Implantation of the zygote in the uterine wall is completed approximately 1 week after fertilization, and differentiation (specialization) of cells is apparent as the inner cell mass and trophoblast or outer cell mass form. The inner cell mass becomes the actual fetus, whereas the outer cell mass gives rise to the embryonic membranes, the amnion and placenta. The period from 3 to 8 weeks is termed the *embryonic stage*, and this is a critical time in the development of all the organs and structures in the fetal body. During this period termed organogenesis, cells divide rapidly, move, and differentiate to form the basic functional elements of the various organs systems and external structures such as the limbs and eyes. By the end of 8 weeks, all organs are formed. For example, the primitive fetal heart is beating at 4 weeks. Note all times relate to that which has elapsed since fertilization, thus the CNS is forming within 1 week of the woman's first missed menstrual period.

Exposure of the embryo to any teratogen (any substance or situation that causes a developmental abnormality) during this early stage usually causes major widespread damage to the developing structures and leads to serious congenital abnormalities (see Fig. 21-6, which outlines the effects of teratogens on the organs at various times during the pregnancy). Common teratogens include drugs, viruses, alcohol, and radiation. It is preferable to avoid all medications, including herbal remedies and those available without prescription during pregnancy or to consult with a physician to determine a safe alternative. Viruses such as rubella (German measles) and erythema infectiosum (fifth disease) are known to cause damage to the embryo and fetus. For example, during the first trimester, maternal rubella affects infants in 90% of cases, causing spontaneous abortion (loss of the embryo or fetus) or major congenital anomalies.

Major abnormalities rarely occur from exposure after 20 weeks. Erythema infectiosum, acquired during the first half of pregnancy, causes severe anemia in the fetus and possible death. Cigarette smoking by the mother usually results in a child with low birth weight and increased irritability and may also result in stillbirth. There is also an increased risk of placenta previa and abruptio placentae with exposure to tobacco. Because alcohol can easily pass through the placental barrier, there is risk of damage to the fetus during the entire pregnancy. Fetal alcohol syndrome, which varies in severity, impairs a child's neurologic and intellectual development as well as causing unique physical characteristics (e.g., typical facies) and growth retardation. Increased intake of folic acid before and during pregnancy has greatly reduced the incidence of neural tube defects such as spina bifida and anencephaly (see Chapter 14 and Figure 14-26 for information on spina bifida).

After 8 weeks, the term *fetus* is used and most organs have completed basic formation. Teratogens have less effect on development during this period because cell damage occurs primarily in certain tissues that are actively differentiating at the time of exposure. Continued growth and development result in completion of many specialized structures such as the lungs. Elementary functions can be observed as the limbs move and amniotic fluid is swallowed. However, *functional* impairment, particularly in the central nervous system, can occur with exposure to teratogens at this stage of development. During the last trimester in utero, the fetus gains weight, and organs such as the lungs mature. With improvements in technology and neonatal care, the fetus may be able to survive (remain viable) outside the uterus as early as 22 to 23 weeks after conception. Birth at such a premature age is often accompanied by complex medical problems as the child adapts to live outside the uterus.

Monozygotic or identical twins form when the developing embryo divides to form two separate, genetically identical embryos. This occurs in approximately 1:100 births for unknown reasons. Dizygotic or fraternal twins form when two ova are fertilized by two different sperm, resulting in two genetically dissimilar embryos.

Physiological Changes During Pregnancy

Pregnancy is a normal process in the life cycle. The standard period for pregnancy is divided into three trimesters, each approximately 3 months long and each involving significant changes in the mother and the developing fetus. In some individuals, these changes may precipitate complications or aggravate preexisting pathologies in the mother. Good prenatal care at an early stage and throughout the pregnancy is essential to minimize the risk of potential complications.

Diagnosis of Pregnancy

Laboratory diagnosis of pregnancy is based on the presence of human chorionic gonadotropin (hCG) in the mother's plasma or urine, using enzyme-linked immunosorbent assay (ELISA)–based tests. The hormone hCG, which is secreted by the chorionic villi after implantation of the fertilized ovum in the uterus, can be detected by a simple office or home test. Many typical signs of pregnancy, such as nausea or morning sickness, do not provide confirmation of pregnancy because each could result from other causes.

The *positive* (absolute) signs occur later in the pregnancy and include the fetal heart beat as detected by auscultation or ultrasound, fetal movement detected by someone other than the mother, and visualization of the fetus with ultrasound.

The *estimated date of delivery* (EDD) or *estimated date of birth* (EDB) can be calculated easily using Nägele's rule if the first day of the last menstrual period (LMP) is known. Three months are subtracted from that date, and then 7 days are added to the resulting figure. For example, if the LMP began on October 20, one would subtract 3 months (July 20) and add 7 days, giving an EDB of July 27. Various charts and wheels are available to provide the dates quickly. For women with longer cycles or irregular menstrual cycles, the formula must be adjusted. First pregnancies are often slightly longer.

Gestation refers to the length of time since the first day of the LMP, and equals 280 days (40 weeks) or 10 lunar months. Gestational age is 2 weeks longer than the actual age of the child from the time of *fertilization*—266 days or 38 weeks.

Gravidity and parity are terms used to describe a woman's history of pregnancy and childbirth. Gravidity refers to the number of pregnancies; for example, a *primigravida* is a woman who is pregnant for the first time. Parity refers to the number of pregnancies in which the fetus has reached viability (approximately 22 weeks of gestation). A *multipara* has completed two or more pregnancies to the point of fetal viability. Coding systems are available to document histories. For example, a five-digit system records, in sequence, the number of pregnancies, the number of deliveries, the number of premature deliveries, the number of abortions of any type, and the number of children living. The history of a woman in her second pregnancy who has one child living and no other experiences would be recorded as 2-1-0-0-1.

Amniocentesis is the withdrawal of a small amount of amniotic fluid, including some sloughed fetal cells, from the uterus after 14 weeks. The fluid can be checked for its chemical content and the cells cultured for chromosome analysis. Amniocentesis is recommended when there are signs of abnormality, perhaps from an early ultrasound examination, maternal blood screening, or a history of genetic disorders; it may also be used when the mother is more than 35 years of age to check for Down syndrome. There are some risks because the test is invasive. This test may also be used later in pregnancy to check fetal lung maturity. An alternative process is chorionic villus sampling (CVS), which can take place earlier in pregnancy and is useful for chromosomal examination and diagnosis in high-risk clients.

Physiological Changes and Their Implications

Hormonal Changes

Levels of estrogen and progesterone in the maternal blood are increased during pregnancy as the placenta increases its production of these hormones, which are essential to the development of the uterus, maintenance of pregnancy, and preparation of the breasts for lactation (milk production). Hyperplasia of the thyroid gland and increased production of thyroxine also occur (see Chapter 16 for more information on thyroid hormones), which increases the mother's metabolism.

Reproductive System Changes

Estrogen causes a tremendous increase in the size of the uterus owing to hypertrophy of the muscle cells, some hyperplasia, and an increase in fibrous tissue. The number of blood vessels in the uterus is also greatly increased to ensure the adequacy of the blood supply to the fetus. As the fetus and uterus grow, they exert pressure on the surrounding structures (Fig. 22-1). For example, pressure on the bladder and bowel may alter elimination patterns, and upward pressure on the diaphragm may restrict lung expansion, leading to shortness of breath on exertion.

THINK ABOUT 22-1

Explain how the pressure of a large uterus would affect the filling of the bladder and the frequency of urination. How would these changes affect other activities?

Other changes in the reproductive system include increased vascularity of the cervix and vagina, resulting in a softening of the tissues (Goodell's sign) and a typical deeper purplish color of the mucosal lining (Chadwick's sign). Cervical mucus is more abundant and thick and forms a cervical plug to protect the uterine contents

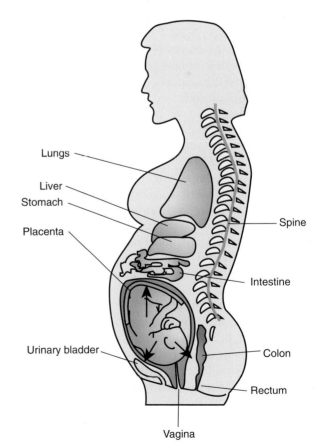

FIGURE 22-1 Sagittal section of a pregnant woman demonstrating the effects of the expanding uterus.

from foreign material and microbes. Vaginal secretions increase and become more acidic (pH 3.5 to 6.0), which is a deterrent to some infecting organisms but, when combined with increased glycogen content, predisposes to yeast or monilial infections during pregnancy. The breasts become larger as the ducts and glands develop preparatory to milk production, and fatty deposits in the breast tissue increase. Bluish veins on the breast surface become more prominent and the breasts are tenderer.

Weight Gain and Nutrition

The average weight gain during pregnancy is 11 to 14 kg, or 25 to 30 lb, much of which occurs in the last trimester. The increased size of the uterus and its contents (the placenta, amniotic fluid, and fetus), the enlarged breasts, additional blood volume, and stored nutrients or fat all contribute to the weight gain. There is an increased demand for protein, carbohydrate, fat, vitamins, and minerals to promote healthy tissue development during pregnancy. The metabolic rate of the mother increases in the latter half of pregnancy. However, any caloric intake beyond that required is stored as adipose tissue (fat).

Extra weight during pregnancy comes from (estimates, somewhat different in each pregnancy):
- Baby: ≈8 pounds
- Placenta: 2-3 pounds
- Amniotic fluid: 2-3 pounds
- Breast tissue: 2-3 pounds
- Blood supply: 4 pounds
- Stored fat for delivery and breastfeeding: 5-9 pounds
- Larger uterus: 2-5 pounds
- Total: 25 to 35 pounds

The fetus stores iron in the last trimester to provide for its needs during the first few months after delivery. Adequate calcium is required for fetal bones and teeth. It is a myth that calcium is drawn from the mother's teeth to supply the fetus, but changes in salivary secretions can promote dental caries. Food cravings often include foods that are high in sugars; consumption of such snacks can increase the risk of caries. Even beneficial foods such as dried fruits or raisins can be a problem. Prenatal care should include a consultation with a dentist or dental hygienist to ensure good oral hygiene.

Digestive System Changes

Nausea and vomiting are common in the first trimester because of the hormonal changes that occur in pregnancy. Changes in eating patterns often reduce discomfort. Frequent small meals, avoidance of fatty or spicy foods, and a reduced fluid intake with meals are suggested. Medication is recommended only in severe cases. The combination drug doxylamine-pyridoxine has been studied extensively and appears to be a safe treatment during pregnancy. Severe uncontrollable vomiting, or *hyperemesis gravidarum*, may lead

to dehydration and electrolyte imbalances and may affect nutrition at a critical point in fetal development. Hospital care is often necessary to maintain fluid and electrolyte balance.

The relaxation of smooth muscle in the stomach and intestines by progesterone results in decreased motility in the digestive tract; slower emptying of the stomach; reflux of stomach contents into the esophagus (*heartburn*); and feelings of bloating and abdominal discomfort. The pressure of the expanding uterus interferes with digestive function also. Constipation is common owing to decreased gastric motility and iron supplements. If chronic, constipation may lead to hemorrhoids, which are dilated veins in the anal canal. These can become very painful and may bleed or become infected. A diet high in fiber is recommended to avoid constipation and straining during defecation.

THINK ABOUT   22-2

a. Suggest a reason for maternal weight loss during the first trimester of pregnancy.
b. List three potential effects of excessive intake of foods associated with food cravings.

Musculoskeletal Changes

Marked postural changes occur in the mother as pregnancy progresses. The pelvic joints relax or loosen as hormones prepare the pelvis for delivery, resulting in a loss of stability and a *waddling gait*. The increased abdominal weight leads to a shift in the center of gravity and a tendency toward lordosis or increased lumbar curvature. These changes may lead to backache, particularly if the back and abdominal muscles are weak. Continued regular moderate exercise during pregnancy is helpful in maintaining good posture as well as cardiovascular fitness.

THINK ABOUT   22-3

Suggest several ways of reducing or preventing backache during pregnancy.

Cardiovascular Changes

Blood volume, including the relative volumes of both fluid and erythrocytes, is greatly increased to meet the metabolic needs of the fetus. For example, blood flow to the uterus and kidneys must increase to supply more oxygen to the fetus and uterine tissue and remove wastes. Vascular resistance tends to decrease because smooth muscle in the arterioles is somewhat relaxed as a result of increased progesterone. The heart rate may increase slightly, and blood pressure frequently drops slightly in the first two trimesters but then rises again to normal levels during the last trimester.

The increased blood volume leads to congestion and edema in many tissues. For instance, there may be nasal congestion, which affects breathing. Gingivitis, or inflammation of the tissues around the teeth (gums), is common, causing bleeding. Fatigue or stress may impede daily oral hygiene, resulting in more severe *pregnancy gingivitis* and caries.

The increased production of red blood cells for the fetus requires increased iron intake by the mother. Iron supplements are frequently required. Because of a relatively greater increase in fluid, the hematocrit decreases slightly, and the woman appears to have a low hemoglobin level (physiologic anemia).

Varicose veins frequently develop during pregnancy (see Chapter 12 and Fig. 12-33 for more information on varicose veins). Either the superficial or the deep veins of the legs may be involved. The superficial veins appear as large, distended purplish veins. Varicose veins result from restriction of blood flow in the veins to the heart due to the pressure of the uterus, particularly in women who must stand for long periods of time or who are predisposed to this condition by defects in the vein walls or valves. Varicosities can cause sensations of heavy or aching legs. Legs should be elevated whenever possible, and restrictive clothing such as tight stockings should be avoided to enhance the flow of venous blood. The risk of dangerous blood clots and emboli to the lungs is increased, particularly after delivery.

When a pregnant woman lies in a supine position, the inferior vena cava may be compressed by the heavy uterus, resulting in decreased venous return to the heart and less cardiac output, leading to potential hypotension, or low blood pressure. Lying on the left side usually facilitates maternal blood flow back to the heart and increases output to the placenta and the fetus. A supine position will also affect the blood pressure and pulse, giving false readings.

THINK ABOUT   22-4

Using your knowledge of normal blood pressure controls, explain why blood pressure does not rise when blood volume increases during pregnancy.

Potential Complications of Pregnancy

Ectopic Pregnancy

Commonly called tubal pregnancy, an ectopic pregnancy occurs when the fertilized ovum (zygote) is implanted outside the uterus. In most cases of ectopic pregnancy, implantation occurs in the fallopian tube. The incidence has been increasing over the past 20 years, perhaps because of an increase in pelvic inflammatory disease that may scar the tube, restricting movement of the zygote to the uterus. Spontaneous abortion may follow in the early stages of pregnancy or the embryo may continue to develop, eventually causing the tube to rupture. This may lead to severe hemorrhage or peritonitis (a serious infection in the peritoneal cavity) with loss of the fallopian tube. The pregnant woman experiences severe pelvic or abdominal pain as blood irritates the peritoneal membranes. Ectopic pregnancy is considered a medical emergency and requires prompt treatment, usually surgical removal of the embryo and associated tube, to prevent hemorrhage and shock. It is currently not possible to maintain a tubal pregnancy to the time the fetus would be viable outside the uterus.

Preeclampsia and Eclampsia: Pregnancy-Induced Hypertension

Pregnancy-induced hypertension (PIH) refers to a state of persistently elevated blood pressure (more than 140/90) that develops after 20 weeks of gestation and returns to normal after delivery. A specific cause has not been determined, although numerous risk factors have been identified. Pregnancy-induced hypertension, if not controlled, may lead to damaged blood vessels in tissues such as the kidneys and retina of the eye, or to stroke or heart failure. The decreased blood flow to the uterus may cause premature degeneration of the placenta and presents a risk to the fetus. The efficacy of low doses of aspirin (ASA) in controlling PIH continues to be investigated.

Preeclampsia and eclampsia are more serious conditions in which the blood pressure is higher, and kidney dysfunction is indicated by proteinuria, weight gain, and generalized edema (face, hands, feet, and legs). In some patients with preeclampsia, a complication develops. This condition is known for its manifestations by the acronym HELLP (for *H*emolysis, *E*levated *L*iver enzymes, and *L*ow *P*latelets). In a few cases, HELLP progresses to coagulation disorders such as disseminated intravascular coagulation, as indicated by excessive bleeding. Also, preeclampsia may progress to eclampsia, in which the blood pressure becomes extremely high and generalized seizures (grand mal) or coma develops. Immediate hospitalization is required for adequate treatment of eclampsia.

THINK ABOUT   22-5

Compare the signs of PIH with those of eclampsia and explain how eclampsia endangers the pregnant woman and her fetus.

Gestational Diabetes Mellitus

Diabetes mellitus develops in 2% to 5% of women during pregnancy (see Chapter 16 for more information on diabetes). This condition involves increased glucose intolerance and leads to increased glucose levels in blood and urine. Glucose levels should be closely monitored in women in whom there is a family history of diabetes or who have previously had high birth weight infants. Dietary management is important, and insulin may be necessary in some cases. Oral hypoglycemic drugs are contraindicated as potentially teratogenic.

There is a higher risk of fetal abnormalities if blood glucose is increased in the first trimester, as well as an increase of other complications and stillbirth. The newborn born to a woman with diabetes is usually larger in size and may experience problems regulating blood glucose immediately after birth. Gestational diabetes may resolve after the pregnancy, but in many cases diabetes develops in that individual at a later time.

Placental Disorders

Placenta previa occurs when the placenta is implanted in the lower uterus or over the cervical os (the passage between the uterus and the cervix). In the case of placenta previa when the uterus expands and contracts near the end of pregnancy, the placenta is torn and bleeding occurs. The sign is bright red bleeding that is painless. Diagnosis is confirmed by ultrasound. Although in some cases the leak may close, any hemorrhage during pregnancy places both mother and fetus at risk and requires immediate assessment and intervention.

Abruptio placentae refers to premature separation of the placenta from the uterine wall, resulting in bleeding that may or may not be evident vaginally, depending on where the tear occurs. The blood is often dark red, and abdominal pain is common. Abruptio placentae occur more commonly during the last trimester.

THINK ABOUT 22-6

Using your knowledge of normal cardiovascular function, explain why any hemorrhage is serious for both mother and fetus.

Blood Clotting Disorders

Thrombophlebitis and Thromboembolism

Thromboembolisms, or blood clots, are common following childbirth and usually develop in the veins of the legs or pelvis (see Chapter 12). To prevent the formation of clots in the legs, the new mother is encouraged to be up and walking immediately after sedation or anesthesia has worn off even in a Cesarean section birth. Thrombus may form spontaneously (phlebothrombosis), usually because of stasis of blood or increased coagulability. In some cases, the clot forms over an inflamed area in the vein wall (thrombophlebitis). If a piece of the thrombus breaks away (an embolus), it will flow with the venous blood to the right side of the heart and then

into the lungs, where it will lodge in a pulmonary artery or smaller branch, obstructing blood flow in the lungs. This is a *pulmonary embolus* (see Chapter 13 for more information), which can be very serious and can affect respiratory and cardiovascular function. It is important not to massage a leg that is painful or red until the risk of thrombus has been eliminated. Antiembolic stockings and bed rest may be helpful, as well as careful management of the coagulation problem.

Disseminated Intravascular Coagulation

Disseminated intravascular coagulation (DIC) is not a primary problem, but is a serious complication of events such as abruptio placentae and preeclampsia. In DIC, an increased activation of the clotting mechanism occurs, resulting in diffuse blood clots and excessive consumption of all clotting factors. Diagnosis is confirmed by the low serum levels of clotting factors. This situation leads to hemorrhage as the clotting factors are no longer available for normal clotting. The formation of multiple thrombi in the tissues causes organ damage in later stages, but the signs of DIC are related to hemorrhage in early stages. Bleeding may occur from the uterus, at injection sites, from the nose or mouth, under the skin (purpura), or internally.

THINK ABOUT 22-7

Differentiate the location and effects of a thrombus from an embolus.

Rh Incompatibility

Blood incompatibility can develop when the Rh factor antigens on fetal red blood cells differ from those on maternal red blood cells. Rh incompatibility can be more serious when it leads to hemolytic disease of the newborn (erythroblastosis fetalis). Rh incompatibility results when the mother is Rh negative and the fetus is Rh positive (Fig. 22-2). During the first pregnancy there are usually no problems unless the mother has been exposed to Rh-positive blood at some prior time through a blood product or abortion. At the end of the first pregnancy, when the placenta tears during delivery, some Rh-positive fetal blood enters the maternal circulation, stimulating the formation of antibodies to Rh-positive cells in the mother. During subsequent pregnancies, the maternal Rh antibodies cross the placenta to the fetus. The resulting antigen-antibody reaction in the fetus destroys the fetal red blood cells. Hemolysis of red blood cells leads to severe anemia or low hemoglobin and possible heart failure and death in the child. Hemolysis also causes high serum bilirubin levels in the child, resulting in jaundice (yellow color in the eyes and skin) and potential neurologic damage (kernicterus) as bilirubin enters brain tissue.

Rh FACTOR INCOMPATIBILITY OF MATERNAL–FETAL BLOOD

(ERYTHROBLASTOSIS FETALIS, OR HEMOLYTIC DISEASE OF THE NEWBORN)

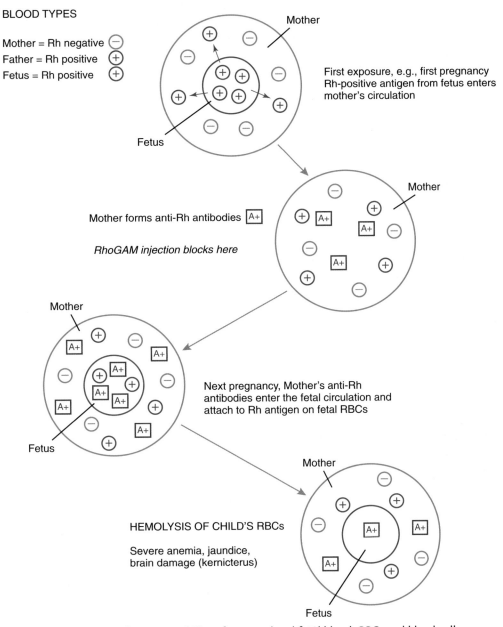

FIGURE 22-2   Rh incompatibility of maternal and fetal blood. *RBCs,* red blood cells.

If the fetus experiences severe hemolysis in utero, an early birth or intrauterine transfusion may be recommended. After birth, an exchange transfusion may be required. When the neonate is jaundiced, phototherapy (exposure of the newborn's body to fluorescent or blue light) can reduce serum bilirubin levels by promoting conjugation of bilirubin and excretion in the bile.

Routine screening of maternal blood for Rh antibodies (indirect Coombs' test) is carried out early in pregnancy and at regular intervals during the pregnancy. If the mother has *not* become sensitized and developed antibodies, for example, during the first pregnancy, she can be given passive immunity at the time of delivery to suppress the immune response temporarily. This is done by administering Rh immunoglobulin (RhoGAM) to the mother within 72 hours of delivery. This process prevents sensitization of the mother as a result of fetal red blood cells entering her body during labor and delivery.

Infection

Localized wound infections are usually contained if they are treated quickly. *Puerperal infection* (childbed fever) is infection of the reproductive tract at any time during the 6 weeks following birth. It may be endogenous (because of vaginal flora) or exogenous (because of causes in the environment). Cervical lacerations or episiotomy repairs are vulnerable to infection. Common organisms include group B hemolytic *Streptococcus*, *Escherichia coli*, *Staphylococcus aureus*, *Mycoplasma*, and *Chlamydia trachomatis*.

A predisposition to *endometritis* (inflammation of the uterine lining) can be caused by the separation of the placenta, which leaves raw tissue open to easy access of organisms from the vagina. Any retained placental fragments also promote infection. Signs of infection include fever, vomiting, lower abdominal pain, and foul smelling discharge from the vagina. The infection may spread to cause *pelvic cellulitis* (infection in the connective tissues or broad ligament of the pelvis) or *peritonitis* (infection of the peritoneal membranes) (see Chapter 17). Peritonitis results from infection that spreads directly along the fallopian tubes into the peritoneal cavity and is a serious complication of childbirth. Peritonitis is manifested by severe pain, high fever, tachycardia, and abdominal distention. Scar tissue resulting from infection that involves the fallopian tubes or ovaries may cause infertility. Pelvic abscess, a localized infection, may persist following peritonitis.

Adolescent Pregnancy

The adolescent period is a time of growth, change, and maturation in many areas of the body (see Chapter 23). The teenager has increased nutritional needs to meet the demands of her own growth, and, in addition, dietary intake, physical activity, and hormonal changes are more erratic during this period. Pregnancy at this time carries an increased risk of complications. The teenage gravida may not seek prenatal care early in the pregnancy, and this results in inadequate nutrition to support the growth needs of the teen and fetus as well as lack of identification of potential problems of pregnancy. The young woman's pelvis may be too small to allow for passage of the fetal head, increasing risk during labor and delivery. Anemia is a common problem if prenatal vitamin supplements with iron are not taken. Factors such as maternal smoking, alcohol use, and drug intake are more common in adolescent pregnancies and often negatively affect outcomes for the fetus. These should be identified as quickly as possible and support provided for discontinuation of the high-risk behavior. Psychosocial factors are often present and require support and counseling during the pregnancy.

Babies born to adolescent mothers frequently weigh less than normal or are preterm, and labor and delivery may be difficult owing to immature pelvic structure. For the mother, pregnancy-induced hypertension (high blood pressure) is a common complication. If the young mother receives and accepts prenatal guidance and support, the pregnancy often progresses with minimal complications.

CASE STUDY A

Gestational Diabetes Mellitus*

C.S. was a healthy, active teenager, other than experiencing irregular menstrual cycles and severe dysmenorrhea (painful menstruation). She had gained weight during her college years. Family history indicated that a paternal great-grandmother had diabetes.

Current history included two miscarriages at 3 months' gestation and one at 5 months following amniocentesis. At age 36, following a course of fertility drugs, C.S. became pregnant, but developed high blood pressure in the first trimester. Routine testing at 3 months' gestation revealed elevated blood glucose and protein in the urine as a result of gestational diabetes and kidney dysfunction. Insulin injections and daily oral ASA were prescribed, as well as weekly appointments with the obstetrician. A weight loss of 30 pounds occurred during the pregnancy.

1. Using your knowledge of normal physiology, explain how glucose and protein can be present in the urine.
2. List the potential risks with gestational diabetes.
3. Why was insulin prescribed?

   Delivery was induced 4 weeks before term because of persistent elevated blood pressure. A healthy male child, weighing 5 pounds 11 ounces, was delivered.

   Postpartum, blood glucose remained high, but was controlled by diet and exercise.

   A second pregnancy at age 38 again led to elevated blood pressure, proteinuria, and diabetes, which was controlled by insulin injections and close monitoring.
4. Suggest several possible complications of high blood pressure during pregnancy.
5. Why is close monitoring important during these pregnancies?

   A healthy female child, weighing 8 pounds 5 ounces, was delivered at term. Following this pregnancy, blood pressure and blood glucose remained elevated. Treatment included dietary modifications, exercise, and oral hypoglycemic drugs (see Chapter 16).

---

*This case study is continued in Chapter 16.

CHAPTER SUMMARY

Numerous normal changes occur in the mother's body during pregnancy, related to elevated levels of estrogen and progesterone as well as to the demands of the developing child. Mild nausea and abdominal discomfort, increased blood volume, relaxation of the pelvic joints, and postural effects are common occurrences. In some cases, however, these changes may exacerbate or precipitate a maternal disorder such as hypertension, or a maternal disease or infection may predispose the fetus to additional risks or disease.

- Hyperemesis gravidarum requires medical supervision to prevent dehydration and acidosis.

- Pregnancy-induced hypertension and preeclampsia developing in the latter part of pregnancy require close monitoring to prevent complications for mother and child.
- Blood glucose levels in the mother must be checked to detect gestational diabetes.
- Rh incompatibility occurs when an Rh-negative mother carries an Rh-positive child. The consequences (hemolysis of fetal red blood cells) can be avoided by treating the mother at delivery to prevent an immune response and development of maternal antibodies.

- Thromboembolism and pulmonary embolus are risks for some women after delivery, particularly those with varicose veins or increased blood clotting tendencies.
- Adolescent pregnancy incurs additional risks because of the mother's immature body.
- Teratogens, including drugs, chemicals and alcohol, viruses, and radiation, cause major damage to the embryo during the first 8 weeks, often before pregnancy is suspected. All potential teratogens should be avoided during childbearing years.

STUDY QUESTIONS

1. State possible signs of pregnancy resulting from physiologic changes in the woman.
2. Suggest some guidelines for fluid and food intake that would optimize fetal development and minimize complications or discomfort for the mother. Include a rationale for each.
3. Explain how a good fitness program is helpful during pregnancy.
4. Differentiate among abruption, previa, and ectopic pregnancy in terms of cause, time of occurrence, and signs.

5. Explain how each of the following affect the pregnant woman and fetus: PIH, eclampsia, and gestational diabetes.
6. Explain why the adolescent gravida is at greater risk of complications of pregnancy.
7. Suggest several signs or symptoms of the development of postpartum infection.

ADDITIONAL RESOURCES

Beers HB, Berkow R: *The Merck Manual of Diagnosis and Therapy*, ed 18, Whitehouse Station, NJ, 2006, Merck Research Laboratories.

Lowdermilk DL: *Maternity & Women's Health Care*, ed 9, St. Louis, 2007, Mosby.

Web Sites

http://www.womenshealth.gov *The National Women's Health Information Center*

http://www.marchofdimes.com/professionals/professionals.asp *March of Dimes medical references, tests and research*

http://www.webmd.com/baby/guide/healthy-weight-gain

CHAPTER 23

Complications of Adolescence

CHAPTER OUTLINE

LEARNING OBJECTIVES

After studying this chapter, the student is expected to:

1. Identify the body mass index, risk of metabolic syndrome, and potential problems associated with obesity.
2. Describe the changes in the postural abnormalities kyphosis, lordosis, and scoliosis.
3. Discuss the bone infection osteomyelitis and the importance of early treatment.
4. Describe the effects of juvenile rheumatoid arthritis.
5. Compare the eating disorders anorexia nervosa and bulimia nervosa.
6. Explain the cause and potential effects of acne.
7. Describe the disease infectious mononucleosis.
8. Describe the following disorders involving the reproductive system: chromosomal abnormalities, testicular cancer, and menstrual abnormalities.

KEY TERMS

adhesions	effusion	lipoprotein metabolism	pustule
amenorrhea	emaciated	menarche	sebaceous
androgens	epiphyseal plate or disc	metabolic syndrome	sebum
anemia	esophagitis	metaphysis	sinus
anomalies	glucose metabolism	monosomy	type 2 diabetes
arrhythmias	gonadotropins	osteoporosis	
body mass index	gonads	periosteum	
caries	insulin resistance	puberty	

Review of Changes During Adolescence

Adolescence is a time of major physiologic, psychological, and sociologic changes, a time of transition into adulthood. It is also a time when certain diseases, developmental or infectious, tend to develop. The period of adolescence is generally considered to begin with the development of secondary sex characteristics around the age of 10 to 12 years and to continue until physical growth is completed at about age 18. The term *puberty* indicates the onset of reproductive changes,

beginning with the appearance of secondary sexual characteristics and the first menstrual cycle in females. Both the timing and the extent of change vary greatly among individuals. In recent years, perhaps because of improved nutrition, maturation has tended to occur at an earlier age.

The biologic changes typical of adolescence result primarily from hormonal activity stimulated by the hypothalamus and pituitary gland. Gonadotropin releasing hormone (GnRh) from the hypothalamus stimulates and increases the release of gonadotropins from the pituitary. Gonadotropins (LH and FSH) support the further development of the ovaries and testes. In the female, the ovaries release ova and the sex hormones estrogen and progesterone, and in the male, the testes begin to produce sperm and to release testosterone. Although these sex hormones are produced in small quantities by the adrenal cortex during all stages of life, the larger quantities now available from the gonads are responsible for the unique types of growth and development that are characteristic of the teen years.

Linear growth is accelerated during the typical adolescent growth spurt. In most males the growth spurt occurs later than in females and usually lasts longer because epiphyseal closure is delayed in males. In recent generations both males and females have achieved a greater average height. Any growth retardation usually is apparent before adolescence, but if it is evident at this time it can be confirmed by x-rays illustrating an abnormally thin epiphyseal plate or disc. Other skeletal changes include the development of a broader pelvis in females and an increase in the width of the shoulders and chest in males. Because of the anabolic actions of the male sex hormones (androgens) or testosterone, males develop more skeletal muscle mass than females during puberty. This is obvious in the shoulder and chest areas. In a newer form of substance abuse, synthetic androgens, the "muscle-building" steroids, are taken by some adolescents to improve body image and athletic performance, without regard for dangerous side effects on the heart and liver. The growth changes of adolescence do not occur simultaneously. Limb growth occurs first, then hip and shoulder development, and increase in skeletal muscle mass is last. This is why the adolescent may appear awkward and gangly for a time until proportionate and complete maturation is accomplished.

Additional factors influencing growth during this period include nutrition, genetic factors, and activity levels. It is most important that calcium and vitamin D intake be adequate during this period. It has become evident that the risk of osteoporosis later in life is influenced by maintaining sufficient calcium intake from childhood and throughout life. Unfortunately, dietary intake often becomes erratic during this period just when demand is higher for iron, protein, and other nutrients. Therefore it is essential for the adolescent to maintain basic nutritional requirements.

With increasing body dimensions, there is an associated increase in blood volume and in the strength of cardiac contractions, although the pulse rate diminishes. Both *cardiovascular* and *pulmonary* functions reach adult values during adolescence, but usually they do not keep pace with musculoskeletal growth, leading to decreased exercise tolerance and marked fatigue at times in active teens. The basal metabolic rate gradually declines to adult levels during this period.

> **THINK ABOUT 23-1**
>
> Predict three factors that could interfere with normal development during adolescence.

Obesity and Metabolic Syndrome

Recent research has shown that the ability to burn fat during exercise declines after puberty. This metabolic change along with changes in activity and diet can lead to obesity during adolescence. Not only is obesity a significant factor in the teen's self-image, it also constitutes a major threat to their health and leads to pathophysiologic changes in metabolism that predispose the teen to diabetes and cardiovascular disease as well as permanent joint damage.

Overweight refers to and excess amount of body weight that may be a result of muscles, bone, fat, and water.

Obesity refers to an excess amount of body fat. Overweight and obesity are due to a caloric imbalance. This imbalance may be due to more calories consumed than expended, and can also be affected by various genetic, behavioral, and environmental factors.

Obesity is determined by calculating the body mass index (BMI). The BMI is an international standard and is calculated based on the child or adolescent's age as well as height and weight. Standard charts are provided within the back covers of this text. Adolescents are considered clinically obese if the BMI is at the 95th percentile or greater for their age. Adolescents whose BMI is between the 85th percentile and the 94th percentile are clinically "at risk for obesity." Note that the amount of fat normally differs with gender and age until after age 20, thus adult BMI charts are not applicable to adolescents. Figure 23-1 illustrates the

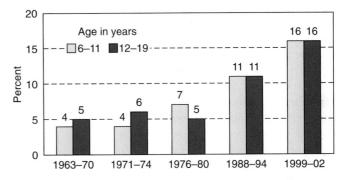

NOTE: Excludes pregnant women starting with 1971–74. Pregnancy status not available for 1963–65 and 1966–70. Data for 1963–65 are for children 6–11 years of age; data for 1966–70 are for adolescents 12–17 years of age, not 12–19 years.
SOURCE: CDC/NCHS, NHES and NHANES

FIGURE 23-1 Prevalence of obesity among adolescents in the United States 1963-2002. *(From CDC/NCHS, NHES, and NHANES.)*

prevalence of adolescent obesity in the United States over several decades.

Alarm has been expressed regarding the recent increase in obesity in children and teens. In the 6- to 11-year age group, the number of obese children has doubled between 1980 and 2000, whereas the number in the 12- to 19-year group has tripled. Obesity in children 6 to 11 years (in the United States) has risen from 7% in 1980 to 18% in 2010. Obesity in the 12-19 age group has risen from 5% in 1980 to 18% in 2010. Accompanying this significant trend is a marked increase in children and young adults with type 2 diabetes mellitus, elevated blood cholesterol/lipid levels, and increased blood pressure. The prevalence of psychological problems is also higher in obese children. Because many obese children continue to be obese adults, these conditions will lead to a higher incidence of cardiac problems, strokes, and musculoskeletal problems such as osteoarthritis. The increased obesity in children and young adults appears related to increased intake of high fat and high carbohydrate snacks, high sugar soft drinks, and "fast foods" in conjunction with decreased exercise and activity related to excessive time spent watching television or playing computer games. It is recommended that nutritious, healthy snacks and meals as well as increased regular physical activity be encouraged. This will also promote general health, growth, and development of the body. A child's body mass index (BMI) calculated from the height and weight should be monitored if unusual weight gain is noticed.

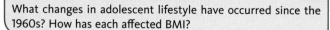

THINK ABOUT 23-2

What changes in adolescent lifestyle have occurred since the 1960s? How has each affected BMI?

Metabolic syndrome is defined in various ways, but three factors are common to all definitions: presence of significant abdominal fat mass resulting in an increased waistline measurement, changes in glucose metabolism and changes in lipoprotein metabolism. Changes in cardiac output, hypertension and/or type 2 diabetes may also be present. (See Chapter 12 for discussion of coronary artery disease and Chapter 16 for discussion of diabetes.) Metabolic syndrome occurs in 1% to 4% of children and adolescents and in 49% of significantly and clinically obese young people. Obesity is the primary cause of the syndrome and any weight loss is significant in preventing complications.

The underlying cause of metabolic syndrome is the release of insulin antagonists by adipose tissue. An increased proportion of body fat results in insulin resistance and changes in metabolism. Specific changes resulting from insulin resistance are discussed in Chapter 16. These changes are a major risk factor for the development of cardiovascular disease and type 2

diabetes. The incidence of cardiovascular diseases such as hypertension and congestive heart failure is higher in individuals with metabolic syndrome and onset is as early as the teens in adolescents with the syndrome. The same is true of type 2 diabetes. Earlier onset of cardiovascular disease and/or type 2 diabetes leads to earlier complications and significantly shortened life expectancy. The current generation of adolescents may be the first to have a shorter life expectancy than their parents.

THINK ABOUT 23-3

1. How does obesity and change in self-image affect the teen's diet and exercise?
2. Why does the teen need to consume a balanced diet rather than trying the most recent fad diet?
3. How can physical activity be increased in daily life activities without the use of expensive equipment or fitness club memberships?

Musculoskeletal Abnormalities

During the growth spurt, muscular development lags behind skeletal growth; thus, less support is available for the weight-bearing areas. Coordination may be impaired at times. Adequate warm-up before exercise or competitive sports is essential to reduce the risk of injury. Postural abnormalities can easily develop during this growth period. Other factors, such as developmental abnormalities in children with Down syndrome or cerebral palsy, may be further aggravated during this period (see Chapter 14). If a correction of a postural abnormality is not undertaken in the early stage, the curvature will progress throughout the adult years, leading to complications.

Kyphosis and Lordosis

Kyphosis, often called hunchback or humpback, is an increase in the convexity of the thoracic spine (Fig. 23-2). Although it often develops in mature adults secondary to disorders such as osteoporosis (bone demineralization) and tuberculosis, a milder and reversible form, commonly of postural origin, occurs during the adolescent growth spurt. Teens frequently hunch over, particularly if they are taller than their peers or are self-conscious about breast development. Also, skeletal muscle support may be temporarily inadequate. Marked kyphosis can interfere with lung expansion and ventilation. Exercise and postural change can usually reverse mild deformities, although severe deformity may require surgery or a brace for correction.

Lordosis is an exaggerated concave lumbar curvature, or "swayback." Again, it may accompany musculoskeletal disease, but frequently it develops because of poor posture during the adolescent growth spurt. Obesity

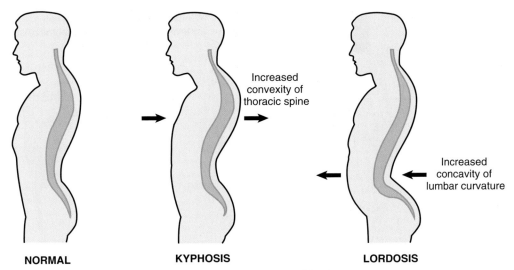

Increased
convexity of
thoracic spine

Increased
concavity of
lumbar curvature

NORMAL   **KYPHOSIS**   **LORDOSIS**

FIGURE 23-2 Kyphosis and lordosis.

aggravates the tendency toward lordosis because the center of gravity for the body is altered, and postural compensation causes the change in vertebral alignment.

Scoliosis

Scoliosis is a lateral curvature of the spine affecting either the thoracic or lumbar area, or both, and it may be accompanied by rotation of the vertebrae (Fig. 23-3). The curvature becomes greater during growth spurts. Screening programs, offered in many schools, aid early diagnosis. Otherwise, it may be noticed when clothes do not fit properly, or the uneven shoulder elevation may become apparent when the child bends forward.

Scoliosis may be classified as structural or functional. *Structural* scoliosis is a primary spinal deformity, of which 80% are idiopathic (without known cause), although a genetic factor appears to play a key role. In the idiopathic form, females are more frequently affected than males (5:1). Congenital scoliosis results from developmental defects such as hemivertebrae, this deformity altering spinal alignment. Sixty percent of congenital scoliosis cases occur in girls, some of whom have additional congenital defects such as urinary tract abnormalities. Another form, degenerative scoliosis, may develop in older individuals with osteoporosis or osteoarthritis, which create an unstable vertebral column. *Functional*, nonstructural, or postural scoliosis is secondary to another problem such as unequal leg length or spinal nerve compression. Unequal spinal muscle supports related to partial paralysis, trauma, muscular dystrophy, cerebral palsy, or spinal tumors may lead to loss of the normal curvature.

Early effects of abnormal spinal curvature include:
- Loss of alignment of the hip and shoulder
- Rotation of the vertebrae, which affects the pelvis and thorax. The ribs can become rigid in an abnormal

position; if severe, this rotation and fixation can restrict ventilation.

In teenagers with milder postural scoliosis, exercise and bracing may be helpful in restoring the normal curvature of the back. However, surgical correction with instrumentation and fusion of the vertebrae is often required, causing restriction of the individual's activity for long periods of time. Unfortunately, even when corrected, complications, including a return of the abnormal curvature, may occur later in life.

THINK ABOUT 23-4

a. Compare the abnormal curvatures associated with kyphosis, lordosis, and scoliosis by preparing a chart with a simple line drawing and a brief description of each.
b. Bend your head and shoulders forward and down. Attempt to take a deep breath. What happens?
c. Describe the potential complications of scoliosis if it is not treated in the early stage.

Osteomyelitis

This infection of the bone may occur at any age most commonly as a complication of trauma such as fractures (see Chapter 9). However, it is common in the adolescent period, associated with minor trauma, particularly in younger males. Often a history of minor trauma, a soft tissue injury, precedes this condition. A bruise or sprain leaves the area vulnerable to blood-borne organisms from another site, such as a skin boil, an abscess, or sinusitis. In adolescents the common causative organism is *Staphylococcus aureus*, but any pathogen can be the culprit. The most common site of infection in adolescents is the metaphysis (the area between the end and central shaft of a long bone) of the femur or tibia in the leg. Certain conditions such as sickle cell anemia also

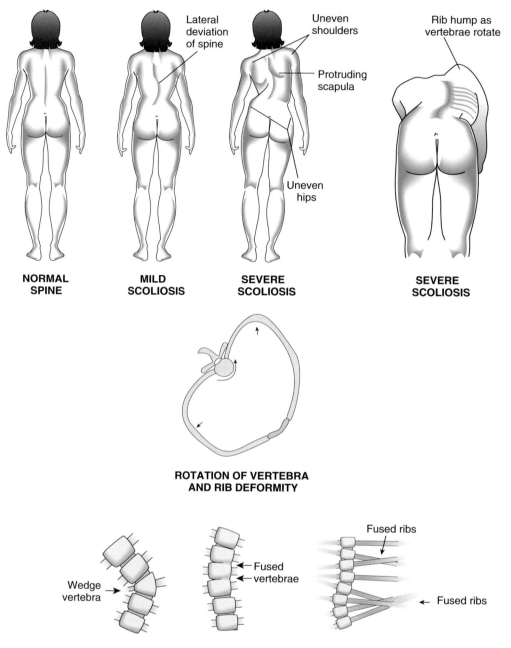

NORMAL SPINE

Lateral deviation of spine

MILD SCOLIOSIS

Uneven shoulders

Protruding scapula

Uneven hips

SEVERE SCOLIOSIS

Rib hump as vertebrae rotate

SEVERE SCOLIOSIS

ROTATION OF VERTEBRA AND RIB DEFORMITY

Wedge vertebra

Fused vertebrae

Fused ribs

Fused ribs

SOME CONGENITAL DEFORMITIES CAUSING SCOLIOSIS

FIGURE 23-3 Scoliosis.

predispose adolescents to bone infection, as do, of course, open injuries and fractures.

The course of osteomyelitis involves:

- A local accumulation of purulent exudate or pus develops, which destroys the bone in the area (Fig. 23-4). This exudate creates pressure within the rigid bony structure and causes severe pain owing to pressure on the nerves and the periosteum, or outer covering of the bone, may be lifted or torn off if the pressure becomes excessive.
- Stimulation causes the surrounding bone to develop new bone growth around the infected site, walling off an area of infection and necrotic bone, which then becomes more difficult to treat effectively.
- If the pressure of the exudate tears the periosteum on the surface of the bone, a sinus or passage through the soft tissue may develop, spreading the infection to adjacent tissue.
- Possible joint involvement. Usually the epiphyseal plate acts as a barrier to joint involvement, although the infection can spread through the joint capsule to cause infectious arthritis. If the epiphyseal plate or periosteum is damaged, the future growth of the child may be affected.

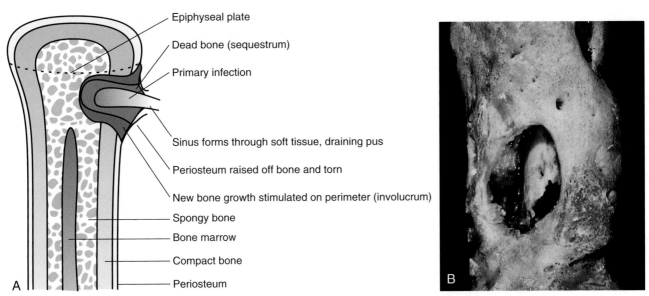

Epiphyseal plate
Dead bone (sequestrum)
Primary infection
Sinus forms through soft tissue, draining pus
Periosteum raised off bone and torn
New bone growth stimulated on perimeter (involucrum)
Spongy bone
Bone marrow
Compact bone
Periosteum

A

B

FIGURE 23-4 **A,** Osteomyelitis. **B,** Femur with osteomyelitis. Resected femur illustrating draining osteomyelitis. The drainage tract (sinus) in the subperiosteal shell of a new viable bone (involucrum) reveals the necrotic cortex (sequestrum). *(B from Kumar V, Abbas AK, Fausto M: Robbins and Cotran Pathologic Basis of Disease, ed 7, Philadelphia, 2005, Saunders.)*

Manifestations of osteomyelitis include the local signs of inflammation—swelling, redness, and warmth at the site, and pain that increases with movement. Usually there are systemic signs of infection as well, including fever, leukocytosis, malaise, and irritability.

Treatment requires aggressive drug therapy with bone-penetrating antimicrobials appropriate for the causative organism. If chronic infection develops, surgery may be necessary to remove necrotic and infected tissue in order to allow healing.

The prognosis is improved when treatment takes place in the early stage of infection.

THINK ABOUT 23-5

a. List all the manifestations of osteomyelitis.
b. Suggest reasons why osteomyelitis might not be diagnosed in an early stage.
c. Give several reasons why early treatment is important.

Juvenile Rheumatoid Arthritis

Juvenile rheumatoid arthritis (JRA) is a group of autoimmune diseases that cause chronic inflammation in the connective tissue in areas such as the joints in children. It is somewhat similar in pathology to adult rheumatoid arthritis (see Chapter 9), but it has certain distinctive qualities. For example, onset is more marked and large joints, such as knees, wrists, and elbows, are more frequently involved, and more systemic effects are apparent. Juvenile rheumatoid arthritis is classified in three subgroups, depending on the joints affected, the types of antibodies found in the blood, and the other effects. One form is termed Still's disease, distinguished by its systemic effects and acute onset with high fever, skin rash, and enlarged spleen.

The specific cause is not known, although there is a genetic factor and links to an infectious agent or environmental factor have been suggested. A study is in process recording cases occurring in siblings. It affects 1:1000 children and is more common in two age groups, children aged 2 to 5 years and those aged 9 to 12 years. Many cases are mild and remain undiagnosed for some time. One or more pairs of joints may be involved, depending on the specific type of JRA that is present.

The synovial membrane of the joint is inflamed, resulting in swelling and effusion (fluid) in the joint with gradual erosion of the cartilage. Affected joints are red and swollen in the initial or acute stage; they are often tender to touch and stiff after rest. Joint pain does not seem to be severe, but mobility is impaired by the persistent swelling, stiffness, and occasional muscle spasms. If the inflammation persists, adhesions can form, causing fixation and deformity of the joint.

Specific diagnostic tests are helpful but not diagnostic in JRA because the rheumatoid factor is usually not present in the child's blood. Joint swelling or discomfort lasting more than 6 weeks is an indicator. General signs of inflammation such as leukocytosis are present and antinuclear antibodies (ANA) are frequently found in the blood. Other conditions such as infection or trauma must be ruled out.

The course may be marked by remissions and exacerbations, or the signs may persist continuously. The disease may last for a few months or for years. Complications such as hip involvement or iridocyclitis (inflammation of the eye) may occur.

Treatment includes nonsteroidal anti-inflammatory drugs (see Chapter 5) and glucocorticoids if needed. Glucocorticoids may be required for severe inflammation or if organs such as the heart are affected. Disease-modifying anti-rheumatic drugs (DMARDs) such as methotrexate may be used in small doses to slow the progress of the disease and prevent joint damage. Physiotherapy and exercise, particularly swimming, are important to maintain the flexibility, alignment, function, and proper development of the joints. Growth may be impaired during the time of active disease, related to immobility or to glucocorticoid treatment, but often a catch-up growth spurt follows recovery. In some cases unequal limb growth related to joint involvement may occur, and the individual may never reach his or her original growth potential.

The prognosis is positive for the majority of children, with more than 50% experiencing complete remission, and only a small number developing severe joint deformities and motor disability.

THINK ABOUT 23-6

a. Explain several ways in which arthritis affects mobility.
b. Explain how long-term arthritis of the legs might affect a child's growth.

Eating Disorders

In Western cultures, eating disorders such as anorexia nervosa and bulimia are a common problem in adolescents and young adults, primarily females. Because more children now tend to obesity in early childhood and adolescence, increasing numbers of teens are focusing on their bodies and desire to change their bodies. With eating disorders, the major medical concern is the effect of poor nutrition on growth and development and on the child's general health status. The incidence of eating disorders is increasing, but often the affected person makes a great effort to conceal the problem, making it more difficult to detect and treat in the early stages. In addition to the physical problems, the psychological and behavioral factors in these disorders need to be addressed. The two major problems are anorexia nervosa and bulimia nervosa; they may occur separately or, more frequently, they may overlap.

Anorexia Nervosa

Anorexia nervosa is an extreme loss of weight because of self-starvation, in the absence of another disease. The onset of anorexia occurs in two peak periods, first in the

early teen years (ages 12 to 14) and again later in the 16- to 17-year age range, with females being most often affected. The psychological component is strongly evident in these patients, who typically are young women who are perfectionists and high achievers. This psychological component, combined with a history of family conflict, a confused perception of body image and sexuality, and a morbid fear of "fatness," leads to anorexia. Research is also focusing on possible hypothalamic abnormalities related to hunger as well as other physiologic dysfunctions.

The basic problem in anorexia nervosa is a refusal to eat, resulting in severe malnutrition, including protein and vitamin deficits. The affected person may also induce vomiting, take excessive amounts of laxatives, and exercise strenuously to achieve even further weight loss. The anorexic appears markedly emaciated (thin and wasted). Other manifestations include amenorrhea (lack of menstrual cycles), low body temperature and cold intolerance, low blood pressure and slow heart rate, dry skin and brittle nails, and development of fine body hair (lanugo).

It has been demonstrated that low calcium intake at this time can predispose to osteoporosis later in life.

In some cases, anorexia nervosa can be life threatening. Dehydration can be severe, affecting kidney and cardiovascular function (see Chapter 2). Electrolyte imbalances such as hypokalemia and hyponatremia may cause complications such as cardiac arrhythmias (irregular heart rhythms) and cardiac arrest. Hospitalization and long-term psychotherapy with behavioral modification may be necessary to arrest the weight loss and initiate recovery. Many specialized clinics and support groups have been formed to deal with eating disorders.

Bulimia Nervosa

Bulimia is also common in females but occurs more frequently in older adolescents. Bulimia is characterized by binge eating, particularly of carbohydrates, followed by purging. Binge eating consists of ingesting huge amounts of food, usually high in calories, within a very short period of time. This is followed by purging by means of self-induced vomiting and an excessive use of laxatives and diuretics. Compulsive exercising is frequently associated with the disorder. The cycle may be repeated several times during a day or less frequently. Bulimia and anorexia may often overlap.

The bulimic often maintains a relatively normal weight, although appropriate levels of individual nutrients may not be sustained, resulting in problems such as anemia (low hemoglobin levels) and menstrual irregularities. Frequent vomiting causes fluid and electrolyte imbalances, which may cause cardiac arrhythmias, tetany, or severe abdominal pain. Dental personnel should be aware that recurrent vomiting leads to erosion of tooth enamel (usually on the lingual surface of the maxillary teeth) and increased dental caries, tears and ulcers in the oral mucosa, enlarged parotid and submandibular glands, and chronic esophagitis with sore throat and difficulty in swallowing. Self-induced vomiting may leave visible scars on the fingers or back of the hand used to stimulate the gag reflex.

Binge eating disorder is a different condition characterized by intake of excessively large amounts of food, but lacks purging. It is often associated with obesity. Depression and guilt feelings are found frequently.

THINK ABOUT 23-7

Prepare a chart comparing anorexia and bulimia according to eating pattern, body weight, and potential complications.

Skin Disorders

Acne Vulgaris

Acne is a very common skin infection in adolescence and through the teen years, particularly in males, although there is a wide variation between its mild and severe forms. Severe forms can lead to permanent scarring. The lesions of acne affect the sebaceous glands and associated hair follicles on the face, neck, and upper trunk (Fig. 23-5). At puberty these glands increase in activity, resulting in plugged pores and infection.

There are two types of lesions. Comedones, often called whiteheads or blackheads, are noninflammatory collections of sebum (the oily glandular secretion), sloughed epithelial cells, and bacteria, which clog the gland and prevent normal drainage. These lesions usually resolve without scarring. The second type of lesion involves a severe inflammatory response and

infection. The hair follicles swell and rupture, and *Propionibacterium acnes*, a bacterial component of normal flora, breaks down the sebum into irritating fatty acids, resulting in inflammation. Staphylococcal organisms invade, creating a pustule (raised red mass containing purulent exudate). The lesion is often aggravated by irritation caused by the individual's picking at or squeezing the mass. Eventually the lesion ruptures, causing local tissue destruction and possibly spreading to nearby areas. Skin damage and scarring are a common outcome.

Identifying predisposing factors that can be modified in the client's history will help reduce the incidence of new lesions. These include hereditary predisposition, increased androgen levels, premenstrual hormonal fluctuations, the application of oily creams, the use of certain drugs, heavy or irritating clothing, backpacks and helmets, and exposure to increased heat and humidity. Shampooing and cleaning the area more frequently (but avoiding harsh soaps and scrubbing), improving general nutrition, and avoiding oil-based cosmetics are helpful preventive measures. Peeling agents (benzoyl peroxide, tretinoin, and isotretinoin) and antibacterial agents (tetracycline) assist in controlling severe lesions and reducing the cosmetic problem. Dermabrasion may be successful in removing some scars.

THINK ABOUT 23-8

a. Describe the development of an acneiform lesion.
b. Suggest measures that can reduce the severity of acne.

Infection

Infectious Mononucleosis

Infectious mononucleosis is an acute infection affecting lymphocytes caused by the Epstein-Barr virus (EBV, which is in the herpes group). It is common in adolescents and young adults. The infection is usually mild and self-limiting, but occasionally is marked by complications. The agent is transmitted by direct contact with infected saliva (hence the term "kissing disease"), airborne droplets, and blood. Epstein-Barr virus invades epithelial cells in the nasopharynx and oropharynx and penetrates to lymphoid tissue, targeting the B lymphocytes and producing typical antibodies. The incubation period is approximately 4 to 6 weeks.

The manifestations include:
- Sore throat, headache, fever, fatigue, and malaise
- Enlarged lymph nodes (lymphadenopathy) and spleen (splenomegaly)
- A rash on the trunk

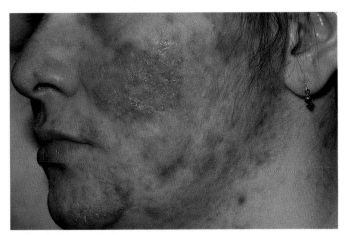

FIGURE 23-5 Acne vulgaris. *(From Kumar V, Abbas AK, Fausto M: Robbins and Cotran Pathologic Basis of Disease, ed 7, Philadelphia, 2005, Saunders.)*

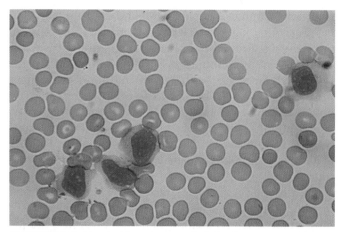

FIGURE 23-6 Atypical lymphocytes in infectious mononucleosis. *(From Kumar V, Abbas AK, Fausto M: Robbins and Cotran Pathologic Basis of Disease, ed 7, Philadelphia, 2005, Saunders.)*

- An increase in lymphocytes and monocytes in the blood, and the presence of atypical T-lymphocytes (Fig. 23-6)
- A positive heterophil antibody test (Monospot test)

Possible complications include hepatitis, ruptured spleen, and meningitis. Because no effective treatment for virus infections is available, supportive measures, particularly bed rest, are indicated. As with many viral infections, recovery may be prolonged, and fatigue and malaise may be persistent. Fitness students and trainers should be aware of an important safeguard against rupture of the spleen; that is, ensuring that the spleen has returned to normal size before an individual participates in sports or strenuous exercise programs.

Disorders Affecting Sexual Development

Chromosomal Disorders

Depending on the manifestations, some genetic disorders are diagnosed early in life, and some are not diagnosed until puberty, when the effects on sexual development become apparent. An example is *Klinefelter's syndrome*, which affects males owing to the presence of an additional X chromosome (XXY instead of XY; see Chapter 21). Although mental retardation is a common finding, most boys are diagnosed at puberty because the testes remain small, sperm are not produced, and secondary male sex characteristics do not develop. *Turner's syndrome*, a monosomy X in which one X chromosome is missing, affects sexual development in females and causes other abnormalities as well.

Anomalies or malformations commonly occur in the heart and genitourinary system; growth is retarded; and at puberty the growth spurt, development of secondary sex characteristics, and initiation of the menstrual cycle are lacking. Hormone replacement treatment is beneficial in these girls.

Tumors

Testicular tumors are not common but do affect young adult males in their twenties and thirties. When this tumor develops in the testes of the adolescent, it is usually malignant (see Chapter 19). As early as possible, adolescents should be checked and treated for undescended testes (see Fig. 19-2), because this condition is frequently the predisposing factor. This cancer manifests as a unilateral hard, heavy mass and often is not painful. Serum markers may be present, depending on the type of tumor. Routine testicular self-examination is helpful in achieving early diagnosis and treatment. Surgical removal of the affected testicle is necessary. Removal of one testicle usually does not affect sexual function or fertility. However if radiation or chemotherapy is required after surgery, sterility is likely; therefore sperm should be banked to provide embryos in the future.

Menstrual Abnormalities

Delayed menarche or primary amenorrhea, the absence of menstruation after age 17, is usually caused by an abnormality in the reproductive organs (structural or hormonal) or an abnormality in the pituitary gland or hypothalamus. Consistent strenuous physical activity, such as training for competitive sports, and certain systemic disorders, such as hypothyroid or diabetes, may also delay menarche.

Dysmenorrhea refers to the discomfort that occurs in varying degrees during the first or second day of menstruation (see Chapter 19). In some girls the pain is incapacitating, and vomiting or fainting may occur. The cramping pain is related to the increased secretion of uterine prostaglandins, which increase muscle contractility and directly irritate the nerve endings, and to the vascular changes and ischemia in the uterine wall that occur as the endometrium is shed. Dysmenorrhea may be treated with hormones or nonsteroidal anti-inflammatory drugs such as ibuprofen (Advil). Popular nonprescription products for dysmenorrhea such as Midol contain aspirin, caffeine, and cinnamedrine, a uterine relaxant. Secondary dysmenorrhea usually is related to infection or other pathologies.

CASE STUDY A

Obesity

M.R., age 12, weighs 26 kg and is 60 in/150 cm tall. She is concerned about her weight, but finds it hard to "diet" because her family constantly snacks while watching TV. She enjoys texting friends and using the computer for chats and surfing the latest musical groups. Her father tells her not to worry about her weight, that men like women with some "meat on their bones." Although she likes swimming, she has stopped going to the local pool since her weight has increased.

1. Using the tables on the inside of the back cover, calculate M.R.'s BMI. What weight category does this BMI represent? Why are specific tables used to calculate BMI in children and adolescents rather than a simple formula of mass divided by height used for adults?
2. What family factors are related to M.R.'s weight?
3. What personal factors are related to M.R.'s weight?
4. M.R. is at high risk of developing metabolic syndrome because of her weight. What potential life-threatening health problems may she experience if she does develop this syndrome?
5. When will such health problems most likely occur?
6. What changes in body function occur in metabolic syndrome and how are these monitored?
7. How can M.R. change her lifestyle to reduce complications? What support would be helpful?

CHAPTER SUMMARY

Adolescence generally refers to the period of time between the development of secondary sex characteristics and the completion of physical growth around age 18. The increased secretion of gonadotropins and sex hormones is primarily responsible for musculoskeletal changes and sexual maturation.

- Obesity is increasingly common in adolescents and is most often accompanied by changes in metabolism of lipids and glucose leading to metabolic syndrome. Metabolic syndrome leads to cardiovascular disease and type 2 diabetes. Complications occur at an early age and limit life expectancy.
- Abnormal spinal curvatures such as lordosis and scoliosis may develop during the adolescent growth spurt. Scoliosis, a lateral curvature of the spine, affects the alignment of the hips, shoulders, and ribs, requiring prompt treatment.
- Osteomyelitis is a serious infection of the bones that may complicate minor injuries. There is a risk of damage to the periosteum or joint, affecting growth.
- Juvenile rheumatoid arthritis is similar in many ways to the adult form, but it affects the large joints more frequently and manifests more systemic effects than does the adult form. Most individuals recover fully.
- Anorexia nervosa, characterized by a refusal to eat, and bulimia nervosa, typically binge eating accompanied by self-induced vomiting and purging, may occur separately or as a combination in a specific patient. A psychological component is frequently present. Complications are common.
- Acne vulgaris is an infection of the hair follicles on the face and neck, which may cause significant scarring.
- Infectious mononucleosis is a communicable infectious disease caused by the Epstein-Barr virus, usually with mild signs and symptoms but with a prolonged recovery period.
- Chromosomal abnormalities affecting sexual development, such as Klinefelter's syndrome, may become obvious at puberty.
- Male adolescents should be checked for maldescent of the testes, a predisposing factor to testicular cancer. This cancer occurs in young men less than age 30.

STUDY QUESTIONS

1. Briefly describe five changes that indicate sexual maturation in the female.
2. Differentiate structural from functional scoliosis and give an example of a cause of each type.
3. Explain how the signs of osteomyelitis differ from the signs of JRA.
4. How do anorexia and bulimia differ from each other?
5. Explain how anorexia and bulimia can have serious consequences.
6. Explain how scars may develop from acne.
7. Describe the cause and transmission of infectious mononucleosis.
8. Why should undescended testes not go untreated?
9. Describe the cause and significance of metabolic syndrome.

ADDITIONAL RESOURCES

Behrman RE, Kliegman RM: *Nelson Essentials of Pediatrics*, ed 4, Philadelphia, 2002, Saunders.

Web Sites

http://www.nih.gov/news/WordonHealth/jun2002/childhoodobesity.htm *Word on Health (National Institutes of Health)*

http://www.niams.nih.gov *National Institute of Arthritis and Musculoskeletal and Skin Diseases*

http://www.cdc.gov/nccdphp/dnpa/healthyweight/assessing/bmi/childrens_BMI/about_childrens_BMI.htm#interpreted%20the%20same%20way *Healthy Weight—it's not a diet, it's a lifestyle! (Centers for Disease Control and Prevention)*

http://www.cdc.gov/healthyyouth/obesity/facts.htm

http://www.cdc.gov/nchs/data/databriefs/db82.htm

Complications of Aging

CHAPTER OUTLINE

LEARNING OBJECTIVES

After studying this chapter, the student is expected to:

1. Describe the metabolic and structural changes in tissues.
2. Discuss the effects of hormonal changes as women and men age.
3. Describe the common changes in the heart and the arteries.
4. Explain the causes and effects of osteoporosis and osteoarthritis in older individuals.
5. Discuss the common changes in nervous system function.
6. Describe common changes in the digestive system and the urinary system.
7. Explain the increased incidence of infections and cancer.
8. Explain how multiple system disorders can interact and cause complications.

KEY TERMS

arteriosclerosis	fractures	neurofibrils	plaques
articular cartilage	frequency	neurotransmitter	presbyopia
atherosclerosis	glaucoma	nocturia	retina
cataracts	incontinence	osteoarthritis	sedentary
cholesterol	intervertebral discs	osteoblastic	senescence
dyspareunia	kyphosis	periodontal disease	xerostomia

The Aging Process

Aging begins after birth but becomes more evident at about 30 years of age. The process is irreversible, but the rate and effects of aging vary greatly among individuals and do not necessarily match *chronologic* age. The typical changes in various organs do not occur at the same time or in any particular order. The extent of the changes also depends on the individual's genetic makeup, lifestyle, and health status. Many diverse research projects are taking place into the physiologic changes related to aging with the goal of delaying changes or reversing them. Much of this research is in developmental biology and includes the study and expression of various genes that have been identified in normal development.

Senescence refers to the period of life from old age to death. Overall, women live longer than men. The average life span is increasing, creating a higher proportion of older individuals in the population. This trend occurs largely because of improved social and living standards, better nutrition, and advancements in health care. Physical exercise that occurs on a routine basis and increases cardiac output and ventilation may slow tissue changes associated with senescence by providing improved nutrition and oxygenation to the tissues. Cognitive activities requiring problem solving such as card games, puzzles and reading seem to reduce senescence in the central nervous system. Social interaction during exercise or games is also significant in maintaining function.

With aging, a general reduction in function occurs throughout the body at the cellular and organ level, and the body is characterized by a decreased capacity to adapt to change. Aging is a natural process, but it is affected by many pathologic processes. *Degenerative changes associated with aging may predispose an individual to certain pathologies, and pathologic changes can hasten aging.* Of particular concern are the organs and tissues that cannot regenerate, such as the brain and myocardium. This chapter covers only some of the more significant effects of aging that are linked to pathologic problems. For additional information, a gerontology reference should be consulted.

There are different theories about the causes of aging. One theory suggests that aging is programmed genetically through the cells and that this control directly limits the cells' reproductive capacity (see Chapter 1). Predetermined cell death is termed *apoptosis*. Other possible factors include wear-and-tear, cellular damage resulting from accumulated wastes and altered protein (amyloid) or lipid (lipofuscin) components, or increased degenerative changes in *collagen* and elastin fibers. In addition, random errors occur during cell mitosis. Some theories suggest that aging is related to resident latent viruses or increased autoimmune reactions in which the body rejects its own tissues, or to environmental agents that affect cells. One concern relates to free radicals such as peroxides, reactive chemicals produced during cell metabolism. Free radicals are known to damage nucleic acids and cells, leading to cancer and other diseases. It is likely that many factors contribute to the aging process, and that these factors may vary in individuals.

Changes in the tissues are obvious. Cells assume less regular arrangements in tissues later in life. Elastic fibers are lost, and the number of collagen cross-linkages or other abnormal structures in tissues and organs increases. Mitosis, or cellular reproduction, gradually slows down, partly in response to the slower metabolic rate, resulting in decreased tissue repair. Some cells such as neurons and muscle cells cannot replicate, and when they die function is reduced in these tissues. Certain cells appear to have limits on the number of times they can replicate, and therefore they are not replaced in older individuals. Other cells accumulate wastes or are altered by environmental factors and become less functional or die, ultimately leading to organ failure. It has become evident that prolonged exposure to numerous environmental factors such as radiation, viral infections, and chemicals over the years leads to an increased risk of cancer and other diseases in older people. Many of these changes also occur in younger individuals, so they are not unique to the aging process.

> **THINK ABOUT   24-1**
> a. List changes in the tissues of the body that occur with aging.
> b. List the signs of aging you have noted in individuals at 30, 50, and 80 years of age.

Physiological Changes with Aging

Hormonal Changes

Generally hormone secretions remain relatively constant with advancing age, but the number of tissue receptors may decrease, thus diminishing the body's response to hormones. This effect is apparent in disorders such as type 2 diabetes mellitus, which is common in older persons. In this condition, sufficient insulin is produced, but because the number of cell receptors is reduced, glucose does not enter the cells (see Chapter 16). In the absence of any specific pathology, the pituitary, thyroid, parathyroids, adrenals, and pancreas appear to maintain relatively normal function, producing hormones in adequate quantities.

The major natural hormonal change occurs in women at about age 50, when the ovaries cease to produce estrogen and progesterone; subsequently, serum levels of follicle-stimulating hormone (FSH) and luteinizing hormone (LH) rise in response to natural feedback mechanisms (see Chapter 19). The effects of the decreased estrogen and progesterone are described in the following sections. Although there is a gradual decrease in testosterone levels in the male, the testes do not totally cease to function.

Testosterone levels in males peak during teen and early adulthood. After the age of 30 testosterone levels decrease about 1% a year. The decline is usually not obvious until later in life.

Reproductive System Changes

Menopause is the term given to the change that occurs in women at around age 50, when the ovaries cease to respond to FSH and LH, resulting in lack of ovulation, cessation of the menstrual cycle, and declining estrogen and progesterone levels. The decreased levels of sex hormones lead to changes such as thinning of the mucosa, loss of elasticity, and decreased glandular secretions in the vagina and cervix. These changes may cause inflammation and dyspareunia, or painful sexual intercourse. The effects can be minimized by topical (local) administration of estrogen creams. There are risks associated with oral hormone replacement therapy; therefore individual case assessment is necessary. The pH of the vaginal secretions becomes more alkaline, thus predisposing older women to recurrent vaginal infections. Breast tissue also decreases in volume. These changes in hormone levels in the early stage of menopause frequently lead to systemic signs such as "hot flashes," which involve periodic sweating or vascular disturbances. Also headaches, irritability, and insomnia are common manifestations. The effects of menopause may be felt for short or long periods of time (several years) and are more marked in some women than others. Approximately 25% of women experience significant effects. If surgical removal of the ovaries is necessary before menopause occurs naturally, similar effects will be evident.

In males, testosterone levels decline gradually, the testes decrease in size, sperm production is somewhat reduced, and the glandular secretions of the prostate are decreased, but the older male is capable of fathering a child. The common problem in older males is *benign prostatic hypertrophy* (BPH) (see Chapter 19), in which the central part of the gland around the urethra hypertrophies, resulting in some degree of obstruction of the urethra. If urinary flow is significantly impaired, surgery may be necessary.

Cancer of the reproductive organs is more common in both males (prostatic cancer) and females (uterine and breast cancer) in later years and may be related to altered hormonal levels. Frequent examinations by a physician in addition to routine self-examination and testing (e.g., mammograms) are essential to lessen the risk of advanced malignancy.

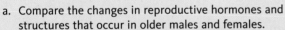

THINK ABOUT 24-2

a. Compare the changes in reproductive hormones and structures that occur in older males and females.
b. Using your knowledge of the normal actions of the sex hormones, suggest some effects of decreased secretion of sex hormones on various body tissues and structures. (You may refer to Chapter 24 for help with hormonal actions.)

Changes in the Skin and Mucosa

Some changes in the skin are related to genetic factors; many are based on exposure to sun and weather. With aging, both the skin and mucous membranes become thin and fragile. The dermis is thinner and subcutaneous tissue is diminished. Fewer capillaries are present and cell proliferation is decreased, resulting in slower wound healing and atrophy of the glands. The numbers of sensory receptors in the skin and mucosa decline. These factors increase susceptibility to injury, bruising occurs frequently, and the mucosal membranes become inflamed or ulcerated.

The skin is often dry and appears wrinkled as elastic fibers are reduced and collagen fibers become less flexible. Obvious lesions include skin tags (small projections of skin) on the neck and axillary areas, keratoses (rough raised masses, often dark in color) over the body, and lentigines or liver spots (dark flat macules), often on the hands and face. The hair becomes gray as melanocytes are reduced in number, and thinning occurs as the number of hair follicles decreases.

Cardiovascular System Changes

Age-related changes occur in the cardiac muscle fibers and the connective tissues in the heart. Fatty tissue and collagen fibers accumulate in the heart muscle with aging and may eventually interfere with impulse conduction and cardiac muscle contraction. The size and number of cardiac muscle cells declines, reducing the strength of cardiac contractions. In the absence of any pathologic changes, the left ventricle appears smaller, because demand is also reduced. Cardiac muscle fibers do not undergo mitosis and cannot be replaced. Heart valves often thicken and therefore become less flexible and efficient. In some individuals, vascular degeneration causes a decrease in the oxygen supply to the heart muscle and reduces the ability of the heart muscle to use oxygen. Thus, cardiac output and cardiac reserve are diminished, decreasing the maximum cardiac output possible with stress. Adequate fluid intake is important to maintain cardiovascular function, as the percentage of fluid in the body declines in older individuals. Again, a regular fitness program is most helpful in maintaining cardiac function.

The common pathologies of the cardiovascular system are associated with degenerative changes in the arteries, both in the heart and throughout the body (see Chapter 12). Loss of elasticity and accumulation of collagen in the arterial walls result in thickening of the arterial walls, thus limiting expansion of the large arteries and obstructing the lumina of smaller arteries. This leads to arteriosclerosis and elevated blood pressure. Also, degenerative changes promote the accumulation of cholesterol and lipid in the walls of large arteries, the condition known as atherosclerosis, particularly when the individual has elevated blood lipid levels. These lipid plaques obstruct blood flow and predispose to thrombus formation. Atherosclerosis is a common cause

THINK ABOUT 24-3

a. Based on your general knowledge, can you suggest ways of restricting the diet to reduce the risk of cardiovascular problems?
b. Suggest different types of exercise appropriate for older individuals and explain how regular exercise can delay the onset of degenerative changes.
c. Explain how the reduced blood supply may affect the skin and mucosa.
d. Describe the outcome of a blocked artery.

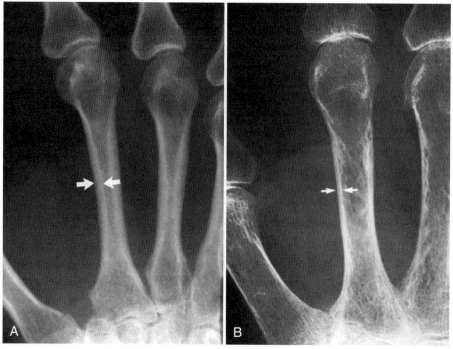

FIGURE 24-1 **A**, Normal metacarpal bone. **B**, Osteoporotic metacarpal bone. *(From Helms CA: Fundamentals of Skeletal Radiology, ed 3, Philadelphia, 2005, Saunders.)*

of angina, myocardial infarctions (heart attacks), peripheral vascular disease in the legs, and strokes. Dietary changes, including reduced cholesterol intake, and regular exercise programs assist in lowering blood lipid and cholesterol levels and lessen the risk of vascular degeneration and high blood pressure.

Musculoskeletal System Changes

Osteoporosis

The important change in bone with aging is loss of calcium and bone mass, which leads to osteoporosis. This condition may occur for many reasons, but the high incidence in postmenopausal women is a concern because of the serious consequences (see Chapters 25 and 9 for additional information on osteoporosis). Fractures of the spine, pelvis, and limbs are common occurrences, requiring hospitalization and limiting mobility. It is recommended that older women have a routine bone density test to check for the "silent" development of osteoporosis. It is now apparent that many men, approximately 1:8, also lose bone mass.

Several risk factors are associated with osteoporosis in older persons, including:
- Hereditary predisposition
- Decreased estrogen levels
- Decreased weight-bearing activity or stress on bone (sedentary or inactive lifestyle or immobility)
- Decreased intake of calcium, vitamins C and D, at all ages, including childhood
- Decreased intestinal absorption of calcium

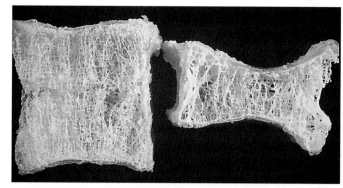

FIGURE 24-2 Osteoporotic vertebral body *(right)* shortened by compression fractures, compared with normal vertebral body *(left)*. *(From Kumar V, Abbas AK, Fausto M: Robbins and Cotran: Pathologic Basis of Disease, ed 7, Philadelphia, 2005, Saunders.)*

- Decreased osteoblastic activity, that is an increased risk with glucocorticoid/cortisol use

Deposition of new bone is reduced, leading to decreased bone mass and density. Note the reduction in the outer layer of compact bone in the metacarpal bone in Figure 24-1. The bones are often porous and brittle, thus precipitating frequent fractures in areas such as the vertebrae and pelvis (Fig. 24-2). Spontaneous vertebral fractures result in decreased height and kyphosis with increased age (see Fig. 23-2 illustrating kyphosis). As the thoracic curvature increases, the individual compensates by increasing the cervical curvature and tilting the head, leading to a typical hunchback posture (dowager's hump) and a shuffling gait. This impairs ventilation and mobility.

Recommendations to reduce the risk and the progression of osteoporosis with aging include:
- Increased calcium intake plus adequate vitamin D for all age groups (the current recommendation for the daily calcium intake for those greater than 50 years is 1500 mg, plus 800 IU vitamin D)
- Walking and other weight-bearing exercise, physiotherapy, or rehabilitation program
- Drugs such as the bisphosphonates (e.g., alendronate sodium [Fosamax]), an inhibitor of bone resorption
- Individualized hormonal therapy, including selective estrogen receptor modulators (e.g., raloxifene/ [Evista]), estrogen/progestin replacement therapy or synthetic calcitonin (Miacalcin) or parathyroid hormone

Osteoarthritis

Degeneration of the cartilage in the joints is a common problem that results in osteoarthritis (see Chapter 9). In this condition, the articular cartilage becomes thin and erosions occur, impairing joint movement and causing pain, particularly in the large weight-bearing joints such as the knees and hips. In some cases, bone spurs or overgrowths develop at points of stress, further restricting movement. Pain increases with walking and other movements. Joint replacement may be necessary.

Herniated Intervertebral Disc

The fibrocartilage in the intervertebral discs in the spine degenerates with age, and a sudden stress on the back may result in herniation of a disc. This herniation causes pressure on the spinal nerves and results in severe back pain (see Chapter 14). If the pressure is not relieved, permanent damage to the nerves can result. Also, as the intervertebral discs become thinner, loss of height becomes apparent.

Other Changes

- Skeletal muscle mass declines with aging owing to both atrophy and a decreased number of fibers. Skeletal muscle fibers cannot be replaced. Loss of muscle and subcutaneous tissue leads to an increased susceptibility to skin breakdown and pressure-related ulcers because of the reduced cushion between skin and bone. Also, there is less "insulation" to retain heat in the body and less "cushioning" against falls or pressure.
- The strength of muscle contractions decreases somewhat, but this also depends on the activity level of the individual.
- Flexibility is reduced as elastic fibers degenerate throughout the body.
- Often movements become slower, stiffness becomes evident, and coordination and balance are reduced. These changes are associated with changes in the

musculoskeletal structures as well as in the neurologic components. Dressing, walking, food preparation, and many other daily activities require a longer time to complete.

Regular moderate, low-impact exercise, such as swimming or Tai Chi, helps to maintain mobility and flexibility, both by increasing the efficiency and activity of muscle and bone and by improving the circulation of blood to the tissues. Good nutrition, particularly protein, minerals, and vitamins, is also important in maintaining the integrity of the basic structures in older people.

> **THINK ABOUT 24-4**
>
> a. Using your knowledge of normal physiology, suggest how improved circulation with exercise could slow the onset of degenerative changes in the musculoskeletal system.
> b. How does pain from osteoarthritis affect the ability to exercise and maintain an appropriate body mass?
> b. Why would severe trauma to skeletal muscle such as a crush injury have permanently disabling effects?

Respiratory System Changes

In aging individuals, ventilation, both inspiration and expiration, is limited for several reasons:
- Elasticity in the lung tissue is reduced.
- The costal cartilage between the ribs and the sternum calcifies, reducing rib movement.
- Skeletal muscle (e.g., intercostal muscles) atrophies and weakens.
- Any skeletal change (e.g., rib shape) may reduce thoracic movement.

Expiration is reduced, and residual volume is increased (see Chapter 13). The more restricted lung movements lead to decreased expansion for deep breathing and coughing. Weaker skeletal muscles also reduce cough effectiveness. When the capability for initiating an effective cough is impaired, secretions tend to accumulate, and the risk of pneumonia increases.

Vascular degeneration in the lungs leads to decreased perfusion and reduced gas exchange in the alveoli. There tends to be a reduced oxygen level rather than an increased carbon dioxide level. Regular physical exercise is effective in maximizing ventilation and circulation. Breathing exercises and oxygen therapy may be helpful in assisting respiratory function in those with respiratory pathologies and supporting physical activity.

Nervous System Changes

Because neurons are not replaced after birth, a natural reduction in brain mass occurs with aging. This does not affect cognitive function in many individuals because there is a considerable reserve of neurons. Loss may occur in different areas of the brain, at different times and to varying degrees. Maintenance of high activity levels and stimulation of the nervous system in the later years appear to assist in maintaining brain function. Exposure to toxic materials such as lead tends to hasten the degeneration.

Some of the degenerative changes observed in the brain tissue include lipid accumulations in the neurons, loss of the myelin sheath, and development of abnormal neurofibrils (masses of tiny, tangled fibrils) and plaques on the cells. Vascular impairment such as arteriosclerosis hastens the degenerative process. Neurofibrils and plaques are present in much higher numbers in those who become mentally incompetent through organic brain syndrome, a condition that includes senile dementia and Alzheimer's disease (see Chapter 14). There also appears to be a decreased cellular response in the brain to neurotransmitter chemicals such as norepinephrine, leading to delays in synaptic transmission.

General changes in function commonly noticed in older persons include slower response time, decreased reflexes, and short-term memory lapses. However, past experiences can greatly facilitate decision making and the learning process. It has been documented that the elderly can learn new information and skills, although the process is slower because the individual incorporates more information and uses more functions of the brain rather than learning by rote.

The autonomic nervous system does not always provide adequate adaptation, resulting in decreased tolerance to extreme hot or cold temperatures. The elderly feel chilled owing to poor blood circulation, decreased metabolism, and decreased activity levels. Often there is reduced temperature sensitivity in the skin when touching hot or cold surfaces.

Changes usually occur in the special senses as well. In the eye, the iris and its associated muscles degenerate, resulting in decreased adaptation by the pupil to light and possible obstruction of flow of aqueous humor, leading to increased intraocular pressure and glaucoma (see Chapter 15). The lens tends to become yellow and less transparent, interfering with color perception, especially blue hues. Night vision is impaired, and many elderly people are unable to drive safely when it is dark. The lens eventually may become opaque as cataracts develop. If vision is lost, surgery may be required to remove the cataract. The lens also becomes larger and less elastic, causing presbyopia (farsightedness) and possibly cataracts. Vascular degeneration may affect the retina of the eye, which contains the nerve cells for receiving images, and this condition causes permanent visual loss.

Hearing loss associated with aging is usually caused by degenerative changes in the inner ear in either the nerve receptor cells of the cochlea or the nerve fibers supplying the ear. In noisy surroundings, it may become difficult to discriminate among sounds, impairing communication and deterring socialization.

The senses of taste and smell often diminish with aging. Taste may be altered by reduced salivary secretions or decreased perception within the central nervous system. The ability to discriminate among odors is reduced. Diminished powers of taste and smell may impair appetite and nutrition.

THINK ABOUT 24-5

Describe four neurologic changes that can be expected to occur in an older individual.

Digestive System Changes and Nutrition

Maintenance of good nutrition is a problem in many elderly. Sometimes the older person feels that less food is needed and components such as meat (protein) are unnecessary at this stage of life. In the mouth, loss of teeth because of periodontal disease (inflammation and infection in the tissue surrounding the teeth) and decreased salivary secretions frequently restrict dietary choices as the older person experiences difficulty in chewing many foods. Often dentures are not satisfactory for chewing as the gums and bone recede. The mucosa thins and blood flow is reduced. The fragile tissues in the mouth are easily irritated by ill-fitting dentures or accumulated food particles. Xerostomia, or dry mouth, is common because the amount of saliva is reduced. Decreased saliva may also result from use of certain drugs or from the mouth-breathing associated with many respiratory problems. Swallowing difficulties resulting from neurologic causes or mechanical obstructions such as scar tissue or hiatal hernia may develop (see Chapter 17). The need for a soft diet and other factors such as lack of socialization, fatigue, restricted mobility, or financial concerns may also limit food choices and interfere with nutritional status.

Obesity is common in some older individuals, particularly those who lead sedentary lives. The basal metabolic rate (BMR) decreases significantly as one ages. This reduction must be accompanied by a decrease in the intake of fats and carbohydrates to maintain an appropriate weight. In some cases, excessive carbohydrate and fat intake may mask the signs of protein, fiber, or vitamin deficits. Obesity increases cardiac workload as well as the likelihood of atherosclerosis and hypertension. Gallstones are also a complication of obesity, as is osteoarthritis affecting the weight-bearing joints. Insulin resistance caused by obesity is an important factor in metabolic syndrome leading to altered glucose and lipid metabolism as well as type 2 diabetes.

Atrophy of the mucosa and glands of the digestive tract frequently reduces digestive secretions and absorption of essential nutrients. Absorption of vitamin B_{12}, calcium, and iron may be impaired but can be replaced by vitamin B_{12} injections plus more easily absorbed forms of calcium and iron. Decreased mucus secretion and thinning of the mucosa predisposes the older person to peptic ulcer development. Unfortunately, signs of ulcers are vague or may be masked by self-medication in the early stages.

Older individuals are predisposed to malignancies in the digestive tract, particularly in the stomach and colon, which may be related to hereditary factors as well as to dietary intake. Carcinogenic substances in the diet are more hazardous when they are associated with constipation because of the prolonged exposure of the tissues to these substances during transit through the gut. Constipation is common in the elderly. Many factors contribute to it, including decreased activity, low fiber and fluid intake, and excessive use of laxatives. Chronic constipation frequently leads to hemorrhoids.

THINK ABOUT 24-6

a. Using your knowledge of normal physiology, list the factors that lead to constipation.
b. Describe several possible pathologic conditions involving the digestive tract in older people.
c. Explain why obesity is undesirable in the elderly.

Urinary System Changes

Kidney function is reduced with aging owing to loss of glomeruli and degeneration of the tubules and blood vessels. The kidneys have a diminished ability to compensate for rapid changes in electrolyte and acid levels and may have a reduced capacity to secrete drugs into the urine, resulting in excessively high levels of drugs in the blood.

A major complication of aging is reduced control of bladder function as the muscles of the urethra and bladder become weaker. Reduced bladder capacity and incomplete bladder emptying result in frequency, nocturia (frequent urination during the night), and infection. In women, the pelvic floor muscles have often been stretched and weakened by childbirth, reducing the ability of the external sphincter to restrict urinary outflow. Also, decreased estrogen levels may decrease smooth muscle tone. Sensory perception of a full bladder is reduced, and this problem, combined with a weakened urethral sphincter, often results in incontinence (involuntary voiding of urine). Incontinence usually results in incomplete emptying of the bladder, which leads to residual urine and frequent urinary tract and bladder infections (cystitis) (see Chapter 18).

Other Factors

Infections are common in the elderly, in whom poor circulation impairs the normal defense mechanisms, and tissue healing is delayed owing to the reduced rate of mitosis. Although the antibody pool is large, the immune response to new microbes is less effective because lymphocytes are slower to respond to antigens and are less active in the later years. Skin breakdown and ulcers may predispose those with immune-deficient states to infection.

Surveys of chronic care facilities indicate a high incidence of urinary tract infections. Men are at risk because of prostatic obstruction and women because of bladder prolapse, incontinence, and thinner mucosa in the bladder. Both sexes tend to have more frequent catheterizations or instrumentation, predisposing to infection.

Cancer is more common in the elderly because the immune system becomes a less effective surveillance unit, and older people have had a higher cumulative exposure to carcinogens (see Chapter 20). The incidence of breast cancer in women and prostate cancer in men rises dramatically with increasing age.

Older people are more subject to *autoimmune* disorders and more *degenerative* pathologies related to wear and tear, many of which are *chronic* progressive disorders. Adaptation to *stressors* is slower in the elderly and more difficult because the systems may be unable to respond to the increased demands.

Multiple Disorders

Multiple disorders are common in the older population. Osteoarthritis may lead to obesity and diabetes; cardiovascular disease may lead to changes in sexual function, cognitive deficits, or respiratory problems. It is important to ensure that the older adult with multi-system disorders is treated for all the interacting problems by all health care workers. If one problem is ignored, it may well lead to exacerbation of the problem and further complications.

Many elderly people take a large number of *medications*, both prescribed drugs and over-the-counter (OTC—no prescription required) medications and herbal remedies. These combinations increase the possibility of undesirable drug interactions, particularly if an individual is consulting several doctors (see Chapter 3). Sometimes patients become confused regarding dosage; therefore written instructions and a system to monitor timing are essential to prevent a missed dose or an overdose. Other problems with medications in the elderly include a higher risk of idiosyncratic or unexpected reactions, toxic effects caused by unpredictable absorption, distribution, and elimination of drugs, and impaired function such as lethargy or lack of coordination. Noncompliance may be an issue. As the tissue receptors and body mass change in the elderly, it is often necessary to adjust the dosage and combinations of medications.

THINK ABOUT 24-7

Suggest three ways by which the changes common to aging may be delayed to some extent.

CASE STUDY A

Complications of Aging

Mrs. H., age 85, is living alone in her family home after the death of her spouse 6 years ago. Recently, she has been using a cane to walk because of "stiff joints" in her knees and hips. Before this, she usually walked for 1 to 2 hours per day in her small community neighborhood, but finds it too tiring and painful these days. She has lost 22 lb (10 kg) and states that she finds it difficult to shop and cook for herself. She states that she takes a vitamin pill each day, but usually has tea and a few cookies or toast when she is hungry. Blood tests reveal hemoglobin of 90 g/L, elevated electrolytes, and elevated hematocrit. She is diagnosed with anemia and dehydration as well as osteoarthritis in several joints. Her physician indicates she is not healthy enough to consider joint replacement at this time.

1. What is the probable cause of Mrs. H.'s anemia and how does anemia affect her health?
2. How might Mrs. H.'s malnutrition affect her ability to fight infection or maintain tissue integrity?
3. What role has pain played in the development of Mrs. H.'s malnourished state?
4. Why does Mrs. H. have an elevated hematocrit and elevated electrolytes?
5. Mrs. H. does not want to take any medications for her joint pain, stating that "I am old and pain is to be expected." How is control of her joint pain related to prevention of future malnutrition?

CASE STUDY B

Alzheimer's Disease

Mr. J. is a 75-year-old widower and quite active. He has a history of elevated blood pressure, which he controls effectively with diet and exercise at the local community center. Recently he has been neglecting his appearance and hygiene and his friends at the community center have noted his absence from many activities. He has missed appointments with his nurse practitioner at the local clinic stating that he thought the appointments were "next week." While playing cards with friends, he becomes angry and throws his cards down, saying, "This is a stupid game!" His adult daughter visits him while on a business trip in a nearby city and notes his confusion and irritability. When the nurse practitioner refers him to a gerontology assessment unit, a preliminary diagnosis of early Alzheimer's disease is made.

1. What are the possible causes of Mr. J.'s irritability?
2. How will early Alzheimer's disease affect his ability to control his weight and blood pressure as he has done in the past?
3. What problems does Mr. J. face if medication is prescribed for his elevated blood pressure?
4. What potential complications could occur if Mr. J.'s weight increases to 20% over the desirable weight?

CASE STUDY C

Multiple Disorders of Aging

Mrs. B.N. is 67 years of age and has had a long history of arthritis, which is treated with anti-inflammatory medication. Her doctor has prescribed a drug to protect her stomach, but the drug is very expensive. She has chosen to take the "arthritis pills" without the "stomach pills" because her stomach feels fine. Recently she has had indigestion, which is relieved somewhat by eating. She also noticed hard, black tarlike stools.

The indigestion becomes very painful and she vomits several times one morning. She is weak and lies down to rest, but her nausea and vomiting continue. When her heart begins to beat as though it "is trying to run away with me," she calls a friend to take her to the hospital. She is examined and a diagnosis of acute gastritis and irregular heartbeat is made. Treatment is started.

1. What fluid and electrolyte imbalances can be caused by vomiting? How are these imbalances related to Mrs. B.N.'s irregular heartbeat?
2. Mrs. B.N. has experienced an irregular heartbeat that reduces cardiac output and may cause blood to pool in the atria of the heart. What are two potential problems that Mrs. B.N. may experience from the altered function of the heart?
3. What has caused the change in Mrs. B.N.'s stools and what potential problem can occur if this continues?

CHAPTER SUMMARY

Aging begins after birth, but the effects vary considerably with the individual, not with chronologic age. With aging, a general reduction occurs in cell and organ function. Possible factors contributing to the aging process include apoptosis, effects of "wear-and-tear," metabolic products accumulating in cells, and increased autoimmune reactions in the body.

- Hormones other than the sex hormones normally continue to be secreted at normal levels. Women demonstrate some tissue degeneration in the reproductive structures. Most men develop some degree of benign prostatic hypertrophy.
- Cancer frequently develops in the reproductive systems of men and women.
- Skin and mucosal membranes become thinner and blood flow is reduced.
- The major change in the cardiovascular system involves arterial degeneration.
- Osteoporosis develops frequently in postmenopausal women related to factors such as decreased estrogen levels, more sedentary lifestyle and diet, as well as genetic predisposition.
- Osteoarthritis or herniated intervertebral disc impairs mobility in many older individuals.
- Ventilation capacity is reduced in the elderly.
- Older persons may experience slower neurologic response times and reflexes, but past experience and

acquired knowledge facilitate decision making and learning.

- Degenerative changes in the eyes and ears often impair vision and hearing.

- Many individuals do not receive adequate nutrition.
- The kidneys are not as capable of retaining fluid, and bladder control may be less effective.

STUDY QUESTIONS

1. Describe appropriate guidelines for a healthy diet for an older individual.
2. Explain the different ways in which regular moderate exercise can benefit an older person.
3. Suggest some reasons why the aging process varies among different individuals.
4. Why are infections more common in elderly individuals?

ADDITIONAL RESOURCES

Abrams WB, editor: *Merck Manual of Geriatrics*, ed 3, Whitehouse Station, NJ, 2000, Merck.

Applegate EJ: *The Anatomy and Physiology Learning System Textbook*, ed 2, Philadelphia, 2000, Saunders.

Guyton AC, Hall JE: *Textbook of Medical Physiology*, ed 11, Philadelphia, 2006, Saunders.

Web Sites

http://nihseniorhealth.gov *National Institutes of Health-seniors health issues*

http://www.nia.nih.gov *National Institute on Aging*

http://www.geron.uga.edu *The University of Georgia College of Public Health Institute of Gerontology*

CHAPTER 25

Immobility and Associated Problems

CHAPTER OUTLINE

LEARNING OBJECTIVES

After studying this chapter, the student is expected to:

1. Describe the possible effect of immobility on skeletal muscle, bone, and joints.
2. Discuss the development of decubitus ulcers.
3. Explain the changes in blood pressure and potential thrombus formation.
4. List the potential problems related to respiratory function.
5. Discuss the common effects of immobility on appetite, bowel function, and urinary function.
6. Discuss the potential effects of immobility on the nervous system and psychological implications.
7. Describe the potential effect of immobility on a child's growth.

KEY TERMS

atelectasis	extensor	osteoblastic	stasis
basal metabolic rate	flaccidity	osteoclastic	supine
contracture	flexor	paraplegia	
decubitus ulcers	hemiplegia	pneumonia	
diplegia	orthostatic hypotension	quadriplegia	

Factors Involving Immobility

Immobility, or lack of movement, may involve only one part of the body such as a fractured arm in a cast. A part of the body may be affected, as occurs with paralysis: one side of the body (hemiplegia), the lower half of the body (paraplegia), or the trunk and all four limbs (quadriplegia). Diplegia refers to symmetric paralysis in any area of the body. In a coma or during an acute illness the entire body may be immobilized. The effects of such inactivity depend on the extent of the immobilization and its duration. Physiotherapy or passive exercise imposed on the involved area of the body can minimize the effects of lack of voluntary movement. Respiratory therapy is significant in preventing infections such as pneumonia.

When the body is supine (lying on the back), the loss of the force of gravity affects many of its natural functions, primarily in the intestines and urinary tract. Other noticeable effects result from the lack of stress normally exerted on bone by skeletal muscle and the decreased circulation of blood. Bed rest also alters respiratory function, metabolism, and renal function.

Musculoskeletal System Effects

Inactive muscle loses strength, endurance, and mass very quickly. Perhaps you have seen an arm or a leg shriveled up with *atrophied* muscle (often called disuse atrophy) after it has been confined to a cast for several weeks. Loss of muscular strength due to immobility progresses at a rate of about 12% each week. After 3 to 5 weeks of immobility due to bed rest almost one-half of the muscular strength is lost. Correct positioning and reduction of abnormal stress on immobilized muscles and joints are important because these structures may stretch or shorten, resulting in abnormal fixation of a joint, altering biomechanics. For example, an ankle may develop contractures when a tight, heavy blanket or improper positioning puts excessive and inappropriate pressure on the foot (Fig. 25-1). Generally flexor muscles are stronger than the opposing extensor muscles (which atrophy more than the flexor muscles), and this imbalance may allow an inactive joint to take an abnormal position if flexibility is not maintained by range-of-motion exercises. With inactivity, tendons and ligaments shorten and lose elasticity. Prolonged immobility causes fibrous tissue to replace muscle cells, leading to muscle wasting and weakening, decreased flexibility, further possibly irreversible deformity (contracture), and loss of function.

The lack of muscular activity impairs venous return, which causes pooling of blood in dependent areas of the body, development of dependent edema, and a decrease in cardiac output, which may cause dizziness or fainting when changing position.

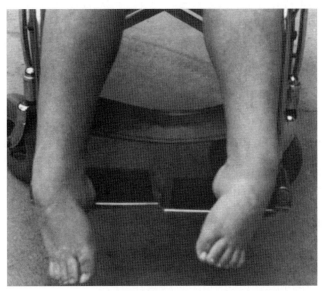

FIGURE 25-1 Contracture of the feet in a patient with muscular dystrophy. *(From Jahss MH:* Disorders of the Foot and Ankle, *vol. 1, ed 2, Philadelphia, 1991, Saunders.)*

Bone deteriorates with inactivity. Bone is a "living" tissue in which new bone is constantly forming (osteoblastic activity) and other bone is being resorbed (osteoclastic activity). Bone demineralization occurs because the lack of weight bearing and muscle action reduces osteoblastic activity or bone formation; however, osteoclastic activity continues. This process leads to loss of bone mass and *osteoporosis* with the potential for spontaneous fractures if undue stress is placed on the bones (see Chapters 24 and 9).

The breakdown of muscle and bone tissue initially results in elevated serum levels of nitrogen wastes such as creatinine and in elevated serum calcium. Hypercalcemia may cause renal calculi or kidney stones if fluid intake is inadequate and the urine becomes too concentrated (see Chapter 18). Also a high serum calcium level can further impede muscle activity because it decreases muscle tone and leads to flaccidity or loss of muscle tone. Passive range-of-motion exercises and weight bearing if tolerated on a regular basis are helpful in preventing these complications.

Tendons and ligaments that connect the muscles to bone and maintain joint structure also require movement to maintain their structure and functionality. After 4 to 6 days of immobility these forms of connective tissue begin to shorten and the density of the tissue increases limiting flexibility and range of motion.

THINK ABOUT 25-1

a. Explain effects of immobility on posture and joints.
b. Explain how immobility can lead to osteoporosis.

Cutaneous Effects

The skin breaks down easily when its circulation is impaired and cell regeneration is reduced. Blood supply is often reduced in places where the skin is stretched over bony projections and there is little fatty or muscular tissue to cushion the weight of the body. Areas that are particularly vulnerable to poor blood perfusion include the ischial tuberosities, sacrum, the greater trochanter of the hip, the heels, and the elbows. Pressure at these points causes ischemia and necrosis of tissue (Fig. 25-2), leading to decubitus ulcers (pressure sores or bedsores). Other factors that promote skin breakdown and development of decubiti include:

- Poor general circulation or anemia
- Edema
- Inadequate subcutaneous tissue in the elderly or debilitated person
- Loss of sensation
- Prolonged static positioning
- Mechanical irritation or friction by clothing, braces, or other equipment
- Excessive moisture from perspiration or urine
- Poor personal hygiene
- Inadequate nutrition or hydration
- Trauma to the skin due to friction against clothing or sheets if a patient is moved without due care or slides down in bed, or if skeletal muscle spasms occur; adhesive tape may irritate the skin directly or indirectly when it is removed

Pressure ulcers are difficult to heal unless the predisposing conditions can be removed.

The affected area first appears red, and then superficial skin breakdown is apparent. Ulceration follows, and the area may become a purplish-red color if the damage is deep. Eventually necrosis destroys deeper tissue, and a large open area develops with full-thickness damage. Local infection is common.

The risk of skin breakdown can be reduced if sensitive areas are protected by sheepskin pads or flotation devices and the patient's position is changed frequently to avoid prolonged pressure in certain areas, thereby maintaining adequate circulation.

> ### THINK ABOUT 25-2
> a. Explain why an elderly person confined to a wheelchair might develop decubitus ulcers.
> b. Suggest several specific ways of reducing the risk of skin breakdown and ulceration.

Cardiovascular System Effects

Initially when a person is fully immobilized, the horizontal body position leads to more blood returning to the heart from the legs. Blood pools in the trunk, especially in the lungs. Initially this increased venous return leads to an increased intracardial pressure, increasing the heart rate and stroke volume.

With *prolonged* immobility and bed rest, venous return and cardiac output are reduced, and the patient is subject to orthostatic hypotension with short periods of dizziness or fainting, pallor and sweating, and rapid pulse whenever the body position is quickly changed. Normally skeletal muscle contractions as part of regular activity assist in returning the venous blood to the heart. Also when the body position changes from supine to upright, reflex vasoconstriction occurs in the skin and viscera to promote venous return. Adequate venous return ensures sufficient cardiac output to supply the brain and prevent a drop in blood pressure and fainting. When a patient becomes mobile after a prolonged period of bed rest, it may take several weeks for the reflex controls to return to normal, ensuring adequate circulation.

Other problems occur when the blood pools in dependent areas. The increased volume of blood in these areas leads to increased capillary pressure and edema (see Chapter 2). A persistent increase in interstitial fluid (edema) leads to reduced arterial flow and capillary exchange of nutrients in that dependent area, thus predisposing the person to tissue necrosis, ulcers, and infection in the area. Even if a small area such as an arm is immobilized, the limb should be elevated to reduce edema.

The stasis or pooling of blood associated with immobility promotes thrombus formation in the veins, particularly in the legs. In addition to sluggish blood flow and decreased venous return, blood clots may be encouraged by compression or damage to blood vessels resulting from pressure related to the body position in bed or a wheelchair. Action of skeletal muscles, such as the contractions of the calf muscles, compresses the major veins in the legs aiding in the venous flow back to the heart. Blood clotting is also encouraged in patients with dehydration or cancer by the increased

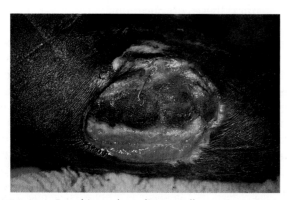

FIGURE 25-2 Decubitus ulcer. *(From Callen J, Greer K, Hood A, et al: Color Atlas of Dermatology, Philadelphia, 1993, Saunders.)*

coagulability of the blood associated with these conditions. The combination of three factors; venous stasis, hypercoagulability and blood vessel damage are known as Virchow's triad and when present, they dramatically increase the chances of a deep vein thrombosis. Thrombi are a threat because a thrombus may break away with movement or massage, resulting in a *pulmonary embolus*, which has serious consequences for respiratory and cardiovascular function (see Chapter 13). Depending on the primary problem, antiembolic stockings, exercises, or anticoagulant therapy may be helpful prophylactic measures.

Respiratory System Effects

Initially when a person is immobilized, there is less demand for oxygen because metabolism is decreased, unless some factor such as infection is increasing the resting rate of metabolism or basal metabolic rate (BMR); therefore the respiratory system can easily meet the body's requirements. Usually respirations become slow and shallow.

When the person is supine in bed, deep breathing and coughing become more difficult because chest expansion is restricted by body weight and the upward pressure of the abdominal contents against the diaphragm. Gas exchange is decreased as thoracic capacity is reduced and ventilation is diminished. Any muscle weakness will impair the effectiveness of respiratory efforts. Many drugs, including sedatives (to promote sleep and reduce anxiety) and analgesics (to control pain), depress neuromuscular activity and the respiratory control center, leading to slowed, shallow respirations.

When a person is immobilized, secretions build up in the airways and are difficult to remove because the cough mechanism is less effective. Ciliary action may be reduced if nutrition is impaired or the patient is a smoker. Other factors leading to increased secretions in the lungs include more viscous mucus due to dehydration and inflammation due to instrumentation, related to surgery or testing procedures. Increased fluids in the lungs further impair lung expansion. Stasis of secretions predisposes the patient to serious respiratory complications. The increased mucous secretions frequently lead to infection (hypostatic pneumonia) or obstruction of the airway and collapse of the lung (atelectasis). Pneumonia and atelectasis may also result from aspiration of food or water intake, which occurs more easily when the patient is immobilized or in a supine position. Normally in the upright position, gravity assists the rapid movement of food down the esophagus.

Respiratory therapy, including breathing exercises, may be helpful and are frequently part of the preoperative preparation. Personal respirometers provide an incentive for patients to improve their ventilation capacity before and after surgery.

THINK ABOUT 25-3

Explain why pneumonia is a common occurrence in immobilized persons.

Digestive System Effects

The major problem associated with immobility and the gastrointestinal tract is constipation. Elimination is affected by the slower passage of feces through the intestine due to muscle inactivity and body position, which results in a harder stool. In people who are ill, the intake of food, fiber, and fluid is often reduced, leading to reduced peristalsis in the intestine and more water absorption from the fecal mass. Weakened muscles make defecation more difficult, as does the awkwardness of using a bedpan in a supine position. The elderly patient is particularly vulnerable to bowel complications. In addition to using appropriate laxatives, an increase in fiber and fluid intake will reduce the problem of constipation in the patient with decreased activity.

When a person is inactive, appetite is often reduced, leading to decreased dietary intake. This may result in a negative nitrogen balance (protein deficit), especially when muscle tissue is breaking down. The protein imbalance contributes to a low hemoglobin level and delays in healing. Unfortunately, the decreased food intake usually aggravates fatigue and depression, which further decrease appetite and ultimately may cause malnutrition and further delays in healing and recovery. New liquid products to deliver adequate calories and nutrients are somewhat easier for the immobilized person to consume. If normal nutrition cannot be maintained orally, it may be necessary to use t1otal parenteral nutrition (TPN), in which the required nutrient solution is administered directly into a vein or via a nasogastric tube.

In some cases immobility can lead to obesity. When a person is inactive, caloric intake can quickly exceed the energy expended. Also there may be an increase in snacking as a result of stress and discomfort.

Urinary System Effects

Stasis of urine in the kidneys or bladder frequently causes infection or renal calculi (stones) to develop in the urinary tract (see Chapter 18). A supine position leads to residual urine in the calyces of the kidney in the dependent area because normal drainage by gravity into the ureter is impeded. It is also difficult to empty the bladder completely into a bedpan when one is supine or the muscles are weakened. Renal calculi are more likely to develop in people with hypercalcemia caused by prolonged immobility or with reduced fluid intake. Bladder infection (cystitis) is common in immobilized people if calculi form or catheters are used to drain the urine.

Another potential effect on the urinary system involves an increase of diuresis, leading to dehydration. A blood shift into the thorax can potentially stimulate release of atrial natriuretic peptide (ANP) from the heart which acts as a powerful diuretic. This blood shift can also stretch the aortic arch and receptors in the carotid sinus, which reduces antidiuretic hormone (ADH) release. This reduction in ADH will reduce the reabsorption of water by the kidneys, which further increases the diuretic effect of the ANP and increasing overall urine output, which can lead to dehydration.

Neurological/Psychological Effects

Prolonged pressure on the skin and underlying tissue as well as resultant tissue damage can activate pain sensations as sense receptors such as exteroceptors, mechanoceptors, or nociceptors are stimulated. Over time the continued pressure can cause serious local tissue damage that can destroy the nerves, resulting in a new sensation of tingling in the affected area and eventually a total loss of feeling in the area. Damage to the nerves and innervation of the muscles can also result in spasms.

In addition to the psychological effects of pain, the person's lack of control over his or her environment can have negative psychological effects. These effects include depression, anxiety, confusion, and forgetfulness. The overall increased levels of stress involved in immobility has been linked to the release of stress hormones such as corticosteroids, which can result in widespread physiologic changes affecting an individual's overall health.

THINK ABOUT 25-4

Explain how immobility may affect the urinary system to produce a systemic as well as local effect.

Effects of Immobility on Children

When children are immobilized for an extended period of time, normal growth is often delayed because the physical movement to stimulate bone and muscle development is lost. Catch-up growth may be possible when mobility returns. Depending on the underlying condition, deformities involving the hips, spine, hands, and feet may develop. Other developmental delays are common when sensory and experiential stimulations are decreased.

CASE STUDY A

Trauma and Immobility

L.D. is a 27-year-old man who has no chronic health problems. He prides himself on keeping fit and enjoys "living on the edge." Last weekend he was thrown from his motorcycle when it spun out on a wet patch of pavement. In the emergency department, he was diagnosed with fractures of the left tibia and ribs. He reported being in pain and having difficulty breathing. He was discharged with a full leg cast and medication for pain to be taken every 4 hours as needed. He was told not to bear any weight on his affected leg and was shown how to walk with crutches.

1. How will L.D.'s broken ribs affect his respiration and what potential problem may occur if L.D. does not follow instructions to breathe deeply and cough?
2. How does the pain medication affect his ability to deep breathe and move?
3. How will L.D.'s lifestyle, health habits, and age affect healing of the damaged tissues?
4. L.D.'s pain medication makes him nauseated. Why is it important for him to maintain a diet high in calcium, protein, and vitamins C and D?
5. L.D.'s skin itches under the cast and he finds this very irritating. On one very hot day, he resorts to inserting his mother's knitting needle under the cast to scratch the skin. Why are skin breakdown and infection greater risks in the cast limb?
6. After 4 weeks L.D.'s cast seems quite loose and it is replaced with a new walking cast. L.D. is distressed to see that the leg is thinner than it was. What is the cause of the change in the size and shape of L.D.'s fractured leg?
7. What problems is L.D. likely to experience when the cast is finally removed from his leg?

CHAPTER SUMMARY

Immobility may involve one part of the body (e.g., a limb) or a major portion of the body, and it may be temporary or permanent.

- Effects on muscle and bone develop within a short period. Skeletal muscle atrophies with loss of strength and mass, osteoporosis occurs, and contractures may arise.
- Skin breakdown or decubitus ulcers develop easily, particularly where pressure causes ischemia after the person remains in one position for a long time.
- Orthostatic hypotension and thromboembolism are two problems associated with cardiovascular function.
- Deep breathing and cough effectiveness may be restricted by immobility, predisposing to stasis of secretions in the lungs, followed by pneumonia.
- Reduced peristalsis associated with immobility frequently leads to constipation.
- Immobility may predispose to urinary stasis, renal calculi, infection and dehydration
- Immobility can cause the stimulation of sensory receptors in the skin and effected tissue leading to pain.
- Growth in children is frequently delayed during periods of immobility.

STUDY QUESTIONS

1. Explain how immobility affects the circulation.
2. Give several reasons why healing may be delayed during a period of immobility.
3. Explain how frequent changes of position would affect:
   a. the amount of interstitial fluid in an area
   b. respiratory function
   c. the skin

ADDITIONAL RESOURCES

Hockenberry MJ: *Wong's Essentials of Pediatric Nursing*, ed 7, St. Louis, 2005, Mosby.

Lewis SM, Heitkemper MM, Dirksen SR, O'Brien PG, Bucher L: *Medical-Surgical Nursing: Assessment and Management of Clinical Problems*, ed 7, St. Louis, 2007, Mosby.

Potter PA, Perry AG: *Fundamentals of Nursing*, ed 7, St. Louis, 2009, Mosby.

Web Sites

http://www.geronurseonline.org *Gerontological Nursing (American Nurses Association)*

http://depts.washington.edu/rehab/sci *Northwest Regional Spinal Cord Injury System (University of Washington)*

http://nsweb.nursingspectrum.com/ce/ce127.htm *Nursing Spectrum*

http://www.nursingtimes.net/ *Nursing Times*

http://www. ncbi.nlm.nih.gov/ *National Center for Biotechnology Information*

CHAPTER 26

Stress and Associated Problems

CHAPTER OUTLINE

LEARNING OBJECTIVES

After studying this chapter, the student is expected to:

1. Describe the stress response.
2. Explain how the stress response is related to diseases.
3. Describe how severe stress may lead to acute renal failure, stress ulcers, or infection.
4. Suggest positive coping strategies.

KEY TERMS

bronchodilation	homeostasis	maladaptive
endorphins	lipolysis	physiologic

Review of the Stress Response

The stress response is a generalized or systemic response to a change (stressor), internal or external, and may be modified in specific situations. The role of stress in disease became more firmly established in the 20th century, when Hans Selye, in 1946, defined his *general adaptation syndrome* (GAS), or "fight or flight" concept. His work revealed that the body constantly responds to minor changes in its needs or environment, such as altered food intake or activity level, and thus maintains homeostasis. The body has built-in mechanisms that quickly compensate for physiologic changes in fluid balance or blood pressure. Minor fluctuations in body functions are normal.

A *stressor* is any factor that creates a significant change in the body or environment. It may be physical or psychological or a combination of the two. A stressor may be a real or anticipated factor, or it may be a short-term or long-term factor. Possible stressors include pain, exposure to cold temperatures, trauma, anxiety or fear, a new job, infection, or indeed, even a joyous occasion. *Stress* is considered to occur when an individual's status is altered by his or her reaction to a stressor. The stress response is the generic but complex response made by the body to any stressor. The body's physiologic response to different types of stressors is the same, although the response may vary in intensity and effects in a given situation or person. An additional, specific response may occur with certain stressors; for example, infection may initiate a fever.

Each person may *perceive* stressors differently. A certain stressor for one individual may be mildly exciting or stimulating, but for someone else the same stressor may be deeply depressing. It may even cause illness in another person. If the individual can cope with the stressor, the body returns to its normal status, but if the person cannot adapt, harmful effects may result from the stress. This may be termed "distress."

Stressors are a normal component of life and can be a positive influence on the body when appropriate coping mechanisms function well. Stressors may stimulate growth and development in many ways. Without any changes or stressors in life, a person would merely exist in a dull, inert, unresponsive form. But if a stressor is extremely severe or is perceived as a very negative influence, or when multiple factors effect change at one time, the body's adaptive mechanisms may not suffice. Then the body systems become more disrupted, maladaptive or inappropriate behavior can occur, and homeostasis is not possible for that person. Factors such as aging or pathologic disorders may interfere with an individual's ability to respond adequately to a stressor. A vicious cycle may develop when the original stressor remains, and the effects of this stressor prevent the body from coping with new stressors. In some cases, more damage results, adding to the stress and lessening the person's coping capabilities even further, thereby decreasing the probability of a return to normal status. In the same way, maladaptive behaviors such as ignoring the stressor or eating unwisely are likely to add additional problems without removing the original stressful factor.

THINK ABOUT 26-1

a. Give examples of non-physical stressors that can result in physiological responses.
b. Describe several coping mechanisms that can be used in dealing with physical stressors.
c. Describe several coping mechanisms that can be used in dealing with psychological stressors.

Selye originally defined three stages in the stress response (GAS). In the alarm stage, the body's defenses are mobilized by activation of the hypothalamus, sympathetic nervous system, and adrenal glands. In the second, or resistance stage, hormonal levels are elevated, and essential body systems operate at peak performance. The final stage, or stage of exhaustion, occurs when the body is unable to respond further or is damaged by the increased demands. Extensive research into various aspects of stress has followed Selye's work. It has been found that the stress response involves an integrated series of actions, including the hypothalamus and the pituitary gland, the sympathetic nervous system, the adrenal medulla, and the adrenal cortex. The locus ceruleus, a collection of norepinephrine-secreting cells in the brain stem, provides the rapid response in the nervous system. Any type of stressor immediately initiates a marked increase in ACTH secretion followed by a great increase in cortisol secretion. The major actions are summarized in Figure 26-1.

Significant effects of the stress response include:
- Elevated blood pressure and increased heart rate
- Bronchodilation and increased ventilation
- Increased blood glucose levels (resulting from glycogenolysis and gluconeogenesis in the liver and protein catabolism in muscle as well as lipolysis)
- Arousal of the central nervous system
- Decreased inflammatory and immune responses (cortisol reduces the early and later stages)

These activities increase the general level of function in critical areas of the body such as the brain, the heart, and the skeletal muscles by such mechanisms as increasing oxygen levels, increasing circulation, and increasing

the rate of cell metabolism. Short-term stressors, mild or moderate, appear to enhance cognitive function and short-term memory. The stress response also results in an increased release of endorphins, which act as pain-blocking agents (see Chapter 4).

In most cases, the body responds positively, the stressor is dealt with, the stress response diminishes, and body activity returns to normal. Additional distress results if the state of stress is severe or prolonged, or if the individual's adaptive mechanisms are impaired for some reason. It may be noticed that when an illness requires additional treatment, such as hospitalization or physiotherapy, extra stressors are added that may overwhelm the patient. For example, hospitalization may give rise to fear and pain or to anxiety associated with separation from the family or job, change in routine and diet, and loss of privacy and control over one's life. In other cases, hospitalization may offer positive relief from the burden of illness.

With major or prolonged stress, intellectual function and memory are frequently disrupted. One factor related to the change is the large amount of glucocorticoids released because memory impairment has been shown to occur in persons taking large doses of glucocorticoids.

THINK ABOUT 26-2

a. Using your knowledge of normal physiology, explain the probable source of the increased glucose level in the blood with stress.
b. Name the organs in which vasoconstriction occurs and blood flow diminishes during a stress response. Name the areas that have increased blood flow.
c. State two ways by which oxygen supplies to the brain may increase during a stress response.
d. List the hormones released during the stress response and two significant actions for each.

Stress and Disease

Greater than 40% of all adults experience adverse effects from stress and 75% to 90% of doctor's office visits are for stress-related problems and complaints. Stress may cause a specific problem such as a headache, which may develop during a stress response or, in some persons, as the stressor is relieved. Prolonged *vasoconstriction* may cause inflammation and necrosis that result in stomatitis (ulcers in the mouth) and necrotizing periodontal disease (Fig. 26-2), or nausea. More severe complications may arise if reduced blood supply impairs function or causes necrosis in the gastrointestinal tract or kidneys. In some patients who have preexisting pathologic conditions, a stress response may become an additive or exacerbating factor, creating an acute complication or adding to the severity of the original disorder. For

PROCESS

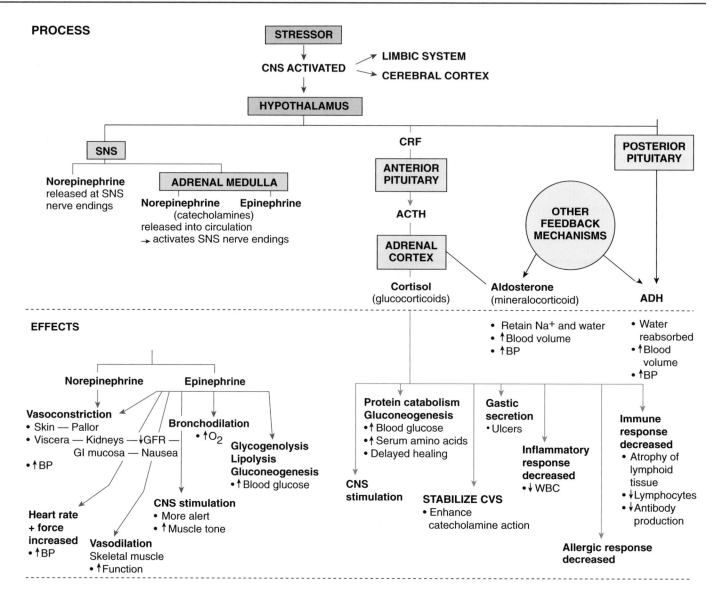

FIGURE 26-1 The stress response. ACTH, adrenocorticotropic hormone; ADH, antidiuretic hormone; BP, blood pressure; CNS, central nervous system; CRF, corticotropin-releasing factor; CVS, cardiovascular system; GFR, glomerular filtration rate; GI, gastrointestinal; SNS, sympathetic nervous system; WBC, white blood cell.

example, elevation of blood pressure or cardiac dysrhythmia (irregular heart rate) resulting from a stress response may seriously aggravate the condition of an individual with a damaged heart.

Stress has been shown to be a precipitating factor in some disorders. Chronic infections such as herpes simplex (cold sores) often erupt when the person is stressed. Acute asthma attacks or a seizure may be triggered in some individuals by a stressful situation. The onset of cancer or an infection frequently follows a serious life crisis, which suggests that the immune system has been depressed.

In many chronic disorders stress is an exacerbating factor. The stressor may be physical or emotional. For example, multiple sclerosis, rheumatoid arthritis, systemic lupus erythematosus, asthma, acne, ulcerative colitis, and eczema are some conditions that usually become more acute when a stressor is present. It is important for a person with a chronic illness to develop improved coping mechanisms and an adequate support system to delay exacerbations or progressive degeneration in chronic illness.

In some diseases such as hypertension, coronary artery disease, and diabetes mellitus, stress is thought

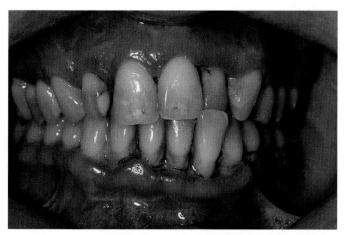

FIGURE 26-2 A possible effect of stress in the oral cavity: inflammation and necrosis (necrotizing periodontal disease seen in young adults at academic examination time). *(Courtesy of Evie Jesin, RRDH, BSc, George Brown College, Toronto, Ontario, Canada.)*

to be an etiologic factor. It has been noted that serum cholesterol is elevated during stress, and the reactive vasoconstriction affects blood pressure and blood vessels when stress is sustained.

A brief selection of stress-related disorders is summarized in Box 26-1.

Potential Effects of Prolonged or Severe Stress

Severe stress may lead to a variety of serious complications, such as renal failure or perforating stomach ulcers. *Acute renal failure* results from prolonged severe vasoconstriction and reduced blood supply to the kidney. Reduced blood supply causes tubular necrosis, obstruction of filtrate flow, and cessation of glomerular filtration or shutdown (see Chapter 18). In some cases, permanent kidney damage results. *Stress ulcers* may develop with severe trauma; a good example is Curling's ulcers, which are associated with burns. Stress ulcers are multiple gastric ulcers, often asymptomatic, but nevertheless dangerous because they frequently manifest with gastric hemorrhage (see Chapter 17). Several factors in the stress response contribute to ulcer formation. Intense vasoconstriction in the gastric mucosa decreases mucosal regeneration and mucus production, decreased motility causes stasis of chyme in the stomach, and the catabolic effects of glucocorticoids delay tissue regeneration—all of which contribute to ulcer formation.

When possible, preventive measures are taken to reduce the risk of complications from severe stress. For example, to prevent acute renal failure, caregivers promote fluid flow through the kidneys by encouraging increased hydration, and physicians order drugs that dilate the renal arterioles and thus protect renal function. To guard against stress ulcers, medications may be administered to protect the gastric mucosa and reduce acid secretions, thereby preventing ulcer development.

BOX 26-1   A Selection of Stress-Related Disorders

Gastrointestinal System
Peptic ulcer, stress ulcers
Ulcerative colitis
Regional ileitis
Nausea, diarrhea
Stomatitis, periodontitis

Nervous System
Multiple sclerosis
Seizures
Depression
CVA (stroke)

Respiratory System
Asthma

Musculoskeletal System
Rheumatoid arthritis

Cardiovascular System
Hypertension
Angina
Congestive Heart Failure

Skin
Herpes Simplex
Eczema
Acne

Urinary System
Acute renal failure
Cirrhosis due to alcohol abuse

Other
Cancer
Infection
Autoimmune Disorders
Obesity

Another potential complication of severe stress is *infection,* which is related to depression of the inflammatory response and the immune system by increased cortisol secretion. Because these body defense mechanisms are reduced, opportunistic infections may develop, and the person becomes susceptible to infection by unusual organisms that are not normally pathogenic (see Chapter 7). The lack of an inflammatory response may mask the signs of infection until it is well established. In time, lymphoid tissue atrophies, and the circulating leukocytes are reduced in number and function. The increased incidence and growth of malignant tumors associated with severe stress have also been linked with the decreased efficiency of the surveillance function of the immune system.

Continued stress may impede the *healing* of tissue following trauma or surgery. Two major factors are involved. First, the increased amounts of cortisol reduce protein synthesis and tissue regeneration, and second, the increased catecholamine levels lead to vasoconstriction, reduced blood supply, and reduced delivery of nutrients to the traumatized area. In some cases, these effects lead to an increased risk of infection and increased amounts of scar tissue at the site of the trauma or the surgery.

Posttraumatic stress disorder (PTSD) has been recognized as a serious consequence of a major disaster. It was first recognized in war veterans, and now has been diagnosed in individuals involved in catastrophic events or personal trauma. This syndrome usually occurs within 3 months of the event, but may cause symptoms years later. Three categories of symptoms may occur: revisiting or reliving the event, avoidance of certain activities and a lack of emotional response, and a dissociative state in which the person is non-responsive. There is also a high risk of the person with PTSD developing a dependence on drugs and/or alcohol. With treatment, symptoms usually resolve in 6 months, but in some cases symptoms persist or reoccur for several years.

THINK ABOUT 26-3

Explain how reduced blood flow in an area can interfere with healing and increase the risk of infection.

Coping with Stress

To prevent stress from becoming a negative influence on the body, it is important for each individual to recognize stress-inducing factors and discover the best way to deal with them, both emotionally and behaviorally. People must take appropriate action to solve the problem or develop improved coping mechanisms if the stressor cannot be removed. For many people, this is easier to say than to do, especially when a stressor becomes overwhelming or when multiple stressors develop. Fatigue, age, inadequate nutrition, insufficient knowledge, or lack of emotional support are among the factors that may interfere with an appropriate response.

A support system, even short term, is essential to minimize the risk of development of pathologic effects caused by stress. Strategies may include:

- Ensuring adequate rest and a healthy diet
- A change in lifestyle in order to adapt to the new situation
- Adopting a regular moderate exercise program that assists in controlling stress, particularly if it is undertaken at a time when stress levels are high:
  - Aerobic exercise such as cycling, swimming, or running is useful to release muscle tension and improve circulation as well as to provide a distraction
  - During aerobic exercise, the body uses more fats for energy, and therefore blood sugar levels remain more stable

- A relatively constant blood supply to the brain prevents mood swings and reduces irritability
- Engaging in distracting activities for a time and then assessing the problem more objectively
- Counseling and support services
- Using relaxation techniques, imagery, biofeedback therapy, and music and art therapy
- Using antianxiety medications (minor tranquilizers such as lorazepam [Ativan] for a short period of time). These medications must be used with caution because even low doses can have adverse side effects such as drowsiness, memory loss, impaired judgement, confusion, nausea, and lack of energy.
- Undertaking a methodical approach, assessing options or goals, and making immediate decisions

Just as each person perceives stressors differently, each must develop an individualized set of coping mechanisms, and these skills will probably have to be modified periodically.

It is well to recognize any tendency toward maladaptive behavior at an early stage in the response to stress. Avoiding sleep, eating junk food, drinking too much coffee, and smoking constantly are behaviors that are more likely to add stress than to alleviate it.

CASE STUDY A

Situational Stress Response

L.D. is a 13-year-old healthy teenager who is very anxious about getting her wisdom teeth removed by the dentist. She is afraid that the dentist will use a needle to "freeze" her mouth. In the past, she has felt light-headed and dizzy when receiving routine immunizations in the doctor's office. Her mother thinks that L.D.'s anxious behavior is silly and tries to reassure L.D. on the drive to the dental office that everything will be fine. The dental office is quite busy and the receptionist states that the dentist has had an emergency patient and there will be a delay before L.D. will be seen. L.D. waits 30 minutes for her appointment.

1. What stressors are present for L.D.?
2. How will the delay affect L.D.'s stress response? What could reduce L.D.'s stress during the wait?
3. When L.D. is finally called by the receptionist, she gets up and immediately feels like she is going to faint. Which change in the nervous system is responsible for her hypotension? Is this part of the usual response to stressors?
4. She is sweating and her pupils are dilated. What specific changes have occurred to cause these manifestations?
5. L.D.'s mother tells her to "calm down" and "be brave." How would this likely affect the stress L.D. is experiencing?

The dentist reassures L.D. that she will use a mask to deliver the anesthetic rather than a needle and L.D. agrees to go ahead with the procedure. L.D. has four teeth extracted and is sent home. At home she experiences pain and stiffness in her jaws.

1. How will continued pain and stiffness affect tissue healing and recovery?
2. What can L.D. do to reduce her stress the next time an invasive procedure is scheduled?

CHAPTER SUMMARY

The basic stress response is the same in all situations, with variations depending on the specific stressor or cause. Stressors are a normal part of life.

- The stress response is considered to include three stages—alarm, resistance, and exhaustion—involving the activities of the hypothalamus, pituitary, sympathetic nervous system, and adrenal glands.
- Stress may cause minor problems such as headache, may precipitate a more serious problem such as a seizure or cancer, or may exacerbate a chronic illness such as ulcerative colitis.
- Severe prolonged stress or multiple stressors may have serious consequences such as development of peptic ulcer or acute renal failure.
- An individual can resolve stressful situations in a positive manner and return to a normal state using appropriate coping mechanisms.

STUDY QUESTIONS

1. List the factors or mechanisms in the stress response that contribute to increased oxygen supplies for the cells and explain how each factor contributes to the stress response.
2. Describe a recent stressor in your life and the stress response that followed it.
3. List some disorders that are stress related.
4. Describe two potential complications of severe stress.
5. Why are maladaptive coping mechanisms such as excessive eating or alcohol intake not helpful?

ADDITIONAL RESOURCES

Web Sites

http://www.cmha.ca/?s=Post+Traumatic+Stress+Disorder& submit=Search&lang=en *Canadian Mental Health Association—Post Traumatic Stress Disorder*

http://www.apahelpcenter.org/articles *American Psychological Association*

http://www.nlm.nih.gov/medlineplus/stress.html *Medline Plus: Stress*

http://www.nimh.nih.gov/ *National Institute of Mental Health*

http://www.mayoclinic.com *Mayo Clinic*

http://www.webmd.com/ *Web MD*

CHAPTER 27

Substance Abuse and Associated Problems

CHAPTER OUTLINE

LEARNING OBJECTIVES

After studying this chapter, the student is expected to:

1. Use the appropriate terminology.
2. Discuss the factors predisposing to substance abuse.
3. Identify possible signs of substance abuse.
4. Describe the problems of drug overdose, withdrawal, pregnancy, psychological effects, and infection.

KEY TERMS

chemical dependency
depressant
euphoria

hallucinogens
hepatotoxin

perception
stimulant

synergism
tolerance

Substance abuse, or chemical dependency, is a newer term used to cover the older concepts of addiction and alcoholism. Substance abuse is a matter of concern to all health care workers. A recent estimate suggests 22.6 million persons use illicit drugs, with marijuana being used by the most people; 17.6 million people experience alcohol abuse problems or alcohol dependency. In the United States in 2009 there were 37, 485 drug deaths, which exceeded the number of motor vehicle deaths.

The World Health Organization estimates that for every dollar spent in substance abuse treatment, $7 are saved in related health care. Social and economic costs are also reduced as people return to productive work in their communities. These statistics do not include individuals abusing legally acquired drugs. This chapter provides a brief introduction to the topic of substance abuse.

The World Health Organization has taken substance abuse into its global health priorities and defines it as the harmful or hazardous use of psychoactive substances, including alcohol and illicit drugs. Abuse of chemicals, whether prescribed or illicit, leads to changes in behavior, sleep patterns, and interpersonal relationships. Employment is often precarious as the individual focuses on obtaining the drug as a priority.

Most of these chemicals cause serious health problems or death if abuse is not addressed. For example, alcoholism leads to cirrhosis of the liver and brain damage. Cocaine causes damage to the heart and brain. Anabolic steroids cause heart disease. People using intravenous drugs can contract hepatitis or human immunodeficiency virus (HIV). Children born to substance abusers are directly and indirectly affected as a result of the parent's substance abuse. Many babies are born addicted and must be supported as they experience withdrawal from the agent. Family dynamics threaten the physical and mental health of the developing child, and there is a higher incidence of substance abuse among children of drug abusers. Complications can easily arise in the health care of substance abusers because their diagnostic tests may be distorted and general assessment clouded, unwanted drug interactions may occur, and pathologic processes may be initiated or aggravated by the inappropriate use of drugs.

Substance abuse has implications for the family and employer of the individual as well as for society. Because access to drugs may be facilitated in the work environment, health care workers themselves may be directly involved in substance abuse. Early recognition of dependency can lead to more successful treatment of the problem. Many professional groups, including the health professions, now provide counseling and therapy for those affected by substance abuse in the workplace.

Terminology

Terminology frequently changes in the area of substance abuse, and there may also be overlap or lack of clarity in some definitions.

- *Substance abuse,* or *chemical dependency,* is a broad term that refers to the inappropriate or unnecessary (nonmedical) use of drugs or chemicals that impairs a person's function in some way to some extent. The substance is desired by the individual because it may cause euphoria, a sense of pleasure ("high"), or may alter one's perception of reality, or decrease one's awareness of people and the environment. Essentially the drug interferes with the brain's "reward system," increasing the craving for the drug as well as promoting tolerance and dependence. Substance abuse is not limited to illegal or street drugs, but may include prescribed drugs or other readily available substances.
- *Habit* means a practice, often involuntary, of using drugs or other substances at regular and frequent intervals. Habit may be associated with either common customs such as constant coffee drinking or cigarette smoking or the use of illegal or street drugs. These terms do not apply to the occasional use on social occasions of a substance such as alcohol when the user feels no need to consume a large amount or to have a drink at regular short intervals.
- *Dependence* includes both physiologic and psychological craving for the substance.
- *Physiologic* dependence means that the body has adapted to the presence of the drug or chemical so that discontinuing the drug results in *withdrawal* signs such as tremors or abdominal cramps.
- *Psychological* dependence refers to a continuing desire to take the drug to be able to function.
- *Tolerance* implies that because the body adapts to the substance, in time, the amount of the substance

taken must be increased to achieve the same effect. The client who has tolerance to a substance will experience withdrawal if use the substance is discontinued.
- *Addiction* is an older term but is still in common use and is employed for the most serious form of substance abuse—the uncontrollable compulsion to use a substance, often with serious consequences for the individual, the family, and society. Substance abuse at this level often involves increased use of the substance, loss of control over use, leading to multidimensional issues, including health, social, psychological, occupational, and legal problems.

THINK ABOUT 27-1

Define the terms tolerance and physiologic dependence.

Abused substances may be classified in many ways, including mode of action and source. Under *mode of action,* commonly abused psychoactive substances include:
1. Central nervous system *depressants* or tranquilizers, such as alcohol
2. *Narcotics* or pain killers, which cause euphoria and drowsiness
3. *Stimulants,* such as coffee or amphetamines
4. *Psychedelics* or hallucinogens, which alter a person's perception and awareness and produce illusions

Some chemicals actually manifest both stimulant and depressant effects. For example, alcohol is really a central nervous system (CNS) depressant, although initially it appears to be a stimulant because it first depresses the higher brain centers used for judgment or the inhibitory neurons.

Abused drugs are also classified by *source.* They include legally prescribed medications. These include but are not limited to: tranquilizers or sedatives that are prescribed and used long after the need for them has passed, medications shared with another person, prescriptions acquired from several sources, and medications combined with other substances such as alcohol or nonprescription drugs to achieve the desired effect. The surge in drug deaths has recently been fueled by increased availability and abuse of prescription painkillers (such as OxyContin) and antianxiety drugs. Prescribed drugs that are considered more addictive or dangerous are restricted by government agencies and are available only for research or with a signed written prescription without refill provisions. Heroin and morphine are regulated this way, as are stimulants such as those prescribed for attention deficit hyperactivity disorder.

Many psychoactive substances are readily available without restrictions, such as sleep-inducing or wake-up pills; cough syrups; spray paints; decongestants; alcohol-based hair lotions; or glues, nail polish removers, aerosols, and solvents for sniffing or inhaling. These generally provide a short "high" followed by depression and disorientation. Such substances are frequently misused and have been responsible for a number of suicides and accidental deaths. As a result, substances of this type are kept behind the counter in stores and must be requested.

Illegal or street drugs are widely available and are both costly and more dangerous for the user because their content is unpredictable. Such usage often leads to overdose or toxic effects caused by adulterating substances. Many street drugs are better known by their common names than by their medical or chemical names. For example, "speed" or "uppers" is the term used for amphetamines, "angel dust" for phencyclidine (PCP), and "snow" or "powder" for cocaine. Methamphetamine is a highly addictive, easily manufactured stimulant, and is known as "crank," "ice," or "crystal." It can be sniffed, injected, smoked, or taken orally. It stimulates the body by increasing dopamine levels in the brain, but subsequently damages dopamine-producing neurons in the brain. A high dose causes elevated body temperature and seizures. Heroin is commonly known on the street as "blow." "Ecstasy" or MDMA, a stimulant, is a *designer* drug, chemically modified to provide special effects and avoid legal restrictions. Ecstasy imparts a feeling of euphoria and energy. A high dose leads to hyperthermia and heart failure. It is commonly known as "X," "K," or "Special K."

The market for illegal drugs has become a matter of concern both economically and socially because of the increased criminal activity and violence associated with drug trafficking. Many street drugs are easily manufactured from inexpensive chemicals in simple "laboratories." Regulations to restrict access to the precursor chemicals required to produce the popular street drugs have been enacted in many countries, in an effort to control the source of street drugs. Street drugs are often diluted with contaminants that may be toxic; this practice is done to increase profits and or to make the substance more marketable on the street. It is important that screening for both the primary compound as well as known contaminants is done when treating a drug-induced emergency.

Discussion continues about the medical benefits compared with the abuse potential, and the legal versus illegal status of marijuana. An active ingredient, dronabinol (Marinol), or delta-9-tetrahydrocannabinol, is available for the controlled treatment of nausea, vomiting, and wasting associated with cancer chemotherapy or AIDS. It is not effective in all patients. Other less definitive areas involve tobacco smoking and the social use of alcohol, in which the concepts of addiction and health risks are not well defined.

Individuals who abuse substances such as alcohol often crave risk or excitement and participate in activities that are inherently dangerous. Driving under the influence or in an impaired state is an example of such behavior. 40% of all traffic related deaths are related to alcohol use/abuse. Social limits on behavior are often dampened by the depressive effects of many chemicals leading to impaired judgment and difficulty controlling feelings of anger. Interaction with law enforcement or emergency medical personnel may be unpredictable and carry increased danger to first responders.

THINK ABOUT 27-2

Differentiate the effects of stimulants from those of psychedelic drugs.

Predisposing Factors

Theories regarding the etiology or cause of substance abuse focus on psychological imbalances, personality deficits, biologic abnormalities, dysfunctional interpersonal relationships, or a combination of these factors. Current research is considering the role of gender differences in addiction, particularly with respect to women. Questions center on whether the abuse of substances is related to physiologic or socioeconomic factors facing women.

Substance abuse has been attributed to:
- Heredity and/or genetics
- Family systems and practices
- Disease
- The ready availability of drugs
- Stress and increased medical use of antianxiety agents
- Increased acceptance of alcohol or marijuana as a recreational tool in all age groups

Environmental/Behavioral Risk Factors

Unfortunately, substance abuse is becoming more common in young adolescents. The public receives mixed messages about substance abuse from the media. In many publications, both advertising and articles on drug use by high-profile personalities lend a glamorous facade to the abuse. This aura of glamor and excitement influences young people, who respond to peer pressure and the need to express independence among their contemporaries. Recent developments among teens include "M and M" parties in which the contents of parents' medicine cabinets are raided and combined at the party. Recent surveys have shown that 55% of those age 12 and older who used prescription drugs for nonmedicinal problems obtained them from friends or family. A handful of the mixture of drugs is taken without any knowledge of what is being consumed. This risk behavior is particularly challenging for health care workers because the combined affects make treatment very difficult. Educational measures to reduce substance abuse have not been very effective, and both peer pressure and the "curiosity" factor remain problems in the abuse of substances by young people.

The rapid changes and increased complexity of society, the increase in family breakdown, and economic factors including homelessness and job loss have also contributed to the increase in substance abuse. Some individuals use drugs to cope with anxiety and stress because drugs alter one's mood or perception of reality. Evidence supports the correlation between increased stress and increased substance abuse, and a return to addiction after a period of withdrawal. People who take narcotic analgesics for prolonged periods of time risk becoming dependent because the drugs are addictive, creating a state of euphoria while relieving pain. Narcotics are helpful when medically treating severe pain, particularly in patients with terminal illnesses. Heroin is rarely used medically because of its very strong tendency to produce dependency. Research on substance abuse continues in an effort to find not only its cause but also factors related to it and improved methods of prevention and treatment.

A more recently developed category of abused substances involves the synthetic anabolic steroids, similar to testosterone, taken by some athletes and bodybuilders. Substance abuse among athletes in competitive sports has been well publicized, and it has spread into the high schools. Abuse also involves many different groups in the general population, and increasingly includes females. Some individuals with eating disorders ingest anabolic steroids in order to build muscle mass and enhance performance. Unfortunately, these drugs cause mood disorders, high blood pressure, serious cardiac damage, and liver cancer. There are effects on sexual function, fertility, and appearance as well.

Date rape drugs have become another form of substance abuse in which the person who administers the drug gets a rush from the illicit behavior and the abused may experience physical and psychological trauma. Alcohol is mixed with certain drugs such as Flunitrazepam (Rohypnol); gamma-hydroxybutyrate, an easy drug to manufacture; or lorazepam, depressing the CNS and rapidly causing a deep sleep. No memory of the events after administration is retained. For this reason, it is difficult to bring charges against the abuser or institute treatment.

Indications/Recognition of Abuse

Recognition of substance abuse is very difficult because the pattern of consumption can vary. A substance may be taken consistently and frequently or in large amounts periodically (for example, binge drinkers).

Some individuals are affected by relatively small amounts, whereas others can function quite well with a high intake. Combinations of chemicals usually exert a more marked effect than one substance, and combinations also tend to cause more toxic effects.

The effects of an individual drug depend on the classification of the drug. Depressants usually decrease the level of CNS function, whereas stimulants increase CNS activity. Generally drugs impair neurologic function in some way; for example, by slowing the reflexes, reducing coordination and judgment, or impairing sensitivity and perception. Information about specific drugs can be found in reference texts on substance abuse or pharmacology. The method of administration may also indicate drug abuse in some people; for example, intravenous use leaves injection marks on the body.

General indications of substance abuse include changes in behavior, appearance (e.g., eyes), personality, daily living patterns, or work habits. In adolescents, this may include a change in friends, academic achievement, interest in sports, or increase in risk-taking behaviors. Frequently, the person may be defensive, angry, or embarrassed if he or she is questioned about drug intake. The pattern of behavior is that any stress will immediately require a "helpful" pill or a drink. Often a cycle develops in which the person takes a depressant to relax or sleep and then needs a stimulant to wake up. As the need for drug support increases, more secretive behavior may ensue; and there may be less personal care of clothes and appearance, more excuses for time and performance lapses, stronger efforts to acquire substitute drugs, and eventually criminal activity. Some individuals may become malnourished or may develop anemia or infection and ignore normal health needs.

It is important for any health care worker to be sensitive to the issue of substance abuse. Caution is advisable when strangers request specific drugs for pain relief; for example, in a dental office. Drugs, including samples and prescription order forms, should not be visible or readily available to clients.

Potential Complications of Substance Abuse

Overdose

Overdose is a common acute problem. Some drugs have a relatively small safety margin, and an increased dose may cause toxic effects or death. Street drugs may be contaminated by other substances, thereby causing unanticipated effects. A common emergency situation develops when a combination of drugs, often including alcohol, results in a stronger reaction (synergism) than the individual components normally cause. Many hospital emergency rooms list alcohol-drug combinations as their major overdose cases and the primary cause of brain damage and death. The barbiturates, which induce sleep, and the narcotics morphine and heroin depress the CNS and compromise respiratory function. These substances may depress respiratory effort to a critical level (very slow and shallow respirations), leading to respiratory failure or cardiac arrest. Antidotes such as naloxone (Narcan), which is given for narcotic overdose, can stimulate the respiratory drive. Although the anti-anxiety drugs such as diazepam do not cause respiratory depression when used alone, they may cause brain damage and coma when combined with alcohol.

Other stimulant drugs, such as Ecstasy, cause marked elevations in blood pressure that frequently result in brain damage.

Withdrawal

Discontinuing a drug on which the body has become physically dependent results in withdrawal symptoms. The signs of withdrawal may be mild or severe depending on the specific drug used and the amount of drug to which the body cells have adapted. Common signs of withdrawal include irritability, tremors, nausea, vomiting and stomach cramps, high blood pressure, psychotic episodes, and convulsions. It is safer to experience withdrawal under medical supervision in a hospital or detoxification center than on one's own.

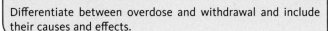

THINK ABOUT 27-3
Differentiate between overdose and withdrawal and include their causes and effects.

Effects on Pregnancy

The pattern of neglect of health and nutrition established in the female substance abuser usually continues during pregnancy, creating serious prenatal concerns for both the woman and her fetus. Many women who are abusing substances do not seek prenatal care because of fear of detection or lack of funds. They often are admitted to the hospital in labor with no prior history of care and generally have a higher risk of perinatal complications.

Many chemical substances, including alcohol, can affect the fetus, resulting in congenital defects. Fetal alcohol syndrome is a serious example of fetal damage. The incidence of fetal alcohol syndrome increases with the dose of alcohol consumed and with any nutritional deficits. No safe level of alcohol consumption during pregnancy has been determined, and generally pregnant women are encouraged to restrict consumption. The newborn child of a woman who has abused alcohol during pregnancy has characteristic physical and facial abnormalities and is cognitively delayed. Alcohol consumption late in pregnancy is likely to cause cognitive and behavioral abnormalities more commonly than physical defects in the child.

Both cigarette smoking and exposure to second-hand smoke decrease blood flow through the placenta. The consequences of maternal exposure to cigarette smoke include an increase in stillbirths, low birth weight for gestational age babies, and increased irritability in the infant after birth. Some drugs such as cocaine and barbiturates lead to addiction in the newborn, who then must undergo withdrawal therapy after birth. Cocaine causes maternal hypertension, decreasing the placental blood supply to the fetus, resulting in developmental defects or premature birth.

Cardiovascular Problems

Cocaine and other stimulants such as amphetamines affect the cardiovascular system, causing irregular heartbeat and increased blood pressure. This may lead to heart attacks, strokes, or heart failure at a young age.

Infection

Systemic infections such as hepatitis B and HIV are common in drug abusers who share needles and other materials when injecting drugs. Local lesions can also form due to local infection of injection sites. These lesions can later become gangrenous leading to potential systemic infections.

Neurological/Psychological Effects

Hallucinogenic or psychedelic drugs such as lysergic acid diethylamide and PCP lead to increased but unreal and distorted interpretation of sensory input into the brain with little control over the experience. The user hopes for a pleasant, euphoric experience (a "high"), but may have an unpleasant episode with a combination of acute fear, panic, and depression, increasing the risk of suicide. Many hallucinogens also have physical effects, including increased blood pressure, nausea, and tremors. "Ecstasy" (MDMA) increases basal metabolism and body temperature and is associated with dehydration and electrolyte imbalances that can lead to cardiac arrest. These drugs also impair the memory and distort the perceptions and judgment, presenting a high risk to those who operate machinery or drive an automobile while under the influence of the drug.

Alcohol

Cirrhosis (Laënnec's Cirrhosis)

Alcoholic liver disease, or Laënnec's cirrhosis, develops in persons with chronic alcoholism or long-term excessive alcohol intake. In 2010 there were 15,990 liver disease deaths due to alcoholism. Alcohol is a hepatotoxin, an irritant that causes metabolic changes in the liver cells, leading first to lipid accumulation in the cells (fatty liver), then to inflammation and necrosis (alcoholic hepatitis), and finally to fibrosis or scar tissue formation (see Chapter 17 for a discussion of cirrhosis). Destruction of the liver takes place insidiously, with only mild signs and symptoms until the condition is well advanced and irreversible.

Nervous System Damage

Chronic alcoholism may cause serious nerve damage in the brain owing to a combination of neurotoxicity and malnutrition. A combination of Wernicke's syndrome, manifested by confusion, disorientation, and loss of motor coordination, and Korsakoff's psychosis, which involves altered personality and amnesia, can occur with long-term abuse.

Treatment for Substance Abuse

A person suffering an overdose or toxic effect should be treated immediately in an emergency room. Withdrawal from an abused substance should be handled in a medical facility, preferably one with experience in dealing with this problem (e.g., a drug detoxification center). Supportive care is required to prevent complications. Clients frequently benefit from psychiatric intervention. Family support services and follow-up are also beneficial. Secondary medical problems such as cirrhosis or pregnancy also require medical supervision.

Treatment for any addiction must be individualized and include a holistic approach to all of the individual's problems. Long-term therapy and support are usually required to maintain abstinence or a significant decrease in use.

Therapy may include methadone maintenance programs for heroin dependency. Methadone is a synthetic opioid that prevents withdrawal symptoms, improves function, and lessens the craving for narcotics in dependent persons. Methadone is administered in prescribed doses in a controlled situation. Methadone programs have been successful in reducing crimes associated with heroin abuse. Newer treatment for opiate addiction may be administered in oral tablets that can be used without daily clinic attendance. Such programs include monthly monitoring of treatment.

Disulfiram (Antabuse) is a deterrent to alcohol use. The drug is taken on a daily basis and causes unpleasant reactions (severe headache, vomiting, difficulty in breathing, and visual problems) when the patient ingests even a small amount of alcohol. Initially observed drug therapy may be employed to establish compliance with the treatment program.

In many persons requiring treatment for substance abuse, malnutrition, particularly protein and vitamin B deficits, is a problem that requires treatment. Counseling and behavior modification therapy are ongoing requirements. Some corporations have developed rehabilitation programs to assist employees with drug dependency, and some of the health professions have established self-help groups for their own members. Support groups such as Alcoholics Anonymous and Narcotics Anonymous are available for those with dependency problems, as are groups for families of affected persons (such as Al-Anon). In addition, many community agencies can provide guidance and resources.

CASE STUDY A

Alcohol Abuse

Mr. M. is a 40-year-old salesperson with a wife and three teen-aged children. He has recently begun to have a beer at lunch and a few drinks after work to reduce his work-related stress. An economic downturn in the housing industry has reduced the need for new home appliances and his income and sales record has been affected. Several other salespeople have been laid off at his firm. He has been told that if his sales and attendance records do not improve he will be fired. He and his wife are constantly arguing about finances and the children's increasing demands for money. His drinking has increased to several beers at lunch and continued drinking after dinner. When he returns to work with alcohol on his breath, he is dismissed from his job. He continues to consume alcohol during the day as he attempts a job search. His wife is very concerned, as are his teenaged children.

1. What is the action of alcohol on the CNS and how has alcohol abuse affected Mr. M.'s ability to deal with customers and his coworkers?
2. Mr. M. states he is a social drinker and "can stop at any time." How accurate is his self-assessment?
3. What stressors are present in Mr. M.'s case?
4. Why does Mr. M. continue to increase his alcohol intake?
5. What changes in liver function can Mr. M. expect if he continues to drink large amounts of alcohol?
6. Mr. M. complains to his wife that all the stress is causing "indigestion." How do stress and alcohol consumption affect GI function?
7. Why is Mr. M. at greater risk of trauma?

   Mr. M. is convinced to see his doctor and is referred to a center that assists alcoholics recover and remain sober. He recovers over the following year and successfully completes job retraining at a local college. Mr. M. is assisted in his job search and settles into work with new colleagues. His relationship with his family improves and he makes several friends among his coworkers. He celebrates his second year of sobriety with his wife.

8. What behaviors increase the risk of Mr. M. reverting to alcohol abuse?
9. What is the long-term prognosis for Mr. M.?

CHAPTER SUMMARY

Substance abuse or chemical dependency in an individual complicates health care because diagnostic tests may be inaccurate, disease may be masked or aggravated, and drug interactions are likely to develop.

- Dependency may be psychological, physiologic, or a combination of these.

- Categories of abused substances include illegal street drugs, prescribed medications, alcohol, and household substances.

  Effects of substances include CNS stimulation or depression or hallucinations.
- Some indicators of substance abuse are behavioral changes; decreased regard for appearance, family, or work responsibilities; or specific physical characteristics.
- Overdose or toxicity is a frequent outcome because the safety margin in the dose is often small, street drugs may be contaminated, and combinations of chemicals are dangerous.
- Withdrawal is best accomplished with medical support.
- Children of substance abusers are frequently born with congenital defects and a dependency to the substance.
- Potential complications for substance abusers include infection, liver disease, malnutrition, CNS damage, and cardiovascular disorders.

STUDY QUESTIONS

1. List several factors that are considered to predispose a person to substance abuse.
2. Describe several signs that may indicate the presence of substance abuse.
3. Describe two potential health problems resulting from substance abuse.
4. Explain several reasons why withdrawal requires medical attention.

ADDITIONAL RESOURCES

Web Sites

http://www.nida.nih.gov/DrugPages/Steroids.html Steroids (Anabolic) (National Institute on Drug Abuse)

http://www.steroidabuse.org *Anabolic Steroid Abuse (National Institute on Drug Abuse)*

http://www.drugabuse.gov *(National Institute on Drug Abuse)*

http://www.mayoclinic.com *Mayo Clinic*

http://www.psych.org *American Psychiatric Association*

http://www.asam.org *American Society of Addiction Medicine*

http://www.csam.org *Canadian Society of Addiction Medicine*

http://www.cdc.gov/ *Centers for Disease Prevention and Control*

CHAPTER 28

Environmental Hazards and Associated Problems

CHAPTER OUTLINE

LEARNING OBJECTIVES

After studying this chapter, the student is expected to:

1. Describe the sources and name examples of hazardous materials in the environment.
2. Describe the effects of hyperthermia and hypothermia.
3. Discuss the effects of radiation.
4. List possible safety measures in the workplace.
5. Describe examples of dangerous insects and animals.
6. Discuss the possible effects of contaminated food and water.

KEY TERMS

demyelination	leukemia	pica	toxicology
detoxification	neuritis	seizures	tympanic membrane
ecosystems	occlusion	solvents	vectors
encephalopathy	paralysis	syncope	
hemolytic anemia	particulate	tinnitus	

Many agents in the environment can cause damage to cells and organs in the human body. Frequently the damage occurs silently as the agent accumulates in the body. Sufficient documentation may have been gathered to enable researchers to discern the correct cause only years later, after signs and symptoms have become apparent. For example, evidence linking cigarette smoking and second-hand smoke to the occurrence of lung cancer has led to widespread bans against smoking in public areas.

The substantial increase in childhood cancers and hypersensitivities, including asthma and anaphylaxis, is cause for serious concern about the environment. The National Center for Health Statistics indicates 6.5 million children and 16 million adults in the United States were diagnosed with asthma in 2005. This constitutes almost 8% of the population in the United States and its territories. Puerto Ricans experienced an incidence rate 125% greater than that in non-Hispanic white people and 80% greater than in non-Hispanic blacks. In the 0- to 17-year age group, boys are affected 30% more frequently than are girls; in adults, this relationship is reversed, with 40% more women than men experiencing asthma. The overall death rate for asthma in the United States is 1.4 deaths per 100,000 people, and these deaths match incidence data closely.

Hypersensitivities to new chemical substances in the environment have greatly increased. The increased number of chemicals in food processing, synthetic materials in buildings and furnishings, and cosmetics and toiletries is of concern. Security of water and food supplies from chemical and microbial contamination is of concern in all areas of the world. Many of these chemicals cannot be metabolized in the body, increasing the level of toxins in the cells. Physical factors also play a role in environmental disease; awareness of the role of sun exposure in combination with chemical exposure is increasing.

Only in recent years have additional safety procedures been instituted in the workplace and the environment to protect individuals from some of these hazards. Regulations have been established by individual groups in the health professions and industry, and by the Occupational Safety and Health Administration (OSHA). In Canada, the federal government has instituted mandatory training about hazardous materials in the workplace (Workplace Hazardous Materials Information System, or WHMIS) and the precautions required for storage, handling, and use. These regulations cover areas such as infection control, protective equipment, exposure to harmful substances, and hazardous material. For example, improved ventilation systems may be required in factories, or soil in certain areas may be tested for contaminants before new housing is constructed. In many places, safety-monitoring groups have been established, and unions and workers cooperate in providing training programs that supply information about the standard symbols used for hazardous materials and the precautions recommended for handling them. To increase awareness of the role of these agents in pathologic processes, a few examples of diseases arising from environmental hazards are presented here. Additional information can be found in toxicology texts or environmental references. Every worker should feel free to question potential risk factors in the workplace or living environment.

Chemicals

Unwanted chemicals may be ingested in contaminated food or water, inhaled into the lungs, or absorbed through the skin. Exposure may occur in the workplace or at home. Food and water may have been contaminated by industrial wastes; for example, freshwater fish may absorb mercury in lakes and rivers. It now appears that farmed salmon may contain toxic chemicals contained in feed. Some water processing plants test for over 300 chemicals, including PCBs, DDT, and dioxin, as well as lead and mercury. It is not unusual for chemical wastes to remain in the original dangerous form; alternatively, they may undergo transformation into more toxic materials or break down into harmless substances. For example, although pesticides may remain in the environment for a long time, some, such as DDT, do not break down into harmless chemicals, and therefore high levels gradually accumulate in the environment. Many ecosystems are disturbed by the use of

pesticides, including those of microorganisms, some of which may become pathogenic, or disease causing. The increased availability of organically grown fruits and vegetables has provided an opportunity for consumers to reduce their exposure to chemicals ingested in food.

Tissue damage may result from a large dose in a single incident, or, more often, damage results from repeated exposure to small amounts of the unwanted material. The chemical may cause damage at the site of entry, or it may enter the blood and circulate to other sites in the body. Frequently this process occurs without the knowledge of the individual. Normally the liver is responsible for detoxification, or inactivation and removal of foreign chemicals from the body. In many cases, however, these chemicals bypass the liver and are stored in certain tissues, gradually accumulating to dangerous levels over years of exposure. Usually there are no obvious signs of this accumulation. For example, hexachlorophene was widely used in hospitals as well as in homes as an antiseptic in soaps and powders until it was discovered that it was absorbed through the skin, particularly broken skin. Heavy use eventually caused brain damage. Now the use of hexachlorophene is restricted. However, new types of antibacterial soaps are being used extensively, and it may be some years before the effects of these new chemicals are documented.

Currently there is increasing concern about children's exposure to plastics in the environment. Chemicals such as phthalates are used to soften plastics and prevent shattering. Toys, bottle nipples, and soothers made of phthalates have been withdrawn from the market in the United States and Canada, but products produced overseas may still contain the banned product. Bisphenol A (BPA) is a hardening agent used in plastic baby bottles and water bottles. This chemical has been recently classified as a toxin by the Canadian government. The concern about such plastics relates to their ability to mimic hormones such as estrogen and act physiologically within the tissues. It is thought that such endocrine disrupters can lead to infertility and promote the growth of endocrine-sensitive cancers.

There is also increasing concern about chemicals and regulation of the menstrual cycle and reproduction in women. Recent surveys link exposure to solvents to increased risks in women for altered menstrual cycles, spontaneous abortions (miscarriages), and stillbirths.

Chemicals may affect the body in different ways. Chemical substances often injure cells directly by damaging the cell membrane and causing swelling and eventual rupture of the cell. This results in inflammation and necrosis in the tissue. Some chemicals alter the metabolic pathways in the cell, leading to degenerative changes. Many chemicals are carcinogenic; that is, they cause mutations of the cell and lead to the onset of cancers such as leukemia. A few examples of dangerous chemicals are described in the following section.

Heavy Metals

Lead and mercury are examples of heavy metals that can accumulate in the tissues with long-term exposure. *Lead* can be ingested in food or water or inhaled and is then stored in bone. Lead is heavily used in industry and is found in lead pipes and batteries. It is also a common childhood poison because children tend to chew on items covered with lead-based paint, such as toys or furniture, and they ingest paint flakes from walls or woodwork. There have been recent widespread recalls of common toys manufactured offshore because of the use of lead paints. Lead has been found to vaporize over time from some imported (and unregulated) vinyl window blinds. Individuals with pica (the craving for nonfood substances such as clay) may also develop high blood levels of lead.

The toxic effects of lead include:
- Hemolytic anemia (destruction of erythrocytes leading to low hemoglobin levels) (Fig. 28-1)
- Inflammation and ulceration of the digestive tract (lead colic)
- Inflammation of the kidney tubules
- Damage to the nervous system such as neuritis (inflammation and demyelination of peripheral nerves) and encephalopathy (edema and degeneration of neurons in the brain). Children manifest lead toxicity with seizures or convulsions, delayed development, and intellectual impairment. Even low doses of lead can cause irreversible brain damage.

Lead poisoning can be detected by bone defects or "lead lines" in the bone as well as on the gingiva or gums adjacent to the teeth.

Acids/Bases

Acids and bases can cause corrosive damage to living tissue which is classified as a chemical burn. The classification of the type of chemical burn follows the same standard system as thermal burns. Acids and bases can be found in numerous household products as well as in labs and manufacturing facilities. In addition to acids and bases, strong oxidizers, reducing agents and solvents can also cause chemical burns.

Treatment will depend on the specific chemical causing the burn. In general first aid involves rinsing off the chemical with water or a neutralizing solution. In some cases involving lipophilic chemicals such as hydrofluoric acid, the burn symptoms may not be immediately obvious but may appear hours later.

Inhalants

Inhalants can be classified as particulate, such as asbestos and silica, or gaseous, such as sulfur dioxide and ozone; or they may arise from solvents, such as carbon tetrachloride. Although local irritation of the eyes and nose is often noticeable when exposure occurs, the inflammation of the respiratory tract and the effect on the central nervous system are not immediately apparent. Some inhaled or aspirated solvents such as carbon tetrachloride diffuse into the circulation and eventually cause inflammation of the liver cells and irreversible hepatic damage as well as pneumonitis. Other inhalants affect the lung tissues directly.

Sources of toxic inhalants include factories, laboratories, mines, insecticides, and aerosols. Paints, glues, furniture, and floor coverings supply irritants in the home. Smog is visible air pollution that contains both noxious gases, such as hydrogen sulfide, and particles from dust and smoke. Beginning in the late 1990s, the poor ventilation in crowded airplanes raised concerns about risks to passengers and crew from inhaled substances and infectious agents as well as lower oxygen levels. Many office and apartment buildings are not supplying sufficient fresh air to the interior.

Iron oxide and silica are examples of inhaled particles that frequently cause lung damage in workers in mines or other industries using these substances. These chemicals can cause episodes of acute inflammation, or they may lead to low-grade chronic inflammation, resulting in fibrosis in the lung. More information on chronic lung disease is found in Chapter 13. Also, chronic cough and frequent infections result from the irritation and inflammation of the respiratory mucosa and may lead to additional damage. Geographic areas with heavy pollution demonstrate an increased incidence of chronic lung disease. Many of these particles are carcinogenic and increase the risk of lung cancer.

Many gases such as sulfur dioxide also cause inflammation in the lungs. Carbon monoxide, which results from incomplete combustion (e.g., automobile exhaust), is not a threat in small amounts for healthy people; but because it displaces oxygen from hemoglobin, it can be dangerous for individuals with cardiovascular or

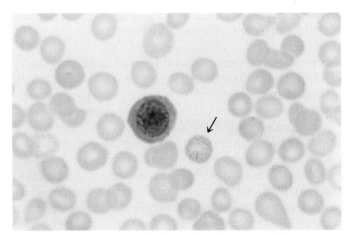

FIGURE 28-1 Red blood cell showing lead poisoning. *(From Stevens ML:* Fundamentals of Clinical Hematology, *Philadelphia, 1997, Saunders.)*

respiratory disease. Carbon monoxide remains bound to hemoglobin for significant periods of time and can lead to a fatal decrease in oxygen supply if exposure is prolonged. Carbon monoxide monitors are available to warn of the presence of the colorless and tasteless gas.

Cigarette smoking predisposes the smoker to lung disease, including emphysema, bronchitis, and lung cancer, and also to bladder cancer, peptic ulcers, and cardiovascular disease. Smoking impairs fertility, and during pregnancy it also affects fetal development, leading to stillbirth or low birth weight infants and an increased risk of complications. These concerns have led to social and political action concerning cigarette smoking and second-hand smoke exposure. Many areas across the country now have laws banning smoking in the workplace and any indoor place other than the home.

Asbestos

Asbestos is still found in older buildings, where it was used for insulation. Exposure of the lungs to asbestos can cause a severe acute inflammation and subsequent scarring, which could lead to chronic problems such as mesothelioma, Malignant mesothelioma is a rare form of lung cancer that develops in the mesothelium and is often caused by exposure to asbestos, (Fig. 28-2). Other asbestos related diseases include asbestosis, pleural plaques, and pleural thickening. Chronic asbestos related diseases often take a long time to manifest which leads to delayed diagnosis and poor prognosis for recovery.

Pesticides

Pesticide illness is a grouping of diseases and complications that can be caused by some type of exposure to pesticides. Depending upon the type of pesticide and amount of exposure these chemicals can cause a variety

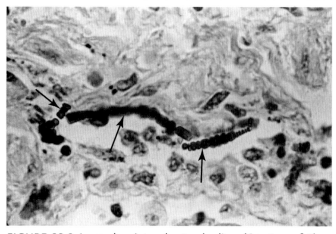

FIGURE 28-2 Lung showing asbestos bodies. *(Courtesy of Shaw RW, MD: North York General Hospital, Toronto, Ontario, Canada.)*

of both acute and chronic adverse health effects. Because their organs and body systems are still in the process of developing infants and small children are especially sensitive to health risks that can arise due to exposure to pesticides.

Signs of acute exposure problems include diarrhea, nausea, vomiting, pinpoint pupils, rashes, headaches, irritation of the eyes, skin or throat. Chronic exposure can, with some chemicals, lead to the aggravation of asthma problems, cause damage to the immune system, as well as increase the risk of certain cancers and birth defects. Treatment for a pesticide illness will usually depend on the specific chemical(s) involved.

> **THINK ABOUT 28-1**
> a. Explain why chronic lung disease such as bronchitis occurs more frequently in highly industrialized regions.
> b. Describe two possible effects of chemical toxicity in the body, giving an example of each.
> c. Explain why young children are at greater risk of pathologic changes resulting from exposure to hazardous chemicals such as pesticides.

Physical Agents

Temperature Hazards

Hyperthermia

Although the body has mechanisms such as vasodilation and diaphoresis for adapting to temperature extremes, hyperthermia, an excessive elevation in body temperature, can occur when the environmental temperature is unusually high, preventing effective cooling of the body. Also, strenuous activity that generates excessive body heat on a hot day or inadequate replacement of the fluid and salt lost in perspiration may lead to hyperthermia. Because of less effective physiologic compensation mechanisms, older people, infants, and cardiac patients are most at risk for overheating, as demonstrated in a severe heat wave in Chicago during the summer of 1995 that resulted in more than 100 fatalities.

Syndromes associated with hyperthermia include:
- Heat cramps with skeletal muscle spasms caused by loss of electrolytes
- Heat exhaustion, with sweating, headache, nausea, and dizziness or syncope (fainting), the most common problem, resulting from loss of water and sodium leading to hypovolemia
- Heat stroke, with shock, coma, and very high core body temperature, the most serious complication. Heat stroke occurs commonly in the elderly, infants, or debilitated persons. Early signs include red, dry skin, headache, dizziness, and rapid weak pulse. It is caused by general vasodilation, a marked decrease in circulating blood volume, and damage to the heart.

Prompt cooling and fluid and electrolyte replacement in persons with these syndromes are essential to prevent brain damage or cardiac failure.

Hypothermia

Exposure to cold temperatures may have localized or systemic effects. There has been an increase in serious cases of hypothermia in colder climates as the number of homeless individuals in these areas has escalated. Children are also vulnerable, because they may not understand the risks.

Localized frostbite usually affects the fingers, toes, ears, or exposed parts of the face. Wet clothing increases the danger. In these areas, vascular occlusion occurs quickly and may lead to necrosis and gangrene. Usually sensation is lost early, and the individual may not be aware of the danger. Close observation of exposed areas for color changes, particularly whitish or bluish spots, is important. Gradual warming of the area without rubbing can minimize the damage.

Systemic exposure to cold temperatures may occur with submersion in cold water, lack of adequate clothing in cold weather, or wet clothing on a windy day, particularly if body movement is reduced. Low temperatures can affect many body tissues, depending on the length of time of the exposure and the actual temperature. Shivering occurs initially in an effort to generate more body heat, and then the body feels numb. Lethargy and confusion become marked. The pulse and respirations become slower, and the person becomes unresponsive. Reflex vasoconstriction and increased blood viscosity lead to ischemia and reduced metabolism. When the core body temperature drops, the capillaries and cell membranes are damaged. This leads to abnormal shifts of fluid and sodium and ultimately to hypovolemic shock (low blood pressure), and cell necrosis ensues. Rewarming must be done slowly and cautiously and must be accompanied by fluid replacement to maintain adequate circulation and minimize cell damage. Often the brain is protected against edema by the administration of corticosteroid drugs during the return to normal body temperature.

THINK ABOUT 28-2

a. Compare the effects of hypothermia and hyperthermia on the circulation.
b. Suggest some reasons why it would be difficult for a person submerged in an icy lake to continue swimming.
c. How does hypothermia affect cell metabolism and oxygen requirements of the brain?

Radiation Hazards

Ionizing Radiation

Ionizing radiation, much of it arising from natural sources such as the sun and radioactive minerals in the soil, is an ongoing hazard. Increasing concern has been voiced regarding the change in the protective ozone layer in the earth's atmosphere and the resultant risk of more radiation. However, the expanded exposure to radiation in homes (e.g., radon gas, a byproduct of the natural decay of uranium in the earth, can seep into a house through soil or water), industry and defense systems, nuclear reactors for generation of electricity, and medicine for diagnostic procedures such as x-ray and tracer studies, as well as for treatment presents the primary risk of exposure for workers and clients. Health care workers who are at risk of exposure to radiation must use lead shields and wear monitoring devices to check individual exposure.

Ionizing radiation includes x-rays and gamma rays as well as particles such as protons and neutrons. These rays and particles differ both in energy levels and their ability to penetrate body tissue, clothing, or lead. Increased distance from the source lessens the amount of radiation to which a person is exposed. Radiation emissions are measured in roentgens. The amount of radiation absorbed by the body is measured in *rads*, or "radiation-absorbed doses." Radiation primarily affects cells that undergo rapid mitosis, such as epithelial tissue, bone marrow, and the gonads (ovaries and testes). With small doses of radiation, cells can sometimes repair the ruptured DNA strands. With larger doses, DNA is altered and often cross-linkages form, leading to mutations in the cell and development of cancer (see Chapter 20 for carcinogenesis). The cells may be destroyed. Exposure to large amounts of radiation leads to radiation sickness, resulting in damage to the bone marrow, digestive tract, and central nervous system. Without intensive care and bone marrow replacement, most victims of radiation sickness die within a few days.

Radiation damage may occur with a single large exposure, usually accidental, or may accumulate with repeated small exposures. The effects of repeated small doses of radiation have not been well studied and there is far less information about the resulting pathology than for massive exposure, such as occurred when atomic bombs were used against cities in Japan in 1945 and in the 1986 nuclear meltdown of the Chernobyl nuclear reactor in Ukraine.

Light Energy

Exposure to both visible light and ultraviolet (UV) rays can cause damage to skin and eyes. Cumulative damage is manifested by the development of skin cancers resulting from ultraviolet rays related to sun exposure, as seen frequently in older individuals. The UV damages the nucleotides in the cell's DNA. Reducing exposure and routine use of skin lotions that block damaging ultraviolet rays, both UVA and UVB, is recommended to reduce the risk of skin cancer. Exposure of the eyes to strong UV radiation can also cause permanent damage depending on the specific wavelength involved. The shorter wavelengths can cause corneal cell damage, UVA and B can cause lens damage, and the longer wavelengths have been implicated in macular degeneration and retinal tissue damage (see Chapter 15)

Visible laser light can also cause severe damage to the eyes. Two types of eye damage that can be caused by a laser beam are tissue thermal burns, affecting structures such as the cornea, and photochemical damage to the retina. Powerful lasers can also cause thermal damage to unprotected skin.

THINK ABOUT 28-3

a. Epithelial tissue is very sensitive to radiation. List specific structures that include epithelial tissue likely to be damaged by radiation.
b. Give several specific examples of radiation sources in your community and workplace.

Noise Hazards

Hearing impairment may result from excessive noise, for example, a single loud noise such as a gunshot or a variety of noise intensities can cause cumulative damage. A sudden, extremely loud noise may rupture the **tympanic membrane** (eardrum) or damage the nerve cells in the inner ear (see Chapter 15) Inner ear damage involving the nerves is usually irreversible. Cumulative damage caused by noise may result directly from noise in the workplace but is often associated with higher noise levels in urban areas and recreational sources such as rock music. Ear protection (e.g., plugs) is now required in most noisy work environments. Because only soft or high-pitched sounds are lost initially, the effects of such trauma are often gradual and go unnoticed until they are well advanced. In some cases, the individual may notice **tinnitus**, or ringing in the ears, which is a more obvious warning of the problem.

Food and Waterborne Hazards

Contaminated food and water are common sources of gastroenteritis, or vomiting and diarrhea. This topic is covered in Chapter 17. Infection can be spread in many ways. Organisms such as *Escherichia coli,* part of normal intestinal flora, are transmitted by the oral-fecal route when personal hygiene or community sanitation is not up to standard. So-called "traveler's diarrhea" is an example of this type of infection. In some regions a high risk of infection is associated with swimming in areas where adequate sewage treatment is not maintained or water runoff drains through cattle pastures. Antibiotic-resistant pathogens, originating from humans or animals treated with antibiotics, have also been found in lakes and rivers. Generally water in deep wells has been filtered underground, and is considered safe. However,

heavily contaminated water may seep into the water table and wells, where untreated water may cause widespread illness.

In the 1990s, several extremely toxic strains of *E. coli* emerged and have continued to cause serious illness, including deaths from kidney damage. Hemolytic uremic syndrome develops when specific strains of *E. coli* invade the bloodstream and cause damage to renal tubules. Many serious outbreaks have occurred in North America. It is imperative that any meat products that have been ground and processed be cooked thoroughly to the recommended temperature.

Institutions frequently have outbreaks of *Salmonella* infection associated with contaminated poultry products or with food handlers who are *carriers* (a person who is a reservoir for the organism and can spread it but shows no clinical signs of infection). Widespread infection may also occur in nurseries or daycare centers when careful handwashing and other infection control techniques have not been maintained. Stool cultures can be used to identify the responsible organism. In many cases such infections are self-limiting, but infants and elderly people are at increased risk and may become dehydrated very quickly.

Other pathogens that have been identified in food-borne outbreaks include *Listeria* and *Shigella*. Listeria is most common in processed meat products such as sausage or ham and is quite common in the environment. This makes control extremely difficult. *Shigella* causes dysentery, a bloody diarrhea that is extremely dangerous. *Shigella* is a bacterium that is transmitted primarily through unwashed hands; only a small loading dose of organisms is needed to cause serious infection.

Melamine is a plastic that has been added to food and milk in some areas of the world to allow dilution of the food with water. Melamine reacts as a protein when tested and can go unnoticed in milk or other food unless specific testing is carried out. Adulteration of food is done to increase profit margins. The result of ingestion of melamine is acute renal failure and possible death.

Biological Agents

Bites and Stings

Bites and stings may cause disease and other physical complications.
1. By direct injection of animal toxin into the human body. Examples of toxins involved in bites include the neurotoxins produced by poisonous snakes or spiders that affect the nervous system, causing **paralysis** and respiratory failure or seizures.
2. By transmission of infectious agents through animal or insect **vectors** to humans. An example of an infection transmitted by an animal bite is rabies or hydrophobia, which is caused by an RNA virus. Rabies is

caused primarily by the bites of wild animals, such as raccoons or skunks, but also occasionally by bites from domesticated animals (cats or dogs) that have been bitten by infected wild animals. Following any bite, the animal is usually impounded and monitored for infection. Rabies leads to nerve paralysis and death if it is not treated quickly. In certain regions, ticks and mosquitoes are threats because they transmit infections such as rickettsial Rocky Mountain spotted fever and Lyme disease, caused by a spirochete also transmitted by ticks.

3. By an allergic reaction to the insect's secretion. An example of an allergic reaction is the response of some individuals to bee or wasp stings: an anaphylactic reaction—a sudden and severe life-threatening hypersensitivity or circulatory allergic reaction. Anaphylaxis is identifiable by respiratory difficulty and shock in someone who has just been bitten (see Chapter 7).

CASE STUDY A

Occupational Hazards of Fighting Forest Fires

E.C. is a 24-year-old professional firefighter in a western region that has had severe forest fires because of hot, dry, windy weather. He has worked overtime for several weeks and is experiencing continual shortness of breath, fatigue, and exercise intolerance, which are unusual for him. E.C. complies with health and safety requirements, including wearing appropriate protective equipment. Community support agencies are on-site to provide water, food, and support as needed.

Fighting forest fires exposes workers to extreme heat, fatigue from working on uneven terrain, toxins used in fire suppression, insecticides, pesticides, particulate matter, and carbon monoxide. Protective equipment reduces exposure to toxic substances, but is not used in down time when exposure can also occur because of wind currents and close proximity to the fire sites.

1. What factors in E.C.'s work situation increase the risk of health problems?

2. What role do the support agencies play in reducing health problems for the firefighters?
3. What are possible causes of E.C.'s exercise intolerance and fatigue?
4. How may the toxins in smoke affect lung function if they irritate the lung tissues?
5. What long-term risks exist for firefighters exposed to smoke from woodland fires?

CHAPTER SUMMARY

Increased awareness of medical problems arising from water and air pollution, contaminated food, and industrial exposure to dangerous substances has sparked increased concern for environmental issues.

- Common chemicals with harmful effects include heavy metals and pesticides, which are appearing in consumer goods manufactured offshore.
- Inhalants such as asbestos are classified as particulates, whereas sulfur dioxide and carbon tetrachloride are gaseous. These substances cause respiratory tract inflammation and may also be absorbed into the circulation to cause damage elsewhere in the body.
- Hyperthermia may cause heat cramps, heat exhaustion, or heat stroke, depending on the rise in body temperature.
- Exposure to cold temperatures may cause localized frostbite with tissue necrosis or generalized hypothermia affecting the circulation and cell function.
- Radiation damage may result from a single exposure or be cumulative. Radiation damages DNA, particularly in cells undergoing mitosis.
- Bites and stings cause disease in three ways, by injection of toxins, transmission of infectious agents, or allergic reactions.
- Ingested toxins cause food poisoning, liver damage, and other manifestations.

STUDY QUESTIONS

1. Explain the potential benefits of reducing the use of pesticides and insecticides.
2. List examples of the dangerous gaseous and particulate components of chemical inhalants.
3. Describe the potential effects of chemicals on the respiratory tissues.
4. Explain how skin cancer is linked to sun exposure.
5. Give several examples of excessive noise in your environment.
6. Name a biologic agent and the associated problem for each of the following:
   a. Transmission of an infection through a bite
   b. Hypersensitivity reaction
   c. Injection of a toxin
7. Define a carrier.
8. Define fecal-oral transmission of infection and give an example.

ADDITIONAL RESOURCES

American Journal of Industrial Medicine (available at: http://www3.interscience.wiley.com/cgi-bin/home), New York, Wiley-Liss.

Web Sites

http://www.who.int/ith/en/index.html *International Travel and health (World Health Organization)*

http://library.hsh.com/?row_id=77 *Environmental Hazards in the Home*

http://www.cdc.gov/nceh/ehhe/ *CDC National Center for Environmental Health*

http://www.cdc.gov/nchs *CDC National Center for Health Statistics*

http://www.firstaid.webmd.com/ *WebMD*

http://www.cdc.gov/niosh/ *National Institute for Occupational Health and Safety*

Appendices

Ready Reference 1

Body Planes, Cavities, Regions, and Fluid Compartments

The following terms are useful in describing body position and movement as well as the location of structures in the body.

Body Planes (Fig. RR1-1)

coronal	a line from side to side, dividing the front and back halves of the body
midsagittal	a line from superior to inferior along the midline, dividing the right and left halves of the body
sagittal	a vertical line from superior to inferior at any point that divides the body into right and left parts
transverse	a line dividing the upper and lower halves of the body

Body Cavities (Fig. RR1-2)

abdominal cavity	below the diaphragm; contains the stomach, intestines, pancreas, and liver
dorsal cavity	cranial cavity and vertebral cavity
pelvic cavity	most inferior cavity, containing the urinary bladder, rectum, and uterus
thoracic cavity	above the diaphragm; contains the heart, lungs, esophagus, trachea, aorta, and venae cavae
ventral cavity	thoracic cavity and abdominopelvic cavity

Body Regions (Figs. RR1-3 and RR1-4)
Body Fluid Compartments (Fig. RR1-5)

There are several fluid compartments within the body that are significant in understanding fluid and

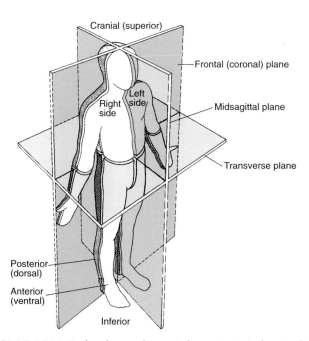

FIGURE RR1-1 Body planes. (*From Solomon EP:* Understanding Human Anatomy and Physiology, *Philadelphia, 1987, WB Saunders.*)

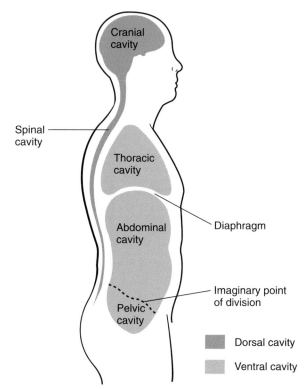

FIGURE RR1-2 Body cavities. (*From Leonard PC:* Building a Medical Vocabulary, *5th ed. Philadelphia, 2001, WB Saunders.*)

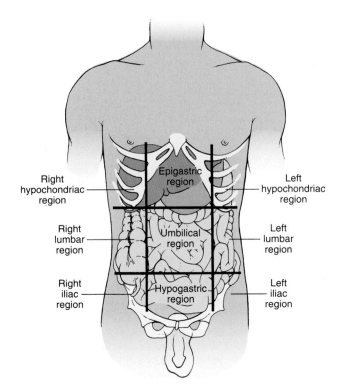

FIGURE RR1-3 Body regions. *(From Dowd SB, Wilson BG: Encyclopedia of Radiographic Positioning, Philadelphia, 1995, WB Saunders.)*

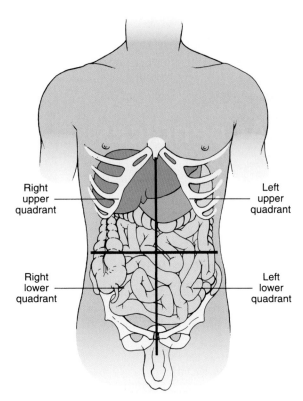

FIGURE RR1-4 Body regions. *(From Dowd SB, Wilson BG: Encyclopedia of Radiographic Positioning, Philadelphia, 1995, WB Saunders.)*

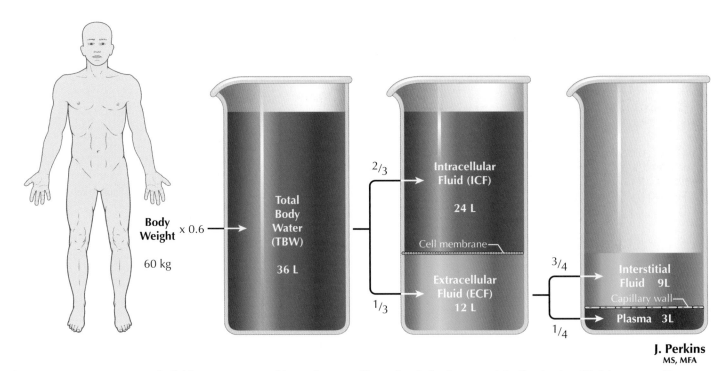

J. Perkins
MS, MFA

FIGURE RR1-5 Body fluid compartments. *(Netter Anatomy Illustration Collection, copyright Elsevier, Inc. All rights reserved.)*

TABLE RR1-1 Fluid Volumes of Fluid Compartments in the Adult

Compartment	Volume (liters)	% of Body Weight (varies with BMI)
Intracellular (ICF)	28	40
Interstitial (ISF)	11	15
Intravascular	3	5
Total Body Water (TBW)	42	60

TABLE RR1-2 Distribution of Electrolytes in Body Fluids in mEq/L

Electrolyte	Intravascular	Interstitial (ISF)	Intracellular (ICF)
Bicarbonate	25	27	12
Calcium	4	3	4
Chloride	112	118	4
Magnesium	1	1	34
Phosphate	2	2	40
Potassium	4	4	150
Protein	17	Trace to absent	54
Other	6	7	90

electrolyte dynamics. It is important not to confuse these physiological compartments with cavities that are anatomical structures. The fluid compartments contain differing proportions of total body water and differing concentrations of specific electrolytes (Tables RR1-1 and RR1-2).

Intracellular Fluid Compartment	the compartment and fluid within cells and bounded by cell membranes
Extracellular Fluid Compartment	the compartment outside of cells including:
• *Interstitial Fluid Compartment*	the fluid between cells
• *Vascular Fluid Compartment*	the fluid within lymph capillaries and blood vessels

Common Body Movements (Fig. RR1-6)

Ready Reference 2

Anatomic Terms

Prefix or Root (Combining Form) Used in Anatomic Terms

ab	away from
ad	toward
adeno	gland
ante	before, forward
anti	opposed
auto	self
bi	two
caud	lower part or tail
cephal	top or head
cervic, cervico	neck
circum	around
contra	opposite, against
crani	head
en, endo	in
epi	over, above
ex, exo	out
hemi	half
inter	between
intra	within
mega	large
mono	one
poly	many
post	after, behind
retro	behind
sub	below or under
super, supra	above
version	to turn

Directional Terms

afferent	moving toward
anterior	front or abdominal surface
contralateral	opposite side
distal	far from the center or point of attachment
dorsal	back surface
efferent	moving away
external	outside
inferior	lower part, beneath
internal	inside
ipsilateral	same side
lateral	toward the side
medial	toward the midline
posterior	toward the back
prone	lying on the abdominal surface
proximal	near the center or point of attachment
superior	above, upper part
supine	lying flat on the back
ventral	front or abdominal surface

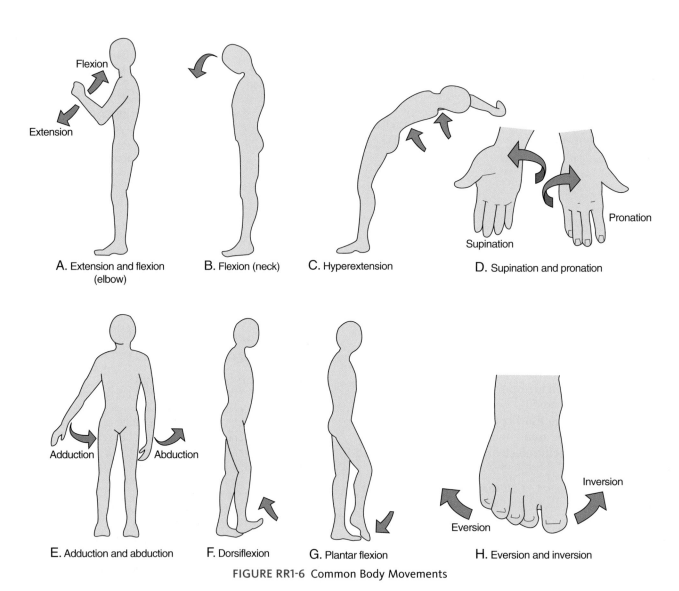

A. Extension and flexion (elbow)

B. Flexion (neck)

C. Hyperextension

D. Supination and pronation

E. Adduction and abduction

F. Dorsiflexion

G. Plantar flexion

H. Eversion and inversion

FIGURE RR1-6 Common Body Movements

Ready Reference 3

Conversion Tables (Tables RR3-1 and RR3-2)

TABLE RR3-1   Measurement Conversion Table

Common Units

nano	one billionth	nanogram	ng	10^{-9} g
micro (μ)	one millionth	microgram	μg	10^{-6} g
milli	one thousandth	milligram	mg	10^{-3} g
kilo	one thousand	kilogram	kg	10^{3} g
centi	one hundredth	centimeter	cm	10^{-2} m
		millimeter	mm	10^{-3} m

Conversion Factors

To Convert	Multiply by
centimeters to inches	0.39
inches to centimeters	2.54
meters to feet	3.28
feet to meters	0.305
fluid ounces to milliliters	30
milliliters to fluid ounces	0.03
liters to quarts	1.06
quarts to liters	0.95
gallons (US) to liters	4.4
grams to ounces	0.035
ounces to grams	28
pounds to grams	453.6
kilograms to pounds	2.2
grains to grams	0.065
calories to joules	0.23

Some Equivalents

1 grain (apothecary) = 65 mg (metric) = 0.035 ounce

15 grains = 1 g

437.5 grains = 28.3 g = 1 ounce

453.6 g = 1 pound or 16 oz

1 kg = 35.2 ounces or 2.2 pounds

1 dram (apothecary) = 4 mL

30 mL = 1 fluid ounce

1 liter = 2.1 pints or 1 quart

Equivalents for Household Measures

1 teaspoon = 4 mL

1 tablespoon = 15 mL or 0.5 fluid ounce

1 cup = 240 mL = 8 fluid ounces = 0.5 pint

1 quart = 960 mL = 4 cups = 2 pints

1 fluid ounce = 30 mL

1 liter = 1.06 quart

1 inch = 2.5 cm

TABLE RR3-2   Temperature Conversion Chart

To Convert Fahrenheit to Celsius:

Subtract 32 from the number of °F and multiply by 5/9:
$(X°F - 32) \times 5/9 = Y°C$

To Convert Celsius to Fahrenheit:

Multiply the number of °C by 9/5 and add 32:
$(Y°C \times 9/5) + 32 = X°F$

Equivalents	°F	°C
	95.0	35.0
	96.0	35.5
	97.0	36.1
	98.0	36.7
Normal body temperature	98.6	37.0
	99.0	37.2
	100.0	37.8
	101.0	38.3
	102.0	38.9
	103.0	39.4
	104.0	40.0

1 °C = 1.8 °F

0 °C = 32 °F (freezing point of water)

20 °C = 68 °F (room temperature)

100 °C = 212 °F (boiling point of water)

Ready Reference 4

Common Abbreviations and Acronyms

ABGs	arterial blood gases
ABO	blood types, A, B, and O
ACE	angiotensin-converting enzyme
ACh	acetylcholine
ACTH	adrenocorticotropic hormone
ADH	antidiuretic hormone
ADLs	activities of daily living
AED	automatic external defibrillator
AFP	alpha-fetoprotein
AIDS	acquired immune deficiency syndrome
ALL	acute lymphocytic leukemia
ALS	amyotrophic lateral sclerosis
ANA	antinuclear antibodies
aPTT or APTT	activated partial thromboplastin time
ARDS	adult respiratory distress syndrome
ARF	acute renal failure
ASA	aspirin, acetylsalicylic acid
ATP	adenosine triphosphate
BBB	bundle branch block (heart)
BM	bowel movement
BMR	basal metabolic rate
BP	blood pressure
BPH	benign prostatic hypertrophy
BSA	body surface area
BSE	breast self-examination

CA	cancer
Ca^{++}	calcium ion
CABG	coronary artery bypass graft
CAD	coronary artery disease
CAT or CT scan	computerized axial tomography or computed tomography
CBC	complete blood count
CCU	coronary care unit
CDC	Centers for Disease Control and Prevention, USA
CEA	carcinoembryonic antigen
CF	cystic fibrosis
CHF	congestive heart failure
Cl$^-$	chloride ion
CNS	central nervous system
COPD	chronic obstructive pulmonary disease (also COLD, chronic obstructive lung disease)
CPR	cardiopulmonary resuscitation
CRP	C-reactive protein
C&S	culture and sensitivity test
CSF	cerebrospinal fluid
CVA	cerebrovascular accident (stroke)
CVP	central venous pressure
D$_5$W	intravenous solution of 5% glucose in water
D&C	dilation and curettage of the uterus
DIC	disseminated intravascular coagulation
DNA	deoxyribonucleic acid
DNR	do not resuscitate
DPT	diphtheria, pertussis, and tetanus vaccine
Dx	diagnosis
EBV	Epstein-Barr virus
ECF	extracellular fluid
ECG	electrocardiogram
ECT	electroconvulsive therapy
EEG	electroencephalogram
ELISA	enzyme-linked immunosorbent assay (antibody or antigen test)
EPS	extrapyramidal signs
ESR	erythrocyte sedimentation rate
ESWL	extracorporeal shock-wave lithotripsy
FUO	fever of undetermined origin
GABA	gamma-aminobutyric acid (neurotransmitter)
GFR	glomerular filtration rate
GVHD	graft-versus-host disease
Hb or Hgb	hemoglobin
HbA	hemoglobin A
HbA1c	glycosylated hemoglobin A
HbF	fetal hemoglobin
HBV	hepatitis B virus
HCG	human chorionic gonadotropin
HCl	hydrochloric acid
HDL	high-density lipoprotein
HIV	human immunodeficiency virus
HLA	human leukocyte antigen
HPV	human papillomavirus
HSV	herpes simplex virus
IBD	inflammatory bowel disease
ICF	intracellular fluid
I&O	intake and output of fluids
ICP	intracranial pressure
IICP	increased intracranial pressure
ICU	intensive care unit
IDDM	insulin-dependent diabetes mellitus

IgG	immunoglobulin G (gamma globulin)
INR	international normalized ratio (prothrombin time)
IOP	intraocular pressure
IRDS	infant respiratory distress syndrome
ISF	interstitial fluid
JRA	juvenile rheumatoid arthritis
K$^+$	potassium ion
LDL	low-density lipoprotein
LLQ	left lower quadrant
LMP	last menstrual period
LOC	level or loss of consciousness
LP	lumbar puncture
MAOI	monoamine oxidase inhibitor (antidepressant drug)
MD	muscular dystrophy
MHC	major histocompatibility complex
MI	myocardial infarction (heart attack)
MMR	measles, mumps, and rubella vaccine
MRI	magnetic resonance imaging (test)
MS	multiple sclerosis
Na$^+$	sodium ion
NaCl	sodium chloride, salt
NIDDM	non-insulin-dependent or type 2 diabetes mellitus
NMR	nuclear magnetic resonance test
NPO	no food or fluid (nothing) by mouth
NSAID	nonsteroidal anti-inflammatory drug
OA	osteoarthritis
OD	overdose or right eye
OS	left eye
OTC	over-the-counter (availability of drugs, e.g., ASA [aspirin])
Pao_2	partial pressure of oxygen in arterial blood
Pco_2	partial pressure of carbon dioxide
pH	hydrogen ion concentration (acidity)
PID	pelvic inflammatory disease
PKU	phenylketonuria
PMN	polymorphonuclear leukocyte (polys, neutrophil)
PMS	premenstrual syndrome
PSA	prostate specific antigen
PT	prothrombin time, pro time
PTCA	percutaneous transluminal coronary angioplasty
PTT	partial thromboplastin time
PVC	premature ventricular contraction
PVD	peripheral vascular disease
RAS	reticular activating system
RBC	red blood cell (erythrocyte)
RFA	radio frequency ablation (destruction)
RLQ	right lower quadrant
ROM	range of motion
SIDS	sudden infant death syndrome
SLE	systemic lupus erythematosus
SOB	shortness of breath
STD/STI	sexually transmitted disease/infection
T&A	tonsillectomy and adenoidectomy
TB	tuberculosis
TBC	thrombocyte (platelet) count
TBW	total body water
TIA	transient ischemic attack
TMJ	temporomandibular joint
TPA	tissue plasminogen activator
TPN	total parenteral nutrition

TPR	temperature, pulse, respiration
URI	upper respiratory infection
UTI	urinary tract infection
VS	vital signs
WBC	white blood cell (leukocyte)
WHO	World Health Organization

Common Pharmaceutical Abbreviations

Rx	take
M or mitte	send (amount)
sig	label
ac	before meals
cc	with meals
pc	after meals
PO	by mouth, orally
SL	sublingual, dissolve under tongue
IM	intramuscular injection
SC or SubQ	subcutaneous injection
IV	intravenous injection
stat	immediately
bid	twice daily
tid	three times daily
qid	four times daily
hs	bedtime
prn	as needed
q4h	every four hours
q8h	every eight hours
OD	right eye
OS	left eye
gtt	drop
tab	tablet
cap	capsule

Ready Reference 5

Common Diagnostic Studies and Tests

The diagnostic tests described in this section are basic tests that are usually available and most often used to diagnose and monitor diseases and the effectiveness of treatment. A brief description is included for some of the procedures. Additional, specialized tests may be offered in certain institutions. New techniques and more accurate equipment are constantly being developed. Test results are now available more rapidly with the use of multiple analyzers and computers. However, older procedures and equipment may be used by some centers.

Endoscopic Examination

Endoscopy is used to visualize lesions or structures directly by inserting a tube into the body through an opening (e.g., trachea) or through the body wall. This procedure may facilitate a diagnosis or be used to obtain a specimen (tissue or fluid) for further examination and diagnosis (e.g., a biopsy) or perform simple surgery (e.g., remove cartilage debris from a knee joint). Examples of endoscopic examinations include bronchoscopy, gastroscopy, cystoscopy, proctosigmoidoscopy, arthroscopy, and laparoscopy.

Imaging Studies
Radiograph or X-ray Film
Ionizing radiation provides an image on film of bones and soft tissues that varies in density with the absorption of the x-rays striking the tissues (see Fig. 9-3 and Fig. RR5-1).
- *Plain x-ray films* are used as a preliminary screen for problems such as fractures or pneumonia.
- *Contrast medium* may be used (e.g., barium swallow or barium enema) to illustrate digestive tract abnormalities in more detail. In angiography various contrast media are used to examine the blood vessels. Myelograms utilize a dye to visualize the spinal cord and nerve roots.
- In *mammography,* low-dose X-ray films are used to detect lesions in breast tissue.
- In *bone density scanning (DEXA),* two X-ray beams are used simultaneously to measure the thickness of bone. The dose rate of radiation is much less than a plain X-ray.

Computed Tomography (CT scan, formerly computerized axial tomography or CAT scan)
A cross-section of tissues is provided by a scanning machine taking X-ray films in a series of shots from all directions (360 degrees); these measure differences in tissue density. A computer processes and compiles the readings to produce an image (Fig. RR5-2).

Ultrasonography (ultrasound)
High-frequency sound waves that bounce off body structures are used to obtain images by ultrasonography (Fig. RR5-3). The echoes reflect differences in the structures, which are analyzed and then visualized. This test is useful because it does not involve radiation, is noninvasive, is considered safe during pregnancy (can be used to measure fetal size and development), and is relatively inexpensive. It is limited by the fact that sound waves cannot penetrate deeply.
- *Doppler ultrasound* assesses the blood flow in arteries and veins by measuring sound waves reflected from moving red blood cells.
- *Echocardiography* measures the efficiency of heart valves and heart function (see Fig. 12-25) echocardiogram illustrating mitral stenosis).

Magnetic Resonance Imaging (MRI)
MRI makes use of a magnetic field surrounding the body and the hydrogen (water) content of the body. Radio waves provide the energy source. Relative tissue densities are calculated by computer to produce an image. MRI is noninvasive and safe because it does

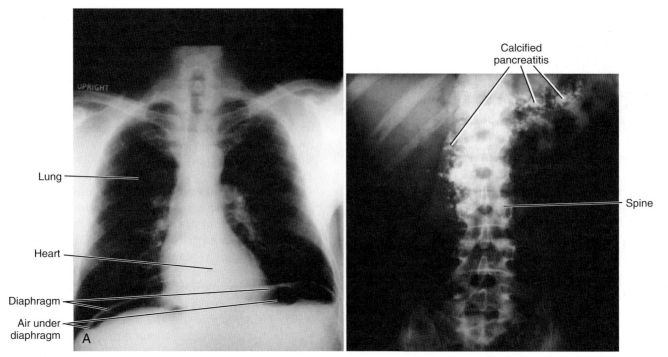

FIGURE RR5-1 X-rays. **A,** X-ray of chest shows air under the diaphragm, which has leaked out of a ruptured stomach; heart and lungs are normal (frontal view). *(Courtesy of Dr. Christine MacAdam, Department of Medical Imaging, North York General Hospital, Toronto, Ontario, Canada.)* **B,** X-ray of the spine (frontal plane) shows evidence of calcification from previous pancreatitis. *(Courtesy of Dr. Christine MacAdam, Department of Medical Imaging, North York General Hospital, Toronto, Ontario, Canada.)*

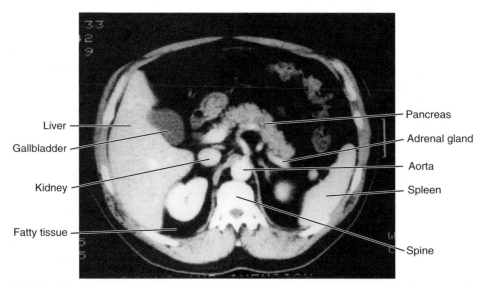

FIGURE RR5-2 Computed tomography (CT) scan shows cross-section of organs. *(Courtesy of Dr. Christine MacAdam, Department of Medical Imaging, North York General Hospital, Toronto, Ontario, Canada.)*

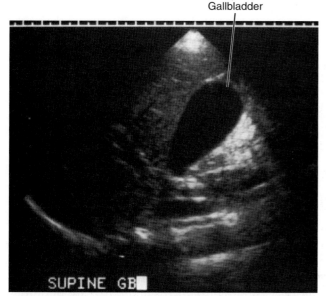

Gallbladder

FIGURE RR5-3 Ultrasound of gall bladder and liver. *(Courtesy of Dr. Christine MacAdam, Department of Medical Imaging, North York General Hospital, Toronto, Ontario, Canada.)*

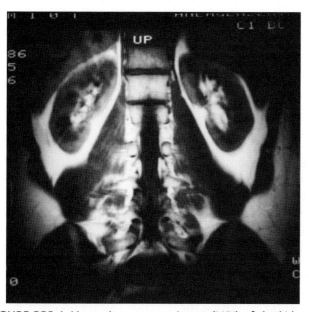

FIGURE RR5-4 Magnetic resonance image (MRI) of the kidneys (frontal plane). *(Courtesy of Dr. Christine MacAdam, Department of Medical Imaging, North York General Hospital, Toronto, Ontario, Canada.)*

not use ionizing radiation or injected contrast media. It provides more detailed visualization and can project past bone; therefore, it is particularly useful for visualization of neurologic and cardiovascular abnormalities (Fig. RR5-4).

Nuclear Scanning

Nuclear medicine tests involve tracking the distribution of a radioactive tracer substance (radiopharmaceutical, radionuclide, or radioisotope) in the body. A substance that is normally used in the body, such as iodine or phosphate, is labeled with a very small amount of radioactive material and administered (orally, by injection, by inhalation) to the patient. A scanning procedure traces gamma ray emissions as it follows the radioactive material through the body to the appropriate tissue; for example, iodine to the thyroid gland or phosphate to bone. Abnormalities of distribution of the tracer substance or of tissue function can be detected by this process. A computer transforms the scan into an image. For example, a "hot spot" indicates increased uptake of the radioactive material and could be used to identify an overactive thyroid or the presence of a metastatic bone cancer. By contrast, a malignant thyroid tumor is usually "cold" with less radioactivity. An embolus obstructing blood flow would be illustrated by an area without radioactivity in the lung or heart (radioactive thallium scan). The radioactive material is soon excreted by the patient.

Positron Emission Tomography (PET)

Positron emission tomography (PET) involves radioisotopes used with a scanner and computer to provide a cross-sectional functional image of a tissue such as the brain. This method is used to determine biochemical changes in the tissue and thus functional changes such as oxygen uptake in the tissue.

Determinations of Electrical Activity

Electrocardiogram (ECG, EKG)

By attaching electrodes to the chest and limbs of a patient, the conduction system of the heart can be assessed. The rate, rhythm, and characteristics of the contractions can be recorded by the machine. Typical abnormal patterns assist in the diagnosis of myocardial infarctions, cardiac dysrhythmias, electrolyte imbalances, and digoxin toxicity (see Fig. 12-17).

Holter monitoring uses a portable ECG device to monitor cardiac activity in ambulatory patients while they perform and keep a log of their daily activities. The patient wears a small recording device attached to electrodes on the chest for a 24-hour period, and any cardiac abnormalities can be correlated with the daily routine.

Stress test (exercise electrocardiography)

Electrocardiographic measurements and blood pressure are monitored during a period of controlled exercise on a treadmill or stationary bicycle to determine the cardiac response to increased workload. The test is useful in detecting early coronary artery disease, checking post-MI cardiac function, and assessing the effectiveness of medication. It may also be used before establishing an individual's fitness or exercise program.

Electroencephalogram (EEG)

The electrical activity of the neurons in the brain is determined by electrodes attached to the scalp; the activity is then recorded as waves by the machine.

Abnormal patterns may result from seizure disorders, tumors, or injuries. Absence of electrical activity in all parts of the brain may be used to confirm brain death.

Pulmonary Function Tests

Both pulmonary volumes and capacities (e.g., tidal volume, total lung capacity—see Fig. 13-3 and Table 13-1) can be measured using a spirometer, a machine into which the patient breathes through a mouthpiece. These tests assist in diagnosing specific respiratory disorders, response to treatment, or progression of chronic disorders.

Blood Tests

Hematology testing

Blood is checked for its components and its blood clotting capability (hemostasis). Depending on the particular test, blood may be procured from a vein or a small puncture on the fingertip (see tables in the inside front cover).

- *Complete blood count (CBC)* is used to check the count and characteristics of all formed elements or cells (erythrocytes, leukocytes, and thrombocytes) as well as hemoglobin and hematocrit. This examination is useful in the diagnosis of anemias or leukemias.
- *Hemoglobin (Hgb)* indicates the amount of hemoglobin in the blood for oxygen transport, independent of the number of red blood cells.
  - *Glycosylated hemoglobin (HBA1c)* measures the amount of glucose bound to hemoglobin. This reflects the blood glucose levels over a period of time, e.g., months.
- *Hematocrit (HCT)* indicates the percentage of erythrocytes in a specific volume of blood. The number of WBCs is not significant in measuring the cell volume. Hematocrit can indicate fluid imbalance or anemia.
- *White blood cell differential count,* often referred to as a "differential count," determines whether there has been a change in the proportions of leukocytes and may provide a clue to the cause of a problem. For example, an increase in eosinophils usually indicates an allergic response.
- *Bone marrow aspiration* may be used to confirm abnormalities related to the production of blood cells such as megaloblastic anemia or leukemia. Specimens may be taken from the anterior iliac crest or sternum.
- *Blood culture and sensitivity* may be performed if bacteremia or unknown infection is present.
- *Blood clotting tests* evaluate various clotting times (e.g., prothrombin time) and serum levels of the clotting factors (e.g., fibrinogen). These tests may be used to determine deficits of individual factors or monitor anticoagulant treatment.
- *Hemoglobin electrophoresis* is used to detect the presence of abnormal hemoglobin (e.g., HbS).
- *Serum-ferritin* level indicates the level of iron storage.

- *Glycosylated hemoglobin* test (HbA1c) is used to monitor control of diabetes mellitus over the past 90 to 120 days.

Blood chemistry tests

Automated electronic systems are now in widespread use. They make use of computerized multiple analyzers that can run a number of tests rapidly. Depending on the outcome, additional tests may be required in specific situations.

Blood chemistry tests evaluate:
- Arterial blood gases (ABGs) for acid-base balance or oxygen levels, including serum pH, PO_2, PCO_2, SO_2 (oxygen saturation), CO_2 and O_2 content, bicarbonate, base excess and base deficit, and serum pH
- Serum hormone levels (e.g., ACTH or thyroid—T_3 and T_4)
- Lipid levels, including serum cholesterol and triglycerides, lipoproteins such as high-density lipoprotein (HDL) and low-density lipoprotein (LDL)
- Serum electrolytes (e.g., K^+, Na^+, Cl^+)
- Glucose (fasting blood sugar or glucose tolerance test)
- Serum enzymes and isoenzymes (to determine the site of infarction or inflammation or monitor the spread of a malignant tumor)
- Serum levels of bilirubin (direct, indirect, and total)
- Urea or ammonia to check kidney and liver functions

Special methods such as chromatography may be used for amino acid determinations.

Immunodiagnostic Tests

Major changes are occurring in the area of immunodiagnostic testing as improved methods are developed to assess serum antigen and antibody levels. Current methods make use of precipitation or agglutination reactions, immunofluorescence tests, or enzyme-linked immunosorbent assay (ELISA). Immunologic testing is used for many purposes, such as the diagnosis and monitoring of the course of hepatitis, diagnosis of HIV infection, screening for infection during pregnancy (the TORCH test), ABO blood typing, and assistance in the diagnosis of diseases resulting from immunologic abnormalities (e.g., antinuclear antibodies in systemic lupus erythematosus or rheumatoid factor in rheumatoid arthritis).

Skin tests, scratch, or patch tests, are simple local tests based on immune responses. They are used to check for specific allergies or exposure to microbes (e.g., Mantoux test for tuberculosis).

Chromosomal and Genetic Analysis

Chromosome analysis, including techniques used in cytogenetics and molecular biology, is used to examine the chromosomes and/or DNA to determine chromosome or genetic abnormalities in affected individuals or carriers, to determine paternity, or in forensic science. DNA identification is used routinely, and information is being recorded in computer data banks. Gene mapping and subsequent development of tests for various genetic defects is a current major project. White blood cells are commonly used for this type of testing, but other sources of cells, such as fetal cells in amniotic fluid, may also be used.

Therapeutic Drug Monitoring
Serum drug levels are checked in patients in whom there is a narrow therapeutic range of a drug and risk of toxicity or who have severe renal or liver disease or potential drug interactions. Examples of drugs monitored are digoxin, lithium, lidocaine, and phenobarbital.

Urine Tests
Routine urinalysis is used to check the physical and chemical characteristics of a freshly collected urine specimen. Physical examination of the specimen includes its appearance and specific gravity. Color of urine may be altered by drugs or diet. Chemical analysis includes pH and presence of abnormal constituents such as protein or ketones, as well as electrolyte levels and wastes such as urea.

Microscopic examination determines the presence of cells or urine casts. Tests such as creatinine clearance are used to determine the glomerular filtration rate. Pregnancy tests make use of urine levels of human chorionic gonadotropin. Patients who have diabetes mellitus or are on certain diets may monitor their own urine for ketones.

Cerebrospinal Fluid Tests
Cerebrospinal fluid is collected by means of a lumbar puncture (see Fig. 14-11). The pressure is measured, and the fluid is examined for appearance, protein and glucose levels, and the presence of cells or microorganisms.

Fecal Tests or Stool Analysis
A fecal specimen is checked for its physical characteristics such as color and consistency. Presence of occult blood is determined by the guaiac test. Stool cultures are used to check for parasites as well as other microbial content. Chemical tests include tests for lipids, enzymes such as trypsin, or mucus. Microscopic examination assesses factors such as the presence of leukocytes (abnormal).

Microbiologic Tests
Any body fluids or exudates from lesions may be examined for the presence of microorganisms, which then may be identified. Body fluids may include sputum, blood, urine, stool, semen, gastric aspirate, or cervical scrapings. Microscopy may involve the use of different types of microscopes (dark-field, phase-contrast, electron), depending on the site from which the sample was obtained and the type of microbe suspected. Stains such as Gram's stain may be used to assist with identification. Cultures, using a medium suitable for the specific organism, and sensitivity tests to determine the most effective drugs, are common procedures (see Figs. 6-2 and 6-15). Organisms such as viruses require living tissue for culture, a more complex and time-consuming procedure.

Ready Reference 6
Example of a Medical History
The *purpose* of a medical history is to obtain information regarding a patient's health status, then to assess the implications of this information for planning and implementing healthcare interventions. Goals include the:
- Establishment of general considerations required for treatment of an individual
- Identification of any medical condition that could be complicated by actions of the healthcare provider
- Identification of a medical condition, medication, or other treatment that might require special precautions or modified treatment on the part of the healthcare provider
- Identification of any condition that could create a risk for staff or other patients
- Assurance that any changes in the patient's condition or treatment are recorded
- Promotion of accurate and effective communication among all parties
- Need to cover any legal requirements concerning risk factors for each patient

There are many different forms available for a medical history. These may be modified to meet the needs of a particular health profession.

There are essentially three parts to a medical history. First, a basic form is often completed by the patient before the first appointment. Then, the healthcare professional may ask questions, record observations, and make notes regarding specific items in the patient's history or regarding the patient's current complaint. The patient's responses may prompt more questions or additional information may be needed. Lastly, a section for updating records may be included. A typical form is shown in Figure RR6-1.

PATIENT:NAME _____   **DATE** _____

          ADDRESS _____

          TELEPHONE NUMBER: HOME _____   BUSINESS _____

DATE OF BIRTH: _____

SEX   F   M

MARITAL STATUS _____   OCCUPATION _____

FAMILY PHYSICIANS NAME _____   PHONE NUMBER _____

When did you last see your family doctor? _____

Date of last physical examination? _____

Date of last chest x-ray? _____

Last hospitalization. Purpose _____   Date _____

List any medical condition you are currently being treated for _____

List any drugs you are taking _____

List any other treatments you may be taking at this time _____

List any allergies _____

Please check any conditions you have experienced

Angina   _____

Heart attack   _____

High blood pressure   _____

Other heart problem   _____

Any blood or bleeding problems   _____

Frequent infections   _____

Stroke   _____

Seizures   _____

Eye problems   _____

Hearing problems   _____

Dizziness, vertigo   _____

Mobility problems   _____

Headaches   _____

Cough, sinus problems   _____

Breathing problems   _____

FIGURE RR6-1 Medical history form.

Tuberculosis   _____

Peptic ulcer   _____

Intestinal disorder   _____

Liver disease, jaundice   _____

Any dietary restrictions   _____

Recent weight loss/gain   _____

Diabetes   _____

Thyroid   _____

Other hormonal problems   _____

Kidney or bladder problems   _____

Arthritis and joint problems   _____

Osteoporosis   _____

Skin rashes or lesions   _____

Cancer   _____

Pregnancy   _____

Smoker   _____

Other concerns: _____

SUGGESTIONS FOR ADDITIONAL QUESTIONS

Current disorder and treatment

     How long have you had this condition?

     What medications or treatment are you receiving?

     Do you have a specialist for this?   Name?   Phone?

Drugs

     How long have you been taking this medication?

     Do you have any unwanted effects from this drug?

     Do you take any "over-the-counter" medications, such as vitamins, pain killers, laxatives, or herbal remedies?

Heart:

Chest pain (do you have chest pain, *when(triggers?)*, how long does it last? how long have you been having this? do you take nitroglycerin, *do you have nitroglycerin with you?*)

Heart attack (When, how long were you hospitalized, bypass surgery, drug treatment such as anticoagulants, any special precautions now?)

High blood pressure (controlled? what is it now? do you take it yourself? medication, any dizziness or fainting?)

Irregular heart rate (when? medication? *do you have a pacemaker?*)

Heart valves (Have you had rheumatic fever, congenital heart defect, artificial valve, take "blood thinners"?)

Heart failure (*breathing* problems, can you climb stairs? Are you uncomfortable lying down? do you need extra pillows for sleeping, legs swelling?)

Blood problems (Do you have anemia? Type?, *Bleeding problems?, frequent infections*)

Do you take penicillin before a dental appointment? (Information on prophylactic drugs to prevent infective endocarditis and the high risk groups is published by the American Heart Association—www.americanheart.org)

Other concerns?

Nervous System

Stoke—How long ago? Whar residual effects did it have? Eg. mobility, speech, memory

Seizures (type, frequency, precipitating events, medication?)

Mental health—(specific disorder, treatment)

Visual problems (glaucoma, cataract, glasses or contact lenses?)

Hearing problems (hearing aid?)

Dizziness, vertigo (when, predisposing factors?)

Headaches (type, when, medication?)

Fainting (when?)

FIGURE RR6-1, cont'd   *Continued*

Respiratory Problems
Recurrent cough/cold; sinus
Asthma (frequency of acute attacks, precipitating factors, inhaler?)
Smoker (for how long? amount?)
Chroinc respiratory disorders—asthma, bronchitis, emphysema (for how long? medication, effects?)
Tuberculosis (when, how diagnosed, active, medication)

Gastrointestinal System
Appetite (is it good, snacks, fluid intake)
Diet (any restrictions?)
Recent significant weight gain/loss
Peptic ulcer (discomfort, diet, medication)
Intestinal disorder (type, chronic diarrhea, colitis)
Liver disease (hepatitis, cirrhosis, jaundice)

Endocrine function
Diabetes (type, controlled by, acute and chronic complications, when was last meal and insulin taken)
Thyroid (hypo or hyperthyroid, treatment?)
Take glucocorticoids regularly?
Other hormonal problems?

Urinary system
Kidneys (disorder? control?)
Bladder (frequency, infections?)

Musculoskeletal
Arthritis—rheumatoid, osteoarthritis, gout, ankylosing spondylitis (where, therapy)
Artificial joint (type, when?)
Osteoporosis (cause, complications, treatment)
Mobility—limitations, stairs

Skin
Skin rashes—contact/irritants (tape), allergies
Infections (Herpes)
Chronic disorders (Eczema, psoriasis, other, factors, treatment)

Other concerns or observations
General infections (current, recurrent or chronic, frequency? type? STD, fungal, viral)
Immunizations (Have you had all recommended immunizations? Influenza?)
Cancer (site, when, chemotherapy, radiation)
Pregnancy (any problems, limitations?)
Surgery—what, when, any problems

Precautions _____

_____

RECORD UPDATE
Date _____
Changes in health status _____

Concerns and Precautions _____

FIGURE RR6-1, cont'd

Ready Reference 7

Disease Index

Acne vulgaris A staphylococcal infection involving the sebaceous glands and hair follicles, common in teenagers; Chapter 23

Acromegaly Caused by increased secretion of growth hormone in the adult and resulting in broader bones and soft tissue growth; Chapter 16

Acute necrotizing fasciitis Rapidly invasive and destructive multimicrobial infection of soft tissue; Chapter 8

Acute respiratory failure The end stage of many respiratory problems when severe hypoxemia and/or respiratory acidosis results, interfering with nervous system function; Chapter 13

Addison's disease A deficit of adrenocortical hormones leads to hypotension, hypoglycemia, and cardiac arrhythmias; Chapter 16

AIDS Active infection with HIV which meets the criteria established by the CDC and WHO; Chapters 7, 10 and 14

Allergic rhinitis Hay fever, an allergic response to inhalants causes sneezing and profuse watery nasal discharge; Chapter 7

Alzheimer's disease A form of dementia, with progressive loss of cognitive function and personality changes; Chapter 14

Amenorrhea Absence of menstruation, which may result from many factors; Chapter 19

Amyotrophic lateral sclerosis A progressive degenerative condition involving loss of upper motor neurons in the cerebral cortex and lower motor neurons in the brainstem and spinal cord leading to paralysis; Chapter 14

Anaphylaxis Life-threatening, systemic hypersensitivity reaction causing circulatory shock and airway obstruction; Chapter 7

Anemia, aplastic Bone marrow failure results in pancytopenia, with resultant anemia, increased bleeding tendencies, and high risk of infection; Chapter 10

Anemia, iron deficiency Decreased hemoglobin production (microcytic, hypochromic erythrocytes) due to iron deficit; Chapter 10

Anemia, pernicious Autoimmune reaction leads to decreased absorption of vitamin B_{12} due to lack of intrinsic factor. This results in megaloblastic RBCs that are prematurely destroyed; Chapter 10

Anemia, sickle cell A genetic defect in hemoglobin causes sickling and hemolysis of RBCs under hypoxic conditions. This causes multiple thrombi and infarctions throughout the body; Chapter 10

Angina pectoris Transient chest pain resulting from myocardial hypoxia when demands on the heart increase or if oxygen supply to the heart is impaired; Chapter 12

Ankylosing spondylitis A progressive inflammatory condition involving the spine, leading to fibrosis and ankylosis; Chapter 9

Anorexia nervosa An eating disorder in which extreme weight loss results from self-starvation; Chapter 23

Aortic aneurysm A localized dilation in the aorta, which may rupture; Chapter 12

Aphasia A group of speech and language disorders resulting from brain damage; Chapter 14

Appendicitis Obstruction and inflammation in the appendix with possible rupture; Chapter 17

Arteriosclerosis Degeneration of small arteries causing hardening of the walls and narrowing of the lumen with decreased blood flow; Chapter 10

Aspiration Liquids and solids may cause obstruction and inflammation in the airway; Chapter 13

Atelectasis The collapse or nonaeration of part or all of a lung; Chapter 13

Atherosclerosis Development of lipid plaques with attached thrombi in large arteries, causing obstruction; Chapter 10

Atopic dermatitis (eczema) Chronic inflammatory skin condition related to genetic and hypersensitivity factors; Chapter 7

Basal cell carcinoma Skin cancer, slow-growing, commonly on exposed areas of the body; Chapter 20

Benign prostatic hypertrophy Hyperplasia of prostatic tissue compressing the urethra; Chapter 19

Bladder cancer An invasive tumor in the bladder wall, often related to exposure to chemicals or recurrent infections; Chapter 18

Brain tumor Benign and malignant tumors are space-occupying lesions, resulting in increased intracranial pressure; Chapters 14 and 20

Breast cancer A common malignant tumor in women, frequently metastasizing at an early stage; Chapters 19 and 20

Bronchiectasis A secondary respiratory problem in which dilated bronchial walls allow pooling of secretions and recurrent infections; Chapter 13

Bronchiolitis A viral infection in the bronchioles and small bronchi in young children; Chapter 13

Bronchitis Chronic inflammation and recurrent bacterial infections damage bronchial walls, leading to obstructions and hypoxia (COPD); Chapter 13

Bulimia nervosa An eating disorder characterized by binge eating, followed by purging; Chapter 23

Burns A thermal (heat) or non-thermal (chemical or electrical) injury to the body causing acute inflammation and tissue destruction; Chapter 5

Cancer, oral cavity Squamous cell carcinoma commonly on the floor of the mouth or tongue; Chapter 17

Candidiasis Common fungal infection, which may involve the mouth, esophagus, vagina, or skin; Chapters 7, 17, 19, and 27

Cardiac arrhythmias Abnormalities in the conduction system of the heart cause irregular rhythms and decreased cardiac output; Chapter 12

Cataracts Progressive clouding of the lens of the eye; Chapter 15

Celiac disease A malabsorption disorder related to intolerance to gluten and atrophy of the intestinal villi; Chapter 17

Cellulitis Infection, often staphylococcal, of the dermis and subcutaneous tissue; Chapter 8

Cerebral aneurysm A dilated area on the circle of Willis that may rupture and cause brain damage; Chapter 14

Cerebral palsy A group of disorders caused by brain damage during the perinatal period, and classified by the type of motor impairment; Chapter 14

Cerebrovascular accident A CVA or stroke is an infarction of brain tissue resulting from a thrombus, embolus or hemorrhage, and causing permanent loss of brain tissue; Chapter 14

Cervical cancer An invasive cancer linked to viral infections of the cervix. It can be diagnosed in situ by a Pap test; Chapter 19

Chlamydial infection A common sexually transmitted disease that may cause PID in women; Chapter 19

Cholelithiasis Formation of gallstones, consisting of cholesterol or bilirubin, which may obstruct the biliary tract; Chapter 17

Cirrhosis Gradual destruction of liver tissue with loss of function and ultimately liver failure; Chapter 17

Cleft lip and palate Developmental defects of the mouth and nose caused by failure of tissues to fuse at the midline; Chapter 17

Colorectal cancer A tumor, signs of which depend on the location. Signs may be occult blood in the stool, change in bowel habits, or obstruction; Chapter 17

Condylomata acuminata (genital warts) A sexually transmitted disease caused by human papillomavirus; Chapter 19

Congestive heart failure (CHF) Inability of the heart to pump sufficient blood to meet the needs of the body. This may result from heart damage or increased demands on the heart. Cardiac output is reduced and backup congestion in the tissues or organs develops; Chapter 12

Conjunctivitis Inflammation or infection of the conjunctiva of the eye; Chapter 15

Contact dermatitis Skin rash resulting from hypersensitivity reaction or direct irritation following direct exposure to a substance; Chapters 7 and 8

Creutzfeldt-Jakob disease A type of dementia caused by an infectious prion; Chapter 14

Cryptorchidism Maldescent of the testes after birth; Chapter 19

Cushing's syndrome Excessive glucocorticoids in the body cause catabolic effects on tissues, increased risk of infection and hypertension; Chapter 16

Cystic fibrosis Genetic disorder affecting the exocrine glands, causing thick mucus to obstruct the bronchioles in the lungs, pancreatic and biliary ducts. Respiratory infections are common; Chapter 13

Cystitis Infection of the bladder usually due to *E. coli*; Chapter 18

Dental caries Tooth decay caused by bacterial action on sugars; Chapter 18

Depression A groups of mood disorders based on changes in neurotransmitter activity; Chapter 14

Detached retina A tear in the retina deprives retinal cells of nutrients which, if prolonged, may cause permanent loss of vision; Chapter 15

Diabetes insipidus A deficit of antidiuretic hormone resulting in excessive loss of fluid and dehydration; Chapter 16

Diabetes mellitus A relative deficit of insulin leads to hyperglycemia and multiple metabolic abnormalities; Chapter 16

Dislocation The separation of two bones at a joint with loss of articulation and deformity; Chapter 9

Disseminated intravascular coagulation (DIC) A complication of many disorders, DIC causes excessive blood coagulation, consumption of clotting factors, leading to hemorrhage; Chapters 10 and 22

Diverticular disease Outpouching of the intestinal wall, often multiple, which may become inflamed or infected and may cause obstruction; Chapter 17

Down syndrome A chromosome disorder, trisomy 21, causing multiple defects in physical and intellectual development; Chapter 21

Dumping syndrome Removal of the pyloric sphincter results in uncontrolled gastric emptying, which leads to intestinal distention and hypovolemia following meals; Chapter 17

Dwarfism May be caused by a deficit of growth hormone; Chapter 16

Dysmenorrhea Painful menstruation, both primary and secondary; Chapter 19

Dysphagia Difficulty in swallowing due to neurological or structural problems; Chapter 17

Eczema (atopic dermatitis) Chronic inflammatory skin condition related to genetic and hypersensitivity factors; Chapter 7

Emphysema The destruction of alveolar walls decreases oxygen diffusion and loss of elasticity in the lungs impedes expiration, leading to over-inflated lungs (COPD); Chapter 13

Endometrial cancer Carcinoma of the uterus is usually indicated by bleeding in older women; Chapter 28

Endometriosis Endometrial tissue is present outside the uterus and responds to hormonal changes; Chapter 19

Epiglottitis Bacterial infection and inflammation may obstruct the airway; Chapter 13

Epispadias Urethral opening on the dorsal surface of the penis; Chapter 19

Esophageal cancer Squamous cell carcinoma frequently caused by chronic irritation; Chapter 17

Fibrocystic breast disease Nodules in breast tissue that change with cyclic hormonal levels. Some types should be monitored; Chapter 19

Fibromyalgia A syndrome of symptoms including chronic pain in soft tissues of the body, sleep interruptions, fatigue and in some cases depression; Chapter 9

Flail chest injury Multiple rib fractures cause loss of chest wall rigidity and paradoxical movements of the flail section during ventilation, resulting in hypoxia and circulatory impairment; Chapter 13

Fracture A break in a bone, of which there are various patterns; Chapter 9

Furuncle (boil) Staphylococcal infection in a hair follicle; Chapter 8

Gastric cancer An ulcerative cancer often arising in the mucous glands; Chapter 17

Gastritis, acute Inflammation or infection of the gastric mucosa causing nausea or vomiting, sometimes with pain; Chapter 17

Gastritis, chronic Chronic irritation causes atrophy of the gastric mucosa, including loss of secretory glands; Chapter 17

Gastroenteritis Acute inflammation or infection of the stomach and intestines causing pain, vomiting and diarrhea; Chapter 17

Gastroesophageal reflux Intermittent flow of gastric contents into the esophagus related to an incompetent sphincter or increased abdominal pressure; Chapter 17

Glaucoma Increased intraocular pressure due to increased aqueous humor. May damage the retina and optic nerve; Chapter 15

Glomerulonephritis (acute poststreptococcal) Antistreptococcal antibodies cause inflammation in the glomeruli of the kidney causing increased permeability and decreased GFR; Chapter 18

Goiter Enlargement of the thyroid gland associated with both hyperthyroid and hypothyroid conditions; Chapter 16

Gonorrhea A common sexually transmitted disease that may cause PID in women; Chapter 19

Gout Deposits of uric acid and urate in the joint cause inflammation and damage to the cartilage; Chapter 9

Guillain-Barré syndrome Reversible inflammation and degeneration of the spinal nerves, causing paralysis and loss of function in an ascending pattern; Chapter 14

Hay fever (allergic rhinitis) An allergic reaction involving the nasal mucosa, causing increased watery secretions and sneezing; Chapter 7

Head injury Various types of injury may damage brain tissue directly or through increased intracranial pressure; Chapter 14

Hemophilia Classic hemophilia is a genetic disorder characterized by excessive bleeding resulting from a deficit of clotting factor VIII; Chapter 10

Hepatitis, infectious Viral infection of the liver by one or more of the hepatitis virus group, causing inflammation and necrosis; Chapter 17

Hepatitis, toxic Inflammation and necrosis of the liver due to chemicals or drugs; Chapter 17

Herniated intervertebral disc Rupture or stretching of the annulus fibrosis of the disc causes pressure on spinal nerves and pain; Chapters 14 and 24

Herpes simplex Recurrent, viral infection usually around the mouth (HSV-1) or genitalia (HSV-2); Chapters 8, 17, and 19

Herpes zoster Infection in adults by varicella virus involving a unilateral cranial or spinal nerve; Chapter 14

Hiatal hernia Part of the stomach protrudes above the diaphragm either temporarily or permanently, causing reflux and inflammation; Chapter 17

Histoplasmosis A fungal infection frequently in the lungs that may spread to other sites; Chapter 13

HIV infection Presence of human immunodeficiency virus (HIV) and antibodies in the blood, without signs of active infection; Chapter 7

Hodgkin's lymphoma A malignancy involving the T-lymphocytes that first develops in a single lymph node, then spreads in an orderly fashion; Chapter 11

Huntington disease An inherited disorder with onset in adulthood where progressive atrophy of the brain affects motor and cognitive functions; Chapter 14

Hydrocele Excessive fluid around the testes; Chapter 19

Hydrocephalus Excessive cerebrospinal fluid accumulates, compressing the brain tissue; Chapter 14

Hydronephrosis A disorder secondary to obstructions in the urinary tract, causing backup of urine and compression of renal tissue; Chapter 18

Hyperparathyroidism Often due to an adenoma, it causes hypercalcemia and osteoporosis; Chapter 16

Hypertension, essential Consistently elevated blood pressure of unknown origin; Chapter 14

Hypertension of pregnancy Elevated blood pressure, proteinuria, and edema occurring in pregnancy. Formerly termed pre-eclampsia or eclampsia; Chapters 12 and 22

Hyperthyroidism Increased secretion of thyroid hormones causes hypermetabolism; Chapter 16

Hypoparathyroidism Hypocalcemia causes weak cardiac contractions and tetany; Chapter 16

Hypospadias Urethral opening on the ventral surface of the penis; Chapter 19

Hypothyroidism If severe and untreated, causes cretinism in the infant and child, myxedema in the adult; Chapter 16

Impetigo Highly contagious staphylococcal infection around the mouth, commonly occurring in children; Chapter 8

Inappropriate ADH syndrome Excess antidiuretic hormone (ADH) causes retention of fluid; Chapter 16

Infant respiratory distress syndrome Insufficient surfactant production in premature infants prevents adequate lung expansion, resulting in severe hypoxia and fluid accumulating in the alveoli; Chapter 13

Infectious arthritis Infection and inflammation, sometimes destructive, and usually involving a single joint; Chapter 9

Infectious mononucleosis A viral infection affecting lymphocytes, common in adolescents and young adults; Chapter 23

Infectious rhinitis (common cold) Viral infection (rhinovirus, adenovirus) of the upper respiratory tract; Chapter 13

Infective endocarditis Microorganisms damage heart valves, both previously deformed and normal; Chapter 12

Influenza Viral infection involving the upper and lower respiratory tract, frequently complicated by pneumonia; Chapters 6 and 13

Intestinal obstruction May be structural or functional (paralytic ileus) and manifested by pain and vomiting; Chapter 17

Juvenile rheumatoid arthritis A group of autoimmune diseases causing inflammation in joints and other connective tissue in children; Chapters 9 and 23

Kaposi's sarcoma A skin cancer now frequently associated with AIDS; Chapter 8

Keratitis Inflammation or infection of the cornea of the eye; Chapter 15

Keratoses Benign skin lesions associated with aging or sun damage; Chapter 8

Kyphosis Increased convexity of the thoracic spine; Chapter 23

Laryngotracheobronchitis (croup) Viral infection of the upper respiratory tract, including the larynx, in young children, causing a characteristic barking cough; Chapter 13

Leiomyoma (fibroid) Benign tumor of the uterus; Chapter 19

Leukemia A form of cancer in which one or more leukocytes is an immature, nonfunctional neoplastic cell developing in the bone marrow and peripheral blood, leading to increased risk of infection and hemorrhage; Chapter 10

Liver cancer Secondary tumors are common, the primary cancer is usually hepatocellular cancer related to hepatitis or cirrhosis; Chapter 17

Lung cancer Primary and secondary cancers are common in the lungs. Primary cancer is predisposed by cigarette smoking and insidious in onset; Chapter 13

Macular degeneration Age-related degeneration of the macula lutea in the retina of the eye causes loss of vision in older persons; Chapter 15

Malignant melanoma A skin cancer typically arising from a nevus or mole, which metastasizes at an early stage; Chapter 8

Metabolic syndrome Obesity, hypertension, Type 2 diabetes and lipid abnormalities which together are associated with early mortality, Chapters 12, 16 and 23

Ménière's syndrome Periodic episodes of excess endolymph formation in the inner ear, causes loss of hearing and vertigo, eventually permanent damage; Chapter 15

Meningitis An infection of the meninges covering the brain and spinal cord causing increased intracranial pressure; Chapter 14

Multiple myeloma A form of cancer involving the plasma cells, which invade the bone marrow, destroying bone in the vertebrae, ribs, pelvis, and skull; Chapter 10

Multiple sclerosis A group of chronic progressive disorders, resulting from demyelination in the brain, spinal cord, and cranial nerves; Chapter 14

Muscular dystrophy A group of inherited disorders causing progressive degeneration of skeletal muscle; Chapter 9

Myasthenia gravis An autoimmune disorder that interferes with the neuromuscular junctions, commencing in the face and neck; Chapter 14

Myocardial infarction (MI, heart attack) Obstruction of a coronary artery causes necrosis of heart tissue, impairing pumping ability and/or conduction; Chapter 12

Nephrosclerosis Degenerative changes in the arterioles cause ischemia and necrosis of kidney tissue as well as increased blood pressure; Chapter 18

Nephrotic syndrome A kidney disorder secondary to many systemic disorders as well as kidney diseases, that causes marked proteinuria and lipiduria; Chapter 18

Non-Hodgkin's lymphoma A malignancy involving primarily B-lymphocytes with multiple lymph node involvement; Chapter 11

Osteoarthritis Non-inflammatory progressive degeneration of the articular cartilage in joints, particularly the knees and hips. Impairs mobility; Chapters 9 and 24

Osteomyelitis Infection of the bone, often associated with trauma; Chapter 23

Osteoporosis Loss of bone density and mass leading to fragile bones and spontaneous fractures; Chapters 9 and 24

Osteosarcoma Malignant tumor in bone of child or young adult; Chapter 9

Otitis media Infection of the middle ear cavity; Chapter 15

Otosclerosis Fixation by abnormal bone growth of the stapes to the oval window in the middle ear, causing progressive loss of hearing; Chapter 15

Ovarian cancer Asymptomatic hidden tumor usually diagnosed after metastasis; Chapters 19 and 20

Ovarian cyst Various types and sizes of cysts may form on the ovaries; Chapter 19

Paget's disease Progressive replacement of bone by fibrous tissue and abnormal bone in older persons; Chapter 9

Pancreatic cancer Adenocarcinoma often causes inflammation and obstruction of the ducts; Chapter 17

Pancreatitis Severe inflammation of the pancreas and surrounding tissues associated with autodigestion by pancreatic enzymes; Chapter 17

Panic disorder An anxiety disorder in which attacks occur with increased neuronal activity or changes in neurotransmitters; Chapter 14

Parkinson's disease A progressive degenerative condition affecting mobility, that results from loss of extrapyramidal function; Chapter 14

Pediculosis Infection by lice on the body, scalp, or pubic area; Chapter 8

Pelvic inflammatory disease Ascending infection of the female reproductive tract involving the fallopian tubes and ovaries; Chapter 19

Pemphigus An autoimmune disorder causing blisters to form on the skin; Chapter 8

Peptic ulcer Erosions in the mucosa of the stomach or proximal duodenum because of decreased tissue resistance or increased gastric secretions; Chapter 17

Pericarditis Inflammation or infection of the pericardium, causing effusion and impaired filling of the heart, or painful friction rub; Chapter 12

Periodontal disease Infection and damage to the gingiva, bone, and ligaments around the teeth; Chapter 17

Peritonitis Inflammation or infection of the peritoneal membranes leading to hypovolemia, pain, and possibly septicemia; Chapter 17

Pheochromocytoma A benign tumor of the adrenal medulla that causes increased secretion of catecholamines and hypertension; Chapter 16

Pituitary adenoma A benign tumor affecting the secretion of one or more pituitary hormones and increases intracranial pressure; Chapter 16

Pleural effusion Fluid collects in the pleural cavity due to inflammation, infection, or trauma, reducing lung expansion; Chapter 13

Pneumoconioses Chronic progressive restrictive lung disorders with fibrosis caused by chronic exposure to environmental irritants such as asbestos; Chapter 13

Pneumonia Infection in the lung by pneumococcus, viruses, or other microbes. Congestion interferes with oxygen diffusion and ventilation; Chapter 13

Pneumothorax Air in the pleural cavity results from injury or spontaneous tears in the pleura, causing atelectasis. Various types of pneumothorax may affect circulation and the unaffected lung; Chapter 13

Poliomyelitis A viral infection involving motor neurons in the spinal cord and medulla, often causing weakness or paralysis. Post-polio syndrome is now symptomatic in many persons with a history of polio in childhood; Chapter 14

Polycystic kidney A group of genetic disorders in which gradually enlarging cysts progressively destroy kidney tissue; Chapter 18

Polycythemia vera Increased production of erythrocytes causing increased blood volume, viscosity and blood pressure; Chapter 10

Pre-eclampsia Elevated blood pressure and kidney dysfunction during pregnancy; Chapter 22

Premenstrual syndrome A group of manifestations present the week before onset of menses; Chapter 19

Primary fibromyalgia syndrome Group of idiopathic disorders affecting muscles and tendons, causing pain and stiffness; Chapter 9

Prostate cancer Usually adenocarcinoma of the prostate gland, common in older men; Chapter 19

Prostatitis Inflammation or bacterial infection of the prostate gland; Chapter 19

Psoriasis Chronic inflammatory skin condition, characterized by rapid cellular proliferation; Chapter 8

Pulmonary edema Fluid collecting in the alveoli and interstitial spaces for many different reasons, interfering with oxygen diffusion and lung expansion; Chapter 13

Pulmonary embolus Thrombus or other material traveling through the venous circulation to block blood flow through the lung, interfering with respiratory function or circulation; Chapter 13

Pyelonephritis Ascending infection of one or both kidneys; Chapter 18

Pyloric stenosis A developmental defect or acquired obstruction involving the pyloric sphincter, preventing gastric emptying; Chapter 17

Rabies Viral infection of the CNS caused by a bite by a rabid animal; Chapter 14

Regional ileitis (Crohn's disease) Chronic inflammatory disorder affecting the ileum, interfering with absorption of nutrients and a potential cause of obstructions; Chapter 17

Renal cell carcinoma Adenocarcinoma usually first indicated by painless hematuria; Chapter 18

Renal failure, acute Sudden loss of all kidney function, potentially reversible, resulting in anuria, acidosis, and elevated serum urea; Chapter 18

Renal failure, chronic Gradual permanent loss of nephrons from primary kidney disease, with end-stage azotemia, acidosis, and fluid-electrolyte imbalance affecting many systems; Chapter 18

Repetitive strain injury Repeated forceful movements damage muscles, tendons, or nerves; Chapter 9

Reye's syndrome Cerebral edema and liver dysfunction, usually following viral infections treated with ASA in children; Chapter 14

Rheumatic fever A systemic inflammatory disorder resulting from an immune reaction, causing permanent damage to heart valves and sometimes the cardiac conduction system; Chapter 12

Rheumatic heart disease Damaged heart valves and dysrhythmias caused by rheumatic fever. Impairs cardiac function; Chapter 12

Rheumatoid arthritis A systemic inflammatory disorder, considered to be of autoimmune origin, causing progressive damage to joints; Chapter 9

Rh incompatibility When the mother is Rh negative and the fetus is Rh-positive, the antigen-antibody reaction causes hemolysis of fetal erythrocytes; Chapter 22

Rickets Soft bone and leg deformity in a child due to lack of vitamin D and phosphate; Chapter 9

Scabies Invasion of the skin by a mite; Chapter 8

Schizophrenia A group of mental disorders characterized by typical alterations in the brain and behavior; Chapter 14

Scleroderma A progressive skin disorder with possible systemic effects, characterized by collagen deposits and inflammation; Chapter 8

Scoliosis Lateral curvature of the spine, often developing in adolescence; Chapter 23

Seizure disorders A group of disorders characterized by different types of recurrent localized or generalized seizures that result from sudden excessive uncontrolled neuronal activity in the brain; Chapter 14

Severe acute respiratory syndrome (SARS) An emerging viral infection (coronavirus) that causes severe congestion in the lungs and hypoxia. Mortality is high; Chapter 13

Shock Decreased circulating blood volume because of impaired pumping by the heart, loss of blood volume, or general vasodilation. This leads to decreased blood pressure and general hypoxia; Chapter 12

Sinusitis Bacterial infection of one or more paranasal sinuses; Chapter 13

Spermatocele A cyst between the testis and epididymis; Chapter 19

Spina bifida Congenital defect in which the posterior spinous processes of the vertebrae do not fuse, in many cases allowing the meninges, CSF, and nerve tissue to protrude; Chapter 14

Spinal cord injury The effects depend on the level of injury and the extent of the permanent damage to the spinal cord; Chapter 14

Squamous cell carcinoma A skin cancer usually related to sun exposure; Chapter 8

Stress ulcers Multiple gastric ulcers resulting from severe ischemia; Chapter 17

Syphilis A sexually transmitted disease with systemic manifestations; Chapter 19

Systemic lupus erythematosus (SLE) A chronic autoimmune disease causing inflammation and damage in multiple systems; Chapter 7

Testicular cancer A rare tumor affecting young males; Chapter 19

Tetanus An infection by a spore-forming bacillus that causes severe, possibly fatal, muscle spasms; Chapter 14

Tetralogy of Fallot A congenital heart defect that includes four cardiac abnormalities: pulmonary stenosis, ventricular septal defect, dextroposition of the aorta, and right ventricular hypertrophy. Leads to mixing of oxygenated and unoxygenated blood in the systemic circulation and thus systemic hypoxia and cyanosis; Chapter 12

Thalassemia A genetic defect in hemoglobin causes premature hemolysis of RBCs and severe anemia; Chapter 10

Thrombophlebitis Inflammation in a leg vein often associated with thrombus formation; Chapters 12 and 22

Tinea Fungal infection of the feet, scalp, or body; Chapter 8

Torsion of the testes Rotation of the testes on the spermatic cord; Chapter 19

Transient ischemic attacks (TIAs) Result from temporary reduction of blood supply in an area of the brain, causing brief loss of function; Chapter 14

Trichomoniasis A sexually transmitted infection that remains localized; Chapter 19

Ulcerative colitis Chronic inflammation and ulceration of the rectum and colon with remissions and exacerbations; Chapter 17

Urolithiasis (renal calculi) Kidney stones most frequently composed of calcium or uric acid, which may obstruct flow of urine; Chapter 18

Urticaria (hives) Skin rash resulting from hypersensitivity to ingested substances; Chapter 8

Uterine prolapse Various degrees of descent of the cervix or uterus into the vagina; Chapter 19

Varicose veins Dilated and tortuous areas of superficial or deep veins in the legs. May cause edema and impaired arterial circulation; Chapter 12

Variocele Dilated vein in the spermatic cord; Chapter 19

Ventricular septal defect A congenital deformity, a hole in the septum between the ventricles, results in a left-to-right shunt of blood; Chapter 12

Verrucae (warts) A skin lesion caused by human papillomavirus, often on the hands or feet; Chapter 8

Wilms' tumor A congenital tumor of the kidney occurring in young children. It presents as a large abdominal mass; Chapter 18

Ready Reference 8

Drug Index

Acetaminophen (Tylenol) Analgesic for mild pain, antipyretic; Chapter 4

Acetylsalicylic acid (ASA, Aspirin) Antiinflammatory, analgesic for mild pain; antipyretic; reduces platelet adhesion and blood clotting; Chapters 4, 5, 12, and 9

Acyclovir (Zovirax) Antiviral agent-herpes simplex; Chapters 8 and 17

Albuterol (Ventolin) Bronchodilator, inhaler; Chapter 13

Alendronate (Fosamax) Inhibits bone resorption in osteoporosis; Chapters 9 and 24

Almotriptan (Axert) Analgesic in the treatment of migraine; Chapter 22

Amantadine (Symmetrel) Antiviral, influenza; Chapters 6 and 13

Amitriptyline (Elavil) Antidepressant; Chapter 14

Amoxicillin (Amoxil) Antibacterial, prophylaxis for endocarditis; Chapters 6 and 12

Amphotericin B (Fungizone) Antifungal drug; Chapter 13

Atorvastatin (Lipitor) Cholesterol-lowering agent; Chapter 12

Azathioprine (Imuran) Immunosuppressant; Chapter 7

Azithromycin (Zithromax) Antimicrobial; Chapter 19

Captopril (Capoten) Antihypertensive; Chapter 12

Cefotaxime Sodium (Cefotaxime) Third-generation cephalosporin antimicrobial; Chapter 6

Celecoxib (Celebrex) Non-steroidal anti-inflammatory analgesic; Chapter 9

Cimetidine (Tagamet) Decrease gastric acid secretion in peptic ulcer; Chapter 17

Ciprofloxacin (Ciloxan) Antibacterial; Chapter 6

Clarithromycin (Biaxin) Antibacterial; Chapter 17

Clindamycin (Dalacin) Antibacterial; Chapters 6 and 12

Codeine For moderate pain; Chapter 4

Cyclobenzaprine (Flexeril) Skeletal muscle relaxant; Chapter 9

Diazepam (Valium) Antianxiety, antiepileptic, relief of skeletal muscle spasm; Chapters 9, 14 and 26

Digoxin Congestive heart failure, antiarrhythmic; Chapter 12

Diltiazem (Cardizem) Reduce cardiac conduction and contractility; Chapter 12

Dimenhydrinate (Dramamine, Gravol) Antiemetic; Chapter 17

Diphenhydramine (Benadryl) Antihistamine, reduce allergic reactions; Chapter 7

Docusate sodium (Colace) Stool softener, laxative; Chapter 17

Donepezil (Aricept) Treat early stages of Alzheimer's disease; Chapter 14

Enalapril (Vasotec) Antihypertensive; Chapter 12

Eletriptan (Relpax) Analgesic for migraine; Chapter 22

Epinephrine General vasoconstrictor, increases heart rate and force, bronchodilator; Chapter 7, 12 and 13

Fluoxetine (Prozac) Antidepressant; Chapter 14

Furosemide (Lasix) Diuretic, for edema; Chapter 12

Glyburide (DiaBeta) Oral hypoglycemic; Chapter 16

Griseofulvin (Fulvicin) Antifungal; Chapters 6 and 8

Haloperidol (Haldol) Antipsychotic agent; Chapter 14

Heparin Anticoagulant; Chapters 10 and 12

Hydrochlorothiazide (Hydro DIURIL) Diuretic, antihypertensive; Chapter 18

Ibuprofen (Advil, Motrin) Relieves pain and inflammation (NSAIDs); Chapters 4 and 5

Isoniazid (INH) Antitubercular drug; Chapter 13

Levodopa (Sinemet, Larodopa) Relief of Parkinson's disease; Chapter 14

Loperamide (Imodium) Antidiarrheal; Chapter 17

Lorazepam (Ativan) Antianxiety drug; Chapter 26

Meperidine (Demerol) Narcotic analgesic; Chapter 4

Metformin (Glucophage) Oral hypoglycemic; Chapter 16

Metoprolol (Lopressor) Antihypertensive, anti-anginal, antiarrhythmic; Chapter 12

Nifedipine (Adalat) Antihypertensive, antianginal, peripheral vasodilator; Chapter 12

Nitrofurantoin (Furadantin) Antibacterial; urinary tract infections; Chapter 18

Nitroglycerin Prevent and treat angina; Chapter 12

Nystatin (Mycostatin) Antifungal agent; Chapter 17

Omeprazole (Prilosec) Reduces gastric acid secretion; Chapter 17

Oseltamivir (Tamiflu) Antiviral—influenza; Chapter 6

Pancrelipase (Cotazym) Pancreatic enzyme replacement, e.g., cystic fibrosis; Chapter 13

Penicillin Antibacterial, primarily gram-positive microbes; Chapter 6

Phenobarbital Sedative; Chapter 14

Phenytoin (Dilantin) Anticonvulsant; Chapter 14

Prednisone Glucocorticoid, anti-inflammatory, reduces allergic reaction; Chapters 5 and 7

Pregabalin (Lyrica) Central-acting analgesic for fibromyalgia; Chapter 9

Promethazine (Phenergan) Sedative, antihistamine, antiemetic; Chapters 7, 17 and 26

Propantheline (Pro-Banthine) Gastrointestinal antispasmodic; Chapter 17

Pyridostigmine (Mestinon) Treat myasthenia gravis; Chapter 14

Psyllium hydrophilic mucilloid (Metamucil) Laxative—bulk; Chapter 17

Ramipril (Altace) Antihypertensive; Chapter 12

Ribavirin (Virazole) Antiviral agent—hepatitis C; Chapter 17

Selegiline (Eldepryl) Treat Parkinson's disease; Chapter 23

Simvastatin (Zocor) Decrease cholesterol and LDL levels; Chapter 12

Spironolactone (Aldactone) Potassium-sparing diuretic; Chapter 18

Streptokinase (Streptase) Thrombolytic agent; Chapters 12, 13 and 14

Sulfasalazine (Salazopyrin) Antiinflammatory/antibacterial; Chapter 17

Tamoxifen (Nolvadex) Blocks estrogen receptors; Chapter 19

Tetrabenazine (Xenazine) Reduces choreiform movements; Chapter 14

Tetracycline Antibacterial, broad spectrum; Chapter 6

Timolol Reduces intraocular pressure in glaucoma; Chapter 15

Trifluoroperazine (Stelazine) Antipsychotic; Chapter 14

Trimethoprim-sulfamethoxazole (Bactrim) Antibacterial; Chapter 18

Warfarin (Coumadin) Anticoagulant, prophylaxis for thrombi; Chapter 12

Zanamivir (Relenza) Antiviral-influenza; Chapter 13

Zidovudine (Retrovir) Antiretroviral agent (HIV); Chapters 6 and 7

Ready Reference 9

Additional Resources

Specific resources may be found at the end of each chapter.

TEXTBOOKS

Anatomy and Physiology

Applegate EJ: *The Anatomy and Physiology Learning System,* ed 4, Philadelphia, 2011, WB Saunders.

Guyton AC, Hall JE: *Textbook of Medical Physiology,* ed 12, Philadelphia, 2011, WB Saunders.

Thibodeau GA, Patton, KT: *Structure and Function of the Body,* ed 14, St Louis, 2012, Mosby.

Tortora GJ, Derrickson BH: *Principles of Anatomy and Physiology,* ed 13, New York, 2011, Wiley.

Pathophysiology

Copstead-Kirkson LE, Banasik, JL: *Pathophysiology,* ed 5, Philadelphia, 2013, WB Saunders.

Kumar V, Abbas AK, Fausto N: *Robbins and Cotran Pathologic Basis of Disease,* ed 8, Philadelphia, 2010, WB Saunders.

McCance KL, Huether SE: *Pathophysiology: The Biologic Basis for Disease in Adults and Children,* ed 6, St Louis, 2010, Mosby.

Medicine

Abrams WB: The Merck Manual of Geriatrics, ed 3, Online at http://www.merck.com/mkgr/mmg/home.jsp.

Andreoli TE, et al: *Andreoli and Carpenter's Cecil Essentials of Medicine,* ed 8, Philadelphia, 2011, WB Saunders.

Porter RS: *The Merck Manual of Diagnosis and Therapy,* ed 19, Whitehouse Station, NJ, 2012, Merck & Co.

Callen JP, Greer KE, Paller AS, Swinyer LJ: *Color Atlas of Dermatology,* ed 2, Philadelphia, 2000, WB Saunders.

Heymann DL: *Control of Communicable Diseases Manual,* ed 19, Washington, DC, 2009, American Public Health Association.

Kliegman RM, Behrman RE: *Nelson Textbook of Pediatrics,* ed 19, Philadelphia, 2012, WB Saunders.

Kliegman RM, Marcdante K, Jensen, HB, Behrman RE: *Nelson Essentials of Pediatrics,* ed 6, Philadelphia, 2011, WB Saunders.

Papadakis M, et al: *Current Medical Diagnosis and Treatment 2014,* ed 53, New York, 2014, Lange Medical Books/McGraw-Hill.

Perkin GD: *Mosby's Color Atlas and Text of Neurology,* ed 2, London, 2002, Mosby.

Pharmacology

Burnham T: *Drug Facts and Comparisons,* St. Louis, Facts and Comparisons, (drug index with monthly updates).

Favaro MKA, Favaro J: *Introduction to Pharmacology,* ed 12, Philadelphia, 2012, WB Saunders.

Gillis MC: *Compendium of Pharmaceuticals and Specialties,* Ottawa, Ontario, Canada, Canadian Pharmacists Association, (annual).

Haveles EB: *Applied Pharmacology for the Dental Hygienist,* ed 6, St Louis, 2011, Mosby.

Krinsky DL, LaValle JB, Hawkins EB, Pelton R, Willis NA: *Natural Therapeutics Pocket Guide,* ed 2, Hudson, OH, 2003, Lexi-Comp.

Mosby's Drug Consult 2007, St Louis, 2007, Mosby.

Skidmore-Roth L: *Mosby's 2013 Nursing Drug Reference,* St Louis, 2013, Mosby.

Skidmore-Roth L: *Mosby's Handbook of Herbs and Natural Supplements,* ed 4, St Louis, 2010, Mosby.

Other Topics

Bergquist LM, Pogosian B: *Microbiology: Principles and Health Science Applications,* Philadelphia, 2000, WB Saunders.

Engelkirk Pand Burton G: *Burton's Microbiology for the Health Sciences,* ed 9, Philadelphia, 2010, Lippincott Williams & Wilkins.

Greenwood D, Slack RC, Peutherer JF: *Medical Microbiology: A Guide to Microbial Infections: Pathogenesis, Immunity, Laboratory Diagnosis and Control,* ed 17, New York, 2007, Churchill Livingstone.

Little JW, Falace D, Miller CS, Rhodus NL: *Little and Falace's Dental Management of the Medically Compromised Patient,* ed 8, St Louis, 2013, Mosby.

Mahon CR, Manuselis G: *Textbook of Diagnostic Microbiology,* ed 4, Philadelphia, 2011, WB Saunders.

Malarkey LM, McMorrow ME: *Saunders Nursing Guide to Laboratory and Diagnostic Tests,* ed 2, Philadelphia, 2012, WB Saunders.

Pagana KD, Pagana TJ: *Mosby's Diagnostic and Laboratory Test Reference,* ed 11, St Louis, 2013, Mosby.

Dictionaries and Medical Terminology

Chaner DE: *The Language of Medicine,* ed 9, Philadelphia, 2011, WB Saunders.

Dorland's Illustrated Medical Dictionary, 32nd ed. Philadelphia, 2011, WB Saunders.

Miller-Keane MT, O'Toole M: *Miller-Keane Encyclopedia and Dictionary of Medicine, Nursing and Allied Health,* 7th ed. Philadelphia, 2005, WB Saunders.

Mosby's Medical, Nursing and Allied Health Dictionary, ed 9, St Louis, 2013, Mosby.

Journals

American Scientist; Published by Sigma Xi, The Scientific Research Society, Research Triangle Park, NC
Heart and Lung: Journal of Critical Care
Journal of Allergy and Clinical Immunology
Journal of the American Medical Association (JAMA)
Journal of Bacteriology
Journal of Clinical Oncology
Journal of Emergency Medicine
Lancet
Nature: International Journal of Science, London, England
New England Journal of Medicine
Scientific American

Journals Published by Professional Groups

American Journal of Nursing
American Journal of Occupational Therapy
Clinical Acupuncture and Oriental Medicine
Clinics in Sports Medicine
Journal of the American Dietetic Association
Journal of Dental Hygiene
Physical Medicine and Rehabilitation Clinics
Respiratory Care Clinics

Web Sites

http://www.ama-assn.org: *American Medical Association.*
http://www.americanheart.org: *American Heart Association.*
http://www.amsci.org: *American Scientist Journal.*
http://www.asha.org: *American Speech-Language-Hearing Association.*

http://www.asm.org: *American Society for Microbiology.*
http://www.cancer.org: *American Cancer Society.*
http://www.cdc.gov: *Centers for Disease Control and Prevention.*
http://www.fda.gov: *United States Food and Drug Administration.*
http://www.healthfinder.gov: *United States Department of Health and Human Services.*
http://www.lungusa.org: *American Lung Association.*
http://jama.ama-assn.org: *The Journal of the American Medical Association.*
http://www.mayoclinic.com: *Mayo Clinic.*
http://aip.completeplanet.com.
http://www.nature.com: *Deep web link to health informtion refers complete planet site.*
http://www.nci.nih.gov: *National Cancer Institute.*
http://content.nejm.org: *The New England Journal of Medicine.*
http://www.nhlbi.nih.gov: *National Heart, Lung, and Blood Institute.*
http://www.niaid.nih.gov: *National Institute of Allergy and Infectious Diseases.*
http://www.niams.nih.gov: *National Institute of Arthritis and Musculoskeletal and Skin Diseases.*
http://www.niddk.nih.gov: *National Institute of Diabetes and Digestive and Kidney Diseases.*
http://www.nih.gov/icd: *National Institutes of Health (research site).*
http://www.nlm.nih.gov/medlineplus: *United States National Library of Medicine.*
http://www.sciam.com: *Scientific American (journal).*
http://www.scienceonline.org: *Science (journal).*
http://www.who.int: *World Health Organization.*
http://www.wfnals.org: *World Federation of Neurology.*

Abscess a localized pocket of infection or purulent exudate surrounded by inflammation.

Accommodation the lens of the eye adjusts its shape for distance.

Acetylcholine (Ach) a neurotransmitter.

Achlorhydria lack of hydrochloric acid in the gastric secretions.

Acidosis an increased number of hydrogen ions; a blood pH of less than 7.4.

Acute a disease with sudden onset of signs and short course.

Adenocarcinoma malignant tumor arising from glandular epithelial cells.

Adenoma benign tumor made up of glandular epithelial cells.

Adhesion a band of fibrous scar tissue forming an abnormal connection between two surfaces or structures, e.g., binding two loops of intestine together.

Adrenergic related to the sympathetic nervous system transmitters, norepinephrine (noradrenaline) and epinephrine (adrenaline).

Afferent toward the center; e.g., afferent nerves carry impulses toward the central nervous system.

Agenesis lack of an organ or structure because of a developmental error.

Agglutination clumping together of cells or particles.

Albumin a plasma protein responsible for maintaining osmotic pressure of the blood.

Aldosterone a mineralocorticoid hormone that increases the reabsorption of sodium and water in the renal tubules.

Alkalosis a decreased number of hydrogen ions; a blood pH greater than 7.4.

Allele one of two forms of a gene at corresponding sites on a chromosome pair; the code for phenotype or characteristic manifested in an individual.

Allergen an antigen that can initiate an allergic reaction.

Alopecia hair loss.

Amenorrhea the absence of menstrual periods.

Amnesia loss of memory.

Amniocentesis removal of a small amount of amniotic fluid from around the fetus for examination and diagnosis.

Amputation the removal of a body part, often a limb or part of a limb, to remove a tumor, prevent spread of infection, or relieve pain.

Anabolism the building up or synthesis of complex compounds from simple molecules.

Anaerobic metabolism and function without oxygen.

Analgesic a substance that relieves pain.

Anaphylaxis a life-threatening systemic allergic or hypersensitivity reaction, with respiratory obstruction and decreased blood pressure.

Anaplasia undifferentiated primitive cells of variable size and shape, associated with cancer.

Anasarca severe generalized edema.

Anastomosis a connection between two blood vessels or tubes.

Androgen steroid hormone that enhances male characteristics, e.g., testosterone.

Anemia a decrease in circulating hemoglobin and oxygen-carrying capacity in the blood because of decreased erythrocyte production, decreased hemoglobin production, excessive hemolysis, or loss of blood.

Anencephaly congenital condition where most of the brain and skull are absent.

Anesthetic a substance that reduces sensation, locally or systemically.

Aneurysm an outpouching or abnormal dilated area in a blood vessel.

Angiogenesis the development of new capillaries.

Angiography an examination of blood vessels using radiographs with a contrast medium.

Angioplasty repair of a blood vessel.

Angiotensin-Converting Enzyme (ACE) an enzyme that converts angiotensin I to angiotensin II, a potent general vasoconstrictor and stimulus for aldosterone secretion.

Anion a negatively charged ion such as chloride, Cl^-.

Ankylosis fixation or immobility at a joint.

Anomaly an abnormal structure, often congenital.

Anorexia loss of appetite.

Antagonism opposing action.

Antibiotic a substance derived from microorganisms that is used to treat infection.

Antidiuretic Hormone (ADH) increases absorption of water in the renal tubules.

Antigen a substance that causes the production of antibodies.

Antimicrobial an agent that kills or inhibits growth and reproduction of microorganisms.

Antineoplastic a substance or process that destroys neoplastic cells.

Antioxidant a substance such as vitamin E that reduces oxygenation and production of damaging "free radicals" during cell metabolism.

Antiseptic reduces the number of microorganisms on the skin.

Anuria absence of urine production.

Aphasia loss of the ability to communicate, speak coherently, or understand speech.

Apnea lack of breathing.

Apoptosis normal programmed cell death in tissues.

Arrhythmia loss of normal heart rate and rhythm; dysrhythmia.

Arteriosclerosis hardening and loss of elasticity of the arterial wall with narrowing of the lumen.

Arthroscopy examination and possible treatment of a joint through insertion of a small instrument.

Ascites abnormal accumulation of fluid in the abdominal cavity.

Asepsis the absence of pathogens.

Aspiration inhaling liquid or solid material into the lungs *or* withdrawing fluid or tissue from a cavity or organ.

Asymptomatic no signs or symptoms.

Asystole absence of cardiac contractions; cardiac arrest or standstill.

Ataxia impaired coordination, imbalance, staggering gait.

Atelectasis collapse and nonaeration of part or all of a lung.

Atherosclerosis development of obstruction by cholesterol plaques and thrombus on the walls of large arteries.

Athetoid involuntary writhing movement of limbs and body.

Atopic inherited tendency to hypersensitivities.

Atresia blind-end to a tube; loss of the lumen.

Atrophy degeneration and wasting of tissue, organs, or muscle due to decrease in cell size.

Atypical unusual, not characteristic.

Aura a sensation, e.g., visual or auditory, usually preceding a seizure or migraine headache.

Auscultation listening for sounds, perhaps with a stethoscope, within the body, e.g., lungs, heart, intestines.

Autoantibody antibodies to self-antigens such as cells or DNA.

Autoclave an appliance to sterilize instruments or materials with steam at high temperature and pressure.

Autodigestion abnormal destruction of tissues by activated digestive enzymes.

Autoimmune the development of antibodies to self-antigens.

Autoinoculation the spread of infection, e.g., by fingers, from one site to a second site on the body.

Autopsy an examination of part or all of a body, including organs, after death (postmortem) to determine the cause of illness and death.

Autoregulation automatic regulation or reflex control of blood flow in an area depending on the local needs.

Azotemia excess urea and other nitrogen wastes in the blood, as in renal failure.

Bacteremia bacteria present in the circulating blood.

Bactericidal chemical that destroys bacteria.

Bacteriostatic substance that reduces the growth and reproduction of bacteria.

Baroreceptor a sensory nerve receptor that is stimulated by a change in pressure, perhaps blood pressure.

Basal Metabolic Rate (BMR) the amount of energy (measured by oxygen requirements) to maintain essential function in the body at rest.

Benign nonthreatening, mild, or nonmalignant.

Bifurcation the division of a tube or vessel into two channels or branches.

Bilirubin a product from the breakdown of hemoglobin, excreted in bile.

Biopsy the removal of a small piece of living tissue for microscopic examination to determine a diagnosis.

Bolus a round mass of food ready to be swallowed; a dose of concentrated drug administered intravenously all at once.

Borborygmus the rumbling or gurgling sounds from gas in the intestine.

Bradycardia abnormally slow heart rate.

Bradykinin a chemical mediator released during inflammation causing vasodilation.

Bronchoconstriction contraction of smooth muscle in the bronchioles, narrowing the airways.

Bronchodilation relaxation of smooth muscle in the bronchioles, widening the airway.

Bruit an abnormal sound heard by auscultation, e.g., blood flow in an aneurysm.

Cachexia extreme loss of weight and body wasting associated with serious illness.

Calcification deposits of calcium in tissues.

Calculus a stone developing in the body, e.g., kidney or bile.

Carcinogen a substance that causes cancer by changing normal cells.

Cardiomegaly a heart that is larger than normal size.

Caries (dental) destruction of the tooth surface; a cavity or erosion in the enamel surface of a tooth.

Carpopedal Spasm a strong muscle contraction of the hand or foot.

Carrier a person hosting an infectious pathogen, who shows no signs of the disease, but could transmit the infection to others.

Catabolism the breakdown of complex molecules into simple molecules during metabolism.

Cataract an opacity of the lens of the eye.

Catheter a small tube inserted into the bladder to remove urine; a tube inserted into a blood vessel or other structure to allow drainage or maintain an opening.

Cation a positively charged ion such as sodium, Na^+.

Chemical Mediator a chemical released in the body during an inflammatory response or immune response.

Chemoreceptor a sensory nerve receptor stimulated by chemical changes such as pH.

Chemotaxis the movement of cells toward or away from an area of the body in response to chemical signals; e.g., phagocytic cells move to an area of tissue injury.

Cholestasis obstructed flow of bile in the liver or biliary tract.

Chorea involuntary repeated jerky movements of face and limbs.

Chorionic Villus part of the placenta that can be tested for genetic defects in the fetus.

Chromosome made up of genes, the genetic code of the living cell, consisting of DNA.

Chronic a condition with insidious or slow onset, mild but continuous manifestations, and long-lasting, often progressive effects.

Chyme thick, semifluid mixture of partially digested food passing out of the stomach into the duodenum.

Clonic Movements consisting of rapid, alternating contraction and relaxation of skeletal muscle.

Coagulation the process of changing a liquid into a solid, e.g., blood forming a thrombus.

Cognitive intellectual abilities, e.g., memory, thinking, problem solving, judgment, initiative.

Cohesion tendency to stick together or be attracted.

Colic sharp severe pain resulting from strong, smooth muscle contraction, e.g., intestinal.

Collagen the common protein making up connective tissue and bone.

Collagenase an enzyme that breaks down collagen fibers.

Colostomy surgical creation of an artificial opening from the colon onto the abdominal surface.

Coma unconscious state; person cannot be aroused.

Communicable Disease a disease that can be transmitted from an infected person, directly or indirectly, to other susceptible hosts.

Complement a series of inactive proteins circulating in the blood; when activated, they can destroy bacteria or antigens, or participate in the inflammatory response.

Compliance the ability of the lungs to expand and recoil *or* the patient's willingness to follow a prescribed treatment.

Congenital present at birth.

Contamination the presence of a pathogen on a body, clothing, or inanimate object.

Contracture shortening of a muscle or scar tissue causing immobility and deformity of a joint or structure.

Contralateral opposite side of the body.

Contusion tissue injury or bruise; bleeding into tissues.

Corticosteroid the steroid hormones from the adrenal cortex, including the glucocorticoids (cortisol) and mineralocorticoids (aldosterone).

C-reactive Protein (CRP) appears in the blood with inflammation and necrosis.

Crepitus the noise heard when the ends of a broken bone rub together *or* when fluid is present in the lung.

Culture growth of microorganisms on a specific nutritious medium in a laboratory.

Cyanosis bluish color of skin and mucosa that occurs when a large proportion of hemoglobin is unoxygenated.

Cyst a closed sac or capsule lined with epithelium, containing fluid.

Cytology the study of cells.

Cytotoxic a substance that damages or destroys cells.

Débridement surgical removal of dead tissue and foreign material from a wound.

Decubitus (Ulcer) skin breakdown from prolonged pressure on skin and tissue over a bony prominence leading to compressed blood vessels and ischemia.

Dehydration a deficit of water in the body.

Dementia progressive loss of intellectual function, loss of memory, personality change.

Demyelination loss of the myelin sheath from a nerve surface, interfering with conduction.

Denude stripping off skin, leaving bare.

Dermatome an area of skin innervated by a specific spinal nerve.

Detoxification the removal of a toxic or poisonous material and or neutralization of its effects on a person.

Dialysis a procedure to remove wastes and excess fluid or adjust blood to normal values in cases of renal failure.

Diapedesis the passage of leukocytes through intact capillary walls to a site of inflammation.

Diaphoresis excessive perspiration.

Differential Count the proportion of each type of leukocyte in a blood sample.

Differentiation increased specialization of cells for certain functions.

Diffusion the movement of molecules from an area of high concentration to low concentration.

Diplopia double vision.

Disinfectant a chemical that may destroy or inhibit the growth and reproduction of microorganisms.

Disorientation mental confusion with inadequate or incorrect awareness of time, place, and person.

Diuresis excessive amount of urine.

Dyscrasia abnormality of the blood or bone marrow; abnormal cell characteristics or numbers.

Dysentery severe diarrhea, often bloody, with cramps.

Dyspareunia pain or discomfort in the pelvis during sexual intercourse.

Dysphagia painful or difficult swallowing.

Dysplasia disorganized cells that vary in size and shape with large nuclei.

Dyspnea difficulty breathing.

Dysuria painful urination.

Ecchymoses reddish blue discoloration of skin or mucosa because of bleeding.

Ectopic away from the normal position, displaced.

Edema the accumulation of excess fluid in cells, tissue, or a cavity, resulting in swelling.

Efferent moving away from the center; e.g., efferent nerve fibers carry motor impulses to muscles.

Effusion the accumulation of fluid leaking from a blood vessel into a cavity or potential space.

Electrocardiogram (ECG) a record of conduction in the heart.

Embolus a mass, e.g., blood clot, air, fat, tumor cells, that breaks away into the circulation and obstructs a blood vessel.

Embryo the early stage of an organism's life; in humans, the developmental stage between implantation in the uterus and 8 weeks.

Encephalopathy impaired function of the brain.

Endarterectomy removal of the intima and any obstructive material in an artery.

Endemic a disease that is always present in a specific region.

Endogenous originating from within the body.

Endorphins morphine-like substances produced in the body that block pain stimuli at sites in the brain and spinal cord.

Endoscope an illuminated optic instrument that can be inserted into a body cavity, tube, or organ to visualize any changes (bronchoscope, cystoscope, laparoscope).

Endospore (Spore) a latent form that certain bacteria can assume under adverse conditions, in order to survive extreme temperatures, drying, or chemicals.

Endotoxin a toxin released from the walls of certain Gram-negative bacteria following lysis.

Enteric related to the intestine.

Enterotoxin a toxin from certain bacteria that damages the intestinal mucosa.

Enzyme-Linked Immunosorbent Assay (ELISA) a test to detect certain antibodies.

Epidemic a disease occurring in higher numbers than usual in a certain population within a given time period.

Epistaxis nose bleed.

Erythema redness and inflammation of the skin or mucosa due to vasodilation.

Erythrocyte Sedimentation Rate (ESR) the rate at which RBCs settle out of a blood specimen (containing anticoagulant); an elevation in ESR is a general characteristic of inflammation.

Etiology cause or origin of a disease or abnormality.

Euphoria an exaggerated feeling of well-being or unrealistic elation.

Eupnea normal, regular, quiet breathing.

Exacerbation an acute episode or increased severity of manifestations.

Excoriation an abrasion or injury to the skin.

Exogenous originating from outside the body.

Exteroreceptors sensory receptors located close to the body surface and are sometimes referred to as cutaneous receptors.

Exotoxin toxin excreted by a bacterium, e.g., neurotoxin or enterotoxin.

Exudate a fluid that accumulates and may leak from tissue, e.g., a serous exudate due to allergy, a purulent exudate, or pus associated with infection.

Fascia sheet of fibrous connective tissue separating and supporting muscle.

Fecalith a hard mass of feces, often impacted, in the intestine.

Ferritin a storage form of iron.

Fetus the human child in utero between 8 weeks and birth.

Fibrinogen the plasma protein that is formed into solid fibrin strands during the clotting process.

Fibrinolysis the breakdown of fibrin.

Fibrosis growth of fibrous or scar tissue related to collagen deposits.

Fimbria a hair-like projection on some bacteria.

Fissure a crack or split in the surface of skin or mucous membrane.

Fistula an abnormal tube or passage formed between structures, e.g., between the esophagus and trachea or between the rectum and skin.

Flaccidity lack of tone in muscle; weakness and softness.

Foramen an opening in bone or membrane.

Free Radical a byproduct of cell metabolism that damages cell membranes, proteins and DNA.

Fulminant rapid, severe, uncontrolled progress of a disease or infection.

Ganglion a collection of nerve cell bodies, usually outside the central nervous system.

Gangrene necrotic tissue infected by bacteria.

Gene a unit of DNA (a nucleic acid sequence) in a particular location on a specific chromosome.

Genetic inherited.

Genotype the genetic makeup of a cell or individual.

Gestation the time between conception and birth.

Gingivitis inflammation of the gums in the mouth.

Globulin a group of proteins in the blood.

Glucocorticoid the steroid hormones from the adrenal cortex, e.g., cortisol (hydrocortisone), that increase blood glucose levels and act to decrease inflammation and allergic reactions.

Gluconeogenesis the production of glucose from protein or fat.

Glucosuria glucose in the urine.

Glycemic Index the rate at which an ingested carbohydrate elevates blood glucose levels.

Glycogen a polysaccharide, made up of glucose molecules, stored in skeletal muscle or the liver.

Glycoprotein a combination of protein and carbohydrate.

Gram Stain a stain for bacteria that differentiates the cell walls of Gram-positive bacteria from that of Gram-negative bacteria; used for identification and choice of drug treatment.

Granulation Tissue newly developed fragile tissue, consisting of fibroblasts and blood vessels, formed during healing.

Granuloma a nodular destructive mass associated with some chronic inflammation or infection.

Gynecomastia abnormal breast enlargement in men.

Hallucination a sensory perception, e.g., visual or auditory, that is not real but results from nervous system excitation.

Hemarthrosis bleeding into a joint cavity.

Hematemesis vomiting blood; may be called "coffee-grounds" vomitus because it appears brown and granular.

Hematocrit percentage of erythrocytes in a blood sample.

Hematoma a blood clot formed following bleeding into a tissue or organ.

Hematuria blood in the urine; may be microscopic (small amount) or gross (large amount, darkening the color).

Hemiparesis weakness on one side of the body.

Hemiplegia paralysis on one side of the body.

Hemolysis destruction of erythrocytes with release of hemoglobin.

Hemoptysis frothy sputum containing streaks of blood, usually bright red; spitting up blood.

Hemostasis blood clotting or controlling bleeding.

Heparin a substance present in the body to prevent blood clotting.

Hepatomegaly enlarged liver.

Hepatotoxin a substance that damages the liver.

Heterozygous having two different alleles at corresponding points on a chromosome pair.

Hirsutism excessive body hair in a male pattern.

Histamine a chemical released from mast cells and basophils during immune reactions; causes vasodilation and bronchoconstriction.

Holistic an approach to health care that includes the physical, mental, emotional, and spiritual needs of the patient.

Homeostasis a relatively stable or constant environment in the body, including blood pressure, temperature, and pH, maintained by the various control mechanisms.

Homozygous having two identical alleles at corresponding points on a chromosome pair.

Hypercapnia increased level of carbon dioxide (CO_2) in the blood.

Hyperemia increased blood flow in an area, resulting in a warm, red area.

Hyperkalemia abnormally high level of potassium ions (K^+) in the blood.

Hypernatremia abnormally high level of sodium ions (Na^+) in the blood.

Hyperplasia an abnormal increase in the number of cells resulting in an increased tissue mass.

Hyperreflexia excessive reflex responses.

Hypertension a persistent elevation of blood pressure.

Hypertonic a solution with a greater concentration of solutes or higher osmotic pressure than that inside the cells present in the solution.

Hypertrophy increased size of an organ or muscle due to increased size of individual cells.

Hyperuricemia excessive uric acid in the blood.

Hypoalbuminemia abnormally low serum albumin levels.

Hypoproteinemia abnormally low level of plasma protein in the blood.

Hypotension low blood pressure and decreased tissue perfusion.

Hypovolemia decreased blood volume.

Hypoxemia insufficient oxygen in the arterial blood.

Hypoxia a decreased or insufficient level of oxygen in the tissues.

Iatrogenic caused by a treatment, procedure, or error.

Ictal related to a seizure (postictal—following a seizure).

Icterus jaundice.

Idiosyncrasy an unusual reaction by an individual to a normally harmless substance.

Idiopathic no known cause.

Immunocompetent a person who can produce a normal immune response.

Immunodeficiency (Immunocompromised, Immunosuppressed) reduced ability of the immune system to produce an immune response to defend the body.

Immunoglobulin a protein with antibody activity.

Incidence the number of new cases of a disease in a certain population within a time period.

Incontinence lacking voluntary control over urination or defecation.

Incubation Period the time between the initial exposure to the infectious agent and the appearance of the first signs of infection.

Infarct, Infarction an area of dead tissue caused by lack of blood supply.

Inflammation the response to tissue damage, indicated by redness, swelling, warmth, and pain.

Insidious a disease whose onset is marked only by vague or mild general signs.

In Situ cell growth and reproduction, such as cancer, remaining at the original site, not invasive or spreading.

Interferons a group of antiviral glycoproteins produced by viral-infected cells.

Interleukin protein (cytokine) primarily produced by T cells, active in the inflammatory and immune responses and leukocyte communication.

Intraarticular into the joint cavity or joint space.

Intractable resistant to treatment, e.g., pain that cannot be relieved by drugs.

Ipsilateral same side of the body.

Ischemia decreased blood supply to an organ or tissue.

Isoenzymes cell enzymes, specific to certain organs, that differ slightly in structure, but have similar functions.

Jaundice yellow color of the sclera of the eye and skin due to excessive bilirubin in the body fluids for any reason.

Karyotype a visual demonstration of the pairs of cell chromosomes arranged in order of size.

Keloid abnormal healing causes overgrowth of collagen and mass of fibrous tissue.

Ketone or Ketoacid chemical byproduct of lipid metabolism.

Kyphosis increased convex curvature of the spine in the thoracic region; "hunchback".

Labile unstable, changing.

Laryngospasm closure of the larynx obstructing the airway.

Latent present but hidden and inactive.

Lesion an abnormality in the structure of a tissue or organ.

Leukocytosis an above-normal number of leukocytes (WBCs) in the blood.

Leukopenia a decreased number of leukocytes in the blood.

Lichenification hardening and thickening of the skin; leather-like.

Lithiasis presence or formation of stones or calculi, e.g., cholelithiasis—gallstones.

Lordosis exaggerated concave curve of the lumbar region of the spine.

Lymphadenopathy a disease affecting the lymph nodes.

Lymphoma malignant neoplasm of lymphoid tissue.

Lysis destruction of a cell.

Lysosome a membrane-bound vesicle in a cell containing digestive or lytic enzymes, including lysozyme.

Lysozyme enzymes found in some cells and in body fluids such as tears, sweat, or saliva, which can destroy some microorganisms.

Macroangiopathy degenerative changes in the walls of large arteries.

Malabsorption impaired absorption of nutrients from the intestines.

Malaise a general feeling of discomfort or unease, of being unwell.

Mast Cells located in the tissues, they release chemicals such as histamine, heparin, and bradykinin in response to injury or foreign material.

Mediastinum the area of the thoracic cavity between the lungs, in which is located the trachea, esophagus, and large blood vessels.

Megaloblast abnormally large, nucleated, immature erythrocytes.

Melena black, tarry stool caused by bleeding in the digestive tract.

Metabolic Syndrome syndrome associated with obesity including hypertension, type 2 diabetes and hyperlipidemia.

Metabolism the chemical processes occurring in living cells, consisting of anabolism (synthesis or building up of new compounds) and catabolism (breakdown of complex substances).

Metaplasia replacement of one mature cell type by another mature cell type.

Metastasis spread of cancer cells to distant sites by the blood or lymphatics; secondary malignant tumor.

Microcirculation blood flow in the very small blood vessels, e.g., capillaries.

Micrometastasis spread of malignant cells not yet detectable.

Microorganism very small living organism, not visible to the naked eye, usually single-celled.

Microscopic visible only when magnified by lenses in a microscope.

Mitosis a process of cell reproduction resulting in two daughter cells with the same DNA as the parent cell.

Morbidity the rate at which a disease occurs; the proportion of a group affected by a disease.

Morphologic the physical size, form, structure, and shape of cells or organs.

Mortality the number of deaths in a group for a specific disease.

Murmur an abnormal sound heard in the heart, caused by a defective valve or opening in the heart.

Mutation a change in the genetic makeup (DNA) of a cell, which will be inherited.

Mycosis fungal infection.

Necrosis death or destruction of tissue.

Neonate newborn child.

Neoplasm abnormal growth of new cells, benign or malignant.

Neuritis inflammation of a nerve.

Neuropathy degeneration of nerve fibers.

Neurotoxin a bacterial toxin that affects the nervous system function.

Neurotransmitter a chemical released upon stimulation from vesicles at the end of the axon of a neuron, in order to stimulate the receptor site.

Neutropenia a deficit of neutrophils in the blood.

Nevus a darkly pigmented lesion on the skin; a mole.

Nociceptor receptors for pain stimuli.

Nocturia urination required during sleep at night.

Nosocomial an infection acquired while hospitalized.

Nuchal Rigidity a stiff neck, often associated with meningitis or brain hemorrhage.

Nystagmus involuntary rhythmic movements of the eyes in any direction.

Occlusion an obstruction or blockage.

Occult hidden, difficult to detect.

Occurrence the incidence and prevalence of disease.

Oliguria abnormally small volume of urine output.

Oncogenic a substance or situation that causes cancer.

Oncology the study of cancer.

Opioid natural or synthetic substance that binds to opioid receptors in the central nervous system, relieving pain; related to opium derivatives such as morphine or codeine.

Opportunist a microorganism, normally nonpathogenic, that causes infectious disease when the person's resistance is reduced, microbial balance is upset, or the microbe is transferred to another part of the body.

Organogenesis the formation and differentiation of organs and systems during embryonic development.

Orthopnea difficult or labored breathing when recumbent that is usually relieved by an upright position.

Orthostatic Hypotension a drop in blood pressure occurring when a person rises from a supine to a standing position.

Osmosis the force that draws water through a semipermeable membrane from a solution of lower solute concentration to a solution of higher concentration.

Osmoreceptors sensory nerve receptors stimulated by changes in fluid and electrolyte concentrations.

Osteodystrophy a general defect in bone development related to altered calcium and phosphate metabolism.

Ototoxic a substance causing damage to the inner ear or auditory nerve.

Palliative providing comfort and relieving pain and other symptoms of a disease without effecting a cure.

Pancytopenia decrease in all blood cells, erythrocytes, leukocytes, and thrombocytes.

Pandemic a worldwide increase in the numbers of people affected by a disease.

Paraneoplastic Syndrome additional disorders such as Cushing's syndrome resulting from some malignant tumors.

Paraplegia paralysis of the lower limbs.

Parasite an organism that lives on or in another living organism.

Parenteral the injection of substances into the body, e.g., intramuscularly or intravenously.

Paresis muscle weakness or mild paralysis.

Paresthesia abnormal sensations.

Paroxysmal Nocturnal Dyspnea awakening in severe respiratory distress, usually associated with pulmonary edema.

Pathogen a disease-causing microorganism.

Pathogenesis the early stages in the development of a disease.

Pathogenicity ability of microorganism to cause disease.

Perforation a hole through the wall of a tube or hollow structure.

Perfusion the flow of blood in the microcirculation to supply oxygen and nutrients to cells.

Periodontal Disease inflammation and damage to the structures anchoring the teeth, including the periodontal ligament, gingiva, and alveolar bone.

Permeable Membrane permits certain substances to pass through.

Petechiae tiny, pinpoint hemorrhages under the skin.

Phagocyte a cell that can surround, ingest, and destroy microorganisms, cell debris, or foreign substances, e.g., a macrophage.

Phenotype the characteristics manifested by a person depending on genetic and environmental factors.

Phlebotomy incision into a vein and collecting of blood.

Photophobia increased sensitivity of the eyes to light.

Pili hair-like appendages on some bacteria for adhesion to tissue and transfer of DNA.

Placebo a medication that lacks active ingredients, prescribed for psychological effect or as part of research studies.

Plaque a flat raised covering or scale.

Plasma the liquid portion of blood, after cells are removed.

Polysaccharide a carbohydrate made up of many sugars; e.g., glycogen, starch.

Polyuria an abnormally large volume of urine excreted within a given time period.

Potentiate to increase the strength or effect.

Precursor a substance that can be used to form other materials.

Prevalence the total number of new and existing cases of a disease in a specific population at a given time.

Prion an infectious abnormal protein particle; does not contain DNA.

Probability the likelihood or chance of occurrence.

Prodromal the initial period in the development of disease before acute symptoms occur.

Prognosis the probable outcome of a disease.

Prophylactic a measure or drug to prevent disease.

Proprioceptors receptors that provide information about body movement, orientation, and muscle stretch.

Prostaglandins (PGs) a group of chemical substances in the body that can exert a variety of effects, such as vasodilation, muscle contraction, and inflammation.

Prosthesis an artificial replacement for a body part, e.g., a limb or heart valve.

Protease an enzyme that breaks down a protein into amino acids.

Proteinuria an abnormality whereby protein is found in the urine.

Pruritus itching sensation.

Pseudohypertrophy abnormal enlargement of tissue or organ due to excessive fat and fibrous tissue.

Ptosis drooping eyelid.

Pulse Pressure the difference between systolic and diastolic pressures.

Pulsus Paradoxus abnormal decrease in systolic pressure during inspiration.

Purpura reddish-blue discoloration of the skin due to bleeding; bruise.

Purulent like pus (microbes, WBCs, and cell debris); thick, yellowish material in tissue often resulting from bacterial infection.

Pyrexia fever.

Pyrogen a substance that causes fever, a rise in body temperature.

Pyuria pus in the urine.

Radioisotope a radioactive form of an element, giving off radiation (beta or gamma) in the body, used in diagnosis and therapy.

Radiosensitive responsive such as cells damaged by radiation.

Radiotherapy treatment of cancer with radiation from an external source (gamma rays), such as radioactive cobalt or an internal implant of radioactive material.

Rales a bubbly or crackling sound in the lungs caused by air mixing with fluid in the airways.

Reflux backward movement of fluid, e.g., from the stomach into the esophagus and mouth.

Regeneration tissue repair through replacement by identical functioning cells.

Regurgitation a reverse flow to the normal, e.g., vomiting.

Reservoir a site where pathogens can survive or multiply.

Resident Flora (also called microflora, indigenous flora, normal flora, microbiota) the variety of nonpathogenic microorganisms that normally permanently colonize various parts of the body.

Retroperitoneal behind the peritoneal membrane against the abdominal wall.

Retrovirus a virus containing RNA and the enzyme reverse transcriptase, required to convert RNA to DNA that is then integrated with host cell DNA.

Rhonchus a harsh noise heard in the lungs resulting from air passing through partial obstruction by thick mucus or exudates.

Sclerosis abnormal hardening of tissue.

Scotoma a defect in the visual field.

Sedative a substance that exerts a calming effect on a person.

Sedentary inactive lifestyle.

Seizure (Convulsion) sudden, involuntary movement with loss of awareness, caused by uncontrolled neuronal discharge in the brain.

Senescence related to aging, growing old.

Septicemia, Sepsis systemic infection arising from bacterial toxins in the circulating blood or bacteria reproducing and spreading through the circulating blood.

Serous watery secretion.

Serum the liquid portion of the blood, lacking cells and clotting factors.

Spasm a strong, involuntary muscle contraction.

Splenectomy removal of the spleen.

Splenomegaly enlarged spleen.

Stasis slowing of the normal flow of fluid.

Steatorrhea fatty, bulky stool resulting from malabsorption.

Stem Cell a basic cell that may divide to give rise to a variety of specialized cells, e.g., the blood cells.

Stenosis narrowing of a tube, valve, or opening (stricture).

Sterile absence of all forms of microorganisms.

Steroid hormones based on a cholesterol structure produced in the adrenal cortex or gonads.

Stomatitis inflammation and ulceration in the mouth.

Stricture abnormal narrowing of a duct or tube.

Stridor an abnormal high-pitched, crowing sound caused by obstruction in the trachea or larynx.

Stupor a state of extreme lethargy, unawareness, and unresponsiveness.

Subluxation partial dislocation of a joint.

Substernal Retraction the chest wall under the sternum moves inward during inspiration.

Supine lying down on the back.

Syncope fainting, temporary loss of consciousness.

Syndrome a group of signs and symptoms characteristic of a specific disorder.

Synergism a combination of substances or agents that produce an effect greater than expected.

Tachycardia excessively rapid heartbeat.

Tachypnea rapid, shallow respirations.

Tenesmus spasms or straining associated with forced or painful elimination of urine or stool.

Teratogen a substance or condition that impairs normal development of the embryo or fetus in utero, causing a congenital abnormality.

Tetany repeated skeletal muscle contractions or spasms, seen in the extremities and face, related to increased irritability of the nerves, often associated with hypocalcemia.

Therapeutic beneficial treatment.

Thrombocytopenia abnormally low number of thrombocytes or platelets.

Thrombus a blood clot attached inside a blood vessel.

Tinnitus abnormal ringing sound or noise in the ears.

Total Parenteral Nutrition (TPN) administration of a nutritionally complete fluid (protein, glucose, vitamins, etc.) into the superior vena cava.

Toxin a substance that can harm the body or interfere with its function; poisonous.

Transcutaneous Electrical Nerve Stimulation (TENS) electrical stimulation of nerve endings through electrodes placed on the skin, for relief of pain.

Transillumination the passage of light through a structure to determine if an abnormality is present.

Trisomy Cells contain an extra chromosome, for a total of 47; named for the pair where the extra chromosome occurs, e.g., trisomy 21.

Turgor indicates tension of the skin based on pressure within the cells; a measure of dehydration.

Ulcer an open, crater-like lesion on the skin or mucous membranes.

Ulcerogenic producing or aggravating ulcers.

Universal Precautions safety precautions at two levels, recommended to protect health care workers from infection, based on the assumption that all patients and all body fluids are sources of infection.

Uremia the end result of renal failure when waste products accumulate in the blood and fluid/electrolyte imbalance develops.

Uveitis inflammation of the uveal tract of the eye (iris, ciliary body, and choroid).

Vaccine attenuated or killed microorganisms administered to induce antibody production.

Vector an animal or insect that transmits disease.

Vesicle a small thin-walled sac containing fluid; e.g., a blister.

Viable ability to sustain life.

Virulence the degree of pathogenicity or disease that a microbe is capable of causing.

Visceroceptors receptors that are located internally and provide information about the environment around the viscera.

Wheeze a high-pitched whining sound typical of obstruction in the bronchioles and small bronchi.

Xerostomia dry mouth with reduced saliva secretion.

Index

Page numbers followed by "f" indicate figures, "t" indicate tables, and "b" indicate boxes.